# DISABILITY EVALUATION

# DISABILITY EVALUATION

**STEPHEN L. DEMETER, M.D., M.P.H., F.A.C.P., F.C.C.P., F.A.A.D.E.P.**
Professor and Head of Pulmonary Medicine
Northeastern Ohio Universities College of Medicine
Rootstown, Ohio;
Head of Division of Preventive Medicine
Akron General Medical Center
Akron, Ohio

**GUNNAR B.J. ANDERSSON, M.D., Ph.D., F.A.A.D.E.P.**
Professor and Chairman
William A. Hark, M.D.–
Susanne G. Swift Professor
Department of Orthopedic Surgery
Rush-Presbyterian-St. Luke's Medical Center
Chicago, Illinois

**GEORGE M. SMITH, M.D., M.P.H., F.A.A.D.E.P.**
G. M. Smith Associates, Inc.
Bethesda, Maryland

*with 150 illustrations*

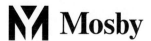 Mosby

St. Louis   Baltimore   Boston   Carlsbad   Chicago   Naples   New York   Philadelphia   Portland
London   Madrid   Mexico City   Singapore   Sydney   Tokyo   Toronto   Wiesbaden

American Medical Association
Physicians dedicated to the health of America

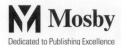 Mosby
Dedicated to Publishing Excellence

American Medical Association
Physicians dedicated to the health of America

*Vice President and Publisher, Medicine:* Anne S. Patterson
*Editor:* Laura DeYoung
*Associate Developmental Editor:* Jennifer Byington Geistler
*Editing Assistant:* Alicia E. Moten
*Project Manager:* Linda Clarke
*Senior Production Editor:* Allan S. Kleinberg
*Manufacturing Supervisor:* Andrew Christensen
*Designer:* Carolyn O'Brien
*American Medical Association Editors:* Jane Piro and Kathy Richmond

Printed in the United States of America
Composition by W. C. Brown
Printing/binding by Maple Vail Press

Mosby–Year Book, Inc.
11830 Westline Industrial Drive
St. Louis, Missouri 63146

**Library of Congress Cataloging-in-Publication Data**

Disability evaluation / [edited by] Stephen L. Demeter, Gunnar B.J.
    Andersson, George M. Smith.—1st ed.
        p.   cm.
    Includes bibliographical references and index.
    ISBN 0-8151-2400-7 (alk. paper)
    1. Disability evaluation   I. Demeter, Stephen L.   II. Andersson,
Gunnar, 1942–   .   III. Smith, George M. (George Marlowe) 1934–
    [DNLM: 1. Disability Evaluation.   W 925 D611 1996]
RC963.4.D56  1996
616.07′5—dc20
DNLM/DLC
for Library of Congress                                                95-25683
                                                                         CIP

97  98  99  00/9  8  7  6  5  4  3  2

**JOHN ALLEN, Ed. M.**
Chief Executive Officer
Rehabilitation Consultants for Industry
Oak Brook, IL

**HARVEY L. ALPERN, M.D., F.A.A.D.E.P.**
Assistant Clinical Professor of Medicine
University of California at Los Angeles
Los Angeles, CA

**GUNNAR B.J. ANDERSSON, M.D., Ph.D., F.A.A.D.E.P.**
Professor and Chairman
William A. Hark, M.D. –
Susanne G. Swift Professor
Department of Orthopedic Surgery
Rush-Presbyterian-St. Luke's Medical Center
Chicago, IL

**THOMAS J. ARMSTRONG, Ph.D.**
Professor
Center for Ergonomics, Industrial and Operations
 Engineering
University of Michigan
Ann Arbor, MI

**GERALD M. ARONOFF, M.D., F.A.A.D.E.P.**
Medical Director
Presbyterian Orthopaedic Pain Center
Presbyterian Orthopaedic Hospital
Charlotte, NC;
Assistant Clinical Professor
Tufts Medical School
Medford, MA

**PETER S. BARTH, Ph.D.**
Professor of Economics
The University of Connecticut
Storrs, CT

**CHRISTOPHER BELL, J.D.**
Partner
Jackson, Lewis, Schnitzler & Krupman
Washington, D.C.

**DONALD S. BLOSWICK, Ph.D.**
Associate Professor
Department of Mechanical Engineering
Director
Ergonomics and Safety Program
Rocky Mountain Center for Occupational and
Environmental Health
University of Utah
Salt Lake City, UT

**MARGARET BRYANT, J.D.**
Jackson, Lewis, Schnitzler and Krupman
New York, NY

**DON B. CHAFFIN, Ph.D.**
Johnson Professor and Director
Center for Ergonomics
University of Michigan
Ann Arbor, MI

**MOIRA CHAN-YEUNG, M.D., F.R.C.P.C.**
Professor
Department of Medicine
University of British Columbia;
Respiratory Division
Vancouver General Hospital
Vancouver, British Columbia, Canada

**MARK S. COHEN, M.D.**
Assistant Professor and Director of Orthopedic
 Education
Director of Hand and Elbow Program
Department of Orthopaedic Surgery
Rush-Presbyterian-St. Luke's Medical Center
Chicago, IL

**ALAN L. COLLEDGE, M.D.**
Medical Advisor
Occupational Health Services
Salt Lake City, UT

**MICHAEL COOPER, J.D.**
Jackson, Lewis, Schnitzler and Krupman
New York, NY

**EDWARD M. CORDASCO, M.D., F.A.C.P., F.C.C.P.**
Clinical Professor of Medicine,
Case Western Reserve University;
Director of Occupational and Environmental
    Respiratory Center
St. Lukes Solon;
Emeritus Staff
Cleveland Clinic Foundation
Cleveland, OH

**STEPHEN L. DEMETER, M.D., M.P.H., F.A.C.P.,
F.C.C.P., F.A.A.D.E.P.**
Professor and Head of Pulmonary Medicine
Northeastern Ohio Universities College of Medicine
Rootstown, OH;
Head of Division of Preventive Medicine
Akron General Medical Center
Akron, Ohio

**DONALD F. EIPPER, M.D.**
Associate Professor of Internal Medicine
Nephrology Section
Northeastern Ohio Universities College of Medicine
Rootstown, OH

**JAMES M. ELEGANTE, J.D.**
Attorney
Parson, Behle and Latimer
Salt Lake City, UT

**DONALD ELISBURG, J.D.**
Consultant
Potomac, MD

**MARTIN FRITZHAND, M.D., F.A.A.D.E.P.**
Assistant Clinical Professor of Urology
University of Cincinnati Medical School
Cincinnati, OH

**JOHN D. FRYMOYER, M.D.**
Dean
College of Medicine
University of Vermont
Burlington, VT

**STEVEN R. GARFIN, M.D.**
Professor of Orthopedics and Rehabilitation
University of California
San Diego, CA

**ARAM GLORIG, M.D.**
Consultant
House Ear Institute
University of Southern California
Los Angeles, CA

**JUDITH GOODWIN GREENWOOD, M.P.H., Ph.D.**
Director of Research and Information
West Virginia Workers' Compensation Division
Charleston, WV;
Clinical Associate Professor, Community Medicine
West Virginia University
Morgantown, WV

**TEE L. GUIDOTTI, M.D., M.P.H.**
Professor of Occupational and Environmental
    Medicine
Director of the Occupational Health Program
Department of Public Health Sciences
University of Alberta, Faculty of Medicine
Edmonton, Alberta, Canada

**SCOTT HALDEMAN, M.D., Ph.D., F.R.C.P.(C)**
Associate Clinical Professor of Neurology
University of California
Irvine, CA

**JAMES E. HANSEN, M.D.**
Emeritus Professor of Medicine
Division of Respiratory and Critical Care Physiology
    and Medicine
Harbor-UCLA Medical Center
University of California at Los Angeles
Torrance, CA

**PHILIP HARBER, M.D., M.P.H.**
Professor of Medicine
Director of Occupational and Environmental Medicine
University of California at Los Angeles
Los Angeles, CA

**ROWLAND G. HAZARD, M.D.**
Orthopaedics and Rehabilitation
University of Vermont
Burlington, VT

**RICHARD J. HERZOG, M.D.**
Associate Professor of Radiology
The University of Pennsylvania
Philadelphia, PA

**GEORGE B. HOLMES, Jr., M.D.**
Assistant Professor
Department of Orthopaedic Surgery
Director of Foot and Ankle Surgery
Rush-Presbyterian-St. Luke's Medical Center
Chicago, IL

**DAVID L. HORWITZ, M.D., Ph.D.**
Vice President, Medical and Regulatory Affairs
SciClone Pharmaceuticals
San Mateo, CA

**KAREN JACOBS, Ed.D., OTR/L, FAOTA**
Clinical Assistant Professor
Occupational Therapy
Boston University
Boston, MA

**ERIC L. JENISON, M.D.**
Professor of Clinical Obstetrics/Gynecology
Northeastern Ohio Universities College of Medicine
Rootstown, OH;
Director
Gynecology and Oncology
Akron General Medical Center
Aultman Hospital
Akron, OH

**RICHARD E. JOHNS, Jr., M.D., M.S.P.H.**
Medical Director
Alliant Techsystems
Magna, UT

**BARBARA JUDY, R.N.**
ADA Coordinator
West Virginia University
Morgantown, WV

**ARTHUR H. KEENEY, M.D., D.Sc.**
Dean Emeritus
Distinguished Professor of Ophthalmology
Department of Ophthalmology
University of Louisville School of Medicine;
Consulting Medical Staff
University of Louisville Hospital
Louisville, KY

**JEFFREY D. KLEIN, M.D.**
Orthopaedic Surgery
Hospital for Joint Diseases Orthopaedic Institute
New York, NY

**J. BRUCE KNEELAND, M.D.**
Associate Professor of Radiology
Hospital of the University of Pennsylvania
Philadelphia, PA

**PHILIP LEVY, M.D.**
Senior Clinical Lecturer in Internal Medicine
University of Arizona School of Medicine;
Phoenix Endocrinology Clinic Ltd.
Phoenix, AZ

**THOMAS A. LoIUDICE, D.O., F.A.C.P., F.A.C.G.**
Professor of Medicine
Northeastern Ohio Universities College of Medicine
Rootstown, OH;
Chief
Section of Gastroenterology
St. Thomas Hospital Medical Center
Akron, OH

**JAMES V. LUCK, Jr., M.D.**
President
Chief Executive Officer
Medical Director
Orthopaedic Hospital
Los Angeles, CA

**JOHN H. MATHER, M.D.**
Chief Medical Director
Social Security Administration
Baltimore, MD

**LEONARD N. MATHESON, Ph.D.**
Director
Employment and Rehabilitation Institute of
    California
Santa Ana, CA

**THOMAS MAYER, M.D.**
Medical Director
Pride Research Foundation;
Clinical Professor
Department of Orthopedic Surgery
University of Texas Southwestern Medical Center
Dallas, TX

**JOHN A. McCULLOCH, M.D., F.R.C.S.C.**
Professor of Orthopaedics
Northeastern Ohio Universities
    College of Medicine
Rootstown, OH

**JOHN D. McLELLAN, Jr., J.D.**
Attorney
Alexandria, VA

**MARK N. OZER, M.D.**
Clinical Professor
Department of Neurology
Georgetown University Medical School;
Medical Director, Stroke Recovery Program
National Rehabilitation Hospital
Washington, DC

**KENNETH C. PALS**
Board of Regents
International Workers' Compensation College;
Senior Associate
Crouse Dorgan Consultants, Inc.
Edmonton, Alberta, Canada

**LAWRENCE P. POSTOL, J.D.**
Seyfarth, Shaw, Fairweather and Geraldson
Washington, D.C.

**DAVID ROBBINS, M.D., M.P.H.**
Clinical Associate Professor
Department of Psychiatry
New York Medical College
Valhalla, NY;
Adjunct Assistant Professor
Department of Psychiatry
Cornell University
New York, NY

**ANTHONY A. ROMEO, M.D.**
Assistant Professor
Department of Orthopaedic Surgery
Rush-Presbyterian-St. Luke's Medical Center
Chicago, IL

**JEFFREY A. SAAL, M.D., F.A.C.P.**
Clinical Associate Professor
Department of Functional Restoration
Stanford University Medical Center
Menlo Park, CA

**JOEL S. SAAL, M.D.**
Clinical Instructor
Department of Functional Restoration
Stanford University Medical Center
Menlo Park, CA

**ROBERT THAYER SATALOFF, M.D., D.M.A., F.A.C.S.**
Professor of Otolaryngology
Thomas Jefferson University
Philadelphia, PA

**BRIAN SCHULMAN, M.D.**
President
Occupational Psychiatry
Bethesda, MD

**CHRISTOPHER A. SHEPPARD, M.D.**
Associate Professor of Clinical Internal Medicine
Department of Internal Medicine
Northeastern Ohio Universities College of Medicine
Rootstown, OH;
Chief of Neurology
Akron General Medical Center
Akron, OH

**GEORGE M. SMITH, M.D., M.P.H., F.A.A.D.E.P.**
G. M. Smith Associates, Inc.
Bethesda, MD

**LEONARD J. SWINYER, M.D.**
Clinical Professor of Dermatology
University of Utah
Salt Lake City, UT

**JAMES S. TAYLOR, M.D.**
Head, Section of Industrial Dermatology
The Cleveland Clinic Foundation
Cleveland, OH

**PAUL D. TEYNOR, M.D.**
Intermountain MRO Services, Inc.
Salt Lake City, UT

**MOSHE TOREM, M.D.**
Professor and Chairman
Department of Psychiatry
Northeastern Ohio Universities College of Medicine
Rootstown, OH;
Chairman
Department of Psychiatry and Behavioral Sciences
Akron General Medical Center
Akron, OH

**RALPH O. WALLERSTEIN, M.D., M.A.C.P.**
Clinical Professor of Medicine
University of California, School of Medicine
San Francisco, CA

**RONALD J. WASHINGTON, M.D., F.A.A.D.E.P.**
Dallas, TX

**KARLMAN WASSERMAN, M.D., Ph.D.**
Chief
Division of Respiratory and Critical Care Physiology
    and Medicine
Harbor-UCLA Medical Center
Torrance, CA

**KENNETH M. WILLNER, J.D.**
Senior Associate
Paul, Hastings, Janofsky & Walker
Washington, DC

**TIMOTHY WOLFE, B.S., R.P.F.T.**
Pulmonary Laboratory
Saint Lukes Medical Center
Cleveland, OH

**LEE C. WOODS, M.D.**
Staff Physician
Orthopedic Hospital
University of Southern California
Los Angeles, CA

**DENNIS J. WRIGHT, M.D.**
Assistant Professor of Surgery
Northeastern Ohio Universities College of Medicine
Rootstown, OH

To Baze,
The love of my life,
My best friend,
My wife

and

(with respect to the Society of Jesus)
"Ad Dei Gloriam Majoram"

*Stephen L. Demeter*

To my wife, Kerstin, for her never-ending
encouragement and support

*Gunnar B.J. Andersson*

To my wife, Marcia, and my children,
Janine, Lisa, and Matthew, for their
inspiration, encouragement, and
compassionate patience.

*George M. Smith*

Disability management represents an area of medicine that has a large financial impact upon the financial status of not only this but other countries. Despite the large expenditures of money, time, personnel, and resources there exists no single, comprehensive compendium of information on disability evaluation. The ideal compendium would include information on the financial impact of disability, the role of physicians in diagnosing and quantifying impairment, the role of lay professionals (most notable lawyers) in translating medically derived impairment into legally allowable disability for financial disbursement, and an analysis of the social and legal constructs upon which disability determination is based. This book has been developed along these lines and contains sections devoted to each of these important issues.

Depending upon one's definition of disability, between 35 and 46 million Americans can be labeled as disabled. Since no standardized or generally accepted definition exists, it is difficult to arrive at meaningful and accurate figures. The cost of disability to this country, generated by those individuals, takes many forms. These include costs due to exclusion from the work place, costs engendered by providing medical care for those individuals, earning replacements for those individuals from insurance and government and industrial stipends, costs incurred by medical evaluations necessary to document impairment and disability, legal costs required for the same issues, and ancillary costs used to translate impairment into disability. In 1980, these aggregate costs of disability were estimated to be $177 billion, or approximately 6.5% of the gross domestic product.

The principal audience for this book is physicians, attorneys, and other health care workers who assess individuals with medical conditions that preclude them from the work place on either a temporary or permanent basis, either totally or partially. Much time and effort has been devoted to assembling authors who are not only knowledgeable about the impairment process but also experts in this field. These individuals include some who have worked on, and developed sections of, the *Guides to the Evaluation of Permanent Impairment*, published by the American Medical Association, people holding similar positions for the Social Security Administration, well known and respected authors who have published in their field, and members and teachers of disability organizations including the American Academy of Disability Evaluating Physicians.

The clinical chapters are devoted to explaining why things were done in certain fashions in the various disability rating systems. They allow the physician to understand why certain tests are included as discriminating and/or determining tests for impairment and why others were excluded. They allow the physician to understand why certain clinical examinations are accepted, acceptable, or rejected. They allow the physician to have a firm grasp of the background information necessary to properly use the rating systems. These rating systems, many times, take the appearance of "cookbooks". This book then allows for a broad and rich understanding of the rationale behind these formulae.

No less importantly, the sections on rating systems allow the users of the medical information to understand why physicians do what they do and how they do it. They allow these users to understand the scope and range of a physicians' report, to assess its reliability and validity, and provide rationale for either acceptance or rejection of the information provided by the physician. They allow for understanding and comprehension by translating "medicalese" into more understandable language.

Other sections of this book complement the medical information. These sections are written for the physician and nonphysician alike. They provide an understanding of the function of ancillary personnel who are important for the disability process. All too often, physicians and nonphysicians alike have little understanding of the roles of these professionals. Other sections provide an analysis and explanations of the laws and regulations that deal with disability. Like anything else, if one does not understand the rules, one cannot produce satisfactory results. The process of impairment evaluation within a framework of laws and regulations is still imperfectly understood by most physicians. By including a discussion of these laws, this book provides the background information necessary to enhance the physicians' understanding of their role and allows nonphysicians to define not only the physicians' role but their own role in the disability arena. Lastly, a variety of introductory chapters are provided for a richer and deeper understanding of the development of disability systems and the social impact of disability issues.

Perhaps the most important reason for the existence of this book is the enhancing and strengthening of the disability process in not only this but in other countries. Impairment evaluations have, too often, been the "poor stepchild" of the medical profession. Until recently, physicians have had little opportunity to receive training in this field. There is a saying in the computer industry: "Garbage in, garbage out" (or GIGO). Unfortunately, many times impairment evaluations and disability determinations are dependent upon, and result in, GIGO. From the financial perspective alone, a book such as this one is needed to improve the disability process. On a more humanistic level, improvement in the impairment evaluation and disability process is necessary to ensure that an impaired individual is fairly treated, properly managed, and appropriately compensated.

There are many individuals who have helped with the development of this book that need to be acknowledged. Recognition must first go to Tallamadge Hiebert, Ph.D., M.D., who, to my knowledge, is the first individual to demand respect for and enhance the awareness of disability as an important element of the medical profession and demand that this become a scientific discipline. Appreciation goes to my editors at Mosby, including Laura DeYoung and Jennifer Byington Geistler, who have been so gracious with their time and support for this book. Lastly, my secretarial and supporting staff, Judy McCormick, Marlene Sieben, and Deborah Krassow must also be recognized.

It is said that all great men stand upon the shoulders of those who came before them. While making no pretense to being a great man, I have nevertheless stood on many broad shoulders. Those individuals responsible for my development include the Sisters at Incarnate Word Academy, Parma Heights, Ohio, especially Sisters DeLourdes, Bernadette, and Peters; and the fine teachers that I had at St. Ignatius High School, Cleveland, Ohio; at Northwestern University, Evanston, Illinois; and at the University of South Florida in Tampa, Florida. Recognition must also go to the fine teachers that I had at The Ohio State University College of Medicine, including Nye Larrimer, M.D.; during my residency training at Mount Carmel Medical Center in Columbus, Ohio, including Robert Murnane, M.D., and Donald Traphagen, M.D.; and during my fellowship training at the Cleveland Clinic Foundation in Cleveland, Ohio, including my good friend, and mentor, Edward Cordasco, M.D. Special note and recognition must also be given to D. Carlton Gajdusek, M.D., winner of the 1978 Nobel Prize in Medicine, who has influenced me more profoundly than he will ever know. Carl Zenz, M.D., Sc.D., and Tee Guidotti, M.D., M.Ph., have also provided support and encouragement in my later years of professional life.

I gratefully acknowledge my parents, Steve and Arline Demeter, who provided the thirst and opportunity for knowledge. Without them, I would not be who I am today. My sister, Dianne Sampas, and brother, David, have provided support throughout the years. Most especially, my gratitude goes to my wife, Geraldine, whose patience, understanding, and support have been necessary for me to exist as a man and a physician. My children, Beth and Stephen, have provided the time and opportunity and gracious understanding to allow me to work on this project.

*Stephen L. Demeter*

# CONTENTS

# PART I

# BASIC CONCEPTS

# CHAPTER 1

# APPROACH TO DISABILITY EVALUATION

*Stephen L. Demeter*
*George M. Smith*
*Gunnar B. J. Anderson*

## OBJECTIVES

This book is intended to serve as a primary reference source for disability-oriented medical evaluation protocols and techniques. Disability evaluation encompasses both medical and nonmedical aspects of evaluation and is effectively accomplished only when both components are properly managed. Readers, both physician and nonphysician, are offered a broad understanding of the conceptual framework and operational settings within which disability evaluations take place. The editors have structured this book to help physicians and medically-based readers understand the nonmedical components of disability assessment by reviewing the background and mechanics of the impairment evaluation process for each organ system, then providing a matrix for matching specific job skills with functional capabilities. For nonmedical users of medical information, the book offers sufficient understanding of the nature, purpose, content, and limitations of the medical impairment examination and the disability evaluation to enable them to ask physicians appropriate questions, to understand physicians' answers, to determine if more information is needed, and to have confidence in the validity of the medical information given. The concepts and methodologies set forth in this book are designed to minimize the barriers claimants face and to promote an atmosphere of trust and mutual respect among the parties involved in that person's claim.

Recognizing the breadth of the objectives just described, the book is divided into three parts:

*Part I* focuses on the origins and evolution of the current social, legal, and administrative concepts regarding disability systems in general, specific types of disability systems, and the medical practice of impairment evaluation.

*Part II* sets forth the medical specifications for disability-oriented impairment evaluations. Case examples are peppered throughout this section to give a "real world" look at the physician/patient exchange.

The American Medical Association *Guides to the Evaluation of Permanent Impairment*, although not a worldwide standard for physicians, will be used in these examples to establish conclusions.[1]

*Part III* looks beyond the outcome of the medical evaluation and focuses on the resources available to assist in restoring persons to maximum useful function and, ultimately, employment. The concepts of employment law and the provisions and impact of the Americans with Disabilities Act and the Family and Medical Leave Act are also detailed.

Appendix A defines common terms used in the disability management arena. Appendix B provides names, addresses, and phone numbers for various resource organizations.

## COMPONENTS OF THE DISABILITY EVALUATION PROCESS

Precise definitions, communication, and role awareness are essential parts of the disability evaluation. Each of these areas will be discussed.

### Definitions

#### Need for Precise Definitions

A disability could be defined as a non- or altered-ability to successfully accomplish a given task. Such a definition would ill suit the purposes of this book. Nor would it help to distinguish what it is that is being evaluated during the disability process. We are not particularly interested in defining and describing all the limitations that nature has imposed on each individual. We are interested solely in those deviations that are important for tasks of the workplace. Further, we are not interested in all the deviations in capability that serve to segregate an individual's place in the workplace, only those created due to a departure from prior capabilities caused by a departure from an individual's "normal" state of health. For example, in the first instance, we do not address the issue of why a person cannot be a championship marathon runner or a yoga mystic. We do address why an individual cannot sustain remunerative employment at a specific level. In the second instance, we do not address the issue of why the average person cannot play at the level of a concert pianist. We do address the issue of why the concert pianist can no longer perform at this level.

## Disability

"Disability" (or "nonability") arises out of an individual's inability to perform a task successfully because of an insufficiency in one or more areas of functional capability: physical function, mental function, agility, dexterity, coordination, strength, endurance, knowledge, skill, intellectual ability, or experience. "Disability" is not necessarily related to any health impairment or medical condition, although a medical condition or impairment may cause or contribute to disability. "Disability" requires a conceptual definition; it is "the gap between what a person *can* do and what the person *needs* or *wants* to do."[1] The medical condition may limit the individual's capacity for physical or mental activity or may lead to restrictions placed on the individual's activities to prevent further harm.

Disability may be temporary or permanent, depending on the ability to treat the medical condition. In addition, there are degrees of disability, usually termed partial or complete. Any number of factors affect these determinations because disability refers to the fit between ability and function in a job. Therefore, to determine the degree of disability, the physician must weigh the medical impairment, the demands of the occupation, and how these two interact: Can the job be modified to fit the individual's abilities? Can the worker be retrained or rehabilitated to the point where he or she can perform that job or another job? Many variations are possible.

Confusion occurs in dealing with the language of laws, regulations, or policies and procedures, which ordinarily speak of the consequences of disability rather than accurately defining the disabled state. Examples include the following:

*Private Disability Insurance:* "Disabled for the substantial and material duties" of an occupation.

*Workers' Compensation Law:* "If the injury causes temporary, total disability, the disability payment is two-thirds of the average weekly earnings."[2]

*Social Security Disability System:* "Disabled for substantial, gainful activity."

*Family and Medical Leave Act:* Has a "disability" that makes the individual unable to work.[3]

While each of these "definitions" conveys a sense of what "disability" means within that system, none offers specific operational criteria that can be applied to determine whether or not an applicant for disability benefits is disabled.

### Impairment versus Disability

Impairment is defined as the loss of a physiologic function or of an anatomic structure. Intellectual impairment involves diminished or lost cognitive function. Evaluation of impairment is addressed in the American Medical Association *Guides to the Evaluation of Permanent Impairment.*[1] In the AMA *Guides*, "impairment" is defined as "a deviation from normal in a body part or organ system and its functioning."[1] "Disability" is defined as "an alteration of an individual's capacity to meet personal, social, or occupational demands or statutory or regulatory requirements, because of an impairment."[1] Impairment assessment is deemed a medical evaluation, while disability is determined in an operational setting, such as the workplace or in a structured, functional capacity evaluation where observations are made of the individual's capacity to carry out particular tasks or perform specified functions. Therefore, an "impaired" person is not necessarily "disabled."[1]

A *disability*, for the purpose of this book, is defined as a medical impairment that prevents remunerative employment. An *impairment* is defined as the inability to successfully complete a specific task based upon insufficient intellectual, creative, adaptive, social, or physical skills. A *medical impairment* is defined as an inability to successfully complete a specific task which the individual was previously capable of completing or one which most members of a society are capable of completing due to a medical or psychological deviation from an individual's prior health status or from the status expected of most members of a society.

### Communication

In communication, a thought or idea is expressed by the sender and delivered to a receiver. For that thought or idea to be properly interpreted by the receiver, both sender and receiver must have a common frame of reference or speak the same language. In relation to disability evaluations, physicians and nonmedical personnel must be able to communicate about medical problems and limitations, using the same definitions as they apply to the workplace.

Physicians are trained to assemble and analyze medical information, communicating with each other within a framework of established medical diagnostic criteria and generally accepted medical principles and practice. They use highly technical and specialized

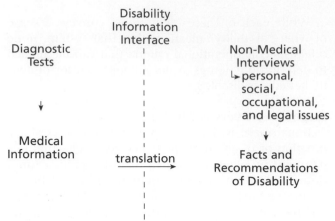

FIGURE 1-1    Medical (impairment) information obtained in a disability-oriented medical evaluation must be translated into nontechnical terms to be instrumental in deciding the presence or degree of disability. (Adapted from material by G. M. Smith Associates, Inc., Bethesda, Md.)

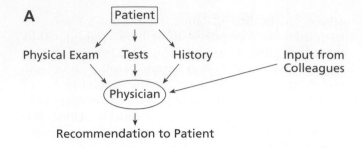

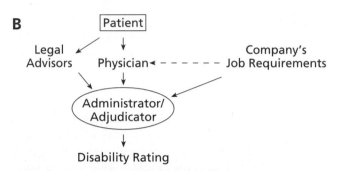

FIGURE 1-2    The physician's change in role. **A,** The physician is the primary decision maker in the traditional medical evaluation. **B,** The administrator or adjudicator is the primary decision maker in the disability evaluation.

medical language to communicate with each other and with other health-care professionals. When communicating with nonmedical users of medical information, they must speak in nontechnical terms. The information that flows each way across this information interface must be understandable, supportable, reasonable, and useful. All parties who work with disability evaluation depend on each other for the system to work efficiently and properly. Figure 1-1 illustrates the dynamics of this type of communication.

### Role Awareness

Physicians, in a standard medical evaluation, are the primary decision makers (Fig. 1-2, *A*). In the disability evaluation process, the physician's role as primary decision maker is yielded to other participants in the evaluation process. Figure 1-2, *B*, shows the administrator as the central authority when determining disability. Unless physicians are aware of this change in role, they may be frustrated or confused about "Who's in charge?" "What do they want?" and "Why is my report being challenged?"

## FORMULATION OF THE REPORT

Physicians must become more than casually acquainted with the specific provisions and procedures of the employment and workers' compensations laws and regulations in the states where they practice, the Social Security Act, the Americans with Disabilities Act, the Family and Medical Leave Act, and the regulations published by the federal agencies administering these statutes. By becoming knowledgeable re-

garding these matters, physicians will be able to assess the requests and reasons for a disability-oriented medical evaluation, ask appropriate questions of the requestor, understand the needs of the requestor, and provide a report that is complete, accurate, supportable, and responsive to the stated needs.

By the same token, those on the nonmedical side of disability management must understand the role, functions, thought-processes, and limitations of the physician so that they can formulate questions and have realistic expectations regarding the evaluation's outcome. The request for a disability-oriented medical evaluation must explain enough regarding the evaluation's objectives for the physician to assess those objectives, translate them into a medical-evaluation protocol appropriate for that system, and provide a responsive report. The user of the medical information must also understand the technical medical statements the physician uses in formulating conclusions and recommendations. Clear communication is of utmost importance. This book is intended to facilitate optimum communication.

### References

1. *Guides to the evaluation of permanent impairment,* ed 4, Chicago, 1993, American Medical Association.
2. Workers' Compensation Laws of California, Labor Code S4653, p. 280.
3. Family and Medical Leave Act of 1993.

# CHAPTER 2

## HISTORY OF DISABILITY AS A LEGAL CONSTRUCT

*Judith Goodwin Greenwood*

As long as humankind has existed there has inevitably been impairment and disability. The life-giving processes of gestation and birth themselves can result in physical and mental incapacities that impede an individual's full, normal function. Natural disasters such as earthquakes and hurricanes cause injuries and impairment as do accidents of all kinds from home to work, from recreation to transportation. Violent aggression from single-encounter assaults to ethnic conflicts and full scale wars can also create disability. Even without all this, the process of life and aging itself guarantees that if we live long enough, impairment of some sort will occur.

Throughout history disability and impairment have been unwanted human conditions; therefore, they have been the subject of miraculous recoveries (Jesus healed the lame and the blind) or they have caused ostracism and even punishment (disabled and impaired persons in concentration camps were the first to be exterminated in Nazi Germany). Between the extremes of miraculous cures and extermination, from ancient to modern times, impairment and disability have been addressed through religious and secular charity. It is only in modern times that they have been accorded legal status. But unlike other human conditions, such as poverty, gender, childhood, old age, and race, that have been accorded legal status, disability has challenged and continues to challenge definitive categorical boundaries. All over the world, particularly in the developed countries, governments and adjudicating bodies struggle to determine who is disabled. The definitions of disability expand and contract more along political and ideological lines than according to any clear physical determinations.

To trace the history of disability as a legal construct, I will discuss the development of the English Poor Laws, the development of the German invalidity and pension system, the development of state workers' compensation laws, and the federal Social Security Disability Insurance program in the United States. In conclusion, I will discuss the present and future outlook on disability.

## THE ENGLISH POOR LAW DEVELOPMENT

The English Poor Law of 1601 was passed in response to the decline of feudalism and community bonds that existed for the protection of all, not only against outsiders seeking to acquire property or to wreak revenge, but for the protection of individuals with special needs: children, the elderly, and the infirm and impaired. Within the feudal system, charity from community members took care of deserving people with special needs. The new economic system, however, brought with it a new class of people: unemployed wanderers or vagrants who turned to begging or charity together with people of special needs, such as orphans, the blind, and the physically defective. These two categories—vagrants and the infirm or persons with special needs—could overlap as some disabled persons may have been intermittent workers who moved from job to job as their conditions permitted.

The English Poor Law of 1601 was a culmination of earlier laws in the sixteenth century that initially provided voluntary funds for those unable to work. When those funds proved insufficient, compulsory contributions were sought within towns and parishes. With these compulsory contributions it became necessary to identify clearly those persons in need who would qualify for assistance. Thus, local government replaced religious charity. While the codified Old Poor Law (as the Poor Law of 1601 came to be known) was national legislation, the parish remained the administrative unit. The law was enforced by both local justices and church wardens who assessed and collected a household contribution (or tax) and determined the distribution of funds among the needy.

The question of legitimacy for poor relief was paramount. As Deborah Stone has observed:

> The phenomenon of vagrancy was virtually an obsession with social theorists and law makers all over Europe in the sixteenth, seventeenth, and eighteenth centuries. It is unlikely, therefore, that the specific causal theories elaborated for the English case tell the whole story. (Enclosure or conversion of public grazing land to private property was probably the one phenomenon unique to England, at least in scope.) Bad harvests, currency debasement, price inflation, and the conclusion of wars may have temporarily exacerbated an existing situation, but the problem was clearly fundamental and pervasive. And whatever its actual magnitude in terms of actual numbers of vagrants, it was serious enough to command enormous intellectual, economic, and political effort. (p 30)[16]

To control the vagrancy problem and to provide for persons in need, English policy makers in the early seventeenth century with the Old Poor Law and again in the nineteenth century with the New Poor Law made work ability and locality predominant issues. Workhouses were set up for those poor persons able to work. Poor children and orphans were apprenticed to craftsmen. "Settlement Laws" restricted movement of the poor between parishes, but also gave parishes the power to remove young family members from "families overburdened with children" and to send orphans to apprenticeships.

The issue of work ability and need for some relief for the poor came to a head with the New Poor Law of 1834, which stated the "principle of least eligibility" wherein a poor person's economic situation had to be below that of an independent laborer of the least means in order to qualify for a workhouse. Need for assistance outside of or beyond a workhouse (then referred to as "outdoor relief") was based on inability to work according to various categories of conditions: the sick, the insane, the "defective" (blind, deaf and dumb, then later "lame" and "deformed"), the aged and infirm, and children. All except children became part of the developing concept of sanctioned disability and classified as unable to work.

Thus categorization and means testing became an essential part of English welfare policy from the seventeenth century onward. The concept of need was drawn ever more stringently into opposition with work ability. Certification of legitimacy for assistance became the imperative in separating the ablebodied from those who were poor because of some specified condition of physical or mental impairment that prevented work.

With regard to the ablebodied, the New Poor Law restrained labor mobility either by forcing lower-class laborers to accept low wages to avoid the workhouses or by confining poor ablebodied persons of "least eligibility" to workhouses, often under harsh conditions.

## THE GERMAN INVALIDITY AND PENSION LAW OF 1889

In Germany, as in England, taking care of the needs of those persons who were unable to take care of themselves fell to the church when society was primarily agrarian. As industry developed in the German states in the mid-1800s, the Catholic church, which was not affiliated with the states as was the Protestant church, became particularly active in charitable work helping individuals displaced by the emerging economic order. As industry was developing, Otto von Bismarck ascended to political power, first as prime minister to King Fredrick William IV of Prussia, then as chancellor to William, who became emperor of a unified Germany under the name of Wilhelm I. The unification of the separate German states was consummately forged by Bismarck.

Chancellor Otto von Bismarck, a conservative, determined that social insurance was the way to instill patriotism and loyalty to the new German state as well as to quell political activism in the rival Social Democratic party. In contrast to the English Poor Laws, the German social legislation of the 1880s was not a codification of earlier laws directed at controlling vagrancy and the needs of the poor, but part of a planned and concentrated effort of state-sponsored social welfare that was concerned with social hierarchy and labor mobility. As noted in the last section, the shift in Europe from a feudal and community resource-based economy to a wage-based manufacturing economy required governments to focus on the work ability of its citizens. Three laws comprised Bismarck's approach.

In 1883 national health insurance was introduced for a large segment of workers. In 1884, after three draft laws, a plan to compensate workers for lost wages when injured on the job was enacted with costs paid fully by employers. (Bismarck had to give up his idea of a federal contribution due to opposition from other conservatives.) In 1898, when addressing work disability, the government decided that disability was a function of lost earning capacity and job opportunity, and not, as narrowly interpreted in the English Poor Laws, a categorical incapacity to work.

The concept of disability as a function of lost earning capacity allowed the German state to promote regional job mobility for persons with skills needed in the economy of other localities, but at the same time to protect individuals who already held jobs requiring similar education and experience. The interest of the nation-state was to provide comparable jobs for displaced workers or to provide disability pensions. While acceptable alternative job options for educated, clerical (white collar) workers were relatively narrow, the available job market for manual (blue collar) workers was considerably broader. Thus, as German law developed, white-collar workers were considered separately from blue-collar workers. Earning capacity again determined the difference: white-collar workers had to demonstrate a loss of half their earning capacity to qualify for a disability pension, while blue-collar workers had to demonstrate a two-thirds loss of earning capacity. The concept of disability was clearly and carefully tied to both occupational and social structure and was used to preserve a person's sense of security within the social system.

Again I turn to an analytic observation made by Deborah Stone, who has studied and written in detail on disability as a special status for public assistance:

> Disability in German policy, as in English policy, serves to demonstrate the boundaries between the work and need system, but the boundaries are defined very differently. In Poor Law policy the purpose of the categories was to help people in the work-based system as long as possible so as not to lose their productivity. Disability was thus defined very narrowly, and restricted (originally) to a small set of recognizable conditions that permanently incapacitated a person or totally incapacitated him or her temporarily. The Poor Law concept allowed people out of the work-based system and into the need-based system only when they were absolutely devoid of productive ability. In German social insurance, the effect of the category was to preserve very fine distinctions in the internal occupational hierarchy. The German definition of disability thus let people out of the work-based system when keeping them in would disrupt the social hierarchy. (pp 66–67)[16]

Two very different ideologies in philosophies of welfare are evident. Prior to 1870, Germany had been a loose confederation of separate principalities until Prussia with Bismarck at the helm exerted leadership in a drive toward unification and industrialization. Thus in the German system, social insurance was instituted as a material benefit given by the state to its citizens, and the cost of providing the insurance was viewed as a political expediency to maintain their loyalty if an appropriate work status could not be maintained.

On the other hand, in England where the events of history allowed a slower shift from an agrarian to an industrialized, mercantilist economy, any "outdoor relief" or direct government subsidy was seen as a drain on resources that could otherwise have gone to productive development. Stone notes that in late eighteenth century England, Jeremy Bentham, the philosopher-industrialist, developed an idea of how the blind could indeed knit and how children "would be harnessed to a seesaw apparatus designed to pump water as a byproduct of their play."[16] Productivity of any kind, not social status and earning capacity, was the issue.

## RECOGNITION OF DISABILITY IN THE UNITED STATES

### Workers' Compensation

The first legal recognition of disability in the United States developed out of the tremendous industrial expansion that started after the Civil War and extended into the early twentieth century. Injuries and fatalities related to work were very common and accepted as inevitable. There were spectacular catastrophes, including the death of 362 miners in a mining explosion in West Virginia in 1907, and 164 women in New York in the Triangle Shirtwaist fire in 1911.[15] Whether there was death or injury, the only recourse employees or their families had was to bring a tort action against the employers in court to claim damages.

Employers, however, had three common law defenses known as the "unholy trinity" that were difficult to overcome: assumption of risk (employees supposedly knew the risks of the job before accepting employment), the fellow-servant rule (coworker negligence), and contributory negligence by the employee. Nevertheless, as traumatic work-related injuries and fatalities mounted in the early twentieth century, judges allowed more and more cases to be brought to trial, and more and more frequently juries were holding employers culpable and determining monetary awards. Still, many injured employees and their families did not have the resources to go to trial; consequently many employees and their families were left destitute. There was a growth of social concern for a remedy to the poverty caused by work-related injuries and fatalities. At the same time, employers were increasingly faced with the uncertainty of potential liability for injuries and the unpredictability of jury awards if a lawsuit was brought.

A political consensus grew for finding a clear and certain remedy to the dual problem; state after state, beginning with Wisconsin in 1911, mandated an employer-financed insurance program. At first the program was limited to the most hazardous occupations, and it compensated workers and their families for lost wages resulting from work-related injury or death. Workers lost their right to sue the employer for damages, but gained assurance of a certain level of wage-replacement benefits and coverage of medical expenses if they were injured, while employers accepted limited liability for all work-related injuries and deaths. Within this original "no-fault" system, injured workers were considered to be victims of inevitable industrial accidents and, as conceived in Germany, society or the state had an obligation to offer some limited form of wage-based social insurance. Unlike the German form, however, there was initially little or no concern within state workers' compensation programs for using insurance benefits as a way to maintain social hierarchy and labor mobility. Like the original English Poor Law, prevention of poverty, not disability and its social management, was the driving concern for the development of workers' compensation programs in the United States.

By 1920, 42 of the 48 states and the District of Columbia had workers' compensation laws in place. The state-by-state process of legislating workers' compensation laws has been called the "most dramatic event in the twentieth century history of American civil justice."[5] For 25 years after its inception, workers' compensation was the only social disability income program in the United States.

The glory was short-lived, however. The decade of the 1920s saw a workers' compensation system in relative decline compared to the aspirations of reformers and early proponents of the system. Programs became dominated by disputes over whether certain injuries were work-related or over the exact extent of disability or impairment and the corresponding amount of benefits. Also, politically-appointed administrators who lacked appropriate legal expertise and objectivity in labor-management relations contributed to the developing adversarial climate. The basic concept of workers' compensation as a self-contained program for the provision of wage-replacement benefits and for the adjudication of disputes between employers and employees regarding those benefits became fixed. By the mid-1930s when the debate heated up over wider disability coverage through Social Security, workers' compensation was not considered a model program because leading reformers saw little distinction between occupational disability and nonoccupational impairment. They also expressed skepticism over the quality of medical care that was provided for the injured worker by the large number of company doctors.

## Social Security Disability

The two-decade Social Security debate over wider disability coverage, lasting into the 1950s, was not about whether entitlement to benefits was appropriate, but about the definition of disability and how disability was to be determined. At the time, disability clauses in private insurance carrier life insurance policies usually stated disability as being "wholly" and "totally" incapable of working. However, the courts generally interpreted these statements with some leniency, taking the position that a person need not be totally helpless. (p 74)[16] For a variety of reasons including judicial interpretation, poor underwriting practices, and industry competition, the commercial insurance carriers had experienced significant losses in disability coverage, and their experience increased the skepticism and fears of conservatives about adding disability coverage into the Social Security program.

The liberals, however, pursued a strategy of incrementalism. Social Security historian Martha Derthick observes that "incremental change in whatever institutional setting has less potential for generating conflict than change that involves innovation in principle." (p 314)[6] Thus disability insurance through Social Security came about in a gradual process. The first step was taken in 1954 when disabled persons were exempted from making Social Security contributions but still remained eligible for an old-age pension at age 65. Disability was then defined as the "inability to engage in any substantial gainful activity because of any medically determinable physical or mental impairment that can be expected to be of long, continued, and indefinite duration."[13]

In 1956, the law was amended to provide disability benefits to individuals between the ages of 50 and 65 who, because of disability, were unable to work according to the above definition. In 1958, the law was amended so that monthly benefits were payable to dependents of disabled workers. In 1960, the age 50 limitation for eligibility was removed, and in 1965, the duration of disability was changed to what it remains today: disability needs to have lasted, or be expected to last, for a continuous period of not less than 12 months.[14] In 1972, benefits were substantially increased, and Medicare benefits were made available to beneficiaries who received disability benefits for two years or longer. Over this nearly two decade period, not only did Congressional amendments to the Social Security Act liberalize the rules and regulations for determining disability, but liberal judicial interpretations resulted in the disability program taking on "some of the features of an unemployment compensation program." (p 36)[12] This meant that there must be a lack of readily available employment opportunities for an individual, along with physical or mental impairment. A theoretical ability to engage in "substantial gainful activity" of any kind, anywhere, was deemed by the courts insufficient to disprove disability.

Through all the incremental development of the federal disability program, however, physical or mental impairment along with its measurement has remained the anchor of decision making. Impairment and its measurement provided political expediency for the proponents of the Social Security Disability Insurance program because it allowed them to present disability as a relatively narrow and measurable concept to skeptical conservatives. While presenting disability as synonymous with impairment may have been the path of least resistance to win over support initially, it has led to the confusion of the entire disability construct that is an amalgam of a number of factors with impairment being only one of them. Nevertheless, with impairment established as the benchmark of disability, medical providers who were asked to measure impairment assumed a controlling role in a major social insurance program with the attendant anomaly of their becoming gatekeepers for the provisions of non-medical social insurance benefits.

## THE IMPAIRMENT/DISABILITY MATCH/MISMATCH

As previously discussed, making impairment the defining condition of disability imbued the concept of disability with a false sense of a definite boundary. *Impairment* is associated with *disability* only insofar as it is a necessary and contributory factor; in itself it is not sufficient to cause disability. The consideration that an individual who is impaired is not, as a consequence, necessarily disabled was clearly developed in the third edition of the AMA *Guides to the Evaluation of Impairment* and is reiterated in the fourth edition.[1] Disability compensation through both workers' compensation and Social Security, however, rests on the premise that disabled persons automatically because of their illnesses or impairments would be employed, or have opportunities for better employment, if their illness or impairment did not exist. This premise is flawed. A person with impairments is not necessarily disabled.

A number of public policy researchers on disability have concluded that disability is not a problem that can be categorically resolved through medical impairment rating systems. As Howards, Brehm, and Nagi have pointed out, disability, unlike impairment that is defined as a measure of physical or mental deficits, is a relational concept that involves a variety of situational, behavioral, and attitudinal factors that are not easily measurable. Disability and non-disability, they

point out, is the false dichotomization of a continuum. (pp 118-122)[10] Health factors related to employment and unemployment simply cannot be isolated clearly and consistently from all other factors. Several years earlier, Berkowitz, Johnson, and Murphy had argued that:

> . . . policy makers should give a much higher priority to policies designed to affect the interaction between households and employers. The evidence we have described . . . in previous chapters points to this juncture as a critical segment in the disability process. It shows that physical limitations are not for most persons the controlling influence on whether or not they are disabled . . . All . . . facts point to the conclusion that the work environment is as likely a candidate for public action as the individual. (p 143)[3]

Analyzing the Social Security and workers' compensation models of disability determination in 1984, I recommended a shift from a medical frame of reference to a socioeconomic frame of reference for work-related disability:

> A new approach to contending with work-related disability would place the burden of responsibility on employers for preventing or intervening on disabling situations, rather than on physicians for evaluating and treating disabling conditions. Effort is needed on the part of employers and unions to work out early return to work policies and procedures. Political leaders need to institute companion laws requiring insurers and benefit transfer programs to maintain return to work incentives. (p 600)[7]

As Deborah Stone repeatedly points out throughout her excellent analysis of disability as a special social status, the real issue at the heart of disability is recognition of need for social monetary support versus individual responsibility for earning wages. The popular conception of disability is much broader than the legal conception. Many more people consider themselves disabled than the actual number of those who receive disability benefits of one kind or another. (For instance, in the 1990 Census, 8.2% of the working U.S. population reported themselves as having a work disability, while only 4.2% said they were actually prevented from working [Table 4, p 185].) Thus disability as a popular conception is different from disability as an administrative legal concept that is focused on measurable impairment. The popular concept will shift according to socioeconomic dynamics that include unemployment and labor market conditions as well as age, education, and other factors including work ethic.

Thus social insurance programs seek to balance larger socioeconomic interests such as economic growth and protection of monetary resources with perceived individual needs and rights to those resources. As Stone astutely observes, "Disability programs are thus always in the position of selecting out applicants who do not meet program criteria: rarely are they in the position of soliciting applicants or persuading people to look at themselves as disabled." (p 144)[16]

Because the popular concept of individual disability is broader than the administrative legal concept, judicial interpretation tends to rebalance the scale in favor of individual need and rights when issues of entitlement are disputed. Modest, even minor, impairments that arguably are disabling can become significant when more immediate socioeconomic and demographic factors contribute to an individual's difficulties.

Clearly, disability is an unstable concept constantly beset by structural tensions within any social disability system. Not only is pressure for expansion exerted by individuals with perceived needs, but also by all who profit from the system as well. Physicians and other providers can expand the duration and definition of disability with questionable tests and treatments for which they receive payment, and attorneys set fees that are contingent on proving that the individual is disabled. Neither physicians, the official gatekeepers of the impairment boundary, nor attorneys, who are better served by the popular conception of disability than by the stricter administrative legal concept, have any professional interest in securing a firm boundary for disability. The only real beneficiaries against the expansion of disability are the insurers and financiers.

## A PRESENT AND FUTURE OUTLOOK ON DISABILITY

This chapter has traced the historical progression of the social response to disability in Western Europe and the United States through the mid-twentieth century as illustrated below: (p 1250)[8]

Secularization–17th century–Late 19th century

Bureaucratization–Late 19th century–Mid-20th century

Medicalization–Mid-20th century

Particularization–Late 20th century

The secularization of disability beginning with the development of the English Poor Law progressed into the bureaucratization of disability that took form with the German Invalidity and Pension Law, and they continued with the state workers' compensation programs in the United States and the whole administrative apparatus for the Social Security Disability Insurance program. The medicalization of disability began, along with the bureaucratization of disability and reliance on physician certification of disability, through measurement of impairment, but it reached its peak with the Social Security Disability Insurance program and the administratively required clinical methods of evaluating physical or mental impairment.

As accumulated social policy and medical research have shown, however, the medical impairment model has proved insufficient for understanding and dealing with disability. This insufficiency is illustrated by the recent Boeing study on back pain. A longitudinal prospective medical study was conducted on 3020 aircraft employees to identify risk factors for reporting acute back pain at work. There was a four-year follow-up of 279 workers who subsequently reported back problems. Other than a history of current or recent back problems, psychosocial factors and perceptions of work, especially a lack of job satisfaction, were significantly more predictive of reported back pain than physical examination measures, physical capacities, and physical work characteristics.[2,4]

The emerging outlook on disability is one of particularization in terms of all that is involved, including not only impairment, but a combination of attitudinal, behavioral, and situational factors. Disability must be addressed, if it is to be successfully addressed, in terms of its details. Resources and services must be particularized to individual needs and simplified rather than determined according to bureaucratic rules and regulations or medical evaluations alone. While bureaucratic services for monetary compensation and medical services for diagnosis and treatment will always be needed, the need for a variety of disability prevention and management services is emerging as disability becomes understood as a complex of diverse particulars in relationship to one another.

In workers' compensation especially, the particularization of disability is likely to offer hope for some real changes in outlook. As noted earlier, the distribution and adjudication of benefits has been the central focus of workers' compensation administrations over the better part of the twentieth century. This focus relates to the basic power inequality inherent in the employer-employee relationship that can be, and often is, exploited by employers whose essential interest is in productivity and profit margin. Without enlightened self-interest (which fortunately is emerging in some high-technology industries) or some external incentive, many employers will not adopt management practices that assure a safe and satisfying work place. Too often employers regard the filing of a workers' compensation claim as simply negative behavior on the part of the employee, rather than the result of poor safety practices and job dissatisfaction as was found in the aforementioned Boeing study.

Emily Speiler, Professor of Labor Relations Law at West Virginia University and a former workers' compensation administrator, has written an impressive and scholarly review article on the lack of real safety incentives in current workers' compensation programs while at the same time cost-containment activities have become abundant as workers' compensation costs have rapidly escalated.[15] Her essential query is: Where does the injury prevention/cost containment connection come from? The complete answer, a complex analysis of labor relations law and workers' compensation economics, can be summarized as follows. Employers, either by choosing what seems the easiest path or through ignorance, seek to control their workers' compensation costs by controlling the reporting of claims rather than by actually working to prevent injury-based claims, which they believe requires more effort with regard to having viable safety programs and creating a climate of job satisfaction.

The bureaucratization and medicalization of the disability concept made it all the easier to spread the blame between the employees who file claims, the agencies that manage the claims, and the providers who treat work-related injuries and illnesses. Particularizing the *process* of disability shifts the focus from filing a claim to the actual occurrence of an injury or illness episode and the response to its occurrence. The shift is bringing about a new safety consciousness along with early disability management efforts when a work-related injury or illness does occur. The basic management-labor compromise that supports workers' compensation is now evident in some notable state reform efforts. Speiler writes:

> Safety rhetoric is now ubiquitous. Not only unions, but workers' compensation insurers, insurance departments, workers' compensation administrators, academic commentators, and employers organizations are all beating the safety drum. Safety legislation has emerged as a primary political focus of workers' compensation reform in the 1990s; it has become the language of political compromise. The current state legislative reforms reflect this new consensus. (pp 249-250)[15]

She then concludes her review by discussing the new safety and health provisions, all of which are aimed at achieving prevention of injuries as well as their disabling consequences.

A recent Michigan disability prevention study involving a random sample of 220 Michigan businesses from seven different industries demonstrates the probable good of such state reform efforts by showing that those employers who move aggressively with policies and practices designed to prevent injuries and their disabling consequences have significantly lower workers' compensation costs. In fact, within a given industry, costs can vary up to ten times between employers with effective management policies and practices that promote safety and job satisfaction and those who have few such policies and practices.[11] As well as safety practices, one other important employer practice found in the Michigan study was having aggressive return-to-work programs with modified work assignments for injured workers. Such a proactive approach is effective disability management.

The movement toward disability prevention and early-injury management is critically important in light of the expanding dynamic of disability described in the previous section. In her concluding analysis of the expansion of disability as social status, Stone discusses three dimensions of the legal disability construct that, once met, invite new circumstantial conditions to be claimed as disabling. (pp 172-186)[16] First, if one is disabled by official standards, it is because of an injury or some external force or agent not related to the person. This is the "no-fault" premise of disability that frees both the individual and the employer from responsibility and provides the morally worthy dimension of monetary compensation. Incapacity, the second dimension of disability, is determined by functional performance criteria of physical and mental exertion or by loss of wages or earning capacity. Third, clinical findings of abnormality are used to explain and establish incapacities. As diagnostic methods expand, so do the clinical findings of more and more abnormalities, and more and more vulnerable individuals who find it difficult or dissatisfying to work are put to tests of performance that are often inaccurate or misunderstood. Thus more and more incapacities are magnified through the accident/external agent argument and deemed to be legally work-related and work-preventing disabilities. Regarding disability in general, Irving Zola has stated:

> Studies have increasingly appeared that note a large number of disorders escaping detection . . . two-thirds to three-fourths of all existing conditions. Such data as these give an unexpected statistical picture of illness. Instead of its being relatively infrequent or abnormal, the empirical reality may be that illness . . . is the statistical norm. (p 243)[17]

Thus it comes that we are all impaired to some extent at some time, and social insurance programs are at risk for more and more individuals who have clinically explainable incapacities that appear to be caused by external forces and who are morally worthy of compensation. Workers' compensation programs have been particularly vulnerable to expanding disability. As I have stated elsewhere:

> The line between the obvious traumatic workplace injury and the gradual disability brought on by lifestyle and aging has blurred tremendously. The more blurred it has become, the more litigious the workers' compensation system has become. As some point, the irrationality of blaming the workplace for more and more personal liabilities must become patently obvious to policymakers. (p 25)[9]

Mental stress, heart conditions, and back pain are particularly relevant examples.

Putting injury prevention and disability management ahead of disability evaluation begins to rebalance the social welfare scale and the use of resources and services. Fair and equitable compensation of impairment for those who cannot work for wages, either temporarily or permanently, will always be necessary in an industrial society. But the "no-fault" principle of compensation must be balanced with industrial and corporate responsibility for the prevention of injury and disability. Otherwise, as Stone points out, "the keepers of the categories will have to elaborate even more situations in which people are legitimately needy, until the categories become so large as to engulf the whole." (p 192)[16] As such, impairment and disability must begin to be viewed as a manageable part of the human condition rather than a legal status or concept.

## References

1. American Medical Association: *Guides to the evaluation of permanent impairment*, Chicago, 1988, 1993.
2. Battie MC, Bigos SJ: Industrial back pain complaints: a broader perspective. *Orthop Clin North Am* 22:273-282, 1991.
3. Berkowitz MF, Johnson WG, Murphy EH: *Public policy toward disability*, New York, 1976, Praeger.
4. Bigos SJ, Battie MC, Spengler DM, et al: A prospective study of work perceptions and psychosocial factors affecting the report of back injury. *Spine* 16:1-6, 1991.
5. Darling-Hammond L, Kneisner TJ: *The law and economics of workers' compensation*, Santa Monica, Calif., 1980, Rand Publications.
6. Derthick M: *Policymaking for social security*, Washington, D.C., 1977, Brookings Institution.
7. Greenwood J: Intervention in work-related disability: the need for an integrated approach. *Soc Sci Med* 19:595-602, 1984.
8. Greenwood J: Disability dilemmas and rehabilitation tensions: a twentieth century inheritance. *Soc Sci Med* 20:1241-1252, 1985.
9. Greenwood J: A historical perspective on workers' compensation in the context of national health policy debate. In Greenwood J, Tericco A, editors: *Workers' compensation health care cost containment*, Horsham, Pa., 1992, LRP Publications.
10. Howards I, Brehm HP, Nagi SZ: *Disability: from social problem to federal program*, New York, 1980, Praeger.
11. Hunt HA, Habeck RV: *The Michigan disability prevention study*, Kalamazoo, Mich., 1993, W. E. Upjohn Institute for Employment Research.
12. Rockman S: *Judicial review of benefit determination in the social security and veterans administration*. Report to the Committee on Grants and Benefits, Administrative Conference of the United States, Washington, D.C., Aug. 1970.
13. Social Security Amendments: P.L. 761, Title 1, Section 215(i), Par. 3, Washington, D.C., 1954.
14. Social Security Amendments: P.L. 89-97, Title 3, Washington, D.C., 1964.
15. Speiler E: Perpetuating risk: workers' compensation and the persistence of occupational injuries. *Houston Law Review* 3:119-264, 1994.
16. Stone D: *The disabled state*, Philadelphia, 1984, Temple University Press.
17. Zola I: *Missing pieces*, Philadelphia, 1982, Temple University Press.

# CHAPTER 3

# ECONOMIC COSTS OF DISABILITY

*Peter S. Barth*

The purpose of this chapter is to explore a set of issues relating to the economics of disability. In particular, the focus is on the costs imposed by disability. Like a number of other social sciences, the economics profession has not been timid about extending its reach into subjects that are customarily the domain of others. Consequently, serious studies that examine "the economics of . . . " extend into many fields that traditionally have not been exposed to economic analysis. Since the economics of disability have begun to receive attention only within the past few years, the field still must be considered as formative and incomplete.

Before the costs of disability can be estimated, some acceptable definition of *disability* is needed. Unfortunately, this is no simple issue. At one level, a definition is needed in order to understand who it is that is disabled and the degree to which they have some condition. Consequently, an appropriate definition should be one that is capable of being measured. Chapter 1 described the concepts of impairment and disability from a medical and legal perspective. This chapter will address the concepts of disability from an economic standpoint. The concept of disability changes with each perspective. As seen in Chapter 1, no universal definition of disability exists. When various writers, economists, or business persons discuss the financial impact of disability, there is no common consensus about its definition. This confusion can lead to financial inaccuracies in any data collected about disability costs.

An analogy can be drawn here with the development of the concept of poverty at the outset of the Great Society. The decision was made early to create a measurable definition of poverty. This enabled the Johnson administration to accomplish several things. First, it established that the extent of the problem was substantial, justifying a War on Poverty. Second, the measurements that followed the definition identified the socio-demographic characteristics of the poor (i.e., by defining "poverty," target groups could be established). Third, a precise definition allowed measurement to be made of the changes in the number of poor that occurred as economic conditions changed, and as policies were implemented. That same definition is used today to establish eligibility for certain public entitlement programs (e.g., programs are available for persons with income levels at or below 150% of the poverty threshold). From this basis, various disability data are collected and collated. An operational definition of *disability* from an economic viewpoint results.

One such source of data is the National Health Interview Survey (NHIS), which has been carried out for three decades. It consists of a representative sample of the civilian, noninstitutionalized population.[1,20] Approximately 120,000 individuals are included in each sample survey. Persons are asked if an impairment or health problem prevents or limits their activities and whether that condition is chronic (lasting 3 months or more). Respondents are classified according to the degree of activity limitation. Those with the least severe limitations are persons with limitations that are not in their major activity. Those with the most severe limitations are unable to carry out their major activity. The concept of *major activity* is defined according to one's age so that for children it is attending school, for those aged 18–69 it includes working or keeping house, and for those aged 70 and older it is living independently.

Each of these concepts (i.e., chronic condition, limits, major activity, age cut-offs) can be subject to some second guessing. Further, that it is based on self-reporting is itself of some concern. Yet the concepts do permit measurement, and the degree of stability in the approach permits comparisons to be made over time.

The NHIS data suggest that over 33 million persons have limitations, with almost 10 million of them unable to carry out their major activity.[1,20] Additionally, about 2.2 million disabled persons reside in institutional facilities. Disability rates as defined are higher for males, blacks, low-income, and older individuals.[1,23]

While a need for measurement creates a quantitative source to define disability, this definition need not be synonymous with the medical and legal definitions. The economic impact of an impairment on disability depends upon several factors including one's occupation, the state of the labor market, and a person's willingness and ability to make an occupational shift. Further, with changes in any of these factors, disability could disappear or reappear, while the individual's health status remains stable.

It is difficult to quarrel with the recent report that concluded that disability statistics are "a patchwork of data that reflect the complexity of the concept of disability" or that "it is clear that the number of persons with disabilities depends on the definition of disability."[20] The report cites the NHIS estimate of 35 million, yet notes that another reputable source, the Survey of Income and Program Participation (SIPP), has estimated the number at 46 million. The point is that any estimates of the costs of disability depend directly upon the estimated incidence in the population, which in turn depends upon the definitions and concepts used.

## CONCEPTUALIZING COSTS

Estimating the costs of disability requires establishing both the number of disabled people as well as the average cost of disability. This exercise can be carried out for reasons that extend beyond any academic challenge. Estimates that appear to demonstrate a high cost of disability might suggest a significant public policy burden. Estimates that seem low would provide less justification for new and expanded programs to curtail disability through workplace safety or to assist impaired workers. This is not to impugn the motives of those carrying out such studies. Rather, it is to explain the substantial degree of interest that greets each new set of cost estimates.

Researchers who attempt to estimate the costs of disability or of particular illnesses or conditions have used one of two approaches. One approach, the *prevalence method,* relies upon cumulating the costs incurred, however conceived, of all the persons with a condition in a given year. In this calculation, the time of onset of the condition is of no concern. What matters is that the condition exists in that year. Alternatively, one could calculate the lifetime costs incurred by those who first develop a condition this year. The second approach, the *incidence method,* derives the present value of lifetime costs by summing the present cost and the discounted value of all future costs. Each approach, though they are conceptually and calculation-wise quite different, responds to the question of what are the costs of a specific health condition.

Economists may measure costs in different ways, but they are consistent as to how they conceive of them. Typically, an economist asks how much output, or product, is expended or is foregone due to the presence of disability. A foregone output, for example, is the partial or total loss of their work-connected earnings. Another foregone output is the partial or total loss of earnings from family and household members due to their inability to earn because of the time devoted to caring for the disabled person. The major expended outputs are the medical, hospital, pharmaceutical, attendant, equipment, and refurbishing expenses needed to care for the impaired or ill individual. Note that the sources of the funding for this last category are not relevant under this operational concept of disability. Providing these services and products means that real resources are being expended, regardless of whom the ultimate payers are.

Persons not familiar with this method of calculating costs should note some of its features. First, since younger and older persons are generally not members of the labor force, the costs of their disability tend to be lower, because their disability does not result in any direct diminution of output. However, if others are forced to reduce their working time in order to assist such persons, their output would fall as gauged by their reduced earnings (foregone output).

Second, disability for young persons can result in direct reductions in future output. One could estimate, therefore, the lifetime direct costs of a disabled person by calculating the reduced or lost earnings in future years. All future losses must be subjected to some time rate of discount, leading to lower cost estimates for younger disabled persons. If many of the disabled are quite young, the incidence method would show a higher social cost than would the prevalence approach.

Third, it is likely that some household members may feel compelled to enter the workforce as a result of the loss of earnings to another member of that household who has become disabled. In such cases it is not appropriate to parallel the treatment given to household members who have reduced their working time to assist the disabled person. That is, one should not reduce the estimated costs of disability because a family member's earnings have increased. Clearly, the earnings increase in that case has come at the expense of either time lost from household duties or from time previously at leisure, both of which have real value.

To estimate the costs of health care treatment and rehabilitation add all expenditures made on behalf of the disabled person (regardless of who pays the bill) and subtract those expenditures that would have been made for conditions other than those pertaining to the disability.

It should be apparent that efforts to carry out these calculations involve employing a variety of assumptions, and that overall estimates may be quite sensitive to the assumptions selected. Assumptions aside, the underlying data tend to be fragmented and not entirely consistent, suggesting that these estimates must be approached cautiously.

An excellent analysis by Chirikos, using the prevalence approach, places the aggregate costs of disability in 1980 at $177 billion, about 6.5% of gross domestic product.[6] The methodology he employed parallels the description above. He acknowledges that his estimates could be adjusted if more data were available. Since his assumptions appear to be consistently cautious, his estimate can be regarded as a reasonable lower bound of disability costs that year.

Using a set of techniques that are similar to those used by Chirikos, but employing an alternative data set, different assumptions, and limiting the group to those aged 18 to 64, Hill reports the direct costs of disability in 1984 to be $145 billion.[16] Though the Chirikos estimate of the direct costs in lost time and earnings for the disabled only was for 1980, adjusting that estimate for the subsequent 33% growth in the consumer price index, would place his estimate in 1984 dollars at about $91 billion. Clearly, the differences between the Chirikos and Hill estimates highlight the margins of approximation that exist, even when highly competent researchers undertake this type of effort.

The estimates by Chirikos find that 51% of the costs of disability derive from the medical care and other goods and services provided to the disabled. About 39% of the overall total stems from the lost earnings (foregone output) of the disabled, and about 10% from the labor market losses of household members of persons with disabilities. About 65% of the labor market losses were for males.

Chirikos acknowledges that he ignores those who sustained no earnings loss because of expenditures made to overcome the consequences of an existing impairment. Moreover, there is no estimate of the costs of pain and suffering, yet these are real costs that courts and juries are regularly called upon to evaluate. That they are difficult to assess in the aggregate suggests that a wise course is simply to note their existence without seeking to attach some precise value. Indeed, the difficulty is magnified when one recognizes that the suffering may extend to household members of the person disabled and that courts do award damages, for example, for loss of consortium to those affected by another person's disability.

Because pain and suffering are so difficult to evaluate, and because there are economic incentives to embellish or to diminish their scope, it is understandable that substantial suspicion surrounds claims for damages that they cause. One way to measure the value of pain and suffering is to calculate the amount that one would spend to avoid incurring them. Though this is an indirect approach, it can be measured. The bottom line is that pain and suffering substantially contribute to the costs that individuals, and thereby society, incur due to disability and excluding them leads to an underestimation of the aggregate economic impact of disability.

Where perfectly functioning labor markets are assumed to exist economists can comfortably argue that workers' earnings perfectly reflect their productivity. Though such perfection may exist at best in the long run, and at worst in textbooks only, this conventional treatment seems more appropriate than other methods. It allows one to measure the value of any output foregone by the degree to which a worker sustains reduced earnings. Typically, where disability leads to unemployment, reduced hours of work, or a lower level of wages, the cost is evaluated based on the overall earnings decline, as a proxy for the lost output to society. This conceptualization stems from the economist's traditional framework that considers full, or near to full, employment as the equilibrium state.

Disability does result in reduced productivity at times even without any decline in earnings. Though such a situation is not likely to occur in businesses that seek to survive over the long run, such temporary phenomena are possible. For example, other employees may pitch in and assist a worker with a problem that reduces his or her productivity. This may involve stepping up their own work effort (which means no overall loss of productivity has occurred) or it may mean that they aid in covering-up any shortfall in a co-worker's normal output (here a loss of product does occur). Reductions in output without any consequences in earnings may also represent poor monitoring by the managers of employee performances. In either case, an underestimate of the costs of disability seems likely where the measure is loss of earnings, yet employees continue to receive their predisability earnings despite operating at reduced levels of productivity. There are no global estimates of the costs of such hidden productivity losses.

As an example of the hidden productivity loss concept, a recent study by Greenberg et al of major depression, bipolar disorder, and dysthymia places their overall economic costs to society at $36.2 billion annually (excluding the costs attributable to death by suicide).[12] The authors assume that the reduced productivity of continuing employees with these conditions yielded a 20% reduction in worker output, resulting in an economic cost of $12.1 billion. This figure exceeds the costs of work days actually lost, and is about equal to the estimated annual costs of hospitalization, outpatient care, and drugs associated with these illnesses. The study is notable for two reasons. First, it attempts to place a dollar value on the hidden or obscured cost that is associated with certain illnesses and disabilities. Second, this valuation helps to contribute to a very high overall estimate for a single set of conditions, suggesting that the work of Chirikos or Hill may substantially undervalue the costs of disability.

## ALTERNATIVE COST METHODS

Though economists measure an item's cost in terms of the real resources used or foregone by it, the public view of costs is often quite different. Noneconomists usually focus on expended resources or the calculation of the costs of health care and rehabilitation, where actual dollars are exchanged for specific services and products. In this case, the two measures of costs are essentially the same.

Transfer payments, a major source of dollars spent, are not considered economic costs though they are often treated as such by noneconomists. A transfer payment is a payment from one agent to another that is not a payment for a product or a service rendered. Insurance benefits, both private and social, are transfers when money is paid out. Payments by government to those with perceived economic needs are transfer payments. Welfare recipients may derive their needs as a consequence of disability, but these are not the economic costs of disability. Instead, one household has money transferred to it to spend, resulting in someone else having less available for that purpose, for example, a taxpayer. Since one person's gain is balanced against someone else's loss, no real resources are lost to society.

That economists do not consider transfer payments as economic costs does not diminish the interest in the dollar payments due to disability. A recent study by the Bureau of Economic Research (Rutgers University) estimated that cost transfers to the disabled in fiscal year 1986 exceeded $86 billion (Table 3-1).[16]

The leading source of cash transfers was Social Security Disability Insurance (SSDI) at $20.1 billion or 89% of the $22.5 billion in Social Insurance Disability payments. Privately obtained disability insurance paid out almost $11 billion in 1986. Indemnity benefits under workers' compensation ($12.4 billion), disabled veterans' compensation ($5.7 billion), automotive bodily injuries ($9.3 billion), and other bodily in-

**TABLE 3-1**   CASH TRANSFERS (IN BILLION DOLLARS) FOR DISABILITY—FISCAL YEAR 1986

| | |
|---|---|
| Social Insurance | $22.5 |
| Private Disability Insurance | 10.8 |
| Indemnity Payments | 45.0 |
| Income Support (Welfare) | 8.2 |
| Total | $86.5 |

From Hill MA: The economics of disability. In Thompson-Hoffman S, Storck IF, editors, *Disability in the United States: a portrait from national data*, New York, 1991, Springer.

juries ($17.6 billion) amounted to $45 billion (52% of the total). Welfare payments, primarily provided by supplemental security income payments to the blind and the disabled, were over $8.2 billion.

This full-scale accounting of cash transfers needs an updating since both the nominal and real benefits have increased as has utilization. Workers' compensation and Supplemental Security Income payments have probably doubled in the interim and SSDI benefits have grown at a slower, but still explosive, rate, particularly since 1990.

In addition to the cash payments transferred, the 1989 study estimates that medical care costs for the disabled were about $79 billion in 1986, with about 58% accounted for by payments by the individual recipients, or by their privately provided health insurance programs. Medicaid accounted for 20% and Medicare for 11% of these costs with the balance from sources such as workers' compensation and the veterans' medical program. Clearly, the costs of health care for the disabled have grown since 1986 at least at the pace of overall health system costs. (From 1986 to 1993, health care prices grew by about 68%.)[11]

The final category of outlays for direct services to the disabled is estimated to have been at $3.5 billion in 1986. About one half of this amount was expenditures for educational and vocational rehabilitation. The total of cash transfers, medical care, and direct services expenditures for persons aged 18–64 in 1986 was estimated at $169 billion. The figure is consistent with other estimates. For example, in hearings on the Americans with Disabilities Act (ADA), the Commissioner of the U.S. Equal Employment Opportunities Commission (EEOC) testified that "one dollar in every 12 that the Federal Government spent was a direct payment to a disabled person or to a disability program. What had started out as a minor cost has escalated into a major drain on our economy."[9] Since federal outlays in Fiscal Year (FY) 1987 were $1004 billion, Commissioner Kemp estimated that $85 billion was spent on disability at the federal level alone.

## CHANGING INCIDENCE OF DISABILITY

The economic costs of disability are a product of the incidence of disability and average cost per disabled person. Differences in survey methodologies and definitions mean that a simple conclusion regarding the incidence rate of disablement in the population is perilous. The changing age composition of the population becomes a significant element in evaluating any changes in incidence rates over a long-term period. A changing political climate along with varying incentives available to claimants renders interyear comparisons of successful applications for SSDI and SSI (for blindness and disability) poor indicators of changing disability rates. Several excellent studies of the changing incidence rates can be found in Chirikos, Haveman and Wolfe, Wolfe and Haveman, and Ycas.[5,15,24,25]

Ycas, in 1991, stated that "overall work disability rates have not changed a great deal over time. They probably rose in the mid-70s and since may have tended to decline. All this variation is vastly smaller than one would expect from the doubling and halving of disability benefit award rates."[25] The release of the 1990 decennial census findings appears to confirm Ycas' conclusion. In 1990, 12.8 million persons, aged 16–64, had a work disability.[18] Of these, 6.6 million, more than half, were defined as severely disabled (i.e., unable to perform work of any type). Nationally, the rates of severe and non-severe work disability decreased by 3.9% and 4.7% respectively from 1980 to 1990, and the incidence of work disability declined from 85.2 to 81.5 per 1,000 persons.[18]

The comparison of work disability rates from the 1980 and 1990 decennial censuses suggests three notable observations. First, though rates are down, the declines are sufficiently small to characterize the two data points as fairly level. That is true for the aggregate as well as the components (i.e., the severely and nonseverely work disabled). However, these rates as reported were not age adjusted. With the increasing age of the population in this group of persons aged 16–64, a growing incidence rate is to be expected.

The overall near stability in disability rates roughly parallels the stability in expenditures for SSDI from 1980 to 1990, although intradecade swings were quite substantial. In 1990, expenditures for SSDI were 63% above 1980 levels with consumer prices rising at a rate of 59%.[11,22]

In inflation-adjusted dollars, between 1980 and 1990, there was a very slight increase in the level of expenditures for SSDI, and there was a slight decline in the rate of work disability. With a larger population level, the data are broadly consistent. However, that does not match the experience under workers' compensation programs where benefits grew by 118% between 1980 and 1989.

The economic downturn of the early 1990s, along with the changing political environment, may have altered this condition of apparent long-term stability. From December 1990 to December 1993, the number of SSDI recipients grew by 23%.[22] From Fiscal Year 1990 to 1993, SSDI expenditures increased more than 38%. Over that 3 year period, the consumer price index rose by less than 11%.[11]

A second striking characteristic of the census findings is the wide interstate variability in incidence rates of disability. For example, according to the 1990 decennial census, Alaska, New Jersey, and Connecticut had rates of 6.6, 6.2, and 6.4% respectively.[18] By contrast, the rates in West Virginia, Kentucky, and Arkansas were 12.6, 11.4, and 11.2% respectively. It seems readily apparent that the very large interstate variations are correlated with the economic environment of the states and the nature of each state's main industry. States with low income levels, high unemployment rates, shifting industrial bases, and low levels of human capital appear to be those, typically, with higher disability rates.

A third observation is that those states with higher incidence rates of disability in 1990 tended to be those with higher rates in 1980 as well. It seems quite evident that the economic character of work disability, itself a consequence of regional labor market conditions, is a critical dimension of the incidence, and ultimately the costs, of disability in the United States.

## WHO PAYS FOR DISABILITY?

When considering the expenditures made on account of disability, one needs to ask who is footing the bill. Surprisingly little work has been done to address this question. What follows are observations, though any of the issues raised below can be explored in greater depth.

Both workers' compensation and SSDI are economic mainstays of disabled workers and their families. The goal of either program is to replace the earnings lost for covered workers who meet certain eligibility criteria. Yet neither program seeks to replace the full earnings loss due to disability; as a consequence, some of the financial burden of disability is shouldered inevitably by the disabled. Most workers' compensation programs aim to replace two-thirds of lost gross earnings. All programs have initial waiting periods that are uncompensated, and all have statutory caps on weekly compensation benefits. Permanent disability benefits are very rarely compensable for a lifetime and only a few states provide any cost-of-living adjustments for long-term benefits. Not infrequently, workers must also pay for the costs of litigating for the benefits they receive.

SSDI benefits are payable only after a 5 month waiting period, have ceilings on benefits, and provide health care benefits only 24 months after cash benefits begin. Offsets exist in order to limit any stacking of benefits under this program with workers' compensation. Offsets under private disability insurance programs also typically limit any stacking of those benefits with either worker's compensation or SSDI.

Benefits under workers' compensation, SSDI, and private disability insurance are usually linked by formula to an employee's predisability earnings. Yet with the partial exception of health care benefits and Social Security old age retirement benefits, a work disability will substantially jeopardize an employee's supplemental benefits. Totally disabled workers do not have health care for themselves or their families provided by workers' compensation (except for the disabling condition of the employee) and all other supplemental benefits of the employment can cease. Recipients of SSDI are able to gain eligibility eventually for Medicare, and the Social Security old age benefits are not reduced due to prior disability. However, other supplemental benefits, such as privately funded retirement contributions, cease.

It seems clear that a sizeable gap exists between losses incurred by the disabled and the transfer payments typically provided. The gap is especially large in the case of persons who lose time from work while disabled, and particularly where a full job loss results from the condition.

## SUMMARY

One cannot estimate the costs of disability without a definition of disability that is measurable. Economists are generally in agreement that the costs of disability represent the resources used, plus those not used due to the presence of an impairment. This is consistent with the manner in which economic costs are generally calculated. Changing labor market conditions can profoundly affect the calculations of costs.

In a society that is increasingly sensitive to considerations of cost-effectiveness, measures of costs of disability take on considerable importance. The public's interest in the costs of disability is likely centered on the direct expenditures made on behalf of the disabled by government, and perhaps, by others. Relatively little interest appears to exist in the matter of the economic burden of disability that is borne by the individual.

## References

1. Adams PF, Benson V: Current estimates from the National Health Interview Survey, National Center for Health Statistics. *Vital Health Statistics* 10:181, 1991.
2. American Medical Association: *Guides to the evaluation of permanent impairment*, ed 3, revised, Chicago, 1990, AMA.
3. Andreoni D: *The cost of occupational accidents and diseases*, Geneva, 1986, International Labour Office.
4. Berkowitz M, Hill MA: Disability and the labor market: an overview. In Berkowitz M, Hill MA, editors: *Disability and the labor market: economic problems, policies and programs*, Ithaca, N.Y., 1986, ILR Press.
5. Chirikos TN: Accounting for the historical rise in work disability prevalence. *Milbank Q* 64:271-301, 1986.
6. Chirikos TN: Aggregate economic losses from disability in the United States: Preliminary assay. *Milbank Q* 67: Suppl. 2, Part 1:59-91, 1989.
7. Chirikos TN, Nestel G: Economic determinants and consequences of self-reported work disability. *J Health Econ* 3:117-136, 1984.
8. Colvez A, Blanchet M: Disability trends in the U.S. population 1966-1977: analysis of repeated causes, *Am J Public Health* 71:464-471, 1981.
9. Committee on Education and Labor, U.S. House of Representatives, 101st Congress: *Legislative history of Public Law 101-336: Americans with Disabilities Act*, Vol. 2, Washington, D.C., 1990, USGPO.
10. Committee on Labor and Human Resources and the Subcommittee of the Handicapped, U.S. Senate, 101st Congress on S. 933, *Americans with Disabilities Act of 1989*, Washington, D.C., 1989, USGPO.
11. Economic Report of the President, Washington, D.C., 1994, USGPO.
12. Greenberg PE, et al: The economic burden of depression in 1990. *J Clin Psychiatry* 54:405-418, 1993.
13. Greenberg PE, et al: Depression: a neglected major illness. *J Clin Psychiatry* 54:419-426, 1993.
14. Haveman RH, Wolfe B: The decline in male labor force participation (Comment). *J Political Economy* 92:532-549, 1984.
15. Haveman RH, Wolfe B: The disabled from 1962 to 1984: trends in number, composition and well-being. Institute for Research on Poverty, Special Report No. 44, Madison, Wisc., 1987.

16. Hill MA: The economics of disability. In Thompson-Hoffman S, Storck IF, editors: *Disability in the U.S.: a portrait from national data*, New York, 1991, Springer.

17. Leonard JS: Disability policy and the return to work. In Weaver CL, editor: *Disability and work: incentives, rights, and opportunities*, Washington, 1991, AEI Press.

18. Prevalence of Work Disability in the United States—1990. *Morbidity and Mortality Weekly Report* 42:757-772, 8 Oct. 1993.

19. Parsons DO: Measuring and deciding disability. In Weaver CL, editor: *Disability and work: incentives, rights, and opportunities*, Washington, D.C., 1991, AEI Press.

20. Pope AM, Tarlov AR: *Disability in America: toward a national agenda for prevention*, Washington, D.C., 1991, National Academy Press.

21. Rice DP, et al: The economic cost of illness: a replication and update, *Health Care Financing Rev* 7:61-80, 1985.

22. *Social Secur Bull* 56(4), Winter 1993.

23. Storck IF, Thompson-Hoffman S: Demographic characteristics of the disabled population. In Thompson-Hoffman S, Storck IF, editors: *Disability in the United States: a portrait from national data*, New York, 1991, Springer.

24. Wolfe BF, Haveman R: Trends in the prevalence of work disability from 1962 to 1984 and their correlates. *Milbank Q* 68:53-80, 1990.

25. Ycas M: Trends in the incidence and prevalence of work disability. In Thompson-Hoffman S, Storck IF, editors: *Disability in the United States: a portrait from national data*, New York, 1991, Springer.

26. Yelin EH: *Disability and the displaced worker*, New Brunswick, N.J., 1992, Rutgers University Press.

# CHAPTER 4

# OVERVIEW OF VARIOUS DISABILITY SYSTEMS IN THE UNITED STATES

*John D. McLellan, Jr.*

In this chapter we will discuss disability systems that have been established by Congress to meet the needs of specific groups not generally covered under state disability laws. Two of these systems are workers' compensation programs providing the full range of workers' compensation benefits to: (1) federal employees, the Federal Employees' Compensation Program, and (2) longshore and harbor workers, the Longshore and Harbor Workers Compensation Program. Another workers' compensation system, the Black Lung Program, was established solely to provide disability benefits to qualified coal miners who have sustained a disabling black lung medical condition due to their employment in or around coal mines. For further information on workers' compensation programs in general, see Chapter 6.

We also discuss the disability benefits provided by the Department of Veterans Affairs to many military veterans and their families. Attention will be given to how non-workers' compensation law and the Federal Employers' Liability Act work to assist railroad employees and seamen (crew members) in obtaining disability damages from their employers, and other disability benefits available to these two groups.

The discussion herein is meant briefly to acquaint the reader with the identified programs. It does not intend to be a detailed how-to guide of processing individual claims through the different systems. For up-to-date information on claims processing the reader should contact the agency administering the program and/or the sources listed in the end notes to this chapter.

## FEDERAL EMPLOYEES' COMPENSATION PROGRAM

### History and Background

The United States Congress, 25 years before the enactment of a federal workers' compensation law, showed an interest in protecting injured employees by finding ways of maintaining their pay during disability caused by job injury. In 1882, a program was enacted to continue the pay of federal workers in "hazardous occupations" who sustained injury. "Hazardous occupations" was defined to include primarily workers in life-saving situations (Coast Guard and occupations on the navigable waters). Full salary for up to two years was provided but no medical benefits. In the event of death in such employment the worker's family would receive the workers' pay for two years.

Later, but before the turn of the century, Congress authorized the Postmaster General to continue the salary of postal employees during the period of disability caused by injury on the job.

Then in 1908 Congress passed what is often referred to as the first workers' compensation law for federal employees. This law again was for only those employees in "hazardous occupations," but the expanded definition included about 25% of federal employees. Compensation was paid for job injury disability. In essence the compensation was a continuation of the full pay of the employee for the first year and then at 50% for the second year.

This law, while certainly an improvement over the past minimal attempts, still left the great majority of federal workers without protection against loss of wages because of injuries. Congress quickly corrected this coverage gap by passing the Federal Employees' Compensation Act of 1916[1] that, with amendments, comprises the basis of the present Federal Employees' [Workers'] Compensation [FEC] program. All federal employees were covered except, initially, for "Federal Officers." Compensation for wage-loss was originally provided at 66⅔% of the injured or killed workers' pay. At the same time compensable *wages* were set at $100, meaning that, at the beginning, no injured worker received more than $66.67 a week in compensation. For the first time "reasonable medical care" was provided in addition to the income-maintenance compensation payments. "Injuries" covered were then, and are today, "personal injuries," which it was held from the outset includes not only traumatic injuries but, also, what we today refer to as "occupational disease and illness".

The FEC program was run initially by an independent U.S. Employees' Compensation Commission composed of three commissioners who also administered the Longshore and Harbor Workers Compensation Act (LSA) passed in 1927. In 1946 these functions were placed in the new Bureau of Employees' Compensation (BEC) in the recently formed Federal Security Agency. In 1950 BEC was placed in the Department of Labor. BEC was abolished in 1974 and its functions placed in the new Office of Workers' Compensation Programs (OWCP) in the U.S. Department of Labor (DOL).[2]

## Federal Employees' Compensation Act

The Federal Employees' Compensation Act (FECA) is the workers' compensation law covering federal civilian employees and their dependents. FECA emphasis is on providing *continuing income maintenance payments* during periods of wage-loss caused by disability due to a work injury sustained "while in the performance of duty". (Lump-sum awards or settlements are not available.[3]) In addition, the FECA provides full medical care for such injury and, in the event of injury-related death, benefits to survivors. FECA claims are received, adjudicated, and paid by the federal government.[4]

## Administering Agency

The Office of Workers' Compensation Programs (OWCP), Employment Standards Administration, Department of Labor administers the FEC program. Civilian employees of the federal government, including the Postal Service, are covered. Certain other individuals may be covered under defined circumstances. For instance, state and local government law enforcement officers (not employees of the federal government) who are injured while assisting in the enforcement of criminal laws of the United States may be entitled to FEC benefits to supplement, not replace, state workers' compensation benefits.[5]

## Definitions of Disability and Disability Compensation[6]

As stated above, the emphasis in the FEC program is to provide regular income-maintenance payments (compensation) for workers who sustain loss of earnings or decreases in wage earning capacity due to *disability* resulting from *personal injury* sustained *while in the performance of duty*. The payments continue for the duration of such disability. There is no overall maximum number of weeks or monetary amount that limits payments. When the employee qualifies for government retirement the disabled employee may elect (revocable) to continue on FEC or to take government retirement. FEC payments would continue until such time as the employee is found to have no further disability—no further wage-loss, loss of earnings or earning capacity—due to the effects of the accepted injury. Lump-sum payments to injured workers to settle the government's liability to make continuing payments for disability are not available for the reason that the FEC is intended as a wage-loss program with the benefits being paid on a continuing periodic basis during the continuance of disability.[7]

"Disability" means the incapacity, because of employment "injury", to earn the wages the employee was receiving at the time of injury.[8]

"Injury" or "personal injury" means a wound or condition of the body induced by accident or trauma, and *includes a disease or illness* proximately caused by the employment for which benefits are provided under the Act.[9] Injuries or deaths specifically not covered are those caused by the willful misconduct of the employee or caused by the employee's intention to bring about the injury or death of the employee or another and those proximately caused by the intoxication by alcohol or illegal drugs of the injured employee. Note that the definition of injury is straightforward in the sense that neither *unusual* effort on the part of the employee nor exposure to *unusual* employment conditions has to be shown to establish a covered injury.

"While in the performance of duty" has been construed by the *Employees' Compensation Appeals Board (ECAB)* as consistent with the phrase "arising out of and in the course of employment," which is commonly found in state workers' compensation laws. "In the course of employment" deals essentially with the work setting, the locale, and time of the injury, whereas "arising out of the employment" encompasses not only the work setting but also a causal concept, the requirement being that an employment-related factor caused the injury.[10]

"Traumatic injury" means a wound or other condition of the body caused by external force, including stress or strain, which is *identifiable as to time and place of occurrence* and member or function of the body affected. The injury must be caused by a specific event or incident or series of events or incidents *within a single work day or work shift*.[11]

"Occupational disease or illness" means a condition produced in the work environment over a *period of longer than a single work day or shift* by such factors as systemic infection; continued or repeated stress or strain; or exposure to hazardous elements such as, but not limited to, toxins, poisons, fumes, noise, particulates, or radiation, or other continued or repeated conditions or factors of the work environment.[12]

"Continuation of pay (COP)"—When a covered employee sustains a *traumatic* injury, the employee is entitled to receive full pay (regular pay check) during the period of injury-caused disability for up to 45 calendar days. The COP payments are taxed as is the regular pay.

After the 45 days the still-disabled employee would be entitled to appropriate *compensation*.[13]

"Compensation" and "disability compensation" mean the money payments made under the FECA to compensate an injured worker for the disability (lost wages) or permanent impairment (schedule award) sustained as a result of a traumatic injury or occupational disease or illness. For traumatic injuries, compensation would be paid for disability after the 45-day continuation of pay (COP) period. For occupational disease/illness compensation would begin at the earliest eligible date following pay loss (three waiting days).

The amount of the compensation paid *(weekly compensation rate, total disability, and schedule awards)* is computed at 75% or 66⅔% of the workers' pay rate on the date of injury. The 75% is for workers who are married or have dependents. The 66⅔% is for those who are not married and have no dependents.

The compensation rate for partial disability (injury-related loss of earnings or earning capacity) is based on 75% (or 66⅔%) of the difference between the pay rate on the date of injury and the lower earnings or earning capacity after the injury.

Schedule awards are provided for permanent impairment of certain specified members or parts of the body (the head and back are not included) after maximum medical improvement has been achieved. These awards are paid for a specified number of weeks based on the extent of impairment as determined using the current AMA *Guides*[14] and are paid whether or not there is any *disability* (injury-related loss of earnings).[15] See the paragraphs below for an illustration of this point.

Johnny Fed falls at work during his normal working hours and breaks his leg. It is considered an injury while in the performance of duty, and he is found entitled to FEC benefits. The injury prevents him from doing his job as a Navy shipyard worker. He is placed on Continuation Of Pay (COP) for the temporary total disability (total loss of earnings) caused by this "traumatic injury". He is entitled to COP for up to 45 calendar days of medically-supported disability.

After the 45 days he is entitled to receive compensation for total disability or partial disability depending on whether he continues with total- or partial-injury-related disability (loss of earnings). When maximum medical improvement has been reached and it appears that Johnny Fed will have a permanent impairment in his injured leg the treating physician will be asked to supply an opinion as to the extent of injury-caused impairment based on the current AMA *Guides to Physical Impairment*.[16]

If it is found that there remains a 25% permanent impairment in the injured leg, Johnny would be entitled to receive 72 weeks compensation (288 weeks is statutorily provided for 100% loss of use, impairment of a leg; 25% of 288 weeks is 72 weeks). If he has returned to work, he would still be entitled to these payments. If he continues to be disabled, Johnny's total- or partial-disability compensation will stop while he is paid the 72 weeks' compensation.

If at the end of the 72 weeks he is still disabled, constituting a total or partial loss of wages or earning capacity due to the effects of his injury (he cannot go up and down ladders in the shipyard), he could be put back on disability compensation for the duration of his disability. His employing government agency (the Navy) has a responsibility to place Johnny in employment suited to his capabilities and qualifications, and Johnny has a responsibility to accept this suitable employment. If the Navy succeeds in returning him to employment in which he suffers no wage loss compared to his earnings at the time of injury, his compensation for wage loss (total or partial disability) would cease. It also would cease if he returns to employment elsewhere (government or private employment) with no wage loss. If he returns to employment but at lower wages, he is entitled to compensation for partial disability based on the difference between what he was paid at the time of the injury and what he receives in his current job.

If Johnny Fed had suffered an injury to his leg after climbing ladders over more than one day (not a specific incident in one day but caused by his climbing ladders over more than one day), his injury would have been classified as an "occupational disease or illness"—not a "traumatic injury". He would not be entitled to COP (traumatic injuries only) but would receive "compensation" for his disability (wage-loss) during the duration of that injury-related total or partial disability. His entitlement to schedule awards would be the same as for a traumatic injury.[17]

## Medical Benefits

Full medical care is provided for "injury" (under any of the above definitions) sustained while in the "performance of duty" while in service to the United States. This includes examinations, treatments and all services, appliances, and supplies prescribed or recommended by qualified physicians that in the opinion of OWCP are likely to cure, give relief, reduce the degree or the period of disability, or aid in lessening the amount of compensation. The employee is permitted an initial choice of treating physician. A change of physicians will be authorized only upon approval of OWCP after the employee submits an explanation for the change.[18]

The term *physician* includes physicians (M.D. and D.O.), podiatrists, dentists, clinical psychologists, optometrists, and chiropractors, within the scope of their practice as defined by state law. Chiropractors are included but only to the extent that their reimbursable services are limited to treatment consisting of manual manipulation of the spine to correct a subluxation as demonstrated by an x-ray to exist. There is no dollar maximum on medical care.

Medical bills, except those from hospitals and pharmacies, must be signed or stamped by the physician before submittal. Bills may not be paid if submitted more than one year beyond the calendar year in which the treatment was received, or the calendar year in which the claim was first accepted as compensable by OWCP, whichever is later. The employee must advise the treating physician of the employing agency's willingness to accommodate where possible the employee's work limitations and restrictions and return to work when the employing agency offers duties within the limitations and restrictions warranted by the medical condition.

## LONGSHORE AND HARBOR WORKERS' COMPENSATION PROGRAM

### History and Background

The Longshore and Harbor Workers' Compensation Act[19] was passed by Congress in 1927 to provide injury protection to those workers (not seamen) performing duties on the navigable waters of the United States. It was made necessary because the U.S. Supreme Court had ruled earlier that a state could not apply its workers' compensation law so as to protect workers working on the navigable waters of the United States since, the court held, this was the exclusive jurisdiction of the United States [Federal Government].[20]

The Longshore and Harbor Workers' Compensation Act (LSA) is a workers' compensation law covering workers on or adjacent to the navigable waters of the United States. Persons covered include any person engaged in maritime employment, including any longshore worker or person engaged in longshoring operations, and any harbor worker, including those engaged in ship repair, shipbuilding, and ship-breaking activities upon the navigable waters of the United States or adjoining pier and dock areas. The law does not cover a master or member of a crew of any vessel.

The LSA has been extended to cover some other groups of workers not covered by other workers' compensation laws, such as employees engaged in certain operations conducted on the Outer Continental Shelf of the United States; civilian employees of nonappropriated fund instrumentalities (PXs, Officers' Clubs, etc.) of the Armed Forces; employees outside the United States on U.S. Defense Bases; and employees outside the U.S. carrying out "public work contracts" or other U.S.-funded contracts.

The LSA is similar to many state workers' compensation laws that provide wage loss and schedule loss benefits for injuries arising out of and in the course of employment. Full medical care is also provided as are death benefits for survivors of a work-injury death. Lump-sum awards or settlements are available. The benefits are paid by the employers themselves (as authorized self-insurers) or through employer-obtained insurance.

The Office of Workers' Compensation Programs (OWCP), Employment Standards Administration, U.S. Department of Labor administers the LSA program through offices located in many of the port cities of the United States. The OWCP monitors the response of employers to the LSA requirements for providing benefits and medical care. It also furnishes the mechanism to resolve disputes.

### Definitions of Injury and Disability

The LS program provides for income-maintenance (compensation) payments for *disability* resulting from a covered *injury*. The LS program uses the AMA *Guides* as its rating source.

Injuries that can be shown to have occurred on the job while the employee was in performance of duty are generally covered without question. Specifically not included are injuries caused solely by the intoxication of the employee or by the willful intention of the employee to injure or kill himself or another.[21] There are specific presumptions written into the LSA; it is presumed, in the absence of substantial evidence to the contrary, that the claim comes within the provisions of the Act, that sufficient notice has been given, and that the injury was not occasioned by the intoxication of the injured employee or the willful intention of the employee to injure or kill himself or another.[22]

### Payment of Compensation[23]

Typically an injured worker would receive compensation for total disability based on two-thirds of the worker's weekly pay at the time of the injury. This compensation would continue during the medically supported total disability. If the worker has a partial loss of earnings or is otherwise considered partially disabled, the worker would be paid two-thirds of his actual or computed loss of earnings.[24]

Maximum weekly compensation rate is 200% of the current national average weekly wage as determined each year by the Secretary of Labor.

If the injury is to a member (e.g., arm, hand, leg, foot), when maximum medical improvement is reached the compensation for time loss would stop (if it had not stopped sooner because the employee could or did return to work) and the worker would be evaluated for schedule loss (extent of permanent impairment). The AMA *Guides* may be used in this evaluation, but its use is not required by the law or regulations except in hearing-loss cases and occupational illness of a retired worker.

Compensation for serious disfigurement of the face, head, or neck or of other normally-exposed areas likely to handicap the employee in securing or maintaining employment is provided to a maximum of $7,500.

Once the schedule loss is paid the worker is not entitled to additional compensation for wage loss.

Workers who have a back- or head-injury disability will not normally be entitled to a schedule award but are entitled to continued compensation based on two-thirds of the loss of earnings.

Note that the benefits for occupational disease are the same as for injury except where the disease becomes manifest after the employee retires. In such a case compensation is paid for impairment rather than wage replacement and therefore paid as a permanent partial disability benefit as determined in accordance with the AMA *Guides*.[25]

## Medical Treatment and Examinations

The worker may select a physician (not limited to MDs) of his or her choice. Full medical care is provided by the law and is to be paid by the employer or the employer's insurance carrier. There is no overall maximum as to the total amount that may be paid, but the OWCP office having jurisdiction may use a local fee schedule such as a local state workers' compensation fee schedule to determine whether the individual medical charges are reasonable.

Physicians asked to treat these patients receive a Form LS-1 completed by the employer that authorizes treatment. The back side of that form is to be used by the treating physician as the initial medical report, and the report is to be received by the employer within 10 days.

Physicians asked to examine or evaluate workers for disability should give sufficient medical informa-

tion in the physician's report so that the OWCP claims official can make a determination whether the injury-related medical condition precludes the worker from returning to his usual work or some other type of employment, or is unable to do any employment. In evaluating the worker for a schedule loss (permanent impairment) it would seem best for the physician to use the AMA *Guides*. The ultimate decision as to extent of impairment and disability is made by OWCP claims official. That official is to consider other factors in addition to the medical evaluation reports in arriving at his or her decision.[26]

## BLACK LUNG BENEFITS FOR COAL MINERS AND THEIR FAMILIES[27]

### History and Background

In 1969 Congress showed its concern for the safety and health of coal miners not only by establishing safety and health standards for this occupation, but also by taking the unusual step of setting up an income-maintenance program to provide for disabled workers in an area usually thought to be the province of State workers' compensation laws, namely, occupational disease. The sole occupational disease provided for was coal miner's black lung disease. The benefits (medical and compensation) were meant to apply to coal miners in states that were determined to not have in effect an adequate workers' compensation system to protect coal miners disabled with black lung disease. The determination of adequacy of the states' workers' compensation to protect coal miners with black lung is made by the Secretary of Labor, Department of Labor.[28]

The Department of Labor through the Division of Coal Mine Workers' Compensation (DCMWC), of the Office of Workers' Compensation Programs (OWCP), administers the Black Lung Program through offices located in coal-producing areas of the United States. Social Security Offices are authorized by DCMWC to receive black lung claims and to forward them to DCMWC for processing and adjudication.

Some black lung benefit claimants may be required to process their claims through the state workers' compensation system where their coal mine employment was located when such system has been found adequate by the Secretary of Labor.

### Entitlement

The Black Lung Program benefits are provided to *miners* who are totally disabled due to pneumoconiosis (black lung) and to certain survivors of a miner who died due to or while totally or partially disabled by pneumoconiosis under the authority of Title IV of the Federal Coal Mine Health and Safety Act of 1969, as amended.[29] An applicant or claimant for benefits therefore must establish that the definition of miner has been met and that the miner has a prescribed disability due to the defined pneumoconiosis (black lung).

"[A] *Miner* . . . is any person who works or has worked in or around a coal mine or coal preparation facility in the extraction, preparation, or transportation of coal, and any person who works or has worked in coal mine construction or maintenance in or around a coal mine or coal preparation facility . . ."[30]

*Total Disability*—"A miner shall be considered totally disabled if the . . . pneumoconiosis . . . prevents or prevented the miner: (1) from performing his or her usual coal mine work; and (2) from engaging in gainful employment in the immediate area of his or her residence requiring the skills or abilities comparable to those of any employment he or she previously engaged with some regularity over a substantial period of time."[31]

*Pneumoconiosis* is a chronic dust disease of the lung and its sequelae, including respiratory and pulmonary impairments, arising out of coal mine employment. For the purposes of this definition, a disease "arising out of coal mine employment" includes any chronic pulmonary disease resulting in respiratory or pulmonary impairment significantly related to, or substantially aggravated by, dust exposure in coal mine employment. The definition includes coal workers' pneumoconiosis, anthracosilicosis, anthracosis, anthrosilicosis, massive pulmonary fibrosis, progressive massive fibrosis, silicosis, or silicotuberculosis, arising out of coal mine employment.[32]

The claimant in filing an initial claim with an office of DCMWC will be referred by letter to a medical specialist who will be asked to perform the designated testing and examinations necessary to put together the medical documentation needed by DCMWC to determine whether the diagnosis of pneumoconiosis has been established. The cost of this examination, including travel costs, is paid by DCMWC and is not to be paid by the claimant. The claimant may request that DCMWC authorize this medical evaluation through a qualified physician of the claimant's choice.

The DCMWC letter[33] to the evaluating medical specialist will typically ask for one or more of the following: (1) chest x-ray (single view, posteroanterior only); (2) pulmonary function tests; (3) arterial blood-gas study (as specifically defined); and (4) physical examination.

## BENEFITS FOR VETERANS AND THEIR FAMILIES[34]

### History and Background

Congress has responded to the needs of its veterans going back to the veterans of the Revolutionary War and the War of 1812. The present laws providing for veterans are administered by the Department of Veterans Affairs (VA). There are two major disability programs providing monetary benefits to veterans and their families of military conflicts of the United States including the Civil War, the Indian wars, and other defined conflicts up to the present: (1) Service-connected Disability Compensation and (2) Non–service-connected Disability Pension. In addition to monetary benefits, medical benefits are likewise provided.

The Department of Veterans Affairs administers the VA benefit program through 58 regional VA offices located throughout the United States. Monetary payments to compensate for "impairment in earning capacity" due to defined service-connected and defined non–service-connected disability are paid based on a detailed Schedule for Rating Disabilities found in Part 4, Title 38 of the *Code of Federal Regulations*. Use of the schedule assists in arriving at a percentage rating of covered disability upon which the level of payable benefits is determined.

> "This . . . schedule is primarily a guide in the evaluation of disability resulting from all types of diseases and injuries encountered as a result of or incidental to military service. The percentage ratings represent as far as can practically be determined the average impairment in earning capacity resulting from such diseases and injuries and their residual conditions in civil occupations. Generally, the degrees of disability specified are considered adequate to compensate for considerable loss of working time from exacerbations or illnesses proportionate to the severity of the several grades of disability. For the application of this schedule, accurate and fully descriptive medical examinations are required, with emphasis upon the limitation of activity imposed by the disabling condition."[35]

### Eligibility[36]

To receive benefits the person applying must establish basic eligibility as a veteran or the dependent or survivor of a veteran. Once this is established the person must meet the entitlement requirements for the specific benefits applied for. A very general overview of some of the qualifying requirements will be given below. For more specific and detailed entitlement information the patient or physician should contact the local VA office.

A *veteran* is a person who served in the *active military, naval, or air service,* and who *was discharged or released therefrom under conditions other than dishonorable.*[37] While "undesirable" or "bad conduct discharge" from a Special Court Martial *may* disqualify benefit entitlement it seems clear that a *"Bad Conduct Discharge" from a General Court Martial* or a *"Dishonorable Discharge"* definitely *will bar* benefits.

Active military, naval, or air service includes (1) active duty; (2) any period of active duty for training during which the individual was disabled or died of disease or injury incurred or aggravated in the line of duty; and (3) any period of inactive duty training during which the individual was disabled or died of disease or injury incurred or aggravated in the line of duty.

A showing of service during wartime is necessary to qualify for some benefits such as pensions. Specific periods are defined from the Civil War and Indian wars through the present time. Length of service may determine entitlement to and extent of some benefits, but length of service rules do not apply to service-connected disability compensation benefits.

"Willful misconduct" is a statutory bar to benefits. For instance, disabilities resulting from a person's willful misconduct are not compensable; drug addiction and primary alcoholism are considered misconduct, but hepatitis, cirrhosis of the liver, and AIDS are *not* considered willful misconduct.

### Service-Connected Disability Compensation[38]

This program provides compensation for disabilities incurred in or aggravated during a period of military service. This could be a battlefield injury or a football injury incurred during active service. For a disability to be service connected it should be shown that: (1) it is directly related to the service (this could be done through military medical records showing that the condition was diagnosed during military service); (2) it was aggravated during service (a condition prior to that military service became worse during military service); or (3) a statutory presumption applies. For instance, the condition was manifested—not necessarily diagnosed—(*a*) *within one year* of discharge (One Year Rule) for *chronic diseases,* including arteriosclerosis and arthritis (defined conditions), and *certain other diseases* including tropical diseases such as cholera, dysentery, malaria, filariasis; or, (*b*) *at any time* for diseases specific to Prisoners of War such as beriberi, psychosis, any anxiety state, dysthymic disorder, or depressive neurosis.

Also, a service-connected disability could be a condition secondarily related to a service-connected condition (i.e., proximately caused by or linked to a service-connected condition) or an injury that occurred in a VA medical facility.[39]

Determining service-connected disability benefits involves arriving at the appropriate percentage of covered disability by fixing (determining) the diagnosis (see codes and rating schedule[40]), fixing (determining) the symptoms (will affect the degree of disability), and then comparing them against the VA Schedule for Rating Disabilities.[41]

The percentage of (covered) disability thus obtained is intended to reflect the average impairment of earnings capacity, but the result does not necessarily meet this goal. Good medical documentation and support on the veteran's part will make the case here. In a case where there are multiple disabilities, percentages are not added arithmetically, but by the use of the Table of Combined Disabilities.[42] Percentages are set in increments of ten, but may be zero.

With the above determined percentage rating, the level of benefit payments is fixed by statute. Special or increased monthly compensation in special need cases may be available (above the 100% amount).

Increased compensation is payable when disability rated at less than 100% (sole cause) results in unemployability. A veteran unable to secure or follow substantially gainful occupation as a result of service-connected disabilities *only* may be paid at 100% rate. To qualify, the veteran's disability status must be either (*a*) one disability rated at 60% or more; or (*b*) two or more disabilities, one of which is rated at least at 40%; *and* (*c*) sufficient additional disability to bring the combined rating to 70% or more; or (*d*) if the above percentages are not met, in rare cases the Director of Compensation and Pension Service may allow a claim. Evidence must be submitted to establish unemployability. This includes statements of employers and vocational rehabilitation evaluations. Marginal employment up to national poverty level may not bar unemployability benefit. The VA Form 21-8940 is used.[43]

### Non–Service-Connected Disability Pension[44]

VA pension benefits were designed to supplement the income of disabled veterans who, because they gave up career opportunities to serve their country during a time of war, were unable to advance their careers or accumulate enough resources to support themselves adequately after they became disabled. Need and permanent and total disability are crucial factors.[45]

There are three pension programs: Improved (effective January 1, 1979), Section 306 (effective July

1, 1960 to December 31, 1978), and Old Law (before July 1, 1960). Most VA pensioners have the Improved pension. Under this plan the maximum benefit level is reduced by the recipient's (all family) income on a dollar-for-dollar basis for the monthly pension. If the family income exceeds the specified limit, the pension may be totally offset. There may be some offset in the other two plans also. "Countable income" for VA pension purposes does not include Supplemental Security Income payments or welfare benefits.

There are several basic eligibility criteria for a pension. The veteran must: (1) be discharged under conditions other than dishonorable; (2) have wartime service of 90 days; (3) have disabilities that are: (*a*) permanent (i.e., impairment is reasonably certain to continue throughout the life of the disabled person) and (*b*) total (i.e., 100% under the Schedule for Rating Disabilities) [total disability may be assigned with a less-than-total schedular rating under certain defined conditions]; (4) have limited countable income and net worth that does not provide adequate maintenance; and (5) the disability must not be due to the willful misconduct of the veteran.

There may be an Increased or Special Monthly Pension for persons with special needs.

Detailed information on what is required to meet the VA eligibility criteria is available from the local VA office.[46]

## Medical Examinations Conducted to Assist in Determining VA Impairment and Disability (see also Chapter 11)

Since the amount of monetary payments made to the veteran is largely based on the reports of medical evaluations, and the results are compared with the requirements and standards set by the VA's Schedule for Rating Disabilities found in Part 4, Title 38 of the *Code of Federal Regulations,* it is essential that the evaluating physician have a knowledge of what is required. The physician requested by a veteran to examine and provide such an evaluation needs an up-to-date copy of the VA's *Physician's Guide,* or at least a copy or computer printout of the latest update of the particular chapter of the *Physician's Guide* that covers the condition for which the physician is to examine. The physician can obtain this document from a VA service officer. Title 38, Part 4 of the *Code of Federal Regulations* is available from the Government Printing Office or a VA office. Local public or legal libraries may also be able to obtain a copy. See Chapter 11 for further discussion.

## RAILROAD WORKERS AND SEAMEN

Neither railroad workers nor seamen have had the protection of the type of coverage for work injuries afforded by state and federal workers' compensation laws. They have, however, been provided coverage under the Federal Employers' Liability Act, 45 U.S. Code Annotated §§ 51–60, which extended and enhanced their common-law rights to proceed in court against their employer to obtain damages for job injuries.

### Railroad Workers

#### History and Background
Workers on the railroads in the late 1800s found themselves in a very hazardous occupation (described in Chapter 6) with little hope for an adequate recovery in their common law court actions aimed at getting money from their railroad employers to pay the medical expenses and to compensate for their loss of earnings due to their work injuries. These victims of the hazardous employment environment found their quest for damages constantly defeated in the courts by the use by the railroads of the available common-law defenses of (1) contributory negligence, (2) negligence of a fellow servant, and (3) assumption of risk. If the railroad could show that in some way the injury was in part caused by the employee's own negligence or the negligence of one of the employee's fellow workers or that the employee voluntarily assumed the risk of the (hazardous) job then the claim for damages would not succeed, leaving the employee's family to shoulder the burden of this injury and wage loss as best they could.

Congress, in 1908, let it be known clearly that the railroads should shoulder a greater share of the cost of railroad employee injuries by passing the Federal Employers' Liability Act.[47] This law provided specifically that the railroads would be liable in damages to its workers who suffered work injuries and effectively modified or did away with the common-law defenses that were the impediments to successful recoveries.[48]

#### Present-Day Protection
The Employers' Liability Act provides the basis for work-injury damages, payable to injured railroad workers and their families, and is enforceable in court. While there is no workers' compensation law as such covering these workers, there is a program providing a form of income maintenance during periods of short-term sickness and unemployment, whether job related or not. This program, funded by railroad employers, is administered by the Railroad

Retirement Board (RRB),[49] an independent agency of the federal government.

A railroad employee injured in railroad employment and disabled for work can claim and receive the sickness and unemployment benefits to which the employee may be entitled while at the same time pursuing an action for damages under the Federal Employers' Liability Act. However, RRB may be entitled to reimbursement, from any monies received under FELA, for some or all benefits paid. Long-term disability is covered under the railroad workers' disability retirement program also administered by RRB.

## Seamen

### History and Background[50]

Seamen (crew members[51]), while never having experienced the advantages of a workers' compensation law, have been held by tradition or general admiralty or maritime law, perhaps going back to the Middle Ages, to be entitled to income maintenance during a period of illness or disability. This entitlement was termed "maintenance and cure." This concept was accepted by U.S. courts as part of the general maritime law of the United States. In cases where a seaman fell sick or suffered injury while in service of his ship, the vessel and her owner were found liable for *maintenance and cure* in addition to liability to the seaman for an indemnity (damages) for injuries received by the seaman as result of the *unseaworthiness* of the ship and her appliances. The seaman, however, could not recover damages or indemnity for injuries sustained through the negligence of the master or member of the crew.[52]

The maritime tradition and general maritime law requiring *maintenance and cure* of the vessel and her owner was placed into an international convention in 1936 (Shipowners' Liability Convention), which was then made applicable in the United States by a Presidential Proclamation signed by President Franklin D. Roosevelt on September 29, 1939 (54 Stat 1693). The Convention provisions pertinent to a shipowner's maintenance and cure as thus officially adopted into U.S. law provide, in part, that medical care and maintenance at the expense of the shipowner comprises: (1) (*a*) medical treatment and the supply of proper and sufficient medicines and therapeutical appliances, and (*b*) board and lodging; (2) the shipowner shall be liable to defray the expense of medical care and maintenance until the sick or injured person has been cured, or until the sickness or incapacity has been declared of a permanent character; and (3) where the sickness or injury results in incapacity for work the shipowner shall be held liable (*a*) to pay full wages as long as the sick or injured person remains on board; and (*b*) if the sick or injured person has dependents, to pay wages in whole or in part as prescribed by national laws or regulations from the time when he is landed until he has been cured or the sickness or incapacity has been declared of a permanent character.[53]

Subsequently, Congress passed the Jones Act,[54] which extended to seamen (crew members) the same privileges that railroad workers had obtained through the passage of the Federal Employers' Liability Act (FELA).[55] In fact, the FELA was specifically extended by the Jones Act to seamen to give seamen the right to sue for damages where the seaman suffered injury due to the negligence of the master or a member of the crew. This act gives to seamen or their personal representatives a right of action against the employer for negligence. The remedy is the same as that of railroad workers under the Federal Employers' Liability Act (FELA), and the common-law defenses are similarly modified.

### Present-Day Protection

Although seamen (crew members) have no protection under a workers' compensation law as such, an injured seaman has three potential causes of action (enforceable in court) against his employer: (1) the right to recover maintenance and cure to which he is entitled irrespective of negligence of fault, unless the injury was brought about by his own wilful misbehavior; (2) the right, under general maritime law, to recover indemnity for injury caused by the unseaworthiness of the vessel; and (3) the right, under the Jones Act (46 USCS @ 688), to recover indemnity for a personal injury suffered in the course of his employment and due to the negligence of the shipowner.[56]

## References

1. Title 5 U.S. Code, Part 8100.
2. See *A History of the Federal Employees' Compensation Act*, Willis J. Nordlund, 1992, U.S. Dept. of Labor, Employment Standards Administration, Office of Workers' Compensation Programs, Washington D.C., 20210.
3. Title 20, *Code of Federal Regulations* 10.311, 1993.
4. 20 *CFR*, Parts 1 to 71. 20 *CFR* refers to Title 20 of the *Code of Federal Regulations*. The number after *CFR* refers to the specific part or section of the title. The regulations governing the administration of the FECA are found at 20 *CFR*, Parts 1 to 71. The *CFR* is published by the Government Printing Office and is available at designated libraries throughout the United States.
5. 20 *CFR*, Parts 1 & 10.

6. For a valuable guide to the FECA see *Federal Employees Compensation Act: Practice Guide,* by Howard Graham, J.D., 1994, Clark, Boardman, Callaghan.

7. 20 *CFR,* 10.311 (1993).

8. 20 *CFR,* 10.5(a) (17).

9. 20 *CFR,* 10.5(a) (14).

10. See *Digest and Decisions of ECAB,* Volume 42, and Index Digest Supplement XVII, otherwise cited as 42 ECAB 69 (U.S. Government Printing Office) and the cases cited therein.

11. 20 *CFR* §10.5 (15).

12. 20 *CFR* Part 10.5 (16).

13. 5 U.S.C. 8118.

14. *Guides to the Evaluation of Permanent Impairment,* ed 4, American Medical Association, 1993, Chicago.

15. 5 U.S.C. 8107.

16. Ibid.

17. See 20 *CFR,* Part 10, generally especially §§10.100–10.130, 10.207–10.304.

18. See Medical Treatment generally, 20 *CFR* §§10.400–10.457.

19. Longshore & Harbor Workers' Compensation Act (LSA), 33 U.S. Code, Chap. 18, §§901–950. The regulations applying to this Longshore Program are found at 20 *CFR,* Parts 701–704.

20. *Southern Pacific* v. *Jensen,* 244 U.S. 205 (1917).

21. 33 U.S.C., §903.

22. 33 U.S.C., §920.

23. For a good short practical guide to the Longshore Act and its application see *Introduction to Longshore and Harbor Workers' Compensation Act* by Bernard J. Sevel, Esq., Baltimore, Maryland, which is contained in the Maryland *Workers' Compensation Manual* published by MICPEL, Baltimore, MD 21202.

24. A worker with an injury-caused permanent impairment of the back may be entitled to compensation for permanent partial disability, loss of earning capacity, even though he returns to work with no actual loss of earnings. See *Travelers* v. *McLellan,* 288 F.2d 250 (1961).

25. See the LSA Regulations in general at 20 *CFR,* Part 702.

26. See 20 *CFR,* §§702.401–702.422, for Medical care under the LSA.

27. Federal Coal Mine Health & Safety Act of 1969, Subchapter IV, as amended. This subchapter may be cited as the "Black Lung Benefits Act". 30 U.S.C., §§901–945; 20 *CFR,* §§718–727.

28. For more on the background & history see *Larson's Workmen's Compensation Law Treatise,* Arthur Larson and Lex K. Larson, Matthew Bender & Co., §§41.90–41.98 (1994). (This is the reference for the full 11 volume Treatise, not the shorter Desk Edition.)

29. 20 *CFR,* §718.1.

30. See *CFR* §725.202 for the complete definition.

31. Total disability defined in detail at 20 *CFR* §718.204.

32. 20 *CFR,* §718.201.

33. The letter to the physician by DCMWC is usually designated "Ltr. CM-954" and has detailed forms attached indicating the specific medical information needed (i.e., Form CM-433, CM-954a for chest x-ray; Form CM-907, CM-954a for ventilatory study; Form CM-988 for the physical examination; Form CM-1159, CM-954a for arterial blood-gas study).

34. Department of Veterans Affairs, DVA (VA) Benefits. Title 38 U.S. Code, §§1–End. Title 38, *Code of Federal Regulations,* §§0–End. For an excellent reference see the *Veterans Benefits Manual* (VBM), National Veterans Legal Services Project, 2001 S Street NW, #610, Washington, DC 20009, which has proved helpful in dealing with this complex subject.

35. 38 *CFR,* §4.1.

36. See generally 38 *CFR,* Part 3–Adjudication.

37. 38 U.S.C., §101(2).

38. Ibid. See also I *VBM,* Chap. 3.

39. See 38 U.S.C., §351.

40. 38 *CFR,* Part 4.

41. Ibid.

42. Ibid, esp. §4.25.

43. Ibid.

44. See generally, 38 *CFR,* Part 3, and I *VBM,* Chap. 5.

45. I *VBM,* §5.1.

46. I *VBM,* §5.1.2.

47. For the FELA see generally Title 45, U.S. Code Annotated (West Publishing Co.), §§51–60, for background, history, text, and pertinent court cases.

48. The FELA provided in part that railroads (common carriers) in interstate or foreign commerce are "liable in damages to any person suffering injury while he [or she] is employed by such carrier . . . for such injury or death resulting in whole or in part from the negligence of any of the officers, agents, or employees of such carrier, or by reason of any defect or insufficiency, due to its negligence, in its cars, engines, appliances, machinery, track, roadbed, works, boats, wharves, or other equipment." [45 U.S.C.A, §51] that ". . . the fact that the employee may have been guilty of contributory negligence shall not bar recovery, but damages shall be diminished by the jury in proportioned to the amount of negligence attributed to such employee: [but there is no contributory negligence in any case] where the violation by such common carrier of any statute enacted for the safety of employees contributed to

the injury or death of such employee." [45 U.S.C.A., §53] that ". . . such employee shall not be held to have assumed the risks of his employment in any case where such injury or death resulted. . . from the negligence of . . . [railroad employees, or where there was a violation of a safety statute by the railroad]." [45 U.S.C.A., §54]

49. Railroad Retirement Bureau, Main Office, 844 N. Rush St., Chicago, IL 60611 (Phone: 312/751-4500). Other offices in major railroad cities. See their *Sickness Benefit Handbook for Railroad Employees* (UB-11) for benefit information.

50. For background and history generally see 46 U.S.C.A., §688, Notes.

51. "There seems to be no significant distinction between the concepts of 'seaman' and 'crew member'." *Workmen's Compensation,* Arthur Larson and Rex Larson, Desk Edition, Matthew Bender, 1994 @ §90, citing *Gahagan Constr. Corp. v. Armao,* 165 F.2d 301.

52. *Pate* v. *Standard Dredging Corp.,* 193 F.2d 498.

53. See generally *Annotation, Supreme Court's Views as to a Seaman's Right, Under Maritime Law, to Maintenance and Cure;* Allan L. Schwartz, J. D.; 43 L.Ed. 2d 912, Lawyers Cooperative Publishing Co., 1993, and Norris, *The Law of Seamen,* 3d ed, as quoted therein.

54. The Jones Act is in actuality the Merchant Marine Act, 41 Stat. 1007 (1920), 46 U.S.C., §688 (1952).

55. See railroad workers above. FELA, 45 U.S.C.A., §51.

56. Norris, *The Law of Seamen,* 3d ed, @ 557 as quoted in 43 L.Ed. 2d 912.

# CHAPTER 5

# OVERVIEW OF THE CANADIAN DISABILITY SYSTEM

*Kenneth C. Pals*
*Tee L. Guidotti*

All workers' compensation systems have the same basic intent and the same basic features that reflect the purpose of the system: to adjudicate, to compensate, and to rehabilitate the injured worker. All such systems require the employer to pay all costs related to these essential functions. The agencies established as carriers under the systems all have a fiduciary responsibility to both the employer to keep costs under control, and to the injured worker to provide compensation while off work and for rehabilitation to return to work. All systems create a third party to act as the honest broker, usually called the Workers' Compensation Board (WCB). It is not surprising that there are more similarities than differences between the various workers' compensation systems in the United States and in Canada.

However, there are differences in Canada compared to the United States in both the structure of workers' compensation agencies and the processes by which they operate. These differences are most obvious at the level of appeals but are also reflected in costs and in operating philosophy.

This chapter is intended to provide the reader with a general understanding of the workers' compensation systems in Canada, with an emphasis on important differences from systems in the United States, differences that may affect the management of claims.

## JURISDICTION AND LEGISLATION

In Canada, workers' compensation is a provincial responsibility. This means that there is no federal role in the workers' compensation system other than its own responsibility to federal employees. Federal employees are covered by provincial systems under the Federal Government Employees Compensation Act, and their claims are managed by the provincial WCBs on behalf of the federal government as an employer. Otherwise, there is no federal legislation in the area of workers' compensation. The ten provinces and the two territories each have their own legislation and their own workers' compensation corporations. (In this chapter, "province" and "provincial" will refer to both provinces and territories.) These are "crown corporations", created by the province or territory, but managed in the public interest at arm's length from the provincial government. The majority were created in the 1920s.

Public and private employers in Canada are required to purchase coverage from the WCBs, which function as exclusive funds. The age and exclusivity of these funds explains why a disproportionate number, six out of the largest twelve, of larger publicly-mandated funds in North America are Canadian.

Workers' Compensation Acts in the various provinces usually provide only a basic framework for the structure and guidelines for the operation of the WCBs, although there is a great deal of variation in details. Most Canadian WCBs are organized much like corporations in the private sector, with a Board of Directors, a chief executive officer, and divisions responsible for claims management and employer services. Board members are appointed by the provincial government. Each WCB formulates its own policies and procedures, adjudication rules, decisions and orders, and assessment (insurance premium) schedules. The WCBs manage their own funds, anticipate future liabilities, and create reserves out of current earnings to fund these future liabilities. The WCBs always have an operating division responsible for claims management, medical assessment, and rehabilitation services. These divisions award pensions in cases of permanent disability and loss of earnings.

Within this general framework, there is variation. Some Canadian WCBs, such as those in British Columbia, Alberta, and New Brunswick, maintain their own physical rehabilitation facilities. The WCBs of British Columbia, Quebec, and Yukon Territory are also responsible for occupational health and safety in the province.

## BENEFITS

Workers who have been injured on the job are entitled to a percentage of earnings lost as a result of the injury as well as rehabilitation services, medical treatment, and a pension if the injury is permanently disabling or results in a permanent loss of earnings. Workers' compensation benefits are not taxable. They are based on a percentage of preinjury income, up to a maximum of covered earnings. Alberta, Saskatchewan, Ontario, Quebec, and the Northwest Territories pay 90% of net earnings (after deductions); British Columbia, Prince Edward Island, Nova Scotia, and the Yukon Territory pay 75% of gross earnings; Manitoba pays 90% of net for 24 months followed by 80% of net; New Brunswick pays 80% of net for 39 weeks followed by 85% thereafter; and Newfoundland pays 75% of net. The maximum covered earnings ranged from a low of $27,000 in Prince Edward Island to a high of $53,900 in Ontario.

Impairment rating schedules vary among jurisdictions. Two provinces (Manitoba and New Brunswick) use Bell's Tables, named after a medical officer at the WCB in Ontario who developed them. Four jurisdictions (Prince Edward Island, Newfoundland, Yukon Territory, and the Northwest Territories) use the American Medical Association Guides to the Evaluation of Permanent Impairment, although a given jurisdiction may or may not use the most current edition. Six (British Columbia, Alberta, Saskatchewan, Ontario, Quebec, and Nova Scotia) use schedules that incorporate both Bell's Tables and the AMA Guides.

There is a trend among Canadian WCBs to move away from medical impairment as the basis for determining the amount of a disability pension. Instead, the amount of the pension is based on loss of earnings. This recognizes the reality that one worker may be able to maintain earnings capacity despite a major medical impairment, particularly in jobs that are sedentary or professional in nature, while others may experience earnings loss with a relatively minor medical impairment, particularly in jobs that require manual dexterity or special skills.

Another trend in Canada is the shift from a *linear* approach of handling claims from injured workers, approaching the problem as one of keeping the assembly line moving, to a *case management* approach. The case management approach emphasizes communication and coordination. The case manager functions as a coordinator to ensure that all entitlements are provided at minimal inconvenience to the injured worker and ensures smooth communication among all parties with a legitimate interest. This results in better communication between the injured worker, the WCB, the treating professionals, and the employer. Coordination ensures that the injured worker receives appropriate rehabilitation services as efficiently as possible. The ultimate goal is the earliest possible return to work without placing the injured worker at risk. The worker is placed at the center of the decision-making process and is given responsibility for selfcare whenever possible.

Canadian WCBs generally spend less of their assessment revenue on health care payments than WCBs in the United States. In 1991, the six largest WCBs in Canada spent under 14% of assessment revenue on medical benefits compared to over 30% among the six largest American state funds.

## INSURANCE BUSINESS AND COSTS

In all Canadian provinces and territories, the WCBs operate as exclusive carriers. In the United States, most states are open to many insurance carriers. Only six states have exclusive funds. Among the rest, 25 (a recent increase) have competitive state funds in addition to private insurance carriers, and 17 have no state funds at all.

Self-insurance is not common in Canada, unlike the United States. In four jurisdictions (Alberta, Saskatchewan, Yukon Territory, and the Northwest Territories), only the federal government is self-insured. Other provinces allow their provincial governments, municipalities, public utilities, airlines, and railroads to self-insure. Ontario has over 500 self-insurance accounts, mostly government agencies.

Assessment rates, which are insurance premiums paid by the employer, are set at a fixed cost in cents or dollars per one hundred dollars of assessable payroll. These assessment rates are set for particular industries and may be modified up or down by "experience rating," which takes into account the experience with claims from a particular employer. In 1994, the average assessment rate for all industries among WCBs in Canada was about $2.30. The average was over $2.50, however, if the assessments are weighted by payroll (which gives proportionate weight to Ontario and Quebec, the two provinces that account for 65% of payroll in Canada and which have a concentration of manufacturing jobs). The lowest average assessment rate is $1.61, in Yukon Territory, and the highest is $3.18, in Newfoundland.

Employers are grouped into industry classifications according to their risk. They are then further subdivided by industrial activity. A given WCB in Canada may have as few as 5 or as many as 13 industrial classifications and may set as few as 36 or as many as 520 individual rates within this classification. The complexity tends to reflect the diversity of the local economy. In 1994, the lowest assessment rate in Canada was $0.10 in Saskatchewan for the Finance and Insurance class, Banks and Trust rate. The highest rate was $38.15 in Nova Scotia for the Trade Contractors class, Steeplejack/Scaffolding rate.

Rates for the same industry may vary widely among WCBs, depending on the local economy, injury rates, labor relations, legislation, occupational health and safety programs, and the fiscal policies of the WCB. Grocery stores are assessed $0.69 in New Brunswick and $3.26 in Ontario. Residential construction contractors pay $2.50 in Yukon Territory and $8.74 in Quebec; the Canada-wide average is $5.58.

Experience ratings or merit rebates are used in nine of the twelve Canadian WCBs. These plans have the effect of shifting a greater part of the required assessment revenue from the group as a whole to the employers who are actually experiencing the most claims and who are therefore incurring the most costs to the system. Experience rating plans are usually balanced, so that discounts provided to employers with a favorable experience are equal to surcharges on employers with excessive claims. The potential range of experience rating adjustments is typically between 20% and 40% of the assessment rate, although Ontario and Quebec can exceed that range for specialized plans that are aggressively targeting particular industries. A related strategy was introduced by Alberta several years ago under the name "The Window of Opportunity Program." Employers in selected industries who agreed to participate in an intensive audit and occupational safety initiative were given the option of postponing payment of their experience rating adjustment surcharge or part of their assessment. If they showed substantial improvement during this period, the deferred payment was forgiven.

Administrative costs are much lower in Canada. (All figures that follow are converted to U.S. dollars at an exchange rate of US$1.00 = Cdn$1.37.) On average, Canadian WCBs return $0.83 to injured workers for every dollar of revenue, compared to $0.72 in the U.S. The difference in costs is particularly striking as published Canadian costs include the appeals mechanism and U.S. costs do not. Employers pay $2.30 per $100 of assessable payroll in Canada; this figure includes both administrative costs and the cost of the appeals system. Employers in the United States pay $1.79 per $100 of assessable payroll but this figure does not include administrative costs and the costs of litigation or appeals, which can be as much as 25% or more above this base cost, bringing the overall costs into rough parity.

The future costs likely to be incurred from claims resulting from workers who are currently insured must be projected, using actuarial principles, and a reserve of money set aside to fund this future liability. For many years, the principle guiding the management of future liability in Canada has been that "today's employers pay the total, long-term cost of today's accidents." In principle, this liability cannot be allowed to carry forward in the future to be a burden on employers tomorrow. However, unfunded liability has been allowed to occur and has become an increasing concern. In 1992, the 12 Canadian WCBs had combined revenues from employer assessments and investment income of $5.0 billion and assets of $13.4 billion. Applied against liabilities of $24.9 billion, there is a combined unfunded liability of almost $11.5 billion, distributed unevenly among the WCBs. Saskatchewan, Yukon Territory, and the Northwest Territories had excess assets over liabilities, but these are small WCBs compared to the other provinces. Since 1992, Alberta has almost eliminated its unfunded liability but Ontario's has grown.

Concern over the high unfunded liabilities has become a major preoccupation with the management of WCBs, and most systems now have financial plans to achieve full funding within 5 to 20 years. However, because each WCB is separate and responsible according to its own legislation, there is no single uniform or standard approach to managing unfunded liabilities or even to the calculation of actuarial liability. The achievement of a common standard for Canadian WCBs in this area is an ongoing joint project of the Association of Workers' Compensation Boards of Canada and the Canadian Institute of Actuaries.

## APPEALS MECHANISMS

There is greater variation in the appeals mechanism than in the structures of the WCBs themselves in Canada.

The first level of appeal in most jurisdictions is an internal, relatively informal process conducted by specialists in workers' compensation. Hearings are not casual but they do not adhere to the rules of procedure in courts or those customary for formal workers' compensation appeals bodies. Instead, they are more in the nature of conferences to resolve problems before they pass over into the formal appeals process. The claimants speak for themselves if they wish, or they may have an advocate. This first level of appeal has the authority to overturn decisions of the WCB corporation.

The second level of appeal is more formal and constitutes a quasi-judicial hearing with a designated body vested with the authority to resolve the disputed claim. This body is, at least in theory, one step removed from the WCB corporation and its division responsible for claims management.

In nine jurisdictions (British Columbia, Alberta, Manitoba, Ontario, Quebec, New Brunswick, Nova Scotia, Newfoundland, and the Northwest Territories), the appeals body is separate from the WCB corporation. In these provinces, the appeals body is appointed by the government separately from the WCB and has the power to overturn decisions of the WCB corporations. Members of the appeals bodies are representative of workers and employers; they are not usually lawyers.

In the remaining three jurisdictions (Saskatchewan, Prince Edward Island, and Yukon Territory), appeals are handled by the WCB itself, with the Board of Directors of the corporation sitting as a board of appeals. Prince Edward Island is considering legislation that will create a distinct appeals body and will probably adopt this in 1995.

Decisions of bodies empowered to hear appeals are not open to question or to review in a court of law, unless the appellant can convince the court that there was a violation of process under the Workers' Compensation Act or that the decision was arbitrary and patently unreasonable. This pattern is generally similar to the restricted access to the courts in U.S. workers' compensation systems, based on the doctrine of exclusive remedy. Litigation is, at least theoretically, reserved for procedural issues and perceived denial of due process.

However, WCBs are also empowered in many provinces to question the decisions of appeal bodies on grounds of conflict with legislation and perceived contradictory policies. Certain jurisdictions (Alberta, Manitoba, Ontario, Newfoundland, and the Northwest Territories) allow the Board of Directors of the WCB corporation to review the decision of the appeals body when that decision is based on a matter of policy or the application of the Act. These provinces give the WCBs the authority to request and in some cases the power to direct the appeals body to reconsider or to stay its decision. This only happens when there is a perceived conflict with the basic legislation of the workers' compensation system or the fundamental policies of the system. There are some further variations. In British Columbia and Quebec, the chief executive officers of the WCB corporations may refer a decision of the first level of appeal to the second level for similar reasons.

Lawyers are not involved in Canadian WCB appeals to the extent that they are in U.S. appeals. If claimants choose to be represented by a lawyer, they are responsible for their own legal fees.

Canada-wide figures are not available on the flow through the appeals systems. However, the appeals process is illustrated by the experience of one province, Alberta in 1992, which is probably representative of Canada as a whole. The province, with a population of about 2.6 million people and about 650,000 workers, generated 33,500 claims to the WCB for lost-time injuries and illnesses. At the initial level of claims submission and adjudication, there was no involvement of lawyers or other advocates. Approximately 2,400 (7%) claims were appealed to the first level of appeal, which is internal to the WCB, as described above, and in which experienced specialists in workers' compensation review the claim. Seven hundred (2%) claims were appealed to the second level. Among the appellants, 30% represented themselves rather than using an advocate; of those using an advocate, 50% were represented by an Appeals Advisor appointed by the WCB to serve as the claimant's advocate, 30% were represented by a lay advocate such as a union steward, and 20% were represented by a lawyer. Thus, the total number of lost-time claims that involved a lawyer was 450, fewer than 1.5% of the total.

## PREVENTION

In British Columbia, Quebec, and Yukon Territory, the WCB also has legislated responsibility for occupational health and safety; using this model is currently under discussion in Alberta. Even so, most of the other Canadian WCBs are engaged to some extent in injury-reduction programs. The most common mechanism is for the WCB to reimburse the provincial government for all or a portion of the cost of the provincial occupational health and safety agency. Experience ratings systems are also a common means of motivating employers to reduce the number of injuries and the length of time lost.

Industry safety associations are important vehicles for achieving injury reduction and for managing occupational safety programs in some provinces. Alberta and Ontario have provisions in their legislation to fund industry safety associations. Some of these associations appear to have achieved substantial results. The Alberta Construction Safety Association, for example, was formed in 1988 and within six years the reported injury frequency in the Alberta construction industry had fallen by half. These programs have raised awareness within their target industries and have led to the introduction of safety and loss-prevention programs.

Effective claims management by employers goes hand-in-hand with injury prevention. Employers can reduce their claims by preventing injuries in the workplace. Effectively tracking claims and investigating the cause of injuries can help in this effort. Managing claims and rehabilitating and rehiring injured workers also reduce the cost to the system and the time lost attributable to the employer. Unfortunately, many employers have a policy against expedited return-to-work and will not accept workers on modified work terms. In the long run, however, early return to work and injury prevention are considered to be the most effective strategies for reducing compensation costs.

## ACKNOWLEDGMENTS

We thank the Association of Workers' Compensation Boards of Canada for providing most of the data presented in this chapter.

# CHAPTER 6

# WORKERS' COMPENSATION

*Donald Elisburg*

Workers' compensation is a disability program to provide medical and economic support to workers who have been injured or made ill from an incident arising out of and in the course of employment. It is a complex $70 billion a year program in the United States that involves nearly 60 different systems.

In each case, the major task is to determine whether there was an injury or illness and whether the injury or illness arose out of and in the course of employment. Many legal treatises have been written on the determination of the phrase "arising out of and in the course of employment." In this chapter, it is considered a requirement that causation be determined to fall within the workers' compensation system, and that the phrase set forth above is the criterion against which this determination is to be measured.

Subsequent to the diagnosis of the impairment or illness and the determination of causation is the determination of impairment and disability. It is not enough for a worker to have sustained the injury according to the terms of permanent disability benefits. While the worker is under medical care, the system will usually pay for the temporary effects. The larger problem is one of the long term determination of impairment or disability.

It is not sufficient to simply determine that the injury/illness resulted in an "impairment" of function. For purposes of compensability, the issue is one of disablement. That is, does the impairment result in an inability to perform certain functions related to the job? If so, then there is disability in whole or in part that is usually translated into a percentage of wage loss.

## STATE VS. FEDERAL COVERAGE

For reasons that appear to have been historical and economic, workers' compensation is one of the few protective labor standards that has been largely a state-based effort; judging from recent political experience, it is likely to remain so in the near future.

From an historical perspective, with the exception of child labor and womens' hours of work regulations, workers' compensation in the United States was the initial protective labor standard enacted by state legislatures to provide worker protection. Much of what we now call the workplace safety net—collective bargaining, safety and health regulations, pension protection, employment discrimination and wage protections—is a series of laws that were promulgated after the workers' disability programs. Virtually all of these laws were the product of the 1920s-1970s in the pre-New Deal, New Deal, and post-WWII environment that focused on federal solutions. And while each of these areas incorporates state programs, there is little question that the federal government was the driving force behind these laws (see Chapter 2).

The federal involvement has proceeded along two paths. The initial federal legislation was the Federal Employers Liability Act (FELA) to provide injury compensation for railroad workers. This federal role preceded the state efforts at providing workers' compensation to other segments of industry. The second path for the federal legislation was aimed at workers' compensation protection limited to groups of workers that did not fit the state programs, where the state programs simply were not responsive, or where there was exclusive federal jurisdiction.

## POLICY QUESTIONS

In recent years the workers' compensation disability systems, now estimated to have an annual cost in excess of $70 billion, have come under intensive scrutiny and study. There are innumerable books, articles, and commissions analyzing the problems state-by-state. Since the early 1970s, there have been numerous efforts at reforming the state and federal systems. These efforts have had mixed results with the consensus in 1994 suggesting a need for deep seated changes in the current workers' compensation programs if there is to be a true measure of reform.[6,25]

Any student of this system, and those engaged in policy analysis, must address a number of serious questions when considering corrections to the system:

- What constitutes fair and adequate compensation?
- How can the cost of medical care be controlled?
- How should long-latent disease claims be handled?
- What is the proper role of litigation?
- What can be done to restore injured workers to employment?
- How can the system be made more equitable across various jurisdictions?

## TORT SYSTEM AND FELA

The plight of workers in the United States at the end of the 19th century has been well documented (see Chapter 2). Injured workers and their survivors, for the most part, had no right to compensation when their injuries or deaths were work-related. Relief, if any, was through the common-law tort system of personal injury action. As plaintiffs, workers were subject to defenses including contributory negligence, fellow-servant rules, and assumption of risk. Few workers could overcome these hurdles and recoveries were few and small.

Otto Bettmann (*The Good Old Days—They Were Terrible!*, Random House, New York, 1974, pp. 70–71) described those times in vivid terms: "Aside from the steel mills the railroad industry was the most lethal to its workers, killing in 1890 one railroader for every 306 employed and injuring one for every 30 employed. Out of work force of 749,301 this amounted to a yearly total of 2451 deaths, which rose in 1900 to 2675 killed and 41,142 injured. It should be noted that these casualty lists cover only railroaders in the line of duty: civilian casualties in train collisions and level-crossing accidents were another matter. The *New York Evening Post* concluded that the deaths caused by American railroads between June 1898 and 1900 were about equal to British Army losses in the three-year Boer War.

. . . In the high-risk job category the circus stuntman and test pilot today enjoy greater life assurance than did the brakeman of yesterday, whose work called for precarious leaps between bucking freight cars at the command of the locomotive's whistle. In icy weather, it often became a macabre dance of death. Also subject to sudden death—albeit to a lesser degree—were the train couplers, whose omnipresent hazard was loss of hands and fingers in the primitive link-and-pin devices. It took an act of law in 1893 to force the railroads to replace these man-traps.

. . . Industry's cavalier attitude to safety had a predictable effect on lower-echelon bosses. One railroad-yard superintendent refused to roof a loading platform, even though in the cold his men had contracted rheumatism and asthma. His observation: "Men are cheaper than shingles . . . There's a dozen waiting when one drops out."

. . . Whether a worker was mutilated by a buzz saw, crushed by a beam, interred in a mine, or fell down a shaft, it was always "his own bad luck." The courts as a rule sided with the employer; in any event, few accident victims or their kin had the money to bring suit. Companies disclaimed responsibility, refused to install protective apparatus, and paid no compensation. Their only concession to human life was to pay for burying the dead!

In American industry no workers were at greater risk than those working on the railroads.

The Federal Employers Liability Act, FELA, was enacted amidst a general outcry by railroad workers and others for protective legislation. Congress, in its first venture into the realm of worker disability, enacted the initial FELA in 1906 and the present version of FELA in 1908. It was an effort to provide workers with some ability to obtain injury compensation through the courts by modifying the negligence standards and eliminating or modifying certain of the railroads' defenses such as contributory negligence, the fellow-servant rule, and assumption of risk. In a major change, contributory negligence gave way to comparative negligence. The significance is that, under FELA's comparative negligence test, injured workers are not denied compensation if they had contributed to the fault for the accident. Rather, their compensation can be reduced according to the percentage of the fault that was theirs. Furthermore, FELA provides that if the railroad had violated a safety standard, any degree of fault by injured workers is disregarded in determining compensation.[6,16,25]

The FELA was amended at various times to provide more liberal interpretations, and changes in 1939 eliminated any remaining doctrine of assumption-of-risk. The basic FELA statute was used in 1920 when Congress enacted the Jones Act to provide similar protection for seamen. Clearly, the two statutes were designed to cover workers where Congress saw a national industry, i.e., railroads, and maritime on the navigable waters over which the federal government had exclusive control.[7,12,16]

In actual practice, the FELA is the product of decades of judicial interpretation. The Supreme Court has ruled on its effect numerous times and, in the context of a fault-based system, has determined that the required proof of negligence by the railroad is extremely liberal (only a "scintilla" of negligence is needed). The coverage of the Act to workers is also extremely broad (for example, occupational illnesses are fully covered).[6,16,25]

The FELA and Jones Act can be characterized as workers' compensation systems in that the railroads and ship owners have developed extensive claims filing procedures, investigations, and examinations to handle the vast bulk of claims under these laws. A review of a typical FELA or Jones Act file would contain essentially the same information about the injured workers' medical and economic circumstances as in the typical state or federal workers' compensation file.

Participants have developed guidelines for economics and impairment. In a typical FELA case, the injured worker will file a claim that will be processed through the system as though it were a workers' compensation claim. In cases of dispute, the injured worker will seek counsel and proceed through an elaborate system of administrative process within the railroad personnel or claims department, both before and after a proceeding is filed in court. The cases are brought under extremely liberal venue with an option of federal or state courts and the right to a jury trial. Perhaps the most distinguishing feature of the FELA is the ability to have a jury determine whether there was negligence by the parties and for the jury to determine the extent of the damages. Also, by statute, the FELA does not have a schedule of awards, nor a formula for determining benefit levels.[6,15,16,25]

## WORKERS' COMPENSATION

About the same time that Congress began to struggle with the FELA, there was activity in the states to provide a disability compensation system that would be a no-fault approach modeled on the social experiments in Germany and Great Britain in the 1880s and 1890s.

Credit is generally given to Bismarck for the enactment of the first workers' compensation system in the 1880s in Germany (see further discussion in Chapter 2). Other historians have traced the first such systems in Europe to the 1830s. Clearly, the historical product of the industrial revolution and industrialization of America was the strong desire to eliminate the country's terrible cost in human lives during its rise as an industrial power.[21]

## DEVELOPMENT OF THE STATE-BASED WORKERS' COMPENSATION SYSTEM

The push for workers' compensation programs took hold in the progressive states such as Wisconsin,

Ohio, and New York. After many false starts and much litigation, the no-fault workers' compensation schemes were started. These workers' compensation statutes imposed a fixed liability without fault by specifying benefits and eliminating defenses. The constitutional issues brought by employers complaining of unjust taking of benefit payments and impairment of contract (i.e., "no-fault" liability) were settled with the New York statute.[8]

Interestingly, the state-by-state approach was not achieved easily. It was not until 1949 that Mississippi finally enacted a workers' compensation statute. And even today, not all workers are protected by a workers' compensation scheme. In a number of states, agricultural and small-employer exemptions, along with those provided in Federal programs, still leave large numbers of workers without protection and force them to go to the courts for the same relief workers were limited to a century ago. It is also noteworthy that in three states, Texas, South Carolina, and New Jersey, workers' compensation is not even compulsory.[2]

Thus, while a comprehensive scheme of workers' compensation has been enacted in every state, the process has taken more than 50 years and is still not complete. It is also true that while the concept of workers' compensation was to provide adequate and uniform benefits, the achievement of that result has been extremely painful, difficult, inconsistent, and elusive.

From the inception of the state systems, there has been a struggle first to provide adequate benefits, and then to maintain these benefits in line with increases in wages and costs of care. For example, most state laws provide for a benefit level of 66⅔% of the workers' wages. However, the imposition of caps on total benefits has frequently resulted in many workers of average or higher wages receiving less than 50% of their salary, and in some states the caps are so low that, even at the maximum, benefits are at poverty levels.[26]

Additionally, the early state laws did not provide uniform coverage of all occupations and many state laws did not adequately cover occupational diseases. These continuing problems will be discussed later in this chapter.

## DEVELOPMENT OF THE FEDERAL-BASED WORKERS' COMPENSATION SYSTEM

While the states were enacting workers' compensation statutes for the industry in their individual states, the federal government was also under pressure to provide a better injury program for its own workers (see also Chapter 4).

## Federal Employees Compensation Act

In 1916 the Congress enacted the Federal Employees Compensation Act (FECA) to provide a workers' compensation program for its own employees. Since the doctrine of sovereign immunity protected the federal government from lawsuits, the federal system never was required to replace an existing tort system. Basically, Congress provided full coverage to all employees in a system that was much less adversarial than that which developed under the FELA and the state-based no-fault systems. As a self-insurer, the federal government was not obliged to set up a system that functioned with private carriers or insurance funds. In addition, from the enactment of the statute, Congress made the administrative decision final with no appeals to the courts. The issue confronting the federal government and the protection of some two million federal employees has been one of tinkering with the administrative process and the need for Congress to increase periodically the benefit schedule.

In the 1970s Congress improved the FECA by making it conform to the recommendations of the National Commission on State Workmen's Compensation Laws. In addition, a growing backlog of cases convinced Congress to provide an experiment permitting the government to continue an injured worker's pay while the case was being processed. This innovative approach presented difficulties in administration in the 1970s, particularly as the caseload continued to grow substantially.[7,18]

## Longshore and Harbor Workers' Compensation Act and Extensions

The federal government's exclusive jurisdiction over the navigable waters and the limitations of the Jones Act to "seamen" left a class of workers unprotected under a workers' compensation program. Longshoremen and harbor workers who were injured while on the navigable waters of the United States, such as on ships at dock, had no protection from the state systems and were not covered by the Jones Act.

To remedy this problem, the Longshore and Harbor Workers' Compensation Act was passed in 1927 to cover these workers. There were also other groups in federal situations that did not have workers' compensation coverage. Thus, the Longshore Act was extended to employees of private employers in the District of Columbia (1928) and later to workers on military bases outside the United States with the Defense Base Act, and to workers on oil drilling rigs on the Outer Continental Shelf. The Longshore Act has also been applied by contract in airline collective bargaining involving overseas flights.

In 1972, the Longshore Act was extensively revamped to increase and index benefits as well as to extend coverage "shoreside" to longshoremen and shipbuilding workers. The impact of these amendments will be covered in the discussion of current problems of the compensation systems.[7]

## Black Lung Benefits Act

As previously stated, the federal government's role, with the exception of covering railroad workers and seamen, has largely been to provide compensation systems to those workers not otherwise eligible for state protections.

One significant exception to this approach was the black lung legislation. In the 1960s the public and Congress became aware of a serious problem with respect to coal miners and the failure of existing state workers' compensation laws to cover the occupational disease of coal workers' pneumoconiosis or "black lung." Partly as a result of the definition of disease, and partly as a result of statute of limitations on discovery of this long-latent disease, hundreds of thousands of afflicted miners had no program of compensation.

Congress reacted by providing a series of programs to create a compensation program for coal miners with this illness. Initially a federal payment program, the Black Lung Benefit program was extended in the 1970s to coal mine operators, first on a responsible operator basis, and then to a coal-industry-funded program. Because of its extensive application, a number of railroad workers may also be eligible for benefits under this statute. The enormous number of claims, a congressionally-mandated liberal eligibility program, and administrative difficulties made this an extremely costly and controversial program. It also provided massive relief to thousands of coal workers and their families who had no other source of benefits or medical care.[7]

## EFFORTS TO REFORM NO-FAULT WORKERS' COMPENSATION

For 60 years the no-fault workers' compensation system, both at the state and federal level, developed and operated with very little influence or interest from the Congress or the Executive Branch. While the relief provided by these programs was minimally acceptable, it was clear that all was not well with the system. More workers were falling through the cracks than were being helped by this aspect of the safety net.

When Congress enacted the Occupational Safety and Health Act of 1970, it created a National Commission on State Workmens' Compensation Laws. The Commission undertook a comprehensive examination of the existing state systems. Its findings were not encouraging. It found the systems in disarray, with low benefits, inadequate coverage and medical care, poor or no rehabilitation, poor administration, and excessive litigations. The Commission made more than 84 recommendations for improvement, including 19 recommendations said to be "essential" to the future of the state-based workers' compensation system. It did not endorse already-existing federal standards, but suggested that they be considered if the states did not achieve compliance by 1975.[20]

Subsequently, there was much activity in many states with a number of recommendations adopted. In addition, the Department of Labor began to provide assistance to these state programs; Congress upgraded the Longshore Act and the FECA to conform to the federal standards; and the Department of Labor created an Inter-Departmental Task Force to continue the Commission's work in a number of areas.[17]

Compared to the situation in 1972, much has changed in the last two decades. However, in taking stock of the last 20 years of reform, a number of structural problems addressed by the National Commission still remain. Indeed, in the last few years, the economic climate has resulted in a campaign of "backwards" reform, as states reduced benefits, medical protection, and the ability of workers to obtain adequate compensation through the state systems.[11,14,19]

## Some Improvement

Clearly, the total system has in many respects responded positively to the needs as cited in the various commissions and reports.

- Most states have increased benefits for workers. Unfortunately, those states that have not reached the National Commission's recommendations provide a benefit level that, as explained below, frequently forces the injured worker into penury.
- There has been a recognition of the need to compensate for certain occupational diseases by eliminating most of the barriers relating to statutes of limitations and proof of causation.
- While there is better handling of permanent partial-disability evaluation and payments, this remains the most litigious part of the program in many states.
- There is definitely more medical care of a higher quality available.
- There are improved rehabilitation services, as well as more interest in assisting workers to return to work by employers, although this

concept is still not fully accepted by all employers.
- In many areas of the country there is improved professional administration of the system.

## Substantial Failures Undermine Improvements

There has been no broad public consensus about reforming no-fault workers' compensation programs, and therefore no fundamental change. It is generally felt by practitioners and scholars involved in reform efforts that the "improvements" have not accomplished the goal of a fair system.

- The constant and frequently-failed efforts to secure equitable benefits, coverage, administration, medical care, and rehabilitation calls into question whether the systems are fundamentally flawed; or whether in today's economy these systems are relics of the past and not responsive to the needs of the workers, employers, or the public.
- It is incongruous that one of the singular achievements of the 1970s, the elimination of caps on medical treatment, is now being criticized because the cost of medical treatment under workers' compensation is now the most significant issue in considering whether the system is still affordable to employers.
- Expanding the workers' compensation coverage to include occupational disease has been heralded as a great advancement for worker disability protection. However, the medical treatment costs of occupational diseases such as stress-related cases, repetitive motion injuries (such as carpal tunnel syndrome), heart attack and stroke are causing friction in the system as carriers and employers claim that many of these cases are non-work-related. Repetitive motion injuries are reported in epidemic proportions as a consequence of the introduction of new methods of automation that may be ergonomically unsound, and with the increased emphasis on productivity that speeds up production lines regardless of the health effects on workers. The result is a ten-fold increase in these claims over the last decade.[10,13]
- It is also apparent that large bureaucracies do not necessarily beget effective or efficient systems— but at the same time, otherwise good systems have been strangled because of insufficient administrative support.
- The notion of basing benefits on a "wage loss" formula, that is, a comparison of the workers' present earning capacity against the capacity

before injury, was highly favored among reformers in the late 1970s. Recently, however, the administration of wage loss programs and the resultant extensive litigation over these determinations have caused such programs to become an albatross of the 1990s.

These substantial failures in the state systems have meant that any improvement of the claimants' access to the workers' compensation systems have been uneven. Some of the most serious difficulties claimants face include the following:

### Barriers to Entrance

Some states still have barriers to entrance, through limiting statutes of limitation or in rejecting coverage for occupational diseases including stress-related disorders, cumulative trauma (repetitive motion such as carpal tunnel condition), strokes, heart attacks, and toxic exposures with long latencies. The frequent difficulty in establishing causation and work-related tests have the potential for excluding many workers from the protection of these programs.[4,7] Complex judgmental questions need to be asked. For example: Did the mental condition, such as depression, arise from a work-related incident? Did the heart attack result from a single event or from a cumulative series of events at work? Did the carpal tunnel condition arise from repetitive motion on the poultry-processing line? False claims have also been a serious problem.

### Economic Insufficiency: Low Benefits and Medical Cost-Sharing

Despite 20 years of effort, many states have yet to achieve the recommended benefit levels of the National Commission. In a number of jurisdictions efforts have been made to reduce the benefits that already exist.

Various experiments in benefits based on wage loss have proven to be counter-productive. The maximum cap on benefits still results in many high-skilled workers receiving less than the 66⅔% of their wage considered the minimum by the National Commission. For example, the weekly maximum in Mississippi is $244, Arkansas $267, Georgia $250, Nebraska $265, and Puerto Rico $65, while the average weekly earnings of skilled workers in the United States is $386. Many states also have limits on total benefits, either in number of weeks of eligibility or in total dollar payments.[2,24,26]

While most states have full medical protection, the escalating costs of medical care have resulted in enormous pressures on the system to reduce costs. As stated previously, medical care represents about 40%

of the costs of workers' compensation and is rising at an average annual rate of 13%. One of the most difficult issues is whether to require workers to pay for part of the cost of their medical care, with a deductible and co-pay, as they do for their employee health benefits, a concept that is fiercely resisted by workers and their representatives.[3,27] Dealing fairly with issues of medical cost control and containment will be a severe problem for the reformers in the foreseeable future.

### Barriers to Claims Resolution

Appropriate administration has not kept pace with reform. Even states with a good reform effort, such as California and New York, have experienced unacceptable delays due to poor or underfunded administration.

Many states are barely automated, and many states have not yet developed a comprehensive data collection program that is essential to a well-run workers' compensation agency.[1] Doctors also may have inadequate means of reporting workers' compensation problems.

## LITIGATION

While the state-based system may be conceptually no-fault, it is still overwhelmingly an adversary process with its concomitant litigation expense and delay. A recent study conducted in California reflects that nearly every seventh workers' compensation claim in California was litigated, and when medical-only claims are excluded, 45% of all indemnity cases go to litigation.[5]

Difficulties in gaining entrance to the system and controversy over disability levels contribute to the extensive level of litigation. In many states, such as New Jersey and California, the system is so complex that an attorney is necessary to file even an initial claim, thereby causing claimants to pay lawyers' fees of up to 20% of the recovery just to help them through the system.

The resistance of private carriers or the self-insured employers to pay claims promptly and the constant challenge to medical findings has stripped workers' compensation programs of trust by the claimants. Programs for claimant assistance or other measures to limit the need for lawyers have not yet found their way into most state programs, with Ohio being one of a few states who currently have a program for claimant assistance in place. Accordingly, the litigation and high transaction costs that result have seriously impacted the system.

## REHABILITATION ADMINISTRATION

The goal of the workers' compensation programs is to provide benefits, medical care, and assistance so that injured workers may return to their job. Responsive rehabilitation programs are needed to accomplish this goal. These topics are reviewed later together with the concepts of physical rehabilitation, vocational rehabilitation, and the Americans with Disabilities Act (see Chapters 46, 47, and 50). Access to these programs is uneven, with the federal system being less of a problem than in most of the states.[22,23] The concept of return-to-work is an ideal one that may not be practical based on the skills necessary for the original job and the nature of the injury and subsequent impairment. However, many impaired workers can be returned to gainful employment. Physical and vocational rehabilitation maximize this return potential. Job retraining, under vocational rehabilitation, completes this process. With ADA-mandated work accommodation now required, employers will find an ever-increasing need to use these resources to assure a worker-job congruence, with emphasis on the essential components of a job.

## THE FEDERAL SYSTEM IS BETTER IN SOME WAYS . . . BUT ALSO HAS PROBLEMS

### Longshore and Harbor Workers' Compensation Act (LHWCA)

In the 1972 and 1984 amendments to the LHWCA, Congress provided an exceptionally comprehensive benefit and medical program. In particular, benefits are indexed and occupational disease claims enter into the system with little resistance. However, as the Longshore Act is still a private insurance or self-insurance program, a high level of claims are appealed or litigated.[9]

### Federal Employees' Compensation Act

This program, which was last upgraded in 1974, struggled for many years with administrative problems resulting from a rapid increase in claims in the 1970s. By far one of the best programs for benefit and treatment, the program represents the federal government's determination to remain an enlightened employer. The basic non-adversary approach has worked with the federal workforce and is somewhat unique because of the special benefits the federal government gives to this workforce, such as high wages, substantial fringe benefits, and a history of job

security. It is unlikely, however, that this type of system would lend itself to the private sector, because of the differences in employer-employee relationships between public- and private-sector employees. Large companies, especially those with self-insured programs, are more able to devise a non-adversary method of resolving claims.

### Black Lung Benefits Act

This federal program is really a quasi-compensation program. Originally cast as a benefit program for miners with black lung disease, it has since developed into a workers' compensation type program with the implementation of medical protocols and other standards relating to workplace causation. The concept of an industry fund is compelling, but it is also an extremely litigious program and should be noted is a *single illness* program. For all other injuries and illnesses, coal miners are required to file under their state laws. The trust fund concept to deal with occupational diseases that result from the possibility of many employers' potential involvement in the workers' exposure may be useful to consider as a model for a program of state-based funds or federal funds to handle any workers becoming ill from such toxic exposures.

## CONCLUSION

Workers' compensation programs exist to protect workers who are injured or become ill on the job or their families if they are killed. There are approximately 60 different systems of workers' compensation in the United States, each with its own peculiarities and special problems.

The increasingly high costs of medical treatment, benefit payments, and legal fees have created an extremely litigious program in many jurisdictions, thus creating even more costs to the system. Various solutions involving health and safety prevention programs, improved administration, improved medical cost containment and managed care, integration with other disability programs, changes in the coverage and benefits, and better rehabilitation and return-to-work programs have been proposed. The enormous amount of money at stake suggests that no easy solutions are to be found to reform this complex system. What would an ideal system encompass? The elimination of the multiple systems would be an excellent start. The concept of a universal system would eliminate the need for specialized training of attorneys and physicians, the incidence of errors inherent when multiple, mandated pathways are used to achieve the same goal, and the redundancy and costliness of administrative structures. A return to the no-fault concept would reduce the need for attorney assistance and return the entire award to the injured worker. Speedier impairment evaluations by physicians would also be a by-product of returning to the no-fault concept. This would result in easier entry into the return-to-work programs. Lastly, an enlightened concept of the value of rehabilitation and return-to-work (especially considered under ADA) on the part of government, employers, and the injured employee would serve to minimize the enormous cost of dealing with work-site injury and illness.

## References

1. "Administration Requirements for State Workers Compensation Agencies," Washington, D.C., 1991, AFL-CIO NAM Task Force.
2. *1993 Analysis of Workers Compensation Laws*, Washington, D.C., 1993, U.S. Chamber of Commerce.
3. Boden LI, DeFinis JM, Fleischman CA: *Medical Cost Containment in Workers' Compensation: A National Inventory*, No. WC-90-4, Cambridge, Mass., November 1990, Workers Compensation Research Institute.
4. Burton JF Jr and Schmidle TP, editors: *John Burton's Workers' Compensation Monitor*, Horsham, Pa., 1990-91, LRP Publications.
5. "California Workers' Compensation Institute Bulletin," No. 91-12, San Francisco, 26 Sept. 1991, California Workers' Compensation Institute.
6. Cost Containment & Reform Activity Report, Vol. 1, Issue 3, July 1991; Vol. 1, Issue 4, Sept. 1991, Boca Raton, Fla., National Council on Compensation Insurance.
7. DeCarlo DT, Minkowitz M: *Workers Compensation Insurance and Law Practice: The Next Generation*, Fort Washington, Pa., 1989, LRP Publications.
8. DeCarlo DT, Minkowitz M, p. 5-6, op. cit.
9. Discussions with staff of U.S. Department of Labor Office about workers' compensation programs, September 1991.
10. Elisburg DE: "Union Perspective on Cumulative Trauma," *Cumulative Trauma Disorders in the Workplace: Costs, Prevention, and Progress*, Washington, D.C., 1991, Bureau of National Affairs.
11. Elisburg DE: "Workers' Compensation, Twenty Years of Reform," Speech before the International Association of Industrial Accident Boards and Commissions, Sept. 1990.
12. Elkind AB: "Should The Federal Employers' Liability Act Be Abolished?" *FORUM*, Chicago, 1981, American Bar Association, Tort and Insurance Section.
13. Ellenberger J: "Cumulative Trauma Disorders: A View From Labor," Proceedings, American Bar Association Tort and Insurance Section Midwinter Meeting, April 1991.
14. Ellenberger J: "Workers' Compensation Challenges: Organized Labor's View," *Challenges for the 1990s*, WC-90-3, Cambridge, Mass., July 1990, Workers' Compensation Research Institute.
15. "Federal Employers' Liability Act," U.S. House of Representatives, Committee on Energy and Commerce, Subcommittee on Transportation and Hazardous Materials, 101st Congress, 1 Nov. 1989.
16. Havens AI, Anderson AA: "The Federal Employers' Liability Act: A Compensation System in Urgent Need of Reform," *Federal Bar Journal* 34(7): Sept. 1987.
17. Interdepartmental Workers' Compensation Task Force Report, U.S. Department of Labor, 1980. This series of reports contains a wealth of background information on state workers' compensation systems, particularly focusing on occupational disease, Washington, D.C., Government Printing Office.
18. Nordlund WJ, editor: *Proceedings of a Conference Celebrating the 75th Anniversary of the Federal Employees' Compensation Act*, sponsored by U.S. Department of Labor and Rutgers University, July 1992.
19. Recent legislative changes to the workers' compensation laws in Texas, Colorado, and Florida are examples of reduction in benefits, limits on medical care, and related issues.
20. *Report of the National Commission on State Workmen's Compensation Laws, 1972*. This report with its *Compendium* and many additional studies stands as a ready reference to the wide variance and complexities of the state systems, and the many problems with the collective system, No. O-496-632, Washington, D.C., 1973, Government Printing Office.
21. Rosenblum M, editor: *Compendium On Workers Compensation*, The National Commission on State Workmen's Compensation Laws, Washington, D.C., 1972, Government Printing Office.
22. Schiff MB, Miller DL: "The Americans With Disabilities Act: A New Challenge for Employers," *Tort and Insurance Journal* 27 Fall 1991.
23. Swoboda F: "Motion-Injury Experts Await Impact of Disabilities Act," *Washington Post*, 3 Nov. 1991, p. H2.
24. U.S. Department of Labor, Bureau of Labor Statistics: "The Employment Situation: September

1994," Washington, D.C., U.S. Department of Labor, 7 Oct. 1994.

25. Victor RA, editor: *Challenges for the 1990s,* No. WC-90-3, Cambridge, Mass., July 1990, Workers' Compensation Research Institute.

26. "1994 Workers' Compensation and Unemployment Insurance Laws," 1 Jan. 1994, Washington, D.C., AFL-CIO Publication No. R-36-0394-15.

27. "Workers' Compensation on the Critical List," *Forbes Magazine,* 30 Sept. 1991.

# CHAPTER 7

# SOCIAL SECURITY DISABILITY SYSTEMS

*John H. Mather*

The Social Security Administration (SSA) has national responsibility under public law 74-271 for the administration of both the Social Security Disability Insurance (SSDI) program (Title II) and the Supplemental Security Income (SSI) program (Title XVI). Title II (SSDI) provides coverage for cash benefits for those disabled workers (and their dependents) who have contributed to the Social Security trust fund through the Federal Insurance Contribution Act (FICA) tax on their earnings. Title XVI (SSI) provides for a minimum income level for the needy, aged, blind, and disabled. A person qualifies under the SSI program because of financial need. Under Title XVI, financial need is demonstrated by a limit of income and resources to a level that is equal to or less than the amount specified in the law.

## STATUTORY DEFINITIONS OF DISABILITY

Under both programs the definitions of disability and blindness are essentially the same. The law defines disability as "the inability to engage in any substantial gainful activity by reason of any medically determinable physical or mental impairment which can be expected to result in death or has lasted or can be expected to last for a continuous period of not less than 12 months." (Section 223(d)(1)(A))

The law further states that a child under age 18 will be considered disabled for purposes of eligibility for SSI, "if he suffers from a medically determinable physical or mental impairment of comparable severity" to that which would make an adult disabled. (Section 1614(a)(3)(A))

To meet these definitions, an individual's impairment or combination of impairments "are (to be) of such severity that he is not only unable to do his previous work but cannot, considering his age, education, and work experience, engage in any other kind of substantial gainful work which exists in the national economy." (Section 223(d)(2)(A))

## Substantial Gainful Activity

The term *substantial gainful activity* (SGA) means any work activity that involves significant and productive physical or mental activities and is performed (or intended) for pay or profit—currently, up to $500 per month for disabled persons and $850 per month for the blind.

## Medically Determinable Physical or Mental Impairment

The term *medically determinable physical or mental impairment* means that the impairment may be either physical or mental in nature and that it must be demonstrated through the symptoms, by observable clinical signs, and laboratory findings reported by acceptable medical sources, including licensed physicians, licensed or certified psychologists, and licensed optometrists.

## Comparable Severity

The term *comparable severity* means that a child's physical or mental impairment(s) so limits the ability to function independently, appropriately, and effectively in an age-appropriate manner that the impairment(s) and limitations resulting from it are comparable to those that would disable an adult. (CFR 416.909) Specifically, the impairment must substantially reduce, or if the child is younger than a year old, be reasonably expected to substantially reduce, the child's ability to:

1. Grow, develop, or mature physically, mentally, or emotionally and, thus, to attain developmental milestones at any age-appropriate rate; or
2. grow, develop, or mature physically, mentally, or emotionally and, thus, to engage in age-appropriate activities of daily living in self-care: play, recreation, and sports; school and academics; vocational settings; peer and family relationships; or

3. acquire the skills needed to assume roles reasonably expected of adults. (CFR, Part 416.924)

## DESCRIPTION OF SSDI AND SSI PROGRAMS

### Social Security Disability Income

Under SSDI, monthly benefits are payable to people younger than 65 years of age who have worked long enough and recently enough under Social Security. Every person who pays into Social Security contributes to the Social Security Disability Trust Fund. After a certain period of time working in employment covered under Social Security (see below), a person gains insured status and is entitled to a disability benefit if he becomes severely impaired and cannot work. Medicare coverage is available to those who have received SSDI benefits for 24 months.

Under Title II, there are three basic categories of impaired individuals who can qualify for benefits on the basis of disability. These are:

1. Disabled workers younger than 65 years of age if the worker has been employed or self-employed long enough and recently enough under Social Security. Most workers need Social Security work credits for at least five of the ten years preceding the onset of disability to have disability protection. Some older workers, however, may need additional credits depending on their age at the time they become disabled. For the worker who becomes disabled before 31 years of age, the requirement ranges down with the worker's age to as little as 18 months of work.

2. A person continuously disabled since childhood (before 22 years of age) if one of the parents who is covered under Social Security retires, becomes disabled, or dies. These "childhood disability" payments may continue for as long as the individual continues to be disabled. The individual need not have contributed to Social Security to qualify.

3. A disabled widow or widower 50 to 60 years old if the deceased spouse was covered under Social Security. This also applies to certain disabled surviving divorced wives in the same age range. Disabled widows and widowers need not have worked under Social Security. However, they are eligible only if the disability occurs before or within seven years after the spouse's death or, in the case of a widowed mother or father, before or within seven years after the end of entitlement to benefits as a parent with an entitled child in care.

### Supplemental Security Income

SSI disability payments are made to needy people who are younger than 65 years of age and have limited income and few resources. These payments are made from General Revenue funds. Most SSI recipients qualify for Medicaid, a state-run medical assistance program.

Under Title XVI, there are four basic categories of disability claims:

1. An adult (older than 18 years) who is disabled. The definition of disability for the disabled adult under SSI is essentially the same as for the disabled worker or childhood disability claimant under Title II. Both medical and vocational factors are considered in determining disability.

2. An adult who meets the definition of statutory blindness. Under the SSI law, a person who is legally blind does not have to meet the duration requirement. Payment can be made on the basis of temporary blindness.

3. A child (younger than 18 years) who is disabled. The requirements for disability are such that there must be an impairment or impairments of comparable severity to that which is considered disabling for an adult. However, since a child is not normally considered to engage in work activity, vocational factors are not considered. Instead, with children, interference with normal growth and development is a prime consideration.

4. A blind child who meets the definition of statutory blindness. As with adults, there is no duration requirement for children who meet the definition of statutory blindness.

### Program Activity

Each year, more than three million persons nationwide apply for SSDI benefits and/or SSI disability payments.

In 1994 Social Security and SSI disability payments were made to more than four million disabled individuals and their families. These programs provide cash payments and health care coverage when a worker or eligible needy individual is unable to work for at least a year due to a physical or mental impairment. These payments continue as long as the person is unable to work due to impairment. The SSA also has a number of work incentives that provide continued benefits and health care coverage for disabled persons who want to work. Special rules make it possible for impaired people receiving SSDI or SSI benefits to work and still receive monthly cash payments and Medicare or Medicaid. The SSA calls these rules "work incentives".

## ADJUDICATION OF A CLAIM

### The Application Process

Disability claims are processed through a network of some 1300 Social Security field offices, the central office, and 54 state agencies, generically known as Disability Determination Services (DDS). The case flow is as given below.

### Social Security Field Office

An application for disability benefits is obtained by an SSA representative, in person, by telephone, or by mail. The application includes a description of impairment, names and addresses of the claimant's medical sources, dates of treatment, and other information that relates to the alleged disability.

The SSA field office then verifies non-medical eligibility requirements, which include earnings and coverage information. The field office assists the applicant to obtain evidence to substantiate information related to age, the periods and nature of employment, marital status, and if spouse's/children's benefits are involved. The field office may also assist the applicant to develop medical or lay evidence in support of his claim. When the field office verifies that the non-medical eligibility criteria are met, the case is forwarded to the state agency.

### State Disability Determination Services (DDS)

The DDS are fully funded by the federal government, and are the state agencies responsible for collecting and providing medical evidence sufficient to render an equitable determination on whether the claimant is or is not disabled or blind under the law, and to determine when disability began and if the disability has ended.

The DDS obtains, if possible, medical evidence from the claimant's medical sources. If that evidence is insufficient to render a determination, the DDS will purchase a consultation examination from the treating source, or from an independent source.

The medical evidence is then reviewed by a team composed of a physician (in the case of mental impairments, a clinical psychologist may be used) and a disability examiner. Together, they determine eligibility. The state agency sends a determination notice to the claimant. A determination is also made as to whether the applicant is a candidate for vocational rehabilitation (VR). If so, a referral to the VR agency is made.

After the disability determination has been made, the case is forwarded to a SSA field office for further action.

### Medical Basis of Disability

To qualify for payments under either Title II or Title XVI disability programs, an individual must have a *medically determinable impairment*. This means an impairment that has medically demonstrable anatomical, physiological, or psychological abnormalities. Such abnormalities are medically determinable if they manifest themselves by clinical signs or laboratory findings apart from symptoms. Abnormalities that manifest themselves only as symptoms are not medically determinable. *Symptoms* are the claimant's own perception of his physical or mental impairments. *Signs* are anatomical, physiological, or psychological abnormalities that can be observed through the use of medically acceptable clinical techniques. In psychiatric impairments, signs are medically demonstrable abnormalities of behavior, affect, thought, memory, orientation, and contact with reality. *Laboratory findings* are manifestations of anatomical, physiological, or psychological phenomena demonstrable by replacing or extending the perceptiveness of the observer's senses and include chemical, electrophysiological, roentgenological, or psychological tests. Statements of the applicant, including his own description of the impairment, are alone insufficient to establish the presence of a physical or mental impairment.

### Sequential Evaluation Process

There is a sequence in evaluating claims for disability that directly reflects the requirements of the law and regulations. This step-by-step procedure is known as the "sequential evaluation process". Initial steps in the process include a determination as to whether the claimant fulfills the basic eligibility requirements of insured status under SSDI and the "means test" under SSI. Also, a medically determinable impairment that is judged to be severe must exist.

In both adult and childhood claims, the next step in the process involves a determination as to whether an allowance can be made that meets or equals any listing in the Listing of Impairments.

### Listing of Impairments

The Listing of Impairments is published by the SSA under the title *Disability Evaluation Under Social Security (Listing of Impairments)*. It is periodically updated, with the most recent revision in 1994.[3]

The Listing of Impairments is organized by body system as a set of medical evaluation criteria. For each body system the medical evaluation criteria are preceded by key concepts used in evaluating impairments under the system and a description of the type of medical evidence needed. Under each system there appears a Category of Impairments. Each category lists alternative sets of symptoms, signs, or laboratory findings. The Listing of Impairments is similar to the medical criteria in the AMA's *Guides to the Evaluation of Permanent Impairment.*

The Listing is divided into two parts. Part A contains medical criteria that apply to persons 18 years and older (considered adults). The medical criteria in Part A may also be applied in evaluating impairments in persons younger than 18 years if the disease processes have a similar effect on adults and younger persons. Part B contains additional medical criteria that apply only to the evaluation of impairments of persons younger than 18 years. Certain criteria in Part A do not give appropriate consideration to the particular effects of the disease processes in childhood, i.e., when the disease process is generally found only in children or when the disease process is different in its effect on children than on adults. In evaluating disability for a person younger than 18 years, Part B will be used first. If the medical criteria in Part B do not apply, the medical criteria in Part A will be used.

The medical criteria in the Listing describe impairments in terms of specific signs, symptoms, and laboratory findings that are presumed severe enough to preclude an individual from working a year or longer or, in the case of a child, performing age-appropriate activities. The Listing describes more than 100 of the most common diseases and disorders (and the necessary diagnostic criteria) that are so serious or life-threatening that if the claimant meets one of them and is not engaging in substantial gainful activity, the claimant is deemed to be disabled. If an individual has an impairment that does not meet the specific criteria described in the Listing but has an impairment of severity equal to a listed impairment, and is not working at a level of substantial gainful activity, the claimant is also presumed to meet the definition of disability. This concept of meeting or equaling the Listing also is intended as a means of liberalizing the diagnostic criteria. No claimant is denied a determination of disability solely on the basis of not meeting or equaling the Listing.

### Additional Factors in Determining Disability

Adult applicants whose impairment is less severe than one listed or is not of equivalent severity may, in some instances, be found disabled if the demand of the jobs in which the applicants might be expected to engage, based on age, education, and work experi-ence, exceed the claimants' remaining capacity to perform. Individuals may be found disabled if there is sufficient documentation to support a conclusion that they are unable to engage in substantial gainful work (an administrative decision). Substantial gainful work is any work of a nature generally performed for remuneration or profit, involving the performance of significant physical or mental duties, or a combination of both. Work may be considered substantial even if it is less demanding or less responsible than the individual's former work, and it may be considered gainful even if it pays less than his former work. Specific guidelines and grids are used to integrate this information to reach a conclusion.

Childhood applicants whose impairment is less severe than one listed or is not of equivalent severity may, in some instances, be found disabled if the child is unable to function on a sustained basis appropriate to their ages. Determination of disability in a child gives consideration to expected age-appropriate activities and achievement of developmental milestones with a specific assessment of developmental and functional domains. The domains describe the child's major sphere of activity, such as physical, cognitive, communicative, and social/emotional levels and skills.

## GATHERING OF MEDICAL AND OTHER EVIDENCE

Each person who files a claim for disability under the SSA must submit a sufficient amount of medical and other evidence to support the claim. The medical evidence is secured from sources who have treated or otherwise evaluated the claimant.

### Treating Source

In the role as the treating source, the physician/ psychologist provides from existing files and patient records the medical evidence of record (MER) normally required in each disability claim. SSA guidelines emphasize the importance of the treating source's evidence in the decision-making process.

The medical evidence provided by the treating source needs to be as complete and as timely as possible in order for SSA to give the claimants an accurate and prompt decision on their disability claims. In most cases, the treating source's MER is all that the SSA requires to make the disability decision.

### Consultative Examiner for the Disability Determination Services (DDS)

In the absence of sufficient MER, the SSA, through the state DDS, may request additional examinations.

These consultative examinations (CEs) are performed by licensed physicians, licensed osteopaths, or licensed or certified psychologists. While states maintain extensive CE panels and are looking continually for additional CE sources, the treating sources are the preferred CE source if qualified, equipped, and willing to perform the CE for the fee schedule payment. Fees for CEs are set by each state and may vary from state to state.

The DDS in each state can provide more information about performing medical or psychological CEs.

## Medical Evidence of Record (MER)

The essential elements of a good MER are objective medical findings in the form of copies of original clinical records by the claimant's treating physicians and psychologists, hospitals, clinics, the Department of Veterans Affairs, and similar sources of medical treatment. These records should include comprehensive information on symptoms, signs, and laboratory findings that will establish if the claimants have medically determinable impairments severe enough to prevent them from working for a year or more or that may result in their death.

In most cases, this initial medical evidence is all that is needed by the SSA to make a disability determination. The MER provided by the treating source is preferred because it is based on a long-term relationship and consequently the records are more complete. The treating source is familiar with the patient (the claimant) and can often trace or establish the beginning and course of the impairment's response to treatment and prognosis. The SSA guidelines emphasize the importance of the treating source's evidence in the decision-making process.

## Contents of a Medical Report

In order for an MER to furnish the SSA with sufficient medical evidence, it should include:
1. Medical history.
2. Clinical findings such as results of physical or mental status examination.
3. Laboratory findings such as blood pressure and x-rays.
4. Diagnosis (statement of disease or injury based on its signs and symptoms).
5. Treatment prescribed, with response, side effects, and prognosis.
6. Medical source statement of prognosis based on the medical source's own medical findings.

Medical evidence, including clinical and laboratory findings, should be complete and detailed enough to allow the SSA to make the disability determination.

In addition, the report should enable the SSA to be able to determine the nature and limiting effects of the impairment, its probable duration, and the claimant's remaining capacity to engage in work-related physical or mental activities.

## Medical Source Statement

In each case, the SSA requests an additional statement from the treating physician, psychologist, or consultative examination provider. It is called a medical source statement and details what the claimant can still do despite the impairments. This is the opinion that can be rendered as to the claimant's functional capacities, if known. It should describe such work-related activities as sitting, standing, walking, lifting, carrying, handling objects, hearing, speaking, and traveling. In cases involving mental impairments, the SSA needs to include a statement about the claimant's capacity for understanding and memory, sustained concentration and persistence, social interaction, and adaptation.

## ADMINISTRATIVE REVIEW PROCESS

### Appeals Process

A determination that a person is not disabled may be appealed. There are four levels of appeal:

### Reconsideration
If claimants wish to appeal an initial determination, they may file a *request for reconsideration* at the district office within 60 days of receiving the notice of initial determination. State agency staff not involved in the initial file development make a *reconsidered determination*.

### Hearing
Claimants that are dissatisfied with the reconsideration may request a hearing before an Administrative Law Judge (ALJ) from the Office of Hearings and Appeals (OHA) within 60 days of receiving the notice of reconsideration. The ALJ will render a *decision* based only on the evidence of record, if it is desired by the individual. Generally, applicants appear at a scheduled hearing where, for the first time, they can review the evidence in the file and orally present a case. They have the right to representation by an attorney or lay person. The ALJ can arrange consultative examinations, subpoena witnesses, and seek assistance from physicians (*medical experts*) and vocational counselors (*vocational experts*) under contract with the SSA before issuing a decision.

## Appeals Council

If dissatisfied with the ALJ's decision, the claimant may request, within 60 days of receipt of the decision, an Appeals Council review. The Appeals Council, located in Falls Church, Virginia, does not hold hearings, and the applicant submits documentation or written arguments. Generally, when the Appeals Council agrees with the ALJ's unfavorable decision, it denies the claimant's request for review and does not issue a new decision. If so, the ALJ'S decision becomes the final action of the Secretary of Health and Human Services. The Appeals Council can grant the request for review and remand the case to the ALJ for rehearing or reverse the ALJ's decision.

## Federal Court Review

A claimant displeased with the action of the Appeals Council may, within 60 days of the date of receipt of the action, file an appeal in a federal district court. If the claimants or the SSA are dissatisfied with the decision of the District Court, either may appeal to the Court of Appeals and, ultimately, to the United States Supreme Court.

## Continuing Disability Reviews

SSDI benefits and SSI disability payments are made to people whose impairments are expected to prevent them from working for at least a year or that may result in death. The cases of all beneficiaries are periodically reexamined to see if they are still disabled and otherwise continue to meet the requirements for benefits.

The frequency of the reviews depends on the severity of the condition and the expectation of improvement. If improvement is expected, the first review generally will be held within 6-18 months after the decision is made that a person is disabled. If improvement is possible but cannot be predicted, the case will be reviewed about once every three years. If improvement is not expected, the case will be reviewed once every five to seven years.

During the review, an SSA representative will ask the beneficiary if the condition has improved. The representative will ask for documentation of the claimant's current condition, including the names, addresses and phone numbers of doctors, hospitals, and clinics that have treated the beneficiary since the last review. If the beneficiary has worked since the last review, the representative will need information about the dates, pay, and duties of the work.

The case will then be sent to the state Disability Determination Services (DDS). A team, including an experienced disability examiner and a physician or psychologist, will carefully review all of the information and the evidence the beneficiary has provided and will request detailed medical reports from the sources indicated.

In most cases, the information from treating sources should be enough to make a determination. However, if the medical evidence is not sufficient or current, the beneficiary may be asked to have a special examination at the government's expense. If an examination or tests are needed, an appointment will be scheduled with the treating source, another private physician or psychologist, or other medical source. The beneficiary will be notified in writing of the date, place, and time.

The law indicates that disability benefits and payments will be stopped only if the evidence shows that the beneficiary's impairment has medically improved and also shows that the beneficiary can work. It specifies how medical improvement is to be considered in determining if a beneficiary is still disabled. The process is designed to give beneficiaries an opportunity to show that they are still disabled and to ensure that their benefits are not stopped incorrectly. All evidence about the beneficiary's impairment during the past 12 months will be collected. If the beneficiary has more than one impairment, consideration will also be given to the combined effect of the impairments on his ability to work.

If the impairment has not medically improved and the beneficiary is not working, normally benefits will continue.

The SSA has several rules that can help people who are medically disabled but who still try to work. The rules are different for SSDI and SSI. If the beneficiary is receiving Social Security benefits, he may be able to work up to nine months during a trial work period and still receive benefits. Other rules continue cash benefits and Medicare coverage while he attempts to work on a regular basis. If the person is receiving SSI payments, he may continue to receive monthly payments even if their earnings increase, as long as other aspects of their eligibility remain unchanged. If cash payments stop because total income exceeds the SSI income limits, the SSI recipient may still be eligible for Medicaid.

A person who gets a notice that he is no longer disabled under the law may appeal the determination; he has special rights not available to those denied upon initial application for disability benefits. The individual may meet face-to-face with the decision maker during the first level of appeal (reconsideration). Benefits may be continued through the first two levels of appeal if this is requested within 10 days after a decision notice is received.

## CONCLUSION

When medical providers are asked for opinions about claimants applying for Social Security disability benefits, they should carefully consider the limitations of their knowledge and expertise in framing responses. They may prefer to state only the impairments established by objective medical signs and laboratory findings. For example, if the medical provider feels sufficiently competent to render an opinion, he might estimate anticipated functional restrictions. In providing such information, each provider of evidence fulfills a vital, effective function in the disability determination process. The ultimate decision about who is or is not disabled, with appropriate medical and vocational input, should be left to the SSA.

### References

1. "Childhood Disability under the Social Security SSI Program," SSA Pub. No. 64-048.
2. "Consultative Examination," SSA Pub. No. 64-025.
3. "Disability Evaluation under Social Security (Listing of Impairments)," SSA Pub. No. 64-039.
4. "Evaluating Disability under Social Security," SSA Pub. No. 64-045.

# CHAPTER 8

## MEDICAL-LEGAL INTERFACE

*Lawrence P. Postol*

The interface between physicians and the legal world is not always an easy one. Confusion between the professions requires that care must be taken anytime the law and medicine interface. Both are complex fields, with many important decisions being made, and neither field is an exact science. However, if the physician has a minimum level of understanding of the legal system, and the lawyer has an adequate understanding of the medical facts and the limits of medical science, the medical-legal interface can be a successful one.

### THE ROLE OF THE PHYSICIAN IN THE LEGAL WORLD

Some physicians are too fearful of interacting with the legal world, and some are not cautious enough. Those physicians who see a potential lawsuit at every corner, and thus refuse to give a written opinion, or hesitate to call a faker a faker, are too cautious. Those who assume they can do whatever they want, relying either on bluffing or on their malpractice insurance, are also mistaken. Both the lack of caution, and overcautiousness, come from a lack of knowledge of the legal world.

While, in theory, anyone who can pay the $10 filing fee can sue another, lawsuits are rarely filed unless there is some minimal basis for the claim, decided through legal advice. Thus, while the physician can never guarantee that he will never be sued, he can take some steps to reduce greatly the risk of becoming a defendant in litigation.

Conversely, if a physician is so cautious he never gives a definitive opinion, he is useless to the legal system. The key for the physician, in addition to focusing on the medical questions, is to understand the legal issues, how the physician's opinion interfaces with them, and what the physician's role is in answering the legal issues.

### Testifying in Court

It is important to recognize that when a physician testifies in court, he is usually offering a medical opinion as an expert witness. The courts have grappled with minimum standards for an expert witness's opinions, so that "junk science" can be excluded from the courtroom. Thus, a physician must have a minimum scientific basis for his opinion, before he will be allowed to testify in court.

The United States Supreme Court recently addressed when an expert opinion, and in particular, when a medical expert, can offer an opinion into evidence. In *Dabert V. Merrell Dow Pharmaceuticals Inc.*, __ U.S. __, 113 S. Ct. 2786 (1993), the Supreme Court was faced with the admissibility of medical experts' opinions that prenatal ingestion of bendectin can cause birth defects. The Court held that a medical expert's opinion is admissible only if it is based on "scientific validity," that is, if it is based on scientific methods that have tested its validity. Put another way, the person offering expert opinion must have "a reliable basis in the knowledge and experience of his discipline." The Supreme Court noted that trial judges, in order to test scientific validity, must initially determine whether the theory or technique in question "can be (and has been) tested," whether it has been "subjected to peer review and publication," its "known or potential error rate," the "existence and maintenance of standards controlling its operation," and finally, whether it has attracted "widespread acceptance" within a relevant scientific community. The Court emphasized that the heart of scientific methodology is "testing [theories] to see if they can be falsified." The Court also noted that "a known technique that has been able to attract only minimal support...may properly be viewed with skepticism." Of course, the expert's theory must be properly applied to the facts of the claim in dispute: that is, the theory must be relevant to the claim.

In most cases, the medical opinion will not be questioned as to its admissibility, as in a diagnosis of cancer. However, when a physician testifies in a controversial area, especially on causation, he can expect that his opinion will be challenged as to whether it is even admissible, that is, whether it can even be presented to the jury, to be weighed against other experts' opinions.

## Definitions

Lawyers use legal terminology that is often foreign to physicians. It is curious that a lawyer often requests that a physician acting as an expert witness spend hours explaining the details of the doctor's professional opinion to the lawyer, yet the lawyer rarely takes the time to explain certain simple, but critical, legal terminology to the physician who is acting as an expert witness. The following are some of the legal terms that a physician might encounter in dealing with lawyers.

*The Law*—"The Law" is a term lawyers often use to refer to the controlling rules of the litigation. The law is made up of statutes, regulations, and common law. Statutes and regulations are written documents that explicitly define certain rules and duties, although they are often subject to differing interpretations. The common law is simply prior judicial decisions (precedents) that impose obligations and liability on certain persons. For example, if a shop owner is negligent in not shoveling the sidewalk and a person slips on it and falls, the shop owner is liable for the damages to that person. While certain legal principles are fairly uniform, the law does vary from state to state, and from state courts to federal courts.

*An Expert*—An expert is defined in most jurisdictions as any person who by "knowledge, skill, experience, training, or education" has "scientific, technical or other specialized knowledge" that will aid the judge or jury in determining the facts at issue in a lawsuit. The knowledge must be of a type not normally possessed by the general public, or for which the expert has some specialized expertise such that his opinion will aid the judge or jury. An expert may be retained simply to assist an attorney in preparing his case, or he may provide testimony at the hearing.

*Discovery*—A party is entitled to "discover" the relevant facts of a case and the evidence the other party has before the trial. Cases are not to be tried by surprise. The primary mechanisms for obtaining discovery are interrogatories (written questions), requests for production of documents, depositions (a lawyer questioning a witness in the presence of a court reporter and the opposing lawyer), and subpoenas. It is

important to note that, if an expert is hired but his opinion is not going to be used at trial (for example, where his opinion does not support the party's position), his opinion is usually not discoverable.

*Interrogatories*—A party may pose written questions to the other party in litigation; these questions are called *interrogatories*. The interrogatories may relate to the facts of the case as well as potential evidence at the trial. For expert witnesses, a party may send an interrogatory requesting the following information about the expert witness: to state the subject matter on which the expert is expected to testify, and to state the substance of the facts and opinions to which the expert is expected to testify and a summary of the grounds for each opinion.—*Federal Rule of Civil Procedure 26 (a) (2) (B)*.

*Deposition*—A deposition is an oral examination of a person, taken outside the courtroom, and before the trial. A party may take the deposition of any witness, including expert witnesses, to discover what they will say at trial. If a witness is unavailable at trial, his deposition testimony may be offered into evidence. In addition, if a witness testifies at trial, his deposition can be used to impeach him if he makes statements that are inconsistent with his prior deposition testimony.

A deposition may be taken at any location, but it is usually held at an attorney's office or the witness's place of business. The attorneys for both sides, as well as a court reporter, will be present, and the court reporter will transcribe the attorney's questions and witness's answers. If an attorney objects to a question, he states his objection so that the judge can rule on the objection at a later date when the judge reads the deposition testimony. The witness must still answer the question, unless the attorney who represents him instructs him not to answer the question, as when a privileged attorney-client matter is involved.

*Request for Production of Documents and Subpoena*—A party may ask the other side to produce certain documents. Similarly, a subpoena can be sent to non-parties to compel them to produce documents, appear at a deposition or trial, and give testimony.

*Evidence*—Evidence is the testimony that has been heard at trial and the documents admitted at trial. The judge or jury must base their decision only on the evidence admitted. In selecting a physician's writings for admission into evidence, counsel and the physician should be certain that these writings properly explain their client's position.

*Hearsay*—Hearsay is a statement that is offered into evidence by someone other than the person who made the statement; it is normally not admissible.

Thus, a paper written by John Doe cannot be offered into evidence by Dick Smith. There are certain exceptions to the hearsay exclusion rule. Of critical importance, business records that are made in the ordinary course of business are admissible into evidence. Moreover, an expert can base his opinion on facts that are not in evidence, if the facts are "of a type reasonably relied upon by experts in the particular field in forming opinions or inferences upon the subject." However, whatever facts an expert relies upon must be disclosed to the other side if a proper discovery request is made.

### The Physician As An Expert Witness

A physician may be questioned by a lawyer as to the treatment he gave in the ordinary course of business. In such a case, he is a mere witness, like a bystander witnessing a car accident. For example, a physician may treat a patient for carpal tunnel syndrome, and only learn after the fact that the patient has a workers' compensation claim. Nevertheless, the physician can be called as a witness to describe his care and treatment of the injury. More often than not, however, the medical provider will know ahead of his treatment that there is a legal issue, and that he will be called as an expert witness. The minimum skills required of an expert are the "knowledge, skill, experience, training, or education" needed to qualify to give an "expert" opinion on the issue in the case. Any expert witness, including a physician, is judged by his credentials, independence, and ability to convince a judge or jury that his opinion is correct.

When a physician is called as an expert witness by one party, the physician can expect that the other side will have its own expert witness who will disagree with the opinion of the first expert. Judges and juries usually resolve the "battle of the experts" by selecting the expert who has the most impressive credentials, who appears to be least biased, and whose opinion seems most logical and rational. It is with this background in mind that attorneys select a physician as an expert witness.

The lawyer will try to select someone who is a true "expert"—an individual who practices full-time in the medical field in question and who is recognized by his peers as a true authority. Preferably, the physician will have written extensively on the relevant subject and will have performed research in the field in question. Appointments by associations or organizations of fellow professionals to positions of prestige are important. Certification by recognized boards is a minimum qualification. Awards and honors are helpful. Affiliations with universities and teaching positions are impressive to judges and juries, who assume the universities attract the "best and the brightest" and that such teachers keep up with current scientific knowledge. In short, whatever demonstrates a thorough knowledge of the field, and recognition of such knowledge by others, is helpful.

The issue of bias is always raised with respect to experts because he is being paid for his time, and the misperception is that his opinion has been bought. In order to combat this problem, lawyers look for experts who appear to have some independence. Thus, most lawyers try to avoid hiring "professional witnesses"—those individuals who spend a great deal of their time testifying in litigation as experts. The lawyer would rather try to find an individual who does not testify frequently. In addition, when a physician has previously testified on a medical issue, it helps if he has testified on both sides of the fence—for both plaintiffs and defendants—thus showing his independence. Of course, the attorney must be careful to make sure that the expert does not have any prior damaging testimony that conflicts with his opinion in the case at hand.

Attorneys favor a physician who is recognized by his peers as a true expert; such a position helps explain to the judge or jury why the lawyer has called him as a witness and thus helps refute the charge that he is a mere "hired gun". Similarly, the attorney wants a physician whose charges are reasonable. If an expert's fees are quite high, then there is the impression that his opinion is in fact for hire.

Finally, a physician is worthless as an expert witness unless he can communicate his knowledge to a judge and jury. The judge and jury will follow an expert's opinion only if they understand it and are persuaded by it. Thus, a physician must be able to explain technical knowledge to non-medical persons in a fashion that they can understand. Moreover, the presentation must appear to be based on adequate knowledge, be given in an unbiased manner, and withstand a non-medical person's test of reasonableness—does it sound right and make sense? If an opinion is given in a manner in which it "just doesn't sound right or make sense," the judge or jury will simply reject it. The physician must have the ability to teach the judge or jury about his field of medicine in a convincing manner.

### Attorney–Expert Relations

When an attorney requests a physician to testify as an expert witness in a case or provide assistance to the attorney in litigation, the attorney should communicate the nature of the physician's duties and the attorney's expectations. The attorney must give directions in a neutral manner so that the physician's independence will not be compromised. The physician must assure that he has all available relevant information, including all past medical records and reports, depositions, and claim-related documents and correspondence, and that his research is thorough and his opinion unimpeachable.

Physicians often receive calls from attorneys at a very late stage of litigation, and the parameters of an attorney-expert relationship are not well defined. Certain ground rules should be spelled out at the beginning of the relationship. The amount of the fee to be paid by the attorney, and when it will be paid, should be established. Most physicians charge an hourly rate and send a bill after they have testified, although for prolonged cases, interim billing is appropriate and avoids surprises. Moreover, the physician may want to give an estimate of how much time he thinks he will need to prepare his opinion, so that the attorney will not be shocked by the bill.

The physician must remember that whatever information he obtains or relies upon in forming his opinion will be subject to discovery by the other side. Thus, the physician does not want any explicit directions from the attorney as to the final outcome of the expert's opinion, for fear it will appear that he is being led around by the attorney. Similarly, the physician does not want to review any document which will "prejudice" his opinion, such as the attorney's client's position paper. Rather, the physician should expect only to receive all information relevant to his inquiry, and that the outer limits of his investigation should be set forth by the attorney. Of course, this should include *all* of the medical records of the case.

A physician must be thorough in his investigation and analysis. The physician must make sure he has obtained all relevant documents, performed all appropriate tests, and fully researched available medical literature. A good attorney will help a physician obtain all appropriate information and assure that the investigation has been thorough. In preparing for trial, the attorney will often play devil's advocate in a mock questioning session and test the physician's opinion.

A question often arises as to whether the opposing attorney can talk to the patient's physician. If the physician is hired by the patient's attorney and is initially retained as an expert witness, the answer is no, except via a formal deposition with the patient's attorney being present. If the physician's treatment occurred before the litigation was filed and was in the ordinary course of business (a treating physician), then most jurisdictions would hold that the opposing attorney can engage in an *ex parte* interview with the doctor, if the doctor is so inclined, in the same manner that any witness in a litigation can be inter-

viewed. In this circumstance, as a treating physician, he is not an expert witness for either his patient or for the party the patient is suing. Thus, like a witness to a car crash, either side's attorney can try to interview the doctor and get a witness statement/report from the doctor. Some other courts, however, have taken a contrary view, ruling that the physician/patient relationship is special, and thus those courts do not allow *ex parte* contacts, but rather limit the patient's adversary to a formal deposition in order to determine the doctor's opinion.

## The Physician's Report

The physician acting as an expert witness presents his opinion in two forms: the report and the "direct" examination testimony at the trial when he is questioned by the attorney who hired him. Since this presentation is the key to the physician's assistance to the lawyer, the presentation must be well prepared and flawless.

The physician must be extremely careful in preparing his written report, because once he has put something in writing, he will be discredited if he later varies from his report. Moreover, the physician usually only has one opportunity to prepare a report, since a good opposing attorney will discover if any drafts of the report were prepared. For these reasons, many attorneys prefer to receive oral reports and request that the physician either not prepare a written report or do so only after conferring with the attorney. On the other hand, if there is extensive contact with the attorney, the inference is that the attorney unduly influenced the physician's opinion. Each attorney will have his own approach for dealing with this situation. Usually, however, a skilled and experienced attorney will trust the expert to prepare his report without interference. If however, the report is harmful to the attorney's case, he will not use it and will simply hire another physician as his expert witness. The report of an expert witness who was retained for, but not used in, litigation is normally not discoverable by the other side.

## Direct Examination of the Physician

Whether a report is prepared or not, the physician may testify at trial. The attorney will ask the physician questions, and the expert will answer them. One cannot "lead" one's own witness, so the questions cannot suggest the answer. Thus, the attorney and expert must rehearse the physician's testimony so that there will be no surprises and the testimony is clear and convincing.

Where there is an expert on the other side, the physician will have to not only convince the judge or jury of the appropriateness of his opinion but also that his opinion is more credible than the views of the opposing expert. This can be achieved by explaining the thoroughness of his investigation, detailing the literature that supports his analysis, pressing the logical nature of his opinion, and attacking (in a low key manner) the opponent's expert's opinion by highlighting the flaws in his investigation and analysis.

## Cross-Examination

Every expert witness will be cross-examined by the other side's attorney, who will do everything to discredit the expert witness. The opponent's attorney will attack the physician's credentials, independence, thoroughness, and analysis. The attorney in his cross-examination may become hostile and even angry with the physician. It is at this point that the good expert witnesses are separated from the bad ones. The good expert will keep his composure and calmly not only repel the attack, but use the opportunity to reinforce in the mind of the judge or jury the propriety of his opinion.

The opposing attorney will do his best, through questioning, to demonstrate that the physician is stupid, ill-informed, did not have all relevant facts necessary to evaluate the situation, was improperly paid off by the attorney who hired him, and provided an analysis that is illogical and contrary to established scientific principles. To achieve this result, the opposing attorney will use any prior writings or testimony of the physician as well as any available scientific literature.

During the cross-examination, the physician must not lose sight of the key factors that are used to evaluate him: credentials, independence, and expertise. Thus, the physician should be prepared for all questions and respond with informed answers. The physician does not want to appear to be trying to avoid a question, to be hiding anything, or to be ignorant. He must not argue or "fence" with the attorney, but rather must directly answer the attorney's questions without appearing to be an advocate. A dispassionate and direct answer is called for by the physician. A witness is allowed, however, to answer fully any question. Thus, if an answer gives a false or misleading impression, the physician can and should fully answer the question by not only providing the information requested but by adding his explanation of why the information is incomplete or gives a false impression. In this manner, the expert witness can not only stand up to the questioning but can use the cross-examination to continue to press for the acceptance of his opinion.

Finally, the physician should realize that no matter how prepared he is, he may still encounter a surprise question. At this point, the physician must remember that his job is to answer the question in a direct, straightforward manner, and that the lawyer's job is to win the case. Thus, no matter what the question and its apparent adverse inference, the expert witness must always follow the cardinal rule for every witness: be truthful and candid. No witness has ever failed when he has followed this simple rule. Juries can see when a witness tries to avoid a question or gives an incredible answer. Such a response taints the expert's entire testimony.

## THE PHYSICIAN'S STATUS IN ANSWERING MEDICAL-LEGAL QUESTIONS

The first thing a physician must do is clarify his status. If the physician is a treating physician, then there is a physician/patient relationship, which means that the physician owes a duty of care to the patient and that communications between the physician and patient are confidential, although, as noted below, the confidentiality can be waived. If the patient goes directly to the physician, there is no question as to the existence of the physician/patient relationship. However, ofttimes an examinee may come via a referral from an employer or insurer, and yet there may still be a physician/patient relationship. For example, in approximately half the states, under workers' compensation laws, the employer selects the treating physician. Nevertheless, the selected physician owes the same duty of care to the injured worker as to any other patient. If the physician has any question as to whether he is a treating physician or provider, the source of the referral should be consulted as well as the patient. It is important that all three (the physician, referral source, and patient) have the same understanding.

Ofttimes the physician is not hired by the patient, but rather is conducting an examination for another party. This occurs in pre-employment physicals and in the so-called independent medical examination (IME). When a physician performs an IME, he is an expert witness for the person or entity who retained him. If a person puts his medical condition into issue (e.g., a car accident lawsuit or a workers' compensation claim) then the defendant/employer is entitled to have a physician of his choice examine that person. In such situations, the physician owes his duty to the hiring entity, and not the examinee. The physician must, however, clarify his status with the individual. Thus, the physician should inform the individual that there is no physician/patient relationship and that he will not report his findings to the individual (any privilege extends only to the referring party).

If the physician is clearly not treating the examinee and the physician has no duty toward the worker (e.g., pre-employment physicals or an IME), it is of critical importance that the patient be informed of this information up front and that he sign a document recognizing and agreeing to this arrangement. For example, the patient might sign a statement as follows: "I recognize that Dr. XXX is performing a pre-employment physical examination of me at the request of YYY Inc. I understand that Dr. XXX is not my physician, I am not his patient, and he owes no duty to me to look for, or disclose, any medical condition I may have. I further understand and release Dr. XXX to disclose any findings to YYY Inc. and I agree that these findings will not be disclosed to me since the examination conducted by Dr. XXX was at the request and expense of YYY Inc."

Often, a theoretical issue is raised as to what if the physician, performing an IME, discovers a correctable life-threatening condition. Can he inform the patient of it? Obviously, most defendants and employers would never restrict the IME physician from giving the patient this information. However, if the IME physician has any concern, he should make it clear to the defendant or employer, when he is retained, that he can disclose such information to the examinee.

## POTENTIAL MALPRACTICE LIABILITY

Physicians in the disability world, like any other physician, commit malpractice if their treatment or actions do not follow a reasonable standard of care. Of particular concern are (1) the failure to notify a worker of an adverse condition or of a risk of future problems, and (2) the premature return to the job or without adequate work restrictions.

Workers' compensation is the exclusive remedy only between the employee (the first party) and the employer and its agents/other employees (the second party). If any third party negligently contributes to a worker's injury, the employee may sue that third party in civil court, outside the workers' compensation system. For example, if a crane collapses at work and injures a worker, the worker can recover workers' compensation from the employer and sue the manufacturer of the crane for building a defective crane. The most famous lawsuits of this type are by insulators who handled asbestos in their jobs. Millions of dollars have been recovered from the manufacturers of the asbestos. In the same manner, a physician who negligently injures a worker when treating a work injury can be sued for malpractice. The malprac-

tice action for the occupational physician will be no different from a malpractice action against a physician who improperly cared for a non–work-related illness. Moreover, if the employee does not sue, the employer or insurance carrier, who paid the increased workers' compensation benefits caused by the doctor's malpractice, may be entitled to sue the physician for the increased workers' compensation benefits paid as a result of the physician's malpractice.

## Failure to Notify the Worker of an Adverse Condition or of an Increased Risk

If there is a physician/patient relationship, then the physician owes a duty to the patient to disclose any adverse condition and to notify the patient of any risks of future health problems related to the condition. For the physician involved in a disability evaluation, this area of liability is often overlooked.

When an injury causing an impairment is known to the physician, he may use too narrow a focus when examining the patient. For example, if a chest roentgenogram is being read to determine whether the injured worker suffered a broken rib, there may still be a duty on the part of the physician to look for any coin lesion that might represent a tumor. Certainly, the physician does not want to be in the position where the lesion is discovered a year later, and when the chest roentgenogram taken for the work injury a year earlier is reviewed, the lesion can clearly be seen. To a trial jury, that failure is clearly malpractice.

On the other hand, if the physician is treating the worker for a sprained small toe, he is under no obligation to take a chest roentgenogram and look for other abnormalities. Physicians must, of course, use common sense. They must recognize that workers can suffer illnesses and injuries outside the work place. The patient must be looked at not only as a worker but as, yes, a *patient*. In addition, the physician should carefully document the patient's complaints and what the physician did and did not investigate. Indeed, unless it is absolutely clear, the physician should inform the patient that the examination and treatment are limited to the work injury, or the disability at issue, and that the physician did not perform a complete physical examination.

Similarly, the physician should be careful to advise the patient of any risk that the current condition involves. For example, if a worker is recovering from disc surgery, and the worker is being returned to manual labor, the risk of a recurrent disc problem should be carefully explained to the patient. As with all patients, the doctor should assume nothing. Rather, care should be taken to explain the condition fully to the patient and explain in detail (and preferably in writing) what the patient can and cannot do and the risks involved. Of course, the physician should also advise the patient of what "problem signs" to look for that may indicate the need for further medical evaluation.

### Premature Return to Work or Inadequate Work Restrictions

The physician should be especially concerned with the possibility that a worker will allege that the physician returned the employee to work prematurely or with inadequate work restrictions. In the context of a workplace injury, employers are motivated to return the injured worker to work as soon as possible, with the minimum level of work restrictions possible. Conversely, some employees want to stay out of work as long as possible and, when they return to work, they want their duties to be as light as possible. The effort some employees put into not working can surprise even the most hardened soul in this field.

Suffice it to say that the prudent physician should avoid being caught between these two tensions. The physician should carefully document any actions taken and explain them to the employee as well as to the employer. If the employee objects to the physician's actions or shows signs of being a malingerer, the physician may want to refer the patient for a second opinion so that the return to work cannot reasonably be challenged.

A second opinion has the advantage of "covering" the initial physician's opinion. With a second opinion in hand, the physician is no longer "out on a limb" alone. Moreover, if the physician is an in-house doctor, for workers' compensation litigation, the employer will often want a second opinion from an independent outside physician. Although a second opinion is not needed in every case, the experienced physician can usually spot the problem cases: excessive subjective complaints, extreme reluctance to return to work, desire for overly severe work restrictions, an unusually long history of minor injuries, engagement in physician-shopping, etc. In such cases, wise employers realize that a second opinion is money well spent in order to prepare for the unavoidable litigation over the disability claim.

### LIABILITY FOR UNAUTHORIZED RELEASE OF INFORMATION (LIBEL AND SLANDER AND CONTRACTUAL INTERFERENCE)

As with any physician, a physician evaluating a disability has a general duty to keep information concerning patients confidential. Of course, when a worker files a workers' compensation claim or a lawsuit to recover for an injury, this usually waives any privilege of confidentiality and allows the employer/defendant to be informed of the patient's treatment. Indeed, in most jurisdictions, in the case of work injuries, the treating physician must file medical reports with the industrial commission and the employer. Similarly, in many jurisdictions, state statutes require that gunshot wounds or contagious diseases must be reported.

In the absence of a waiver or statutory duty to disclose information, the physician has a duty to protect the patient's confidences and the confidentiality of any treatment given. The physician's breach of this trust can result in liability for invasion of privacy and/or breach of the patient-physician relationship.

Although the physician may have a defense for disclosure based on a duty imposed by law to file a report, or a duty to the public interest, the physician should be sure of his position before making the disclosure. It is generally safer to obtain a consent form, after disclosing to the patient all relevant facts, including to whom the disclosure is being made and what records will be disclosed. A second option is to have the employer or defendant obtain a subpoena for the records.

The hardest cases are ones where there are conflicting duties towards the patient and the public, and there are no clear statutory or regulatory directives as to which duty should prevail. Unfortunately, when the physician must act, it will be only later that the court will tell the physician if he made the right choice. As a general rule, common sense is the best guide.

In emergency situations, the physician should make the minimum disclosure necessary to protect others. Thus, if emergency personnel are about to treat a cut on an AIDS patient, the physician should advise the personnel that OSHA requires medical workers to use gloves and that they should take similar "universal" precautions. However, if it can be avoided, the physician should not disclose that the reason for the precautions is AIDS.

Physicians should also be aware of federal and state regulations that protect certain medical records, even limiting the release with consent of alcohol and drug abuse records. Physicians must also remember that they, like anyone else, can be sued for libel and slander. Although mere opinions are not actionable and testimony in court is privileged, physicians should always be cautious about how they make negative statements and to whom.

Truth is always a defense to an action for libel (written defamation) and slander (oral defamation), but it can often be an expensive process to litigate the truth of a statement. Thus physicians must be careful of what they say and to whom. Generally, libel and slander laws only protect one's reputation. For example, if a physician makes a false statement that injures the worker's reputation (e.g., that the worker is a liar), then the defamatory statement, if untrue, is actionable. On the other hand, diagnostic opinions generally would not affect one's reputation and thus would not be actionable under the law of libel and slander.

However, in the psychiatric arena, the fields of medicine and libel law overlap. Courts have held that psychiatric reports that a state that a worker is mentally unfit to work are actionable since "being nuts" reflects on one's reputation and ability to work. Whether this principle would be extended to calling a worker "a malingerer" or simply physically unfit to work is unclear.

The physician's statement, even if defamatory and untrue, may still be protected if privileged. Thus, there is an absolute privilege for any testimony in a court of law. Moreover, there is generally a qualified privilege if a statement is made in a reasonable manner and for a proper purpose. Generally, a physician's statement to an employer as to the fitness of a worker to perform his job enjoys a qualified privilege. This privilege is "qualified" because it is lost if the physician acts with malice—knowing the statement is false or with reckless disregard for its truth.

Thus, generally, physicians cannot be sued for their opinions concerning a worker's ability to work unless the statement made was false and was made with recklessness. This is a hard standard for a worker to meet. Nevertheless, physicians should make sure they have taken steps such that their conduct is far from reckless, and thus they will not have to prove the truth of their statements via expensive litigation.

Physicians can also be sued for negligent interference with a contractual relationship, which is a relatively new but developing doctrine. Thus, even if there is no physician/patient relationship, the physician may still owe a duty to the worker not to interfere negligently with the worker's relationship with the employer. For example, if a physician performing an examination of a worker for a job application is negligent and incorrectly states that the worker is in poor health, the physician could arguably be held liable to the worker for negligence interference with the worker's contractual relationship—getting a job with the employer. Therefore, the physician, as stated in the AMA *Guides*, should only evaluate impairment and leave disability decisions to the proper authority.

## Insurance Coverage

Many physicians do not worry about their potential liability because they have malpractice insurance. There are two problems with this attitude. Firstly, a claim may cause an increase in the doctor's insurance premium or even cancellation of the policy. Secondly, not all claims are covered by all policies. An insurance policy is a contract. The insurance company says it will defend against and pay certain types of claims when certain conditions are met. Thus, a physician must carefully examine the policy (read the fine print) to see what is and is not covered and what the limits are. This is much like a homeowner's policy, which may not cover damage from floods, or an automobile insurance policy that does not cover the driver if they are legally drunk or only pays a maximum of $300,000 in all cases.

If a physician has a malpractice policy, it may not cover libel or slander. It may not cover the physician when they act as an independent medical examiner, or when a report is written based on a review of records without seeing the patient. This may not be considered the practice of medicine so as to trigger coverage. Rather, an errors or emissions policy may be needed. The physician should read their policy carefully and have any questions answered in writing by the insurance company. It is critically important that the physician know what coverage has and has not been bought.

## RETURNING A WORKER TO WORK

One of the critical and most demanding tasks of a medical provider is deciding when a worker can return to work. A premature return to the job can result in an aggravation of the original injury and longer impairment. An unnecessarily delayed return results in increased workers' compensation costs and an unhappy employer. The balance is achieved when the physician understands the patient and communicates effectively with the employer.

In the rush to have a high-volume practice, some physicians sometimes forget that not all patients are alike. Some employees like their work and want to be with their friends on the job; they are eager to return to work. Some patients are "macho" and believe it is manly to work while being hurt, much like a football player plays while being hurt. Some workers just want to get out of the house and away from their spouse.

Other workers are overly concerned with their health and have unfounded, but real, fears about becoming reinjured. They wrongly equate minimal pain with permanent injury. Some are unrealistically unwilling to accept the slightest amount of pain, despite the fact that their work is no more physically stressful than getting dressed in the morning and engaging in the normal activities of life.

Finally, there are those workers who believe that they deserve a free ride because they were injured and those who simply want to cheat the system—the fakers. It is almost beyond belief the efforts some people make *not* to work. If their energies could be channeled into their job, they would be highly productive workers. Some workers will stay out of work without pay for over a year without any adverse condition, just so they can obtain a workers' compensation settlement. They believe that their cheating and lying is justified because they were hurt and deserve money.

A physician loses credibility and effectiveness if he does not understand that these different types of persons exist. The physician's care and opinions must take into account the individuality of the patient. For the "macho" worker, the physician must take care not to recommend injurious activities. The physician must carefully explain to the employee why he must remain out of work and why, when he returns, he will need light duty restrictions for a short time. The key is to emphasize that if he tries too much too early, he may reinjure himself and become permanently disabled.

For the hypochondriac (and most of us have a degree of this at one time or another), the physician must explain to the worker why it is safe for him to return to work and how the activity of work is actually a form of therapy that will help the recovery. The physician should explain how the light-duty restrictions will protect the worker and that minimal pain should be tolerated.

For the faker, the physician should inform the employer of this fact and release the employee to return to work. Of course, the physician should be sure of his opinion, but this is often easy enough to verify by observing the patient and questioning persons in contact with the patient. The physician should not avoid the issue by simply referring the patient to another doctor or a pain clinic.

In working with employers, the most critical step is for the physician to recognize the nature of the employee and explain this to the employer. Most employers do not want to treat their employees unfairly. Rather, they want to do the right thing. However, many physicians believe whatever their patients say and do whatever the patient wants, which has caused many employers to lose faith in the credibility of physicians.

A physician should not simply hand out disability slips whenever a worker asks that his time be covered and still expect the respect of the employer. Yet, some physicians cover time out despite a lack of objective findings, and when the doctor did not even see the patient during the covered time period. Similarly, a physician should not excuse a worker from a job without knowing the actual physical demands of the job. Likewise, advice on work restrictions should be clear and realistic. Do not say a worker cannot bend; he has to bend to go to the bathroom. Rather, say excessive bending would be unwise, or better yet, quantify it, such as suggesting no more than five spine flexions per hour.

Employers understand rational and clear medical analysis. Yet, most doctor's are afraid to communicate with the employer, or they simply refuse to take the time to do so. This not only results in an unhappy employer, but it can reduce the effectiveness of the physician's care. In returning a worker to the job, the doctor must know what the job is, as well as what light-duty alternatives and work restrictions are practical. Communication with the employer is the key. Often the worker is a poor historian and communicator. A two-minute call to the employer can give the physician invaluable information and result in a satisfied employer.

If a physician engages in prudent medical care, and explains the reasons for his decisions to the patient and employer, all except the fakers will be happy. However, if a physician simply believes all subjective complaints of a patient, in the absence of any objective findings, then the employer will be unhappy and in the long run the physician will have done a disservice to his patient.

In returning a worker to work, the physician must also consider the Americans with Disabilities Act (ADA) requirements on the employer (see Chapter 52). In order to reduce workers' compensation costs and prevent injured workers from getting used to being at home but on the payroll (so-called "workers' compensation syndrome"), many employers reserve light-duty work for employees injured on the job. Other employers, often irrationally ignoring the economic effect of workers' compensation liability, refuse to take injured employees back if they have any work restrictions. Many employers will not accommodate work restrictions if they are for a personal injury or illness not covered by workers' compensation. The ADA has changed all of this.

The return to work of an injured worker used to be simple. The worker returned to his employer with a light-duty slip or work restrictions from his physician. The employer might refuse to take back any worker with such restrictions or might claim that there was no work within the work restrictions. There were no means for the employee to challenge the employer's decision. The ADA now requires much more. Firstly, the employee can challenge—in court—the employer's decision, even the physician's work restrictions. Secondly, the employer must make reasonable accommodations that will allow the employee to return to work despite his work restrictions. While the employer need not create light-duty jobs *per se*, the reasonable accommodations of part-time or modified work schedules, job-restructuring, and reassignment to vacant positions come close to being equivalent to such a light-duty mandate.

To assure compliance with the ADA, the following procedure is recommended. Physicians must provide substantial detail and quantification in their work restrictions. Full-page forms are available that quantify by-the-hour activities such as standing, walking, and sitting. When a worker brings in his work restrictions, the employer should send the worker to his manager/supervisor. The manager/supervisor should then compare the restrictions to the worker's written job description and circle those aspects of the job that prevent the worker from performing. The manager/supervisor should then send the circled job description to the physician and ask him to: (1) confirm that the manager/supervisor's interpretation of the work restrictions is correct and that the doctor thus agrees the worker cannot safely perform the circled duties; and (2) ask the physician to confirm that his work restrictions are based on the ADA safety standard—designed only to preclude probable injuries, not merely possible minor injuries.

The physician should confirm that the correct standard was used, and the employer should confirm that any of the circled precluded tasks are essential functions of the job. The manager/supervisor (or the personnel, safety, or medical department) must then consider reasonable accommodations that would allow the worker to perform the essential functions of the job (for a discussion of the concept of "essential functions," see Chapter 50). Only when the employer determines how few tasks the worker cannot perform can that evaluation be made.

For example, a common work restriction is "no bending." If a supervisor applied the restriction literally, he would disqualify a worker who had to bend once a day to pick up a pencil. Subsequently, if the case went to trial, and the physician took the witness stand, he would in all likelihood testify that he really meant no excessive bending; or no bending with the back, and that bending with the knees is fine; or no bending and lifting heavy objects. It is best to clarify this before the employer spends $50,000 in legal fees preparing for trial.

The next step, which most companies have never considered, is reasonable accommodations. Someone must evaluate them, even though that task does not fall neatly into the framework of the traditional management departments—personnel, safety, medical, or production. Continuing with the example of the "no bending" restriction, possible reasonable accommodations might include: (1) purchasing a crane to lift objects; (2) having an assistant put an object on the workbench; (3) reassigning the lifting to another worker (if it is a nonessential function); or (4) buying a back support so that the worker can safely bend. All these options must be considered and discussed with the worker. It is wise, of course, to document all such efforts to consider and make reasonable accommodations.

## OCCUPATIONAL PHYSICIANS AND NURSES STATUS: CO-EMPLOYEE IMMUNITY AND THE PHYSICIAN-PATIENT RELATIONSHIP

Many medical providers are in-house nurses or doctors; they are employees of the injured worker's employer. Thus, the injured worker and the physician are co-employees. Under normal circumstances, an injured worker's exclusive remedy against the employer and its agents and employees (i.e., co-workers) is the workers' compensation remedy. Neither the employer nor co-workers can be sued for negligence; thus, being an employee may reduce the medical provider's risk of a lawsuit by co-worker employees.

This general rule has normally been applied to company doctors and nurses who are true employees of the employer of the injured worker. Thus, even if the company physician-employee errs in treating the injured worker, the worker cannot sue the physician for malpractice. Rather, the sole remedy is workers' compensation benefits. Company physicians should not, however, blindly assume that this general rule applies to them. At least four states currently recognize exceptions to this rule, and instituting these exceptions appears to be a trend.

Both California and Georgia courts recognize the dual capacity doctrine. Under this doctrine, the company physician-employee is said to have two separate capacities: (1) as a company employee (i.e., co-workers of the injured worker) and (2) as the injured workers' physician. In this second capacity, the injured worker may sue the company physician if he commits malpractice.

At least two other jurisdictions have used a combination of the dual capacity doctrine and semantics to hold company physician-employees liable for malpractice. Both Indiana and Louisiana have held that a physician, in terms of malpractice liability, is always an independent contractor (as opposed to an employee) because a corporation cannot practice medicine and thus direct the work of the physician. As an independent contractor, the physician cannot benefit from workers' compensation exclusivity.

The dual-capacity independent contractor doctrines highlight one of the potential pitfalls that exist in all jurisdictions: even in those jurisdictions that apply the co-worker immunity to company physician employees, the company physician must be a true employee of the corporation. For example, the mere fact that the patient was referred to the physician, or that the company requested an opinion from the physician, does not make the physician a company employee. Rather, the physician would be merely an independent contractor, and thus still liable for any malpractice. To be an employee, withholding taxes, Social Security taxes, and similar employee status actions would have to have been applied to the physician. On the other hand, at least one court has held that the mere fact that the company physician is a part-time employee does not mean the co-worker immunity is inapplicable.

Similarly, the company physician may be able to argue that, although not an employee of the employer, he was its agent, and, as such, the workers' compensation exclusivity bar applies. The question then becomes whether the physician was a mere agent of the employer, or whether the actions were taken independently of the employer, and in the status as a physician.

There is, however, one exception to the workers' compensation exclusivity bar that must be recognized because it applies to everyone. Workers' compensation is a replacement system for negligence lawsuits. It is not designed to replace liability for intentional torts. Thus, the exclusivity bar does not prevent an action for an intentional tort. The classic example is an employee who, dissatisfied with a recent raise, strikes the foreman. The employee's assault is an intentional tort, and thus the foreman can sue the employee. Moreover, for intentional torts, the victim can recover punitive damages as well as compensatory damages. Of concern to physicians, libel and slander is an intentional tort.

In addition, willful and wanton disregard for safety concerns is also considered, in some jurisdictions, to be an intentional tort. Thus, employers have been held liable, outside the workers' compensation system, for ignoring unsafe levels of airborne lead particles and fraudulently concealing the hazards of asbestos, as well as for intentionally concealing the fact that the worker had asbestosis and that further exposure was harmful. Although in most cases the employer is the target of the lawsuit, a company physician who has aided in defrauding the workers can be and has been named as a defendant.

Even if the physician does not benefit from the co-worker workers' compensation exclusivity bar, it is possible to escape liability if there is no physician/patient relationship. For example, some courts have held that when a physician performs a pre-employment physical for an employer and gives no report or advice to the worker, there is no physician/patient relationship with the worker, and thus the worker cannot sue the physician for malpractice. That is, if there is no physician/patient relationship, the physician owes no duty to the worker, and the worker has no reasonable expectations of the physician. Of course, the physician's actions may create other causes of action, such as for libel and slander or negligent interference with a contract (between the employer and the worker).

Occupational physicians thus need to be aware of the applicable legal doctrines in their state, and must then define clearly their relationship with the patient and the employer: (1) Is the physician an employee of the employer or an independent contractor? (2) Is the physician the employer's agent or the patient's treating physician? (3) What, if any, other duties does the physician owe the employee?

## CONCLUSION

If a physician understands the legal issues at stake, and his role in resolving them, he will be much more effective in providing his opinion, and significantly reduce his exposure to potential liability.

# CHAPTER 9

# THE PHYSICIAN AS A WITNESS

*Kenneth M. Willner*

With the passage of the Americans with Disabilities Act (ADA), physicians find themselves in ever greater demand as expert witnesses, as disability discrimination cases are added to the already burgeoning medical malpractice, workers' compensation, and Social Security disability caseloads. Inexorably, more and more physicians will be drawn into the litigation arena. Many will find that their practice and training have not prepared them for this as well as they would like. This chapter discusses the issues that arise in litigation, as they affect testifying physicians, and will outline some concomitants of testimony. In addition, this chapter addresses some points of particular relevance to expert-witness testimony in disability discrimination litigation.

## WHAT IS A MEDICAL EXPERT WITNESS?

An expert witness is a person who, by virtue of specialized knowledge or skill, can assist the judge or jury in evaluating the evidence or determining a fact in issue. This broad definition applies not only to the obvious candidates, such as physicians and scientists, but also to any person with specialized skills, such as a real estate agent or banker testifying about land values.[1,2] A medical expert witness assists with the medical and physiological issues raised in a case. An expert can testify about scientific or technical principles, as well as the application of those principles to the facts of the case—even when the expert has no firsthand knowledge of the facts.[3] Indeed, physicians ordinarily will not be called upon to testify about facts from their own personal knowledge (unless the expert also happens to be the treating physician or is permitted by the court to examine the patient); instead, the physician will be asked to form opinions as to the patient's medical condition based on the observations of others as recorded in medical records. In this respect, an expert's testimony differs markedly from so-called lay (non-expert) witness testimony. Lay witnesses are restricted to their own observations and the inferences that are rationally based on them.[4]

Physicians may base their conclusions on any type of facts or data that physicians reasonably rely upon, even if the facts or data would not ordinarily be admissible in court (e.g. because of the hearsay rule, see Chapter 8). For this reason, attorneys often ask their experts to "rely on" and testify about extraneous documents that the litigant has been unable to get into evidence with a lay witness.[5] While this tactic can assist the attorney with the litigation, it can lead to a difficult cross-examination of the expert, who will have to testify as to some credible reason why the extraneous matter supports his or her conclusions and why it is of the variety that physicians ordinarily rely on.

The question of what kind of evidence an expert can reasonably rely on was very recently muddied in 1993 in a Supreme Court decision that, ironically, was intended to clarify the issue, *Daubert v. Merrell Dow Pharmaceuticals, Inc.*[6] Following 80 years of application of one (fairly ambiguous) standard, the Court has now replaced it with another, even more ambiguous, one. Under the old standard, drawn from *Frye v. United States*,[7] courts admitted only expert testimony based on "generally-accepted" scientific principles. The Court discarded this standard in *Daubert*, decreeing instead that expert testimony in federal courts need only "be supported by appropriate validation—that is, 'good grounds' based on what is known."[8]

Some have worried that this standard will open the floodgates for the admission of so-called "junk" science, mere fancy masquerading as scientific principle. Not to worry, the Supreme Court assures us, federal judges will sit as "gatekeepers" to assure that "the reasoning or methodology underlying the testimony is scientifically valid and . . . that reasoning or methodology properly can be applied to the facts in issue."[9]

It remains to be seen whether the judiciary will be able to effectively screen out "unreliable" science. In any event, the decision as to what medical or scientific evidence is reliable is no longer strictly in the hands of the medical or scientific community—a judge is free to admit so-called expert opinions based on theories that have not been generally accepted if the judge is satisfied that the opinions rest on "good grounds." If a judge admits such questionable evidence, it will fall to the opposing expert to point out to the jury the flaws in these arguments and supporting evidence.

## LITIGATION PROCEDURES

From a lawyer's perspective there are two kinds of expert witnesses: (1) testifying experts, who will present their conclusions to the judge or jury, and (2) consulting experts, who will render confidential assistance to counsel behind the scenes. Some cynical types would say that these categories truly break down as follows: A testifying expert is a person who has reached a conclusion that supports the result desired by counsel; a consulting expert is a person who has reached the contrary conclusion. Those who subscribe to this cynicism seriously underestimate the value that an expert can provide to a case, even without testifying. A consulting expert can provide counsel with invaluable insights into the issues in a case and how to address them in the litigation. Such an expert should view his or her role as two-fold: helping counsel to understand the medical issues, and educating counsel as to what additional information is needed and where to find it so that the attorney and the testifying expert may evaluate those issues fully.

A medical expert's role in litigation will often start with an informal consultation with the lawyer. The lawyer will want to know about the physician's education, board certification, residencies, internships, fellowships, and practice, and about his or her prior experience as a witness. Typically, the lawyer will explain the circumstances of the case to the physician in the form of a hypothetical situation, and then try to get a feel for the methodology the physician would use to address the questions at issue, and for how articulate the doctor would be in a trial. The attorney is interested in four things: (1) the expert will reach a favorable conclusion, (2) the basis of the conclusion will be valid, (3) the expert will be able to explain the findings to the judge and jury in an authoritative, articulate and persuasive manner, and (4) the expert is backed up by credentials that will impress the judge or jury.

If this preliminary screening goes well, the attorney will send the expert the materials the lawyer thinks the physician needs to reach his or her conclu-

sions. An attorney, of course, is not a medical expert, and a physician should not assume that the lawyer knows what the expert needs. It is imperative therefore for the physician to explain to the lawyer what information is needed, and to question counsel in detail about what information counsel has and what further information can be obtained from other sources. Needless to say, it can be quite embarrassing for a witness to have new information handed to him or her during cross-examination, and then to have to explain why he or she did not consider it in reaching conclusions.

After analyzing the evidence, the expert should draft a written report. Indeed, the new amendments to the Federal Rules of Civil Procedure now require written reports.[10] In writing the report, the physician should keep in mind that the report is really a trial exhibit. It should clearly state the expert's conclusions[11] and their bases in a way that is both authoritative and understandable to the average juror. If the report is lengthy, it should begin with an executive summary because it is a fact of life that the reader may not make it all the way through the report.

In writing a report, the physician should not keep drafts. If kept, drafts will be obtained by the adversary's expert,[12] and every phrase or conclusion that the expert later thought better of will be fodder for cross-examination.

After the report, the next litigation step is a deposition, a lengthy session in which opposing counsel will ask the expert confusing questions while arguing with the other lawyers. The opposing counsel will question the expert in depth about his conclusions and the basis for them. In addition to trying to gain an understanding of the expert's position, opposing counsel will try to get the expert to make admissions that will undercut the expert's opinions or support the opposing expert's conclusions. The expert should beware of "summary questions," which often inaccurately summarize testimony and are designed to reduce complicated or subtle issues into simplistic one-sentence "sound bites" that can be used effectively in cross-examination at trial. These questions often start with: "It is your testimony that . . . " or "It would be fair to say that . . . " or "In summary, the basis of your opinions is . . . "

Opposing counsel will often try to get a witness to retreat from his or her conclusions by hammering away at any weakness or simply by asking the same question over and over again until the witness gives a different answer. *Stick to your guns!* If the attorney asks the same question more than once (and the expert answered it fairly the first time), it tells the expert that the first answer was harmful to the other side's case, and the attorney wants the expert to change it. The expert should not change his or her conclusions just because the opposition does not like them!

It is important to remember that the goal of a deposition is to avoid damaging admissions; it is not to win the case then and there. The case will be won at trial on the basis of trial testimony or on a summary judgment based on affidavits. At the deposition, an expert should be conservative and thoughtful. There is no need to "go out on a limb" at that point. The opposing counsel will have weeks, if not months, before the trial to investigate ways to cut off any limb the expert climbs onto.

Perhaps the most important part of a deposition takes place before the testimony starts: preparation. The expert should know the material inside and out, and should know the opposing expert's theories just as well. The expert should be prepared to explain both the strengths of his or her own case and the flaws in the opposition's. Counsel should take the time to explain the likely lines of questioning and to point out the opposition's theories of the case. A deposition lacking in surprises is one also lacking in damaging admissions.

Last, and most important, is the trial. This is when the case is truly won or lost. This is the time for home-run hitting by the expert. Trial testimony should exude confidence and authority. It should emphasize not only the expert's conclusions but also the rationale underlying them. It is the explanation that will ultimately persuade the judge or jury that one expert's conclusions are more likely to be correct than another's.

Effective trial testimony calls for extensive preparation. Do not be shy about rehearsing the direct examination with counsel—or with family members or any willing listener. Trial testimony should be as simple as possible, and always geared for the level of the judge or jury. The expert's audience is the judge or jury. Always direct testimony to them, not counsel. At the trial, the expert should repeat his or her conclusions and rationale often, especially at the very beginning and end of the examination, when the factfinder's attention and retention are most likely.

## TYPICAL ISSUES IN DISABILITY DISCRIMINATION CASES

While a physician's testimony in a disability discrimination case has much in common with other types of cases, the new disability discrimination law will also raise new and difficult issues. The medical issues in these types of cases break down roughly into two broad categories: (1) What is the plaintiff's medical condition? and (2) How do the plaintiff's physical limitations affect his or her ability to perform essential job duties?

### The Plaintiff's Condition

While it would seem that an attorney would have little to add in a discussion of how a physician should evaluate a person's physical condition, one point bears raising. A physician witness should be careful to limit testimony to his or her own area of expertise. Surprisingly, some physicians are willing to assume the role of a specialist in litigation even though they would not hesitate to refer the same question to a true specialist in circumstances of patient care.

In one case, for instance, the question before the court was whether an amputation prevented an applicant for an airline pilot job from flying with an acceptable degree of safety. The plaintiff's attorney retained an aviation-medicine specialist who did not consult with a physical medicine specialist regarding the amputation. Even though the plaintiff's physician had not examined or evaluated a patient with a similar amputation for many years and had never seen such a patient attempt to pilot an aircraft, he went on to examine the plaintiff's amputation, evaluate his adaptation to a prosthesis, and testify about the effect of the amputation on the plaintiff's ability to fly.

This situation provided ample material for cross-examination in which the defense demonstrated that the physician lacked the expertise to testify about the essential aspects of the plaintiff's condition and abilities.

In contrast, the defendant's attorney also retained an aviation-medicine (and occupational-medicine) specialist, who then referred the plaintiff to a physiatrist for an examination and report. The physiatrist, who did not testify, is a good example of a consulting expert who played an important litigation role. The aviation-medicine expert further consulted with airline industry experts about the physical demands of the job as they specifically relate to the amputated limb. Thus armed with the input from appropriate specialists, the defendant's aviation-medicine expert was able to articulate the specific reasons why the amputee posed an unacceptable risk to the safety of airline passengers. In contrast, the plaintiff's expert was discredited, because he testified about matters outside of his expertise.

### Application of Physical Limits to the Patient's Job

In the same example, the plaintiff's physician also fell into the trap of testifying unaided about the plaintiff's "ability" to perform complex job duties. While a physician can testify, on the basis of an examination or records, about the physical limits imposed by an impairment (such as reduced range of motion, strength, or coordination), the question of ability generally is not wholly medical. It requires, for example, an evaluation of skill and experience, and thus input from other occupational experts. The apocryphal story of the piano-playing patient is illustrative: after a physician removes the cast from the patient's now-healed broken hand, the patient asks whether he will be able to play the piano. The doctor replies that he will, and the patient responds: "That's GREAT; I never could before I broke my hand."

The plaintiff's expert testified that the plaintiff was "able" to fly safely. However, he was unaware of and did not consider (nor was he qualified to evaluate) important nonmedical evidence, such as the plaintiff's history of flying accidents. Nor could he withstand cross-examination about his qualifications for or experience with evaluating flying skill and "ability." A physician in this position should either limit testimony to a medical evaluation of the plaintiff's condition or consult with other experts to learn about the demands of the plaintiff's job and to seek an evaluation of the plaintiff's necessary skills, before testifying about "ability." A physician should consider the same issues when responding to questions about whether a person's impairment can be accommodated and whether a specified accommodation is sufficient to permit the person to perform essential job duties. These questions require input from occupational experts, not only physicians (see Chapters 46 to 51).

A similar issue arises with respect to whether a person meets the ADA definition of a person with a disability (see Appendix A and Chapter 50). A person is disabled under the statue if they have a mental or physiological disorder that substantially limits one or more major life activities.[13] Major life activities are the basic activities that the average person can perform with little or no difficulty, "such as caring for oneself, performing manual tasks, walking, seeing, hearing, speaking, breathing, learning, and working. A person is substantially limited in these activities if he or she is unable to perform, or is "significantly restricted as to the condition, manner or duration" of performing, one or more of them, taking into account the nature, severity and duration of the impairment. A person is substantially limited in the major life activity of working only if the person's condition significantly restricts him or her from performing a broad class of jobs; the inability to perform a particular job, even if it is the one chosen by the person, does not constitute a disability."[14] In testifying about this issue, the physician can address the limits imposed by a plaintiff's medical condition, but must be careful in testifying about the impact of those limits on major life activities. More than one expert has been embarrassed on cross-examination by videotapes, movies, or other records of a plaintiff performing activities the expert said the plaintiff could not do.

Another related issue facing medical experts in disability discrimination cases arises from the ADA defense that employers need not employ a person if, as a result of a impairment, the person poses a "direct threat" to the health or safety of the individual or others in the workplace.[15] The ADA regulations expressly require an employer to assess the individual's ability to perform essential job functions safely, based on "a reasonable *medical* judgment that relies on the most current medical knowledge and/or on the best available objective evidence."[16] Thus, medical expert testimony on this subject is very important to support such a defense.

However, the regulations miss the point that in many cases "ability" and "safety" are not exclusively medical determinations. Often, as described above, input from other occupational experts will be required to evaluate ability. In other cases, where the job requirements and conditions are not in dispute, a physician may testify unaided about medical risks. For example, medical testimony alone should suffice in a case involving the risk of hypoglycemia, heart attack, or seizure experienced by a driver with diabetes, heart disease, or epilepsy, or by a person with a back condition who must lift heavy weights. Of course, the question of whether the risk of harm, once established, is unacceptably high is really a public policy decision, not a medical one.

These issues will, no doubt, keep physicians employed as expert witnesses for years to come.

## References

1. Federal Rule of Evidence 702, Note of Advisory Committee.
2. Federal Rule of Evidence 702.
3. Federal Rule of Evidence 702, Note of Advisory Committee.
4. Federal Rule of Evidence 701.
5. Federal Rule of Evidence 703.
6. __ U.S. __ , 113 S.Ct. 2786 (1993).
7. 293 F. 1013, 1014 (D.C. Cir. 1923).
8. __ U.S. at __ , 113 S.Ct. at 2798-9.
9. Black B, Singer JA: *From Frye to Daubert: a new test for scientific evidence,* 1 Shepard's Expert and Scientific Evidence Quarterly at 25 (citing *Daubert,* __ U.S. at __ , 113 S.Ct. 2786 (1993)).
10. Federal Rule of Civil Procedure 26(a) (2) (effective December 1, 1993).

11. In prior years, experts were required to present their conclusions in the form of "opinions." While this is still the predominant practice, it is no longer required (Federal Rule of Evidence 702, Note of Advisory Committee.)

12. *See In re Air Crash Disaster at Stapleton Int'l Airport,* 720 F. Supp. 1442, 1444 (D. Colo. 1988) ("all materials possessed by an expert in relation to a case in which he is expected to testify are discoverable").

13. 29 C.F.R. §1630.2 (g) (1).

14. *Id.* at §1630.2(i).

15. 29 C.F.R. §1630.15(b) (2).

16. *Id.* at §1630.2(r) (emphasis added).

# CHAPTER 10

# CONTRASTING THE STANDARD MEDICAL EXAMINATION AND THE DISABILITY EXAMINATION

*Stephen L. Demeter*

Most physicians approach impairment ratings and disability evaluations (DEs) by extrapolating from the knowledge and experience gained in their own specialty. Impairment ratings and disability examinations are emerging, if not as a specialty in their own right, then as a field requiring specialized knowledge and skills. This chapter explores the fundamental differences between the standard medical examination (ME) that a practitioner performs in his or her own specialty area and the disability examination (DE) required in that field.

## SIMILARITIES

See the box on this page for similarities between a disability evaluation and a standard medical examination/practice.

## History

The history is the single most important facet of every patient encounter. It has been stated that 90% of all diagnoses are based on the history alone. For the ME, physical examinations and laboratory tests rarely change the initial impressions and are used primarily to confirm and quantitate diagnostic abnormalities. This is also true for a DE, although to a lesser degree because the diagnosis of a problem is not really the goal in a DE as it is in the standard ME. A physician often assumes the role of a detective in the standard ME. In the DE the physician works to obtain an impairment rating wherein the diagnosis is often known, and proceeds to evaluate the functional impact of the impairment. Thus the history takes on the role of documenting an injury or quantitating the effects on a person's life-style or capabilities.

Depending on the type of examination performed and the expected treatment recommendation, some MEs also focus on documentation and quantitation (for example, is surgery needed for a patient with spinal stenosis?) and some DEs are oriented toward arriving at a proper diagnosis (does a person exposed to potentially toxic fumes have a resultant asthma or is hyperventilation syndrome the cause for the shortness of breath?), relating it to the patient's ability to do work (should the person be considered unable to perform this particular task?). In general the history either assists in diagnosis or provides documentation and quantitation.

## Physical Examination

A sound and skillful physical examination is a necessary component of both the ME and the DE. As with the history, the evidence obtained with a physical examination supports or denies a diagnosis, documents abnormalities, and quantitates pathological changes. In the DE, however, the next step, that of evaluating the impact of an impairment, is the focus. In addition, for a DE, certain examinations may be limited to conform to a particular rating system (see later discussion).

---

### SIMILARITIES BETWEEN A DISABILITY EVALUATION AND A STANDARD MEDICAL EXAMINATION/PRACTICE

1. Gather the patient's history.
2. Perform a physical examination.
3. Order appropriate laboratory tests.
4. Apply the information obtained in steps 1 to 3.
5. Report the information from steps 1 to 3.
6. Act ethically.
7. Establish a practice.

## Laboratory Testing

As with the history and physical examination, laboratory tests assist in making a diagnosis, documenting a problem, or quantitating an abnormality. During a DE the types of tests ordered and performed may differ from those used in an ME, according to the rating system used.

## Applying Information

Regardless of the emphasis, knowledge is obtained about the individual's abnormalities and limitations, and the expected future of that individual vis-a-vis those abnormalities and limitations. The critical difference between the DE and the ME lies in the application of that knowledge, not its acquisition.

## Reporting Information

Once knowledge is derived, a report is prepared to summarize the knowledge and finalize the conclusion. In the standard ME these conclusions may be mental, verbal, or written down in a listing of diagnostic conclusions or therapeutic recommendations; alternately, a written report may be prepared. The DE uses the written report exclusively.

## Ethical Considerations

The earliest and best-known standard of medical ethics is found in the Hippocratic Oath. Physicians are expected to act compassionately and always in the best interest of their patients; to be honest and sincere; and to be knowledgeable about their particular field and its limitations, willing to refer patients to other physicians when their limitations are exceeded. Just as a physician is morally bankrupt if he or she intentionally falsifies diagnoses or makes recommendations for inappropriate treatment, so too is the physician who provides a biased report which overestimates or underestimates an impairment rating in his or her role as a plaintiff's or defense physician when performing a DE. The end result of a DE is usually a monetary award for the examinee rather than an operative or therapeutic intervention, but the requirement to be honest applies as much in a DE as in an ME. An inequitable monetary outcome from a purposely biased DE may affect a person as profoundly as any false diagnosis made in an ME and should be equally condemned.

## Establishment of a Practice

Physicians accept compensation for applying their knowledge and skills in patient care. Toward this end, practices are established. Many physicians supplement their medical practice by performing DEs, and some physicians specialize in this area. Semi-retired physicians, especially those formerly involved in fields where the cost of malpractice insurance is high, are particularly drawn to this area.

## DIFFERENCES

In addition to the subtle changes in the emphasis in an otherwise similar situation, true differences between MEs and DEs exist and are detailed here. See the box below.

## Goals

As noted earlier, although both the DE and the ME start with a history, physical examination, and laboratory testing to arrive at a diagnosis and/or assessment, the ME has the goal of formulating a therapeutic recommendation, whereas the DE moves toward an impairment rating and an evaluation of the functional impact that results. Occasionally the physician performing a DE will be asked to comment on the effects of treatment, provide an assessment of permanency, or make recommendations regarding future treatment (medical or surgical) or the effects of reha-

---

### DIFFERENCES BETWEEN A DISABILITY EVALUATION AND A STANDARD MEDICAL EXAMINATION/PRACTICE

1. Goals
2. Opportunities for examination
3. Treatment recommendations
4. Work history
5. Rating system requirements
6. End results
7. Peripheral issues
8. Reliance on nonmedical personnel
9. Specific issues addressed
10. Extrapolation regarding causation
11. Legal responsibilities and malpractice coverage
12. Source of referrals

bilitation. However, none of these elements are the same as the recommendations regarding therapeutic approaches or treatments formulated by the treating physician. The treating physician takes an *active* role with regard to the recommended treatment and *actively* reassesses the results of treatment and then further recommends either continuation or alteration in the treatment plan. The physician doing a DE merely extrapolates from the knowledge acquired through the examination to predict future outcomes, a *passive* role. Thus, once information is acquired, there is a wide divergence regarding its application, with the physician assuming an active role in the ME and a passive one in the DE.

## Opportunity for Examination

An ME is rarely limited to a single examination, whereas this is normal for the DE. This important difference creates a situation where the disability examiner must, by necessity, be more thorough than a medical examiner, who will generally have further opportunities to ask the patient questions that were missed, overlooked, or underemphasized while taking the initial history, to perform additional elements of the physical examination, or to obtain additional laboratory tests. The disability evaluator must rely on the expectations of the requesting party to address adequately concerns over the adequacy, completeness, or comprehensiveness of the examination. For example, in performing "entry-level" evaluations for the Bureau of Worker's Compensation, the examination is completed within 15 to 20 minutes and addresses only a single issue. In contrast, examinations providing the basis for testimony in cases expected to go to trial can take as long as 3 or 4 hours for the history and physical examination alone. Clearly, performing an in-depth examination is appropriate for the latter situation but would be inappropriate for the former. A good rule to remember when performing DEs is *to do what is expected*, which requires a preknowledge of the depth necessary for completing a competent examination as determined by the requesting party. This should be clarified with the requesting party before the examination is performed.

## Treatment Recommendations

As already discussed, the major difference between the standard ME and the DE is whether the physician adopts an active or a passive role in relation to the examinees' medical problems, a crucial legal difference. Any recommendations given by the physician to the examinee regarding the findings derived from the DE can be considered as "treatment" and should

be avoided. No prescriptions are given. These issues are more completely developed in Chapter 8. The reader may wish to read this chapter thoroughly and/or consult an attorney or malpractice carrier.

## Work History

Work histories are important in an ME, particularly in attempting to establish a causation for a particular problem or illness. However, they assume a more important and vital role in the DE. Except for very brief DEs, the examinees should list all jobs that they have ever held (starting with babysitting or delivering papers as a teenager). The examinee can prepare this part of the history before the examination or after checking in with the receptionist. This list is reviewed with the examinee to clarify dates, job titles and/or descriptions, and exposures and/or injuries. This information is crucial in correlating an impairment rating with the future employment evaluation, which constitutes the DE.

## Rating System Requirements

In addition to establishing the expectations of the referring source, it is vital that the physician be aware of which rating system will be used. The various systems have varying rules about specific elements in the history or physical examination. Of greater importance, however, are the restrictions placed on the laboratory tests that are accepted, acceptable, and paid for. Additionally, mandatory prerequisites are often set before some tests are performed.

### Illustrations of ratings systems

An individual comes to you for a pulmonary impairment rating and a DE. If the individual is being tested for the Social Security System, the name of the manufacturer of the spirometer and the model number must be included in the report (see Chapter 27). The paper speed, height of the graphs, and conditions of the test are all clearly stated in the *Social Security Handbook*.[1] The following points are noted:

1. A volume-time curve is recommended even though this is an outdated test. When a flow-volume loop is used to measure the forced vital capacity and the forced expiratory volume ($FEV_1$), volume calibrations at 30, 60, and 180 L/min must be performed and included in the report. (These regulations represent an improvement in the testing protocol because flow-volume loops were considered totally invalid tests as recently as the previous, 1992, edition of the listings.[2])

2. If the examinee is wheezing or if the airflow rates are low, a spirometric test is acceptable only after

a bronchodilator has been given. To use prebronchodilator data is unacceptable when determining impairment.

The American Medical Association *Guides* allow the use of only those machines approved by the American Thoracic Society, but flow-volume loops are acceptable. Postbronchodilator results are also only used under circumstances similar to those found in the Social Security System.[3] However, the third edition (revised) of the AMA *Guides* states that "an individual should be evaluated after he or she has received optimum therapy or is in optimum health,"[4] while the fourth edition states, "a patient may decline treatment with a surgical procedure, a pharmacological agent, or other therapeutic approach. The view of the *Guides* contributors is that if a patient declines therapy for a permanent impairment, that decision should neither decrease nor increase the estimated percentage of the patient's impairment."[4] This issue was not addressed in the 1992 Social Security System *Listings,* but the 1994 edition states that the spirometric values to be used exist "during the individual's most stable state of health."[1] Thus a person who just finished smoking a pack of cigarettes or who refuses to take prescribed bronchodilators could be evaluated under the fourth edition of the AMA *Guides* and the 1992 Social Security *Listings,* but not under third edition of the AMA *Guides* and only under the 1994 Social Security *Listings* if this represents that person's stable state of health (as long as the spirometric rules were followed regarding bronchodilator administration).

Arterial blood gas levels can be valuable measures of pulmonary impairment. They represent a crucial component of an examination performed under the Black Lung Law, are deemed usually unnecessary under the AMA *Guides,* and are performed only "in a clinically stable condition on at least two occasions, three or more weeks apart within a 6 month period"[1] under the Social Security System. Furthermore, the $PaO_2$ is stratified according to the $CO_2$ content, altitude of the testing facility, and presence or absence of obesity in the examinee under the Social Security *Listings,* by the $PaCO_2$ only in the Black Lung Regulations, and by none of these measures in the AMA *Guides.*[3]

In assessing impairment resulting from coronary artery disease, the Social Security System will only pay for the ECG or a thallium stress test, although it will accept the results of a coronary angiogram if independently obtained. Very specific requirements are found with regard to treadmill speed, the ECG strips, and interpretations. The AMA *Guides* are less strict on technical details.

Thus, the physician must be aware of the proscriptions, limitations, and requirements of the various components of the history, physical examination, and laboratory tests based on the rating system used for each DE. Lack of awareness can create improper and insupportable results.

## End Results

The end result of a DE is a rating that expresses the impact of the patient's impairment on the person's life. In an ME, the diagnosis serves as the springboard to therapeutic recommendations. It must again be emphasized that the rating derived from a DE directly reflects the rating system used as determined by the requesting source. The types of examination used in deriving this rating are system-specific, as is the final result—the rating itself

## Peripheral Issues

There are circumstances where the requesting source will appreciate, request, or expect peripheral information. Examples include a detailed job description (especially the present job) and personal and demographic information concerning the examinee (place in family; information on parents or siblings, including medical problems, education, jobs, and home life; present family; prior families/marriages; economic information; prior occupation-related injuries or litigation; education and training; hobbies; travel; or physical status of the home). Knowledge of the expectations of the referring source as well as the nature of the DE helps in deciding how deeply to delve into these aspects.

## Reliance on Nonmedical Personnel

Disability is directed toward the concept of the ability to sustain remunerative employment. Impairment is a limitation caused by a medical problem. Therefore a truly comprehensive disability report may include evaluations performed by nonmedical personnel, such as industrial hygienists, occupational safety experts, environmental engineers, social workers, occupational rehabilitationists, physical rehabilitationists, vocational rehabilitationists, and accountants (see Chapters 46 to 49). Rarely will a physician need to include these contributions in an ME, although these circumstances arise occasionally and the physician should be aware of these professionals' contributions.

## Specific Issues Addressed

It must be remembered that the physician is requested to examine and report on one or more specific issues. These should be explored and documented to the depth appropriate to the request. Other issues, medical or otherwise, may be inappropriate for the final report.

## Extrapolation Regarding Causation

What does one do when examining an individual with a low-back problem when that problem (injury) represents only one of many similar problems? How does one determine an impairment rating for the second of four low-back injuries? How much of this impairment was caused by the situation in question? For example, how much of an individual's pulmonary problems was caused by his working in a coal mine and how much by his 2-pack-a-day cigarette smoking habit? These questions, obviously, separate a DE from an ME, where no such issues ever arise. There are no simple solutions to the dilemmas of causation involving multiple injuries or factors. Occasionally old records or laboratory tests help, but guesses can be the only answer—educated guesses based on all the knowledge, skill, and experience that physicians, specializing in certain areas, as well as in the area of disability examination, can offer. The resolutions to these requests involve honest, ethical, and educated estimates.

## Legal Responsibilities and Malpractice Coverage

As mentioned earlier, the disability evaluator must never cross the line and become a treating physician. Such an action places the physician into the legal and malpractice liability role that the treating physician assumes. Therefore a medical malpractice insurance policy may not be of value in a disability evaluating practice; a general policy or specific liability coverage may be more appropriate. These legal issues are beyond the scope of this chapter, and the physician should consult Chapter 8, a lawyer, or his or her malpractice carrier.

## Source of Referrals

A medical practice relies on patient, physician, or third-party referrals in order to maintain an adequate patient base. A disability examination practice has similar requirements, but the referral sources are generally different, including governmental agencies (Social Security Department, state Workers' Compensation boards, the Veterans Administration, or the Federal Aviation Agency, for example), insurance companies, and attorneys. As in a medical practice, referral sources are maintained by providing satisfactory work. However, the results of examinations must not be biased to satisfy the referring source. Vigilance and honesty are the only safeguards against such a bias.

## References
1. Social Security Administration: *Disability evaluation under Social Security,* 1994, U.S. Department of Health and Human Services.
2. Social Security Administration: *Disability evaluation under Social Security,* 1992, U.S. Department of Health and Human Services.
3. American Medical Association: *Guides to the evaluation of permanent impairment,* ed 4, Chicago, 1993, American Medical Association.
4. American Medical Association: *Guides to the evaluation of permanent impairment,* ed 3 (rev), Chicago, 1990, American Medical Association.
5. Department of Labor, Employment Standards Administration: *Standards for determining coal miners' total disability or death due to pneumoconiosis,* Fed Reg 1980 (February 29); 45:13678-13712.

# CHAPTER 11

# THE DISABILITY-ORIENTED MEDICAL EVALUATION AND REPORT

*George M. Smith*
*Stephen L. Demeter*
*Ronald J. Washington*

Just as there are major orientation differences between the medical examination and the disability evaluation, the reports generated by each procedure differ significantly in orientation. The guidelines offered in this chapter are comprehensive and may be used as a general background reference or as checklists, depending on the preferences and needs of the physician and the referral source.

The first principle in preparing a disability report focuses on communication with the referral source regarding the purpose of the evaluation, the expectations concerning the issues to be addressed, and the technical requirements of the disability system within which the evaluation will be conducted. The second principle focuses on reviewing the medical and nonmedical documents generated and defining the lifestyle of the examinee (both occupational and nonoccupational) within which questions about disability or employability have arisen. The box on page 74 provides a checklist of the specific steps to be taken in following these two principles.

In communicating with the referral source, the physician must clarify the objectives of the evaluation, the specific questions to address, and what expectations can reasonably be achieved. For example, while a physician may be able to determine that a particular examinee's medical condition could have been caused by an injury related to a particular set of circumstances, unless the physician has direct knowledge regarding the occurrence of those circumstances, it is impossible for that physician to affirm defensibly that the circumstances did indeed cause the medical condition. Moreover, unless the physician has full knowledge regarding an employer's willingness or unwillingness to accommodate an employee's functional limitations, the physician cannot defensibly affirm that the employee has a job-specific disability, assuming the alterations on the employer's part are the only inhibiting factor.

With adequate preparation, the content and process of the medical evaluation may be structured in terms related to the decision criteria, so that the kinds of medical information needed for that particular examination are provided.

## THE MEDICAL COMPONENT

The evaluating physician's primary medical task is to define thoroughly and accurately the examinee's current health status. First, the evaluating physician analyzes the medical information contained in the clinical records, which reflect past evaluations and treatments. The object is to determine whether there is a medical foundation on which to base the diagnosis and management of the examinee. To review, analyze, and appropriately comment on past and present medical history, the examining physician must have access to existing medical records, reports, and results of tests and diagnostic procedures dating from at least the onset of the medical condition for which the evaluation is being performed. Omission of these records renders the disability report incomplete and potentially places the acceptability of the conclusions in jeopardy. The disability report must be complete with records supplied by the treating physicians. Differences in clinical findings, especially any recent findings, must be addressed and properly accounted for.

If the information contained in the records is insufficient to justify a diagnosis or a medical management plan and additional clinical information must be acquired, the desired approach is to record all positive and pertinent negative findings through the medical history, the physical examination, and the tests and diagnostic procedures. The box on page 75 provides a checklist of the elements essential to a complete medical evaluation.

## STEPS IN PREPARING A DISABILITY-ORIENTED MEDICAL REPORT

I. Verify the purpose(s) of the evaluation with the requestor(s)
  A. Employability determination
    1. Postoffer, preplacement medical evaluation
    2. Approval of medically-based absence
    3. Medically-based job modification/accommodation of a "disability"
  B. Disability determination
    1. Workers' compensation
      a. Temporary or permanent
      b. Partial or total
    2. Short-term disability
    3. Long-term disability
    4. Personal injury
    5. Medical malpractice
    6. Social Security disability benefits
    7. Other federal program
  C. Verify the requirements of applicable law and regulations and/or the provisions of the disability insurance policy
    1. Definition of disability
    2. Report format/special forms, if any
    3. Requirements for special information
    4. Requirements for special certifications by the evaluating physician
II. Review disability and nonmedical records
  A. Workers' compensation records
    1. Accident/incident report
    2. Employer's first report of injury
    3. Employee's claim form
    4. Physician's first report
    5. Previous workers' compensation claim files

6. Medical records and reports, including reports of independent medical evaluation(s)
  B. Other disability insurance records
    1. Disability claim form
    2. Attending physician's statements
    3. Individual's supplemental statements
  C. Investigative reports
  D. Legal records
    1. Depositions
    2. Workers' compensation decisions
    3. Court decisions
  E. Personnel records
    1. Employment application
    2. Past and current job descriptions
    3. Performance appraisals
    4. Attendance records
    5. Employee relations records
      a. Counseling memos
      b. Written notices and warnings
      c. Termination notice
III. Review medical records
  A. Medical office records
  B. Hospital records
  C. Emergency room records
  D. Reports of medical specialty evaluations
  E. Reports of other disability evaluations
  F. Laboratory test results
  G. Results of diagnostic procedures
  H. Results of special tests
  I. Consultation reports
  J. Reports of independent medical evaluations

## CONTENT OF THE DISABILITY-ORIENTED MEDICAL EXAMINATION

I. Medical history based on a review of records and an interview with the examinee, noting
   A. Time and circumstances of onset
   B. Clinical findings on physical and/or mental status examination both initially and on successive evaluations
   C. Results of prior tests and diagnostic procedures
   D. Initial and follow-up treatment, analyzing types, responses, and changes
   E. Current symptoms with particular attention to recent recurrence or change

II. Examination
   A. Mental status examination
   B. Physical examination

III. Laboratory tests as medically warranted (and approved by the requestor)

IV. Special tests and diagnostic procedures as medically warranted (and approved by the requestor)

V. Medical specialty evaluation(s) as medically warranted (and approved by the requestor)

Once the history is established, the examining physician must ensure that the clinical examination addresses all the relevant clinical issues. Part Two of this book details the clinical evaluation of each body system. Careful attention to the information contained in the clinical chapters will maximize the evaluating physician's ability to achieve the objective of thoroughness in the medical aspects of the evaluation. Although the evaluating physician may be a medical specialist performing an evaluation that focuses on a particular body part, system, or function, the individual should always be considered as a whole.

## THE NONMEDICAL COMPONENT

In the clinical setting, an attending physician is usually called on to focus attention principally on medical technical issues. Only peripherally will he or she be involved in employability or disability matters, usually when asked to complete a work release/work restriction form, a report for a workers' compensation claim, a Social Security disability form, or an attending physician's report for a disability insurance company. However, the physician performing a disability evaluation is *expected* to address any and all medical technical issues that arise during the course of a medical evaluation, to fulfill the ultimate objectives of the disability-oriented medical evaluation, to protect the interests of all parties concerned with the outcome, and to understand and respond to the requirements and needs of the disability system through which the request for evaluation was made (see the box on pp. 76-77).

## THE REPORT

A properly-constructed report for a disability-oriented medical evaluation includes all of the elements of a comprehensive clinical evaluation report and addresses the needs of the disability system. When more than one disability system is involved, although the clinical content of the medical component of the report will not change, it may be appropriate for the evaluating physician to produce a separate report for each system. The box on pages 78-80 provides a comprehensive listing of elements in the report.

It should be noted that a reasoned analysis of the medical information in conjunction with appropriate nonmedical information is essential to determine whether the individual is employable or, within the framework of one or more disability systems, whether the individual meets the criteria for the award of disability benefits. Thus the report contains two major subdivisions: one documents and analyzes the medical findings of the evaluation (both past and present) and one analyzes the impact and consequences of the examinee's medical condition on life activities. Accepted standards of medical record-keeping mandate the inclusion of both positive findings and pertinent negative findings. Thus, in reviewing medical records, when particular information is not recorded, such as a report of neurologic findings in connection with an office visit for evaluation for low-back pain, the evaluating physician may justifiably conclude that the attending physician omitted the information because he or she did not conclude that the complaints were associated with a medical condition serious enough to warrant its consideration. Explaining the clinical meaning of such omissions may well strengthen the evaluating physician's conclusions regarding the severity of the individual's medical condition.

*Text continued on p. 80.*

# UNDERSTANDING AND RESPONDING TO THE NEEDS OF THE REFERRAL SOURCE

I. What functions does the medical advisor/consultant/evaluating physician perform for the referral source?
   A. *Professional/technical function*—Assess and explain the probative value of medical information
   B. *Clinical function*—Perform a disability-oriented medical evaluation when appropriate
   C. *Communications functions*—Analyze and explain, both orally and in writing, enough about medical issues and their relationship to nonmedical issues so that the referral source feels comfortable with the information and confident in making necessary decisions

II. What critical questions must the medical advisor/consultant/evaluating physician ask of the referral source?
   A. What are the issues of this case?
   B. What is the purpose of the evaluation?
   C. What are you asking me to do?
   D. What questions do you want me to answer?
   E. Will you ask me to help you prepare for and assist in depositions of the claimant's physicians?
   F. Is it likely that I will be deposed?
   G. Will there be a trial if the case is not resolved?
   H. If so, will there be a jury?
   I. Will you ask me to serve as a witness if there is a trial?
   J. If so, will I be a fact witness or an expert witness?

III. What critical question must the medical advisor/consultant/evaluating physician answer personally?
   A. Beyond the information requested, what information does the referral source need?

IV. What information does the evaluating physician need?
   A. Dates
      1. Date of birth
      2. Date of hire
      3. Date of the incident
      4. Onset of the medical condition
      5. Date of onset of (alleged) disability
      6. Date of the first medical examination
      7. Critical employment-related dates
   B. Definitions
      1. Workers' compensation/Insurance
         a. Medical condition
         b. Partial disability
         c. Total disability
         d. Residual disability
      2. *Federal*—Americans with Disabilities Act Accommodation: modification of a job or work situation that enables an individual to meet the same job demands and conditions of employment as any other individual in a similar job
      3. AMA *Guides to the Evaluation of Permanent Impairment*
         a. *Impairment*—loss of, loss of use of, or derangement of a body part, system, or function
         b. *Disability*—impact of the impairment on capacity to meet personal, social, or occupational demands or to meet statutory or regulatory requirements
      4. *Occupational disability*—a medical condition precludes travel to and from work, being at work, or assignment of appropriate tasks and duties while at work, with or without accommodation
   C. Clear statement of the burden of proof the claimant must meet
      1. Law
      2. Regulations
      3. Insurance policy contract

# UNDERSTANDING AND RESPONDING TO THE NEEDS OF THE REFERRAL SOURCE—cont'd

4. Employer's policy
5. Labor management agreement

D. *Relevant medical information from primary clinical source documents*—Documents containing information obtained or communicated for the purpose of documenting the medical history and clinical findings and for managing a patient's clinical care
   1. Emergency room records or other first encounter records
   2. Medical office records
   3. Hospital inpatient records
   4. Consultation reports
   5. Physical therapy/occupational therapy records
   6. Reports of the results of laboratory tests
   7. Reports of the results of diagnostic tests and procedures
   8. Any other documents related to medical management of the claimant

Note 1—Letters to addressees not involved in managing the clinical management of the claimant (e.g., claims examiners, lawyers, disability evaluating physician) are *not* medical source documents. They have the quality of testimonial statements only.

Note 2—Reports of independent medical evaluation(s) or disability evaluation(s) by a physician who is not a treating physician *are not* primary clinical source documents.

Note 3—Unless you are a treating physician, your report is *not* a primary medical source document.

E. Relevant information from nonmedical primary source documents

1. Injury report
2. Employer's first report
3. Physician's first report
4. Personnel records
   a. Employment application/employment history
   b. Performance appraisals
   c. Counseling memos/disciplinary actions
   d. Awards and commendations
   e. Dates of changes in employment situation
      (1) Promotion/demotion
      (2) Transfer
      (3) New supervisor
      (4) New work assignment
5. Legal documents
   a. Complaints
   b. Briefs
   c. Interrogatories
   d. Depositions
   e. Affidavits
6. Case-related correspondence

V. *When is a disability-oriented medical evaluation necessary?*—When the medical advisor/consultant/evaluating physician agrees to carry out a medical evaluation for a specific purpose

Note—If you perform an evaluation:

1. Verify the examinee's understanding of the purpose of the evaluation
2. Ensure that it is clinically complete with respect to the medical condition regardless of what is asked for

# CONTENT OF THE DISABILITY-ORIENTED MEDICAL EVALUATION REPORT

I. Introduction
   A. Identifying information
   B. Referral source
   C. Purpose of the evaluation
   D. For each disability system:
      1. Cite applicable law and/or regulations
      2. Cite the criteria for disability/employability
   E. Date of the initial evaluation and the dates of all follow-up visits
   F. List of all records, reports, x-rays, results of special tests and diagnostic procedures, laboratory test results, with source and date for each
II. Results of the clinical evaluation
   A. History of the medical condition(s)
      1. Method by which the history was obtained
      2. Identity of the history taker(s)
      3. Narrative description of the history, including reference to all positive and pertinent negative results:
         a. As extracted from the records and reports
         b. As obtained from the examinee
      4. Comments regarding agreement and discrepancies within and between the sources
   B. Findings from physical examination and mental status examination
      1. Positive and pertinent negative clinical findings
      2. Validation signs (as appropriate)
      3. Ability to dress and undress, get on and off the examining table
      4. For each body part, system, and function, report observations which are required under the criteria of the disability system of record
   C. Findings from laboratory tests and diagnostic procedures
   D. The results of medical specialty evaluations
III. Clinical impressions
IV. Assessment of current health status
   A. Explain the basis for a conclusion that the clinical information is or is not sufficient to assess the individual's current health status
   B. Explain whether each medical condition has become static or well-stabilized with reference to past records and current findings to support each conclusion
   C. If improvement or deterioration of any medical condition is expected, explain the basis for the conclusion, the expected course of the condition, and the time frame within which the improvement or deterioration is likely to take place
   D. Performance-related impact
      1. Activities for which performance capacity is called into question based on the medical condition
      2. Activities for which reconditioning would be necessary because of limited strength or endurance
   E. Risk-related impact
      1. Activities that would be likely to result in injury or harm to the examinee or aggravation of the medical condition
      2. The likelihood of sudden or subtle incapacitation
   F. Impact on employability, including whether the medical condition(s) precludes
      1. Travel to and from work
      2. Being at work
      3. Assignment of tasks and duties
   G. Impact on life activities
      1. Personal activities
         a. Self-care (personal hygiene, dressing, food preparation and eating, etc.)
         b. Personal business (maintaining a bank account, paying bills, entering into contracts such as leases, loans, or insurance)
      2. Social activities
      3. Leisure and recreational activities
V. Medical management plan
   A. Recommendations for further diagnostic testing
   B. Referral for medical specialty evaluation
   C. Periodic reevaluation of active treatment
   D. Rehabilitation/reconditioning

## CONTENT OF THE DISABILITY-ORIENTED MEDICAL EVALUATION REPORT—cont'd

E. Follow-up evaluation

VI. Synthesis of information

   A. Review and analyze documentation
      1. Note consistency of information from various health care providers
      2. Evaluate sufficiency of the information on which diagnoses and medical management plans are based
      3. If the examinee was employed, include
         a. Why examinee stopped working
         b. If still absent from work, why examinee has not returned
   B. Analyze the accumulated medical information
      1. Medical history
         a. Historical interview, clinical findings, treatment, and response
         b. Any conspicuous omissions of information
      2. Conclusions
         a. The examinee's medical condition has or has not become static or well-stabilized
         b. The examinee is or is not likely to suffer subtle or sudden incapacitation
         c. The examinee is or is not likely to suffer injury, harm, or aggravation of the medical condition by engaging in specific work-related and non–work-related activities
         d. Risk avoidance or therapeutic value is associated with restricting the individual from particular activities, both on and off the job
      3. Life situation factors
   C. Assess the medical and nonmedical information in relation to the following factors
      1. Likelihood that the circumstances could have caused or contributed to the onset or aggravation of the medical condition
      2. Consistency or inconsistency in records, reports, history, and previous clinical findings
      3. Validity of the diagnosis with respect to established medical diagnostic criteria
      4. Appropriateness of the treatment and medical management with respect to generally-accepted medical principles and practices
      5. Assessment of the degree to which the medical condition has or has not adversely affected the examinee's non–work-related life activities (driving, use of public transportation, shopping, self-care, leisure activities)
      6. Likelihood that the individual will suffer sudden or subtle incapacitation, noting
         a. How soon
         b. How sudden
         c. How severe
         d. The probable consequences in terms of injury or harm to the individual or others and aggravation of the medical condition
         e. The degree to which the medical condition has or has not become static or well-stabilized
      7. The need for further treatment and the nature of such treatment
      8. Likelihood that the medical condition will improve
      9. Possible restrictions or job modifications to
         a. Enable the individual to carry out essential job functions
         b. Reduce to an acceptable level the risk of sudden or subtle incapacitation; injury, harm or aggravation of the condition; or injury or harm to others (see discussion of "direct threat" in Chapter 50)
      10. Degree to which the individual meets the criteria of the disability system under which the evaluation is conducted

VII. Conclusions and recommendations, including a reasoned explanation for their basis
   A. The burden of proof with respect to disability, employability, or accommodation is met

*Continued.*

**CONTENT OF THE DISABILITY-ORIENTED MEDICAL EVALUATION REPORT—cont'd**

   1. Identify specific items of information that conform to the specific elements required for proof
   2. Estimate the expected duration of the individual's inability to meet job demands and conditions of employment, personal or social demand, or the requirements of law or regulation
   3. State the medical basis on which to recommend medical follow-up actions, if appropriate and warranted
B. The burden of proof is not met. Explain what information would have been supportive in relation to the specific elements of the burden of proof and reaffirm their absence or insufficiency in the documentation

While the clinical content of the medical portion of the report is independent of the purpose for which the report is written, it is appropriate, and in some cases necessary, for the physician to record medical observations that go beyond strictly clinical needs to satisfy the requirements of a particular disability system. In addition, it may be necessary to modify the nonmedical portion of the report to be acceptable to a specific disability system. For example, while a workers' compensation system (Chapter 6) may require information assessing "permanent partial disability," the Social Security system (see Chapter 7) requires information indicating whether the examinee meets the criteria set forth in the *Listings* or is able to engage in substantial gainful employment. The physician's conclusions must be explained credibly in each case, but the explanation must be tailored to the system being used.

Finally, to meet the needs of nonmedical users, the report must use nontechnical terms to explain the validity and probative value, or significance, of the medical information with respect to the criteria for disability, employability, or accommodation, while being responsive to the administrative or legal issues involved. The user must understand the rationale underlying the conclusions and be able to adopt that rationale in formulating a plan of action. Recommendations regarding the specific writing of the report are given in the box on page 81.

# RECOMMENDATIONS FOR PRODUCING A WELL-WRITTEN REPORT

1. Use short paragraphs.
2. Provide space (two or three lines between headings).
3. Avoid surplus words such as compound prepositions and word-wasting idioms when simple, concise words suffice.
4. Employ active verbs. Passive verbs require a supporting verb (was) followed by a preposition (by). Reserve the use of the passive verb for situations when the actor is unknown or for added emphasis.
5. Generally, use short sentences, especially in comparing items. Vary sentence length somewhat for variety, which improves readability.
6. Guide your reader. Begin sentences with names and dates. Place new information or important facts at the beginning of a sentence or paragraph.
7. Arrange your words with care, following the normal English word order of subject first, then verb, and then object. Avoid wide gaps between the subject, the verb, and the object.
8. Present material in tables when appropriate. Tables present complicated bits of information clearly and concisely.
9. Use commonly-understood English phrases and clearly defined terms. For example, instead of using terms like inspection, palpation, percussion, and auscultation, choose verbs (inspect, palpate, percuss, auscultate). Lay language is preferable: I observe, I see, I feel.
10. Avoid language quirks and habits. Maintain neutrality and objectivity.
11. Document all sources of information, both medical and nonmedical. Present these materials chronologically, identifying the date, source, recipient, and subject matter.
12. Carefully proofread and edit your report. Typographic errors and other easily-corrected mistakes diminish the impact of the report. Rephrase passages that seem unclear on the second reading. Make sure that your report has successfully translated medical language into good English.
13. Use headings, underlining, and bold-face print for emphasis and organization. Strive for a professional format that presents information clearly.
14. Provide a list of references as needed. If appropriate, enclose a copy of one or two articles with appropriate passages highlighted. This adds power and credibility to your report.

# CHAPTER 12

# BIOSTATISTICS AND EPIDEMIOLOGY

*Stephen L. Demeter*

This chapter briefly reviews some concepts and terms used in biostatistics and epidemiology applicable to the following sections of this book. Once these powerful ideas are mastered, a deeper and richer understanding of the ideas they describe can be gained.

## DISTRIBUTION CHARACTERISTICS

*Mean, median, mode,* and *standard deviation* are terms applying to the distribution of results.

The *mean* is the average of a range of values and is denoted by the symbol $\bar{y}$ where $\Sigma y$ is the sum of values in a sample containing n values. Mathematically, $\bar{y}$ equals the sum of the values ($\Sigma y$) divided by the number of values ($n$). Assume a study yields 19 observations ($n = 19$) and the observed values ($y$) are as follows:

1 2 2 2 3 3 3 4 4 6 6 6 7 7 7 7 8 8 9

The sum of these values, or $\Sigma y$, is 95. To find $\bar{y}$, you must divide the sum (95) by the number of values (19), yielding 5 (Fig. 12-1).

The *median* is the value that lies in the middle of the sample. It is calculated by multiplying the number of values plus one by 0.5. If $n$ is odd, the median is the $(0.5)(n + 1)$ value; if $n$ is even, the median lies between the two middle values. For example, if $n = 19$, the median lies at the $(0.5)(19 + 1)$ value, or the 10th $y$, which is 6. If $n = 20$, the median lies at the $(0.5)(20+1)$ value, which would be at the 10.5 value. Since there is no 10.5 value, the median is determined as the average between the $y$ value at position 10 and the $y$ value at position 11.

The *mode* is the most frequently occurring value in the sample. In Figure 12-1, the mode is 7.

The mean, median, and mode do not necessarily equal each other. When they do equal each other, the distribution is said to form a *normal curve* (Figure 12-2, *A*). When the mean, median, and mode are not equal, the curve is skewed to the left or right (Figure 12-2, *B* and *C*). The greater the difference between the mean and the median, the greater the skewing of the curve.

The *standard deviation,* designated *s* or *SD,* reflects how much each value in the sample deviates from the mean, or average, value. Mathematically, it is derived using the following formula:

$$\sqrt{\frac{\Sigma(y - \bar{y})^2}{n - 1}}$$

Most inexpensive calculators can easily calculate the standard deviation.

What does the standard deviation reveal about the distribution of values in a sample? Why is the standard deviation commonly identified in biological and medical studies? The standard deviation reveals the "spread" of the values, which leads to an analysis of whether the findings have statistical significance or result from chance. For a normal distribution curve, 68% of the observations fall within 1 SD of the mean, 95% within 2 SD, and 99.7% within 3 SD (Figure 12-3).

Other statistical terms and expressions, including Student's *t*-test and chi-square values, will not be discussed here. The reader is referred to biostatistics texts for this information.

## EPIDEMIOLOGIC TERMS

Epidemiology is defined as the study of disease occurrence in a given population. This discussion will focus on the terms needed to understand the ideas presented in this text. These terms include, most importantly, sensitivity, specificity, incidence, and prevalence; other terms and the formulas where they are defined are listed in Table 12-1. The concepts represented by these terms allow the application of statistical values to population groups (Table 12-2).

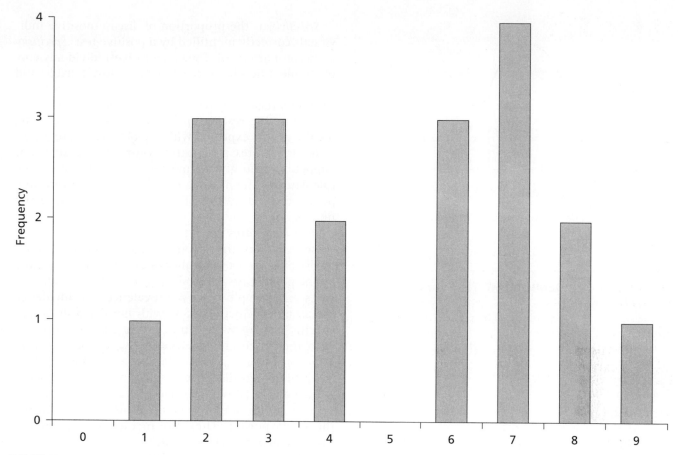

**FIGURE 12-1**    Frequency distribution (*n* = 19, mean = 5, median = 6, mode = 7, standard deviation = 2.47).

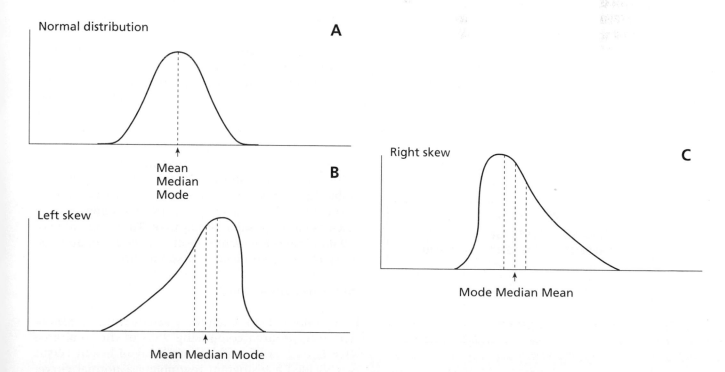

**FIGURE 12-2**    Normal and skewed distributions. **A,** Normal distribution. **B,** Left skew. **C,** Right skew.

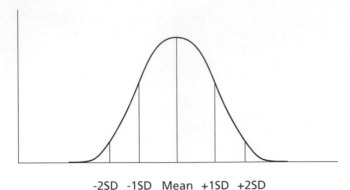

-2SD  -1SD  Mean  +1SD  +2SD

**FIGURE 12-3**    Standard deviations of a normal distribution.

**TABLE 12-1**    EPIDEMIOLOGIC TERMS
AND FORMULAS*

| NAME | FORMULA |
|---|---|
| Total positive tests | $a + b$ |
| Total negative tests | $c + d$ |
| True positives | $a$ |
| True negatives | $d$ |
| False positives | $b$ |
| False negatives | $c$ |
| Sensitivity | $a/(a + c)$ |
| Specificity | $d/(b + d)$ |
| Positive predictive value | $a/(a + b)$ |
| Negative predictive value | $d/(c + d)$ |

*See Table 12-2 for $a$, $b$, $c$, $d$.

**TABLE 12-2**    $2 \times 2$ TABLE

| SCREENING TEST | FINAL DIAGNOSIS DISEASE PRESENT | DISEASE ABSENT | TOTAL |
|---|---|---|---|
| Positive | $a$ | $b$ | $a + b$ |
| Negative | $c$ | $d$ | $c + d$ |
| Total | $a + c$ | $b + d$ | $a + b + c + d$ |

*Sensitivity* is the proportion of disease-positive individuals correctly identified by a positive test. *Specificity* is the proportion of disease-negative individuals correctly identified by a negative test. How reliable and valid a test is relates to its sensitivity and specificity. Decisions regarding whether to accept the data gathered in testing rest on epidemiologic studies comparing the events expected with the observed outcomes.

*Incidence* rates reflect the occurrence of an event happening in a given time period. Incidence can be calculated as the number of *new* cases in a given time period divided by the population at risk during the time period.

*Prevalence* rates reflect the cumulative number of these events at any given time. Prevalence is found by dividing the *total* number of events at a given time by the population at risk during that time period.

As an example of how prevalence and incidence are used, if factory workers with herniated discs in a specific factory were studied, the denominator for both incidence and prevalence would be the total number of workers in that factory at risk for developing a herniated disc. We can assume this number is 100, and that 10 workers had preexistent disc disease and an additional 10 developed disc disease during the study period. Then the incidence rate (or the number of new cases during the period of study) would be 10/100, which is 10%, whereas the prevalence (or total number of cases at any given time) would be (10 + 10)/100, or 20%.

### *r* Values

The *r* value addresses the issue of validity and is used in developing a predictive model. The r value is the slope of the line resulting when one value is compared with another (or comparing *x* and *y*). Comparing weight gain with caloric intake, study results would be plotted as shown in Figure 12-4. The slope of the line gives the *r* value, ranging from +1.0 (perfect correlation) to −1.0 (perfect inverse correlation), with a value of 0 showing absolutely no correlation. Table 12-3 translates the slopes or *r* values into usable terms of statistical association. (NOTE—Values can be used as either positive or negative. Thus an *r* value of +0.6 indicates a *moderate* positive association, and one of −0.6 a *moderate* negative association.)

### Statistical Significance

In a normal curve, all the *y* values within 2 SD are found in an area comprising 95% of the total area (see Fig. 12-3). If a population study of height versus sex yielded a histogram resembling a normal curve,

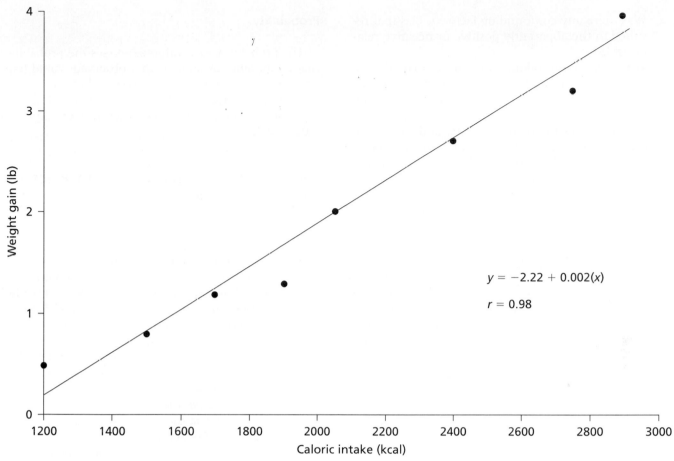

**FIGURE 12-4**     Regression line.

**TABLE 12-3**     *r* VALUES

| ABSOLUTE VALUE OF *r* | DEGREE OF ASSOCIATION |
|---|---|
| 0.8–1.0 | Strong |
| 0.5–0.8 | Moderate |
| 0.2–0.5 | Weak |
| 0–0.2 | Negligible |

any given result could be expressed as being within or outside 2 SD. These findings would then have statistical significance depending on where they fell.

### Null Hypothesis and *p* Value

The null hypothesis states that any differences between two groups result from random variation or chance rather than a statistically meaningful associa-tion. When a study is performed, the null hypothesis must be stated and then either accepted or rejected on statistical grounds. The expressions used for either acceptance or rejection are significance level and probability (*p*) value.

We may develop the hypothesis that a CT scan is a useful test for diagnosing a herniated disc. A study is performed and the results analyzed. The null hypothesis states that there is no association between the CT scan findings and the proven pres-ence of a herniated disc. There can only be one of three results:

1. The CT scan correctly identifies a herniated disc in all (or almost all) circumstances.
2. It correctly identifies it in only some circum-stances, but not enough to make it a worthwhile or valid test.
3. There is no correlation between the two (the null hypothesis).

To be able to make these descriptive statements, one must turn to a statistical analysis. This statistical analysis also addresses three issues:

1. Is the correlation correct?

2. Was there any confounding factor or bias that resulted in the apparently positive or negative relationship?
3. Was there any random variation that could have produced the positive or negative relationship?

The second issue should not be a concern if the study was properly designed to eliminate all known sources of bias. If the results of many tests, addressing the same hypothesis, yield similar results, the chance of bias is (theoretically) eliminated unless exactly the same bias is present in each and every test.

Statistical analysis attempts to eliminate the third issue as a cause for the observed result. To do this, a test statistic (derived from Student's $t$-test or from the chi-square test) is computed and compared with a predetermined value that provides a tangible meaning to the statistical values derived from the test (termed the critical value). When the test statistic exceeds the critical value, then the null hypothesis is rejected and the test results are accepted as showing a true relationship. The critical value is arbitrarily placed, usually at 5% (that is, all the results fall within 2 SD of expected values). Repeated testing of the same hypothesis is used to accept or reject the association. If repeated testing has not been or cannot be performed, the significance level is examined to determine if the test results should be accepted or rejected. If the significance level is 10%, 25%, or 50%, we should be wary of accepting the results. (When using the $t$-test or the chi-square test, the higher the number, the lower the probability.)

## Probability

The probability or $p$ value expresses the probability that a difference as large as that observed would happen by chance. A $p$ value of 0.05 (or 5%) is usually chosen in most clinical studies. The validity of the test increases as the $p$ value decreases (for example, to 0.01 or 0.001).

## GENERAL PRINCIPLES IN APPLYING STATISTICS AND EPIDEMIOLOGIC CONCEPTS

The following points should be noted:

- The greater the number of experimental observations made, the greater is the reliance on the statistical expression; for example, if a study comprises only 3 results, the fact that all 3 are positive (100%) is less conclusive than if 97 of 100 were positive (97%).
- A $p$ value of 0.051 (greater than the "accepted cutoff" of 0.05) in a large study differs little from a $p$ value of 0.049.
- Because a study shows statistical significance does not automatically mean that this should or would be accepted clinically; for example, a benign but imperfect treatment for a benign disease can be compared with a new treatment that causes death at a $p$ value less than 0.05 but results in a cure for that benign condition. Clinically, the former may be more acceptable since we are dealing with a benign disease.

# PART II

# ORGAN SYSTEMS

# SECTION A
Musculoskeletal System Assessment

# CHAPTER 13

## GENERIC ASSESSMENT SYSTEMS

*Gunnar B. J. Andersson*

Because impairment represents a limitation of function, it is the functional loss that ideally should be quantified during an impairment evaluation. For the musculoskeletal system function is difficult to quantify. Different parts of the body interact differently depending on requirements, and adaptation frequently occurs.

To address this difficulty, three different impairment evaluation methods have evolved that are sometimes used separately and are sometimes combined. It is the purpose of this chapter to discuss the three models, their advantages and disadvantages.

### ANATOMIC SYSTEMS (BASED ON EXAMINATION)

The anatomic approach to disability evaluation started with the recording of amputation, ankylosis, and fixed deformity. Later it came to include weakness, loss of sensation, and measurement of range of motion (ROM). Whereas amputation, ankylosis, and fixed deformity can be accurately, reproducibly, and objectively determined, weakness, loss of sensation, and measurements of ROM are more difficult to measure and are subjective in the sense that they all rely on the participation and cooperation of the person to be evaluated. Further, it can be argued that weakness and ROM are indicators of function and therefore are functional rather than anatomic measures. The reason why additional measures have been added is that amputation, ankylosis, and deformity cover only a small part of impairment disorders, making a pure anatomic system useless for the majority of evaluations. The American Medical Association (AMA) *Guides to the Evaluation of Permanent Impairment*[1,2] initially used a modified anatomic approach that included the measurement of ROM. In the third and fourth editions diagnostic features have been included, especially for the spine. This is an example of how impairment systems develop not along one methodological principle only but by combining different evaluation principles.

### DIAGNOSTIC SYSTEMS (BASED ON PATHOLOGY)

A diagnostic system is based on assigning impairment percentages for certain diagnostic groups. The advantages are simplicity and reproducibility (if criteria for the groups are objective and enforced). Deciding on criteria appears simple on the surface, but consider the difficulty in diagnosing certain spinal conditions such as a herniated disc or low-back sprain. When population groups are studied, anatomic evidence of herniated discs occurs in at least 25% of individuals who have never had back pain or sciatica and have no impairment (see Chapter 15). For clinical (as distinct from anatomic or radiologic) diagnosis, therefore, a herniated disc seen on an MRI is not sufficient to make a diagnosis, but there must also be appropriate symptoms and signs. Further, a narrow spinal canal accentuates the clinical syndrome of disc herniation but can equally correctly be diagnosed as spinal stenosis. Low-back sprain, the most common back diagnosis, is a diagnosis by exclusion, the existence of which many question. Any patient who complains of back pain can be fitted into this category if no other is applicable. The difficulty in developing diagnostic criteria is not the main weakness of a diagnosis-based system, however. Rather, it is the fact that the actual degree of impairment related to a specific diagnosis is highly variable, which is a problem.[7] For these reasons, a diagnosis-based system is probably best used as an adjunct to other measurements. An expanded diagnosis-based system is currently used by the Social Security Administration[9,10] and for Worker's Compensation Disability Evaluation in Minnesota.[8] The former combines diagnosis with history, physical examination, and laboratory tests (as applicable), whereas the latter combines diagnosis with history, physical examination, pain complaints, and x-ray evaluation. The most recent edition of the AMA *Guides* uses two approaches to evaluate spine conditions. The "injury model" assigns the patient to one of eight injury categories. If none of the eight categories is applicable, the evaluator should abandon this approach and use a ROM instead. The ROM model uses a diagnosis-based component, impairment estimates, percents with range of motion estimates and percents, and spinal nerve deficit (sensation, weakness) estimates and percents.

## FUNCTIONAL SYSTEMS

There is currently no pure functional system in use, although this would conceptually be the best method to evaluate impairment and disability. The difficulty lies in measuring function. Several functional indicators can be measured but their relationship to overall function remains uncertain. These include ROM—the most frequently used functional estimate and the easiest to obtain—as well as strength, endurance, and coordination. Various chapters in this book discuss these measures. The California Industrial Accident System includes functional parameters. These are patient estimates, however, without objective verification.[4] The Social Security Administration determines abilities to perform basic work activities and residual functional capacities for work, but depends on medical reports for its review and rarely directly measures physical capacities. Requiring sophisticated objective measures of various functions is impractical and costly, and the methods are still not technically advanced to the level where function can be precisely determined.

## DISCUSSION

The ideal impairment evaluation system would include the features listed in the box on this page. The most important feature is validity, since any system should, of course, actually measure impairment. The rating should also be consistent for the same impairment evaluated by the same evaluator (intra-individual reliability). Further, when the impaired person is evaluated by several evaluators, the rating should be the same (inter-individual reliability). Wide variations in impairment rating between physicians has been reported for spinal conditions.[3-6] Rating variations from 3% to 35% in West Virginia were attributed to such factors as patient's personality, patient's level of education, and social environment. Brand and Lehmann[3] found the variability disturbing and concluded that "any method of rating impairment is arbitrary at best and incorrect and unfair at worst". Clark et al[4] found variation from 0% to 70% in California. Clearly, the level of reproducibility reported by these investigators is unacceptable.

## CHARACTERISTICS OF AN IDEAL IMPAIRMENT EVALUATION SYSTEM

1. Valid (actually measure impairment disability)
2. Reproducible (within and between investigators)
3. Practical (office setting)
4. Discriminating (among levels of impairment)
5. Quantifiable (for administrative and computer purposes)
6. Acceptable to all systems, including workers' compensation, Social Security, government and private insurance
7. Based on current understanding of pathophysiology

Practicality is an important consideration in impairment evaluation because of the large number of persons who are evaluated. Over 4 million Americans receive support from the Social Security Disability Insurance (SSDI) and Supplemental Security Income (SSI) programs; about 1.5 million claims are made each year, and each year there are more than 2 million examinations for workers' compensation disability claims related to the musculoskeletal system alone. Given these numbers, it is important that physicians can perform evaluations in their offices or clinics.

The ability to define different levels of impairment ("to discriminate") is another important feature. As has been previously discussed, this is one of the difficulties in using a pure diagnostic system, because the same disease can cause different degrees of impairment, and the same impairment different degrees of disability. Quantification is another important feature; it is necessary for administrative purposes and to make it possible to computerize the impairment evaluation. Clearly, it would also be advantageous if all authorities requesting impairment evaluations used the same system. This one system could be perfected and all impairment evaluators be better trained. Finally, impairment ratings should reflect pathology whenever possible. Basing an impairment rating on subjective complaints alone, without disease verification, raises issues of fairness.

## SUMMARY

The perfect impairment rating system does not exist in the 1990s. Anatomic systems alone cannot measure impairment in large groups of people where such measurements are required. Diagnostic systems, on the other hand, suffer from a lack of agreement on diagnostic criteria and from inability to discriminate between levels of impairment between individuals with the same diagnosis. Functionally based systems are not realistic at the present time because technology is not sufficiently advanced and validated. Combining different features from the different alternatives is the only realistic solution. Developing methods to quantify pain and to determine function are challenges for the future. Relating impairment to disability is another area requiring further attention. Other chapters in this book will address these issues as they relate to different joint systems.

## References

1. American Medical Association: *Guides to the evaluation of permanent impairment*, Engelberg A, editor, ed 3, Chicago, 1988, American Medical Association.
2. American Medical Association: *Guides to the evaluation of permanent impairment*, Doege TC, editor, ed 4, Chicago, 1993, American Medical Association.
3. Brand RA, Lehmann TR: Low back impairment rating practices of orthopaedic surgeons. *Spine* 8:75, 1983.
4. Clark WL, et al: Back impairment and disability determination: another attempt at objective, reliable rating. *Spine* 13:332, 1988.
5. Greenwood, JG: Low-back impairment-rating practices of orthopaedic surgeons and neurosurgeons in West Virginia. *Spine* 10:773, 1985.
6. Lehmann TR, Brand RA: Disability in the patient with low back pain. *Orthop Clin North Am* 13:559, 1982.
7. McBride E: *Disability evaluation*, Philadelphia, 1963, JB Lippincott.
8. Minnesota Medical Association: *Worker's compensation permanent partial disability schedule*, Minneapolis, 1984, Minnesota Medical Association.
9. Social Security Administration: *Disability evaluation under Social Security*, Washington, D.C., 1979, U.S. Government Printing Office, pp. 1-22.
10. U.S. Bureau of Disability Insurance: *Disability evaluation under Social Security: a handbook for physicians*, Washington, D.C., 1970, U.S. Government Printing Office.

# CHAPTER 14

# RANGE-OF-MOTION EVALUATION

*Thomas Mayer*

## INTRODUCTION

Testing the range of motion (ROM) as a clinical measurement of impairment remains an accepted method of musculoskeletal assessment in the AMA *Guides to the Evaluation of Permanent Impairment.*[4] Recently, challenges to use of this methodology have emerged, centered on: (*a*) the relationship between mobility deficits and impairment; (*b*) age-related changes; (*c*) normative data; (*d*) ability to evaluate patient effort; and (*e*) accuracy of measurements in specific joints or spinal regions. These questions have led to exploration in other directions, based on the fundamental AMA *Guides* principle that impairment evaluation should be based on gauging functional loss.

In some cases, human performance testing involving greater complexity and requiring greater patient cooperation has been advocated for assessing impairment (e.g., strength, endurance, pulmonary function, lifting capacity, or other activities of daily life simulations). On the other hand, the use of the "diagnostic category" has gained greater popularity for a number of reasons.[39] Using the diagnosis as a substitute for performance testing makes the assessment easier, allowing a larger number of treating or evaluating physicians (and other health providers) to perform these assessments. Since determination of impairment usually entails a *nonmedical outcome* (of distributing financial benefits) utilizing a medical "gatekeeper process", operational simplicity represents a compelling objective, particularly to external payors.

However, involvement of a medical gatekeeper introduces equally justifiable concern. An administrative process that is scientifically valid must adhere to sound medical principles, in fact as well as theory. This is especially important if fairness to the vital interests of the patient being evaluated is to be best served. There is obvious validity in the link between impairment and the loss of specific functions such as mobility and strength, even when correlation with a medical diagnosis may be limited. A single diagnosis may be associated with wide variations of functional impairment, handicap, and disability. This is particularly true in controversial, but common, musculoskeletal disorders such as those involving the spine. However, the problems inherent in human performance measurement may be accentuated in controversial cases, particularly when claimants know that rewards will be greater for lesser performance. Range-of-motion evaluation represents a microcosm of the controversy created by the differing goals of the various parties represented in a disability claim, including the employer, the injured worker, the insurance company, the regulatory agency, and the physician.

A rudimentary understanding of the terms *impairment, disability, handicap,* and *employability* is required for full assimilation of these issues. **Disability** is an *administrative* term and refers to an individual's inability to perform certain activities of daily life, such as gainful employment or recreation, which are customarily accessible to the average, healthy individual. **Impairment** is a *medical* term and represents an alteration of the patient's usual health status that is *evaluated by medical means.* **Handicap** occurs as a consequence of an *impairment,* representing a barrier to performance of an activity of daily living, but one which may be overcome by *reasonable accommodation* or *adaptation. Accommodation* refers to modification of the environment to suit the needs of the handicap and decrease the degree of disability. *Adaptation* by the individual achieves the same goal by enhancing residual capabilities to replace those that may have been lost. **Employability** represents another administrative process affected both by *disability* and *handicap.* Any decrease in employability as a consequence of an injury may result in *economic loss* to the patient, leading to a compensatory monetary award whose numerical value must be determined statutorily. One factor in this award is the evaluation of perceived damage to the patient's health status (or *impairment*),

**TABLE 14-1    CONSIDERATIONS IN SELECTING AN IMPAIRMENT METHODOLOGY**

| PRINCIPLE | CONSIDERATIONS |
| --- | --- |
| Objectivity | Validity, intratester reliability, accuracy. Relevance preferred. |
| Consistency | Intertester reliability. Small range of normal human variability preferred. |
| Fairness | Relationship between numerical impairment rating and true alteration of health status and physical function. |
| Accuracy | Precision, signal-to-noise ratio, specificity, sensitivity; potential to discriminate, intraindividual and interindividual alterations in health status. |
| Relevance | Correlation between assessment technique and alteration of health status from "normal." Requires comparison to normal *functioning.* |
| Convenience | Test must be easy to perform, preferably with techniques known to all potential evaluators. Limited educational requirements. Limited time required for assessment. |
| Cost | Minimum desirable by parties requesting assessment but not at the price of significantly increased variability. Shortest possible time commitment of expert evaluators. Minimize variability to minimize disputes generally considered worth paying for. |

for which the physician is generally deemed responsible. Once one determines to place a numerical value on impairment, one requires an administrative methodology which must respond to a number of sometimes contradictory objectives (Table 14-1).

Range-of-motion testing in impairment evaluation is essentially a quantitative component of the physical examination. The most abbreviated musculoskeletal physical examination almost always includes a qualitative assessment of mobility during the initial, interim, and terminal visits to assess progress. When a patient reaches a plateau, it is often assumed that all temporary impairment in the range of motion has resolved. If there is loss of mobility, it is generally be-

lieved that it should be correlated in some way with a component of the *permanent impairment.* In the absence of optimum rehabilitation and effort, this assumption may be untrue. When a *quantitative assessment* is required, in order to provide a numerical component of the administrative process of *disability evaluation,* a deeper understanding of the principles and methodology of mobility assessment is needed.

Evaluation of impairment, as noted above, presumes a temporal factor; that is, there will be a *temporary* component of mobility loss during a period of healing, intervention, and rehabilitation, followed in some cases by a *permanent* component. With acute injury or illness, joint or para-articular swelling affecting soft tissues is frequently accompanied by some temporary loss of motion. Loss of mobility may be one of the only clinical signs leading to a correct diagnosis, particularly in situations in which visualization of superficial structures (to detect in-tissue consistency, color, or temperature changes) may be absent. In most cases, resolution of an acute infection or inflammatory process, if properly treated, results not only in complete symptomatic recovery, but also in full restoration of joint mobility.

However, in situations involving episodic or repetitive trauma, continuous use (or stress), and patients with systemic arthritis or severe joint derangement, para-articular scarring and contracture may occur, and lead to residual stiffness. While this loss of motion may be painless, there is often a correlation between persistent pain and loss of motion with episodes of increasing pain-associated symptoms that correlate with episodic mobility deficits. These correlations of functional loss and synovitis with acute exacerbations are most easily recognized in hemophilic arthropathy or systemic arthritis.[1,31,64]

In the same way, alteration of range of motion at the time of *maximum medical improvement* (or the point at which the condition becomes *permanent and stationary*) may correlate with the degree of permanent impairment sustained by that individual as a treatment outcome. The measurement of mobility may then assist the clinician in evaluating one of the critical functional outcomes of natural healing, medical intervention, and physical rehabilitation.[42]

The complex relationship between *pain* and *loss of motion* is worth exploring in more detail. Pain is a crucial symptom that leads formerly healthy individuals to seek medical assistance and assume the status of *patients* in a majority of cases. In the musculoskeletal system, this relationship is even more pronounced. Yet, because pain is usually perceived exclusively by the subject with the painful condition, the important symptom of pain is the least verifiable symptom a patient can experience. In cases of acute infection or trauma, signs of swelling, heat, or induration may provide objective evidence for subjective pain complaints. In most disability evaluations, however, coming as they do at the termination of medical treatment, a report of pain is usually viewed as entirely subjective, particularly since it is prone to exaggeration. Great effort may be expended on identifying signs of psychological distress, called "nonorganic signs", which may be used (or misused) subsequently to discredit complaints of the claimant.

Loss of motion, on the other hand, has the advantage of being observable and quantitatively measurable. It lacks objectivity only insofar as it is prone to voluntary restriction through suboptimal effort, as in any human performance test. By itself, loss of motion may create functional loss (e.g., joint contractures). However, when joint motion is both restricted and painful, the impairment is compounded. The relationship is further complicated because pain itself may lead to restriction of joint motion, whether voluntarily, involuntarily, or both. Perhaps the greatest paradox and challenge to be dealt with in impairment evaluation is that this varied relationship between pain and loss of mobility presents both the greatest correlational advantage and worst confounder of the process. The future usefulness of this technique, as with any quantitative human performance test, will depend on measurement processes that can stratify, insofar as it is possible, the interrelated impairments due to pain from those due to functional loss.

## PRINCIPLES OF MOBILITY TESTING

### Neutral Zero Method and Terminology

Two parallel goals in musculoskeletal impairment evaluation are to achieve *objectivity* and *consistency*. One crucial factor in meeting these goals is standardized terminology and measurement protocols to enhance both intratester and intertester reliability. The Neutral Zero concept is the most generally accepted of these concepts.[13,25] The principle begins with a *zero starting position*, equivalent to an individual standing erect with hands by the side in a *military-attention* posture. All movement is then recorded from this starting position in the three planes intersecting at 90° angles: *sagittal, coronal,* and *axial.* Figure 14-1 demonstrates the three planes,[4] differing from the neutral zero position only in that the forearms are held in the anatomical supine position.[25]

The most common sagittal plane terms, *flexion* and *extension,* will be addressed first. This terminology may be confusing if one fails to recognize that there is a difference between the *neutral zero position* (from

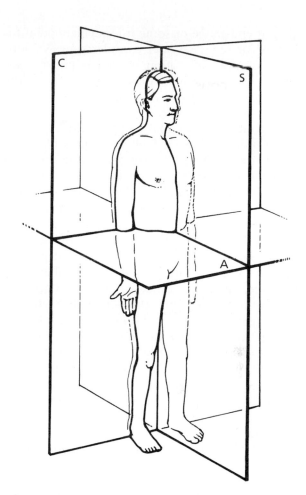

**FIGURE 14-1**    Body planes for measuring motion. *S,* Sagittal plane: a vertical plane that divides the body into right and left parts. *A,* Axial plane: a crosswise plane that divides the body into upper and lower parts and is perpendicular to the sagittal and frontal planes. *C,* Coronal plane: a vertical plane that divides the body into anterior and posterior parts. (Modified from American Medical Association: *Guides to the evaluation of permanent impairment,* ed 4, Chicago, 1993, and Gerhardt J: *Documentation of joint motion,* ed 3 (rev), Portland, 1992, Oregon Medical Association.)

which the numerical starting point is derived) and the *supine anatomic position* (from which the named direction of motion is derived). The difference is only relevant in the upper extremity distal to the elbow (Fig. 14-1). Beginning in the *supine anatomic position,* all sagittal motion is termed *flexion/extension.* One must view the femur as the dividing line, above which *flexion* increases as the volar angle decreases; distal to the femurs, volar angle decrease is termed *extension.* All axial motion is termed *pronation/supination* or *rotation* (either left/right or internal/external). Coronal motion is described by a large number of terms including *abduction/adduction, eversion/inversion, deviation* (e.g., ulnar/radial), or *lateral bend* (e.g., left/right spinal).

Regardless of direction of measurement, the neutral zero position always represents the 0° position, whether at end-range or some intermediate point for the joint(s) or regions under consideration. Numerical values of range of motion are generally expressed in the angle through which a joint passes from the neutral zero position to its terminal position. In some joints, such as the elbow, knee, and fingers, the neutral zero position is essentially in full extension, and all the recorded motion is in flexion. Loss of extension mobility is termed *flexion contracture*. In other joints, the neutral zero position is at some midpoint of the planar range. *Ankylosis* refers to complete joint immobility and is expressed as a specific angle in the terminology of the plane(s) involved (e.g., ankle ankylosed at 10° [plantar-] flexion). More commonly, some residual joint range of motion persists, but the joint is limited in reaching the usual extreme of the range. Since it is generally acknowledged that impairment is greater when the neutral zero position can no longer be achieved, the presence of a flexion contracture in a joint like the elbow, knee, or fingers is of greater significance than loss of terminal planar motion when the neutral zero position is preserved (for example, retained cervical spine motion from 30° flexion to 30° extension). Contractures in joints with a midpoint neutral zero position may also be administratively termed *ankylosis*.[3]

The term *hyperextension* connotes a potentially pathological condition of *hypermobility* which may involve either a genetic predisposition to ligamentous laxity, or ligament and capsular injury creating residual post-traumatic joint instability.[14,74] When an extremity is affected in terms of mobility, a contralateral normal side is often available for comparison. This is not true in the spine, so that a *normative database* must be developed, if deviations from "normal" are to be identified. When quantitative, rather than qualitative, expressions of these deviations are needed, this introduces the requirement to account for normal human variation in performance measurements, including such factors as age, gender, weight, and/or joint laxity. Even occupational variations can be identified in some joints, although it remains unclear whether the presumed occupational influence causes the mobility difference, or there is an accompanying genetic predisposition selecting for the occupation, or both.[54]

Range of motion can be measured either actively (AROM) or passively (PROM). AROM, generally acknowledged as a *safer* method of measurement, requires the patient's voluntary cooperation using active muscle contraction. This method may have the unintended side effect of limiting terminal motion, as when a co-contraction is stimulated. PROM requires the intervention of the examiner moving a joint to a terminal position, which is generally considered more objective because the movement is free of control by the examinee. Distal extremity joints lend themselves more readily to this type of measurement. Even under conditions of maximum effort, AROM may be different from PROM, as is the case when pain inhibits active (increased loading) motion or when muscle weakness prevents full active motion against gravity. Whenever possible, the examiner should evaluate both AROM and PROM.

## Measurement Techniques

Quantitative measurement in most joints, particularly in the extremities, is facilitated by use of the simple two-armed goniometer.[27] As the goniometer is essentially a hinge, it is particularly useful whenever a typical hinge or ball-and-socket joint is being measured in a single plane (Fig. 14-2, *A* and *B*). Measurement is also facilitated by the presence of a

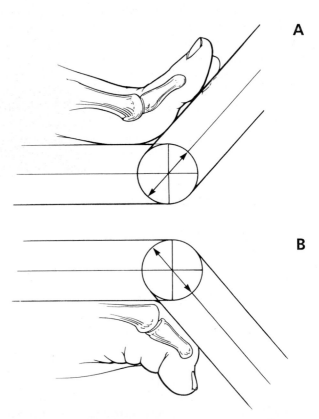

**FIGURE 14-2**    Evaluating the range of motion of a toe, the metatarsophalangeal (MTP) joint of the great toe. **A,** Extension. The goniometer is under the MTP joint, and its angle is read as a baseline. The patient extends (dorsiflexes) the toe maximally, and the angle subtending the maximum arc of motion is read; the baseline angle is subtracted. **B,** Flexion. The goniometer is placed over the MTP joint. The baseline angle is read. The patient plantar flexes the MTP joint maximally. The angle subtending the maximum arc of motion is read, and the baseline angle is subtracted. (From American Medical Association, *Guides to the evaluation of permanent impairment,* ed 4, Chicago, 1993.)

contralateral side, easy palpation of bony landmarks, and experience of the test administrator. In contrast, however, overlying soft tissue, obesity, and lack of contralaterality or regional movements (e.g., the spine) make use of the goniometer less preferable due to decreasing accuracy, relevance, and/or objectivity. For special situations, smaller flat-surface goniometers have been developed (e.g., finger measurements[28]).

Inclinometers are versatile tools that have evolved from the simple carpenter's level. Small, inexpensive versions of these devices, with reasonable accuracy, can be obtained at any hardware store (Fig. 14-3). Since goniometry is ineffective in spine measurement, inclinometers are preferred for use in these regions.[34,36,44,69] A dual inclinometer technique has been developed for measuring each of the specific spinal regions. Subtraction of the motion of the lower inclinometer from the upper inclinometer leads to a true spinal motion measurement (Fig. 14-4).[32,38,44] It is customary to measure true cervical motion from the occiput to T1, thoracic from T1-T12, and lumbar from T12 to the sacrum.

Beyond the simple tools, a multitude of other motion measurement devices have been devised. A magnetic compass may be utilized to measure inclination out of the gravitational plane.[16,36,45] Flexicurves and kyphometers have been used for specialized spinal regional measurements and are designed to overcome some of the limitations of other measurement tools in these areas.[11,29] Various electrogoniometers or electronic inclinometers have been developed as tools for more accurately assessing spinal motion in a gravitational plane. Unfortunately, excellent device accuracy may be offset in routine spinal evaluation by inexperience, lack of training, and other determinants.[38,49,76]

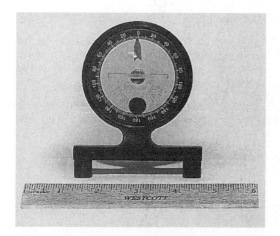

**FIGURE 14-3**    A mechanical inclinometer. (From American Medical Association, *Guides to the evaluation of permanent impairment*, ed 4, Chicago, 1993.)

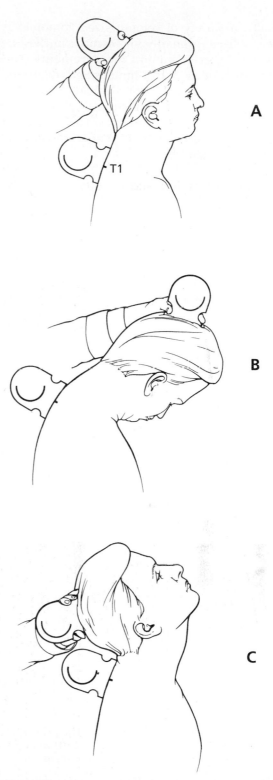

**FIGURE 14-4**    Two-inclinometer measurement technique for cervical flexion and extension. **A,** The subject is sitting with the head in the neutral position, and the inclinometers are held over the occiput and T1. **B,** With the subject flexing the neck fully, determine the lower inclinometer angle. Then subtract the lower angle from the upper angle. **C,** With the patient extending the neck, read the two angles and subtract the T1 angle to determine the extension angle. (From American Medical Association, *Guides to the evaluation of permanent impairment*, ed 4, Chicago, 1993.)

Finally, a variety of computerized goniometers have been utilized, primarily for research purposes, to obtain very precise motion measurements. These include such devices as 3-dimensional digitizers, computerized inclinometers, optical scanners, video combined with light emitting diodes, and various multi-position x-ray techniques. The expense of these approaches precludes their general medical use (see also Chapter 18).[9,17,50,51,62,65,72]

### Accuracy, Reliability, and Validity

The term *accuracy* refers to how close a measured value approaches the "real" or "actual" value. It is limited by the *precision* of the measurement, which is determined by the smallest increment of measurement indicated by the scale on the device (5° on most simple goniometers or 1° on most electronic inclinometers). The *reliability or reproducibility* refers to the ability of a clinical measurement to equal a previous or prior series of measurements. Reliability is a complex concept that depends on a multitude of factors (Table 14-2). Reliability testing is the most common method for assessing the utility of a measurement system, because it is easy to evaluate statistically. Its disadvantage is that it originates from a somewhat imprecise social-sciences conceptual framework, rather than from physics-based measurement principles commonly used in engineering science. *Validity* is another social-sciences concept that refers to the usefulness of a measurement system (as opposed to a device) in evaluating a clinical paradigm. It may consist of many types of validity (such as face validity, content validity, construct validity, and consensual validity).

Considering all of the potential *sources of error*, ±5° is the commonly acknowledged variability that may be encountered before any "real" change in motion can be accepted as valid.[2,3,8] Additionally, it is axiomatic that inclinometers or goniometers should be checked periodically against a *reference standard* such as a wall or floor. While the device accuracy of a simple two-armed goniometer is usually limited only by its precision, its reliability in a measurement system is generally conceded to be good, although intertester reliability is usually less than intratester reliability. This appears to be more a function of test administrator training than an issue related to the device itself.[8,21,28,57,60] Reliability testing for inclinometers provides a confusing mixture of impressions for the reader, since most investigators have failed to recognize that assessment of inclinometric measurements in a *measurement system* like the spine raises all of the possible *sources of error* noted in Table 14-2.

The *device error* for inclinometers is usually found to be very low, with the device accuracy generally determined by its precision. This is usually about ±5° for inexpensive fluid-filled inclinometers, decreasing to 0.5° for electronic inclinometers with optical-electronic scanners. Limitations in reliability testing noted in multiple clinical studies are usually on the basis of sources of error other than the device. Com-

---

**TABLE 14-2** FACTORS IMPORTANT IN TESTING RELIABILITY AND CLINICAL UTILITY INVOLVING DEVICES FOR HUMAN PERFORMANCE MEASUREMENT

| PRINCIPLE | CONSIDERATIONS |
|---|---|
| Device Accuracy/Precision | The ability of the device to repeatably produce the same value. |
| Human/Device Interface | The reliability component based on applying the device appropriately to the individual being measured, depending commonly on factors such as bony landmarks, overlying soft tissues, parallax, skin adhesion, and relationship between skin movement and underlying bony movement. |
| Test Administrator Training | The skill and training of the test administrator recognizing the multiple potential sources of error, usually evaluated by comparing intratester and intertester reliabilities. |
| Normal Human Variability | Variability associated with factors such as age, gender, weight, occupation, training, and culture, that can be anticipated even with perfect device and measurement validity. |
| Errors Unique to Subjects Undergoing Impairment Evaluation | Limited effort and cooperation; secondary gain for poor performance; effect of pain; threat of litigation and adversarial environment. |

mon pitfalls are improper identification of bony landmarks, inadequate warm-up of subjects, improper use of the device with the subject, and lack of recognition of the motion end-point.[7,12,15,19,24,26,32,38,46,53,55,56,63,73,75] In general, examiners interested in maximizing reproducibility of their spinal measurement skills should concentrate on expertise with the device chosen, ability to find bony landmarks, and firm application of the device to the subject's body.

## Normal Human Variability and Databases

Age is definitely a factor in range of motion. Due to intrauterine compression, significant alterations in range of motion of neonates can be demonstrated, particularly in the shoulders, elbows, ankles, knees and hips.[23,30] Generally speaking, mobility is higher in children than in adults, and it progressively declines with age, due to a number of factors including genetics, training, trauma, occupation, and gender.[6,14,59,67,74] Age-related changes tend to occur symmetrically in the extremities if they are not accompanied by factors that act unilaterally, such as injury or arthritis. As such, the importance of age-related change is greater in the spine, where lack of contralaterality implies that quantitative impairment evaluation using range of motion must rely on a normative database. Normal values depend on a multitude of factors, many of which have been assessed and demonstrated.[32,38,40,41] Other studies have tested chronically impaired patients before and after rehabilitation to document the physical progress in overcoming *temporary impairment* to reach their final status of *residual permanent impairment*.[33,35,43] Changes related to age have been well-documented in the literature.[18,19,47,66,70] Gender plays a surprisingly small role in mobility except in cases of ligamentous laxity and normal human variability seen with training effects in females engaged in activities involving stretching. Cultural differences related to childhood positioning or customary postures (e.g., "hunkering" in many Asian cultures) may be the reason for significant variability of motion in lower-extremity joints such as the hip and ankle.[18,32,66]

The concept of "normal values" is especially noteworthy in relation to spine measurements. Normal spine measurements can be very useful for impairment ratings, because the patient's less-than-optimum effort can be anticipated when greater financial reward is associated with poorer performance. Many studies have looked at normal range of motion with a variety of techniques, and are available for the preparation of mobility-based impairment systems.[20,22,37,48,52,54,58,61,67,68]

## Relationship of Motion to Impairment

Impairment evaluation is performed by a physician using medical means, and is most commonly used in determining awards related to permanent injury. In turn, this occurs most commonly in the industrial setting (e.g., workers' compensation cases). An increasing number of workers' compensation venues have chosen to use impairment-based administrative systems, rather than those based on wage loss or demonstration of inability to work (disability-based systems). Since spinal disorders represent a majority of the workers' compensation permanency awards, much of the controversy has focused on human-performance measurements in these situations. These contentious and multifactorial indemnity contests bring a social, rather than a scientific/medical bias, to the debate over the relationship between impairment and range of motion. Such debate really hinges on the relationship between any form of musculoskeletal impairment, regardless of the rating method, and the perceived "disability" involved in the injury for which society will reward the claimant. The complexity of the situation is compounded in a variety of different ways, including attempts to relate spine flexibility in uninjured workers to the possibility of future back-pain complaints and further illustrated by the variable relationship between pain and motion.[5]

Under ideal circumstances, there would be perfect correlation between physical impairment as measured by some functional human performance test and the complaints of pain and work or other type of impairment alleged to exist. This impairment number then might be converted to a numerical rating of disability by using a few well-selected social factors such as age, education, and skills. Unfortunately, such a construct has been and no doubt will continue to be elusive. In a classic study, looking at a multitude of important factors, Waddell et al found a number of variables to coincide with an independent measure of impairment. The majority of the relevant measures were related to active or passive range of motion measurements.[71] However, others have continued to focus attention on the limitations of standardized techniques of range-of-motion measurement in assessing spinal impairment, particularly as related to age changes.[20,35] Further complicating the situation is that increasing age may produce musculoskeletal soft-tissue diseases and injuries on a microtrauma level, which may lead to painful alterations of function without any objective change in AROM or PROM. Declines in mobility with age are usually accompanied by changes in the mechanical properties of ligaments and increasing stiffness associated with these changes.

*Thomas Neal, M.D.*

However, normative testing in older-age populations has generally ignored this potentially correctable stiffness due to inactivity, which is to be differentiated from uncorrectable age-related change.[10]

Even more disconcerting is the episodic nature of "permanent" mobility loss, which increases with inflammation and often is accompanied by greater levels of pain. Disability may also be increased by environmental factors, such as the need to bend, climb, run, or reach overhead, creating episodic increases in impairment or disability. This may occur in an individual who had previously achieved a stable balance in functioning through reasonable accommodation combined with physical adaptation. The social imperatives of protecting impaired workers, yet providing incentives to maintain productivity, can only be achieved by recognizing the advantages and limitations of the most sophisticated functionally-based methodologies for assessing impairment.

## Limited Effort and Cooperation

This chapter has reviewed some of the issues involved in clinical measurement of range of motion for impairment evaluation purposes. Current literature demonstrates that accurate, precise range-of-motion measurements can be obtained if the examiner is familiar with pitfalls in measurement. These pertain to proper use of the device, identification of anatomic landmarks for correct device application, and experience and skill in the use of the measurement system. The examiner must also be aware of normal human variation, as influenced by age, gender, occupation, and culture. In the situation in which range-of-motion measurement is being used for impairment evaluation, another set of factors apply, with which the sophisticated examiner should be familiar (Table 14-2). Since the financial award is intimately tied to the quantitative functional performance measurement, the claimant's motivational disincentives often will prevail over the need for maximum effort. Several methods may be used to neutralize this potential behavior. In the extremities, and even in the cervical spine, gentle PROM can be used to validate AROM. The medical records must be carefully surveyed to be certain that the patient has cooperated adequately with his rehabilitation. Otherwise, the evaluator cannot be certain that the decreased mobility noted at the time of the examination exists and is an actual reflection of *permanency*, rather than being a sign of temporary impairment or the result of voluntarily limiting the range of motion.

It is a paradox that noncompliant and unmotivated patients often receive greater financial rewards, re-

gardless of the impairment evaluation methodology used (diagnosis, surgical procedures, mobility testing, etc.). If the examinee demonstrates suboptimal effort, impairment higher than that expected for the degree of pathology, or limited evidence for rehabilitation compliance, the patient may not be at the state of "maximum medical improvement." In some cases, the claimant may be rehabilitated before being remeasured. If this is not possible, or if the patient has refused or abandoned appropriate rehabilitation, the examining physician must estimate what the range of motion *would have been* had the patient received and cooperated with treatment that resolved the temporary impairment component.

Finally, another useful discriminating validity factor for the physician is to determine whether there is a correlation between the pathologic state (as measured by other factors) and the range of motion. For example, an individual showing only 20% of normal lumbar spine motion and no history of systemic disease, spinal surgery, or previous injury, and who has supposedly been fully rehabilitated, is demonstrating functional changes inconsistent with that degree of pathology. Small deficit variations from normative values may be anticipated in nonoperated cases after completion of treatment. Even in operated cases, when only one or two spinal levels are involved, full mobility of the remaining joints should create only mild deficits of total regional mobility. In the case of spinal fusion, where complete immobility of one or more spinal joints has occurred, more significant loss of mobility may be anticipated. Because these changes also create higher biomechanical loading on adjacent joints, and because these changes have been shown to hasten the degenerative process at the adjacent joints, higher impairment ratings for loss of motion, as well as for the anatomical changes produced, are justifiable.

## SUMMARY

Ultimately, we must question the wisdom and propriety of utilizing *any* functional measure for assessing a nonmedical, indemnity-based construct like impairment or disability. It is not surprising that administrators, attorneys, and legislators are attempting to abandon many of the older methods of disability evaluation to escape the morass of social disincentives to productive behaviors created by rewarding disability. In the past half-century, economic philosophies in the industrialized world have favored relatively-high unemployment, which has made disability a convenient method for providing minimum incomes for displaced workers, irrespective of the cost. Musculoskeletal injury, particularly involving the spine, is a favored route of entry into this system. The shift into using medically determined impairment for social purposes, and turning the physician-evaluator into the gatekeeper for this system, is a parallel development. This use of medical impairment evaluation produces a misleading impression of scientific validation for what is essentially an economic issue. Therefore, the place of range-of-motion measurement for impairment rating remains controversial. The value of range of motion, however, as a scientific measure of real physical impairment remains high. It is useful for making an initial diagnosis, measuring progress of treatment, and recognizing limitations associated with maximum improvement and has far greater ability to discriminate between individual cases than a diagnostic category. It remains unclear whether these medical activities quantifying range of motion can be reconciled with nonmedical socioeconomic forces that seek to place aspects of social policy under a mantle of scientific respectability.

## REFERENCES

1. Altman R: Criteria for the classification of osteoarthritis of the knee and hip, *Scand J Rheumatol Suppl* 65:31-39, 1987.
2. American Medical Association: *Guides to the evaluation of permanent impairment*, ed 3, Chicago, 1988.
3. American Medical Association: *Guides to the evaluation of permanent impairment*, ed 3 (rev), Chicago, 1990.
4. American Medical Association: *Guides to the evaluation of permanent impairment*, ed 4, Chicago, 1993.
5. Battie M, Bigos S, Fisher L, et al: The role of spinal flexibility in back pain complaints within industry: a prospective study. *Spine* 15:768-773, 1990.
6. Baxter M: Assessment of normal pediatric knee ligament laxity using the genucom. *J Pediatr Orthop* 9:546-550, 1988.
7. Boline P, Keating J, Haas M, Anderson A: Interexaminer reliability and discriminant validity of inclinometric measurement of lumbar rotation in chronic low-back pain patients subjects without low-back pain. *Spine* 17:335-338, 1992.
8. Boone D, Azen S, Lin C-M, et al: Reliability of goniometric measurements, *Phys Ther* 58:1355-1390, 1978.
9. Brown R, Burstein A, Nash C, Schock C: Spinal analysis using a three-dimensional radiographic technique. *J Biomech* 9:355-365, 1976.
10. Buckwalter A, Goldberg V, Woo S: *Musculoskeletal soft-tissue aging: Impact on mobility*, American Academy of Orthopaedic Surgeons Symposium, Chicago, 1993.
11. Burton A: Regional lumbar sagittal mobility: measurement by flexicurves. *Clin Biomech* 1:20-26, 1986.
12. Capuano-Pucci D, Rheault W, Aukai J, et al: Intratester and intertester reliability of the cervical range of motion device. *Arch Phys Med Rehab* 72:338-340, 1991.
13. Cave E, Robert S: A method for measuring and recording joint function. *J Bone Joint Surg* 18:455-465, 1936.
14. Cheng J, Chan P, Hui P: Joint laxity in children. *J Pediatr Orthop* 11:752-756, 1991.
15. Clapper M, Wolf S: Comparison of the reliability of the Orthoranger and the standard goniometer for assessing active lower-extremity range of motion. *Phys Ther* 68:214-218, 1988.
16. Dillard J, Trafimow M, Andersson G, Cronin K: Motion of the lumbar spine: reliability of two measurement techniques. *Spine* 16:321-324, 1991.
17. Dopf C, Mandel S, Geiger D, Mayer P: Analysis of spine motion variability using a computerized goniometer compared to physical examination: a prospective clinical study. *Spine* 19:586-595, 1994.
18. Dvorak J, Antinnes J, Panjabi M, et al: Age and gender related normal motion of the cervical spine. *Spine* 17(Suppl):393-398, 1992.
19. Dvorak J, Panjabi M, Novotny J, Antinnes J: In vivo flexion/extension of normal cervical spine. *J Orthop Res* 9:828-834, 1991.
20. Einkauf D, Gohdes M, Jensen G, Jewell M: Changes in spinal mobility with increasing age in women. *Phys Ther* 67:370-375, 1987.
21. Elveru R, Rothstein J, Lamb R: Goniometric reliability in a clinical setting: subtalar and ankle joint measurements. *Phys Ther* 68:672-677, 1988.
22. Fitzgerald G, Wynveen K, Rheault W, et al: Objective assessment with establishment of normal values for lumbar spinal range of motion. *Phys Ther* 63:1776-1781, 1983.
23. Forero N, Okamura L, Larson M: Normal ranges of hip motion in neonates. *J Pediatr Orthop* 9:391-395, 1989.
24. Gajdosik R, Bohannon R: Clinical measurement of range of motion: review of goniometry emphasizing reliability and validity. *Phys Ther* 67:1867-1872, 1987.
25. Gerhardt J: *Documentation of joint motion*, ed 3 (rev), Portland, 1992, Oregon Medical Association.
26. Gill K, Krag M, Johnson G, et al: Repeatability of four clinical methods for assessment of lumbar spinal motion, *Spine* 13:50-53, 1988.
27. Greene W, Heckman J: *The clinical measurement of joint motion*, Chicago, 1994, American Academy of Orthopaedic Surgeons.

28. Hamilton G, Lachenbruch P: Reliability of goniometers in assessing finger joint angle. *Phys Ther* 49:465-469, 1986.

29. Hart D, Rose S: Reliability of a noninvasive method for measuring the lumbar curve. *J Orthop Sports Phys Ther* 8:180-184, 1986.

30. Hoffer M: Joint motion limitation in newborns. *Clin Orthop* 148:94-96, 1980.

31. Johnson R, Babbitt D: Five states of joint disintegration compared with range of motion in hemophilia. *Clin Orthop* 201:36-42, 1985.

32. Keeley J, Mayer T, Cox R, et al: Quantification of lumbar function 5: reliability of range-of-motion measures in sagittal plane and in vivo torso rotation measurement techniques. *Spine* 11:31-35, 1986.

33. Kohles S, Barnes D, Gatchel R, Mayer T: Improved physical performance outcomes following functional restoration treatment in patient with chronic low-back pain: early versus recent training results. *Spine* 15:1321-1324, 1990.

34. Loebl W: Measurements of spinal posture and range in spinal movements. *Ann Phys Med* 9:103, 1967.

35. Lowery W, Horn T, Boden S, Wiesel S: Impairment evaluation based on spinal range of motion in normal subjects. *J Spinal Dis* 5:398-402, 1992.

36. MacRae I, Wright V: Measurement of back movement. *Ann Rheum Dis* 28:584-589, 1969.

37. Mallon W, Brown H, Nunley J: Digital ranges of motion: normal values in young adults. *J Hand Surg* 73A:882-887, 1991.

38. Mayer T, Brady S, Bovasso E, et al: Noninvasive measurement of cervical triplanar motion in normal subjects. *Spine* 18:2191-2195, 1993.

39. Mayer T, Dowdle J: Impairment/disability evaluation. *Am Assoc Orthop Surg Bull* 40(2):12-13, 1992.

40. Mayer T, Gatchel R, Keeley J, et al: A male incumbent worker industrial database. Part I—Lumbar spinal physical capacity. *Spine* 19:755-761, 1994.

41. Mayer T, Gatchel R, Keeley J, et al: A male incumbent worker industrial database. Part II—Cervical spinal physical capacity. *Spine* 19:762-764, 1994.

42. Mayer T, Mooney V, Gatchel R: *Contemporary conservative care for painful spinal disorders: concepts, diagnosis and treatment,* Philadelphia, 1991, Waverly Press.

43. Mayer T, Pope P, Tabor J, et al: Physical progress and residual impairment quantification after functional restoration. Part I—Lumbar mobility, *Spine* 18:389-394, 1994.

44. Mayer T, Tencer A, Kristoferson S, Mooney V: Use of noninvasive techniques for quantification of spinal range-of-motion in normal subjects and chronic low-back dysfunction patients. *Spine* 9:588-595, 1984.

45. Mellin G: Method and instrument for noninvasive measurements of thoracolumbar rotation. *Spine* 12:28-31, 1987.

46. Miller S, Mayer T, Cox R, Gatchel R: Reliability problems associated with the modified Schober technique for true lumbar flexion measurement. *Spine* 17:345-348, 1992.

47. Moll J, Wright V: Normal range of spinal mobility. *Ann Rheum Dis* 30:381-386, 1971.

48. Morrey B, Askew L, Chao E: A biomechanical study of normal functional elbow motion. *J Bone Joint Surg* 63A:872-877, 1988.

49. Paquet N, Malouin F, Richards C, et al: Validity and reliability of a new electrogoniometer for the measurement of sagittal dorsolumbar movements. *Spine* 16:516-519, 1991.

50. Pearcy M: Measurement of back and spinal mobility. *Clin Biomech* 1:44-51, 1986.

51. Pearcy M, Portek I, Sheperd J: The effect of low-back pain on lumbar spine movements measured by three dimensional x-ray analysis. *Spine* 10:150-153, 1985.

52. Petherick M, Rheault W, Kimble S, et al: Concurrent validity and intertester reliability of universal and fluid-based goniometers for active elbow range of motion. *Phys Ther* 68:966-969, 1988.

53. Portek I, Pearcy M, Reader G, et al: Correlation between radiologic and clinical measurement of lumbar spine movement. *Br J Rheumatol* 22:197-205, 1983.

54. Reid D, Burnham R, Saboe L, et al: Lower extremity flexibility patterns in classical ballet dancers and their correlation to lateral hip and knee injuries. *Am J Sports Med* 15:347-352, 1987.

55. Reynolds P: A measurement of spinal mobility: a comparison of three methods. *Rheumatol Rehab* 14:180-185, 1975.

56. Rheault W, Miller M, Nothnagel P, et al: Intertester reliability and concurrent validity of fluid-based and universal goniometers for active knee flexion. *Phys Ther* 78:1676-1678, 1988.

57. Riddle D, Rothstein J, Lamb R: Goniometric reliability in a clinical setting: shoulder measurements. *Phys Ther* 67:688-693, 1987.

58. Roaas A, Andersson G: Normal range of motion of the hip, knee and ankle joints in male subjects, 30-40 years of age. *Acta Orthop Scand* 53:205-208, 1982.

59. Roach K, Miles T: Normal hip and knee active range of motion: the relationship to age. *Phys Ther* 71:656-665, 1991.

60. Rothstein J, Miller P, Roettger R: Goniometric reliability in a clinical setting: elbow and knee measurements. *Phys Ther* 63:1611-1615, 1983.

61. Ryu J, Cooney W, Askew L, et al: Functional range of motion of the wrist joint. *J Hand Surg* 16A:409-419, 1991.

62. Salisbury P, Porter R: Measurement of lumbar sagittal mobility; a comparison of methods. *Spine* 12:190-193, 1987.

63. Shirley F, O'Connor P, Robinson M, MacMillan M: Comparison of lumbar range of motion using three measurement devices in patients with chronic low back pain. *Spine* 19:779-783, 1994.

64. Spiegel T, Spiegel J, Paulus H: The joint alignment and motion scale: a simple measure of joint deformity in patients with rheumatoid arthritis. *J Rheumatol* 14:887-892, 1987.

65. Stokes I, Wilder D, Frymoyer J, Pope M: Assessment of patients with low-back pain by biplanar radiographic measurements of intervertebral motion. *Spine* 6:233-240, 1980.

66. Sullivan M, Dickinson C, Troup J: The influence of age and gender on lumbar spine sagittal plane range of motion: a study of 1126 healthy subjects. *Spine* 19:682-686, 1994.

67. Svenningsen S, Terjesen T, Auflem M, et al: Hip motion related to age and sex. *Acta Orthop Scand* 60:97-100, 1980.

68. Swanson A, Goran-Hagert C, de-Groot-Swanson G: Evaluation of impairment in the upper extremity. *J Hand Surg* 12A:896-926, 1987.

69. Troup J, Hood C, Chapman A: Measurements of sagittal mobility of the lumbar spine and hips. *Ann Phys Med* 9:308-313, 1968.

70. Twomey L, Taylor J: Age changes in the lumbar articular triad. *Aust J Physiother* 31:106-112, 1985.

71. Waddell G, Somerville D, Henderson I, et al: Objective clinical evaluation of physical impairment in chronic low-back pain. *Spine* 17:617-628, 1992.

72. Whittle M: Calibration and performance of a three-dimensional television system for kinematic analysis. *J Biomech* 15:185-196, 1982.

73. Williams R, Binkley J, Bloch R, et al: Reliability of the modified-modified Schober and double inclinometer methods for measuring lumbar flexion and extension. *Phys Ther* 73:26-36, 1993.

74. Wynne-Davies R: Familial joint laxity. *Proc Royal Soc Med* 64:689-690, 1971.

75. Youdas J, Carey J, Garrett T: Reliability of measurements of cervical spine range of motion—comparison of three methods. *Phys Ther* 71:98-106, 1991.

76. Zaki A, Goldberg M, Khalil T, et al: Comparison between the one and two inclinometer techniques for measuring body ranges of motion using the Orthoranger II. In Das, B, editor: *Advances in industrial ergonomics and safety II,* 1990:135-142, New York: Taylor & Francis.

# CHAPTER 15

## THE ROLE OF RADIOLOGIC IMAGING IN IMPAIRMENT EVALUATION

*Richard J. Herzog*
*J. Bruce Kneeland*

During the course of the evaluation of patients who have acute, subacute, or chronic injuries, which limits their occupational capacity or activities of daily living, a clinician will frequently order diagnostic tests to determine if there is objective evidence of tissue dysfunction. Since injuries to the musculoskeletal system are a frequent cause of impairment, it is important for the clinician working with these patients to understand the efficacy of the diagnostic tests that are available to assess these clinical problems. Radiologic imaging studies have been heavily utilized to document objective pathologic changes in the musculoskeletal system, but to use these tests effectively it is necessary to understand their strengths and limitations. The efficacy of these tests is not only affected by the quality of the study but by the expertise of the individual who interprets the examination. The additional data provided by these tests only become useful clinical information when integrated with the patient's history, physical examination, and other diagnostic tests.

The radiologic studies that are frequently ordered in the evaluation of the musculoskeletal disability include standard plain films, magnetic resonance imaging (MRI), radionuclide studies, ultrasound (US), and computed tomography (CT). This chapter will focus on the application of plain films, MRI, US, and CT in impairment evaluation. Both plain films and CT have played a major role in the detection of osseous abnormalities in the body, while MRI has been particularly useful in the assessment of soft tissue injury (e.g., cartilage, muscles, tendons, and ligaments). In addition, MRI is particularly sensitive to detect abnormalities of cancellous bone. The application of US is limited to the assessment of superficial soft tissue structures. A basic understanding of the physics and the technical factors involved in these different modalities is needed in order to facilitate the selection of the appropriate imaging modality for different diagnostic problems.

## PHYSICS AND TECHNICAL FACTORS OF RADIOLOGIC STUDIES

The musculoskeletal system has long been studied with plain film radiographs. In fact the first anatomic images ever taken by Roentgen were of the human hand. Radiographs are projection images in which the contrast arises from the differential attenuation (i.e., scattering and absorption of x-rays by different structures). This type of image demonstrates the anatomy of the cortical and cancellous bone at high resolution, as well as the abnormalities that affect them. The visualization of bony detail results from the strong attenuation of the x-ray beam by calcified structures. Metallic appliances and clips used for surgical procedures on the musculoskeletal system attenuate x-rays even more effectively than calcium and are also well seen. The capacity of this technique to demonstrate abnormalities in the soft tissues of the musculoskeletal system is exceedingly limited due to small differences in attenuation by different soft tissues. Soft tissue abnormalities may be detected as a vague increase in density due to replacement of fat by water-density structures, distortion of the surface contour, and the presence of calcifications or gas. Plain films are inexpensive and readily available. They do, however, carry the small but finite risks associated with the use of any ionizing radiation, in particular, the induction of neoplasms.[43,219,251]

Computed tomography (CT) utilizes x-rays to generate cross-sectional images in which the intensity is proportional to the degree of attenuation of the x-ray beam. As with plain films, the strong scattering of x-rays by the calcium permits a relatively detailed visualization of bony detail in cross-section. In contradistinction to plain films, the extremely pronounced attenuation of the x-ray beam by metallic appliances gives rise to streak artifacts that can obscure large parts of the image. CT gives more detailed information regarding the soft tissues than do plain films, although it is still limited by the relatively small differences in x-ray scattering present among different soft tissues. Differences in soft tissue attenuation can in many cases be increased by the intravenous administration of iodine-containing contrast agents. Iodine strongly attenuates x-rays, and differences in delivery of the contrast agent to a given region (e.g., due to differences in perfusion of the tissues or permeability of the vessels) can result in differences in attenuation of the x-rays that are detectable by CT. The planes of section that can be imaged with CT are limited by both the physical geometry of the gantry and the constraints of patient positioning within the gantry, although there is clearly more flexibility in positioning the extremities than the chest or abdomen. CT also poses the previously noted small but finite risks associated with ionizing radiation.[89]

Ultrasound forms images by transmitting pulses of high frequency sound and detecting the reflected pulses. The images so formed are dependent on both the strength of the reflected wave as well as the distance traveled by the reflected wave. Sound waves do not penetrate the bones and cannot be used to evaluate these structures. They can, however, demonstrate the morphology of the soft tissues of the more superficial soft tissues of the musculoskeletal system. Ultrasound is widely available, relatively inexpensive, and is believed to be completely safe. Ultrasound of the musculoskeletal system, however, although reported to be successful in the hands of some investigators, is technically demanding and has not gained widespread acceptance.[192]

Radionuclide bone scanning, which is usually performed with Tc-99m MDP, provides low resolution projection images, or with the use of single photon emission computed tomography (SPECT), cross-sectional images of the skeletal system. The degree of uptake at a given location is proportional to the blood flow and to the amount of new bone formation. The bone scan is exquisitely sensitive to the presence of any process that increases the amount of new bone formation such as neoplasm, trauma, or osteoarthritic hyperostosis. Its sensitivity to all of these diseases, however, renders it nonspecific as to the nature of the disease present in any given case.[36, 172]

Magnetic resonance imaging is a method of forming cross-sectional images of the body that uses the magnetic properties of the hydrogen nuclei of "mobile" water molecules. Mobile water molecules are those molecules that are not tightly bound to macromolecules. In order to create MR images the subject must first be placed in a strong static magnetic field. This induces a difference in the energy levels of the hydrogen nuclei whose magnetic moments are pointed in the direction of the static field and those

that are pointed in the opposed direction. Transitions between these levels are then induced by irradiating the nuclei with an additional magnetic field that is oscillating at the "resonant" frequency of the hydrogen nucleus. As the excited nuclei return to their original state they emit a brief pulse of energy. This emitted pulse can be detected and constitutes the MR signal. Spatial localization of the MR signal is achieved by superimposing on the strong static magnetic field a relatively weak magnetic field with a known spatial variation called a gradient field. The characteristic "banging" noise associated with MRI results from turning these gradient fields off and on. The signal intensity in MRI arises from the number of mobile water nuclei present per unit of tissue volume and, more importantly, from properties of the nuclei called the *T1 and T2 relaxation times*. These latter two quantities characterize the rate of recovery of the nuclei from the excited to the unexcited states (T1) and the decay of the MR signal (T2). It is the relaxation times that are altered from their normal values by the presence of disease. The precise method used to excite the nuclei determines whether the signal intensity and hence the image contrast are more dependent on differences in T1 (T1-weighted) or on differences in T2 (T2-weighted) among the different tissues. The soft tissue contrast afforded by differences in relaxation times is far greater than the differences seen in the attenuation of x-rays that determines contrast in CT, and for this reason the contrast between normal and abnormal tissue seen with MR imaging is generally much greater. Intravenous contrast agents are used in MR imaging to further enhance contrast. MR contrast agents produce their result by shortening the T1 relaxation times and, as with the CT contrast agents, alter the contrast to different regions based on differences in vascular perfusion or permeability. Another strength of MRI resides in its direct multiplanar capabilities. CT is limited to obtaining scans only in the plane of the gantry. Any additional multiplanar CT images are constructed by a computer algorithm that results in some loss of image detail.[29]

MRI is generally safe for subjects, although certain patients are at risk and must not be imaged. These include patients with cardiac pacemakers, neurostimulatory devices, certain types of intracranial aneurysm clips, radiographically visible metallic fragments within the orbits or spinal canal, and patients with certain types of prostheses. While MRI probably provides the greatest amount of information compared to other radiologic imaging techniques, it is also the most expensive and probably the most complex method of imaging available.[210]

## SPINAL DYSFUNCTION

### Radiographic Abnormalities with Chronic Pain

Since back pain is the second leading cause of work absenteeism, and is the number one cause of workers' compensation claims, it is important to understand the appropriate role of radiologic imaging in the assessment of spinal dysfunction. The goal of any imaging study is to define accurately the pathomorphologic changes in a specific tissue, organ, or part of the body. Objective categorization of pathologic changes facilitates the interpretation and communication of abnormalities detected on a test, and these same criteria can be used on follow-up evaluation to assess the effects of different forms of therapy (e.g., surgical intervention or nonoperative rehabilitation). The reproducibility and the reliability of all objective diagnostic criteria must be rigorously evaluated in prospective blinded studies prior to their implementation.[30,206,212,255]

Patients with neck or low-back pain (LBP) are a challenge to the physician who desires a precise pathoanatomic diagnosis prior to the initiation of therapy. Back pain and neural dysfunction are a frequent symptom complex for many processes afflicting the lumbar spine and paraspinal tissues. For this reason, a clinician assessing a patient after a work-related injury must consider and exclude a large number of potential causes to explain a patient's symptoms. Fortunately, most episodes of back pain are self-limited, and no diagnostic tests are needed. However, if pain persists or becomes worse, it is usually necessary to order a diagnostic test to provide the additional clinical information needed to choose rationally the appropriate therapeutic modality. Prior to ordering any diagnostic test, a clinician must determine how the information provided by the test will affect patient management and mentally compare projected test costs and expected benefits. The more precise the information provided by a diagnostic test, the greater will be its impact on directing patient care. The value of different tests depends on their sensitivity, specificity, accuracy, risk, cost, and availability.

Prior to 1970, plain film radiography was the primary radiologic study available to evaluate patients with neck or back pain. Plain films provide direct information only on the morphology of the osseous components of the spinal motion segments (i.e., the vertebral bodies and the facet joints at each disc level). Any pathologic process that precipitates osseous destruction, degeneration, or remodeling can be detected on plain films if a sufficient amount of bone is affected by the pathologic process. When a worker has symptoms of acute or chronic low-back pain and/or sciatica, disc disease and/or spinal stenosis must be excluded as a potential cause of the worker's symptomatology. Plain film findings that are indicative of disc degeneration include decreased disc height, a disc vacuum phenomenon, end-plate ridges and sclerosis, and a degenerative olisthesis (Fig. 15-1). Unfortunately these changes occur relatively late in the natural history of disc degeneration and most of them represent adaptive changes of the bone to the abnormal biomechanics of a degenerating disc. The only plain film findings indicative of an acute disc herniation would include an acute Schmorl's node, displacement of calcified disc material, or a limbus vertebra (i.e., a fractured vertebral body rim secondary to displaced disc material). But to determine that these represent an acute finding, a prior set of normal spine radiographs would be needed.

In order to determine the value of plain radiographs in the work-up of back or radicular pain, it is necessary to know the spectrum of findings detected on plain films of asymptomatic patients. Frymoyer et al[68] evaluated the plain films of 292 subjects, including 96 with no history of back pain, 134 subjects with a history of previous or current moderate back pain, and 62 subjects with a history of prior or current severe back pain. In the three groups the frequency of transitional vertebrae, Schmorl's nodes, disc vacuum phenomenon, "claw" spurs, and disc space narrowing at the L3-4 and L5-S1 disc levels, were similar. Traction spurs or disc space narrowing at the L4-5 level had a positive correlation to severe low-back pain. Only end-plate spurs increased in incidence with aging. Spurs and disc narrowing had no correlation with occupation. Dabbs et al[44] evaluated disc height on the plain films obtained on 51 asymptomatic and 86 symptomatic subjects. Both groups of patients had evidence of decreased disc height and there was no significant difference between the two groups. Witt et al[254] also compared the plain film findings in patients with and without back pain. There was no difference in the prevalence of disc degeneration or spondylosis comparing the 238 patients with LBP and sciatica to 68 asymptomatic patients. The incidence of both disc degeneration and spondylosis increased with age in the two groups.

In contrast to the studies that have demonstrated limited value of plain films in the assessment of patients with LBP, Torgerson et al[228] evaluated 217 asymptomatic patients between the ages of 40 and 70, and 387 symptomatic patients in the same age range. Fifty-six percent of the symptomatic patients had plain film evidence of disc degeneration compared to 22% of the asymptomatic patients. Even though this difference may be significant, the findings of disc degeneration lack specificity to explain symptomatology

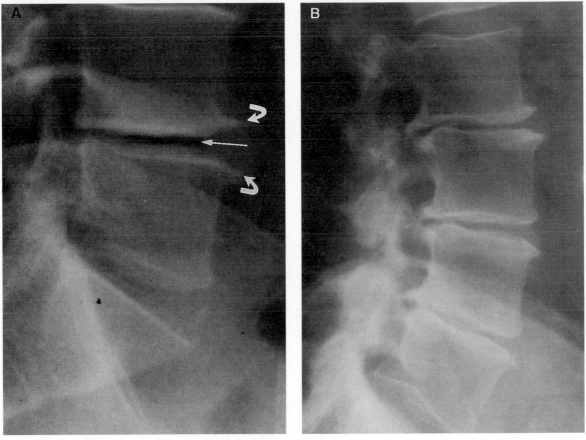

**FIGURE 15-1**    On the spot lateral radiograph of the lumbosacral junction **(A)** at the L4-5 disc level there is decreased disc height, a disc vacuum phenomenon (*straight arrow*), anterior end-plate ridges (*curved arrows*), and end-plate sclerosis. On the full lateral radiograph of another patient **(B)** there is evidence of multilevel disc degeneration with decreased disc height, both anterior and posterior end-plate ridges, end-plate sclerosis, and a minimal retrolisthesis at the L2-3 disc level.

considering their common occurrence in both the symptomatic and the asymptomatic groups. Torgerson et al also found a higher incidence of spondylolysis and spondylolisthesis in the symptomatic patients. In addition, they reported that osteophyte formation had no direct correlation to back pain.

Considering the increasing age of the work force, it is important to determine the value of plain films in the older patient population. Biering-Sorensen et al[15] reported on the plain films findings of 666 60-year-old men and women taking part in a general population survey. Evidence of disc degeneration was significantly more common in individuals reporting low-back pain compared to those without pain. L4-5 disc degeneration was the only radiologic abnormality correlated to work absence due to LBP. The authors calculated the predictive value of a positive or negative finding of L4-5 disc degeneration in relation to LBP within the last ten years. The predictive value of a positive finding was 64% and the predictive value of no disc degeneration was 49%, clearly indicating the limited value of the radiologic findings.

When comparing the data from studies reporting on patients with back or neck pain, the precise characteristics of the cohort group must be specified (e.g., physical condition, social and work history, and psychological status if relevant). The value of plain film studies also depends on the reliability of the interpretation of the spine radiographs. Coste et al[40] have reported on the variability of the interpretations by rheumatologists who were assessing spinal plain films obtained on patients with benign LBP. A significant variability of interpretation was observed for findings considered by the author to be important in the assessment of patients with LBP. There were low levels of agreement in the diagnosis of Schmorl's nodes, apophyseal joint abnormalities, spondylolysis, and structural deviations. The highest levels of interobserver agreement were for the detection of disc abnormalities. The authors concluded that better standardized criteria are needed to improve the reliability of plain film interpretation of the spine. Andersson et al[5] reported on the influence of spinal motion segment orientation and reader variability in the measurement of disc height. Three orthopaedic surgeons and three radiologists, using the same measurement criteria, assessed disc height on lateral spinal radiographs. Differences of up to 50% of the nominal disc height were observed between different readers. Spinal orientation also affected the accuracy of the measurements, and the authors concluded that accurate measurements cannot readily be made on routine spine radiographs.

Considering the limitations of spinal radiographs in the assessment of patients with LBP, in what clinical situations are they indicated? Liang et al[135] performed a cost-effective analysis of plain films in the assessment of primary-care patients with back pain. The cohort group included patients aged from 18 to 60 with acute low-back pain, but no symptoms or signs suggesting serious disease (e.g., cancer or infection). The authors concluded that the risks and costs of obtaining lumbar x-rays at the initial patient visit compared to performing x-rays eight weeks later for patients with persistent symptoms did not seem to justify the relatively small associated benefit of an earlier x-ray examination. This was based on the assumption that the probability of diseases requiring specific therapy was 0.2% in this patient population. The probability of disease may be different in referral practices. Deyo et al[50] also assessed the value of lumbar spine films in a primary-care facility. They developed a selective group of indications for ordering early radiographs that included age greater than 50, significant trauma, neuromotor deficits, unexplained weight loss, suspicion of ankylosing spondylitis, drug or alcohol abuse, history of cancer, use of corticosteroids, temperature greater than 100°F, recent visit for same problem that has not improved, and patients seeking compensation for back pain. Using these criteria, 40% of 227 patients presenting with one of these indications had x-ray findings that could explain their symptoms compared to 12% of the patients who lacked these indications. The indication with the highest diagnostic yield was age greater than 50. While their data support the safety and value of applying selective x-ray ordering criteria, it is apparent that their indications are limited to patients presenting to a primary-care facility and not for impairment evaluation.

When a patient presenting with back or leg pain requires further diagnostic evaluation, the question arises as to what constitutes a complete radiologic study, where should it be performed, and who should provide the diagnostic interpretation of the study. Even with its limited sensitivity and specificity, plain film radiography should be the initial screening exam when radiologic evaluation is indicated. Scavone et al[201] attempted to determine what constitutes an adequate lumbar spine examination. They evaluated 993 radiographic studies performed on 782 patients presenting with a variety of problems. Anteroposterior (AP), lateral, oblique, and spot lateral radiographs constituted the standard study for all patients. The authors initially interpreted only the AP and lateral radiographs on each patient. This was followed by an evaluation utilizing all five radiographs. In 97.9%, the diagnoses could be made using only the AP and lateral radiographs. In 2.4% of the patients the diagnoses were missed. The 19 missed diagnoses included unilateral spondylolysis (68%), bilateral spondylolysis (26%), and a congenital anomaly (5%). The value of oblique radiographs focuses on the evaluation of the pars interarticularis and the facet joints. The authors found that while the oblique views provided the best evaluation of the facet joints, the degenerative changes of the facets could also be seen on the AP and lateral radiographs. The additional information obtained on the oblique views concerning facet degenerative changes did not change patient diagnosis or therapy. The authors concluded that the oblique views should be obtained if there is a questionable abnormality on the AP and lateral views, and possibly in the evaluation of patients with major trauma. The limited x-ray study (i.e., the AP and lateral radiographs) was also appropriate for the evaluation of patients with chronic symptoms.

In addition to the utilization of spinal radiographs for evaluation of patients with acute and chronic back or leg pain, radiographs have also been used as part of the preemployment evaluation to screen job applicants. Bigos et al[16] reported on the value of preemployment x-rays for predicting acute and chronic back injury claims. The prevalence of spina bifida occulta, spondylolysis, spondylolisthesis, transitional vertebrae, Scheuermann's disease, facet tropism, straightening of the lumbar spine, or evidence of degenerative disc disease was determined. The radiographic study included full AP and lateral views of the spine, along with a spot lateral view of the lumbosacral junction. The data indicated that the radiographs were not helpful in predicting who is more likely to make a back claim injury, or to detect the worker who becomes disabled for more than six months. The authors concluded that the radiation exposure is not justified due to the limited predictive value of the preemployment screening radiographs.

The diagnostic value of any imaging study is highly dependent on the quality of the examination. Rueter et al[196] reported on the quality of radiography of the lumbar spine performed in hospitals and other facilities. A critical factor affecting the quality of a radiograph is film processing. If film is underprocessed, then additional x-ray exposure to the patient would be needed to achieve the same density on a film that has been processed normally. Underprocessing also degrades image quality. The authors found that 33% of hospitals, 25% of radiology facilities, and 48% of chiropractic facilities underprocessed lumbosacral spine radiographs. It is evident from this report that there is currently a need to improve the quality of radiographic studies at all facilities performing routine spinal x-rays. This is important considering that the quality of spinal radiographs directly affects the accuracy of x-ray interpretation. Shaffer et al[209] conducted a series of experiments to assess the consistency and the accuracy of sagittal translation measurements from x-rays of varying quality. The authors found that high-quality radiographs were more accurately evaluated than the lower-quality exams. They also demonstrated a high false-positive and false-negative rate using different methods of measurement in the experimental setting, along with inconsistencies in the interpretations of the clinical flexion-extension studies.

While neck pain is not as frequent as back or leg pain as a cause for worker disability claims, it is frequently the symptom of patients experiencing spinal pain after a vehicular injury or a fall. Workers performing overhead activities or who carry loads that may strain the neck muscles may also have debilitating neck or arm pain. There is little question on the value of radiographs as the initial screening exam to detect fractures or malalignment in patients who have experienced major neck trauma (Fig. 15-2). Their value in the assessment of patients with minor trauma or with chronic neck symptoms is less clear. To assess the efficacy of cervical x-rays it is first necessary to determine their accuracy and then to compare the findings on plain films obtained on asymptomatic and symptomatic patients.

Friedenberg et al[65] correlated the findings observed on radiographs of a cadaveric cervical spine to the anatomic findings. Anteroposterior, lateral, and oblique views of the cervical spine were performed prior to dissection. They found a 67% correlation between the radiographic and the anatomic manifestations of disc degeneration. Disc space narrowing was the most common x-ray finding and even minor narrowing of the disc space on the x-ray correlated to anatomic disc degeneration. Posterior osteophytes were most easily seen on the oblique projections, and they were always associated with disc space narrowing. Only 57% of large posterior osteophytes detected on dissection were identified on the spinal radiographs. Evaluation of the apophyseal joints was difficult on the radiographs and only 32% of the anatomic abnormalities were identified on the radiographs. It is evident that cervical spine radiographs,

like lumbar radiographs, lack sensitivity in the detection of early degenerative changes, but they are very specific for degenerative disease once they become positive.

The radiographic findings of the cervical spine in asymptomatic patients were reported by Gore et al.[75] They evaluated the incidence and severity of degenerative changes of the cervical spine on lateral radiographs obtained on 200 asymptomatic men and women. Age correlated significantly to the severity of disc space narrowing, end-plate sclerosis, anterior and posterior osteophytes, and the degree of lordosis. The severity of each type of degenerative change correlated with severity of the other types of degeneration at the same disc level. By the age of 40, 35% of the individuals had evidence of degenerative changes and this increased to 83% by the age of sixty. In the older age groups, evidence of disc degeneration was more prevalent in men compared to women.

Friedenberg et al[66] compared the findings of radiographs performed on 92 asymptomatic and symptomatic patients. Degenerative changes were most common at the C5-6 and the C6-7 disc levels in both groups. Sixty-two percent of the symptomatic patients had changes at the C5-6 level, compared to 35% of the asymptomatic individuals. This difference was statistically significant. Similar to the findings by Gore,[75] degenerative changes in the cervical spine increased with age in the asymptomatic individuals. Comparing the two groups with respect to foraminal stenosis and facet arthrosis demonstrated no significant difference in the severity of the degenerative changes. The authors concluded that the value of cervical spine radiographs in determining the clinical significance of degenerative disease of the spine was limited, and at best, radiographs could provide information on the severity of the degenerative process.

Gore et al[76] evaluated the predictive value of cervical radiographs to detect patients who may develop chronic neck pain after the onset of cervical symptoms. Two hundred five patients with neck pain were followed clinically for a minimum of 10 years after the onset of symptoms. Thirty-two percent of the patients had moderate or severe neck pain on follow-up evaluation. The only clinical feature that was of value to predict outcome was a history of an injury associated with severe neck pain. The presence or severity of the pain was not correlated to the degree of degenerative changes, the sagittal spinal canal diameter, the degree of cervical lordosis, or to any changes in these measurements detected on spine radiographs during the follow-up period. At the time of the initial evaluation, 57% of the patients with injuries and 42% of the patients without injuries had normal cervical x-rays. The authors also compared the radiographic

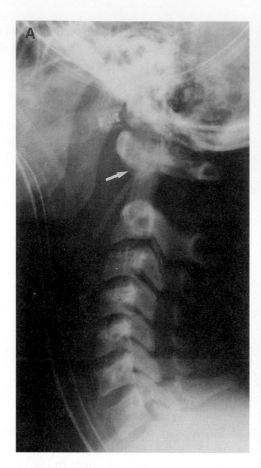

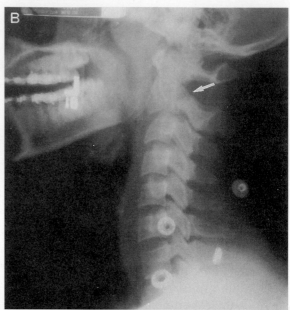

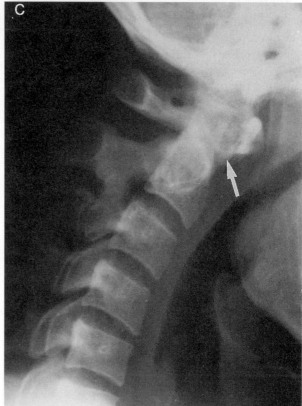

**FIGURE 15-2**    On the lateral radiograph of a patient in a motor vehicle accident **(A)** there is marked distraction and anterior subluxation at the C1-2 motion segment (*arrow*). On another patient **(B)**, who experienced an extension injury, there is a fracture of the posterior arch of C2 (*arrow*). The flexion lateral radiograph on a third patient **(C)**, who was injured in a football game, demonstrates instability at the C1-2 motion segment with increased space between the anterior arch of C1 and the odontoid process (*arrow*).

findings between these symptomatic patients and a group of age matched asymptomatic patients. They found that anterior osteophyte formation was the only degenerative change that was present more frequently in the symptomatic patients who were over the age of 35 and had a history of neck injuries. The authors concluded that the treating physician must

be cautious in making a prediction of final outcome based on the findings of cervical radiographs.

With the cross-sectional imaging capabilities of both CT/MPR and MRI it is possible to evaluate the paraspinal musculature in patients presenting with back pain. Alaranta et al[3] recently evaluated the fat content of lumbar extensor muscles in patients with disabling low-back pain. They found a positive correlation between the fat content of the lower lumbar paraspinal muscles and the severity of self-reported disability in men. It is not possible from their study to determine if the muscle atrophy was the cause or the result of back pain. The possibility of paraspinal muscle compartment syndromes as a potential etiology of back pain has also been reported and both CT[34a] and MRI[52] were used to document edematous changes with the muscles.

## Degenerative Spinal Disease

Plain films provide a global assessment of the severity of degenerative spinal disease, but they are extremely limited in determining the precise location of a pathologic process to explain a patient's symptoms. With the development and implementation of cross-sectional imaging studies (e.g., MRI and CT with multiplanar reconstructions [CT/MPR]), it became possible to evaluate directly the soft tissue and osseous components of each spinal motion segment. Degenerative disc disease, which includes the osseous adaptive changes induced by the biomechanically abnormal disc, is probably the most common etiology of back or leg pain, when a precise etiology can be defined. Kirkaldy-Willis[120] was one of the first investigators who stressed the importance of the progressive nature of disc degeneration and herniation.

Degenerative spinal disease is a continuous subclinical process that frequently does not cause symptoms. Abnormalities detected on CT or MRI studies on asymptomatic individuals[21,23] do not represent false positive findings, but actual structural or pathologic changes of spinal structures that are not evoking symptoms and therefore not clinically important. In other words, the significance of these morphologic changes can only be determined by correlating the test results to the patient's symptoms. Both CT/MPR and MRI provide excellent delineation of morphologic changes of disc degeneration. The major difference between the imaging modalities resides in the ability of MRI to delineate pathoanatomic and physiochemical changes in a degenerating disc prior to alterations of disc contour. Both the nucleus pulposus and annulus fibrosus consist of water, collagen, and proteoglycans, with the major differences between the two being the relative amount of these components, level of hydration, and the particular type of collagen that predominates.[71] With MRI, it is possible to delineate different parts of disc architecture. On T2-weighted images, the high signal intensity in the central position of the disc originates from both the nucleus pulposus and the inner annular fibers.[259] The outer annular fibers demonstrate very low signal intensity, as do the adjacent anterior and posterior longitudinal ligaments[175] (Fig. 15-3). The signal intensity in the disc is related to its state of hydration and the physicochemical state of the disc's tissue.[72,92] With aging, there is gradual breakdown of proteoglycans in the nucleus, gradual desiccation of the mucoid nuclear material, and loss of anatomic delineation between the nucleus and inner annular fibers.[146] Over the age of 30, an intranuclear cleft, which represents ingrowth of fibrous tissue,[2] can be identified in normal discs on T2-weighted MR images.

Both experimentally and clinically, the occurrence of a radial annular tear may be a step in the development of disc degeneration and herniation.[136,260] It is now possible with MRI to delineate small tears in the outer annulus with T2-weighted[260] or gadolinium-DTPA (Gd-DTPA) enhanced T1-weighted images[193] (Fig. 15-4). Annular tears may be present in the periphery of a disc and not communicate with the nucleus pulposus. These tears have been referred to as rim tears and occur at the insertion site of the outer annular fibers into the vertebral body end-plates.[171] Osti et al[170] reported on the possible significance of these peripheral tears as a source of acute back pain. As a disc ages, there may be coalescence of these peripheral tears and delamination of the annular fibers. This may precipitate a generalized bulge of the disc contour due to the loss of the tensile strength of the outer segment of the disc.

If a radial tear develops and communicates with the nucleus pulposus, the disc will begin to degenerate and demonstrate decreased signal intensity on T2-weighted images. Disc herniations result from the displacement of nuclear, annular, or end-plate material through these communicating radial tears. Displacement of the disc material into the region of the outer annular-posterior longitudinal ligament complex will cause altered morphology of the periphery of the disc, resulting in a focal protrusion of the disc beyond the margin of the vertebral body endplates. A contained disc herniation represents displaced discal material that is still bound by the outer annular fibers and/or the posterior longitudinal ligament. Both CT/MPR and MRI provide excellent delineation of these contour changes[111,252] (Fig. 15-5).

In some patients, the development of annular fissures may lead to internal disc disruption[19] or intervertebral disc resorption[105] without the displacement of discal material. MRI is helpful in the evaluation of these patients because it demonstrates altered signal intensity in the abnormal disc. Unfortunately, it is relatively common to detect discs with decreased signal intensity in patients who are totally asympto-

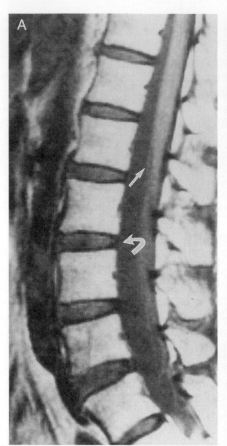

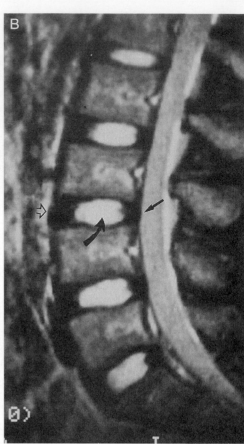

**FIGURE 15-3** On the sagittal T1-weighted image of the lumbar spine **(A)** there is excellent delineation of the conus medullaris (*straight arrow*). The intervertebral disc space is well delineated, but the posterior margin of the disc is not well defined due to the similar signal intensity of the posterior outer annular fibers and the adjacent cerebrospinal fluid (*curved arrow*). On the sagittal T2-weighted image **(B)** there is increased signal intensity in the cerebrospinal fluid and excellent delineation of the posterior margin of the disc (*straight arrow*). There is increased signal intensity within the central portion of the disc (*curved arrow*) that represents a combination of the nucleus pulposus and the inner annular fibers. The anterior annular fibers (*open arrowhead*) are also delineated. (From *Physical Medicine and Rehabilitation: State-of-the-Art Reviews,* Vol. 4, No. 2, Hanley & Belfus, Inc., June 1990.)

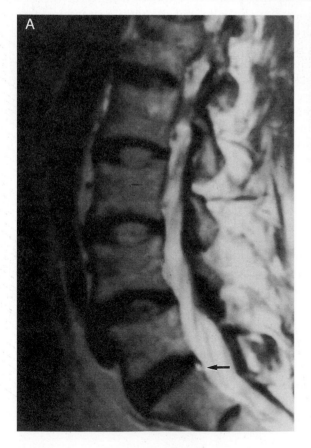

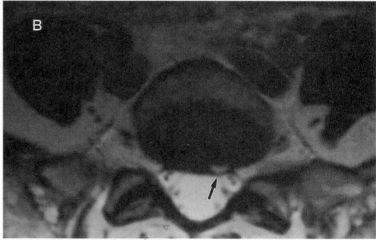

**FIGURE 15-4** On the spin-echo T2-weighted sagittal **(A)** and axial **(B)** images there is a small focus of high signal intensity in the outer annular fibers (*arrow*) representing a small annular tear.

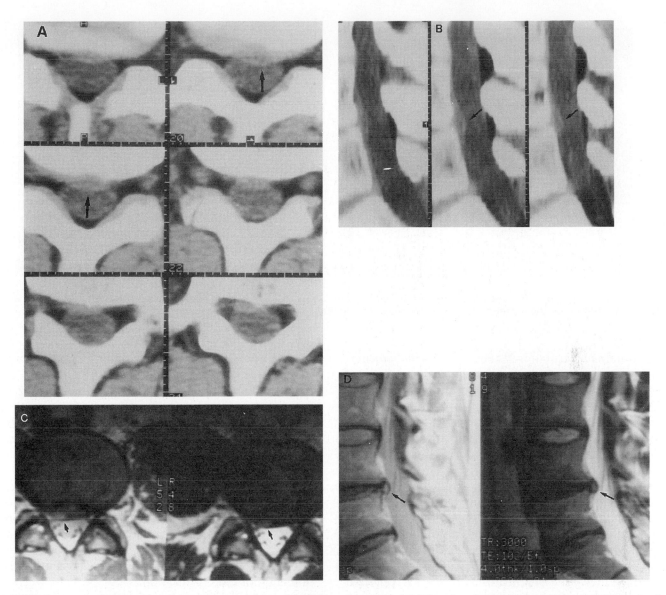

**FIGURE 15-5**    A small contained disc herniation (*arrow*) is delinated on the axial **(A)** and sagittal **(B)** images of a CT/MPR study. On another patient, on the axial **(C)** and sagittal **(D)** images of an MRI study, there is a small contained disc herniation (*arrow*).

matic.[21] For this reason, some patients with persistent back pain who have had an MRI study delineating decreased signal intensity at one or more disc levels are sometimes further evaluated with discography and CT-discography. These studies are performed at some centers for the preoperative evaluation of a patient with multilevel disc degeneration to localize which disc level generates the patient's pain, or for a patient with refractory mechanical back pain who has had a normal MRI study. In addition to the information these tests provide on the abnormal morphology of the disc, the discogram is a provocative test to demonstrate the patient's pain response when the disc is injected. When performing lumbar discography, it is routine to inject the suspected abnormal

disc level and the contiguous disc levels, even when these discs appear normal on the MRI evaluation. There have been several reports documenting discs with normal signal intensity on MRI that were abnormal morphologically on discography.[14,263] Discography cannot detect peripheral annular tears that do not communicate with the nucleus pulposus.[258] While some studies have reported on the advantages of discography, its value in the workup of patients with back or radicular pain is still controversial.[1,6,245]

With the superb soft tissue resolution of MR imaging, it may be possible to determine whether a disc herniation is contained by the outer annular posterior longitudinal ligament complex or has extruded through this complex, becoming an extruded,

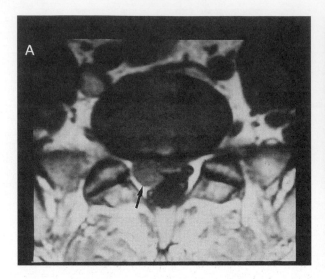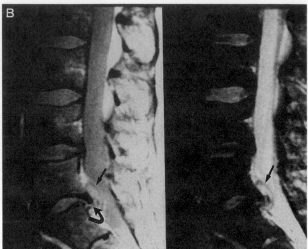

**FIGURE 15-6** At the L5-S1 disc level, a disc extrusion (*straight arrow*) is identified on the MRI axial **(A)** and sagittal **(B)** images. There is interruption of the posterior outer annular/posterior longitudinal ligament complex (*curved arrow*).

noncontained herniation[80] (Fig. 15-6). This information is needed for the successful application of percutaneous discectomy[147] and chemonucleolysis. It is also important as an indicator of surgical outcome for lumbar disc herniation.[102] The diagnosis of disc extrusion from CT studies is dependent on the configuration of the herniated disc.[67,74] Axial images are always needed on either an MRI or CT/MPR study to evaluate neural displacement or impingement and to detect posterolateral or lateral disc herniations.

Herniated disc material may separate from the disc of origin and become a sequestered fragment. MRI is useful in differentiating between a disc extrusion and sequestration. Sequestered disc fragments usually generate increased signal intensity on T2-weighted images compared to the degenerated disc of origin. In one prospective study, the accuracy of MRI in differentiating sequestered disc fragments from other forms of lumbar disc herniation was 85% compared to a 65% accuracy for CT-myelography.[141] The differential diagnosis of a sequestered disc fragment includes epidural abscess,[179] extradural tumor,[222] conjoined nerve root,[176] nerve root sheath tumor or cyst,[77] synovial cysts,[261] and an epidural hematoma.[134]

Following herniation, the disc will continue to degenerate, and on an MRI study, the degenerated disc will demonstrate decreased signal intensity on the T2-weighted sequence. To date, there has been no prospective study in humans to determine the length of time necessary for a normally hydrated disc to become desiccated after it herniates. Therefore, it is not possible to date the exact occurrence of a disc herniation if a prior imaging study is not available for comparison. Even when secondary degenerative changes are identified (e.g., end-plate osteophytes), a disc her-

niation still may represent an acute process superimposed on a chronic degenerative state. In cases of long-standing disc degeneration, fluid containing fissures may be present in the degenerative disc along with ingrowth of granulation tissue.[42] These pathologic changes may result in increased signal intensity in the disc on T2-weighted images, and this should not be confused with an inflammatory process[158] (Fig. 15-7). Calcification or gas in the disc may be difficult to detect on T2-weighted images due to the decreased signal intensity in the severely-degenerated disc and the absence of an MR signal from the calcium or gas. T1-weighted or gradient echo images have been found to be more useful in delineating a vacuum phenomenon or disc calcification.[155]

With the excellent characterization of normal and abnormal discs by MRI and CT/MRP, it is now possible to study noninvasively the natural history of disc degeneration and herniation. Several studies have reported on the high accuracy of these studies to diagnose disc disease.[53,59,63,67,87] In addition, MRI and CT have been utilized to document the resorption of disc herniations in patients treated nonoperatively.[27,32] Bozzao et al[27] demonstrated that 63% of the patients with disc herniations showed at least a 30% reduction in the size of their herniations, and the greatest size reduction occurred with the larger herniations. Bush et al[32] documented that 76% of disc herniations of nonoperatively treated patients showed partial or complete resolution.

Forristall et al[63] compared MRI and CT-myelography in the evaluation of 25 patients with a suspected disc herniation who underwent surgery. Compared to the surgical findings, the accuracy of MRI was 90.3% and CT-myelography 77.4%. Recently, Bischoff et

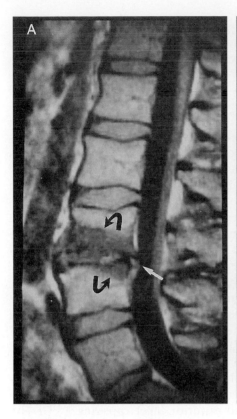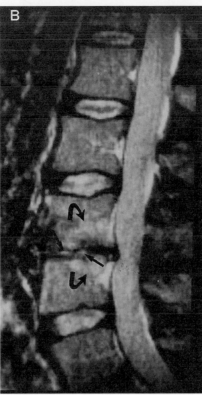

**FIGURE 15-7**    At the L3-4 disc level, on the MRI sagittal T1 **(A)** and T2 **(B)** weighted images, there are changes of chronic disc degeneration. On the T1-weighted sagittal image, there is decreased disc height, posterior protrusion of the disc and spondylotic ridges (*straight arrow*). There is decreased signal intensity in the cancellous bone adjacent to the end-plates (*curved arrows*) due to the presence of fibrovascular tissue. On the T2-weighted sagittal image there is increased signal intensity in the cancellous bone adjacent to the end-plates (*curved arrows*) and in the disc (*straight arrows*) due to the presence of granulation tissue. The vertebral body end-plates on the T2-weighted image are well defined, which helps to differentiate chronic degenerative changes from infection. With infection, the abnormal signal intensity in the vertebral body cancellous bone is usually more extensive that what is identified with chronic degenerative changes.

al[17] compared CT-myelography, MRI, and standard myelography in the evaluation of 57 patients for a disc herniation or spinal stenosis. Compared to the surgical findings, CT-myelography was the most accurate test (76.4%), and plain myelography the most specific test (89.2%), to diagnose a disc herniation. For the diagnosis of spinal stenosis, CT-myelography and MRI were the most accurate (85.3%), and the most sensitive (87.2%), and plain myelography was the most specific (88.9%) However, this study had some methodological limitations and it is only with a prospective study, where all three modalities are performed routinely, that it will be possible to compare the relative accuracy of the different tests.

It is important to remember when evaluating the clinical aspects of different imaging tests of the spine that evidence of herniated discs and spinal stenosis is present in many healthy individuals (Chapter 25). Myelograms, CT imaging, and MRI studies show that disc herniations are anatomically present in 25% or more of asymptomatic individuals. The percentage of abnormal findings increases when the population is older. In a recent MRI study of 98 asymptomatic subjects by Jensen et al,[107] 52% had bulging discs, 27% a disc protrusion (herniation), and 1 subject an extrusion. Stenosis was present in 14%. Only 38% were found to have normal MRI findings. Studies of the cervical spine have obtained similar results.[23,225] Clearly

this means that imaging must be correlated to clinical symptoms and signs for meaningful interpretation.

It is not infrequent that patients who have undergone disc surgery will experience recurrent back pain when they return to work. If conservative management does not relieve the patient's symptoms, an MRI study is the optimal imaging exam to evaluate the operative site. When performing an MR study to evaluate a postoperative patient, the length of time between surgery and the MRI examination is an important factor in determining the significance of MRI findings. In two studies, there was no correlation between the immediate postoperative appearance on an MRI exam and patient's symptoms.[11,194] In the first few postoperative months, the changes detected on an MRI study reflect the reparative response to the operative procedure. An MRI study in the immediate postoperative period may not help to diagnose the etiology of a patient's persistent pain. Even one year after successful disc surgery, an MRI exam may show persistent posterior contour abnormalities of the disc causing mass effect on the thecal sac or nerve roots.[46] Tullberg et al[231] evaluated 36 patients one year after lumbar disc resection and found no consistent correlation between postoperative back or radicular pain and the MRI findings. The value of an MRI study in assessing patients with recurrent back pain or failed back surgery syndrome centers on the differentiation of epidural scar versus disc, after at least two to three months has transpired since disc surgery. Epidural fibrosis is frequently present at an operative site. Recurrent disc herniations are typically contiguous with the disc space, well-marginated, and, compared to the disc of origin, display isointensity or hypointensity on T1-weighted images and isointensity or hyperintensity on T2-weighted images. The intravenous administration of gadolinium-DTPA is particularly helpful in differentiating disc material from fibrosis[35,101] (Fig. 15-8).

As a result of disc degeneration and herniation, there will be altered biomechanics of the motion segment. End-plate degenerative changes are frequently associated with degenerative disc disease. MRI is extremely sensitive to detecting degenerative changes in the adjacent vertebral body end-plates, and Modic[156] has described the pathologic alterations in the vertebral body marrow adjacent to discs undergoing degeneration. With Type I end-plate degeneration, there is decreased signal intensity in the subchondral cancellous bone on a T1-weighted image and increased signal intensity on a T2-weighted image compared to normal bone marrow. The region of altered signal intensity pathologically represents prominent fibrovascular tissue in the marrow adjacent to the vertebral body end-plate. Type II end-plate degenerative changes, which pathologically represent increased fat in the subchondral bone marrow, display signal hyperintensity on T1-weighted images and slight hyperintensity or isointensity on T2-weighted images compared to normal marrow. Type III end-plate degenerative changes represent coarsening and thickening of the subchondral trabeculae, which is depicted on T1- and T2-weighted images as decreased signal intensity. Gradient echo sequences are frequently part of the routine MRI evaluation of the lumbar spine. These sequences are not as sensitive to the signal intensity changes within the disc or in the adjacent vertebral body marrow associated with disc degeneration[154] as are standard spin echo T1- and T2-weighted sequences. On CT/MPR evaluation, only end-plate sclerosis can be delineated, and this is not necessarily correlated to Type III changes identified by MRI. On the T1-weighted image, the MRI signal intensity of the vertebral body is predominantly determined by the amount of fat present in the marrow. It is therefore possible to maintain normal signal intensity in a vertebra with thickened trabeculae if there is still a critical amount of residual fat present in the marrow.

End-plate osteophytosis is frequently associated with disc degeneration. With CT's excellent delineation of osseous structures and its superior spatial resolution, it is more accurate than MRI in the evaluation of the location and size of end-plate osteo-

phytes. CT permits accurate delineation of the position of end-plate proliferative changes in relation to neural structures and differentiation of ridges from disc material. With MRI, it may be difficult to separate an osseous ridge from herniated disc material due to the hypointensity of both structures on T1- and T2-weighted sequences. This is not uncommon in the neural foramina where posterolateral disc herniations are frequently associated with osteophytes projecting off the vertebral body end-plates.

Hypertrophy and hyperplasia of connective tissue of the spinal motion segment are frequently precipitated by disc degeneration. The degenerative tissue may encroach into the central spinal canal and compress the neural structures. Spinal stenosis is defined as a local, segmental, or generalized narrowing of the central or intervertebral canals by bony or soft tissue elements that may lead to encroachment on the neural structures. The narrowing may involve the bony canal alone or the dural sac, or both.[7] The degenerative changes most often associated with central stenosis include osteophytes projecting off the vertebral body end-plates, hypertrophy and bony proliferation of the facet joints, and hypertrophy of the ligamenta flava and anterior facet capsules.[184,204] The purpose of MRI and CT/MPR in the evaluation of a patient presenting with back pain, radiculopathy, or intermittent claudication is not just to demonstrate the presence of stenosis, but to define the relative contributions of each component of the stenotic process (Fig. 15-9).

In the lumbar spine, it has become clear that patients of any age may have disc degeneration superimposed on a stenotic process or may have isolated stenosis as a cause of leg or back pain.[31,86] In order to obtain a true diameter of the central spinal canal, axial images orthogonal to the long axis of the spinal canal or midline sagittal images must be performed. With the excellent spatial resolution of osseous structures, CT/MPR provides the optimal technique to ascertain precise osseous spinal measurements. The classification of spinal stenosis as congenital, developmental, and acquired is extremely helpful when evaluating a small spinal canal.[240,242] Congenital stenosis is due to disturbed fetal development and may occur as one element of a congenital malformation of the lumbar spine. Developmental stenosis is a growth disturbance of the posterior elements, involving the pedicles, lamina, or articular processes, resulting in decreased volume of the spinal canal.[190] A true midline osseous sagittal diameter measuring less than 12 mm is considered relative stenosis and a diameter of less than 10 mm is considered absolute stenosis.[241] This diameter is measured from the middle of the posterior surface of the vertebral body to the point of

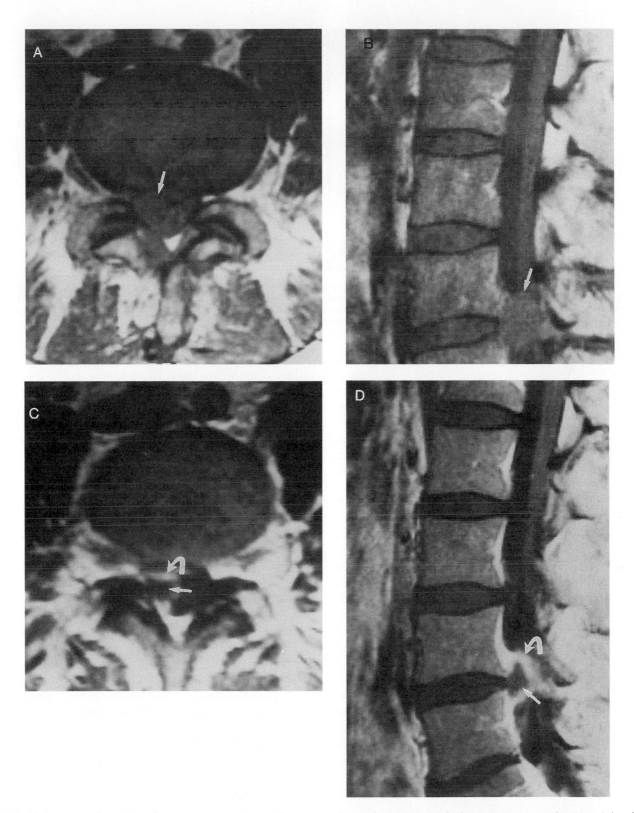

**FIGURE 15-8**     On the MRI study on a postoperative patient presenting with recurrent right leg symptoms, on the T1-weighted axial **(A)** and sagittal **(B)** images, there is a poorly defined soft tissue mass (*arrow*) positioned in the right side of the spinal canal. On the sagittal image the mass is contiguous with the disc space. After the intravenous injection of Gd-DPTA, on the repeat T1-weighted axial **(C)** and sagittal **(D)** images, there is enhancement of the vascularized fibrous tissue (*curved arrow*) surrounding the herniated disc material (*straight arrow*).

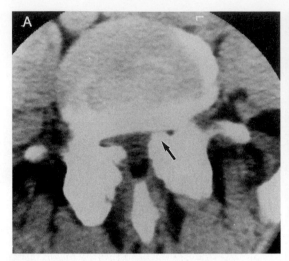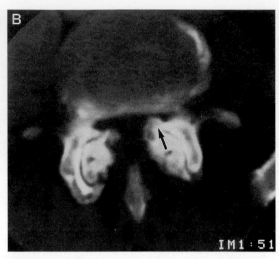

**FIGURE 15-9**    At the L4-L5 disc level, on the axial CT images (**A** and **B**), there are severe degenerative changes of the facet joints with prominent osteophytes causing stenosis of the subarticular and lateral recesses and the central spinal canal. The proliferative changes of the left facet joint (*arrow*) are causing severe stenosis of the left subarticular lateral recess. (From *Physical Medicine and Rehabilitation: State-of-the-Art Reviews,* Vol. 4, No. 2, Hanley & Belfus, Inc., June 1990.)

junction of its spinous process and laminae. With relative stenosis, the reserve capacity of the spinal canal is reduced, thus predisposing the neural elements to impingement or compression by a small disc herniation or mild degenerative changes. Porter et al[177] reported that patients with a small spinal canal, detected with ultrasonography, do not have a greater prevalence of back pain, but if they do experience back pain it will be of greater severity compared to patients with a normal-sized canal. Acquired stenosis is the narrowing of the central or intervertebral canals by degenerative changes of the discovertebral joints, facet joints, and ligamenta flava.[202,204,240]

In a prospective study, 60 patients with suspected lumbar disc herniations and/or spinal central stenosis were studied with first generation MRI, standard CT, and/or myelography, and the results were compared to the findings at surgery. The surgical diagnosis of stenosis agreed with MRI in 77% of the cases, CT in 79%, and myelography in 54%.[157] This study did not differentiate between central and intervertebral canal stenosis, and the CT study did not include multiplanar reformations which are extremely helpful in the evaluation of stenosis.[130,142] Schnebel et al[202] compared MRI with CT-myelography in the diagnosis of spinal stenosis and demonstrated a 96.6% agreement between the two tests.

The importance of intervertebral foraminal stenosis as a cause of radicular symptoms[178] and its significance in failed back surgery has been well-documented.[31] Considering that all neural foramina in the spinal column have a vertical and horizontal dimension, as well as a length (up to 12 mm at the L5-S1 disc level), the foramen is truly a three-dimensional structure (i.e., a canal). Pathologic changes of any

component of the foramen may impinge or compress the exiting nerve root. The foramen at the L5-S1 disc level is unique in its morphometry, and due to its length, it may be stenotic at its entrance, mid, or exit zone. The most common etiology of stenosis at this level is an osteophytic ridge projecting off the inferior end-plate of L5 and less commonly the superior end-plate of S1.[26,184] Degenerative changes of the facet joint or the anterior facet capsule may lead to decreased volume of the posterior and superior compartment of the foramen, potentially causing neural compression. Extraforaminal (far-out) stenosis[253] may also occur at the L5-S1 disc level in young patients with spondylolisthesis or elderly patients with disc degeneration and scoliosis.[83] The stenosis is secondary to the apposition of the base of the junction of the transverse process and pedicle of L5 to the adjacent sacral ala. In addition, osseous ridges may project off the lateral margin of the vertebral body endplates of L5 and S1 and may impinge the L5 nerve root in the paravertebral gutter (far-far out stenosis). The pathoanatomy of the intervertebral foramen can be assessed by both CT/MPR and MRI (Fig. 15-10).

## Spondylolisthesis

Degenerative spondylolisthesis is an important cause of central canal stenosis and most frequently involves the L4-5 disc level.[140] Disc degeneration along with degenerative changes of sagittally oriented facet joints[200] predispose the motion segment to an anterolisthesis that rarely progresses beyond a Grade I slip due to the intact neural arch. The combination of hyperostotic ridges projecting off the anteromedial margin of the facet joints, hypertrophy of the liga-

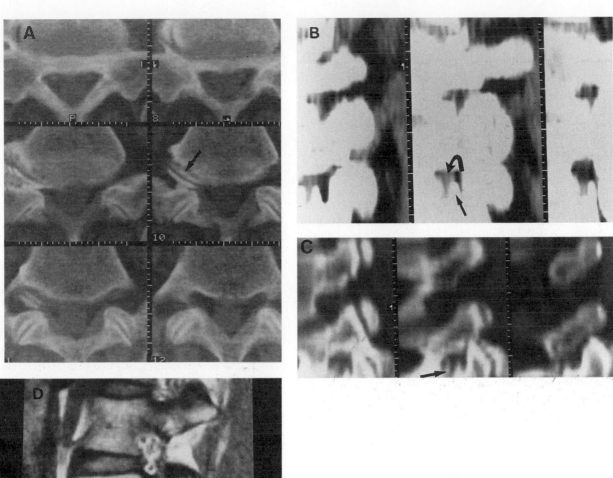

**FIGURE 15-10**    On the axial CT image **(A)**, osseous ridges (*straight arrow*) project into the right neural foramen at the L5-S1 disc level. On the sagittal reformatted images (**B** and **C**), the narrowing of the neural foramen by the osseous ridges (*straight arrow*), along with the compression of the exiting right L5 nerve root (*curved arrow*), are identified. (From *Physical Medicine and Rehabilitation: State-of-the-Art Reviews,* Vol. 4, No. 2, Hanley & Belfus, Inc., June 1990.) On another patient, stenosis of the L5-S1 neural foramen is present on the MRI T1-weighted sagittal image **(D)**. There is protrusion of the disc and osteophytes into the neural foramen (*curved arrow*). A small amount of fat is present around the L5 nerve root (*straight arrow*).

menta flava, annular redundancy, and an anterolisthesis can result in severe central canal and subarticular lateral recess stenosis. There is usually at least mild narrowing of the neural foramina in the cephalocaudal direction secondary to the decreased disc height and the anterolisthesis.

Both disc degeneration and spinal stenosis are frequently detected in patients with isthmic spondylolisthesis. The occurrence of disc herniation has been reported both at the spondylolytic level[223] and at the superjacent motion segment.[79,195] Foraminal stenosis at the L5-S1 disc level is also relatively common due to the decreased cephalocaudal dimension of the canal secondary to the anterolisthesis. This predisposes the L5 nerve root to dynamic impingement and entrapment by osseous ridges encroaching on the foramen.

## Conclusions

Both CT/MPR and MRI are excellent noninvasive imaging studies to delineate pathomorphologic changes of the spinal motion segment. The transformation of the data from these exams into useful clinical information necessitates precise correlation of the exam's results to the patient's clinical condition and any additional diagnostic tests (e.g., EMGs) that have been performed. Proliferative osseous degenerative changes occur concurrently with disc degeneration and herniation. Therefore, it is necessary that all components of the spinal motion segment be completely evaluated in each patient presenting with back or leg pain in order to determine the pathoetiology of their symptomatology. A precise anatomic diagnosis is needed to provide a rational basis for therapeutic decisions. An important question that to date has not been resolved, is which study, CT or MRI, should be ordered when additional information is needed in the evaluation of a patient with spinal symptoms. Thornbury et al[227] recently reported on the relative efficacy of MRI, CT-myelography, and plain CT, to evaluate patients with acute low-back pain that clinically was suspected to be related to neural compression by a herniated disc. Ninety-five patients with acute low-back and radicular pain underwent MRI and either CT (34%) or CT-myelogram (66%). Patients were followed for at least 6-12 months. Fifty-six patients underwent surgery and 39 received conservative treatment. The results of the study demonstrated no statistically significant difference in the diagnostic accuracy of the three modalities to detect a herniated disc that was causing neural compression. The authors concluded that factors such as cost, radiation dose, and invasiveness should influence the selection of modality. They suggest that MRI should replace CT-myelography, but that it should not replace plain CT because of the extra cost of the MRI study. In this study, the cost of a plain CT was $534, for a CT-myelogram $1104, and for an MRI $1135. The recent marked decline in the price of MRI studies would have a significant impact on the study's cost-benefit analysis. While the design of the study was rigorous and well controlled, its results only apply to a narrow spectrum of patients presenting with a very specific clinical problem. Considering the high rate of surgery for the patients in the study (almost 60%), it is evident that they do not represent the spectrum of patients typically presenting with back or radicular pain.

Seventy-four percent of the patients in this study were referred from a neurosurgical clinic. There is still a need to compare the three imaging modalities for the evaluation of back pain, tumor, trauma, arthritis, and infection, prior to recommending which test is optimal in different clinical situations. The age range and symptoms of patients presenting for impairment evaluation are quite broad; therefore the optimal imaging study must be able to detect a broad spectrum of pathologic conditions. Whichever technique is used, clinical correlation is essential to interpret correctly the significance of any findings.

## SOFT TISSUE INJURIES

Injuries to the soft tissues of the body are probably the most frequent cause of musculoskeletal dysfunction secondary to injuries incurred at work, sports, or recreational activities. With the recent development and implementation of MRI, it is now possible to evaluate noninvasively all the soft tissue structures in the body (e.g., muscles, tendons, ligaments, and cartilage) that may be responsible for a patient's symptomatology. Ultrasonography is also used to assess soft tissue disorders of the musculoskeletal system.[84,114] The major advantage of US is its availability, safety, and lower cost compared with MRI. It is limited to the evaluation of tissues that transmit sound waves; thus osseous structures or soft tissues shielded by osseous tissue cannot be evaluated. Compared with the other imaging modalities the efficacy of US is heavily dependent on the operator of the equipment, but this should not preclude its use in the appropriate clinical situations. Considering its cost and availability, the role of US may grow as staff in more centers become proficient in its application. This is already true in many European countries where US is heavily used in the evaluation of musculoskeletal disorders.[9,168] The following sections will present the role of radiologic imaging in the assessment of patients with musculoskeletal injuries.

## MUSCLE INJURIES

### Muscle Contusions and Tears

Muscle injuries may result from a direct or indirect application of force to the muscle. A direct blow to a muscle may cause a muscle contusion with disruption of muscle fibers. Acute disruption of muscle fibers and capillaries may precipitate soft tissue hemorrhage and a hematoma along with a secondary inflammatory response. With the acute pain associated with muscle injury, it may be difficult on a physical exam to determine the precise location, extent, and severity of an injury. Prior to the implementation of MRI, radiologic imaging studies were of little value in the evaluation of acute muscle injuries. On plain films there may be obscuration of the fat planes surrounding an injured muscle secondary to the perimuscular edema. With CT there may be an alteration of the size or contour of a muscle but detection of intramuscular hemorrhage, edema, or a hematoma is difficult. With the excellent soft tissue contrast resolution provided by MRI, it is now possible to obtain the following important clinical information related to a muscle injury: (1) the extent of muscle edema and/or hemorrhage; (2) if a focal hematoma is present, including its size and location; (3) the degree and extent of muscle fiber disruption; (4) if there is complete disruption of the muscle, whether there is associated muscle retraction; (5) whether there is interruption of the overlying fascia and if there is a muscle herniation; (6) the degree of muscle swelling and the detection of a possible concomitant compartment syndrome; and (7) whether single or multiple muscles are injured. Muscle contusions occur most frequently in the lower extremities, particularly involving the quadriceps mechanism.[198]

On an MRI exam, a muscle contusion is detected by abnormal signal intensity and morphology of the muscle. On spin-echo sequences, normal muscle demonstrates intermediate signal intensity on T1-weighted sequences and intermediate to low signal intensity on T2-weighted or STIR sequences. In a contused muscle, the interstitial edema or hemor-

rhage will be detected as high signal intensity on T2-weighted sequences. Since hemorrhage infiltrates through the muscle, and mixes with the interstitial edema, it is not possible to separate it from the edematous muscle tissue. With a grade 1 contusion (i.e., microstructural fiber failure) there may be a slight increase in the size of the muscle and the margins of the muscle may have a feathery appearance due to the extension of interstitial edema into the perimuscular tissue.[47,148] Edematous changes in the adjacent subcutaneous fat are also frequently detected. With a grade 2 muscle contusion (i.e., partial tear) there will be a focus of disrupted muscle fibers in addition to the altered signal intensity from the interstitial edema and hemorrhage (Fig. 15-11). A grade 3 muscle contusion will appear similar to a grade 2 contusion, except there will be complete disruption of the muscle fibers. With a muscle hematoma, there will be a focal accumulation of blood within a muscle. A hematoma demonstrates intermediate or high signal intensity on a T1-weighted sequence, depending on the chemical composition of the hematoma, and high signal intensity on a T2-weighted sequence. The sequelae of a muscle contusion may include muscle atrophy, fibrosis, calcification, or ossification.

The role of plain films and CT in the evaluation of these potential complications has focused mainly on the detection of muscle calcification or ossification. Myositis ossificans is a benign ossifying soft tissue mass typically located within skeletal muscle. A history of prior trauma is present in approximately 50% of the cases, and frequently the episode of trauma is of a minor degree. Plain radiographs show faint calci-

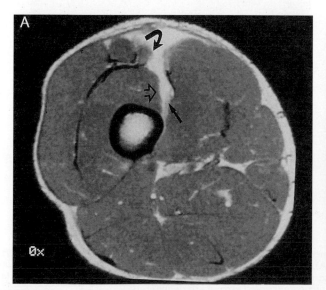
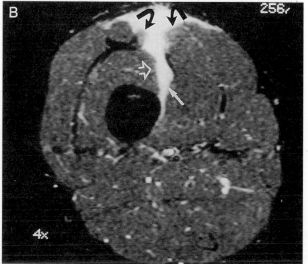

**FIGURE 15-11**    After a direct blow to the thigh, on the proton-density weighted **(A)** and STIR **(B)** axial images, there is a tear of the quadriceps muscle involving both the vastus medialis (*curved arrows*) and the vastus intermedius (*open arrowheads*) muscles. Hemorrhage/edema (*straight arrow*) extends to the femur.

fication within the muscle from 2 to 6 weeks after the onset of symptoms, and a well-circumscribed osseous mass in approximately 6 to 8 weeks. The lesion will then mature over the next six months and become smaller. In the early stages of the lesion, prior to bony maturation, the margins of the ossified mass may be poorly defined on plain films. If there is a history of only a minor injury or no trauma, the possibility of a soft tissue malignancy (e.g., osteosarcoma) is sometimes entertained after obtaining the plain films. If a CT scan is obtained at 4 to 6 weeks, it will demonstrate a rim of mineralization surrounding a central area of decreased attenuation. On an MRI examination, the characteristics of myositis ossificans are highly dependent on the age of lesion. On a T2-weighted sequence, an early lesion usually has well defined margins and has inhomogeneous intermediate to high signal intensity within the lesion. Perilesional edema is also identified with an acute lesion. As the lesion matures, it will develop a rim of mature bone.[126] Mature lesions are well defined with inhomogeneous signal intensity similar to fat. The most important finding on all of these imaging modalities is that the areas of ossification are most mature at the periphery of the lesion and the central core contains the immature cellular components. This is in contrast to a soft tissue osteosarcoma that is most mature centrally and immature peripherally. A few months of watchful waiting will demonstrate the normal maturation of myositis ossificans.

## Muscle Strains

Muscle strains are probably the most common type of injury to the myotendinous unit (MTU). A muscle strain is an acute stretch-induced injury secondary to excessive indirect force generated by eccentric muscular contraction. Muscle strains may occur anywhere in the body, but the most frequent muscles involved are the quadriceps femoris, biceps femoris, semimembranosus, semitendinosus, and the gastrocnemius-soleus complex. Muscles that cross two joints and that have a high proportion of fast twitch fibers are more prone to muscle strains. Muscle strains may also involve the muscles stabilizing the hip, shoulder, and elbow joints. The pain elicited from an acute muscle strain is typically experienced during an athletic activity or immediately at its termination.[163] The pathologic changes in an acutely strained muscle include disruption of the muscle fibers near the myotendinous junction along with edema and hemorrhage. The grade of a muscle strain depends on the degree of fiber disruption and the clinical findings.

The appearance of a grade 1 muscle strain with MRI is similar to the findings of a grade 1 muscle contusion. There may be enlargement of the muscle due to interstitial edema and hemorrhage and on a spin-echo T2-weighted or STIR sequence there will be increased signal intensity within the muscle (Fig. 15-12). Muscle strains are frequently located near its myotendinous junction. The tendon of a multipennate muscle extends into the muscle belly, therefore

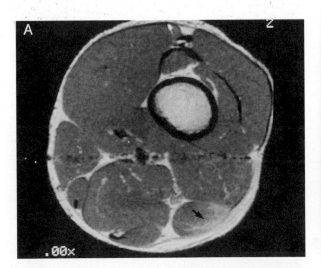 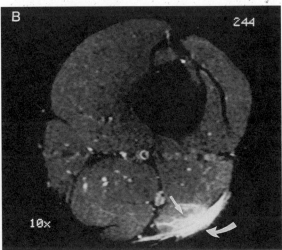

**FIGURE 15-12**   While exercising, the patient experienced the acute onset of pain in the region of the hamstring muscles. On the MRI study obtained after injury, on the T1-weighted axial image **(A)**, there is a subtle increased signal intensity within the periphery of the biceps femoris muscle (*straight arrow*), which is much easier to detect on the axial STIR image **(B)**. On the STIR image the edematous changes in the muscle (*straight arrow*) and in the subcutaneous tissue (*curved arrow*) are delineated.

the symptoms elicited by a strain may be located anywhere within a muscle and not merely at its ends. MRI has provided excellent documentation of the extent and position of these injuries. Fleckenstein et al[62] reported on the MRI appearance of the natural history of acute muscle strains. Acutely, the abnormal signal intensity was identified throughout the muscle, but on follow-up studies the abnormal signal intensity was most prominent in the periphery of the muscle. In one patient there was persistent abnormal signal intensity within the muscle after complete resolution of symptoms.

A grade 2 muscle strain manifests clinically as muscle pain associated with a loss of strength. Pathologically there is a macroscopic partial tear of the MTU. On an MRI study, there will be a partial tear of the muscle fibers associated with edema and/or hemorrhage. With a grade 3 strain there is a complete disruption of the MTU. Plain films provide little useful information in the evaluation of most muscle strains. Only if there is a grade 3 strain that results in gross instability or malalignment (e.g., a quadriceps rupture) will plain films be helpful. CT has also been used to evaluate muscular strain injuries, but it provides less useful clinical information compared to an MRI examination.[215]

In addition to the evaluation of acute or delayed muscle injuries, MRI is an ideal imaging modality to follow the evolution of the inflammatory and reparative processes within a muscle. With MRI it is possible to detect any sequelae from a MTU injury (e.g., muscle atrophy or fibrosis).[78] Clinically it can be extremely difficult to determine when a muscle has completely healed, and if an athlete or worker returns to his athletic activity or job too soon after injury, he may be predisposed to repeat injury. With MRI we have detected acute MTU injuries superimposed on subacute or chronic injuries that may have predisposed the athletes to reinjury.

## Compartment Syndromes

Another recent application of MRI in the assessment of muscle injury is in the evaluation of patients for the possibility of acute or chronic compartment syndromes. An acute compartment syndrome developing after a fracture may be secondary to an accumulation of blood or interstitial edema in a closed fascial compartment. Acute compartment syndromes most frequently involve the lower extremity, but MRI may be of benefit in demonstrating pathologic changes in any muscle. In a patient with an acute paraspinal lumbar compartment syndrome, an MRI study demonstrated increased signal intensity in the symptomatic paraspinal muscles that also had abnormal intracompartmental pressures.[52] Resolution of the abnormal signal intensity paralleled the improvement of the patient's symptoms. MRI has also been used in the evaluation of patients with chronic compartment syndromes. Amendola et al[4] demonstrated that in five patients with a positive clinical history for chronic compartment syndromes and who also had elevated post-exercise pressures, four demonstrated abnormal MRI signal intensity within the muscle. Patients who were initially thought to have a chronic compartment syndrome, but whose pressure measurements were normal, also had a normal MRI examination.

## Conclusions

While MRI is extremely sensitive to detect pathologic changes within a muscle due to accumulation of fluid, it lacks specificity. Any pathologic process that incites an inflammatory response or increases muscle hydration will present with abnormal signal intensity. Other muscular conditions that may appear similar to muscle injury include metabolic myopathies,[106] dermatomyositis,[91,174] diabetic muscular infarction,[164] vasculitis, viral myositis,[90] sarcoid myopathy,[128] and acute rhabdomyolysis.[211] Fibromyalgia, however, presents with a normal MRI.[127] Even a benign procedure such as an intramuscular injection can be detected on an MRI exam as a focus of abnormal signal intensity in the muscle and perifascial tissue.[187] It is quite apparent that the clinical significance of any abnormal finding on an MRI exam can only be determined by close correlation with the patient's history and physical exam. The value of a negative MRI may also be important in reaching an accurate diagnosis or directing treatment.

## TENDON INJURIES

The function of a tendon is to transmit the force from its muscle of origin to the bone where it inserts. Tendons are stressed by muscle contractions and the highest stress on a tendon is generated with eccentric muscle contractions. Excessive acute or chronic stress on a tendon may precipitate fiber disruption and induce pain. Disruption of a tendon may occur anywhere along its length. Avulsion of a tendon from its bony insertion may or may not be associated with a bony avulsion.

There have been a variety of terms used to describe tendon injuries. To classify tendon injuries it is necessary to know whether an injury is related to an acute traumatic event or secondary to chronic overload. The duration of a patient's symptoms must also be considered. An acute injury to a tendon may precipitate fiber failure (i.e., a strain) that is classified as grades 1 to 3 depending on the degree of fiber disruption. Although the term *tendinitis* is frequently used when a patient has pain related to a tendon or to the peritendinous tissue, only an injury that acutely precipitates failure of tendon fibers along with disruption of vascularized peritendinous connective tissue can produce an acute inflammatory response in a tendon (i.e., tendinitis).[131] Tendinitis may be acute, subacute, or chronic depending on the duration of a patient's symptoms. If an acute injury incites an inflammatory response only in the soft tissue surrounding a tendon, (e.g., the peritendon or the paratenon) without disruption of the tendon fibers, then the terms *peritendinitis* or *paratenonitis* are the most appropriate to describe a patient's symptomatology.[131,180]

Chronic microtrauma to a tendon, frequently secondary to chronic eccentric overload, may precipitate intrasubstance fiber failure. There is typically no history of an acute injury and the symptoms have an insidious onset. The chronic pathologic changes identified within the substance of a chronically overloaded tendon include fibrillar degeneration, angiofibroblastic proliferation, fiber necrosis with myxoid and hyaline degeneration, fibrosis, and occasionally chronic inflammation.[185] The term *tendinosis* has been employed to describe these chronic pathologic changes.[136] Tendinosis may represent an abortive healing response of a tendon from chronic overload. It is possible to have changes of tendinitis or peritendinitis superimposed on changes of tendinosis.

A normal tendon is composed predominantly of collagen fibers and it appears as a structure with minimal or no signal intensity on MRI spin-echo or STIR sequences. It is necessary to understand the spectrum of the appearance of normal tendons with MRI, prior to attempting to diagnose pathologic changes.[113,262] Certain tendons (e.g., the posterior tibial tendon[55,205] and the rotator cuff[152]) will demonstrate increased signal intensity within normal segments of the tendon. This may be related to the orientation of a tendon with respect to the direction of the magnetic field used for MR imaging.

With peritendinitis, pathologically there will be increased fluid in the peritendinous tissue secondary to an inflammatory process. This will be detected on an MRI spin-echo T2-weighted or STIR sequence as a focus of high signal intensity surrounding a normal tendon. With tendinosis, a focus of myxoid degeneration or angioblastic proliferation within the substance of a tendon will generate increased signal intensity

within the tendon on a spin-echo T1-weighted or STIR sequence. On a T2-weighted sequence, the abnormal signal intensity may persist, but usually not as bright as it was on the T1-weighted sequence. The signal intensity within a degenerated tendon frequently appears normal on a T2-weighted sequence. Persistent high-signal intensity on a T2-weighted or STIR sequence may be seen if there is inflammatory or degenerative tissue within a tendon. A high-grade partial tear of a tendon provides a mechanism whereby fluid or inflammatory tissue can extend into the substance of a tendon. STIR or other fat suppression sequences have been particularly useful to evaluate tendon disruption.

In addition to the abnormal signal intensity identified within inflamed or degenerated tendons, altered morphology is also frequently identified (e.g., hypertrophy or attenuation of a tendon). A grading system of disorders of the posterior tibialis tendon has been reported.[205] A hypertrophied tendon containing abnormal signal intensity has been classified as grade 1 degeneration or partial tear, an attenuated tendon containing abnormal signal intensity as grade 2 degeneration or partial tear, and a complete tear of the tendon is classified as grade 3.

With the direct multiplanar capabilities of MRI, it is possible to evaluate the condition of any tendon in the body. MRI provides a very sensitive test to detect tendon disorders, but unfortunately it lacks specificity. It is not possible on an MRI study to determine whether a focus of abnormal high signal intensity within a tendon is secondary to acute inflammation or chronic degeneration. If abnormal tendon morphology is also detected (e.g., with an acute partial tendon tear), then it may be inferred that some of the abnormal signal intensity is secondary to an acute inflammatory process. But these acute changes may be superimposed on chronic degenerative changes of a tendon. For this reason, the term *tendinopathy* (i.e., a pathologic condition of a tendon) is probably most appropriate to describe an abnormal tendon detected on an MRI study that demonstrates abnormal signal intensity and is not partially or completely torn. In the assessment of the abnormal signal intensity surrounding a tendon, it is also not possible to determine whether the altered tissue hydration is associated with an inflammatory infiltrate. Therefore, these edematous changes should be described, but not considered as proof for the presence of an inflammatory response.

MRI has had a major impact in the advancement of our understanding of the natural history of tendon failure. With MRI it is possible to detect subclinical injuries (i.e., pathologic changes in a tendon resulting from chronic microtrauma or aging). These injuries by definition do not incite symptoms, but they may

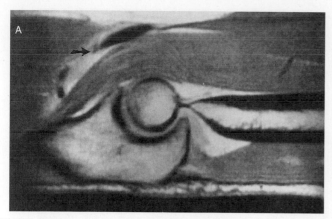

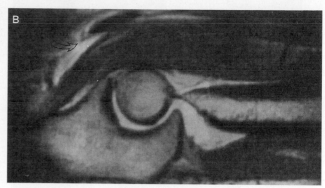

**FIGURE 15-13**        On the MRI evaluation of a patient who fell on an outstretched arm, there is a complete tear of the biceps tendon (*arrow*), on the proton density **(A)** and T2-weighted **(B)** images. (From *Magnetic Resonance Quarterly*, Vol. 9, No. 3, 1993.)

predispose a tendon to future dysfunction or failure. When the tendons of patients with an acute complete tendon rupture are studied histologically, changes of chronic tendon degeneration are usually demonstrated adjacent to the area of an acute rupture. Even a great percentage of nonruptured tendons in healthy individuals demonstrate pathologic changes of chronic degeneration.[112] These abnormalities can be detected with MRI by the demonstration of abnormal signal intensity or altered morphology of a tendon. These abnormal foci detected on an MRI study are not false-positive findings since they represent true pathologic changes in the tendon that do not evoke symptoms. The detection of subclinical tendon injury or degeneration may provide important information with respect to changing training or rehabilitative techniques or to job related activities that may be overloading a tendon.

The location of tendon degeneration and/or tear depends on the etiology of fiber failure. An acute tendon rupture may occur at the myotendinous junction, within the main segment of the tendon, or at the tendon insertion site (Fig. 15-13). The nature of the force, the position of the joint at the time of injury, along with any predisposing factors that may have weakened the tendon, will affect the site of rupture. If failure is secondary to extrinsic impingement (e.g., by a degenerative osseous ridge), the location of tendon failure will occur where the tendon impinges against this extrinsic structure. Chronic overload injuries to a tendon, frequently secondary to eccentric muscle contraction, may cause microstructural damage within the substance of a tendon at its insertion site (e.g., the quadriceps, patellar, or posterior tibial tendons). Extrinsic impingement or intrinsic overload of a tendon may be amplified if there is also instability of a joint that precipitates external friction or in-

creased tension of a tendon when the MTU is active. With MRI it is possible to determine the exact location and extent of an injury to a tendon. Equally important, an MRI exam provides a comprehensive evaluation of all the peritendinous structures that may impinge a tendon and precipitate failure. Ultrasound has been extensively used in the evaluation of tendon degeneration or tears,[110,145] but US provides little or no information about the status of a tendon where it is located beneath an osseous structure. It also has limited use in defining abnormal osseous structures that may cause extrinsic impingement of a tendon. Ultrasound is most valuable in the assessment of a superficially located tendon (e.g., the Achilles[108,109] or patellar tendon).

Chronic intrinsic overload of a tendon is probably the most frequent cause of fiber failure and tendon degeneration in a young or middle-aged individual with tendon dysfunction. Lateral epicondylitis and medial tendinosis are discussed in Chapter 21.

## Achilles Tendon

Dysfunction of the Achilles tendon is a frequent cause of debilitating ankle pain. There is no tenosynovial sheath surrounding the Achilles tendon; therefore, if acute pain is associated with inflammation in the peritendinous soft tissues, it involves the paratenon or peritendon. MRI has proven to be very useful in the evaluation of patients with refractory Achilles pain or an acute rupture. Intrasubstance partial tears or degeneration of a tendon are detected as foci of increased signal intensity on spin-echo and STIR sequences due to the increased hydration of the pathologic tissue. Thickening of the tendon is also usually detected. With a partial tear that interrupts the peripheral fibers of the tendon, or with a com-

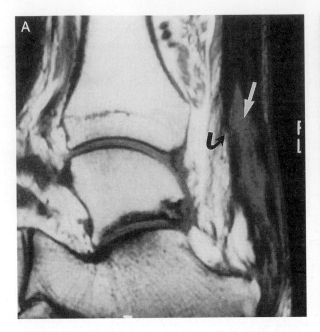

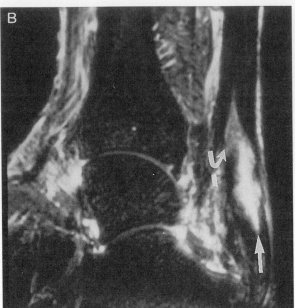

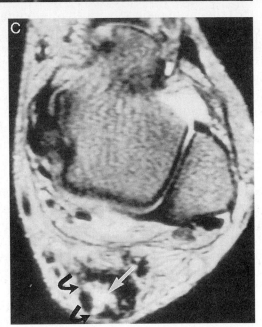

**FIGURE 15-14** During exercising, a runner developed acute pain over the Achilles tendon, in an area where he had previously experienced mild chronic pain. On the T1-weighted **(A)** and STIR **(B)** sagittal images and on the T1-weighted **(C)** axial image, there is diffuse thickening of the tendon along with a long tubular focus of intra-tendinous high signal intensity (*straight arrow*). A partial tear of the peripheral margins of the tendon is also identified (*curved arrows*).

plete tear, focal fiber disruption is identified (Fig. 15-14). The MRI exam can be performed with the patient's foot in both dorsiflexion and plantar flexion to assess the size of the gap between the ends of a torn tendon. Weinstabl et al[248] reported on 28 patients with suspected tendon injury. Of the 13 patients who required operative treatment, all partial and complete tears detected at surgery were correctly diagnosed on an MRI study. Ultrasonography was also performed on 10 of the 28 patients and 1 patient with a partial rupture at surgery had a false-negative US. Kalebo et al[109] recently reported on the diagnostic value of ultrasonography in the assessment of patients with partial ruptures of the Achilles tendon. The overall sensitivity for US was 0.94, the specificity was 1.00, and the accuracy was 0.95 in this highly-selected group of patients. The authors concluded that the advantages of US are its availability, low cost, and real-time imaging capabilities compared to MRI studies.

## Patellar Tendon

Like the Achilles tendon, the patellar tendon is prone to chronic overload injuries.[58] Both US and MRI have been used to evaluate the pathologic changes within the tendon in symptomatic patients. Even though pain and dysfunction of the patellar tendon is usually referred to as patellar tendinitis, pathologic changes detected within the tendon frequently demonstrate changes of fiber disruption,

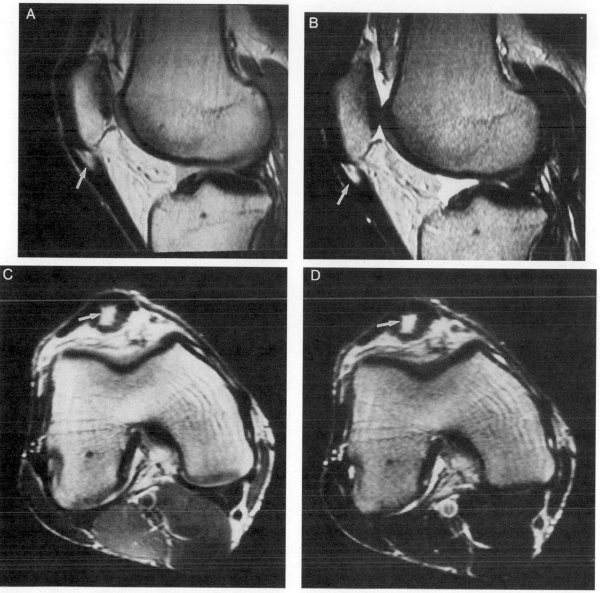

**FIGURE 15-15**    A patient was experiencing chronic pain over the patellar tendon. On the MRI evaluation, on the proton-density **(A)** and T2-weighted **(B)** sagittal images, and on the proton-density **(C)** and T2-weighted **(D)** axial images, there is hypertrophy along with a focal area of high signal intensity in the center of the proximal segment of the tendon at its insertion site (*arrow*). At the time of tendon repair, tissue histology revealed chronic degenerative changes within the tendon at this location.

chronic myxoid degeneration, and focal fibrinoid necrosis.[24] If a patient does not respond to conservative care, an imaging study is frequently ordered to corroborate the presumptive clinical diagnosis and to assist in preoperative planning. With MRI it is possible to determine the exact location and extent of the pathological changes within the patellar tendon (Fig. 15-15).[207] It is difficult to determine the true accuracy or efficacy of US, MRI, or CT, particularly in the detection of small lesions of the patellar tendon. If only large lesions are refractory to conservative therapy, then the detection of small lesions may not be important, but this will have to be proven with a long-term prospective study.

## Rotator Cuff

The rotator cuff is one of the largest tendinous structures in the body and because of its functional demands it is prone to degeneration and failure. The two primary mechanisms of injury to the cuff are extrinsic primary impingement and intrinsic chronic overload. The impingement syndrome presents as painful dysfunction of the shoulder, particularly with overhead activities. The pain is precipitated by entrapment or abrasion of the rotator cuff mechanism (i.e., the rotator cuff and the peritendinous soft tissue) under a degenerated acromioclavicular (AC) joint or under the coracoacromial arch (i.e., the arch formed by the coracoid process, the coracoacromial [CA] ligament, and the acromion). In the supraspinatus outlet, the rotator cuff mechanism may impinge against a thickened coracoacromial ligament, an enthesophyte projecting off the anteroinferior margin of the acromion at the insertion of the CA ligament, or against a curved or hooked acromion. Repetitive abrasion of the rotator cuff mechanism can precipitate bursal inflammation, peritendinous inflammation, or tendon degeneration.[208] Fiber disruption secondary to cuff abrasion will be associated with edema and/or hemorrhage in the cuff and the peritendinous tissues. With MRI it is possible to define precisely the anatomy of the AC joint and the supraspinatus outlet and to detect any evidence of a degenerative process affecting these structures (Fig. 15-16). It is possible to define the location where the cuff may be impinging against areas of bony proliferation or ligamentous hypertrophy. It is also possible to detect evidence of bursal inflammation. Impingement (i.e., to push against) is a physical phenomenon and can be detected by an MRI exam; but the diagnosis of an impingement syndrome, which is a painful symptom complex secondary to the repetitive abrasion and inflammation of the cuff and/or the peritendinous tissue resulting from impingement, can only be made clinically. With continued injury to a cuff, a focal partial tear or full thickness cuff tear may develop. In young patients, degenerative changes of the AC joint

or the acromion are rarely present. Cuff failure is more likely to be secondary to intrinsic overload of the cuff and fatigue failure of the tendon fibers. With the decreased tensile strength of the cuff, further stress may precipitate a partial or full thickness tear. If biomechanical imbalance results from a torn rotator cuff, or is present secondary to primary shoulder instability, secondary impingement of the cuff may also be present and elicit symptoms.

Imaging studies of the rotator cuff are frequently obtained after an unsuccessful trial of conservative therapy for rotator cuff impingement or tear. Prior to the development of US and MRI, plain films were the primary diagnostic imaging tool to evaluate the shoulder for rotator cuff dysfunction. While plain films are helpful in the evaluation of osseous anatomy and pathology, they provide no direct and only limited indirect evidence of rotator cuff pathology. The best indicator for a torn rotator cuff on plain films is when the distance between the humeral head and the acromion is less than 6 millimeters on an AP view of the shoulder with the arm in neutral rotation.[247] Unfortunately this is a very late finding in the natural history of cuff degeneration and when it is present, there is usually a very large or massive tear of the cuff. The supraspinatus outlet view has recently been implemented to assess the shape of the acromion. Since a plain film is a two-dimensional projection of a three-dimensional structure, it is frequently difficult

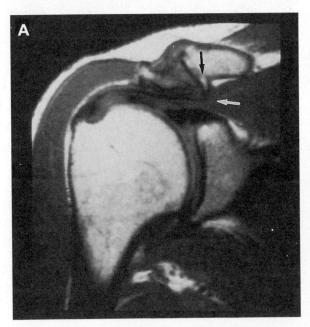
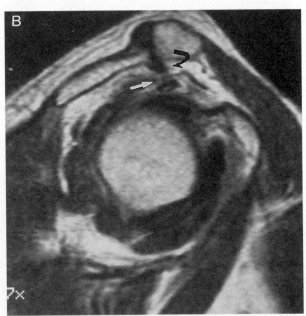

**FIGURE 15-16**    On the MRI examination of a patient experiencing shoulder pain with overhead activity, on the proton-density weighted oblique coronal **(A)** and oblique sagittal **(B)** images, degenerative changes of the AC joint are identified with an osseous ridge projection off the inferior margin of the head of the clavicle (*straight black arrow*) and the inferior surface of the acromion (*curved black arrow*). The supraspinatus myotendinous junction is impinged by the osteophytes (*white arrow*).

to determine the true shape of the acromion. Interobserver variability is also a problem with the interpretation of this projection. Special views have also been developed to detect osseous ridges projecting off the anteroinferior margin of the acromion.[169]

The integrity of the rotator cuff can be assessed by arthrography, which is an invasive procedure. After the instillation of contrast into the should joint, one may detect full thickness cuff tears by the leakage of contrast. The sensitivity of arthrography to detect full-thickness tears measuring over one centimeter is probably over 90%, but the study is less sensitive in detecting small full-thickness tears or partial tears of the articular surface of the cuff. It is insensitive in the detection of partial tears on the bursal side of the cuff that may result from extrinsic impingement. Arthrography provides little information on the status of the cuff fibers (e.g., evidence of degeneration or attrition) and provides no information on the assessment of the coracoacromial arch and the supraspinatus outlet. The detection of a full thickness cuff tear may occur in asymptomatic elderly patients and in asymptomatic individuals who have undergone a surgical repair of the cuff. Calvert[33] performed arthrography on 20 patients after rotator cuff repair and demonstrated leakage of contrast indicating a full-thickness cuff tear in 18 of the patients. Seventeen of the 18 patients were asymptomatic at the time of arthrography.

US and MRI are noninvasive tests performed to evaluate the rotator cuff and the surrounding soft tissue structures. One advantage of US is the capacity to study the cuff with the arm in different positions. This may be particularly useful in the evaluation of patients with shoulder impingement syndrome.[56] There have been several reports on the value of US to detect tears of the rotator cuff.[28,139,250] Weiner et al[250] reported on a group of 225 patients who had preoperative sonography and compared the results of US to the surgical findings. The abnormalities detected on the US included partial and full-thickness cuff tears. US findings were surgically confirmed in 92% of the cases. Misamore et al[153] recently reported a prospective study of 32 patients who had degeneration of the rotator cuff and who required surgery. Preoperatively US and arthrography were both performed. Of the 20 patients who had a full-thickness tear, arthrography detected 100% and US detected 35%. Of the 7 patients with a partial-thickness tear, arthrography was accurate in 3, and US in 2 of the cases. Arthrography was accurate in all 5 patients who did not have a tear and US was accurate in 3 of the cases. Both studies had methodological problems, which introduced potential sources of bias. It appears from the reports in the literature that in some centers US provides useful information for a certain subset of patients. The efficacy of US can not be deduced from these studies as to its application as a screening examination for rotator cuff disorders.

MRI is the optimal imaging modality to provide a comprehensive evaluation of the shoulder in a patient with shoulder dysfunction. The strengths of MRI are its direct multiplanar capabilities, excellent soft tissue contrast resolution, and its ability to evaluate completely both the normal and abnormal osseous architecture of the shoulder girdle. While US has received criticism for its operator dependence, the efficacy of MRI in the assessment of the shoulder is highly dependent on the imaging protocols employed and the expertise of the radiologist interpreting the study. Like all structures in the body, there is a spectrum in the appearance of normal anatomy that must be appreciated.[152,162] The pathoetiology of abnormalities detected on an MRI study can only be determined by precisely comparing the findings on an MRI study to those detected at arthroscopy, arthrotomy, or to tissue histology obtained from cadavers.

The appearance of a normal rotator cuff is similar to that of other tendons in the body. With its high collagen content, it demonstrates minimal signal intensity on spin-echo or STIR sequences. Abnormalities of the rotator cuff are detected by altered cuff morphology along with abnormal signal intensity. Complete assessment of the soft tissues and osseous structures surrounding the cuff is mandatory in order to achieve a comprehensive evaluation of a shoulder. Imaging of the shoulder in three orthogonal planes should be performed on all patients. The axis of the different scan planes is determined by the orientation of the supraspinatus tendon and the scapula. The coronal sequence is oriented parallel to the long axis of the body of the scapula and the supraspinatus tendon. The sagittal sequence is oriented perpendicular to the coronal sequence. Both the coronal and sagittal sequences are oriented obliquely to the coronal and sagittal planes of the body due to the normal rotation of the scapula on the chest wall. Therefore, these sequences are referred to as oblique coronal or oblique sagittal sequences. The axial sequence is oriented perpendicular to the face of the glenoid, and depending on the degree of scapular rotation, it may be necessary to perform an oblique axial sequence with respect to the horizontal plane of the body. Spin-echo T1- and T2-weighted sequences are standard for the evaluation of the shoulder, and additional sequences (e.g., gradient-echo or STIR) may be performed to provide supplemental information.

With a partial tear of the rotator cuff, on an MRI study there will be a focal area of fiber disruption on the bursal or articular surface of the cuff, or within the substance of the cuff. With a full-thickness cuff tear, there will be complete discontinuity of the cuff fibers (Fig. 15-17). Spin-echo T2-weighted sequences are optimal to diagnose partial- or full-thickness tears by the detection of fluid in the cuff defect. Optimally, to diagnose a full-thickness cuff tear, fluid should be detected extending from the articular to the bursal

surface of the cuff along with fluid present in the adjacent subdeltoid bursa. Unfortunately, this is not always detected with a full-thickness tear, particularly when a tear is chronic and has generated a fibrous reaction in the peritendinous tissue. In these cases, assessment of cuff morphology or the detection of cuff retraction may provide the necessary information to

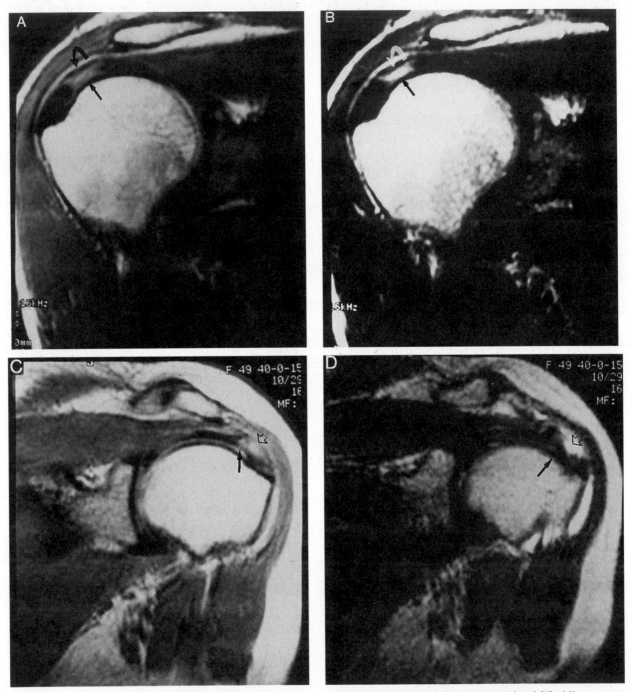

**FIGURE 15-17**    A partial tear of the rotator cuff is identified on the MRI proton-density **(A)** and T2-weighted **(B)** oblique coronal images. There is discontinuity of the articular surface of the cuff (*straight arrow*) but not the bursal side of the cuff (*curved arrow*). On the MRI study performed on another patient with chronic shoulder pain there is a partial tear of the bursal surface of the cuff (*open arrowhead*), on the proton-density **(C)** and T2-weighted **(D)** oblique coronal images. The articular surface of the cuff is intact (*straight arrow*).

reach an accurate diagnosis. With a complete evaluation of a cuff tear in at least two imaging planes it is possible to measure accurately the size and location of a tear. In some reported series the size of a cuff tear appears to have prognostic significance as to which patients will be improved by operative intervention. Full-thickness cuff tears usually first involve the supraspinatus segment of the cuff posterior to the rotator interval. Isolated full-thickness tears of the subscapularis segment of a cuff may be difficult to detect clinically, but MRI provides an excellent means to detect these tears.[70] With MRI it is also possible to determine the degree of cuff retraction and whether there is associated atrophy of the rotator cuff musculature. The status of the rotator cuff musculature may be important in the type of postoperative rehabilitation selected for a patient. The size of recurrent cuff tears also appears to be related to the degree of a patient's dysfunction.[85] The same MRI evaluation performed preoperatively can be employed in the postoperative evaluation of the cuff.

Iannotti el al[103] reported on the efficacy of MRI of the shoulder in the evaluation of 91 patients who required an operative procedure for shoulder dysfunc-

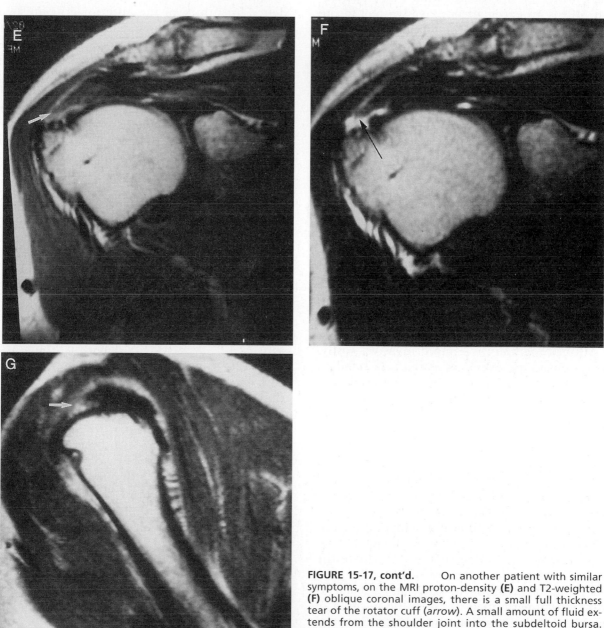

**FIGURE 15-17, cont'd.**    On another patient with similar symptoms, on the MRI proton-density **(E)** and T2-weighted **(F)** oblique coronal images, there is a small full thickness tear of the rotator cuff (*arrow*). A small amount of fluid extends from the shoulder joint into the subdeltoid bursa. While the medio-lateral dimension of the cuff tear can be assessed on the oblique coronal image, a T2-weighted oblique sagittal image **(G)** is needed to evaluate the anteroposterior extent of the tear (*arrow*).

tion and for 15 asymptomatic volunteers. In the detection of a complete cuff tear, MRI was 100% sensitive and 95% specific. Tendinitis was defined arthroscopically as an area of hyperemia on the undersurface of the cuff or as thickening of the subacromial bursa. Degeneration or partial tear of the cuff was defined arthroscopically as fraying or fibrillation of the cuff. For the differentiation between cuff tendinitis and degeneration, the sensitivity of MRI was 82% and the specificity was 85%. In differentiating a normal tendon from one showing signs of impingement, the sensitivity of MRI was 93% and specificity 87%. The authors concluded that high resolution MRI is an excellent noninvasive tool in the diagnosis of disorders of the rotator cuff mechanism. Both the administration and interpretation of the MRI exams in the study were performed by musculoskeletal radiologists with extensive experience with MRI. In addition to this study, there have been several other reports on the high accuracy of MRI to detect fill-thickness cuff tears.[57,96,182,230]

The sensitivity of MRI to detect partial cuff tears is considerably lower than its detection rate for full-thickness tears. In two studies that compared MRI to the findings at arthroscopy, Traughber et al[230] reported that 4 of 9 partial tears were not detected on an MRI study, and Hodler et al[96] reported that only 1 of 13 partial tears was detected on an MRI study. Hodler et al[96] also performed MR-arthrography on these patients and 6 of the partial tears were detected. Both Palmer et al[173] and Karzel et al[116] have recently reported on the improved detection rate of MR-arthrography compared to standard MRI to detect partial- and full-thickness rotator cuff tears. Since MR-arthrography is a more invasive, costly, and time-consuming exam compared to a standard MRI study, its efficacy will have to be proven in well-designed prospective studies before it can be recommended.

## LIGAMENT INJURIES

The most common ligament sprain involves the lateral ligamentous complex of the ankle (i.e., the anterior and posterior talofibular ligaments and the calcaneofibular ligament). Plain films are frequently obtained after an acute ankle sprain to evaluate the integrity of the ankle mortise and to detect the presence of a possible avulsion fracture. Stress radiography can also be performed to assess the integrity of the ligaments if the physical exam is inconclusive[181] and if this information is needed to guide therapy.[10] The accuracy of MRI in the detection of ankle ligamentous tears has been reported in several stud-

ies.[34,188,203,243] The use of thin sections and 3D imaging techniques seems to improve the accuracy of an MRI exam. Prior to obtaining an MRI study to assess the ankle ligaments, it is important to determine how the results of an MRI exam will affect clinical care. The information provided by an MRI study may be useful for preoperative planning, but it provides no indication of the degree of joint instability since it is not a functional examination. To date, there have been no prospective studies to determine the impact of MRI on the outcome of patients with ankle ligamentous dysfunction.

Plain film evaluation is also used to detect evidence for injury of the anterior cruciate ligament (ACL). Positive findings include the detection of bony avulsions or osseous impactions. Overall, plain films are extremely insensitive to detecting ACL injuries. The plain film findings that have a high specificity for ACL tears (e.g., a Segond fracture or gross malalignment of the knee joint) are rarely present with most ACL injuries. Stress radiography[64] may have a role in the assessment of ACL ligamentous dysfunction, but it provides no information on the presence of concomitant knee injuries that may be associated with an ACL tear.

The initial application of MRI in the assessment of ligamentous dysfunction focused on the evaluation of the ACL. In the last few years, there have been many reports documenting the high accuracy of MRI to detect complete tears of the ACL.[73,104,133,151,186,234] With MRI, it is possible to determine the precise location of an ACL tear (e.g., proximal, mid-substance, or distal) (Fig. 15-18). While several studies have reported on the value of secondary signs detected in knees with a torn ACL,[38,144,220,235] the diagnosis of an ACL tear should be primarily based on the appearance of the ACL on the MRI study.[232] Improvement in the detection of ACL tears is accomplished by imaging the knee in three orthogonal planes.[61] In addition to detecting a torn ACL, it is equally important to determine whether there are concomitant injuries to the meniscus, cartilage, bone, or other ligaments of the knee, which may cause similar symptoms and affect knee stability (*vide infra* p. 137). This information is needed when trying to prognosticate the long-term outcome of patients with an ACL injury.[166,214]

Oberlander et al[165] have reported a prospective study that assessed the accuracy of the clinical examination of the knee. The diagnostic accuracy of the clinical exam for intra-articular knee injuries was determined by comparison to arthroscopic findings. An overall correct diagnosis for the clinical exam was present in 56% of the cases, an incomplete diagnosis in 31%, and an incorrect diagnosis in 13%. When a single lesion was present, diagnostic accuracy was

**FIGURE 15-18**     After a ski injury, on the MRI proton-density **(A)** and T2-weighted **(B)** sagittal images, there is a complete tear of the mid-segment of the anterior cruciate ligament (*arrow*).

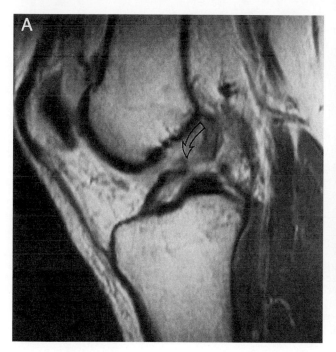

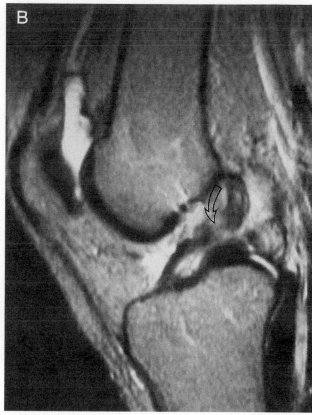

72%, but when more than two abnormalities were present, the accuracy of the clinical exam fell to 30%. Lesions most difficult to diagnose were cartilage fractures, tears of the ACL, and loose bodies. The strength of an MRI exam in the evaluation of an acutely or chronically symptomatic knee is its ability not only to assess the integrity of one structure in the knee (e.g., the ACL) but to provide a comprehensive evaluation of the entire knee. This is particularly important in the clinical situation where pain or locking limits the diagnostic capacity of a physical examination. Complete evaluation of the other ligaments of the knee (e.g., the posterior cruciate ligament,[60,81,82] the medial collateral ligament,[47,149] and the lateral collateral ligament[149,246]) can be achieved with an MRI exam. The same diagnostic criteria applied to ACL tears are applied in the assessment of these ligaments.

In addition to detecting acute ligamentous injuries, it is possible with MRI to assess the degree of ligamentous healing with follow-up studies. We have followed the course of healing of an acute grade 3 MCL injury in several athletes. On the initial study, diffuse maceration of the ligament was detected and not a focal avulsion of the ligament at its bony insertion site. On the MRI study the ligament demonstrated diffuse increased signal intensity on the spin-

echo and STIR sequences. There was no evidence of normal ligamentous fibers spanning from the femur to the tibia. In addition, prominent thickening of the ligament secondary to the fiber disruption and concomitant edema and hemorrhage was present. On the follow-up MRI studies the ligament became well-defined, thickened, and demonstrated decreased signal intensity compatible with collagenous repair (Fig. 15-19). The MRI exam provides direct information documenting the structural restoration of a ligament but cannot determine its functional integrity. In the process of healing, a medial collateral ligament is composed of a greater percentage of Type III collagen and is weaker than a normal ligament composed of Type I collagen. Currently, it is not known whether the MR signal characteristics of Type I collagen are different from Type III collagen.

MRI has also been applied in the evaluation of ACL reconstructive surgery. Both the MRI appearance of a neoligament composed of gracilis and semitendinosus tendons[37,100] and the patellar tendon[183,256] have been reported. The neoligaments typically demonstrate increased signal intensity in the first few months after surgery, reflecting the increased hydration and vascularity of the structure. On follow-up MRI studies, there may be a varied appearance of the morphology and the signal intensity

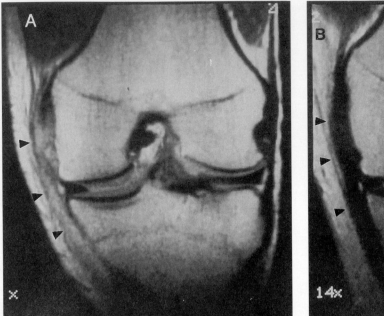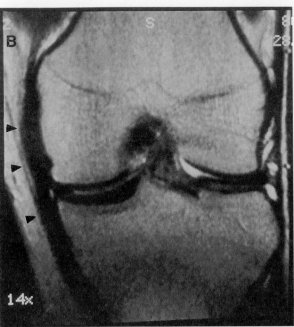

**FIGURE 15-19**    On the MRI evaluation of a patient who experienced an acute valgus injury to the knee, on the proton-density weighted coronal image **(A)** there is diffuse maceration of the medial collateral ligament (MCL) (*arrowheads*). On the follow-up MRI **(B)** obtained approximately eight months after injury, on the T2-weighted coronal image there is a completely healed, hypertrophied MCL (*arrowheads*).

of the ligament. Yamato et al[256] reported on the assessment of 15 patients with a clinically stable patellar bone-tendon-bone autograft from 3 months to 3 years and 3 months after reconstructive surgery. Only in two patients did the entire ligament appear as a band of low signal intensity. Rak et al[183] reported on the MRI evaluation of 37 patients with an ACL reconstruction using patellar bone-tendon-bone autografts. On 43 of 47 MR examinations they identified a well-defined ligament with low signal intensity. The correlation between the clinical exam and MRI was 92% and between the MRI and a second-look arthroscopy was 100%. Coupens et al[41] reported on the follow-up MRI evaluation of the native patellar tendon after it had been used to supply the autograft for ACL reconstruction. They evaluated 20 patients up to 18 months after harvesting the patellar bone-tendon-bone autograft. By 18 months the signal intensity in the residual patellar tendon appeared normal, but there was a significant increase in the thickness of the tendon on all follow-up studies.

## CARTILAGE INJURIES

Damage to articular cartilage due to an acute traumatic injury or to chronic microtrauma may be an important component in the pathoetiology of joint

dysfunction. Prior to the development of MRI, the radiologic detection of cartilage abnormalities on plain films was based on indirect evidence of cartilage damage (e.g., joint space narrowing or secondary osseous degenerative changes). Cartilaginous injury or degeneration can be directly evaluated with arthrography or CT-arthrography. The sensitivity of arthrography is limited, due to the difficulty in evaluating the curved articular surfaces that are present in most joints. The tomographic capability of CT-arthrography improves the detection of cartilaginous lesions[94] but like standard arthrography it has limited applications and is a relatively invasive procedure.

With the excellent soft tissue resolution provided by MRI, it was initially hoped that it would be the ideal study for the assessment of cartilage disorders. In addition to excellent contrast resolution, a high degree of spatial resolution is needed to detect cartilage abnormalities considering that most articular cartilage ranges in thickness from 2 to 3 mm. Since the thickness of the patellar articular cartilage is approximately 5 mm, the initial effort to optimize MRI sequences for the evaluation of articular cartilage has focused on the assessment of normal and abnormal patellar cartilage.

Disorders of patellar articular cartilage are considered a potential source of pain in many patients presenting with knee dysfunction (e.g., young athletes with parapatellar pain syndrome or workers whose jobs require repetitive or long periods of kneeling). Therefore, an accurate noninvasive test to detect these abnormalities would have a significant impact on patient care. The clinical efficacy of MRI in the detection of chondromalacia of the patella was reported by Conway et al.[39] The authors concluded that MRI was relatively sensitive and had a high predictive value in the detection of grades 3 and 4 chondromalacic lesions, even though no statistical analysis of the data was reported. There was also no discussion concerning the preoperative evaluation of these patients or the criteria employed to determine the indications for arthroscopy. McCauley et al[143] evaluated the appearance of the articular cartilage of the patella in 52 patients who underwent knee arthroscopy after an MRI examination. Twenty-nine of these patients had findings of chondromalacia at arthroscopy and the remaining 23 patients had normal patellar articular cartilage. The MRI studies were reviewed retrospectively by two radiologists without knowledge of the arthroscopic findings. An MR diagnosis based on focal signal or contour abnormalities detected on an axial spin-echo proton-density or T2-weighted sequence had a sensitivity of 86%, a specificity of 74%, and an accuracy of 81%. The sensitivity, specificity, and accuracy to detect chondromalacia was higher in the patients without joint fluid compared to patients with effusions. This finding is at odds with other clinical studies,[216] but the imaging techniques used in the different studies are dissimilar. The authors concluded that thinner sections may improve the accuracy to detect chondromalacia, but this will have to be proven with a prospective blinded study.

In addition to the evaluation of hyaline cartilage, one of the initial applications of MRI was in the evaluation of fibrocartilage (e.g., the knee meniscus and the intervertebral disc). The normal knee meniscus is a triangular fibrocartilaginous structure that generates no signal on an MRI study. Abnormal signal intensity within a meniscus is graded 1, 2, or 3, depending on the shape of the abnormal signal and whether it extends to the articular surface of a meniscus. Grade 1 is a globular focus of increased signal intensity that does not extend to the meniscal articular surface. Grade 2 is a linear focus of increased signal intensity that does not extend to the meniscal articular surface, but may extend to the meniscocapsular junction. Grade 3 is any focus of increased abnormal signal intensity that extends to the meniscal articular surface. Several studies have demonstrated the high accuracy of MRI to detect meniscal tears.[25,60,73,104,125] With aging, horizontal meniscal tears are frequently detected in asymptomatic patients,[125] therefore making it more difficult to determine their significance in a symptomatic patient. The standard criteria used to diagnose a meniscal tear on an MRI study are not as accurate in the assessment of the meniscus in older individuals.[95]

The diagnosis of a meniscal tear is more difficult in the postoperative knee because of the altered morphology and signal intensity of the meniscus.[48] An MRI is most valuable if only a small portion of the meniscus has been resected. It is possible to perform an MR-arthrogram with Gd-DPTA to improve the detection rate of postoperative tears, but the MRI study then becomes a relatively invasive and more expensive procedure. In the future, other possible applications of MRI with respect to the meniscus may include kinematic MRI studies to assess meniscal stability, and 3D exams to create templates for meniscal implant surgery.

One question that frequently arises when discussing the optimal MRI examination of the knee is whether a high-field strength MR system (i.e., >1.0 T) is needed for accurate diagnosis. Barnett[12] recently reported on the effect of field strength on the efficacy of MRI diagnosis. The MRI findings in 118 consecutive patients who underwent an MRI examination with a 0.5 T system were compared to the arthroscopic findings. The accuracy for the detection of medial menicus tears was 92%, lateral meniscal tears 93%, and complete tears of the anterior cruciate ligament 97%. These results are not significantly different compared to the use of high-field strength systems. The examination times were longer on the 0.5 T system than on a high-field strength system. Potential sources of bias in this study are that the arthroscopists probably knew the results of the MRI exam prior to the arthroscopic procedure, and the fact that all these patients required arthroscopy indicates that a greater severity of knee dysfunction was present, which may inflate the accuracy of the MRI exam. As noted by the author, it is difficult to eliminate the second potential source of bias if arthroscopy is used as the gold standard.

In a prospective study from England, Spiers et al[217] reported on 58 patients with suspected internal derangement of the knee who had an MRI examination followed by arthroscopy. They found that their preoperative clinical assessment had a sensitivity of 77% and specificity of 43%, and the MRI had a sensitivity of 100% and a specificity of 63%, when compared to the arthroscopic findings. The authors concluded that acceptance of the MRI findings could have resulted in a 29% reduction in the arthroscopic procedures without missing any significant meniscal lesion. Similar results were found by Boden et al[22] and Ruwe et al.[197]

## OSSEOUS INJURIES

In the evaluation of acute skeletal trauma, plain films should be the initial radiologic study obtained to detect the presence of an osseous infraction, and to determine the nature and extent of bony disruption. With acute fractures of the skeletal system that involve cortical bone, standard x-rays are usually adequate to determine whether there is an acute cortical injury. Plain films are optimal to assess angulation, rotation, and distraction of the fracture fragments and to evaluate the integrity of the adjacent joints. At least two orthogonal x-ray views (i.e., 90° perpendicular to each other) are required to accurately assess the extent and alignment of a fracture. To optimize the detection of traumatic changes with plain films, it is important that the relevant clinical history is available at the time of plain film interpretation. Berbaum et al[13] reported on how the knowledge of the location of a patient's symptoms and signs affected the detection rate of fractures. Analysis of receiver-operator characteristic parameters indicated that the clinical information improved the detection rate of fractures. The improvement was based on a improved true-positive rate, without an increased false-positive rate.

With complex fractures, plain films are frequently not adequate to determine the nature and extent of an osseous injury. In these cases, computed tomography is the ideal study to perform, after the initial plain film evaluation. With CT, it is possible to determine the precise number and relationship of the different fracture fragments. It also is excellent in determining whether a fracture extends into contiguous joints, information which is critically needed in presurgical planning. Several studies have reported on the value of CT in the assessment of shoulder,[119] pelvis, tibial,[51] and calcaneal fractures.

Plain films are also the standard examination to follow fracture healing, by detecting the presence and extent of callus formation.[191] Early detection of a delayed union or nonunion is delineated with plain films. If there is a clinical concern about the degree of healing, conventional or computed tomography can be performed to determine the extent of fracture healing. Smith et al[213] reported on the prediction of fracture healing of the tibia by quantitative radionuclide imaging. The test had a sensitivity of 70% and a specificity of 90%. In cases where internal fixation had been applied, the assessment of fracture healing was more difficult.

Chronic osseous microtrauma may result in fractures of the cortical or cancellous bone, if cumulative load exceeds the cell-matrix adaptive capacities. This may occur at the insertion site of tendons into bone (e.g., apophyseal traction injuries[137]) or at sites of mechanical overload related to increased physical activity[54] (e.g., march fractures). Chronic stress fractures are referred to as fatigue fractures if they result from excessive load applied to normal bone or as insufficiency fractures if they result from the application of physiologic stress to weakened bone.[45,117] Bone normally responds to new functional demands by remodeling, but if the rate of tissue disruption exceeds tissue repair, failure may result. Since the pathologic process involves both bone resorption and healing, the stress fractures that develop will initially have indistinct margins and are difficult to detect with plain films. If a stress fracture involves the cortical bone, periosteal new bone formation may be detected at the fracture site. If the fracture involves the cancellous bone, subtle areas of linear sclerosis may be detected in regions of trabecular compaction or callus formation. It usually takes 5 to 6 weeks for an x-ray to become positive after the onset of symptoms, and even then, the findings on plain films may be extremely subtle. If the findings on plain films are indeterminate, additional studies (e.g., CT or bone scintigraphy) may be needed to evaluate the bony changes.[199] CT has proven useful in the assessment of stress fractures of the tarsal navicular,[123] and of the pars interarticularis of the spine. CT has also been employed to differentiate between stress fractures and bone tumors (e.g., osteoid osteomas).

As a result of the active bone remodeling at the site of a stress fracture, a bone scan will usually be positive soon after the onset of symptoms, particularly in a young patient. A positive bone scan will occur with any process that increases bone metabolism and therefore its specificity is limited. In addition, there is limited spatial resolution with a bone scan and it may be difficult to localize precisely the position of an abnormality and to determine if adjacent soft tissues or joints are involved by a pathologic process. There also have been case reports of negative bone scans in patients with stress fractures.[118,221]

MRI is also extremely sensitive in detecting stress fractures or any pathologic process that replaces the normal medullary fat in the cancellous bone by edematous tissue or a cellular infiltrate.[99] In both the inflammatory and reparative phases of a fracture, there will be increased fluid and cellular infiltration at the fracture site. These changes will be detected on a spin-echo T1-weighted sequence as a focus of intermediate signal intensity compared to the high signal of the normal fat, and on a T2-weighted or STIR sequence as a focus of high signal intensity. The strength of MRI compared to a bone scan is its excellent spatial resolution, direct multiplanar capabilities, high soft tissue contrast resolution, and it requires no exposure to ionizing radiation. With an MRI, it is usually possible to localize precisely the position of an abnormality. In cases where other diagnoses are being considered in addition to a stress fracture (e.g., infection or tumor), Gd-DTPA can be used to enhance the value of an MRI study. The results of an MRI study are also immediately available after the completion of an exam, which facilitates optimal patient care.

The major drawbacks of MRI compared to bone scans are its higher cost, lower accessibility, and that it is contraindicated for certain patients. One way to curtail MRI costs is to perform a limited MRI study only, and this has proven to be extremely valuable in the detection of subtle femoral neck fractures in elderly patients.[189] Deutsch et al[49] employed a coronal spin-echo T1-weighted sequence in the evaluation of 23 patients in whom there was a high clinical suspicion of fracture and who had normal plain films. A fracture was demonstrated by MRI in 9 of 9 patients who on follow-up x-rays had fractures, and the MRI excluded a fracture in 14 of 14 patients without fractures. In the same study, radionuclide scans were positive in 4 of 4 patients with a fracture and equivocal in one patient who did not have a fracture. The authors concluded that MRI can provide rapid, cost-effective, and anatomically precise diagnoses of hip fractures in patients with normal or equivocal plain films. Bone scans are also used to detect insufficiency fractures of the femoral neck in older patients,[229] but it may take several days before the scan becomes positive. It also may be difficult with a bone scan to differentiate between a fracture and severe arthritis.

After a direct injury to an extremity, it is fairly common for an individual to experience pain involving an osseous structure. Prior to the application of MRI, the precise etiology of this pain was unclear considering that plain films were usually negative. With the exquisite sensitivity of MRI to detect bone marrow edema, it quickly became apparent that many patients with acute trauma had areas of edematous cancellous bone at the site of an osseous injury.[132,138,150,257] The focal areas of bone marrow edema are most likely secondary to trabecular microtrauma (i.e., bone contusions or bruises) in the cancellous bone. They may occur secondary to an extrinsic impaction injury or may be secondary to bones impacting against one another as a result of acute instability or malalignment.

One of the first injuries where bone contusions were frequently detected was in patients with acute tears of the ACL.[115,159,218] The osseous contusions are typically located in the cancellous bone of the lateral femoral condyle superjacent to the condylar-trochlear sulcus and in the cancellous bone of the posterosupe-

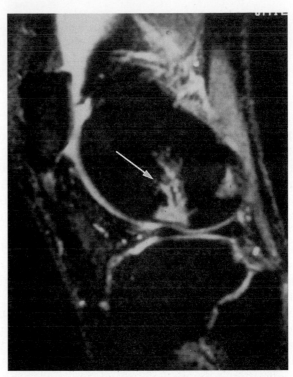

**FIGURE 15-20**    An MRI study was performed on a patient who incurred an acute ACL tear while skiing. The patient presented with lateral joint-line pain, and the clinician suspected a tear of the lateral meniscus. On the STIR sequence there is high signal intensity in the cancellous bone of the lateral femoral condyle (*arrow*). There was no tear of the lateral meniscus on the routine MRI spin-echo sequences or at arthroscopy.

rior segment of the lateral tibial condyle (Fig. 15-20). There are several potential reasons why the detection of these bone contusions is important. Clinically a patient may have lateral joint line pain and the possibility of a torn lateral meniscus must be considered as a potential source of this pain. With an MRI exam, it is not only possible to assess the appearance of the meniscus, but also by demonstrating the presence of a bone contusion it clarifies the etiology of the pain. The fact that the contusion exists also means that the overlying articular cartilage and/or meniscus also sustained a focal impaction force at the time of the injury. Cartilage tears are difficult to detect on an MRI, but the presence of a contusion should alert the radiologist to evaluate critically the articular cartilage overlying the region of the contused bone. Vellet et al[239] reported on a group of 21 patients with acute hemorrhagic knee effusions who underwent an MRI study and arthroscopy. Bone contusions adjacent to the subchondral plate were detected on the MRI in these patients, but at arthroscopy the overlying articular cartilage was normal. When these individuals were reevaluated at 6 to 12 months after the injury with a repeat MRI examination, 67% had developed osteochondral abnormalities. It is possible that when bone contusions are detected at the time of the initial injury, rehabilitation should be directed to prevent further overload to the articular cartilage, perhaps by an extended period of nonweight bearing. It is hoped that this will be investigated by appropriate long-term prospective studies.

By the detection of the position of bony contusions, it is possible to determine the exact location of the bone subjected to an extrinsic force. This information may help clarify the manners and mechanisms of different injuries and help to diagnose the precise etiology of knee pain when the history and physical exam is indeterminate. The diagnosis of patellar dislocation may be difficult if the patella relocates immediately. A patient may present with parapatellar pain and swelling and with a history of the knee giving out. MRI can be particularly helpful in these cases by detecting bone bruises on the anterolateral nonarticular margin of the lateral femoral condyle, and in the medial facet of the patella.[122,129,244] The bony contusions are secondary to impaction of the medial facet of the patella against the lateral femoral condyle when the patella translates medially in the process of relocation. It is also possible to detect injuries of the lateral patellar facet and the lateral facet of the femoral trochlea if they impact against each other as the patella translates laterally. Kirsch et al[122] reported on the findings of transient lateral patellar dislocation in 26 patients. Partial or complete disruption of the medial patellar retinaculum was detected in 96%, a contusion of the lateral femoral condyle in 81%, osteochondral injuries in 58%, lateral patellar tilt or subluxation in 92%, and a joint effusion in 100%. Patellar dislocation had not been suspected prior to the MRI study in 73% of the patients. Axial images revealed the constellation of abnormalities present with transient lateral patellar dislocation. As many of these patients are being imaged for knee dysfunction without the clinical suspicion of transient lateral dislocation, it is mandatory that an axial sequence be part of a standard MRI evaluation for all patients with acute knee dysfunction. From these reports, it appears that the spin-echo[122] and STIR[129] sequences are optimal to detect these abnormalities.

Another important application of MRI in the evaluation of pathologic changes in bone is in the detection of osteonecrosis (ON). STIR and fat suppressed spin-echo T2-weighted sequences are probably optimal to detect marrow edema. The pathoetiology (e.g., atraumatic or traumatic) and the stage of evolution of ON will determine its appearance on an MRI study. Atraumatic ON is an evolving process, whether associated with medications such as steroids, or as part of a

clinical disorder causing ischemia to the femoral head, such as sickle cell or marrow storage diseases. Intermittent ischemia will precipitate microinfarcts with secondary inflammation and repair. The inflammatory and reparative processes are associated with increased fluid in the marrow that may elevate the marrow pressure due to the constraints of the surrounding bone.[109] It appears that the earliest change of ON depicted on a routine MRI is the detection of marrow edema, which explains why the study would be negative in detecting ON secondary to acute vascular disruption.[8] It is possible that both dynamic radionuclide and dynamic MRI studies with Gd-DPTA,[160] which can assess the perfusion status of the femoral head, may be able to detect perfusion abnormalities of the femoral head after a femoral neck fracture. The presence of decreased perfusion to the femoral head does not necessarily mean that ON will develop.

The detection of bone marrow edema on an MRI study is not a specific finding for ON but can be found with other disorders causing increased marrow hydration (e.g., ischemia,[238] fracture, transient bone marrow edema syndrome,[88,237] infection, or malignancy). Once there is osseous repair and/or replacement of the necrotic trabeculae with new bone, a characteristic "double line" can be detected at the interface between the necrotic and viable bone. On an MRI spin-echo T2-weighted sequence there will be a zone of high signal intensity secondary to the reparative tissue, surrounded by a zone of low signal intensity representing the repaired thickened trabecular bone. Any area of fibrosis or mineralized tissue will appear on the T2-weighted sequence as a focus of low signal intensity. Contrast-enhanced MRI studies may help differentiate between viable and nonviable marrow at this stage of ON.[236] With progression of ON, fracture and/or collapse of the femoral head can be detected with MRI, but CT is helpful to delineate small areas of cortical disruption or subchondral fractures. The location and extent of the osteonecrotic bone may be of prognostic value in predicting whether the femoral head will collapse;[167,224] therefore, both sagittal and coronal sequences are needed to calculate the extent of ON. Since MRI is noninvasive, it is possible to follow patients who are at high risk for developing ON,[69,226] or patients who have undergone core decompression,[97,161] to determine the status of their femoral heads. Plain films are insensitive in detecting early ON,[233] and by the time that a subchondral fracture or collapse of the femoral head is detected on a plain film, the value of a core decompression may be limited.

In addition to the detection of ON of the hip, MRI is useful in detecting ON of the knee,[18] shoulder, wrist, or ankle. With the exquisite sensitivity of MRI to detect abnormalities of bone marrow, it was hoped that it could also be applied in assessing patients with reflex sympathetic dystrophy (RSD). Three-phase radionuclide bone scans have a reported 100% sensitivity, 80% specificity, 54% positive predictive value, and 100% negative predictive value for the detection of RSD of the foot.[98] Koch et al[124] reported on the MRI findings of 17 patients with RSD. Ten of 17 were normal on MRI, 6 of 17 had nonspecific soft-tissue changes or bone marrow sclerosis, and 1 of 17 showed changes of abnormal signal intensity. The fact that an MRI is negative with RSD may help elucidate the pathophysiology of RSD. It seems likely that the increased marrow perfusion detected on radionuclide studies may not be associated with concomitant marrow edema.

## CONCLUSION

Musculoskeletal dysfunction occurs when the capacity of the cell-matrix complex to adapt to biomechanical force is exceeded. Whether this is an acute or chronic process will determine the nature of an injury and the secondary tissue response, including inflammation or degeneration. By understanding the initial mechanism of injury and the spectrum of tissue reaction to structural failure, it is possible to predict the manifestations of a myriad musculoskeletal disorders on any type of imaging study. Each radiologic imaging examination, such as plain films, CT, MRI, and ultrasonography, encodes a different physical property of tissue; therefore each study should be used in specific clinical situations. Redundant studies must be eliminated if the costs of health care are to be controlled. Prospective controlled studies must be performed comparing the various imaging modalities to determine their cost-effectiveness. It is also possible that certain imaging studies may decrease medical costs by eliminating more expensive diagnostic procedures such as arthroscopy.[197,217]

## References

1. Abdelwahab F, Gould ES: The role of diskography after negative postmyelography CT scans: retrospective review. *AJNR* 9:187-190, 1988.
2. Aguila LA, et al: The intranuclear cleft of the intervertebral disk: magnetic resonance imaging. *Radiology* 155:155-158, 1985.
3. Alaranta H, Tallroth K, Soukka A, Heliovaara M: Fat content of lumbar extensor muscles and low back disability: a radiographic and clinical comparison. *J Spinal Disorders* 6(2):137-140, 1993.
4. Amendola A, Rorabeck CH, Vellett FD, et al: The use of magnetic resonance imaging in exertional compartment syndromes. *Am J Sports Med* 18:29-34, 1990.
5. Andersson GBJ, Schultz A, Nathan A, Irstam L: Roentgenographic measurement of lumbar intervertebral disc height. *Spine* 6(2):154-158, 1981.
6. Anti-Poika I, Soini J, Tallroth K, et al: Clinical relevance of discography combined with CT scanning. *J Bone Joint Surg* [Br] 72(B):480-485, 1990.
7. Arnoldi CC, et al: Lumbar spinal stenosis and nerve root entrapment syndromes: definition and classification. *Clin Orthop Rel Res* 115:4-5, 1976.
8. Asnis SE, Gould ES, Bansal M, et al: Magnetic resonance imaging of the hip after displaced femoral neck fractures. *Clin Orthop* 298:191-198, 1994.
9. Aspelin P, Ekberg O, Thorsson O, et al: Ultrasound examination of soft tissue injury of the lower limb in athletes. *Am J Sports Med* 20:601-603, 1992.
10. Auletta AG, Conway WF, Hayes CW, et al: Indications for radiography in patients with acute ankle injuries: role of the physical examination. *AJR* 157:789-791, 1991.
11. Balagura S, Neumann J: Magnetic resonance imaging of the postoperative intervebral disc: the first eight months—clinical and legal implications. *J Spinal Disorders* 3:212-217, 1993.
12. Barnett MJ: MR diagnosis of internal derangements of the knee: effect of field strength on efficacy. *AJR* 161:115-118, 1993.
13. Berbaum KS, El-Khoury GY, Franken EA, et al: Impact of clinical history on fracture detection with radiography. *Radiology* 168:507-511, 1988.
14. Bernard TN Jr: Lumbar discography followed by computed tomography: refining the diagnosis of low-back pain. *Spine* 15(7):690-707, 1990.
15. Biering-Sorensen F, Hensen FR, Schroll M, Runeborg O: The relation of spinal X-ray to low-back pain and physical activity among 60-year-old men and women. *Spine* 10(5):445-451, 1985.
16. Bigos SJ, Hansson T, Castillo RN, et al: The value of preemployment roentgenographs for predicting acute back injury claims and chronic back pain disability. *Clin Orthop* 283:124-129, 1992.
17. Bischoff RJ, Rodriguez RP, Gupta K, et al: A comparison of computed tomography-myelography, magnetic resonance imaging, and myelography in the diagnosis of herniated nucleus pulposus and spinal stenosis. *J Spinal Disorders* 6(4):289-295, 1993.

18. Bjokengren AG, Airowaih A, Lindstrand A, et al: Spontaneous osteonecrosis of the knee: value of MR imaging in determining prognosis. *AJR* 154:331-336, 1990.

19. Blumenthal SL, et al: The role of anterior lumbar fusion for internal disc disruption. *Spine* 13(5):566-569, 1988.

20. Boden S, Davis DO, Dina TS, et al: The incidence of abnormal lumbar spine MRI scans in asymptomatic patients: a prospective investigation. *J Bone Joint Surg* 72A:1178-1184, 1989.

21. Boden SD, David DO, Dina TS, et al: Abnormal magnetic resonance scans of the lumbar spine in asymptomatic subjects. *J Bone Joint Surg.* 72-A(3):403-408, 1990.

22. Boden SD, Labropoulos PA, Vailas JC: MR scanning of the acutely injured knee: sensitive, but is it cost effective? *J Arthro Surg* 6(4):306-310, 1990.

23. Boden SD, McCowin PR, Davis DO, et al: Abnormal magnetic resonance scans of the cervical spine in asymptomatic subjects. *J Bone Joint Surg* 72-A(8):1178-1183, 1990.

24. Bodne D, Quinn SF, Murray WT, et al: Magnetic resonance images of chronic patellar tendinitis. *Skeletal Radiol* 17:24-28, 1988.

25. Boeree NR, Watkinson AF, Ackroyd CE, et al: Magnetic resonance imaging of meniscal and cruciate injuries of the knee. *J Bone Joint Surg* (73)-B:452-457, 1991.

26. Bohatirchuk F: The aging vertebral column (macro- and historadiographical study). *Br J Radiol* 28(332):389-404, 1955.

27. Bozzao A, Gallucci M, Masciocchi C, et al: Lumbar disk herniation: MR imaging assessment of natural history in patients treated without surgery. *Radiology* 185:135-141, 1992.

28. Brenneke SL, Morgan CJ: Evaluation of ultrasonography as a diagnostic technique in the assessment of rotator cuff tendon tears. *Am J Sports Med* 20:287-288, 1989.

29. Bronskill MJ, Sprawls P: The Physics of MRI: *1992 AAPM Summer School Proceedings,* American Institute of Physics, Woodbury, 1993.

30. Burstein AH: Editorial. Fracture classification systems: do they work and are they useful? *J Bone Joint Surg [Am]* (75)-A:1743-1744, 1993.

31. Burton CV, et al: Causes of failure of surgery on the lumbar spine. *Clin Orthop Rel Res* 157:191-199, 1981.

32. Bush K, Cowan N, Katz DE, Gishen P: The natural history of sciatica associated with disc pathology: a prospective study with clinical and independent radiologic follow-up. *Spine* 17(10):1205-1212, 1992.

33. Calvert PT, Packer NP, Stoker DJ, et al: Arthrography of the shoulder after operative repair of the torn rotator cuff. *J Bone Joint Surg [Br]* (68)-B:147-150, 1986.

34. Cardone BW, Erickson SJ, Den Hartog, Carrera GF: MRI of injury to the lateral collateral ligamentous complex of the ankle. *J Comput Assist Tomogr* 17:102-107, 1993.

34a. Carr D, Gilbertson L, Frymoyer J, et al: Lumbar paraspinal compartment syndrome: a case report with physiologic and anatomic studies. *Spine* 10(9):816-820, 1985.

35. Cavanagh S, Stevens J, Johnson J: High-resolution MRI in the investigation of recurrent pain after lumbar discectomy *J Bone Joint Surg* 75-B:524-528, 1993.

36. Chandra R: *Introductory physics of nuclear medicine,* Philadelphia, 1976, Lea and Febiger.

37. Cheung Y, Magee TH, Rosenberg ZS, Rose DJ: MRI of anterior cruciate ligament reconstruction. *J Comput Assist Tomogr* 16:134-137, 1992.

38. Cobby MJ, Schweitzer ME, Resnick D: The deep lateral femoral notch: an indirect sign of a torn anterior cruciate ligament. *Radiology* 184:855-858, 1992.

39. Conway WF, Hayes CW, Loughran T, et al: Cross-sectional imaging of the patellofemoral joint and surrounding structures. *RadioGraphics* 11:195-217, 1991.

40. Coste J, Paolaggi JB, Spira A: Reliability of interpretation of plain lumbar spine radiographs in benign, mechanical low-back pain. *Spine* 16(4):426-428, 1991.

41. Coupens SD, Yates CK, Sheldon C, Ward C: Magnetic resonance imaging evaluation of the patellar tendon after use of its central one-third for anterior cruciate ligament reconstruction. *Am J Sports Med* 20:332-335, 1992.

42. Coventry MB, Ghormley RK, Kernohan JW: The intervertebral disc: its microscopic anatomy and pathology: Part II—changes in the intervertebral disc concomitant with age. *J Bone Joint Surg* 27(2):233-247, 1945.

43. Curry TS III, Dowdey JE, Murry RC Jr: *Christensen's physics of diagnostic radiology,* Philadelphia, 1990, Lea and Febiger.

44. Dabbs VM, Dabbs LG: Correlation between disc height narrowing and low-back pain. *Spine* 15(12):1366-1369, 1990.

45. Daffner RH, Pavlov H: Stress fractures: current concepts. *AJR* 159:245-252, 1993.

46. Deutsch AL, et al: Lumbar spine following successful surgical discectomy. *Spine* 18(8):1054-1060, 1993.

47. Deutsch AL, Mink JH: Articular disorders of the knee. *Magn Reson Imag* 1(3):43-56, 1989.

48. Deutsch AL, Mink JH: The postoperative knee. In: Mink JH, Reicher MA, Crues JV, et al: editors, *Magnetic resonance imaging of the knee,* New York, ed 2, 1993, Raven Press, p. 237.

49. Deutsch AL, Mink JH, Waxman AD: Occult fractures of the proximal femur: MR imaging. *Radiology* 170:113-116, 1989.

50. Deyo RA, Diehl AK: Lumbar spine films in primary care: current use and effects of selective ordering criteria. *J Intern Med* 1:20-25, 1986.

51. Dias JJ, Stirling AJ, Finlay DBL, Gregg PJ: Computerised axial tomography for tibial plateau fractures. *J Bone Joint Surg [Br]* (69)-B:84-88, 1987.

52. DiFazio FA, Barth RA, Frymoyer JW: Acute lumbar paraspinal compartment syndrome. *J Bone Joint Surg [Am]* (73)-A:1101-1103, 1991.

53. Edelman RR, et al: High-resolution of surface-coil imaging of lumbar disk disease. *AJR* 144:1123-1129, 1985.

54. Eisele SA, Sammarco GJ: Fatigue fractures of the foot and ankle in the athlete. *J Bone Joint Surg [Am]* (75)-A:290-298, 1993.

55. Erickson SJ, Cox JH, Hyde JS, et al: Effect of tendon orientation on MR Imaging signal intensity: a manifestation of the "magic angle" phenomenon. *Radiology* 181:389-392, 1991.

56. Farin PU, Jaroma H, Harju A, Soimakallio S: Shoulder impingement syndrome: sonographic evaluation. *Radiology* 176:845-849, 1990.

57. Farley TE, Neumann CH, Steinbach LS, et al: Full-thickness tears of the rotator cuff of the shoulder: diagnosis with MR imaging. *AJR* 158:347-351, 1992.

58. Ferretti A, Ippolito E, Mariai P, Puddu G: Jumper's knee. *Am J Sports Med* 11:58-62, 1983.

59. Firooznia H, et al: CT of lumbar spine disk herniation: correlation with surgical findings, *AJR* 5:91-96, 1984.

60. Fischer SP, Fox JM, De Pizzo W, et al: Accuracy of diagnoses from magnetic resonance imaging of the knee. *J Bone Joint Surg* (73)-A:2-10, 1991.

61. Fitzgerald SW, Remer EM, Friedman H, Rogers LF: MR evaluation of the anterior cruciate ligament: value of supplementing sagittal images with coronal and axial images. *AJR* 160:1233-1237, 1993.

62. Fleckenstein JL, Weatherall PT, Parkey RW, et al: Sports-related muscle injuries: evaluation with MR imaging. *Radiology* 172:793-798, 1989.

63. Forristall RM, Marsh HO, Pay NT: Magnetic resonance imaging and contrast CT of the lumbar spine: comparison of diagnostic methods and correlation with surgical findings. *Spine* 13(9):1049-1054, 1988.

64. Franklin JL, Rosenberg TD, Paulos LE, et al: Radiographic assessment of instability of the knee due to rupture of the anterior cruciate ligament: a quadriceps-contraction technique. *J Bone Joint Surg [Am]* (73)-A:365-372, 1991.

65. Friedenberg ZB, Edeiken J, Spencer HN, Tolentino SC: Degenerative changes in the cervical spine. *J Bone Joint Surg* 41(A)-1:61-70, 1959.

66. Friedenberg ZB, Miller WT: Degenerative disc disease of the cervical spine. *J Bone Joint Surg* 45-A(6):1171-1178, 1963.

67. Fries JW, et al: Computed tomography of herniated and extruded nucleus pulposus. *J Comp Assist Tomogr* 6(5):874-887, 1982.

68. Frymoyer JW, Newberg A, Pope MA, et al: Spine radiographs in patients with low-back pain: an epidemiological study in men. *J Bone Joint Surg* 66(A)-7:1048-1105, 1984.

69. Gennuso R, Zappulla RA, Strenger SW: A localized lumbar spinal root arteriovenous malformation presenting with radicular signs and symptoms. *Spine* 14(5):543-546, 1989.

70. Gerber C, Krushell RJ: Isolated rupture of the tendon of the subscapularis muscle: clinical features in 16 cases. *J Bone Joint Surg [Br]* (73)-B:389-394, 1991.

71. Ghosh P, editor: *The biology of the intervertebral disc,* Vol. I, 1988, CRC Press, Boca Raton, Fla., p. 245.

72. Ghosh P, editor: *The biology of the intervertebral disc,* Vol. II, 1988, CRC Press, Boca Raton, Fla., p. 207.

73. Glashow JL, Katz R, Schneider M, Scott WN: Double-blind assessment of the value of magnetic resonance imaging in the diagnosis of anterior cruciate and meniscal lesions. *J Bone Joint Surg* (71)-A:113-119, 1989.

74. Glenn Jr WV, et al: Multiplanar display computerized body tomography applications in the lumbar spine. *Spine* 4(4):282-294, 1979.

75. Gore DR, Sepic SB, Gardner GM. Roentgenographic findings of the cervical spine in asymptomatic people. *Spine* 11(6):521-524, 1986.

76. Gore DR, Sepic SB, Gardner GM, Murray P: Neck pain: a long-term follow-up of 205 patients. *Spine* 12(1):1-5, 1987.

77. Goyal RN, et al: Intraspinal cysts: a classification and literature review. *Spine* 12(3):209-213, 1987.

78. Greco A, McNamara MT, Escher MG, et al: Spin-echo and STIR MR imaging of sports-re-

lated muscle injuries at 1.5 T. *J Comput Assist Tomogr* 15:994-999, 1991.

79. Grenier N, et al: Isthmic spondylolysis of the lumbar spine: MR imaging at 1.5 T. *Radiology* 170:489-493, 1989.

80. Grenier N, et al: Normal and disrupted lumbar longitudinal ligaments: correlative MR and anatomic study. *Radiology* 171(1):197-205, 1989.

81. Gross ML, Grover JS, Bassett LW, et al: Magnetic resonance imaging of the posterior cruciate ligament. *Am J Sports Med* 20:732-737, 1992.

82. Grover JS, Bassett LW, Gross ML, et al: Posterior cruciate ligament: MR imaging. *Radiology* 174:527-530, 1990.

83. Grubb SA, Lipscomb HJ, Coonrad RW: Degenerative adult onset scoliosis. *Spine* 13(3):241-245, 1988.

84. Harcke HT, Grissom LE, Finkelstein MS: Evaluation of the musculoskeletal system with sonography. *AJR* 150:1253-1261, 1988.

85. Harryman DT, Mack LA, Wang KY, et al: Repairs of the rotator cuff: correlation of functional results with integrity of the cuff. *J Bone Joint Surg* (73)-A:982-989, 1991.

86. Hasso AN, et al: Computed tomography of children and adolescents with suspected spinal stenosis. *J Comput Assist Tomogr* 11(4):609-611, 1987.

87. Haughton VM, et al: A prospective comparison of computed tomography and myelography in the diagnosis of herniated lumbar disks. *Radiology* 142:103-110, 1982.

88. Hayes CW, Conway WF, Daniel W: MR imaging of bone marrow edema pattern: transient osteoporosis, transient bone marrow edema syndrome, or osteonecrosis. *RadioGraphics* 13:1001-1011, 1993.

89. Hendee WR: *The physical principles of computed tomography,* Boston, 1983, Little, Brown.

90. Hernandez RJ, Keim DR, Chenevert TL, et al: Fat-suppressed MR imaging of myositis. *Radiology* 182:217-219, 1992.

91. Hernandez RJ, Sullivan DB, Chenevert TL, Keim DR: MR imaging in children with dermatomyositis: musculoskeletal findings and correlation with clinical and laboratory findings. *AJR* 161:359-366, 1993.

92. Hickey DS, et al: Analysis of magnetic resonance images from normal and degenerate lumbar intervertebral discs. *Spine* 11(7):702-708, 1986.

93. Hitselberger WE, Witten RM: Abnormal myelograms in asymptomatic patients. *J Neurosurg* 28:204-206, 1968.

94. Hodge JC, Ghelman B, O'Brien SJ, Wickiewicz TL: Synovial plicae and chondromalacia patellae: correlation of results of CT arthrography with results of arthroscopy. *Radiology* 186:827-831, 1993.

95. Hodler J, Haghighi P, Pathria MN, et al: Meniscal changes in the elderly: correlation of MR imaging and histologic findings. *Radiology* 184:221-225, 1992.

96. Hodler J, Kursunoglu-Brahme S, Snyder SJ, et al: Rotator cuff disease: assessment with MR arthrography versus standard MR imaging in 36 patients with arthroscopic confirmation. *Radiology* 182:431-436, 1992.

97. Hofmann S, Engel A, Neuhold A, et al: Bone-marrow oedema syndrome and transient osteoporosis of the hip: an MRI-controlled study of treatment by core decompression. *J Bone Joint Surg [Br]* (75)-B:210-216, 1993.

98. Holder LE, Cole LA, Myerson MS: Reflex sympathetic dystrophy in the foot: clinical and scintigraphic criteria. *Radiology* 184:531-535, 1992.

99. Hosten N, Schorner W, Neumann, K, et al: MR imaging of bone marrow: review of the literature and possible indications for contrast-enhanced studies. *Adv MRI Contr* 1:84-98, 1993.

100. Howell SM, Clark JA, Blasier RD: Serial magnetic resonance imaging of hamstring anterior cruciate ligament autografts during the first year of implantation: a preliminary study. *Am J Sports Med* 19:42-47, 1991.

101. Hueftle M, et al: Lumbar spine: postoperative MR imaging with Gd-DTPA. *Radiology* 167:817-824, 1988.

102. Hurme M, Alaranta H: Factors predicting the result of surgery for lumbar intervertebral disc herniation. *Spine* 12(9):933-938, 1987.

103. Iannotti JP, Zlatkin MB, Esterhai JL, et al: Magnetic resonance imaging of the shoulder. *Magnet Reson Imag* (73)-A:17-29, 1991.

104. Jackson DW, Jennings LD, Maywood RM, Beger PE: Magnetic resonance imaging of the knee. *Am J Sports Med* 16:29-38, 1988.

105. Jaffray D, O'Brien JP: Isolated intervertebral disc resorption: a source of mechanical and inflammatory back pain? *Spine* 11(4):397-401, 1986.

106. Jehenson P, Leroy-Willig A, de Kerviler E, et al: MR imaging as a potential diagnostic test for metabolic myopathies: importance of variations in the T2 of muscle with exercise. *AJR* 161:347-351, 1993.

107. Jensen MC, Brant-Zawdzi MN, Obuchowski N, et al: Magnetic resonance imaging of the lum-

bar spine in people without back pain. *N Engl J Med* 331:69-73, 1994.

108. Kainberger FM, Engel A, Barton P, et al: Injury of the achilles tendon: diagnosis with sonography. *AJR* 155:1031-1036, 1990.

109. Kalebo P, Allenmark C, Peterson L, Sward L: Diagnostic value of ultrasonography in partial ruptures of the Achilles tendon. *Am J Sports Med* 20:378-381, 1992.

110. Kalebo P, Karlsson J, Sward L, Peterson L: Ultrasonography of chronic tendon injuries in the groin. *Am J Sports Med* 20:634-639, 1992.

111. Kambin P, et al: Annular protrusion: pathophysiology and roentgenographic appearance. *Spine* 13(6):671-675, 1988.

112. Kannus P, Jozsa L: Histopathological changes preceding spontaneous rupture of a tendon: a controlled study of 891 patients. *J Bone Joint Surg [Am]* (73)-A:1507-1525, 1991

113. Kaplan PA, Bryans KC, Davick JP, et al: MR imaging of the normal shoulder: variants and pitfalls. *Radiology* 184:519-524, 1992.

114. Kaplan PA, Matamoros A, Anderson JC: Sonography of the musculoskeletal system. *AJR* 155:237-245, 1990.

115. Kaplan PA, Walker CW, Kilcoyne RF, et al: Occult fracture patterns of the knee associated with anterior cruciate ligament tears: assessment with MR imaging. *Radiology* 183:835-838, 1992.

116. Karzel RP, Snyder SJ: Magnetic resonance arthrography of the shoulder. *Clin Sports Med* 12:123-136, 1993.

117. Kathol MH, El-Khoury GY, Moore TE, Marsh JL: Calcaneal insufficiency avulsion fractures in patients with diabetes mellitus. *Radiology* 180:725-772, 1991.

118. Keene JS, Lash EG: Negative bone scan in a femoral neck stress fracture: a case report. *Am J Sport Med* 20:234-236, 1992.

119. Kilcoyne RF, Shuman WP, Matsen FA, et al: The Neer classification of displaced proximal humeral fractures: spectrum of findings on plain radiographs and CT scans. *AJR* 154:1029-1033, 1990.

120. Kirkaldy-Willis WH: The pathology and pathogenesis of low back pain. *In Managing low-back pain*, New York, 1988, Churchill Livingstone, pp. 49-75.

121. Kirkaldy-Willis H, et al: Pathology and pathogenesis of lumbar spondylosis and stenosis. *Spine* 3(4):319-328, 1978.

122. Kirsch MD, Fitzgerald SW, Friedman H, Rogers LF: Transient lateral patellar dislocation: diagnosis with MR imaging. *AJR* 161:109-113, 1993.

123. Kiss ZS, Khan KM, Fuller PJ: Stress fractures of the tarsal navicular bone: CT findings in 55 cases. *AJR* 160:111-115, 1993.

124. Koch E, Hofer HO, Sialer G, et al: Failure of MR imaging to detect reflex sympathetic dystrophy of the extremities. *AJR* 156:113-115, 1991.

125. Kornick J, Trefelner E, McCarthy S, et al: Meniscal abnormalities in the asymptomatic population at MR imaging. *Radiology* 177:463-465, 1990.

126. Kransdorf MJ, Meis JM, Jelinek JS: Myositis ossificans: MR appearance with radiologic-pathologic correlation. *AJR* 157:1243-1248, 1991.

127. Kravis MMM, Munk PL, McCain GA, et al: MR imaging of muscle and tender points in fibromyalgia. *JMRI* 3:669-670, 1993.

128. Kurashima K, Shimizu H, Ogawa H: MR and CT in the evaluation of sarcoid myopathy. *J Comput Assist Tomogr* 15:1004-1007, 1991.

129. Lance E, Deutsch AL, Mink JH: Prior lateral patellar dislocation MR imaging findings. *Radiology* 189:905-907, 1993.

130. Lancourt, JE, Glenn WV Jr, Wiltse LL: Multiplanar computerized tomography in the normal spine and in the diagnosis of spinal stenosis: a gross anatomic-computerized tomographic correlation. *Spine* 4(4):379-390, 1979.

131. Leadbetter WB: Cell-matrix response in tendon injury. In: Renstrom AFH, Leadbetter WB, editors: *Clinics in sports medicine: tendinitis—basic concepts*, Philadelphia, 1992, WB Saunders, p. 533.

132. Lee JK, Yao L: Occult intraosseous fracture: magnetic resonance appearance versus age of injury. *Am J Sports Med* 17:620-623, 1989.

133. Lee JK, Yao L, Phelps CT, et al: Anterior cruciate ligament tears: MR imaging compared with arthroscopy and clinical tests. *Radiology* 166:861-864, 1988.

134. Levitan LH, Wiens CW: Chronic lumbar extradural hematoma: CT findings *Radiology* 148:707-708, 1983.

135. Liang M, Komaroff AL: Roentgenograms in primary care patients with acute low back pain. *Arch Intern Med* 142:1108-1112, 1982.

136. Lipson SJ, Muir H: Proteoglycans in experimental intervertebral disc degeneration. *Spine* 6(3):194-210, 1981.

137. Lombardo SJ, Retting AC, Kerlan RK: Radiographic abnormalities of the iliac apophysis in adolescent athletes. *J Bone Joint Surg [Am]* (65)-A:444-446, 1983.

138. Lynch TCP, Crues JV, Morgan FW, et al: Bone abnormalities of the knee: prevalence and sig-

nificance at MR imaging. *Radiology* 171:761-766, 1989.

139. Mack LA, Gannon MK, Kilcoyne RF, Matsen FA: Sonographic evaluation of the rotator cuff: accuracy in patients without prior surgery. *Clin Orthop* 234:21-27, 1988.

140. NacNab I: Spondylolisthesis with an intact neural arch, the so-called pseudo-spondylolistheses. *J Bone Joint Surg* 32B(3):325-333, 1950.

141. Masaryk TJ, et al: High-resolution MR imaging of sequestered lumbar intervertebral disks. *AJR* 150:1155-1162, 1988.

142. McAfee PC, et al: Computed tomography in degenerative spinal stenosis. *Clin Orthop Rel Res* 161:221-234, 1981.

143. McCauley TR, Kier R, Lynch KJ, Jokl P: Chondromalacia patellae: diagnosis with MR imaging. *AJR* 158:101-105, 1992.

144. McCauley TR, Moses M, Kier R, et al: MR diagnosis of tears of anterior cruciate ligament of the knee: importance of ancillary findings *AJR* 162:115-119, 1994.

145. Middleton WD, Reinus WR, Totty WG, et al: Ultrasonographic evaluation of the rotator cuff and biceps tendon. *J Bone Joint Surg* (68)-A:440-450, 1986.

146. Miller JAA, Schmatz C, Schultz AB: Lumbar disc degeneration: correlation with age, sex and spine level in 600 autopsy specimens. *Spine* 13(2):173-178, 1988.

147. Mink JH: Imaging evaluation of the candidate for percutaneous lumbar discectomy. *Clin Orthop Rel Res* 238:83-103, 1989.

148. Mink JH: Muscle injuries. In Mink JH, Reicher MA, Crues JH, et al: *Magnetic resonance imaging of the knee*, ed 2, New York, 1993, Raven Press, p. 401.

149. Mink JH: The cruciate and collateral ligaments. In Mink JH, Reicher MA, Crues JV, et al: *Magnetic resonance imaging of the knee*, ed 2, New York, 1993, Raven Press, p. 141.

150. Mink JH, Deutsch AL: Occult cartilage and bone injuries of the knee: detection, classification, and assessment with MR imaging. *Radiology* 170:823-829, 1989.

151. Mink JH, Levy T, Crues JV: Tears of the anterior cruciate ligament and menisci of the knee: MR imaging evaluation. *Radiology* 167:769-774, 1988.

152. Mirowitz SA: Normal rotator cuff: MR imaging with conventional and fat-suppression techniques. *Radiology* 180:735-740, 1991.

153. Misamore GW, Woodward C: Evaluation of degenerative lesions of the rotator cuff: a comparison of arthrography and ultrasonography. *J Bone Joint Surg* (73)-A:704-706, 1991.

154. Modic MT, Masaryk TJ, Ross JS: *Magnetic imaging of the spine*, Chicago, 1989, Year Book Medical Publishers.

155. Modic MT, Masaryk TJ, Ross JS, Carter JR: Imaging of degenerative disc disease. *Radiology* 168:177-186, 1988.

156. Modic MT, et al: Degenerative disc disease: assessment of changes in vertebral body marrow with MR imaging. *Radiology* 166:193-199, 1988.

157. Modic MT, et al: Lumbar herniated disc disease and canal stenosis: prospective evaluation by surface coil MR, CT, and myelography. *AJR* 147:757-765, 1986.

158. Modic MT, et al: Vertebral osteomyelitis: assessment using MR. *Radiology* 157:157-166, 1985.

159. Murphy BJ, Smith RL, Uribe JW, et al: Bone signal abnormalities in the posterolateral tibia and lateral femoral condyle in complete tears of the anterior cruciate ligament: a specific sign? *Radiology* 182:221-224, 1992.

160. Nadel SN, Debatin JF, Richardson WJ: Detection of acute avascular necrosis of the femoral head in dogs: dynamic contract-enhanced MR imaging vs. spin-echo and STIR sequences. *AJR* 159:1255-1261, 1992.

161. Neuhold A, Hofmann S, Engel A, et al: Bone marrow edema of the hip: MR findings after core decompression. *J Comput Assist Tomogr* 16:951-955, 1992.

162. Neumann CH, Holt RG, Steinbach LS, et al: MR imaging of the shoulder: appearance of the supraspinatus tendon in asymptomatic volunteers. *AJR* 158:1281-1287, 1992.

163. Noonan TJ, Garrett WF: Injuries at the myotendinous junction. *Clin Sports Med* 11:783-806, 1992.

164. Nunez-Hoyo M, Gradner CL, Motta AO, Ashmead JW: Case report—skeletal muscle infarction in diabetes: MR findings. *J Comput Assist Tomogr* 17:986-988, 1993.

165. Oberlander MA, Shalvoy RM, Hughston JC: The accuracy of the clinical knee examination documented by arthroscopy: a prospective study. *Am J Sports Med* 21:773-778, 1993.

166. O'Brien WR: Degenerative arthritis of the knee following anterior cruciate ligament injury: role of the meniscus. *Sports Med Arthroscopy Rev* 1:114-118, 1994.

167. Ohzono K, Saito M, Takaoka K, et al: Natural history of nontraumatic avascular necrosis of the femoral head. *J Bone Joint Surg [Br]* (73)-B:68-72, 1991.

168. O'Keeffe D, Mamtora H: Ultrasound in clinical orthopaedics. *J Bone Joint Surg [Br]*, (74)-B:488-494, 1992.

169. Ono K, Yamamuro T, Rockwood CA: Use of a thirty-degree caudal tilt radiograph in the shoulder impingement syndrome. *J Shoulder Elbow Surg* 246-252, 1992.

170. Osti OL, Fraser RD: MRI and discography of annular tears and intervertebral disc degeneration: a prospective clinical comparison. *J Bone Joint Surg [Br]* 74(B):431-435, 1992.

171. Osti OL, Veron-Roberts B, Moore R, Fraser RD: Annular tears and disc degeneration in the lumbar spine: a post-mortem study of 135 discs. *J Bone Joint Surg [Br]* 74(B):678-682, 1992.

172. Palmer EL, Scott JA, Straukse HW: *Practical nuclear medicine*, Philadelphia, 1992, WB Saunders.

173. Palmer WE, Brown JH, Rosenthal DI: Rotator cuff: evaluation with fat-suppressed MR arthrography. *Radiology* 188:683-687, 1993.

174. Park JH, Vansant JP, Kumar NG, et al: Dermatomyositis: correlative MR imaging and P-31 MR spectroscopy for quantitative characterization of inflammatory disease. *Radiology* 177:473-479, 1990.

175. Pech P, Haughton ML: Lumbar intervertebral disk: correlative MR and anatomic study. *Radiology* 156:699-701, 1985.

176. Peyster RG, Teplick JG, Haskin M: Computed tomography of lumbosacral conjoined nerve root anomalies: potential cause of false-positive reading for herniated nucleus-pulposus. *Spine* 10(4):331-337, 1985.

177. Porter RW, Bewley B: A ten-year prospective study of vertebral canal size as a predictor of back pain. *Spine* 19(2):173-175, 1994.

178. Porter RW, Hibbert C, Evans C: The natural history of root entrapment syndrome. *Spine* 9(4):418-421, 1984.

179. Post MJD, et al: Spinal infection: evaluation with MR imaging and intraoperative US. *Radiology* 169:765-771, 1988.

180. Puddu G, Ippolito E, Postacchini F: A classification of Achilles tendon disease. *Am J Sports Med* 4:145-150, 1976.

181. Raatikainen T, Putkonen M, Puranen J: Arthrography, clinical examination, and stress radiograph in the diagnosis of acute injury to the lateral ligaments of the ankle. *Am J Sports Med* 20:2-12, 1992.

182. Rafii M, Firooznia H, Sherman O, et al: Rotator cuff lesions: signal patterns at MR imaging. *Radiology* 177:817-823, 1990.

183. Rak KM, Gillogly SD, Schaefer RA, et al: Anterior cruciate ligament reconstruction: evaluation with MR imaging. *Radiology* 178:553-556, 1991.

184. Rauschning W: Normal and pathologic anatomy of the lumbar root canals. *Spine* 12(10):1008-1019, 1987.

185. Regan W, Wold LE, Conrad R, Morrey BF: Microscopic histopathology of chronic refractory lateral epicondylitis. *Am J Sports Med* 20:746-749, 1992.

186. Remer EM, Fitzgerald SW, Friedman H, et al: Anterior cruciate ligament injury: MR imaging diagnosis and patterns of injury. *RadioGraphics* 12:901-915, 1991.

187. Resendes M, Helms CA, Fritz RC, et al: MR appearance of intramuscular injections. *AJR* 158:1293-1294, 1992.

188. Rijke AM, Goitz HT, McCue FC, Dee PM: Magnetic resonance imaging of injury to the lateral ankle ligaments. *Am J Sports Med* 21:528-534, 1993.

189. Rizzo PF, Gould ES, Lyden JP, Asnis SE: Diagnosis of occult fractures about the hip: magnetic resonance imaging compared with bone-scanning. *J Bone Joint Surg* (75)-A:395-401, 1993.

190. Roberson GH, Llewellyn HJ, Taveras JM: The narrow lumbar spinal canal syndrome. *Radiology* 107:89-97, 1973.

191. Rogers LF, Hendrix RW: Radiography of fracture healing. *Current Imaging* 2:194-200, 1990.

192. Rose JL, Goldberg B: *Basic physics in diagnostic ultrasound*, New York, 1979, Wiley.

193. Ross JS, Modic MT, Masaryk JJ: Tears of the anulus fibrosus: assessment with Gd-DTPA-enhanced MR imaging. *AJR* 154:159-162, 1990.

194. Ross J, et al: Lumbar spine: postoperative assessment with surface-coil MR imaging. *Radiology* 164:851-860, 1987.

195. Rothman SLG, Glenn WV Jr: CT multiplanar reconstruction in 253 cases of lumbar spondylolysis. *ANJR* 5:81-90, 1984.

196. Rueter FG, Conway BJ, McCrohan JL, et al: Radiography of the lumbosacral spine: characteristics of examinations performed in hospitals and facilities. *Radiology* 185:43-46, 1992.

197. Ruwe PA, Wright J, Randall RL, et al: Can MR imaging effectively replace diagnostic arthroscopy? *Radiology* 183:335-339, 1992.

198. Ryan JB, Wheeler JH, Hopkinson WJ, et al: Quadriceps contusions. *Am J Sport Med* 19:299-304, 1991.

199. Satku K, Kumar VP, Chacha PB: Stress fractures around the knee in elderly patients: a cause of

acute pain in the knee. *J Bone Joint Surg* (72)-A:918-922, 1990.

200. Sato K, et al: The configuration of the laminas and facet joints in degenerative spondylolisthesis and clinicocardiologic study. *Spine* 14:1265-1271, 1989.

201. Scavone JG, Latshaw RF, Weidner WA: Anteroposterior and lateral radiographs: an adequate lumbar spine examination. *AJR* 136:715-717, 1981.

202. Schnebel B, Kingston S, Watkins R, Dillin W: Comparison of MRI to contrast CT in the diagnosis of spinal stenosis. *Spine* 14(3):332-337, 1989.

203. Schneck DC, Mesgarzadeh M, Bonakdarpour A: MR imaging of the most commonly injured ankle ligaments: Part II—ligament injuries. *Radiology* 184:507-512, 1992.

204. Schneck DC: The anatomy of lumbar spondylosis. *Clin Orthop Rel Res* 193:20-37, 1985.

205. Schweitzer ME, Caccese R, Karasick D, et al: Posterior tibial tendon tears: utility of secondary signs for MR imaging diagnosis. *Radiology* 188:655-659, 1993.

206. Scott WW, Lethbridge-Cejku M, Reichle R, et al: Reliability of grading scales for individual radiographic features of osteoarthritis of the knee: the Baltimore longitudinal study of aging atlas of knee osteoarthritis. *Invest Radiol* 28:497-501, 1993.

207. Scranton PE, Farrar EL: Mucoid degeneration of the patellar ligament in athletes. *J Bone Joint Surg* (74)-A:435-437, 1992.

208. Seeger LL, Gold RH, Bassett LW, Ellman H: Shoulder impingement syndrome: MR findings in 53 shoulders. *AJR* 150:343-347, 1988.

209. Shaffer WO, Spratt KF, Weinstein J, et al: The consistency and accuracy of roentgenograms for measuring sagittal translation in the lumbar vertebral motion segment: an experimental model. *Spine* 15(8):741-750, 1990.

210. Shellock FG: Safety. In Stark DD, Bradley WG: *Magnetic resonance imaging*, St Louis, 1992, Mosby–Year Book, pp. 522-544.

211. Shintani S, Shiigai T: Repeat MRI in acute rhabdomyolysis: correlation with clinicopathological findings. *J Comput Assist Tomogr* 17:786-791, 1993.

212. Sidor ML, Zuckerman JD, Lyon T, et al: The Neer classification system for proximal humeral fractures: an assessment of interobserver reliability and intraobserver reproducibility. *J Bone Joint Surg* (75)-A:1745-1750, 1993.

213. Smith MA, Jones EA, Strachan RK, et al: Prediction of fracture healing in the tibia by quan-

titative radionuclide imaging. *J Bone Joint Surg [Br]* (69)-B:441-447, 1987.

214. Sommerlath K, Lysholm J, Gillquist J: The long-term course after treatment of acute anterior cruciate ligament ruptures: a 9 to 16 year follow-up. *Am J Sports Med* 19:156-162, 1991.

215. Speer KP, Lohnes J, Garrett WE: Radiographic imaging of muscle strain injury. *Am J Sports Med* 21:89-96, 1993.

216. Speer KP, Spritzer CE, Goldner JL, Garrett WE: Magnetic resonance imaging of traumatic knee articular cartilage injuries. *Am J Sports Med* 19:396-402, 1991.

217. Spiers ASD, Meagher T, Ostlere SJ, et al: Can MRI of the knee affect arthroscopic practice? *J Bone Joint Surg [Br]* 75-B:49-52, 1993.

218. Spindler KP, Schils JP, Bergfeld JA, et al: Prospective study of osseous, articular, and meniscal lesions in recent anterior cruciate ligament tears by magnetic resonance imaging and arthroscopy. *Am J Sports Med* 21:551-557, 1993.

219. Sprawls P Jr: *Physical principles of medical imaging*, Gaithersburg, Md., 1987, Aspen Publishers.

220. Stallenberg B, Gevenois PA, Sintzoff SA, et al: Fracture of the posterior aspect of the lateral tibial plateau: radiographic sign of anterior cruciate ligament tear. *Radiology* 187:821-825, 1993.

221. Sterling JC, Webb RF, Meyers MC, Calvo RD: False-negative bone scan in a female runner. *Med Sci Sports Exerc* 25:179-185, 1993.

222. Sze G, et al: Malignant extradural spinal tumors: MR imaging with gadolinium-DTPA. *Radiology* 167:217-223, 1988.

223. Szypryt EP, et al: The prevalence of disc degeneration associated with neural arch defects of the lumbar spine assessed by magnetic resonance imaging. *Spine* 14:977-981, 1989.

224. Takatori Y, Kokubo T, Ninomiya S, et al: Avascular necrosis of the femoral head: natural history and magnetic resonance imaging. *J Bone Joint Surg [Br]* (75)-B:217-221, 1993.

225. Teresi LM, Lufkin RB, Reicher MA, et al: Asymptomatic degenerative disc disease and spondylosis of the cervical spine: MR imaging. *Radiology* 164:83-88, 1987.

226. Tervonen O, Mueller DM, Matteson EL, et al: Clinically occult avascular necrosis of the hip: prevalence in an asymptomatic population at risk. *Radiology* 182:845-847, 1992.

227. Thornbury JR, Fryback DG, Turski PA, et al: Disc-caused nerve compression in patients with acute low-back pain: diagnosis with MR, CT myelography, and plain CT. *Radiology* 186:731-738, 1993.

228. Torgerson WR, Dotter WE: Comparative roentgenographic study of the asymptomatic and symptomatic lumbar spine. *J Bone Joint Surg* 58(A)-6:850-853, 1976.

229. Tountas AA: Insufficiency stress fractures of the femoral neck in elderly women. *Clin Orthop* 292:202-209, 1993.

230. Traughber PD, Goodwin TE: Shoulder MRI: arthroscopic correlation with emphasis on partial tears. *J Comput Assist Tomogr* 16:129-133, 1992.

231. Tullberg T, Grane P, Isacson J: Gadolinium-enhanced magnetic resonance imaging of 36 patients one year after lumbar disc resection. *Spine* 19(2):176-182, 1994.

232. Tung GA, Davis LM, Wiggins ME, Fadale PD: Tears of the anterior cruciate ligament: primary and secondary signs at MR imaging. *Radiology* 188:661-667, 1993.

233. Turner DA, Templeton AC, Selzer PM, et al: Femoral capital osteonecrosis: MR findings of diffuse marrow abnormalities without focal lesions. *Radiology* 171:135-140, 1989.

234. Vahey TN, Broome Dr, Kayes KJ, Shelbourne KD: Acute and chronic tears of the anterior cruciate ligament: differential features at MRI imaging. *Radiology* 181:251-253, 1991.

235. Vahey TN, Hunt JE, Shelbourne KD: Anterior translocation of the tibia at MR imaging: a secondary sign of anterior cruciate ligament tear. *Radiology* 187:817-819, 1993.

236. Vande Berg B, Malghem J, Labaisse MA, et al: Avascular necrosis of the hip: comparison of contrast-enhanced and nonenhanced MR imaging with histologic correlation (work in progress). *Radiology* 182:445-450, 1992.

237. Vande Berg BE, Malghem JJ, Labaisse MA, et al: MR imaging of avascular necrosis and transient marrow edema of the femoral head. *RadioGraphics* 13:501-520, 1993.

238. Vande Berg B, Malghem J, Labaisse MA, et al: Apparent focal bone marrow ischemia in patients with marrow disorders: MR studies. *J Comput Assist Tomogr* 17:792-797, 1993.

239. Vallet AD, Marks PH, Fowler PJ, Munro TG: Occult posttraumatic osteochondral lesions of the knee: prevalence, classification, and short-term sequelae evaluated with MR imaging. *Radiology* 178:271-276, 1991.

240. Verbiest H: Fallacies of the present definition, nomenclature, and classification of the stenosis of the lumbar vertebral canal. *Spine* 1(4):217-225, 1976.

241. Verbiest H: Results of surgical treatment of idiopathic development stenosis of the lumbar vertebral canal. *J Bone Joint Surg* 59B:181-188, 1977.

242. Verbiest H: Words images knowledge, and reality: some reflections from the neurosurgical perspective. *Acta Neurochirurgica* 69:163-193, 1983.

243. Verhaven EFC, Shahabpour M, Handelberg FWJ, et al: The accuracy of three-dimensional magnetic resonance imaging in the diagnosis of ruptures of the lateral ligaments of the ankle. *Am J Sports Med* 19:583-587, 1991.

244. Virolainen H, Visuri T, Juusela T: Acute dislocation of the patella: MR findings. *Radiology* 189:243-246, 1993.

245. Walsh TR, Weinstein JN, Spratt KF, et al: Lumbar discography in normal subjects. *J Bone Joint Surg* 72-A(7):1081-1088, 1990.

246. Weber WN, Newmann CH, Barakos JA, et al: Lateral tibial rim (segond) fractures: MR imaging characteristics. *Radiology* 180:731-734, 1991.

247. Weiner DS, Macnab I: Superior migration of the humeral head: a radiological aid in the diagnosis of tears of the rotator cuff. *J Bone Joint Surg* (52)-B:524-527, 1970.

248. Weinstabl R, Stiskal M, Neuhold A, et al: Classifying calcaneal tendon injury according to MRI findings. *J Bone Joint Surg [Br]* (73)-B:683-685, 1991.

249. Wiesel SE, Tsourmas N, Feffer H, et al: A study of computer-assisted tomography: the incidence of positive CAT scans in an asymptomatic group of patients. *Spine* 9:549-551, 1984.

250. Wiener SN, Seitz WH: Sonography of the shoulder in patients with tears of the rotator cuff: accuracy and value for selecting surgical options: *AJR* 160:103-107, 1993.

251. Whalen JP, Balter S: *Radiation risks in medical imaging,* Chicago, 1984, Year Book Medical Publishers.

252. Williams AL, et al: Computed tomographic appearance of the bulging annulus. *Radiology* 142:403-408, 1982.

253. Wiltse L: Far-out syndrome. In Rothman LG, Glenn WV, editors: *Multiplanar CT of the spine,* Baltimore, 1985, University Park Press, pp. 384-393.

254. Witt I, Vestergaard A, Rosenklint A: A comparative analysis of x-ray findings of the lumbar spine in patients with and without lumbar pain. *Spine* 9(3):299-300, 1984.

255. Wright JG, Feinstein AR: Improving the reliability of orthopedic measurements. *J Bone Joint Surg* 74-B:287-291, 1992.

256. Yamato M, Yamagishi T: MRI of patellar tendon

anterior cruciate ligament autografts. *J Comput Assist Tomogr* 16:604-607, 1992.

257. Yao L, Sinha S, Seeger LL: MR imaging of joints; analytic optimization of GRE techniques at 1.5 T. *AJR* 158:339-345, 1992.

258. Yasuma T, Ohno R, Yamauchi Y: False-negative lumbar discograms: correlation of discographic and histological findings in postmortem and surgical specimens. *J Bone Joint Surg* 70-A(9):1279-1290, 1988.

259. Yu S, et al: Progressive and regressive changes in the nucleus pulposus: Part II—the adult. *Radiology* 169:93-97, 1988.

260. Yu S, et al: Criteria for classifying normal and degenerated lumbar intervertebral discs. *Radiology* 170:523-526, 1989.

261. Yuy WTC, Drew JM, Weinstein JN, et al: Intraspinal synovial cysts: magnetic resonance evaluation. *Spine* 16(7):740-745, 1991.

262. Zeiss J, Saddemi SR, Ebraheim NA: MR imaging of the quadriceps tendon: normal layered configuration and its importance in cases of tendon rupture. *AJR* 159:1031-1034, 1992.

263. Zucherman J, et al: Normal magnetic resonance imaging with abnormal discography. *Spine* 13(12):1355-1359, 1988.

# CHAPTER 16

# THERMOGRAPHY AND DISCOGRAPHY

*John A. McCulloch*

Thermography and discography are two diagnostics surrounded by considerable controversy in the field of spinal disorders. The purpose of this chapter is to convey a clinical perspective on the two procedures. Since these procedures are often used to support, affirm, or establish a diagnosis of a herniated disc the physician seeking "expert" knowledge in the field needs to be acquainted with details of the field. This chapter provides detailed information which refutes any value that can be based upon these tests.

## THERMOGRAPHY

Thermography originated from studies made by Albert and colleagues[1] in 1964 and Edeiken and co-workers[19] in 1968 suggesting that thermography could detect heat changes in the back when a herniated lumbar disc was present.

### History of Thermography

Since the early 19th century, scientists have been aware of infrared rays, invisible emissions from the sun, and their direct relationship with temperature. The U.S. Army Corps of Engineers issued contracts for the development of infrared scanners for war time aerial use to detect heat (troops, equipment, munitions) on the ground. In 1963, the first infrared imaging machine was demonstrated at the American Medical Association Annual Meeting. Soon after, Edeiken et al[19] published an original work on the use of thermography in detecting herniated lumbar discs. Wexler[13,61,62] soon became the major proponent of this methodology, while Edeiken reassessed its role and decided it was not clinically useful.[18] In spite of Edeiken's change of opinion, the use of thermography for the evaluation of spinal conditions became a "cause." It was supported by clinicians and scientists largely outside of major academic centers and promoted by the legal profession as "a picture of pain to show the jury."[3,38] They drew their support from hundreds of poorly controlled, unscientific studies published[12,37,61,62] almost exclusively in non-peer review journals. Calls for well-controlled scientific studies[22] were ignored. Eventually, studies by Aminoff and colleagues,[2,53,54,55] Getty and colleagues,[44] and Harper and colleagues[25] supported the original observations of Mahoney and colleagues[36] that "thermography as a diagnostic aid in sciatica and peripheral neuropathies was of no diagnostic value." By 1989, the Health Care Financing Administration[26] (HCFA) concluded that the "evidence indicates that thermography is not effective in diagnosing or treating illness or injury."

### The Theoretical Basis for Thermography

There is no question that today's sophisticated infrared thermography machines can accurately measure skin temperature differences in the neck, back, or extremities. What is at issue is the significance of these changes.

#### Physiological considerations

Wexler promoted thermography as a physiological test of sensory and autonomic (dys) function in response to neuronal irritation.[13,58,61] He suggested that thermography was a physiological test of function in contrast to CT and myelography, both of which were static anatomic tests. The basis for his conclusions were as follows:

1. Skin is the major organ for heat regulation of the body.
2. The main determinant of heat loss from the skin is blood flow. Increase the blood flow and the temperature loss through infrared ray emission is increased; when the blood flow is decreased, the reverse happens.
3. Blood flow to the skin is controlled by vasoconstriction of small arteries and veins, determined by impulses of the sympathetic nerves. Increased

impulses from the sympathetic system (fright, flight, and fear) cause the walls of the blood vessels to constrict; as the impulses subside the vessel walls dilate passively, blood flow increases, and heat is dissipated as infrared rays.

4. Peripheral nerves serve as a conduction mechanism for impulses to and from the central nervous system to the skin. They contain motor and sensory fibers, and automatic nervous system fibers. The autonomic nerves exit above the third lumbar segment but autonomic nerves join the peripheral nerve distribution of L3, L4, L5 and S1, far distal to where root encroachment pathology (radiculopathy) occurs.

5. Sensory nerve innervation is provided in a dermatomal distribution, with disturbances originating distally in skin[6] (nociceptor responses) or proximally at the root (e.g., disc herniation). Unfortunately dermatomes have considerable overlap.

6. The sinuvertebral nerve is a branch of the spinal nerve that originates just distal to the dorsal root ganglion and backtracks on itself to reenter the foramen and supply the posterior interface of the disc/vertebral column and the common dural sac. The sinuvertebral nerve contains sympathetic fibers.

7. Irritation of either the sinuvertebral nerve or of the nerve root will present itself as an abnormal heat pattern along the course of a dermatome and this abnormality is easily detected by infrared cameras that detect temperature differences within 0.1°C and in turn produce a colored picture of the extremity depicting temperature valuations.

The theory is attractive because the test (thermography) is noninvasive and risk-free.

## Studies

The following study[39] of thermograms in patients with ruptured discs causing sciatica is presented in order to contribute to the dialogue on the merits of thermography in assessing the patient with sciatica. The setting for this study was the author's private practice of orthopaedics (spine surgery). Two hypotheses advanced by thermographers were tested:

1. Normal patients have symmetrical thermograms of their legs.[56]
2. Patients with radiculopathy have asymmetrical thermograms of their legs.[62]

### Methods and materials

The design of the study was originally proposed by Frymoyer and Haugh:[22]

1. The researchers attempted to perform the test in question using state-of-the-art techniques.

2. The test was performed on groups of symptomatic and asymptomatic subjects who were matched for relevant other variables, such as age and sex, and who were sufficient in numbers for appropriate statistical evaluation.

3. The thermographic reporters were unaware of the disease diagnosis (they were blinded to eliminate observer bias).

4. Comparison of differences in test interpretation by different observers was performed to estimate interobserver reliability.

5. The test results were compared with some other objective standard, which was operative outcome.

### Inclusion criteria

Patients who volunteered for a thermographic assessment met the following *inclusion* criteria:

1. The patient's major complaint was sciatica (rather than back pain).

2. Sciatica was considered to be unilateral leg pain radiating in a dermatomal distribution to below the knee.

3. The duration of the sciatica was ≥3 weeks and ≤1 year.

4. The patient had to have two or four neurological findings (i.e., absence of a reflex, demonstrable motor weakness, atrophy appropriate to the root involved, or a sensory loss in an anatomic distribution).

5. Straight leg raising had to be <50% of the normal limb and/or bowstring discomfort had to be present.

6. The patient had a computed tomography (CT) scan and/or CT myelogram or magnetic resonance imaging (MRI) to support the diagnosis of a herniated disc at the level of, and on the correct side, for the nerve root involvement that had been determined clinically.

7. One year after entry into this study, the patient had to be free of the sciatic discomfort that led to the original presentation (with no subsequent operative intervention).

### Exclusion criteria

Patients were *excluded* from entry into the study according to the following criteria:

1. The patient had a history of prior back surgery.

2. The patient showed any Waddell[58] nonorganic signs.

3. The patient had any lower extremity sign of peripheral vascular disease, varicose veins, or arthritic involvement of the hips, knees, or feet.

4. The patient had undergone lower extremity surgery, such as a meniscectomy, or showed evidence of recent injury to a limb.

5. The patient was diabetic or was using a β-blocker.
6. The patient had a midline disc and/or a cauda equina syndrome.

Control subjects were from three sources: (1) other patients in the same group practice with upper extremity complaints but no back pain or sciatica, (2) relatives accompanying the patient referred to the group practice, and (3) hospital staff. All controls volunteered for the study after reading a general notice (requesting volunteers) posted in the office and the hospital.

Controls were included if there was no history of back or leg pain from any condition. All controls were physically examined to exclude lower extremity conditions. Controls were excluded if they had any of the above exclusion criteria listed for the symptomatic group of patients. Finally, all controls received a detailed informed consent. Controls were matched according to age, sex, height, and weight of the symptomatic group.

Thermograms were performed on both groups using the protocol established by the Academy of Neuromuscular Thermography[37] by a technician/nurse certified by the Academy as qualified to do thermograms (Frank W. Hurst, Jr., The Academy of Neuro-Muscular Thermography, February 8, 1987). Thermograms were performed using a Thermo Vision 782 electronic thermography unit (AGA Corporation, Secaucus, N.J.). The examination was performed in an interior room that was fluorescently lighted, draft-free, and air-conditioned with a baffled unit to maintain comfortable temperature of 68 to 72°F. A temperate-recording device was in place to verify the room temperature.

After a consent form was signed, the patients undressed completely and cooled down for 15 minutes. During this time they could either stand or sit without touching their legs together. A total of three thermograms, with 15-min intervals between each, were completed.

Each set of thermograms consisted of PA views of the spine; anteroposterior (AP), PA, and lateral views of the lower extremities; and dorsal views of both feet, including the toes. After all three sets of thermograms were complete, black and white thermofocusing of the lower spine, before and after alcohol misting, was completed.

All thermograms were numbered according to the sequence in which the patient or the control entered the study. The thermograms were then read blindly by two certified thermographers [P.S. (certification by Thermographic Services, Inc., January 8, 1984) and G.R. (certification by the Academy of Neuro-Muscular Thermography, February 12, 1989)]. The criteria for abnormality was a 1°C difference (cooling) affect-ing at least 25% of the surface area of the dermatome. The affected leg and the dermatome that was abnormally cool were recorded.

Patients and controls were followed by telephone for at least one year after the completion of the study to determine if the symptomatic patients were relieved of their sciatica without any other intervening procedure and to determine if any of the control groups developed sciatica or back pain. Failure of treatment intervention in the symptomatic group eliminated the patient from the study; development of back pain or leg pain in the control group also eliminated the control from the study.

**Results**

Seventy symptomatic patients and 76 controls underwent thermographic assessment during the last nine months of 1987 and the first six months of 1988. After thermographic assessment, all patients underwent microsurgery, percutaneous discectomy, or discolysis in an attempt to relieve their sciatica.

One year later, 14 patients were eliminated from the study: three were lost to follow-up; one had a technically inadequate thermogram (surgical success); one underwent bilateral surgery (surgical success); and nine experienced surgical failure (overall 87% surgical success rate).

This left a total of 56 patients that formed the basis for the blinded study of the value of thermography as a diagnostic aid in patients with clinically, radiologically, and surgically proven sciatica who had a successful treatment outcome to surgical intervention. The procedures used to relieve sciatica are listed in Table 16-1, the demographics of the symptomatic group in Table 16-2, and the levels of involvement in Table 16-3.

**Matching controls**

After eliminating the surgical failures ($n = 9$), the bilateral surgery ($n = 1$), the technically poor thermogram ($n = 1$), and the patients lost to follow-up ($n = 3$), the symptomatic and control groups were matched.

**TABLE 16-1     PROCEDURES TO RELIEVE SCIATICA**

| | |
|---|---|
| Microdiscectomy | 47 |
| Chemonucleolysis | 4 |
| Percutaneous discectomy | 2 |
| Microdecompression and fusion (spondylolisthesis) | 3 |
| Total | 56 |

**TABLE 16-2   DEMOGRAPHICS OF SYMPTOMATIC GROUP**

| | |
|---|---|
| Male:Female | 38:18 |
| Average Age | |
| Male | 40 years |
| Female | 45 years |

**TABLE 16-3   LEVELS OF INVOLVEMENT**

| | |
|---|---|
| L3-4 | 3 |
| L4-5 | 15 |
| L5-S1 | 37 |
| Two-Level (L4-5/L5-S1) | 1 |
| Total | 56 |

**TABLE 16-4   THERMOGRAPHIC INTERPRETATION (CONTROL GROUP)**

| | | |
|---|---|---|
| Reader 1: | Normal, 25; | Abnormal, 31 |
| Reader 2: | Normal, 27; | Abnormal, 29 |
| Intraobserver agreement | | 43/56 (77%) |
| Intraobserver disagreement | | 13/56 (23%) |

Matching was accomplished by listing the controls in alphabetical order and then listing sex, age, height, and weight. The controls were then matched to the symptomatic group first by sex and then by age (±6 years), height (±6 in.), and weight (±30 lb.) All patients had to match in sex and age, and then if an increased height match was made, only an increased weight match would be accepted. In the end there were 56 patients in the symptomatic group and 56 participants in the control group (112 total).

### Results

*Thermographers' postulate 1:*[56] *All normal patients have symmetrical thermograms.*

In the control group, reader 1 (P.S.) read 25 thermograms as normal and 31 as abnormal. Reader 2 (G.R.) read 27 thermograms as normal and 29 as abnormal. The interobserver agreement in this group was 43 of 56 readings (77%) (Table 16-4).

The false positive rate of thermography for reader 1 was $31/56 \times 100 = 55\%$, and that for reader 2 was $29/56 \times 100 = 52\%$.

*Thermographers' postulate 2:*[62] *Abnormal patients have asymmetric thermograms. (a) The thermogram will be cooler on the affected side (leg). (b) The changes will affect at least 25% of the dermatome.*

Reader 1 read 39 thermograms in the symptomatic patients as abnormal and 17 as normal. Of the 39 thermograms read as abnormal, 34 correctly designated the symptomatic limb as the cooler limb. Of these 34, only nine correctly identified the dermatomal distribution of the root impaired by the disc rupture.

Reader 2 read 37 thermograms as abnormal and 19 as normal. Of the 37 thermograms read as abnormal, 28 correctly designated the cooler limb as the symptomatic limb. Of these 28, only six correctly identified the dermatomal distribution of the root impaired by the disc rupture.

The interpretation of the back thermograms was not included in this study of radicular pain.

Using the standard of the cooler limb being the abnormal limb, sensitivity of thermography (ability of a test to be positive when the disease is present) for reader 1 was:

$$34/56 \times 100 = 60\%$$

and for reader 2 was:

$$28/56 \times 100 = 50\%$$

Interobserver agreement was 79% (44 of 56 readings) (Table 16-5).

When dermatomal abnormalities were studied, the sensitivity of thermography in predicting the correct dermatome was:

$$\text{Reader 1: } 9/56 \times 100 = 16\%$$

and

$$\text{Reader 2: } 6/56 \times 100 = 11\%$$

### Discussion

The use of thermography to scan the *legs* in radicular problems was first proposed by Ching and Wexler.[13] They concluded that peripheral (extremity) abnormalities on thermography (cooling) are useful in indicating the significance of any lumbar abnormalities. Subsequent studies by Wexler[61,62] suggested a good sensitivity and specificity to thermography when compared with electromyography (EMG). Other investigators published numerous uncontrolled correlative studies involving thermography and modalities such as CT, myelography, and EMG. The use of thermography soon evolved to produce a pic-

**TABLE 16-5    INTEROBSERVER AGREEMENT (SYMPTOMATIC GROUP)**

|  | READER 1 | READER 2 |
|---|---|---|
| Normal | 17 | 19 |
| Abnormal | 39 | 37 |
| Totals | 56 | 56 |
| Abnormal cold side correct | 34 | 28 |
| Normal or side wrong | 22 | 28 |
| Totals | 56 | 56 |
| Interobserver agreement | 44/56 (79%) | |
| Abnormal side correct, dermatome correct | 9/56 | 6/56 |

ture of pain: "Now we have something convincing to show those twelve people in the jury box."[3] The interest of the senior author, along with that of other investigators, was aroused. On the surface it appeared the authors were looking at an inexpensive, noninvasive, safe test of extremity dysfunction in sciatica. Our first study failed to support the claims of thermography;[36] however, it had some technical weaknesses. In an attempt to satisfy the criticism of the first study, a second study was designed under the guidelines proposed by Frymoyer and Haugh,[22] listed at the beginning of this article. Except for the intraobserver suggestion (No. 4), those criteria have been applied for the valid study design. Symptomatic patients selected for study had unequivocal disc rupture, certified on CT, CT/myelography, and/or MRI to be causing the dominant radicular leg pain, with neurological symptoms and signs and marked reduction in straight leg raising. Not only did they have to have a disc rupture causing classic radicular pain, but they had to undergo successful surgical intervention to remove the disc rupture and be free of leg pain 1 year after surgery. There were no patients with inappropriate clinical symptoms and signs included in the study.[58] This group of study patients represent the purest study group of any patient population in past thermography studies.

Asymptomatic patients were not only symptom- and sign-free of all possible lower extremity conditions, but they must have remained so for 1 year after thermography assessment to be included in the study. This was thought to be a reasonable substitute for radiographic investigation of an asymptomatic patient at the time of study.

It is an attractive theory that disease in the lumbar spine causes enough increased activity in the sympathetic vasoconstrictive system to cause a cold sensation in the affected leg. It is not unusual to obtain this history from a patient with sciatica. To use an infrared camera that relays these temperature changes electronically to a video display unit where a multicolor-coded image is produced is theoretically attractive.

But the clinical role for thermography in this study and others has not been established.[4,6] As stated in a recent Health Technology Assessment Report on Thermography published by the National Center for Health Services Research and Health Care Technology Assessment,[26] "evidence of the technology's clinical effectiveness had not been tested rigorously in prospective, controlled clinical trials." They go on to state that "thermography may only confirm the presence of a temperature difference, but other procedures are needed to reach a specific diagnosis, and thermography adds very little to what a physician already knows based on his history, physical examination and other laboratory studies." The author supports this conclusion.

**Additional Studies**

Aminoff, Olney, and So[2,53-55] have performed three blind studies on the use of thermography in peripheral nerve entrapments, cervical radiculopathies, and lumbosacral radiculopathy. They concluded in all three studies that thermographic findings were "nonspecific, and of little clinical utility." Aminoff and coworkers' studies were criticized on a number of issues, one of them being the failure to use stress tests, although stress tests have never been part of recommended thermography protocol. Additional scientific studies by Getty and colleagues,[44] Harper and colleagues,[25] and Meyers and colleagues,[41] however, clearly demonstrated that thermography was of no use in the determination of the presence or absence of neuropathy or radiculopathy and if abnormal was of no use in the determination of level or side of the lesion.

**DISCOGRAPHY**

Discography is the injection of contrast material into the disc followed by radiographic examination and sometimes CT (Disco-CT). While thermography never enjoyed support in the mainstream spinal community, discography has been firmly embraced by well-respected spine investigators.[9,14-16,23,31,47,51,60,63]

## Acceptable Statements About Discography

Most scientists aware of the pros and cons of discography would agree on the following points:

1. Unlike CT and MRI, discography is an invasive test. It is painful to patients and carries the risk of disc space infection (1-4%).[21]

2. Most discographers use the posterior-lateral approach[40] because it is less irritating to the patients than the midline approach. At the L5-S1 level, the posterior-lateral approach can damage the L5 nerve root.

3. Most discographers would agree that it is necessary to evaluate both the appearance of contrast on radiographs (variously described as morphology and/or nucleogram) and the patients' pain response to the injection. Those studies that have left out the evaluation of pain response are largely invalid studies.[28,43]

4. Discography for the evaluation of cervical or lumbar *radicular* pain has largely been abandoned because (1) it has never been proven of value[30] and (2) CT and MRI are much more accurate in the assessment of radicular pain.[7] Discography is now used primarily in the assessment of axial (back or neck) pain. The abnormal findings so detected are the "contained discogenic disease," "the pain generator," variously known as degenerative disc disease, internal disc disruption, and isolated disc resorption. Patients characteristically have dominant back pain, a normal extremity exam (in regards to straight leg raising and neurological exam), and CT and/or MRI studies that show, at most, a "bulging disc".

5. Discography, for the assessment of back pain, should only be used after the decision has been made to operate (i.e.,to do a fusion). Its sole purpose is to assist the surgeon in deciding on what levels to include in the fusion. This is a conclusion that has never been tested in a scientific study.

6. The other two parameters of discography, namely volume of test material and the pressure of injections, have largely been abandoned except when trying to decide if a disc is contained (high pressure) or noncontained (low pressure for injection). This may or may not be an important consideration when deciding on chemonucleolysis or percutaneous discectomy.

7. The most often quoted study supporting discography is the one by Walsh and co-workers.[59] This study included discograms at three levels on asymptomatic college students (average age 22 years) and was done to determine the validity of Holt's[28] study showing a 37% false-positive rate

in young healthy prisoner volunteers. The authors criticize Holt's study on the following counts:

(a) Holt considered morphology only and did not evaluate pain response.

(b) Holt's patient population of volunteer prisoners was less truthful than the college students.

(c) Holt's discography technique was poor.

(d) Holt used plain x-rays rather than CT/discography.

(e) Holt used very irritating contrast material (Hypaque).

Walsh's study showed a 100% specificity of discography in young college students when pain response was added to disc morphology (nucleogram). They proved that, in asymptomatic young patients, discography would remain negative. But can you extrapolate that to the general population of patients with back pain, which would be much older? What their study did not address was the validity or sensitivity of discography (i.e., the ability of discography to predict not only which level is symptomatic but whether fusion of that level will relieve the patient of his suffering).

## Problems with Discography

The major problem with discography is the lack of any sensitivity studies[64] to support its continuing use. Two studies have been performed by Jackson et al.[27,30] Their first study dealt with the sensitivity and specificity of discography in predicting disc herniations in a difficult patient population referred by other orthopaedic surgeons. The study was done before MRI was generally available and concentrated on the ability to reproduce the patient's extremity pain on provocative testing. They found an 89% specificity (ability of the test to remain negative when a disc rupture was *not* present at subsequent surgery), but only a 43% sensitivity (ability of the test to be positive when a disc rupture was present). In other words, the test was reasonably good in not producing false positives, but poor because there were a large number of false negatives.

The second study[27] was directed at the more frequent use of discography to assist in using it as a test to help decide fusion levels. It was a retrospective determination of discography's ability to select fusion levels in successful 1, 2, and 3 level fusions, two years postoperatively. The conclusion was that "pain reproduction by discography preoperatively is a very poor predictor of clinical outcome postoperatively in patients with solid posterolateral lumbosacral fusions."

Esses et al[20] used an external fixator to help select fusion levels. All patients had provocative discography. They concluded that discography was a less sensitive predictor of surgical results than degenerative changes on routine x-rays, thus supporting the findings of Hess et al.[27] Esses' study can be criticized because:

1. The majority of patients were compensation patients who had been out of work at least 30 months.
2. Over 50% of his patients had had previous surgery.
3. There was successful outcome as measured by relief of pain in only 17 or 27 patients.
4. No statement was made in regards to the ultimate test of successful surgical outcomes in workers' compensation patients—the return-to-work rate.

Only a few studies have used surgical outcome as the "gold standard" to assess the usefulness of discography. One such study was by Colhoun and colleagues[15] who prospectively reviewed the role of discography in successful surgical fusions. They demonstrated that, of the 137 patients in whom discography had revealed disc disease and provoked symptoms, 89% derived significant and sustained clinical benefit from surgery. Of the 25 patients whose discs showed morphological abnormality but had no provocation of symptoms on discography, only 52% had clinical success. The conclusions of this study are difficult to reconcile with the opposite (negative) conclusions of Jackson.[27]

Many studies[42,43,50-52,57,60] are hard to accept in support of discography because:

1. The studies did not use surgical outcome as a determinant in the efficacy of discography.
2. The studies had very low or very high surgical success rates.
3. There were so many variables in the patient population that it was impossible to draw valid conclusions about the usefulness of discography.

A number of studies have attempted to show that even in the presence of a normal MRI (T2 sagittal), discography can produce an abnormal pain response and/or morphology.[8,10,33,35,65] However, on reviewing these articles, the MRIs were of poor quality, not midline cuts, or showed posterior clefts in the annulus; therefore it is difficult to accept these conclusions. In addition, the morphology on discography revealed minor changes compatible with some of the reproduced MRIs. The final criticism of all of these studies is the absence of any clinical outcome criteria.

Finally, if there is agreement that discography has little role to play in assessment of patients with radicular pain, then all those studies with axial and radicular pain mixed are not valid.

Obviously, the role of discography in surgical decision making cries out for valid clinical trials.[45] In setting up these trials, investigators will have to answer the following questions:

1. What is the source of pain on provocative volumetric testing of a degenerative disc? Is it the annulus, the end plate, the facet joints, or surrounding ligaments?
2. How do you explain the production of pain on the injection of hypertonic saline into tissues of normal (asymptomatic) volunteers?
3. Why, as the population grows older and develops more degenerative disc disease, do physicians see fewer patients with low-back pain?
4. If response to disc space injection is most important, what are the parameters that are important to describe the response? Is it the patient's response at the beginning, in the middle, or at the end of the injection? What volume of test material is considered adequate? Should the injection be fast or slow? How many times should the test be repeated in each disc and which response is correct—the one to the first, middle, or last injection? In multiple disc-space testing, how long does the researcher wait after a painful test to test again? Does pain reproduction have to be the exact same pain or just pain in the area where that patient normally has felt pain? Is a sedated patient a valid reporter of pain? If multiple discs are being examined, what is the proper order?

    As can be seen, there are so many variables in patient response to provocative testing that only the most fastidious, pedantic scientists will be able to complete the study.
5. Discography is used for the assessment of fusion levels in axial pain, which by its very nature is a chronic condition before fusion is even considered. How can a test that produces acute pain be used to evaluate a chronic painful condition that is so often modified by intellect, emotion, culture, and environment?
6. If physicians agree that morphology is of limited value (compared to provocation of pain), then the addition of CT (CT/discography[49]) adds little to the value of discography. A number of years ago, when the diagnosis of a foraminal disc was evolving, CT discography did offer guidance, but with the advent of MRI, CT/discography is no longer necessary for the diagnosis of a lumbar foraminal disc.

## CONCLUSIONS

Nachemson[45,46] has called for the discontinuation of discographic studies, except for prospective studies performed in large spine centers. He proposed that they only be done after the approval of human experimentation committees, where the intent is to find out if they can really help in the treatment selection for the chronic low-back-pain patient. While this proposal might seem an unwarranted intrusion on the freedom to practice, it is a criticism and comment that is appropriate. Discography was first introduced in 1948.[34] It is now 46 years later and science has not been brought to bear on the controversy. The prediction can be made that when this occurs, discography will go the way of thermography—into the realm of clinical irrelevancy.

## References

1. Albert SM, Glickman M, Kallish M: Thermography in orthopaedics. *Ann NY Acad Sci* 121:157-170, 1964.
2. Aminoff MJ, Olney RK, So YT: Thermography and the evaluation of neuromuscular disorders. *Semin Neurol* 10:150-155, 1990.
3. Archer SD, Zinn JA: Thermograms: persuasive tools in soft-tissue injury cases. *Trial* Feb:68-71, 1983.
4. Ash CJ Foster MV: Neuromuscular thermography in orthopaedic surgery: a usage poll. *Orthop Rev* 17:589-592, 1988.
5. Ash CJ, Gotti E, Hauk CH: Thermography of the curved living surface. *Missouri Med* 84:702-708, 1987.
6. Ash CJ, Shealy CN, Young PA, et al: Thermography and the sensory dermatome. *Skel Radiol* 15:40-46, 1986.
7. Boden SD, Davis DO, et al: Abnormal magnetic resonance scans of the lumbar spine in asymptomatic patients. *J Bone Joint Surg* 72A:403-408, 1990.
8. Brightbill TC, Pile N, et al: Normal magnetic resonance imaging and abnormal discography in lumbar disc disruption. *Spine* 19:1075-1077, 1994.
9. Brodsky AE, Binder WF: Lumbar discography: its value in diagnosis and treatment of lumbar disc lesion. *Spine* 4:110-120, 1979.
10. Buirski G: Magnetic resonance signal patterns of lumbar discs in patients with low-back pain: a prospective study with discographic correlation. *Spine* 17:1199-1204, 1992.
11. Castagnera L, Lavignolle B, et al: Test de tolerance discale et discomanometrie: intérêt diagnostique et prognostique avant chimionucléolyse. *Acta Orthop Belg* 53:184-194, 1987.
12. Chafitz N, Wexler CE, Kaiser JA: Neuromuscular thermography of the lumbar spine with CT correlation. *Radiology* 157:178, 1985.
13. Ching C, Wexler CE: Peripheral thermographic manifestations of lumbar disc disease. *Appl Radiol* 7:53-110, 1978.
14. Cloward RB, Buzaid LL: Discography: technique, indications, and evaluations of the normal and abnormal intervertebral disc. *Am J Roentgenol* 68:552-564, 1952.
15. Colhoun E, McCall IW, Williams L, Cassar Pullicino VN: Provocation discography as a guide to planning operations on the spine. *J Bone Joint Surg* 70B:267-271, 1988.
16. Collis JS Jr., Gardner WJ: Lumbar discography: an analysis of one thousand cases. *J Neurosurg* 19:452-461, 1962.
17. Edeiken J: Personal communication. M.D. Anderson Hospital and Tumor Institute, Texas Medical Center, Houston, Tex., 1990.
18. Edeiken J, Shaber G: Thermography: a re-evaluation. *Skel Radiol* 15:545-548, 1986.
19. Edeiken J, Wallace JD, Curley RF, Lee S: Thermography and herniated lumbar discs. *AJR* 102:790-796, 1968.
20. Esses SI, Botsford DJ, Kostuik JP: The role of external spinal skeletal fixation in the assessment of low-back disorders. *Spine* 14:594-601, 1989.
21. Fraser RD, Osti OL, Vernon-Roberts B: Discitis after discography. *J Bone Joint Surg* 69B:26-35, 1987.
22. Frymoyer JW, Haugh LD: Thermography: a call for scientific studies to establish its diagnostic efficacy. *Orthopaedics* 9:699-700, 1986.
23. Gibson MJ, Buckley J, Mawhinney R, et al: Magnetic resonance imaging and discography in the diagnosis of disc degeneration: a comparative study of 50 discs. *J Bone Joint Surg* 68B:369-373, 1986.
24. Halligan RM: The hidden truth behind thermography. *For the Defense* 31:12-16, 1989.
25. Harper CM, Low PA, et al: Utility of thermography in the diagnosis of lumbosacral radiculopathy. *Neurology* 41:1010-1014, 1991.
26. Health Technology Assessment Reports: Thermography for indications other than breast lesions. National Centers for Health Services Research and Health Care Technology Assessment. DHSS Publication No. (PHS) 89-3438, 1989.
27. Hess WF, Jackson RP, et al: Pain response by discography as a predictor of clinical outcome of patients with solid posterior lateral lumbosacral fusion. Presented Poster Exhibit, AAOS, New Orleans, Feb. 1994.
28. Holt EP, Jr.: The question of lumbar discography. *J Bone Joint Surg* 50A:720-726, 1966.

29. Hudgins WR: Diagnositc accuracy of lumbar discography. *Spine* 2:305-309, 1977.

30. Jackson RP, Cain JE, et al: The neuroradiographic diagnosis of lumbar herniated nucleus pulposus. *Spine* 14:1356-1361, 1989.

31. Johnson RG, MacNab I: Localization of symptomatic lumbar pseudarthroses by use of discography. *Clin Orthop* 197:164-170, 1985.

32. Karanian ME: Thermography: a plaintiff-oriented technique put on the defense. *For the Defense* 31:6-11, 1989.

33. Konberg M: Discography and magnetic resonance imaging in the diagnosis of lumbar disc disruption. *Spine* 14:1368-1372, 1989.

34. Lindblom K: Diagnostic puncture of intervertebral disks in sciatica. *Acta Orthop Scand* 17:231-329, 1948.

35. Linson MA, Crowe CH: Comparison of magnetic resonance imaging and lumbar discography in the diagnosis of disc degeneration. *Clin Orthop* 250:160-163, 1990.

36. Mahoney L, McCulloch J, Csima A: Thermography in back pain: I—Thermography as a diagnostic aid in sciatica. *Thermology* 1:43-50, 1985.

37. Maultsby JA, Meek JB, Routon J, et al: Thermography: its correlation with the pain drawing. Proceedings of the 1st Annual Meeting of the Academy of Neuro-Muscular Thermography, May 1985. *Post Grad Med* (special edition) March 1986.

38. McAliley S: Thermography: a medical fraud? *Forum* 15:20-27, 1988.

39. McCulloch J, Frymoyer J, et al: Thermography as a diagnostic aid in sciatica. *J Spinal Disord* 6:427-431, 1993.

40. McCulloch JA, Waddell G: Lateral lumbar discography. *Br J Radiol* 51:498-502, 1978.

40a. McCulloch JA: Chemonucleolysis and experience with 2000 cases. *Clin Orthop* 146:128-134, 1980.

41. Meyers S, Cros D, et al: Liquid crystal thermography: quantitative studies of abnormalities in carpal tunnel syndrome. *Neurology* 39:1465-1469, 1989.

42. Milette PC, Melanson D: A reappraisal of lumbar discography. *J Can Assoc Radiol* 33:176-182, 1982.

43. Milette PC, Raymond J, Fontaine S: Comparison of high-resolution computed tomography with discography in the evaluation of lumbar disc herniation. *Spine* 15:525-533, 1990.

44. Mills GH, Davies GK, Getty CJM, Conway J: The evaluation of liquid crystal thermography in investigation of nerve root compression due to lumbosacral lateral spinal stenosis. *Spine* 11:427-432, 1986.

45. Nachemson A: Lumbar discography: where are we today? *Spine* 14:555-557, 1989.

46. Nachemson A: Work for all: for those with low-back pain as well. *Clin Ortrhop* 179:77-85, 1983.

47. North American Spine Society: Position Statement on Discography. *Spine* 13:1343, 1988.

48. Report of the Commission of the Evaluation of Pain. *Soc Secur Bull*, Jan. 1987, Vol. 50, No. 1.

49. Sachs BL, Vanharanta H, Spivey MA, et al.: Dallas discogram description: a new classification of CT/discography in low-back disorders. *Spine* 12:287-294, 1987.

50. Shinomiya K, Nakao K, et al: Evaluation of cervical discography in pain origin and provocation. *J Spinal Disord* 6:422-426, 1993.

51. Simmons EH, Segil CM: An evaluation of discography in the localization of symptomatic levels in discogenic disease of the spine. *Clin Orthop* 108:57-69, 1975.

52. Simmons JW, Emery S, et al: Awake discography: a comparison study with magnetic resonance imaging. *Spine* 165:S216-S221.

53. So YT, Aminoff MJ, Olney RK: The role of thermography in the evaluation of lumbosacral radiculopathy. *Neurology* 39:1154-1158, 1989.

54. So YT, Olney RK, Aminoff MJ: Evaluation of thermography in the diagnosis of selected entrapment neuropathies. *Neurology* 39:1-5, 1989.

55. So YT, Olney RK, Aminoff MJ: A comparison of thermography and electromyography in the diagnosis of cervical radiculopathy. *Muscle Nerve* 13:1032-1036, 1990.

56. Uematsu S, Edwin DH, Jankel WR, et al: Quantification of thermal asymmetry: Part 1—Normal values and reproducibility. *J Neurosurg* 69:552-555, 1988.

57. Vanharanta H, Sachs BL, Spivey MA, et al: The relationship of pain provocation to lumbar disc deterioration as seen by CT/discography. *Spine* 12:295-298, 1987.

58. Waddell G: Clinical assessment of lumbar impairment. *Clin Orthop* 221:110-120, 1987.

59. Walsh TR, Weinstein JN, Spratt KF, et al: Lumbar discography in normal subjects. *J Bone Joint Surg* 72A:1081-1088, 1990.

60. Wetzel FT, La Rocca SH, et al: The treatment of lumbar spinal pain syndromes diagnosed by discography. *Spine* 19:792-800, 1994.

61. Wexler CE: Thermographic evaluation of trauma (spine). *Acta Thermographica* 5:3-11, 1980.

62. Wexler CE: Cervical, thoracic and lumbar thermography: a clinical evaluation. *J Neuro Orthop Surg* 2:183-185, 1981.

63. Wiley JJ, MacNab I, Wortzman G: Lumbar discography and its clinical applications. *Can J Surg* 11:280-289, 1968.

64. Yasuma T, Ohno R, Yamauchi Y: False-negative lumbar discograms. *J Bone Joint Surg* 70:1279-1290, 1988.

65. Zucherman J, Derby R, et al: Normal magnetic resonance imaging with abnormal discography. *Spine* 13:1355-1359, 1988.

# CHAPTER 17

# ERGONOMIC BASIS FOR JOB-RELATED STRENGTH TESTING

*Don B. Chaffin*

## INTRODUCTION

Impairment evaluations are performed by physicians. These examinations provide information about a patient's health status. Disability determinations use impairment evaluation as one of the criteria in assessing a work-related injury. One of the goals of a disability determination is to determine a patient's ability to return to work. This ability is evaluated according to the worker's capabilities and the particular job demands. Capabilities are determined by measuring an individual's total medical impairments, including the degree (total or partial), organ system involved, and the time course (temporary or permanent), as well as an individual's psychosocial capabilities, such as pain tolerance, adaptability, and level of training. The demands of the job are assessed by methods including biomechanics, energy expenditure (see Chapter 28), and time and motion study.

The combination of the worker's capabilities and the demands of the job results in a functional capacity analysis (see Chapters 18 and 51). These determinations not only establish whether an impaired worker can return to his former job but can also help indicate what type of alternate job would be appropriate. This chapter introduces one of the available job evaluation topics—ergonomics.

*Ergonomics* is a word derived from two Greek words, "ergo" meaning work and "nomos" meaning principles or laws. Within industry, ergonomics methods and principles are used to evaluate and design tools, equipment, tasks, and procedures to assure the highest performance possible, while minimizing errors and hazards. Clearly, in application ergonomics requires an eclectic philosophy and knowledge from different disciplines rooted in the life, behavioral, and engineering sciences.

In recent years the occupational applications of ergonomics have emphasized biomechanics as its primary science.[5] This focus on the physical aspects of worker-hardware systems in industry has arisen due to:

1. The increasing recognition that people's musculoskeletal systems are vulnerable to a variety of overstress syndromes that are caused, or at least aggravated by, common manual exertion in jobs.
2. The ability to measure objectively human musculoskeletal exertion capabilities, which has produced a realization that normal, healthy workers vary greatly in their performance capabilities (e.g., approximately 8:1 difference in functional strength capabilities).
3. The emergence of computerized biomechanical models that allow the study and prediction of normal human performance capabilities in different work settings.
4. The development of methods to quantify the physical stresses associated with many different types of manual tasks.

It is this last development that is emphasized in this chapter.

## WHY PERFORM BIOMECHANICAL JOB EVALUATIONS?

The ability to allow a person to return to work, or to be classified as permanently disabled, depends a great deal on the types of jobs available to that person. As summarized by Feuerstein,[13] there are multiple factors that affect return-to-work decisions. Some of these are depicted in Fig. 17-1.

In essence, to return a person to productive work after injury to the musculoskeletal system requires a comprehensive and well-managed program. Information from many experts will need to be gathered at different times in the rehabilitation and evaluation process. This information often will vary greatly as the person's functional capabilities change, and as the employer's work requirements are altered by new production and technical conditions. The acquiring and effective use of this information is not easy. As Sandler[29] wrote:

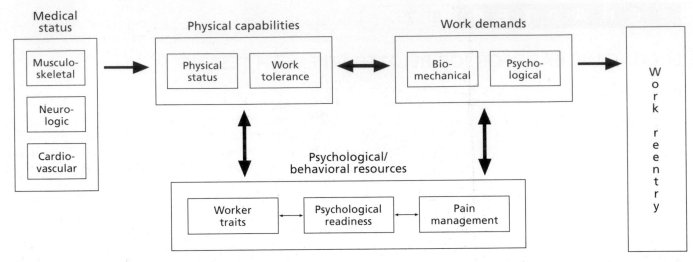

**FIGURE 17-1** Multiple factors potentially affecting return to work following occupational musculoskeletal injury/illness. Conceptual Model of Work Disability. (From Feurestein M: Workers' compensation reform in New York state: a proposal to address medical, ergonomic, and psychological factors associated with work disability. *J Occup Rehab* 3(3):125-135, 1993.)

The difficulty in predicting the eventual outcome of a patient's injury helps fuel to a great extent the costs and abuses in worker's compensation. Additionally, once . . . impairment has been declared by a medical practitioner, it is rarely removed no matter what happens down the road. It is often difficult to know exactly how much a stabilized injury will limit function. Careful functional capacity evaluations against job-specific medical standards will provide fair, consistent, and predictable assessments for such injuries.

The question is not as much about whether specific job information should be considered in a return-to-work or disability decision, but rather what type of job information should be considered and how can it be acquired. Because human strength performance varies so greatly in a healthy population, and is affected by injury and resulting pain-related performance inhibition, knowing a job's strength performance requirement is often critical. Therefore it will be the focus for this chapter, but the conclusions are believed to be much broader. For instance, in some jobs endurance (localized and whole-body), extreme reach, or precision manipulative requirements may influence return-to-work decisions. Though beyond the scope of this chapter, it is hoped that the reader will understand in general how such other job information can be acquired by utilizing a process similar to that described for job-related strength testing.

## USE OF STRENGTH TESTING IN INDUSTRY

Though it is difficult to say when strength testing per se first became popular in industry, Frederick W.

Taylor[31] advocated selection of the best workers for each particular task in his now-famous book *Principles of Scientific Management,* published in 1929. The armed forces have since formally recognized that strength and endurance are required in most combat duties. In this latter regard, "Liftest" was advocated for Air Force personnel selection by Kroemer.[21] Liftest consists of a set of handles that slide in a vertical track. These are lifted by the person being evaluated from near the floor to overhead reach. With repeated trials additional weight is added to the handles until the person can no longer perform the lift. This procedure is reported to simulate many different common lifting tasks in the Air Force, thus having content validity.

Human strength as measured in Liftest and all other such tests is defined as the ability to perform a maximum volitional exertion for a few seconds, with adequate rest between trials to avoid fatigue. Performance in such strength tests is measured as either the peak or average force (or moment) displayed by the person for a few seconds of exertion.[3] The person may apply the force against a stationary load-measuring device in which case static or isometric strength is measured. A formal protocol for this type of testing has been developed by the American Industrial Hygiene Association (AIHA).[3] If movement occurs, as in the Liftest, then the test is a measure of dynamic strength. If the load applied is moved at a constant velocity, which is possible for only a limited part of the motion and for one body segment, then it is referred to as *isokinetic strength* (i.e., near constant velocity). The latter type of test requires expensive equipment to control the velocity. In general, the faster the speed of motion, the lower the resulting dynamic strengths. Figure 17-2 depicts a comparison of dy-

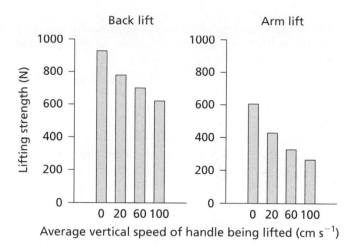

**FIGURE 17-2**    Typical dynamic lifting strength test mean results for 10 healthy males performing maximum isokinetic lifts at different lift speeds. (From Kumar S, Chaffin DB, Redfern M: Isometric and isokinetic back-and-arm-lifting strengths: device and measurement. *J Biomech* 21(1):35-44, 1988.)

namic back- and arm-lifting strengths performed at various speeds.

Isokinetic tests have been developed primarily for clinical use, wherein a designated strength-speed evaluation involving a specific joint is needed to assess treatment effectiveness. A 1994 study by Wheeler et al[33] has shown that in a laboratory, carefully performed isometric and isokinetic trunk-extension strength tests can predict simple lifting capacities ($r^2 > 0.88$). A recent critical review of such applications by Newton and Waddell[27] indicates a lack of good empirical evidence for use of standardized trunk testing to predict risk of low-back injury, however. These same investigators did confirm, as others have, that dynamic trunk strengths are lower in low-back pain patients when compared to healthy individuals, but the overlap in strength distributions between the two groups is so large as to negate the practical use of such tests for prediction of future risk or status of low-back injury.[26]

The Liftest is a form of dynamic, whole-body strength test. Because the load being moved is constant with each trial, it is referred to as an *isoinertial* (*constant mass*) type of test. By incrementally increasing the loads between trials, the testing procedure is referred to as a *psychophysical protocol* (i.e., the physical stress is increased until the person perceives he can no longer tolerate it). This type of testing is becoming standard for functional strength performance evaluations. When careful protocols are used, very good test-retest values are achieved.[9,30] The ability of a standardized isoinertial or isometric lifting test to predict general lifting capability has been shown by Jiang et al[15] and Aghazadeh and Ayoub[1] to be excellent, with $r^2 > 0.77$ for isoinertial tests and $r^2 > 0.72$ for isometric

tests. The ability of various types of tests to predict accurately on-job exertion capability is essential to meet the requirements of the Americans with Disabilities Act (ADA) (see Chapter 50). Such a requirement has further stimulated the development of whole-body work capacity types of strength evaluations.[11]

Whether these newer whole-body work capacity strength tests can predict who is at risk of future musculoskeletal injury remains in question. Isokinetic and isometric testing using standardized (non-job specific) lifting postures have not been able to predict low-back injury.[2,10,25] Earlier studies by Chaffin et al[7] and Keyserling et al[18] using job-specific isometric tests indicated that workers who could not demonstrate the strength to perform specific high-strength elements in their jobs were three times more at risk than their stronger counterparts. The difference in the outcome of these studies appears to be how well the strength tests replicated the high-strength elements in the workers' jobs.

## IDENTIFYING HIGH STRENGTH ELEMENTS IN A JOB

Given that ADA and occupational health and safety outcomes will depend on the data used to define job demands, how can such data be acquired? Traditionally, industrial engineers and work methods practitioners in companies have been held responsible for the following information:[5]

1. Developing a preferred work method (sequence of motions) to be used by a worker to minimize the time required to perform a manual job.
2. Documenting the preferred method, and any conditions that would affect a person's performance.
3. Determining the standard time for the job to be performed by a healthy, normal worker.
4. Preparing training materials and aids to assure a general understanding of the preferred work method.

Detailed studies by time-and-motion-study personnel in many different industries have resulted in formalized classifications of different types of elemental reaches, moves, grasps, and positions. The time that a well-trained worker would require to perform each of these elemental motions has been determined and is well published. These predetermined times are used by time-and-motion analysts to predict job performance times.[19]

The procedure for such analyses requires a time and motion study analyst to identify in published tables similar time values for the following standardized elemental motions:

1. *Reach*—a motion of the unloaded hands or fingers.
2. *Position*—small motion necessary when aligning object to be released at end of motion.

3. *Release*—either a distinct motion of fingers or the release of an object at the end of a motion without such an overt motion.

4. *Disengage*—an involuntary (rebound) motion often required when two objects suddenly come apart under exertion.

5. *Grasp*—an overt motion necessary to gain control of an object.

6. *Eye focus travel*—the time required for the eyes to move and accommodate to provide visualization of an object.

7. *Turn apply pressure*—the manipulation of controls, tools, and objects necessary to turn an object by rotation of the hand about the long axis of the forearm.

8. *Body, leg/foot motion*—the motion of transporting the body with values given per step for varied conditions.

9. *Simultaneous motions*—rules are given so that some motions can be performed together (for example, both the right and left hand reach to an object); therefore only the greater of these two time values is used in standard time prediction.

As one can imagine from this list, a great deal of detailed job information is available from such a job analysis. Though widely used in many industries for estimating production capacities and labor costs, some important biomechanical information still needs to be added for ergonomic purposes, however. For instance, though the load a person moves may be noted, only the average load is needed for time prediction purposes. Biomechanically, the peak load handled is normally the most strength requiring, but it is not often documented in traditional time-and-motion studies. A second limitation arises in that extreme work postures are not delineated. It is when a person must reach down to the floor, or to the side or overhead while applying forces to lift, push, or pull on an object that high biomechanical strength is required. Lastly, traditional time-and-motion study only documents those work elements that comprise 95% of the job (i.e., the time related productive activities). Unfortunately, many peak biomechanical strength requirements are created but go undocumented when a worker performs auxiliary tasks (e.g., replaces stock, lifts and moves defective parts, performs machine maintenance and adjustments).

In essence, traditional time-and-motion study information provides an excellent beginning for a biomechanical job analysis. Too often this valuable information is neglected because ergonomics or health and safety experts will use simple checklists to document the frequency and types of lifting, stooping, walking, or carrying in a job.[5] Such general checklists may suffice for rapid identification of potential exer-

tion related problems in many different jobs, but they rarely contain enough information to discriminate exposures to specific biomechanical stresses.[17]

A third approach to job evaluation has emerged recently. This approach uses videotaping of incumbent workers performing the tasks reported by them and their supervisors to be the most difficult to perform. This direct observation method was found to be more accurate than self-reporting alone of high manual-stress job conditions.[34] If care is taken to assure that the video data can be scaled, that is, size and orientation is known in each frame, adequate postural data can be acquired for biomechanical analyses.[28]

In addition to the postural requirements of a job provided from the videotapes, hand force data must be acquired with particular emphasis on the peak hand forces incurred while a person is in an awkward posture. Normally these data are acquired either by weighing objects that are lifted or using a hand-held force gauge for measuring push-and-pull forces.[5] Care must be taken to assure that both the direction of the hand force as well as its magnitude is determined. As shown in Fig. 17-3, in unencumbered lifting the hand force vector at the beginning of the lift is toward the body. As the lift proceeds, after about 200 to 300 msec when the load is closer to the body, the hand force vector becomes more vertical. It is at this latter location that the peak acceleration of the object causes the hand forces to be the largest (perhaps 30% to 50% larger than the static weight of the object). It is at this point in the lift that the biomechanical analysis should be performed to determine the peak strengths required.

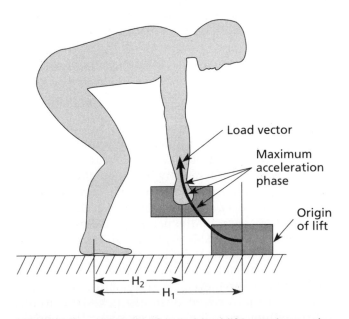

**FIGURE 17-3**   Example of typical load lifting trajectory during an unconstrained floor lift.

## NATIONAL INSTITUTE OF OCCUPATIONAL SAFETY AND HEALTH (NIOSH) LIFTING GUIDE JOB EVALUATION METHOD

If a job's most physically stressful elements are believed to be caused by two-handed lifting tasks, then the NIOSH revised equation for manual lifting evaluation should be consulted.[32] The purpose of the NIOSH analysis procedure is to combine analytically several physical workspace and task factors into the prediction of a Recommended Weight Limit (RWL). The six job factors that must be considered for each lift being performed are:
1. The horizontal (H) distance from the object being lifted to the person as measured from the ankles.
2. The vertical (V) distance of the object from the floor at the beginning of the lift.
3. The distance (D) the object is moved vertically.
4. The asymmetry (A) of the object location relative to the person's lower body and legs when beginning a lift. If the object is directly in front of a person, it would be symmetrically located.
5. The degree of hand grip coupling (C) with the object.
6. The frequency (F) of lifts per minute during one, two, or eight hour periods.

Given job data that describe each of the above factors, simple algebraic equations or tables are provided by NIOSH to estimate the amount of discounting due to each factor. In other words, if one knows the horizontal distance (H) at the beginning of a lift, a table, graph, or equation is provided that gives a modified HM value (which ranges from 0 to 1.0). The modifiers are then used in the following multiplicative equation for computing the RWL (in pounds) for each lift:

$$RWL = 51 \times HM \times VM \times DM \times AM \times CM \times FM$$

If all of the job conditions are optimal, then each modification factor would equal 1.0, and the RWL would equal 51 lb. This would only occur when a worker is standing erect, the load lifted is about 30 in. from the floor, it is compact and lifted close to the body and directly in front of the body, is lifted only a couple inches for a few seconds, and is lifted less than once every five minutes. Clearly, this is not a very common task. Because of the discounting modifiers often having values less than 1.0, it is not uncommon for a typical job that requires lifting of objects from the floor to have an RWL of 15 lb or less.

NIOSH proposes that the RWL value for a lifting task represents the magnitude of weight that can be lifted by about 90% of normally healthy men and women in industry, and creates an L5/S1 spinal disc compression force of less than 770 lb (3400 N). If a weight being lifted on a job exceeds the RWL computed for the lift, then excessive musculoskeletal injuries would be expected, according to Waters et al.[32]

In essence, the NIOSH Lifting Analysis is a comprehensive lifting task evaluation process. It is based on a large amount of published human biomechanical, psychophysical, and physiological data, and thus has good construct validity. For this reason it has been used by many different industries and government agencies to rank or rate the risk of injury in lifting jobs. It does not, however, provide a means to evaluate one-handed lifting, or any other types of manual tasks than lifting (e.g., pushing or pulling exertions are excluded).

## BIOMECHANICAL JOB STRENGTH AND LOW-BACK EVALUATION

Because the NIOSH *Work Practices Guide for Manual Lifting* applies only to lifting with two hands, a more comprehensive job physical stress analysis scheme may be necessary to provide the basis for job-related strength testing. One such scheme relies on a computerized static-strength prediction model described in Chaffin and Andersson.[5] This model compares the load moments produced at various body joints when a person performs manual exertions. Population norms obtained from tests of over 3000 workers in the United States are then used for comparison. By performing this comparison at each body joint, the static-strength model predicts the proportion of the population capable of performing the exertion, as well as predicting compression forces that may be acting on the lower lumbar discs during the simulated exertions.

This computerized strength-prediction methodology provides the means to evaluate a variety of manual exertion data obtained from direct observations of workers. The job analysis procedure is generally the same as that adopted by NIOSH in that a job is first described as a series of physical exertions. What is different, however, is that the analyst must also identify the load vector direction operating on the hands (i.e., "lift" is a vertical downward load vector, "push" is a sagittal plane, horizontal vector toward the body, and "pull" is a sagittal plane, horizontal vector away from the body). In addition, for each task the posture of the torso and extremities at the time of a peak exertion of interest are recorded, usually from measuring body segment angles obtained from stop-action videos or photographs.

An example of the use of this method is shown in Fig. 17-4 for the lifting of a 44-lb (200-N) stock reel. The input and output screens from the *2D Static*

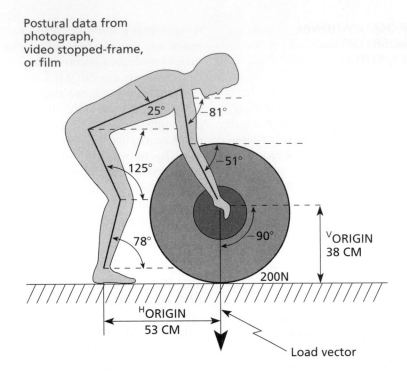

Postural data from
photograph,
video stopped-frame,
or film

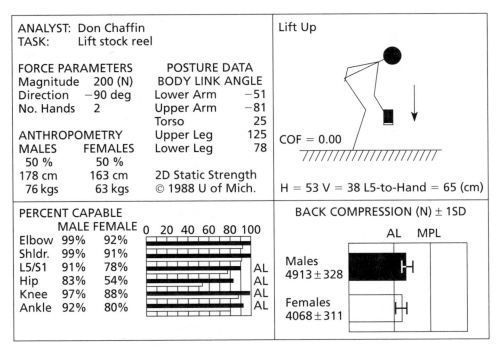

**FIGURE 17-4** The University of Michigan 2D Static Strength Prediction Program™ with the input conditions for evaluating the stock reel lifting task displayed at top and the resulting output screen displayed at bottom. (Courtesy of The Regents of the University of Michigan.)

*Strength Prediction Program*™ developed at The University of Michigan are displayed. The input data required are (1) load magnitude and direction (example: 44 lb [200 N] acting downward at −90°), (2) whether one or two hands are involved (example: two hands are lifting the stock reel), (3) general an-

thropometry of people to be analyzed (example: average weight and stature of men and women are assumed), and (4) the body postural angles relative to a horizontal reference axis. The latter is shown as a silhouette from a photograph in Fig. 17-4, with the reference angles superimposed. Given these input data, the program then outputs several results, shown at the bottom of Fig. 17-4. First is a stick figure drawing of the human kinematic linkage being analyzed. Comparison of it with a photograph, video image, or drawing board manikin provides a qualitative check on the postural-input angles. Also, the vertical and horizontal coordinates of the load or hand center, relative to the ankle, and the L5/S1 disc horizontal to load center distance provide quantitative checks on the postural and anthropometric input values (i.e., Is the load located where one expects it to be relative to that measured from the person being analyzed?).

If the input data are appropriate, the logic described in Chaffin and Andersson[5] is executed, and the program displays (1) a graphical and tabular prediction of the percentage of the male and female populations expected to have sufficient static strength at each major joint, (2) a graphical and tabular prediction of the L5/S1 disc compression forces for men and women, (3) the required static coefficient-of-friction required to not slip, and (4) a statement as to whether the task being performed would result in loss of forward or rearward balance.

Figure 17-4 shows that:
1. The moment strength requirements are greatest at the hips, with only 54% of women and 83% of men having the expected hip extensor strengths.
2. The large H distance and stooped posture cause the predicted compression forces on the L5/S1 disc to be high, over 900 lb (4000 N), which is above the NIOSH Spinal Limit of 770 lb (3400 N).
3. Because it is a vertical lift, the required floor static coefficient-of-friction is 0, and no forward or backward balance problem exists for the posture specified.

Further analysis with the 2DSSPP™ model of successive postures required to lift the 44 lb stock reel up to the stock holder (63 in. above the floor) revealed an interesting trade-off between excessive back stress and shoulder strength demands. Both of these biomechanical outcomes are plotted in Fig. 17-5, with predicted L5/S1 compression forces at the top and the predicted percent of men and women with enough strength shown in the bottom graph. Inspection of the graphs shows that when the load is in the middle position the spinal compression force is at its lowest value and the greatest percent of the population could perform such an exertion. As the load is lifted higher to the stock holder, spinal-compression forces approach (or slightly exceed) the suggested NIOSH

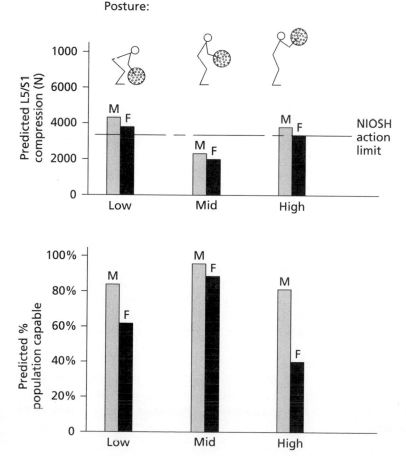

**FIGURE 17-5** Lifting a 44-lb stock reel using UM-2DSSPP™ software with three different lift postures being evaluated. (From Chaffin DB: A biomechanical strength model for use in industry. *Appl Ind Hyg* 3(3):79-86, 1988.)

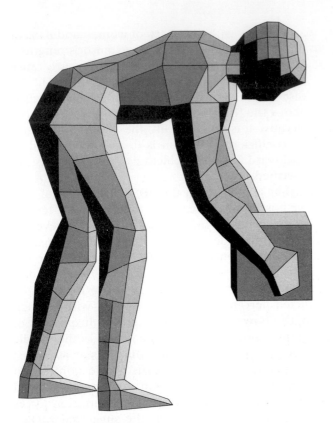

**FIGURE 17-6**    Human graphic used in the UM-3DSSPP™ Job Strength Analysis Program.

hazard level and fewer than 40% of women and only about 80% of men have the shoulder strengths required for such a high lift.

A full three-dimensional static strength analysis model is also available (3DSSPP™) for those exertions performed in postures other than the sagittal plane. Figure 17-6 depicts the human form graphic model developed for this analysis. Both one-handed and two-handed exertions can be simulated and analyzed in a large variety of postures with this model.

Though the static strength prediction programs provide powerful tools for determining the various conditions on a job that demand a great deal of strength, they are static simulations. Marras et al[24] have shown that not only is it important to know what the peak low-back moment requirements are to assign a risk level to a job but that the velocity of the person's torso motion can be a separate risk factor. Indeed, when young, healthy men were asked to lift a load from the floor to a table, they chose a maximal acceptable weight and lifted it dynamically in such a way that peak spinal compression forces were actually double the NIOSH hazard level for a more heterogenous population.[4] In other words, static biomechanical analyses may not be enough to understand all of the complex stresses in a particular exertion.

Though dynamic biomechanical analysis models exist, they either require attaching electronic goniometers to workers or require sophisticated video processing tools to measure the motion dynamics. For these reasons their use in industry has been limited.

## SUMMARY

Given that most experts agree with the concept that disability should be determined by how well a person's functional capability matches required job demands, it is surprising that so many studies attempt to quantify the former with little or no attention given to the latter. In fact it would appear that a large proportion of the medical community would like to neglect job demand information altogether in determining an individual's capacity to work. A review in 1993 of factors used in rating impairment levels for neck and back injuries by Clark and Haldeman[8] disclosed 37 factors believed to be important by a group of California Industrial Medical Examiners. Surprisingly, none of the 37 factors included the need to evaluate the patients' capabilities to perform specific manual jobs. In other words, rating work capacity in clinical practice seems to require only knowledge about the patient, not the job, despite continual recognition by experts regarding the importance of the work environment in disability determinations.[16,20] Quite frankly, as long as the medical community ignores the fact that job demands vary greatly, their ability to make a fair and rational decision about a person's work status will be greatly compromised.

As Lehmann et al[23] have extolled: "Patients must be encouraged to return to work, and employers encouraged to modify injured workers' job tasks to lighter duties until they have recovered sufficiently to return to normal duties." This is the essence of affirmative action. Only by knowing both the person's capabilities and the corresponding job demands can real progress be made. To accomplish this, those that know about people and those that know about the physics of jobs must work together to manage better the injured worker. Not only will the injured worker benefit from such a team approach but perhaps job biomechanical risk factors will be identified and reduced, thus benefiting all workers in the future.

## References

1. Aghazadeh F, Ayoub MM: A comparison of dynamic and static strength models for prediction of lifting capacity. *Ergonomics* 28(10):1409-1417, 1985.

2. Battie MC, et al: Isometric lifting strength as a predictor of industrial back pain reports. *Spine* 14:851-856, 1989.

3. Caldwell LS, et al: A proposed standard procedure for static muscle strength testing. *Amer Ind Hyg J* 35:201-206, 1974.

4. Chaffin DB, Page GB: Postural effects on biomechanical and psychophysical weight lifting limits. *Ergonomics* 37(4):663-676, 1994.

5. Chaffin DB, Andersson GBJ: *Occupational biomechanics,* ed 2, New York, 1991.

6. Chaffin DB: A biomechanical strength model for use in industry. *Appl Ind Hyg* 3(3):79-86, 1988.

7. Chaffin DB, Herrin GD, Keyserling WM: Preemployment strength testing. *J Occup Med* 20(6):403-408, 1978.

8. Clark W, Haldeman S: The development of guideline factors for the evaluation of disability in neck and back injuries. *Spine* 18(13):1736-1745, 1993.

9. Dales JL, Macdonald EB, Anderson JAD: The Liftest strength test—an accurate method of dynamic strength assessment? *Clinic Biomech* 1(1):11-13, 1986.

10. Dueker JA, et al: Isokinetic trunk testing and employment. *J Occup Med* 36(1):42-48, 1993.

11. Dusik L, et al: Concurrent validity of the ERGOS work simulator versus conventional functional capacity evaluation techniques in a workers' compensation population. *J Occup Med* 35(8):759-767, 1993.

13. Feurestein M: Workers' compensation reform in New York state: a proposal to address medical, ergonomic, and psychological factors associated with work disability. *J Occup Rehab* 3(3):125-135, 1993.

15. Jiang BC, Smith JL, Ayoub MM: Psychophysical modeling of manual materials-handling capacities using isoinertial strength variables. *Hum Factors* 28(6):691-702, 1986.

16. Johns RE, et al: Chronic, recurrent low-back pain. *J Occup Med* 36(5):537-547, 1994.

17. Keyserling WM, Brouwer M, Silverstein BA: A checklist for evaluating ergonomics risk factors resulting from awkward postures of the legs, trunk, and neck. *Int J Indus Ergonomics* 9:283-301, 1992.

18. Keyserling WM, Herrin GD, Chaffin DB: Isometric strength testing as a means of controlling medical incidents on strenuous jobs. *J Occup Med* 22(5):332-336, 1980.

19. Konz S: *Work design,* Columbus, Ohio, 1979, Grid Publishing.

20. Krause N, Ragland DR: Occupational disability due to low back pain: a new interdisciplinary classification based on a phase model of disability. *Spine* 19(9):1011-1020, 1994.

21. Kroemer KHE: Development of LIFTEST: A dynamic technique to assess individual capacity to lift material, NIOSH Report 210-79-0041, NIOSH, Cincinnati, Ohio, 1982.

22. Kumar S, Chaffin DB, Redfern M: Isometric and isokinetic back-and-arm-lifting strengths: device and measurement. *J Biomech* 21(1):35-44, 1988.

23. Lehmann TR, Spratt KF, Lehmann KK: Predicting long-term disability in low-back-injured workers presenting to a spine consultant. *Spine* 18(8):1103-1112, 1993.

24. Marras WS, et al: The role of dynamic three-dimensional trunk motion in occupationally-related low back disorders. *Spine* 18(5):617-628, 1993.

25. Mostardi R, et al: Isokinetic lifting strength and occupational injury. *Spine* 17:189-193, 1992.

26. Newton M, et al: Trunk-strength testing with isomachines—part 2. *Spine* 18(7):812-824, 1993.

27. Newton M, Waddell G: Trunk-strength with isomachines, part 1. *Spine* 18(7):801-811, 1993.

28. Paul JA, Douwes M: Two-dimensional photographic posture recording and description: a validity study. *Appl Ergonomics* 24(2):83-90, 1993.

29. Sandler HM: ADA and occupational health: a status report. *Occupational Hazards* 55-56, Oct. 1993.

30. Snook SH: The design of manual handling tasks. *Ergonomics* 21(12):973-985, 1978.

31. Taylor Frederick W: *The principles of scientific management,* New York, 1929, Harper.

32. Waters TR, et al: Revised NIOSH equation for the design and evaluation of manual lifting tasks. *Ergonomics* 36(7):749-776, 1993.

33. Wheeler DL, et al: Functional assessment for prediction of lifting capacity. *Spine* 19(9):1021-1026, 1994.

34. Wiktorin C, Karlqvist L, Winkel J: Stockholm Music I study group: validity of self-reported exposures to work postures and manual materials handling. *Scand J Work Environ Health* 19:208-214, 1993.

# FUNCTIONAL CAPACITY EVALUATION

*Leonard N. Matheson*

Information about the injured worker's functional capacity is a key component of return-to-work planning.[39,41,56,74] Functional capacity evaluation (FCE) is a systematic method of measuring a patient's ability to perform meaningful tasks on a *safe and dependable* basis. Beyond this general purpose, functional capacity evaluation has three specific purposes. The first is to improve the likelihood that the injured worker will be safe in subsequent task performance.[38,54] Routinely, the comparison of an injured worker's capacity to a job's demands is made in an attempt to diminish the risk of reinjury that is associated with a mismatch. Shortfalls in the relationship between a patient's abilities and the environment's demands result in stress[84] or increased risk for injury.[9,15] Numerous researchers[1,11,32,34,75,83] point to the importance of properly matching the worker's capacity to the job's demands. The second is to assist the patient to improve role performance through identification of functional decrements so that they may be resolved or worked around.[41,51,69] Healthcare professionals use this information to steer patients into proper treatment programs and to measure treatment progress. The third is to determine the presence (and, if present, the level) of disability so that the patient's case can be bureaucratically or juridically concluded.[61]

The term *functional* connotes performance of a purposeful, meaningful, or useful task that has a beginning and an end with a result that can be measured. The effect of the patient's impairment on his or her ability to perform meaningful tasks is the focus of functional capacity evaluation.[6,51] As such, functional performance is important to measure because it translates the effect of impairment on disability. Several authors[63-65,85] have described current models of disablement[43] and the rehabilitation process. This chapter reflects adherence to Nagi's model of rehabilitation[63,64] in which function holds a translational role. This model describes pathologic conditions and impairment as factors that, taken within the context of the individual's environmental and personal resources,[6] are the precursors of functional limitation. These factors are addressed by the physician in a medical diagnostic evaluation.[5] If the impairment is sufficiently severe, *functional limitation* can result. Functional limitations are measured by occupational therapists, physical therapists, vocational evaluators, psychologists, and exercise physiologists in a functional capacity evaluation.[51] If the functional limitations are sufficiently severe and are pertinent to role tasks, disability with regard to that role can result. Disability can be described in terms of the role consequences of functional limitations.[27,43,63-65] Disability can be operationally defined as the evaluee's uncompensated shortfalls in responding to role demands.[51] Figure 18-1 represents this definition in graphic terms.

Evaluation of disability is based on the measurement of the functional consequences of impairment in tasks that are pertinent to the particular role under consideration.[65] Thus, in order to evaluate disability, one must measure functional limitations in terms of a particular role.[43] Individuals assume several roles in society, such as spouse, parent, neighbor, worker, teammate, or customer. When the emphasis is on determining the presence or degree of occupational disability, the focus must be on tasks in the worker role and work environment.[80] If the functional consequences are significant and occur in tasks that are critical to the performance of the job, the evaluee can be described as having an *occupational disability.*[51] The extent and type of occupational disability are dependent on the patient's ability to perform these work-relevant tasks. In this chapter, the selection of tasks that are pertinent to the worker role will be addressed.

The term *capacity* refers to the maximum ability or potential of a patient. The use of this term is somewhat misleading because capacity rarely is measured in a performance task unless the patient is highly trained to perform that particular task. Examples of maximum-task performance are found when experienced athletes compete. The individual's maximum level of performance that usually can be measured is termed the patient's *tolerance* for the demands of that task.[51] Further, the *maximum dependable ability* of the patient usually is significantly less than his or her tolerance. Finally, many functional capacity evaluations are concerned only with adequacy for task performance rather than the patient's maximum dependable ability in that task. That is, if the patient is under consideration for a particular job, the task demands of that job may be less than the patient's demonstrated ability. In this circumstance, as the evaluation progresses with increasing loads placed on the evaluee, the evaluation will conclude when the job demand is reached. This may be at a lower performance level than the patient's maximum dependable ability, which is lower than his or her tolerance, which is lower than his or her capacity. The relationship among these variables is described in Figure 18-2.

The term *evaluation* describes a systematic approach to monitoring and reporting performance that requires the evaluator to observe, measure, and interpret the patient's performance in a structured task.[38] FCE should be distinguished from *functional assessment*. Although the terms sometimes are used interchangeably and some functional assessment instruments are used in FCE, they describe different processes. Generally, FCE is based on performance measurement while functional assessment is based on expert ratings from observation or the patient's self-report.[21,25,28,36] The former, which is the focus of this chapter, employs structured performance protocols using test equipment or simulated activities to measure functional performance, while the latter employs structured behavior rating scales to rate observations or self-perceptions.

Because functional capacity evaluation involves measurement of the evaluee in terms of his or her ability to perform work, the scope of these examinations can be quite broad. For example, one of the most widely-respected taxonomies of human performance was developed by Edwin Fleishman[32] and his colleagues based on factor analysis research of the abilities requirements for numerous jobs. In a recent work Fleishman and Reilly[31] describe 52 different abilities that are pertinent to job tasks. Only nine of these abilities involve strength, while an additional ten involve psychomotor abilities that involve response speed and precision. For the purpose of this chapter, the focus of FCE will be narrowed to include physical performance factors in occupational settings that normally are pertinent to musculoskeletal impairment. Further narrowing of focus will be to work demand factors that are pertinent to occupational tasks. It is important to note that this results in a very narrow view of FCE that is necessary because of these space limitations. Even after this narrowing of focus, however, the complexities of functional capacity evaluation can be daunting. This is so because at the interface between the patient's physical abilities and the job's physical demands stand activities such as lifting or handling that have a complex physiologic, psychologic, musculoskeletal, and environmental[80] basis.

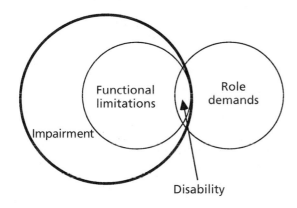

**FIGURE 18-1**     Disability lies at the interface between functional limitations and role demands.

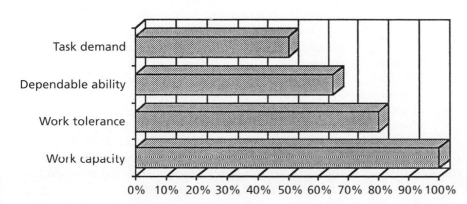

**FIGURE 18-2**     Distinctions among work capacity, work tolerance, dependable ability, and task demand.

| Question | Compared to... | Example output | Duration |
|---|---|---|---|
| Ability to perform key task | Pre-injury ability | "Moderately limited ability to lift" | 1 hour |
| Loss of work capacity | Normal values | "35% loss of lift capacity." | 2 hours |
| Adequacy for job | Specific job demands | "Adequate for demands of fitter at Acme." | 3-6 hours |
| Adequacy for occupation | General occupational demands | "Inadequate for demands of general fitter." | 5-8 hours |
| Maximum dependable ability | General employment standards | "Maximum of 40 lbs infrequent lift." | 3-8 days |

**FIGURE 18-3**     Types of functional capacity evaluation.

## TYPES OF FUNCTIONAL CAPACITY EVALUATION

Functional capacity evaluations involve five different types of evaluation processes, defined by the purpose to which the information derived will be applied. The primary issues that are used to differentiate among the types of FCE are presented in Figure 18-3.

Each of the five types of FCE is described below, arranged along a hierarchy of increasing complexity, time, and expense.

### Functional Goal Setting

If the patient's impairment is sufficiently severe to warrant referral for therapy, measurement of functional status that is pertinent to the impairment in order to set recovery goals is necessary.[53] This evaluation measures the usual functional consequences of the impairment. For example, in the case of a musculoskeletal impairment, range of motion, strength, and work capacity would be measured. Equipment from such manufacturers[1] as ARCON, BTE, Chattanooga, Cybex, Isotechnologies, Lafayette, Loredan, and Smith & Nephew Rolyan is used in this type of evaluation (see the box on p. 171). The information that is collected is used in consultation with the patient to set functional goals. It is also used to provide objective indices of performance to gauge the progress of therapy.

### Disability Rating

If the functional consequences of an impairment are sufficiently severe to result in limitation of the patient's ability to work, measurement of the loss-of-performance ability in key functional areas of work can be used as an estimate of disability.[45,48] Information about the patient's impairment is obtained through a medical examination, while information concerning performance in terms of the key functional areas is obtained through an FCE. Equipment from such manufacturers as Blankenship, EPIC, and Key is used in this type of evaluation. For example, the California Disability Rating System[18,24] uses the percent of lost-lift capacity as the basis of a standard disability rating for injuries that result in work-capacity limitations. After measurement of the loss-of-lift capacity, other issues are addressed, depending on the extent of loss. This system of categorization is presented in Figure 18-4.

The California Functional Capacity Protocol[61] has been developed as a means to measure the functional consequences of soft-tissue injury in order to provide information to the treating physician so that the physician's recommendations concerning work restrictions, which are the basis of the disability rating, will be consistent. Using this model, a disability rating falls into one of eight categories according to a series of functional issues. Each category has been assigned a standard disability rating that is used as one of four variables in a formula that translates the occupational consequences of impairment in terms of an occupational category, taking into account the evaluee's age.

### Job Task Matching

Matching the adequacy of the worker's abilities to the essential functions of the job is the next-most-complex type of functional capacity evaluation. Information concerning the physical demands of a particular job is obtained through a job analysis, whereas information concerning the worker's impairment is obtained through a medical examination.[38,40,41] A comparison of these two sets of information leads to the identification of the physical abilities that require an evaluation of functional adequacy. Equipment from such manufacturers as BTE, EPIC, Isernhagen Work Systems, Loredan, Smith & Nephew Rolyan, and WEST is used in this type of evaluation. This FCE is different from the Disability Rating FCE because the evaluation content is uniquely determined for each evaluee and job in combination.

## MANUFACTURERS AND SUPPLIERS

ARCON
309 McLaws Circle, Suite F
Williamsburg, VA 23185

Baltimore Therapeutic Equipment (BTE)
7456-L New Ridge Road
Hanover, MD 21076

Blankenship
P.O. Box 5084
Macon, GA 31208

Chattanooga Group
4717 Adams Road
P.O. Box 489
Hixson, TN 37343-0489

Cybex
2100 Smithtown Ave.
Ronkonkoma, NY 11779-0903

EPIC
P.O. Box 80864
Rancho Santa Margarita, CA 92688

ERGASYS
25532 Terreno
Mission Viejo, CA 92691

Fred Sammons
145 Tower Drive
Burr Ridge, IL 60521

Isernhagen Work Systems
2202 Water Street
Duluth, MN 55812

Isotechnologies
P.O. Box 1239
Hillsborough, NC 27278

Key Functional Assessments
1010 Park Ave.
Minneapolis, MN 55404

Lafayette Instruments
P.O. Box 5729
Lafayette, IN 47903

Loredan Biomedical
3650 Industrial Blvd.
West Sacramento, CA 95691

MedX
1401 NE 77th Street
Ocala, FL 34479

Smith & Nephew Rolyan
N93 W14475 Whittaker Way
P.O. Box 555
Menomonee Falls, WI 53051

Valpar International
2450 W. Ruthrauff Road
Tucson, AZ 87505

WEST
P.O. Box 2477
Fort Bragg, CA 95437

Work Recovery Systems
2341 S. Friebus, Suite 14
Tucson, AZ 85713

### Occupation Matching

Matching of the patient's functional capacity to the demands of an occupational classification is a separate type of functional capacity evaluation. Information concerning the physical demands of an occupation is obtained from a source such as the *Dictionary of Occupational Titles*.[22,23] The physical demand level is often described in general terms such as those depicted in Figure 18-5.

Information concerning the worker's impairment is obtained through a medical examination that includes an assessment of perceived functional capacity. A comparison of these two sets of information leads to the identification of the level of physical abilities that requires a formal evaluation of functional adequacy. Equipment from such manufacturers as Valpar and Work Recovery Systems is used in this type of evaluation. This type of FCE is more complex than job task matching because the occupational classification contains all job tasks that might be required in the variety of jobs that are found within the classification. It is also more physically demanding because the level of demand within each task has a natural range that is usually somewhat less than the maximum that is actually found in a particular job. However, because the full range of job demands within the occupational classification must be considered, the performance target is the maximum level for the tasks.

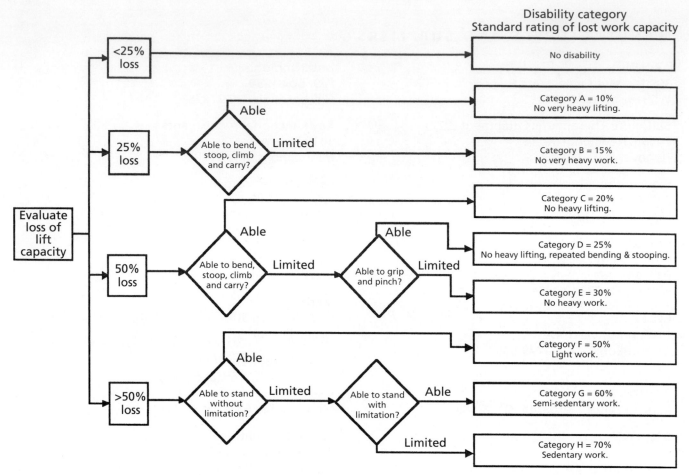

**FIGURE 18-4**    California Disability Rating System Decision Tree.

| PHYSICAL DEMAND LEVEL | OCCASIONAL 0 - 33% of the workday | FREQUENT 34 - 66% of the workday | CONSTANT 67 - 100% of the workday | Typical energy required |
|---|---|---|---|---|
| **SEDENTARY** | 10 lbs. | Negligible | Negligible | 1.5 - 2.1 METS |
| **LIGHT** | 20 lbs. | 10 lbs. and/or walk/stand/push/pull of arm/leg controls | Negligible and/or push/pull of arm/leg controls while seated | 2.2 - 3.5 METS |
| **MEDIUM** | 20 to 50 lbs. | 10 to 25 lbs. | 10 lbs. | 3.6 - 6.3 METS |
| **HEAVY** | 50 to 100 lbs. | 25 to 50 lbs. | 10 to 20 lbs. | 6.4 - 7.5 METS |
| **VERY HEAVY** | Over 100 lbs. | Over 50 lbs. | Over 20 lbs. | Over 7.5 METS |

**FIGURE 18-5**    United States Department of Labor Physical Demand Characteristics of Work chart.

## Work Capacity Evaluation

Matching the patient's functional capacity to the demands of competitive employment is the most comprehensive type of functional capacity evaluation. Because there is no occupational target, the focus of the Work Capacity Evaluation is very broad, encompassing all of the frequently encountered task demands and worker behaviors. Behaviors such as those described in the Feasibility Evaluation Checklist[51] are assessed through observation of performance in a simulated work environment. This checklist includes 21 behavior-anchored rating scales for items such as the ability to accept supervision and work with others, safety in the workplace, and the quantity and quality of the patient's productivity. This type of evaluation uses structured work simulations. These can be purchased from a manufacturer such as Work Recovery Systems or can be constructed based on descriptions found in published resources.[13,51,69]

Selecting the FCE that is appropriate for the evaluee given the context of his or her situation is driven, in part, by the performance-demand targets that are contemplated, given the availability of a job for the evaluee and the specificity of information concerning the job or occupational demands. A decision tree that describes the process through which the evaluee must be directed to receive the proper type of FCE is described in Figure 18-6.

## BASIC COMPONENTS OF WORK DEMAND

Because functional capacity is based on the interaction of the person in a complex environment, certain key attributes of this interaction must be understood. The most basic physical underpinnings of task performance that are normally considered include force, task duration, and work-rest cycles.

## Force

Force is the action on an object that changes its motion. Force is the product of the mass of the object that is experiencing a change in motion multiplied by the acceleration of that motion. Force is commonly expressed in Newtons (N) or pounds. One Newton equals .225 pounds force. The formula for force is:

$$F = m \times a$$

where $F$ is force, $m$ is mass, and $a$ is acceleration. The force that a worker can apply to a task to produce work is dependent on his or her ability to generate power. If force acts on an object in a manner that causes it to rotate about an axis, it is commonly measured in terms of torque. Torque that is measured at the axis of rotation is the product of the perpendicular force on the object multiplied by the distance of the object from the axis.

## Work

Work is the product of force applied over distance, commonly expressed in Newton-meters (Nm), Joules (J), or foot-pounds force (ft-lbf). A Newton-meter (or Joule) is the work that is done when an object of mass one kilogram is moved one meter. A foot-pound is the work that is done when an object of mass one pound is moved one foot. One Newton-meter or Joule equals 0.737 foot-pounds of work. The formula for work is:

$$W = F \times s$$

where $W$ is work, $F$ is force, and $s$ is distance measured in the direction that the force acts.

## Power

Power is the rate at which work is performed, commonly expressed in watts (W), Joules/second (J/sec), or foot-pounds force/second (ft-lbf/sec). Power is the quotient of the work that has been performed divided by the time that was required to perform the work. One watt is equal to 0.737 ft-lbf/sec. The formula for power is:

$$P = W \div t$$

where $P$ is power, $W$ is work, and $t$ is time, commonly measured in seconds.

## Task Frequency

Task frequency normally is measured in terms of units completed per minute. It is important to note that the United States Department of Labor physical-demand characteristics of work system[23] describes task frequency in terms of *percent of the day*. This is a general description of task frequency that is often used for job analyses. Unfortunately, it is not useful for FCE because it does not reflect the consequences of task frequency on the worker.[8,34,59] That is, the individual can accurately be described as having the ability to perform a task, at a certain frequency, for a number of minutes, and repeated a certain number of times each day. In contrast, a statement such as "able to perform a lift from waist to shoulder of 50 pounds for 25% of the work day" does not reflect the physio-

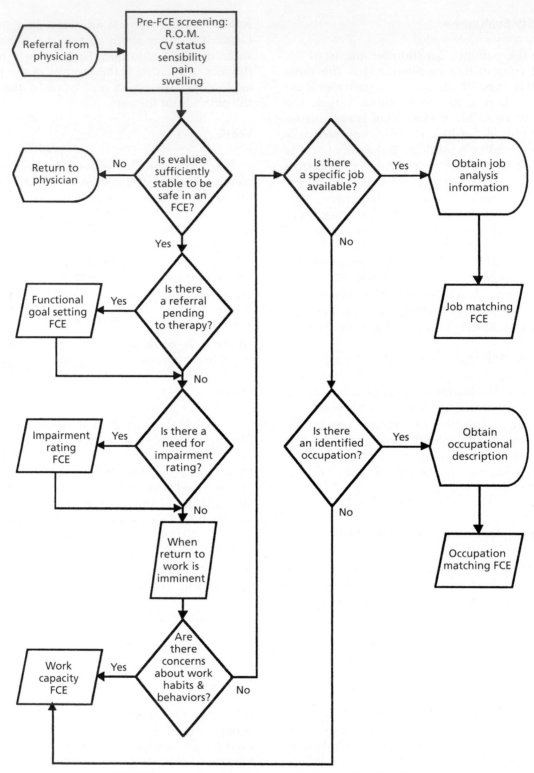

**FIGURE 18-6**     Functional Capacity Evaluation Decision Tree.

logic, biomechanical, or psychophysical bases of work, and is not able to reflect accurately the ability of a patient.

## Task Duration

Task duration is normally measured in terms of seconds or minutes of sustained activity. The individual can be described as having the ability to sustain a task at a certain frequency for a set number of minutes.

## Work-Rest Cycles

Work-rest cycles are normally described by the number of minutes working and resting with a particular pattern of activities during a set period, often two hours. The amount of work that a person can perform is dependent on the combination of work and rest during this cycle.

## BASIC COMPONENTS OF FUNCTIONAL CAPACITY

In the most simple model of functional capacity evaluation, work is considered to be dependent on the person's ability to generate power. The more power that is generated by the patient, the more force that can be brought to bear on the task at hand, thus the more work that can be performed. Power has a physiologic basis that is grounded in the individual's aerobic and metabolic capacity. However, with work tasks, power is applied through the evaluee's biomechanical system and governed by his or her psychophysical limitations. These three coincident domains of function are described in more detail below. Coincidence of these domains indicates that each domain is pertinent in every task.

## Cardiovascular/Metabolic

The performance resources are those that challenge the patient's energy-producing systems. For the patient with a musculoskeletal injury who has remained off of work for more than a few weeks and has not maintained a level of activity that approximates his or her previous work demands, the cardiovascular/metabolic domains often present significant transient limitations.

## Biomechanical

The performance resources are those that challenge the evaluee's anatomical and musculoskeletal system. Skeletal muscles produce torque at the various biomechanical linkages in the body to produce movement and bring force to bear on objects.

## Psychophysical

The performance resources that are available challenge the evaluee's self-perceptions, fears, and built-in work function themes and limits. For the previously injured evaluee, the psychophysical domain will be especially important in tasks that are similar to the task in which a traumatic injury previously occurred.

It is important to recognize which of these domains is always the most limiting. While the presenting issue may appear to require the evaluee's resources primarily in one domain, task performance will be the result of demands on the evaluee in the most limiting domain. This characteristic of FCE must be taken into account in order to attribute accurately functional limitations to a particular impairment.

## SPECIFIC COMPONENTS OF FUNCTIONAL CAPACITY

The focus of the FCE will be on one or more specific components of functional capacity. This will occur as a consequence of selection of those work tasks that are most likely to present the greatest challenge to the evaluee within the context of the presenting impairment. Some of the most common components of functional capacity important include strength, lifting capacity, endurance, range of motion, accuracy of movement, skill, dexterity, and the ability to balance, carry, and climb.

## Strength

After an injury or illness, loss of power due to impairment is one contributor to a loss of work capacity. In a musculoskeletal injury or illness, this is often caused by impairment of a muscle, tendon, ligament, or joint. As a consequence of the impairment, the ability of one or more of these biomechanical units is limited or is made less efficient, causing diminished power generation, which is interpreted as a "loss of strength." Strength can be evaluated by numerous means, depending on the task under consideration. Mainstream equipment for evaluating upper extremity strength includes the B&L pinch gauge, BTE Work Simulator, Dexter ETS from Smith & Nephew Rolyan, Jamar hand dynamometer, Lido WorkSet, MedX Upper Extremity Test, and the WEST 4. Mainstream equipment for evaluating whole-body strength includes the ARCON ST, BTE Lift, ERGASYS, and the

ERGOS from Work Recovery Systems. Mainstream equipment for evaluating lower-extremity strength includes several pieces of equipment from Chattanooga, Cybex, Loredan, and MedX. Mainstream equipment for evaluating back strength includes equipment from Chattanooga, Cybex, Loredan, and MedX.

### Lifting Capacity

The effect of a musculoskeletal impairment is most often measured in terms of the patient's lift capacity. This will be reviewed in more detail later in this chapter. Because of its importance, virtually all of the equipment manufacturers have developed systems to measure lift capacity. Those evaluation protocols that are most widely accepted are available from Blankenship, EPIC, Isernhagen, Key, and WEST.

### Endurance

In a FCE, endurance is termed *sustained activity tolerance,* which is a function of general aerobic and metabolic capacity as well as local muscular capacity (see also Chapter 28). There is an inverse relationship between the ability to sustain a repetitive task and the percent of maximum strength demand. That is, at lower levels of power, the worker can perform more work than he or she is able to perform at higher levels of power because the worker's ability to generate power limits the length of time that power can be sustained. As task demands get closer to the worker's maximum capacity, the length of time that the task can be sustained decreases exponentially. Because this relationship is exponential, the total work that can be performed by a worker is greatest at lower levels of power. Mainstream equipment for evaluating sustained activity tolerance includes the EPIC 5 Manual Material Handling test, the ERGOS Work Simulator from Work Recovery Systems, the Valpar 8, and the Valpar 19.

### Standing Range of Motion

The impaired patient's loss of flexibility is important to consider if it results in a limitation of the physical range in which the evaluee can perform tasks. For example, flexibility of the shoulder may be of crucial importance for a drill press operator or a piano player, but much less important for a psychologist or an insurance salesperson. Mainstream equipment for evaluating standing range of motion includes the EPIC 4 Whole Body Range of Motion test and the Valpar 9.

### Balance, Carry, and Climb

The evaluation of walking balance, carrying, and climbing requires more space than many FCE centers can afford. However, protocols and equipment are available from BTE, EPIC, Isernhagen, Valpar, and Work Recovery Systems.

### Movement Accuracy

The ability of the impaired evaluee to perform tasks quickly and accurately may be reduced after a musculoskeletal injury due to secondary factors such as high levels of pain that interfere with concentration. Movement accuracy is evaluated by such instruments as the Employee Aptitude Survey #9, EPIC 2 Motor Coordination test, and the ERGOS Work Simulator.

### Finger and Hand Dexterity

The ability to move the fingers and hands precisely and with speed is an important component of many jobs. It is diminished by a wide variety of musculoskeletal impairments, including those involving the upper back, cervical spine, and upper extremities. Equipment to measure this component is available from BTE, EPIC, Isernhagen, Key, Lafayette, Valpar, WEST, and Work Recovery Systems.

### Skill

It is important to recognize that "skills lie in the efficient and effective use of capacities as the result of experience and practice."[84] Although skill will only be assessed in a small proportion of FCEs, it can be of paramount importance. Skill is evaluated by numerous instruments from Lafayette, Valpar, and Work Recovery Systems.

### OVERVIEW OF MEASUREMENT

Measurement is the basic task performed by the evaluator in a functional capacity evaluation. Measurement involves the use of numerals as numbers to describe the state of some variable. Unfortunately, the use of numbers is not straightforward. The issue has been reviewed in detail from various vantage points.[58,60,70,73,87]

The information that is gathered in the FCE is *descriptive* and, when standards of performance are available, *normative.*[71] Descriptive results are used to compare the patient's current ability with the patient at a previous point or with the physical demands of work. Normative results are used to compare the patient to a reference population.

Measurement is dependent on the scale that is used. Common scales such as those found on a thermometer, yardstick, or goniometer often are used without thought to the underlying properties of the scale. However, functional capacity evaluation utilizes a wide variety of instruments with various scale attributes. An understanding of these attributes and the limits they impose on the interpretation and use of the information derived in a FCE is important. The four scales are the nominal, ordinal, interval, and ratio.

## Nominal

Numbers represent category labels and are used for classification. Examples include ICD-9 codes or gender and race classifications. Nominal data allow the user to distinguish differences between or among members of separately-classified groups. No value-based mathematical comparisons are permitted.

## Ordinal

Numbers indicate the rank order of measures. The distance between the ranks is unknown and assumed to vary across the span of the scale. Examples from FCE include scores from pain, activity, and depression questionnaires, scores on quantified pain drawings, and scores on functional status questionnaires or manual muscle test ratings.* Ordinal data allow the user to distinguish difference from lesser to greater magnitude along one scale. Ordinal data do not allow the magnitude of the difference to be measured with any degree of precision or unambiguous meaning. Even simple value-based mathematical comparisons must be performed with great care. For example, identical scores in the mid-range on a comprehensive activity questionnaire may be due to an entirely different set of responses from different people. This is a serious problem in FCE because many of the popular behavior rating scales are ordinal.[30] Instruments such as the McGill Pain Questionnaire,[57] Dallas Pain Questionnaire[47] and Oswestry Pain Questionnaire[28] along with Waddell's abnormal illness behavior signs[16,81] are ordinal measures (see Chapter 45). Unfortunately, this limitation often appears to be unrecognized by evaluators and users of the information.

---

*Some functional status instruments that are in an ordinal scale can be transformed into an interval scale through the use of Rasch analysis.[30] This involves an analysis of the instrument's underlying probability structure of responses in order to develop standardized scores that can be interpreted as scores on an interval scale of measurement. An example is the Functional Independence Measure.[25]

## Interval

Numbers indicate the rank order of measures with equal intervals between adjacent items at any segment of the scale. However, the interval scale lacks a meaningful zero point. Value-based mathematical comparisons are permitted along the scale but not between scales. Examples from FCE are heart rate, motor speed, and coordination scores. The difference between a rate of 90 beats per minute (bpm) and 95 bpm is the same as the difference between a rate of 125 and 130 bpm. However, there is no zero reference point on this scale for people who are performing FCE tasks.

Interval data allow the user to distinguish difference from lesser to greater magnitude along one scale and to quantify the difference between scores with precision. When the same variable is measured in more than one subject, interval numbers allow for comparison. However, interval data do not allow quantified comparisons between different measurement variables.*

## Ratio

Numbers indicate the rank order of measures with equal intervals between adjacent items at any segment of the scale and a zero point that indicates absence of the variable that is being measured. Value-based mathematical comparisons are permitted along the scale and between scales. In FCE, variables such as weight and force are examples of ratio scales. Interval data, using ratio numbers, allow the user to distinguish the difference from lesser to greater magnitude along one scale and to quantify the difference between scales with precision at any point on the scale. Thus, proportional comparisons can be made. In addition, proportional changes across more than one scale can be compared. For example, a comparison can be made between pinch strength and grip strength or between grip strength and lift capacity. Both are useful and, because all of these variables are

---

*It is permissible to transform an interval measure to allow interscale comparison by adding or subtracting a constant. For example, a perfect comparison between the two ordinal temperature scales of Celsius and Fahrenheit can be made by accounting for the difference in each scale's zero point. After this adjustment, the Fahrenheit scale increases by 9/5 of the Celsius scale. The primary consideration is whether the constant reflects a meaningful difference between scales. For example, when comparing heart rates between individuals, such a transformation would be permissible to compare the performance of different people if the performance measure were likely to be affected by the underlying fitness level of all subjects and heart rate were an acceptable measure of the underlying fitness level. Only if these assumptions are met is such a transformation permissible.

in the ratio scale of measurement, they can be compared without further consideration or adjustment. Normative data indicate that a 53-year-old man who weighs 180 lbs (82 kg) can grip the Jamar Dynamometer (made by Sammons) with 114 pounds of force and perform an EPIC Lift test from floor to shoulder on an occasional basis with 63 pounds. In clinical practice, the approximate proportion of grip to lift can be a useful comparison that is permissible because each was obtained from a ratio scale.

The scale of measurement is important because the interpretation of the performance is restricted by the nature of the scale.[7,86] For example, if a scale refers to a patient's strength as "fair-plus" (an ordinal measure), a comparison of the patient to others is limited by indicating the patient has more or less strength than another patient, without any ability to quantify the magnitude of difference. Generally speaking, the higher the scale of measurement, the more useful it will be.[71] In the example of strength, a poor-fair-good rating scale can be used to compare the patient to himself or herself over time as he or she progresses in a rehabilitation program. It would be more useful to measure strength using a ratio scale because this will allow a numerical comparison of the evaluee over time in addition to comparison of the evaluee to other people and to the demands of numerous jobs. Because the magnitude of difference is so important in FCE, measures that are based on interval or ratio scales are preferred. If ordinal measures are used, results often are converted to standard scores or percentiles and reported as such.

## MODES OF MEASUREMENT

There are several modes, or method of analysis, of measurement in FCE, each pertinent to a particular type of task. Examples are "time-limited" and "task-limited" measurement, each of which is concerned with the patient's speed of performance. In the former mode, the patient is allowed a set period of time to perform a task with the degree of task completion or number of tasks completed as the performance measurement. In the latter mode, the patient is allowed to complete a set task. The time required to complete the task is the performance measurement.

A focus on measurement of strength performance with regard to lifting tasks will be presented. This is useful because these modes of measurement are similar in many ways to other measures of abilities based on strength. Additionally, lifting as a physical ability is arguably the most important physical demand characteristic of work.[3,9,15,35,59,62,66,75,83]

There are three general classes of strength testing in the evaluation of lift capacity (isometric, isokinetic, and isoinertial). Each is defined by the effect of the test on muscular contraction and is differentiated by the muscles' force of contraction and the rate of shortening (see also Chapter 17).

### Isometric

During isometric contraction, the muscle length is not changed when a load is placed. The force is measured in only one biomechanical position. Isometric activity is not as prevalent in daily tasks as muscular contractions to perform tasks that require movement. The prevalence of isometric tasks is greater for the hand than for any other biomechanical component.

### Isokinetic

Under load the muscle shortens or (if shortened due to prior concentric contraction) lengthens at a fixed rate as a consequence of external control of the velocity of movement of the biomechanical unit. Force is measured throughout the range of movement.

### Isoinertial

The muscle shortens at a variable rate during isoinertial contraction in response to a constant external resistance. As the biomechanical geometry changes to accomplish movement, changes in the muscle length occur at varying velocities. Constant resistance is inferred from the constancy of the mass that is moved because acceleration is assumed to be negligible.

Various technologies have been developed to assess these three general classes of strength tests. The technologies are identified by name in terms of the type of function that each *intends* to assess. It is important to point out that this leads to confusion because of the complexity of the biomechanical system involved in many tasks. The test of the biomechanical system may not be able to isolate sufficiently the level of the muscle's function so that the intended mode of test is actually achieved. For example, while isokinetic testing intends to evaluate the strength of the biomechanical system at a set velocity, accelerative movement occurs early in the task up to the point at which the desired velocity is achieved. Even after that point, there may be a rebound phenomenon before stabilization at the desired velocity is achieved.

Isometric strength is the easiest to test because it ostensibly involves no movement other than the elasticity in the biomechanical units. However, because there are several biomechanical links in the chain that are required if the lifting task is performed while standing, substantial elasticity is present. This can be controlled through proper instructions and the use of equipment that is sensitive to this phenomenon.

Isoinertial strength testing is difficult to achieve because lifting and lowering are performed in an environment in which gravity (an accelerative force) controls resistance. Thus, although acceleration is somewhat standardized through control of the vertical range, inertia is not well controlled from person to person because rates of acceleration vary between people. Within the same person across gradually increasing demand levels, acceleration appears to gradually vary inversely to the increasing load.

### Distinction Between Lift Strength and Lift Capacity

It is important to note that a lifting task usually involves a combination of muscle contractions, depending on the biomechanical segment that is considered. These will change during the task. A "squat lift" from floor to knuckle usually will involve the upper extremities in isometric activity if the worker's style of lift emphasizes lower extremity extension. Conversely, with a lifting style such as that used by competitive weight lifters, this same vertical range might be undertaken with the lower extremities performing isometric stabilization while the upper extremities provide an accelerative force to overcome the inertia imposed on the mass by gravity as it sits at rest. Construct validity has not been demonstrated for strength as it applies to lifting. Similarly, predictive validity of strength as it applies to lifting has been inconsistently supported.[2,3,10,11,42,50,72] However, most of the manufacturers of "iso" equipment advertise the capability of their equipment to predict ability to lift from iso measures. Indeed, most practitioners do not appear to understand (or choose to ignore) this distinction. Given an absence of construct validity or predictive validity, content validity must be used. Content validity relies on the similarity between the evaluation task and the target task. If the evaluation task samples the most significant and salient parts of the target task, it has content validity. Accordingly, lift-strength tasks should be selected that approximate the kinematic (postural) and ergonomic demands of the target task. The use of standard postures is not appropriate if the standard postures do not sample the worker's likely lifting postures.

## LEGAL FRAMEWORK OF FUNCTIONAL CAPACITY EVALUATION

Functional capacity evaluation takes place within the context of professional guidelines as well as numerous state and federal laws. Guidelines for performance testing have been developed and published by the American Psychological Association,[4] American Physical Therapy Association,[77] and the American Academy of Physical Medicine and Rehabilitation.[44] Federal guidelines on which employment decisions are based are found in the Uniform Guidelines for Employee Selection.[26] When the testing procedure involves employment of a qualified individual with a disability, the Americans with Disabilities Act of 1990[27] is pertinent. Additional impairment-specific standards have been published.[37] There is agreement among the various professional and governmental entities that are concerned with performance testing that the selection of a test must be undertaken within the hierarchical context of five standards: safety, reliability, validity, practicality, and utility.

### Safety

When used properly, the test should not be expected to lead to an injury. Most functional tests have the potential to cause harm. Well-designed tests provide exclusionary and performance guidelines and procedural rules that must be followed to minimize this likelihood. Safety is a function of the match between the performance demands and the ability to limit performance appropriately.[37] Determination of the patient's maximum safe and dependable performance level is a professional judgment made by the evaluator based on the patient's performance during the evaluation. This judgment takes into account the signs, symptoms, and behaviors that indicate that the evaluation has progressed to a point at which the safety of the evaluation cannot be maintained with a reasonable degree of certainty. Thus, the professional evaluator's training and experience in using the maximum performance indicators of the test are necessary conditions for functional testing.

### Reliability

The test equipment and test protocol should produce a result that is stable within the test trial, and within evaluators, evaluees, and the date or time of test administration. Reliability can be threatened both externally and internally. External threats are those over which the evaluator has control such as equipment reliability, protocol reliability, and consistency of protocol application. Internal threats are those that reside within the evaluee and include motivation, fear, and pain-avoidance behavior. A functional-capacity evaluation requires that the evaluee put forth maximum voluntary effort in a meaningful task.[69,80] The defined task may require full strength, full velocity, endurance, a target number of repetitions, a maximum rate of responding, or some other "full effort" performance. Characteristics that distinguish performance testing of impaired evaluees from those who are not impaired include activity-related pain, fear of reinjury, test anxiety, and a higher risk of injury. While these factors are difficult to measure with precision, most evaluators agree that they are of significant importance. The functional capacity evaluation must be structured so that it is sensitive to these factors and minimizes their effects.

Intratest reliability (a measure of the patient's consistency of responding) can be assessed by various mathematical means[39,51] using the coefficient of variation statistic as a measure of the consistency of the patient's performance on a repeated-trials task. The coefficient of variation is the standard deviation of a set of at least three scores, divided by the average of the scores, expressed as a percentage. Although the specificity of the coefficient of variation statistic appears to be much higher than its sensitivity for the detection of sub-maximal effort,[17] it is widely used and is built into many FCE test instruments. A more sophisticated indicator of reliability is based on intertest comparisons. In this approach, two or more tests that are biomechanically related are administered, using a protocol that is sensitive to intra-test consistency. (It should be noted that the tests must use a ratio scale of measurement.) This approach is especially powerful if the intratest results have demonstrated high consistency.[51] A case example will describe this approach:

**Case Description**—Mr. Smith is a 39-year-old, 170-pound male auto mechanic with a presenting impairment of low-back soft-tissue injury with activity-related pain. He received palliative physical therapy three times per week for two months before returning to work with his employer on a light-duty basis. He continued in palliative physical therapy for four weeks without making significant progress. Believing he had reached permanent and stationary status, his physician referred him for a Disability Rating FCE. The Cal-FCP was administered by a physical therapist.

**Pertinent Results**—Mr. Smith achieved 30 pounds maximum acceptable weight on EPIC Lift Capacity test #3, which indicates a 58% loss of lift capacity for a male of his age and weight. This also placed him in the range of light physical-demand characteristics. His score of 50 (out of 200) on the Spinal Function Sort (SFS) placed him in the tenth percentile compared with unemployed disabled males in terms of subjective functional capacity, well below the sedentary physical demand characteristics level. His lateral pinch on the B&L Pinch Gauge and grip on the Jamar Dynamometer at position #2 are presented below:

| Test | Right (Dom) | CV% | Left (NDom) | CV% |
|------|-------------|-----|-------------|-----|
| Pinch | 26 lbs | 4% | 25 lbs | 3% |
| Grip | 31 lbs | 5% | 34 lbs | 4% |

**Interpretation and Analysis**—The test results are inconsistent in two ways. The lift capacity results and self-perception score are inconsistent. EPIC Lift test performance places Mr. Smith in the light physical demand characteristics range. A corresponding score of 125 to 135 should have been obtained on the SFS. Thus, his reported limitations are substantially greater than expected given his actual performance test results. The pinch strength and grip strength results also are inconsistent. Pinch strength scores are average. Based on the presumption that it is not possible to "fake good," it is reasonable to expect that a male with average pinch strength would generate grip strength of 120 pounds with the right hand and 115 pounds with the left, based on normative data. Actual grip is one-third of expected. Because this was achieved with an acceptable coefficient of variation, it appears that Mr. Smith may be performing the grip test at less than full effort on a volitional basis.

**Case Result**—Mr. Smith's treating physician constructively confronted him with the inconsistencies reported above and referred him to an activity-oriented work-conditioning program. Initially, he exhibited inconsistencies in FCE testing at this facility although grip strength was found to average 95 pounds on the right and 90 pounds on the left. The therapist assigned tasks from the SFS that she believed Mr. Smith would be able to perform. Under her supervision, Mr. Smith performed these tasks as part of a work-conditioning program. SFS scores improved immediately. Lifting performance improved gradually. After two weeks of treatment, he had improved to a maximum acceptable weight of 45 pounds, which represents a 39% loss-of-lift capacity. After two additional weeks, he attained his usual and customary job target of 60 pounds and returned to full duty. He continued in a supervised exercise program after work for one month and attained a maximum acceptable weight of 70 pounds for full range lifting. This represents a 4% loss of preinjury lift capacity. Thus, he was found to have no permanent residual impairment.

In general, reliability in functional testing has been sparsely studied.[68] With a few exceptions, test protocols in which reliability has been scientifically determined have not been agreed upon. In many other instances, tradition has sufficed for scientific rigor. In one example, Caldwell et al[14] provided guidelines for isometric testing that have been widely referenced and are used as the basis for many strength test protocols. These guidelines were developed for isometric testing of healthy subjects. They were originally presented and have been adopted without any indication that the effect of factors such as the types of instruction were scientifically studied. For example, these guidelines recommend that the evaluator should avoid exhortation of the evaluee during testing. The avoidance of exhortation is widely practiced with these guidelines cited as the original reference. However, Matheson et al[50] found that reliability on both an intra-test basis and a test-retest (inter-rater) basis was not able to be achieved dependably without an exhortative instruction set in isokinetic testing. Other problems with reliability abound. Also with regard to isokinetic testing, Newton and her colleagues[67] report that test reliability is dependent on factors that currently are not common in clinical practice, such as the opportunity to provide a practice session prior to the test session conducted on a subsequent day.

## Validity

The interpretation of the test score should be able to predict or reflect the evaluee's performance in a target task. Whereas reliability reflects the dependability of the measurement, validity reflects the adequacy of the measurement[20] to describe or predict performance. A valid measurement of functional capacity to be used with impaired patients must:

1. Allow the clinician to gauge treatment effect by comparing an initial baseline level of performance with performance at the conclusion of the treatment.
2. Make recommendations for return-to-work by comparing the patient's functional capacity to the job demands.
3. Provide an estimate of impairment for rating purposes by comparing the patient's performance to expected values.

The first two criteria are straightforward. The third is problematic because a reference to expected values is not readily available. In some circumstances, reasonable assumptions can be made about the evaluee's preimpairment functional capacity. For example, if the evaluee is a member of an occupational group for which minimum lift-capacity standards are known, it can be assumed that the evaluee has at least the minimum that is required by the standard. This is a rational approach and frequently is used in medicolegal cases. Another standard that is more easily implemented utilizes a normative database. Unfortunately, normative data for lift capacity tests

that have been designed for use with impaired evaluees are rare.

Any predictive measurement is a combination of the true value plus some amount of measurement error plus some amount of variability due to intervening variables. The greater the degree that the measurement error can be minimized and the intervening variables can be accounted for, the more accurate the prediction. The multiaxial model[79] requires an approach to validity in FCE that is based on testing of a physical performance component[54] with more than one instrument. The overlap and cross-validation between or among instruments not only addresses issues such as the reliability of the evaluee's effort but also allows a more comprehensive picture of the multiple variables that support functional performance. Thus, the validity of the FCE is improved.

Although there is a long history of validity testing in fields such as industrial psychology,[19,32] studies of the validity of functional tests to predict injury or impairment are rare and often produce conflicting interpretations. In clinical use, Newton et al[67] found that discrimination between normals and patients with low-back pain was improved only slightly by functional testing measured isokinetically when compared with clinical evaluation of the physical impairment. However, testing did help to explain the variance concerning work loss after the effects of the clinical evaluation were considered. In general, testing had a lower specificity but a higher sensitivity than clinical observations. Validity concerns are also supported by work by Matheson.[50] With regard to the use of isokinetic back strength to predict lift capacity, validity was not found unless there were special instructions significantly different from those commonly used in the clinical setting. Even with these special instructions, validity was optimal only at isokinetic velocities that were slower than those normally used for back-strength testing of impaired patients.

## Practicality

The cost of the test should be reasonable. Cost is a function of the capital expenditure for the equipment amortized over the life of the equipment plus wage costs and overhead. Although "low tech" approaches to FCE are less expensive initially, a more expensive "high tech" system may be able to provide similar results in less time or with lower-wage staff. Figure 18-7 compares three systems in terms of annual costs based on five levels of use. System A is a "low tech" approach that requires capital outlay of $5,000 and $180 in wage costs per evaluation. System B is a "mid tech" approach that requires capital outlay of $30,000 and $144 in wage costs per evaluation. The savings comes from greater system efficiency that leads to 20% reduction in the evaluator's time needed for evaluation and report preparation. System C is a "high tech" approach that requires capital outlay of $100,000 and $90 in wage costs per evaluation. The savings comes from greater efficiency that leads to a further reduction in the evaluator's time and the use of lower-wage staff due to the highly structured nature of the system. Wage costs were based on a five-hour evaluation with one hour of report preparation. Overhead was calculated at 30% of the wage cost. The equipment was amortized over five years on a straight-line basis.

As Figure 18-7 demonstrates, the effect on cost of the test depends on the cost of the equipment, wages, overhead, and frequency of use. Aside from one study,[52] cost-benefit ratios have been not reported for functional-capacity evaluations. In this study, the cost-benefit ratio was 2.15 for a functional-capacity evaluation performed after active medical treatment had been concluded, prior to entry into vocational rehabilitation. That is, for every $1.00 spent on functional capacity evaluation, $2.15 was saved on rehabilitation services. These savings occurred as patients were identified who could return to their normal jobs without additional rehabilitation. This cost-benefit ratio did not include savings from social welfare costs and lost tax revenues.

## Utility

The usefulness of the procedure is the degree to which it meets the needs of the patient, referrer, and payor. The first four factors in the hierarchy must be adequately addressed in order for utility to be achieved. Of course, without utility, the test is of no value and will not be supported by the market in the long run. Figure 18-8 graphically depicts the relationships among these factors. Safety is the primary concern.

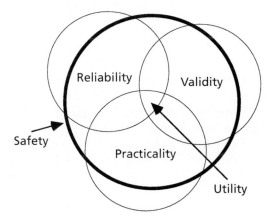

**FIGURE 18-8** Relationship of test factors necessary to achieve utility.

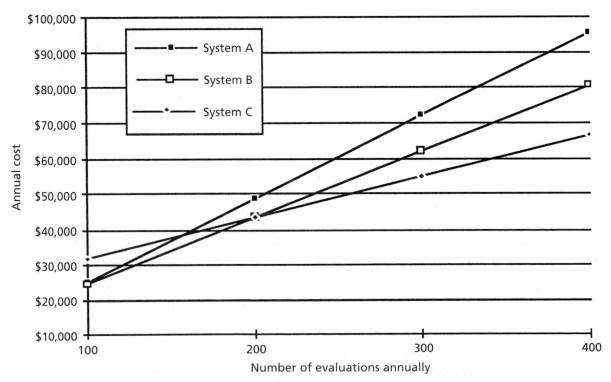

**FIGURE 18-7** Relative cost of three different FCE systems, each requiring different capital outlay and operating costs, depending on the number of evaluations conducted per year.

These factors relate to each other in a dynamic fashion and a decision to emphasize or minimize any one of the factors usually will affect the other factors. This trade-off is important for the evaluator to appreciate. Reliability, validity, and practicality are separate issues that may overlap but must be considered in that order. Where all three overlap within the context for safety, the basic requirements for utility are met. Appropriate FCE practice occurs at the interface of these factors.

## BASIC REQUIREMENTS FOR TEST SELECTION

Beyond the legal framework for functional capacity evaluation, the evaluator must use tests that are *optimal* given the evaluee and the evaluation circumstance. There is no single-most-appropriate test for any one evaluee or for any one evaluation circumstance. Tests must be selected to meet the unique needs of the evaluee-role interface that is described above. In addition to these general guidelines, adherence to the following specific guidelines will ensure an optimal balance of safety, reliability, and validity:

1. Use only standardized test protocols that have all of these characteristics:
    (a) Equipment has been demonstrated to be reliable with adequate maintenance support.
    (b) Test protocol has been demonstrated to be reliable over time on both an intrarater basis and inter-rater basis.
    (c) One or more means of intra-test confirmation of consistency is available.
    (d) One or more means of inter-test confirmation of consistency is available.
    (e) Multiple biomechanical or neuromusculoskeletal variations are able to be selected by the evaluator based on the expected use of the test result.
    (f) Normative data, job demand data, or MTM comparisons are available.
2. Become trained in the use of the test protocols and formally demonstrate skill in the consistent application of these protocols.
3. Select protocols from those identified in No. 1 above that meet the validity needs and practicality restrictions of the assessment process. Consider each test protocol on a patient basis in response to demands of the target role. These demands should be derived from job analysis data. If these are not available, the *Dictionary of Occupational Titles*[22] can be used, although these data are quite general.
4. After collecting the necessary pre-test screening information about the evaluee to rule out con-

traindications for testing, administer the test in the standard manner.
5. Evaluate the *quality* of the data on this basis:
    (a) Screening for intratest variability. If more variability exists than is reported to be normal for the protocol, retest.
    (b) Screening for inter-test variability. If more variability exists than is reported to be normal for the protocol, retest.
6. Interpret the data and provide analysis.

## GENERIC FUNCTIONAL CAPACITY EVALUATION PROCESS

The essential and common components of all functional capacity evaluations are:
1. *Obtain a History*—The patient's medical, social, and vocational status should be recorded in a structured interview. This must be taken prior to the pre-evaluation screening examination. The history should determine the evaluee's perception of his or her own functional limitations and the reason for the FCE. During the history process, an attempt is made to establish rapport and to identify the evaluee's goals. The history should also screen for possible contraindications for testing other than those related to the presenting impairment. This can be facilitated by the use of a health questionnaire. For example, issues such as cardiac, pulmonary, or metabolic disorders should be reviewed. Often, it is useful to ask the evaluee, "Are there any medications you are supposed to be taking that you are not?" to screen for noncompliance.
2. *Perform a Pre-evaluation Screening Examination*—The second component of the FCE is an appropriate screening examination based on the diagnosis of the evaluee. The purposes of the screening examination are:
    (a) To confirm that the evaluee is medically stable.
    (b) To confirm that the evaluee does not have any contraindications for testing.
    (c) To quantify physical impairment for a potential impairment rating, for any post-testing comparisons, or for comparison to measured functional limitations.
The screening examination quantifies impairment and determines which tests are necessary.
3. *Perform Functional Testing*—The third component of the FCE is functional testing. The results of the functional test battery should describe the current functional ability of the injured worker, as well as their limitations, so that reinjury can be prevented.

4. *Interpret Results*—The fourth component of the FCE is one aspect of the process that distinguishes the professional evaluator from the evaluation technician. Interpretation of test results lies within the domain of the professional's expertise and must be undertaken by the professional. Test results that are provided without the interpretation of the evaluator often are meaningless and can be misleading.

5. *Prepare a Report*—Once the findings of the history, prescreening examination, and functional testing have been interpreted, a report should be written. The following areas should be addressed:

    (*a*) Pertinent medical history and diagnosis.

    (*b*) Pertinent social and vocational history.

    (*c*) Pre-screening examination results.

    (*d*) Functional test results:

    (*i.*)    Demonstrated motivation.

    (*ii.*)   Evaluee's perception of function.

    (*iii.*)  Significant functional abilities.

    (*iv.*)   Significant functional deficits.

    (*e*) If there is a job or occupation target, describe how the patient's abilities compare to the demands of the job or occupation.

    (*f*) Recommendations for further testing and other appropriate intervention.

## TECHNOLOGICAL LIMITATIONS

The technological underpinnings of any endeavor dictate its limitations. However, given adequate resources and vigilance, many limitations can be remediated and should be considered only temporary. There are five important technological problems in functional capacity evaluation.

The first technological problem involves the paucity of formal training in evaluation provided to physical therapists and occupational therapists. A survey was conducted in 1993 by Matheson of all of the occupational therapy and physical therapy training programs at colleges and universities in the United States. Only an average of 2 to 3 contact hours in functional capacity evaluation was found in each master's program. Sadly, not all programs offered training. In contrast, entry-level programs for psychologists at the master's level typically require 30 to 50 contact hours for a general overview of psychological testing with substantial additional course work devoted to specific tests. Although there are a few notable exceptions in the medical schools, skimpy offerings of testing courses in the curricula have led to a generally low level of sophistication. This is somewhat overcome by post-graduate work-

shops and seminars but these tend to focus on the clinician's skill development with a particular test rather than on such basic issues as the appropriate measurement scale to use or methods of validation, each of which is an important underpinning of test selection and administration.

The second technological problem has to do with the availability of standardized test equipment. If impairment evaluation is to be standardized and widely available, the equipment must be standardized and widely available. Unfortunately, this is not the case. For example, in the evaluation of grip strength, standardization has been attempted by various bureaucratic entities[12,45] only to be undone by changes in equipment design. The JAMAR Hand Dynamometer is one example of a device that is in widespread use and has undergone modifications with no formal validation of the effect of these changes.[29,33,55] Two JAMAR Hand Dynamometers are pictured in Figure 18-9. The reader will note that the handle configurations are quite different. Trials in the author's laboratory demonstrated differences on the order of 11% to 18% between these two "identical" instruments.

Most clinicians are not aware of these changes. In the most recent edition, 1993, of the *Guides to the Evaluation of Permanent Impairment*,[5] there is no mention of the lack of interchangeability nor is there comment about the need for frequent calibration.

A third technological problem is reactivity in testing. Reactivity reflects changes in performance during one or more administrations of a test that are due to the experience of the administration and reflect neither measurement error nor actual change in the underlying ability. Whether improvements in performance are related to actual physiologic changes such

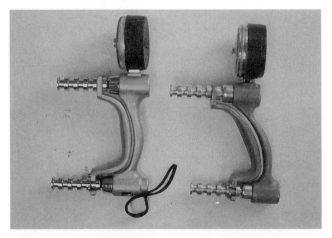

**FIGURE 18-9**    Comparison of two "identical" JAMAR hand dynamometers.

as improvement in the contractile capability of muscle fibers, to the excitation of the fibers, to improved skill or motivation or decreased fear,[82] or to some other factor,[78] performance of chronically-impaired patients often is found to improve after functional testing, without any additional intervention. The original definition of work capacity evaluation as a "systematic process of measuring and developing an individual's capacity to dependably sustain performance in response to broadly defined work demands"[51] purposely paired *measurement* with *development*. The therapeutic effect of functional testing has been reported by Stokes et al,[76] who attributed a significant increase in strength due to learning effect. Kohles et al[46] reported significant improvement after evaluation. Matheson et al[49] found that a measure of functional self-perception improved significantly after testing for chronic back-injury patients if the evaluation took place within one year of injury. Newton et al[67] report that "speed and amount of improvement in the iso measures is greater than could be explained by any known training effect on muscle physiology." These authors point to a training effect that they report is extraneous to the testing situation or to "some learning effect about their low back pain" that may have therapeutic value. The implications for FCE are important. On the positive side, FCE may be viewed under certain circumstances as having a therapeutic effect as a positive experience that provides the impaired patient with information that assists him or her to have a more rational self-perception. On the negative side, reactivity presents yet another challenge to the reliability of FCE test results and suggests the need for more care in the development of test protocols.

A fourth technological problem is the absence of studies[19] to allow for comparison among equipment produced by various manufacturers that purport to test function in similar ways. Without such studies, test results are not comparable except when conducted on the same piece of equipment. This problem is related to the final technological problem, which is the most pressing, dealing with an absence of scientifically derived and widely-recognized testing protocols. The absence of widely-accepted protocols has hampered the development of FCE. For example, the American Physical Therapy Association first published its *Standards for Tests and Measurements in Physical Therapy Practice* in 1991.[77] However, physical therapists are not required to adhere to these standards and may treat them only as guidelines. It is clear that there is a need for all of the major professional organizations involved in FCE to develop similar standards and require adherence.

## SUMMARY

FCE is an important component of the disability evaluation process. It serves to translate the consequences of the impairment into functional limitations that may have role consequences. To the extent that role consequences exist, the evaluee will experience disability. When the role consequences have to do with work tasks, occupational disability may result. Because a serious impairment may threaten a working adult's ability to provide for both the worker and his or her family, a fair and objective FCE is of paramount importance.

## References

1. Abdel-Moty E, et al: Functional capacity and residual functional capacity and their utility in measuring work capacity. *Cl J Pain* 9(3):168-173, 1993.
2. Aghazadeh F, Jiang BC: Some considerations in the use of isometric, isoinertial and isokinetic strength models for predicting lifting capability. *Int J Industr Ergo* 2:101-110, 1988.
3. Alpert J, et al: The reliability and validity of two new tests of maximum lifting capacity. *J Occup Rehabil* 1(1):13-29, 1991.
4. American Educational Research Association, American Psychological Association, National Council on Measurement in Education: *Standards for educational and psychological testing*, Washington, DC, 1986, American Psychological Association.
5. American Medical Association: *Guides to the evaluation of permanent impairment*, ed 4, Chicago, 1993, American Medical Association.
6. American Occupational Therapy Association: *Uniform terminology for occupational therapy*, ed 3, Rockville, MD, 1994, American Occupational Therapy Association.
7. Angoff WH: *Scales, norms, and equivalent scores*, Princeton, NJ, 1984, Educational Testing Service.
8. Atha J: Physical fitness measurements. In Larson LA, editor: *Fitness, health, and work capacity: international standards for assessment*, New York, 1974, Macmillan, pp 449-533.
9. Ayoub MA: Control of manual lifting hazards: I—Training in safe handling. *J Occup Med* 24(8):573-577, 1982.
10. Ayoub MM, et al: Predicting lifting capacity. *Am Ind Hyg Assoc J* 40:1075-1084, 1979.
11. Ayoub MM, et al: Review, evaluation, and comparison of models for predicting lifting capacity. *Human Factors* 22(3):257-269, 1980.
12. Bechtol CO: Grip test: the use of a dynamometer with adjustable handle spacings. *J Bone Joint Surg* 36A:820-824, 1954.

13. Brown C, et al: *Vocational evaluation systems and software: a consumer's guide,* Menomonie, WI, 1994, Materials Development Center, Stout Vocational Rehabilitation Institute, School of Education and Human Services, University of Wisconsin-Stout.

14. Caldwell LS, et al: A proposed standard procedure for static muscle strength testing. *Am Ind Hyg Assoc J* 35:201-206, April 1974.

15. Chaffin DB, Andersson GBJ: *Occupational biomechanics,* New York, 1984, John Wiley & Sons.

16. Chan CW, et al: The pain drawing and Waddell's nonorganic physical signs in chronic low-back pain. *Spine* 18(13):1717-1722, 1993.

17. Chengalur SN, et al: Assessing sincerity of effort in maximal grip strength tests. *Am J Phys Med Rehab* 69(3):148-153, 1990.

18. Clark W, Haldeman S: The development of guideline factors for the evaluation of disability in neck and back injuries. *Spine* 18(13):1736-1745, 1993.

19. Cronbach L, et al: *Dependability of behavioral measurements: theory of generalizability for scores and profiles,* New York, 1972, John Wiley & Sons.

20. De Vellis R: *Scale development: theory and applications,* Newbury Park, 1991, Sage Publications.

21. Deyo RA, Centor RM: Assessing the responsiveness of functional scales to clinical change: an analogy to diagnostic test performance. *J Chron Dis* 39(11):891-906, 1986.

22. Department of Labor: *Dictionary of occupational titles,* ed 4, revised, vol 1 and vol 2, Washington, DC, 1991.

23. Department of Labor: *The revised handbook for analyzing jobs,* Indianapolis, 1991, JIST: the job search people.

24. Division of Industrial Accidents: *Schedule for rating permanent disabilities,* Sacramento, 1978, Department of Industrial Relations.

25. Dodds TA, et al: A validation of the functional independence measure and its performance among rehabilitation inpatients. *Arch Phys Med Rehabil* 74:531-536, May 1993.

26. Equal Employment Opportunity Commission: Uniform Guidelines on Employee Selection Procedures. *Federal Register* 43(166):38290, 25 Aug. 1978.

27. Equal Employment Opportunity Commission: ADA rules and regulations, *Federal Register* 56(144):35726-35756, 26 July 1991.

28. Fairbank JCT, et al: The Oswestry Low Back Pain Disability Questionnaire. *Physiotherapy* 66(8):271-273, 1980.

29. Fess EE: The need for reliability and validity in hand assessment instruments. *J Hand Surg* 11A(5):621-623, 1986.

30. Fisher WP Jr: Objectivity in measurement: a philosophical history of Rasch's separability theorem. In Wilson M, editor: *Objective measurement: theory into practice,* Norwood, NJ, 1992, Ablex:29-55.

31. Fleishman EA, Reilly ME: *Handbook of human abilities,* Palo Alto, CA, 1992, Consulting Psychologists Press.

32. Fleishman EA: On the relation between abilities, learning, and human performance. *Am Psych* 1017-1032, Nov. 1972.

33. Flood-Joy M, Mathiowetz V: Grip strength measurement: a comparison of three Jamar dynamometers. *Occup Ther J Res* 7:235-243, 1987.

34. Fraser TM: *Fitness for work,* Washington, DC, 1992, Taylor & Francis.

35. Garg, A, Ayoub MM: What criteria exist for determining how much load can be lifted safely? *Human Factors* 22(4):475-486, 1980.

36. Granger CV, Wright BD: *Looking ahead to the use of the functional status questionnaire in ambulatory psychiatric and primary care: the functional assessment screening questionnaire.* In Granger CV, Gresham GE, editors: *Physical medicine and rehabilitation clinics of North America: new developments in functional assessment,* Philadelphia, 1993, W. B. Saunders.

37. Hart DL, Isernhagen SJ, Matheson LN: Guidelines for functional capacity evaluation of people with medical conditions. *J Occup Sports Phys Ther* 18(6), 1993.

38. Hart DL: *Test and measurements in returning injured workers to work.* In: Isernhagen SJ, editor: *Work injury management: the comprehensive spectrum,* Rockville, MD, 1994, Aspen Publishers.

39. Hazard RG, et al: Isokinetic trunk and lifting strength measurements: variability as an indicator of effort. *Spine* 13(1):54-57, 1988.

40. Isernhagen SJ: Functional capacity evaluation. In Isernhagen SJ, editor: *Work injury management: management and prevention,* Rockville, MD, 1988, Aspen Publishers.

41. Isernhagen SJ: Functional capacity evaluation and work hardening perspectives. In Mayer TG, Mooney JV, Gatchel R, editors: *Contemporary conservative care for painful spinal disorders,* Philadelphia, 1991, Lea & Febiger, pp 328-345.

42. Jacobs I, Bell DG, Pope J: Comparison of isokinetic and isoinertial lifting tests as predictors of maximal lifting capacity. *Eur J Appl Physiol* 57:146-153, 1988.

43. Jette AM: Physical disablement concepts for physical therapy research and practice. *Phys Ther* 74(5):380-386.

44. Johnston MV, Keith RD, Hinderer SR: Measurement standards for multidisciplinary medical rehabilitation. *Arch PM&R* 73:S3-S23, 1992.

45. Kirkpatrick JE: Evaluation of grip loss. *Calif Med* 85(5):314-320, Nov. 1956.

46. Kohles S, et al: Improved physical performance outcomes after functional restoration treatment in patients with chronic low back pain: early versus recent training results. *Spine* 15:1321-1324, 1990.

47. Lawlis GF, et al: The development of the Dallas pain questionnaire: an assessment of the impact of spinal pain on behavior. *Spine* 14(5):511-515, 1989.

48. Luck JV Jr, Florence DW: A brief history and comparative analysis of disability systems and impairment rating guides. *Orthop Clin North Am* 19(4):839-844, 1988.

49. Matheson L, Matheson M, Grant J: Development of a measure of perceived functional ability. *J Occup Rehab* 3(1):15-30, 1993.

50. Matheson L, et al: Effect of instructions on isokinetic trunk strength testing variability, reliability, absolute value, and predictive validity. *Spine* 17(8):914-921, 1992.

51. Matheson LN: *Work capacity evaluation for occupational therapists*, Rehabilitation Institute of Southern California, 1982.

52. Matheson LN: Evaluation of lifting and lowering capacity. *Vocation Eval Work Adjust Bull* 19(3):107-111, Fall 1986.

53. Matheson LN: Functional goal setting, foundation of the therapeutic relationship. *Am Pain Soc J* 3(2):111-114, 1994.

54. Mathiowetz V: Role of the physical performance component evaluations in occupational therapy assessment. *Am J Occup Therapy* 47(3):225-230, 1993.

55. Mathiowetz V, et al: Reliability and validity of grip and pinch strength evaluations. *J Hand Surg* 9A(2):222-226, March 1984.

56. Mayer TG et al: A prospective two-year study of functional restoration in industrial low back injury. *JAMA* 258(13):1763-1767, 2 Oct. 1987.

57. Melzack R: The McGill Pain Questionnaire: major properties and scoring methods. *Pain* 1:277-299, 1975.

58. Messick S: The standard problem: meaning and values in measurement and evaluation. *Am Psychol* 30:955-966, 1975.

59. Mital A: Psychophysical capacity of industrial workers for lifting symmetrical and asymmetrical loads symmetrically and asymmetrically for 8-hour work shifts. *Ergonomics* 35(7/8):745-754, 1992.

60. Mitchell J: Measurement scales and statistics: a clash of paradigms. *Psychol Bull* 100(3):398-407, 1986.

61. Mooney V, Matheson L: *Soft tissue injury quantification, feasibility study examiner's manual*, Santa Ana, CA, 1994, Employment and Rehabilitation Institute of California.

62. Mundt DJ, et al: An epidemiologic study of nonoccupational lifting as a risk factor for herniated lumbar intervertebral disc. *Spine* 18(5):595-602, 1993.

63. Nagi SZ: Disability concepts and prevalence. Presented to Mary Switzer Memorial Seminar, Cleveland, 1975, National Rehabilitation Association.

64. Nagi SZ: Disability concepts revisited: implications for prevention. In Pope AM, Tarlov AR, editors: *Disability in America*, Washington, DC, 1991, National Academy Press, pp 309-327.

65. National Advisory Board on Medical Rehabilitation Research: *Report and plan for medical rehabilitation research*, Bethesda, MD, 1992, National Institutes of Health.

66. National Institute for Occupational Safety and Health: *Work practices guide for manual lifting* [Technological Report 81-122], Cincinnati, 1981, Division of Biomedical and Behavioral Science, NIOSH.

67. Newton M, et al: Trunk strength testing with iso-machines: Part 2—Experimental evaluation of the Cybex II back testing system in normal subjects and patients with chronic low back pain. *Spine* 18(7):812-824, 1993.

68. Newton M, Waddell G: Trunk strength testing with iso-machines: Part 1—Review of a decade of scientific evidence. *Spine* 18(7):801-811, 1993.

69. Ogden-Niemeyer L, Jacobs K: *Work hardening: state of the art*, Thorofare, NJ, 1989, Slack.

70. Ottenbacher KJ, Tomchek SD: Measurement in rehabilitation research: consistency versus consensus. In Granger CV, Gresham GE, editors: *Physical medicine and rehabilitation clinics of North America: new developments in functional assessment*, Philadelphia, 1993, WB Saunders.

71. Portney LG, Watkins MP, editors: *Foundations of clinical research: applications to practice*, Norwalk, CT, 1993, Appleton & Lange.

72. Pytel JL, Kamon E: Dynamic strength test as a predictor for maximal and acceptable lifting. *Ergonomics* 24(9):663-672, 1981.

73. Rothstein JM, editor: *Measurement in physical therapy*, New York, 1985, Churchill Livingstone.

74. Sachs BL, et al: Spinal rehabilitation by work tolerance based on objective physical capacity assessment of dysfunction: a prospective study with control subjects and twelve-month review. *Spine* 15(12):1325-1332, 1990.

75. Snook SH, Irvine CH: Maximum acceptable weight of lift. *Am Ind Hyg Assoc J* 28:322-329, 1967.

76. Stokes IAF, et al: EMG to torque relationships in rectus abdominus muscle: results with repeated testing. *Spine* 14:857-861, 1989.

77. Task Force on Standards for Measurement in Physical Therapy: Standards for tests and measurements in physical therapy practice. *Phys Ther* 71:589-622, 1991.

78. Troup JDG, et al: The perception of back pain and the role of psychophysical tests of lifting capacity. *Spine* 12:645-657, 1987.

79. Turk DC, Rudy TE, Stieg RL: The disability determination dilemma: toward a multiaxial solution. *Pain* 34:217-229, 1988.

80. Velozo CA: Work evaluations: critique of the state of the art of functional assessment of work. *Am J Occup Therapy* 47(3):203-209, 1993.

81. Waddell G, et al: Symptoms and signs: physical disease or illness behavior? *Br Med J* 289:739-741, 1984.

82. Waddell G, et al: A fear-avoidance beliefs questionnaire (FABQ) and the role of fear-avoidance beliefs in chronic low back pain and disability. *Pain* 52:157-168, 1993.

83. Waters TR, et al: Revised NIOSH equation for the design and evaluation of manual lifting tasks. *Ergonomics* 36(7):749-776, 1993.

84. Welford AT: *Skilled performance: perceptual and motor skills,* Glenville, IL, 1976, Scott, Foresman & Company.

85. World Health Organisation: *International classification of impairments, disabilities and handicaps,* Geneva, 1980, WHO.

86. Wright BD, Linacre JM: Observations are always ordinal; measurements, however, must be interval. *Arch Phys Med Rehabil* 40:857-860, 1989.

87. Wright BD, Linacre JM, Heineman AW: Measuring functional status in rehabilitation. In Granger CV, Gresham GE, editors: *Physical medicine and rehabilitation clinics of North America: new developments in functional assessment,* Philadelphia, 1993, WB Saunders.

# CHAPTER 19

# CUMULATIVE TRAUMA

*Thomas J. Armstrong*

This chapter is concerned with cumulative trauma disorders of the upper limb. These disorders are defined as those disorders that are caused, precipitated, or aggravated by repeated exertions or movements of the body. This definition reflects the philosophy of most workers' compensation laws in the United States (see Chapter 6) and most Western countries. Whether work is a primary cause or an aggravating cause of these disorders is not always clear; however, the way the laws are written, the employer will generally be held responsible unless there is clear and convincing evidence to the contrary. From a disability or an occupational health perspective the question is not "what causes," but "what might cause" cumulative trauma disorders.

## CHARACTERISTICS

The term *cumulative trauma disorder* is a general name used for disorders with similar characteristics.[5] The most commonly-affected tissues of the body include muscles, tendons, and nerves. Frequent diagnoses are myalgia, tendinitis, and carpal tunnel syndrome. A detailed description of the signs and symptoms of these disorders is beyond the scope of this chapter; however, they are often poorly localized, nonspecific, and episodic. Symptoms tend to develop over periods of weeks, months, or even years and recovery similarly requires long periods. These traits often make it difficult to determine the exact time of onset or specific causes of the disorders. Cumulative trauma disorders may go unreported. Workers may not associate their symptoms with specific job-related activities. They may be afraid to report them to management. They can be very resourceful in finding ways of coping so that cases go unreported.

The causes of upper-limb cumulative-trauma disorders are not fully understood, but they are believed to involve multiple factors. The World Health Organization (WHO) has recognized upper limb disorders as being both "personal" and "work related." Personal factors refer to characteristics of the individual (e.g., gender, age, body size and composition, acute and chronic diseases). Work factors refer to characteristics of the job (e.g., work rates, duration, forces, locations, environments). Work-related factors appear to involve common mechanical and physiological mechanisms.[5,101]

Upper-limb cumulative-trauma disorders are a major cause of worker impairment and disability. Some people may refer to cumulative-trauma disorders as the epidemic of the 1990s; however, Ramazzini described these disorders in 1713:[89]

"Various and manifold is the harvest of diseases reaped by certain workers from the crafts and trades that they pursue. All the profit that they get is fatal injury to their health, mostly from two causes. The first and most potent is the harmful character of the materials they handle. . . . The second, I ascribe to certain violent and irregular motions and unnatural postures of the body, by reason of which, the natural structure of the vital machine is so impaired that serious diseases gradually develop therefrom."

Ramazzini went on to describe and trace the causes of these problems among various kinds of workers of his time, such as scribes, bakers, and weavers:[89]

"The maladies that afflict the clerks aforesaid arise from three causes: First, constant sitting, secondly the incessant movement of the hand and always the same direction, thirdly the strain on the mind from the effort not to disfigure the books by errors or cause loss to their employers when they add, subtract, or do other sums in arithmetic."

The modern-day scribe would most likely use a computer, but still would be exposed to "constant sitting," "incessant movement of the hand," and "strain on the mind." Likewise, most bakers no longer hand-mix bread, but they are exposed to similar physical stresses in the handling of ingredients and packaging of products. Also, workers in the upholstery, plastic, and rubber industries are exposed to similar stresses. In addition to "unnatural postures," these stresses include forceful exertions, repeated or sustained exertions, and mechanical contact stresses.

Ramazzini characterized most musculoskeletal disorders as swelling and fatigue, which was disabling in some cases:[89]

> "An acquaintance of mine, a notary by profession, still living, used to spend his whole life continually engaged in writing, and he made a good deal of money by it; first he began to complain of intense fatigue in the whole arm but no remedy could relieve this, and finally the whole right arm become completely paralyzed. In order to offset this infirmity he began to train himself to write with the left hand, but it was not very long before it too was attacked by the same malady."

There may be a tendency to question the validity of worker complaints of pain or other subjective symptoms. There may be suspicion that the workers are motivated by secondary gain. One wonders what secondary gain could have motivated the eighteenth-century workers described by Ramazzini.

Fatigue is an accepted side effect of work in most situations and is not considered compensable; however, chronic muscle, tendon, and nerve disorders should not be accepted and may be compensable. Nearly all human activities involve some pain. The question is how much is too much and when are work or medical interventions warranted. It can be shown that the incidence and severity of pain increases with certain physical activities, but there is not yet a standard for how much pain is excessive.[25,27,91] Only the individual experiencing the pain can say how much is too much for himself or herself. Identification and control of musculoskeletal disorders can be very frustrating if there is no trust between workers, employers, and health care providers. Cailliet[21] describes chronic pain as the "most serious disabling condition of humans" and suggests that pain should be considered a disease, not merely a symptom. He also suggests that trauma and inflammation of soft tissue figure heavily into the cause of musculoskeletal pain:[21]

> "All musculoskeletal pain may be considered a sequela of soft tissue injury, irritation, or inflammation. Trauma in the broadest concept of the term is the greatest cause of soft tissue pain and functional impairment."

Pain may be accompanied by objective physiological signs that can be evaluated using objective tests, including range-of-motion tests, provocative tests, and nerve conduction testing (see also Chapters 44 and 45). Standardized protocols have helped to improve the objectivity of diagnostic criteria for specific muscle, tendon, and nerve disorders.[32,51,56,99] These tests are often used for epidemiological studies.

There have been some attempts to evaluate these tests quantitatively by comparing them with so-called "objective" tests.[35,52] Katz[52] compared the diagnostic results based on the criteria used by the National Institute for Occupational Safety and Health (NIOSH) for carpal tunnel syndrome with those based on nerve conduction studies. Nerve conduction studies are generally regarded as the "gold standard" for diagnosing carpal tunnel syndrome. He found that 67% of all persons meeting the NIOSH criteria[52,68] had carpal tunnel syndrome using objective nerve conduction tests, 58% of those with negative findings had negative nerve conduction tests, and the test could predict only 50% of the population with positive or negative nerve conduction findings. This low sensitivity and specificity raises an interesting question. Are pain-based tests poor or are the objective electrodiagnostic tests they are compared with poor? Normal objective test findings may be a small consolation to a worker in pain. Similarly, a patient with no symptoms and positive nerve conduction tests may be a dilemma to a health-care provider or employer. Undoubtedly, pain and other fatigue-like symptoms will continue to be a major issue in the diagnosis and treatment of upper limb musculoskeletal disorders.

## MORBIDITY PATTERNS

The earliest estimates of the incidence and prevalence of cumulative trauma disorders came from insurance records or clinical case series reports. Zollinger[103] reported some 1927 cases of crepitant tenosynovitis from Swiss insurance records. Obolenskaja and Goljanitzki[78] suggested that high rates of work, 7600 to 12,000 exertions per shift, were a major factor in 189 cases of tenosynovitis of the upper extremities among a group of 700 packers in a tea factory.[57] Conn[26] reported that tenosynovitis accounted for approximately 1% of lost days in the Ohio rubber industry in 1930.

Clinics specializing in services to employers and in-plant medical departments are another source of information about musculoskeletal morbidity patterns. Reed and Harcourt[90] reported that 70 persons with tenosynovitis accounted for 0.54% of all visits to the Indianapolis Industrial Clinic and resulted in 1222 lost days in a 12-month period. Thompson et al[96] reported that 466 of 544 patients with peritendinitis crepitans and simple tenosynovitis seen from 1941 to 1950 at a British hospital and outpatient service were manual workers and agricultural workers. They also reported 40 cases annually with an average absence of 21 days at the Vauxhall Motors Company, which employed 12,000 persons. Hymovich and Lindholm[48] described 66 cases of repetitive trauma disorders reported during a 6-year period among 160 persons employed in the manufacturing of electrical-mechanical products. This corresponds to an incidence rate of 6.6 cases per 100 workers per year or per 200,000 work hours. Fine et al[33] showed that the incidence rates of cumulative trauma disorders at two similar and nearby automobile assembly plants based on required OSHA records were significantly lower than those based on workers' compensation reports (0.03-0.15 vs. 0.29-0.45 cases per 200,000 work hours) and rates based on personal medical absences (0.3-0.4 vs. 3.0-1.8 cases per 200,000 work hours). They found that incidence rates of plant medical visits varied significantly between the two plants (2.0 and 14.0 cases per 100 workers per year) and that at one plant the incidence rate was less than the rate based on personal medical absences. Failure to report all likely cases on the OSHA records has been a cause of OSHA litigation.[28]

Threat of OSHA action and clarification of OSHA record-keeping requirements along with increased awareness of possible work relatedness has no doubt contributed to increased reports of musculoskeletal disorders as a work-related problem. According to the Bureau of Labor Statistics,[19] the incidence of "repeated motion" disorders was three per 10,000 workers per year from 1978 to 1984. Since then it has increased steadily to nearly 30 cases per 10,000 workers per year. Franklin et al[34] reported an incidence rate of 17.4 cases of carpal tunnel syndrome per 10,000 full-time equivalent (FTE) workers in the state of Washington from 1984 to 1986. He reported that the highest rates were among workers in food processing (100-250 cases per 10,000 FTE workers) and those in carpentry, wood products, and logging (60-110 cases per 10,000 FTE workers). Other studies attempt to identify specific causes of cumulative trauma disorders by examining the association between morbidity patterns, work patterns, and worker attributes.

By systematically selecting workers based on work exposure and personal attributes, morbidity patterns can be used to identify common risk factors or to test hypothesized associations between disorders and risk factors. Duncan and Ferguson[30] compared the work behavior of 90 male telegraphers with diagnosed myalgia with that of a group without disorders to test the hypothesis that there is an association between certain work postures and myalgia. Subjects were matched on sex, age, duration of service, and status. They concluded that differences in keyboard design and work height resulting in different operating postures were factors in the myalgia. To test the hypothesis that repetitive work is a factor in tenosynovitis, Luopajarvi et al[65] compared a group of 163 female assembly line packers who performed machine-paced work with up to 25,000 cycles per day with 143 female retail shop assistants who performed nonrepetitive cashier work. The prevalence of hand and wrist tenosynovitis was 56% among the group performing high-repetitive work versus only 14% among the group performing low-repetitive work. By comparing keyboard operators suffering from repetitive strain disorders and job-matched operators without injuries, Oxenburgh et al[84] concluded that repetitive strain injuries were associated with use of keyboards for more than five hours per shift. Using a longitudinal study design, Waersted and Westgaard[97] later reported that short work shifts appeared to delay but not prevent musculoskeletal disorders.

Silverstein et al[92] and Armstrong et al[10] found repetition and force were both associated with the prevalence of carpal tunnel syndrome and hand and wrist tendinitis. Their cross-sectional study design entailed identification of four job categories at each of seven worksites. They then randomly selected at least 20 workers from each job category while maintaining overall gender and age balance across the study groups. They studied a total of 652 workers (89.7% participation rate). The prevalence of carpal tunnel syndrome and hand-wrist tendinitis was determined from interviews and physical examinations of all workers. Avocation activities were investigated, but none were found to be significant.

Nathan et al[74] compared the prevalence of carpal tunnel syndrome using electrodiagnosis among five job classes of "repetition" and "resistance." The prevalence of persons with impaired median sensory conduction increased significantly from the lowest to the highest job-stress class; the prevalence of persons with bilateral slowing increased from the lowest to the second highest job-stress class but decreased for the highest-stress class job. This led them to conclude that carpal tunnel syndrome is not related to work. The low prevalence in the highest job-stress class suggests a "healthy worker" effect in which workers who are adversely affected by physical work stresses associated with a given job leave that job by going onto disability, transferring into another less-stressful job, or quitting—in each case only the survivors are available for study. The results also could be affected by sampling biases, age, and gender, which were not discussed.

Barnhart et al[13] also utilized a cross-sectional study design to evaluate the relationship between repetition and carpal tunnel syndrome among workers at a ski manufacturing plant. They reported a significantly higher prevalence of electrodiagnostic and physical signs among persons performing repetitive work than among those performing nonrepetitive work (15.4% vs. 3.1%).

De Krom et al[29] performed a community-based survey of carpal tunnel syndrome using the population registry of Maastricht, The Netherlands, from September 1983 to July 1985. A questionnaire was used to collect information about the life-style, work, chronic diseases, and symptoms of carpal tunnel syndrome. When comparing persons with symptoms with those without symptoms, they found carpal tunnel syndrome to be associated with working with a flexed or extended wrist, hysterectomy with oophorectomy, menopause, and obesity.

Available morbidity studies show that the prevalence of cumulative trauma disorders increases with increasing exposures to work-related physical stresses; however, it is important to recognize that there appears to be a background prevalence even for the lowest levels of repetition. These data can be characterized as an exposure-response relationship between repetition (Fig. 19-1). The actual prevalence will vary with the disorder under consideration and according to the diagnostic criteria utilized. This relationship is critically important for development of work design specifications. Further studies are required to reach agreement on definitions of risk factors and diagnostic criteria and to then determine the point where risk is significantly elevated. Such studies will need to consider not only the effects of repetition, but also interactions with force, posture, vibration, and other physical work stresses.

Personal factors (e.g., systemic diseases, nutrition, fitness, weight, age, gender, pregnancy) are also important in the cause of these disorders.[2,23,29,34,75] Theoretically, it should be possible to evaluate workers and work for these factors and control them through selection, training, or job redesign. There are several barriers to control through selection. Present U.S. regulations place a high burden on the employer to demonstrate that: (1) the worker has a condition that has a high likelihood of resulting in illness or injury, and (2) it is not possible to accommodate that worker through job modifications.[1] None of the factors are perfect predictors of risk (i.e., their sensitivities and specificities are all below 100%).[45,52] Even if a given

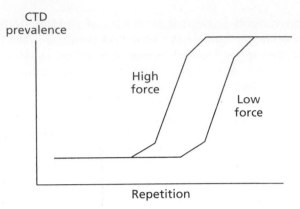

**FIGURE 19-1**   Generic exposure-response relationship for repetition, force, and cumulative trauma disorders.

factor has a high sensitivity and specificity, it will discriminate against some qualified workers. For example, consider a potential population of 100 people. Assume that 10% of the population has a condition that is predictive of a future disorder. If the factor has a sensitivity and specificity both equal to 90%, then it will correctly identify nine of the ten people at risk who would develop disorders, but it would also falsely identify nine out of 90 people who would not develop disorders. If a factor has a sensitivity of 90% but a specificity of only 50%, it would still identify nine of the ten people at risk, but it would also falsely identify 45 people out of 90 as at risk. Most studies of personal risk factors are based on clinical populations. These cases would represent the extreme cases included in the low exposure end of the curve shown in Figure 19-1. It is doubtful that studies to identify persons reliably and legally who will develop cumulative trauma disorders as a result of work, before they are hired, will be available in the foreseeable future.

## MECHANISMS

The mechanisms underlying the development of upper-limb disorders are not fully understood. Armstrong et al[5] proposed a multistage model in which exposure to work activities produces a series of mechanical and physiological events. Mechanical mechanisms involve the transmission of forces through the body to counteract gravity, inertial and drag forces on work objects, as well as the body itself. The tissues of the body, like any material, deform when subjected to a force. The direction and magnitude of the deformation depend on the direction and magnitude of the force and the tissue characteristics.

Figure 19-2 shows a simplified longitudinal view of the wrist. Contraction of the forearm flexor muscles

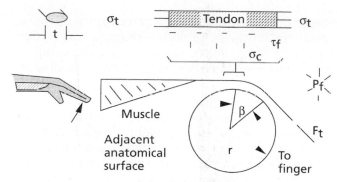

**FIGURE 19-2** The tendons in the wrist can be characterized as a belt stretched around a pulley and subjected to fluid pressure, $P_f$, and tensile, $\sigma_t$, compressive, $\sigma_c$, shear stresses, $\tau_f$.

pulls on the finger flexor tendons; this pull force is transmitted through the tendons to the second and third phalanxes.[18] Newton's second law states that exertion of a force on an object will cause that object to accelerate in the direction of the force and in proportion to its mass. This means that the tendon will move and the phalanxes will rotate toward the contracting muscle. Contraction of the finger flexor muscles causes the joints to rotate in a direction that closes the fist. Contraction of the extensor muscles causes the joint to rotate in a direction that opens the fist. The position of the hand is controlled by a very delicate mechanical equilibrium between those forces that open the fist and those that close the fist.[18] If the moments closing the fist exceed those opening the fist, the interphalangeal joints will rotate in a direction that closes the fist. This rotation will occur until the fingers come into contact with an external object or with another part of the body. As the fingers press against another surface, moments will be produced that oppose those produced by the contracting muscle. This can be seen by tightly closing the fist around a handle or against itself. If the fingers do not encounter another object the joints will rotate until the limits of joint motion are reached. As the joint reaches the limits of its range of motion, it becomes very stiff and resists further rotation. This can be seen by opening the fist to its full extent.

In addition to the forces produced by muscles, acceleration, and passive joint rotation, there are also friction forces on tendon and joint tissues. Friction forces are proportional to velocity. The moving parts of the body, such as tendons, are generally well-lubricated; however, certain disorders result in increased friction. In extreme cases, adhesions may form between tendons and adjacent structures that further impair function.

Forces are classified according to the direction of their action and tissue deformation.[58,85] Pull forces

that act perpendicular to the surface and cause tissue elongation are classified as "tension." Push forces that act perpendicular to the surface and cause tissue shortening are classified as "compression." Forces that act parallel to the surface, such as those produced by friction, are classified as "shear." Shear forces cause angular deformation of tissue. The effect of a force is related to the area over which it is distributed; therefore, forces are normally expressed as a stress or force per unit area. Similarly, deformations are generally related to the size of the object over which the stress is acting; therefore deformations are normally expressed as a strain or the deformation divided by the size of the object. Strains due to compressive and tensile stresses are often expressed as percent shortening or lengthening. Strains due to shear stress are expressed in angular units. The amount of strain produced for a given amount of stress is related to the stiffness of the material. The stiffness of biological tissues increases as they are stretched. Some tissues, such as skin, may stretch several percent before their stiffness increases significantly.[9] This characteristic of skin tends to equalize stress concentrations over the external surface of the body. The stiffness of other tissues, such as tendons, increases very rapidly with the application of a stress.[41] This characteristic facilitates the transmission of force from muscles to the skeletal system.

In addition to the tension forces produced by muscles on the tendon, the tendons are also exposed to compressive forces. The finger flexor tendons in the carpal tunnel are of particular interest because of their possible involvement in carpal tunnel syndrome. These tendons and their adjacent anatomical structures inside the carpal tunnel (Fig. 19-2) have been characterized as anatomical belts and pulleys.[4,58] It can be shown that pressures sufficient to interfere with nourishment of tendon, synovial, and nerve tissues are produced by maximum exertions of the hand. Most workers do not maintain maximum exertions for prolonged periods; however, prolonged exertions at even a few percent of maximum strength are sufficient to affect these tissues adversely. Because these forces are exerted only between the tendon and supporting structure, the nerve is affected by this mechanism only in flexion. Exertion with the flexed wrist forms the basis of the well known "Phalen's" or "wrist flexion" test.[86,93]

Compressive stresses also result from increased fluid pressure. Muscles and tendons are arranged in compartments that can be characterized as fluid-filled sponges encased in a distensible membrane. Fluid pressure is uniformly distributed on the surfaces of the compartment and its contents. Fluid pressure may also be increased by an enlarged fluid volume associated with past trauma.[7] Although the mechanics of these complex structures have not been well described, the magnitude of fluid pressure change is related to the change in compartment shape and volume.[17]

There have been a number of recent studies using fluid-filled catheters to study intracarpal canal pressures. These studies demonstrate that the pressure can be increased by certain postures and repetitive exertions. Pressures as high as 13.3 kPa (100 mm) have been reported in extension of the wrist.[39,63] Wrist extension appears to reduce the cross-sectional area of the carpal canal and draw the ends of the flexor muscles into the carpal canal. Although fluid pressure changes inside the carpal tunnel are not as high as the stress produced by contact between the tendons and the walls of the carpal tunnel, they affect the nerve regardless of posture. Also, increased fluid pressure may occur without exertion of force while a worker is seemingly at rest.

Fluid pressure inside the carpal tunnel can be increased by external contact or pressure. This occurs when the wrist is exerted against an external object such as a hand tool or work surface. These stresses are related to the contact force divided by the area of contact. Lundborg et al[63] demonstrated that pressures of 8 and 12 kPa (60 and 90 mm) produced by pressure on the base of the wrist were sufficient to impair nerve viability and function.

Friction or shear stresses are produced in dynamic exertions at locations where the tendons slide against adjacent anatomical surfaces.[58] Because shear forces act parallel to the surface of the tissue, they are not directly comparable to fluid or compressive stresses. The movement of tendons past adjacent surfaces is lubricated by synovial fluid produced by the synovial sheaths. Synovial fluid also nourishes the tendons and plays a role in repair of tendon damage.

Tensile, compressive, and shear stresses all cause some degree of elastic or viscous deformation in biological tissues. Elastic deformation occurs immediately as a stress is applied or removed. Viscous deformation occurs after the load is applied or removed.[41,73,95] If the recovery time between successive exertions is not long enough for a given force and duration, the recovery will not be complete and the tendon will be stretched further with each successive exertion. Critical recovery times for given work-rest profiles have not yet been determined.

It has been shown that excessive stress will result in mechanical failure or yielding of tendons. In addition to acute mechanical effects resulting from high, prolonged, or repeated exertions, there may be delayed effects involving physiological mechanisms. For example, Z-line disruption can be seen immediately after eccentric muscle loading, but elevation of serum creatine kinase and muscle pain may be delayed.[37,42-44,77]

Wound healing following microrupture of muscle connective tissue or tendons is characterized by three stages:[98] (1) the "inflammatory" stage includes infiltration of polymorphonuclear cells, capillary budding and exudation; (2) the "reparative" stage, which includes accumulation of fibroblasts that produce randomly-oriented and attached collagen fibers, begins in about one week; and (3) the "remolding" stage includes realignment of collagen fibers, with normal alignment beginning in about a month and possibly continuing for several months. This healing process is characterized as extrinsic because it involves infiltration of cells from other tissues. Gelberman and others have put forth an intrinsic healing model for tendons that does not involve external tissues but does involve a series of cellular changes that proceed over a similar time frame.[38]

Mechanical forces interfere with normal physiological processes well before mechanical damage occurs. Exertions above 15% of maximum strength are sufficient to impair muscle circulation and accelerate fatigue.[12,59] Intramuscular pressure and distortion of the vascular bed appear to increase with increasing muscle tension. Studies of skin show that cutaneous circulation will be restricted by much lower tensions than are required for mechanical tissue failure. Kenedi[53] suggested that physiological limits are more meaningful than mechanical limits. Increased intramuscular pressure may also impair perfusion of adjacent tendons and contribute to ischemic tendon damage.[46,47] The mechanisms of nerve entrapments also appear to involve an ischemic mechanism due to external pressure.[63] Pressure may be due to the acute effects of repeated exertions or certain postures, or to a secondary effect due to thickening of the adjacent tissues.[61,86,93,94] Thickening of the flexor synovium in the carpal tunnel is a common finding in carpal tunnel patients.[7,86,102]

In addition to muscles and tendons, ligaments are important load-bearing tissue in certain work activities. Basmajian[14] showed that in certain arm positions the muscles of the shoulder relax and transfer the weight of the upper limb to ligaments. Later studies showed that force-induced pain of these ligaments is a limiting factor of work performance.[15,31] They did not propose the mechanism of pain, but it most likely entailed mechanical strain. Gamekeeper's thumb is perhaps the most extreme example of mechanical failure of a ligament caused by repeated force.[22]

Muscle contraction triggers a series of physiological processes. These processes entail the consumption of substrate (e.g., creatine phosphates, oxygen, glycogen, fatty acids) and the accumulation of by-products, lactates and heat—all of which contribute to fatigue.[15,20,24] Increased intramuscular circulation is required to restore substrates and remove by-products. Sufficient circulation is not possible at high levels of contraction due to disruption of the vascular bed. In addition, muscle contraction entails the release of calcium and potassium into the interstitial spaces; there is evidence that elevated calcium ion concentrations attack cell membranes and increase their susceptibility to damage by free radicals produced during re-oxygenation of hypoxic tissue.[49,62] Further studies are necessary to determine the short- and long-term physiological limits for tendon and nerve loading to plan safe work schedules.

## RECOMMENDATIONS

Sufficient data have not been accumulated yet to develop work-design guidelines based on a given level of risk of a given disorder. In the absence of such data and in the presence of regulations regarding worker safety and health, workers' compensation and nondiscrimination, employers must be vigilant for work factors that "might cause" cumulative trauma disorders and for workers who "might be" experiencing cumulative trauma disorders. Suspect jobs and workers can then be evaluated. The available data provide insight into the development of interventions, but it is essential that all work and medical interventions be evaluated to ascertain their effectiveness.

At the time of this writing, regulations are under development by the U.S. Department of Labor Occupational Safety and Health Administration[79] and the American National Standards Institute (ANSI Z-365)[3] that would specify some of the important components of a control program. Employers should be aware that the absence of a specific standard does not relieve them of their responsibility to provide a safe work place. The General Duty Clause Section 5(a)(1) of the Occupational Safety and Health Act of 1970 specifies that each employer:[81]

". . . shall furnish to each of his employees employment and a place of employment which are free from recognized hazards that are causing or are likely to cause death or serious physical harm to his employees . . ."

In addition Section 8(c)(2), Record Keeping specifies that each employer:[81]

". . . shall make, keep and preserve, and make available to the Secretary . . . such records regarding his activities relating to this Act."

Cumulative trauma disorders are classified "diseases" on the OSHA log.[82,83] Increased incidence of cumulative trauma disorders and the failure to record cases properly have resulted in numerous employer citations by the Occupational Safety and Health Administration.[28] Most general-duty and record-keeping citations have been settled out of court and have resulted in fines and agreements by the company to implement control programs. In addition to the plant being cited, the agreement often includes all other plants owned and operated by the employer. The absence of OSHA or ANSI standards makes it difficult for an employer to know if they are at risk of an OSHA action. Employers may find some guidance from OSHA's Ergonomic Guidelines for the Red Meat Industry published in 1990,[80] which outlines some of the essential components of an ergonomic program. The following recommendations encompass ideas utilized by many employers and presently under consideration by the ANSI Z-365 committee.[72,87]

Each employer should develop a program plan for control of upper-limb cumulative-trauma disorders. The plan should state the objectives and lay out the necessary tasks, steps, and schedules for achieving them. The organizational aspects of an ergonomic program will vary from one work setting to another depending on the size of the work force, the type of work processes involved, the administrative structure of the organization, and the professional services (e.g., health care and engineering) available on site or in the community. The organizational aspects of a generic control program are shown in Figure 19-3.

Each program should include objectives that are as specific as possible and are also achievable. Elimination of all upper-limb disorders may be desirable, but it probably is not achievable. Achieving a rate of upper-limb disorders at the level of those not performing repetitive or stressful hand work is more realistic. Other objectives might specify implementation of a surveillance program, implementation of a training program, a review of jobs for the presence of risk factors for upper limb disorders, and the development of new technologies to reduce work stresses. The plan should also take into consideration the organizational structure and the available resources for the work setting where it is to be implemented. The plan should be periodically reviewed to determine if all the goals are being achieved. If they are not achieved, it should be determined if the goals are appropriate or if other methods are necessary for achieving them. If they are still appropriate, the cause for failing to meet the goals should be determined and remedied.

Active and passive surveillance methods are utilized to identify cumulative trauma disorders. Active surveillance entails the use of questionnaires, surveys, and physical examinations. Several questionnaires and physical examinations have been proposed

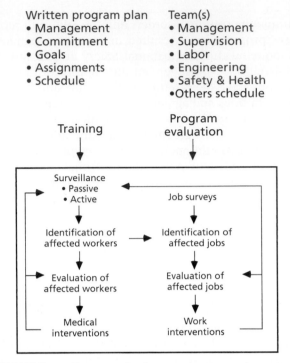

**FIGURE 19-3** Components of a generic ergonomics program that should be tailored to meet the needs of each organization.

that may be adapted to a given setting.[32,51,52,56,68,88] Active surveillance is not just a matter of passing out questionnaires for workers to answer at their convenience. Workers must be given a time, place, and sufficient instructions for meaningful participation. Care should be exercised to avoid biasing the results through the inclusion or exclusion of possible participants. It is also important to avoid leading or suggestive questions.[71] Some investigators eschew questionnaires and interviews in favor of objective tests based on nerve conduction or quantitative sensory testing; however, these so-called "objective" tests only detect disorders of nerves—not those of muscles or tendons. Nerve-conduction testing is considered the most definitive test for carpal tunnel syndrome and is used to determine sensitivities and specificities of other tests (see Chapter 40). At present, other tests compare poorly with nerve conduction testing;[35,52] however, just because a worker does not fit an established diagnostic criterion for carpal tunnel syndrome does not mean that there is nothing wrong with the worker's hands and wrists.

Passive surveillance entails analysis of available data sources (including OSHA records, workers' compensation reports, personal medical claims, and company medical visits). There are several components of an effective passive-surveillance monitoring system. There must be a mechanism for workers to report

problems. Resources vary from plant to plant. Some plants do not have on-site medical resources. In those cases it is necessary to work with the referral health care provider or with local clinics to identify possible causes. Employers need to understand that worker health records are confidential and that the health-care provider may be able to give them only general feedback in which individuals cannot be identified. Reporting will be affected based on either a hostile or a supportive attitude by management toward injured workers. Reporting can also be affected by the attitude of the local medical community. In some communities, health-care providers work closely with local industry by visiting the workplace to observe jobs and discussing possible work restrictions, while in others there may be no such interaction.

Workers need to understand that if persistent discomfort interferes with activities of work or daily living, then they should see a health-care provider for an evaluation. They also should understand that some discomfort may be normal. Workers may need guidance about where to go to report their problems and to get help, but they must not be threatened that reporting will affect their job security or earnings. This can be a problem in plants where wages are based on an incentive system.

OSHA has attempted to facilitate passive surveillance by specifying standardized reporting criteria:[80]

- At least one physical finding (e.g., positive Tinel's, Phalen's, or Finkelstein's test); or swelling, redness or deformity; or loss of motion; *or*
- At least one subjective symptom (e.g., pain, numbness, tingling, aching, stiffness, or burning), *and* at least one of the following:
- medical treatment (including self-administered treatment when made available to employees by their employer),
- lost work days (includes restricted work activity), or
- transfer or rotation to another job.

These reporting guidelines are sensitive because they identify persons with any kind of upper-limb problem that causes them to seek help. They are not very specific because they do not discriminate between various disorders, and they identify unaffected worker as having cumulative trauma disorders.

It is necessary to have a plan for managing workers identified through passive or active surveillance. All possible cases need to be evaluated. In some cases it may be found that the worker has fatigue and requires rest and reassurance. Reassurance may come in the form of an explanation and monitoring of the problem. Other workers may need medical interventions, such as physical therapy, medications, or even surgery. Always the work should be evaluated for possible risk factors, to accommodate the affected worker and prevent future cases.

Specification and interpretation of work restrictions is a common source of frustration for both the health-care provider and the employer. In some cases restrictions are vague, and workers may be laid off or unwittingly given alternative work that is worse that the original. A restriction that says "avoid forceful exertions" may leave an employer wondering what is too forceful. A restriction that says "do not lift more than 20 pounds" does not consider the fact that 20 pounds close to the body is not as bad as 20 pounds at an arm's length from the body. A work restriction should be based on knowledge of the operations at the place of the affected worker's employment. By observing or discussing jobs with management, it may be possible to locate jobs or tasks that entail elements that appear to contribute to a given disorder.

A thorough job analysis should be performed for all affected workers.[6] The analysis should include a description of work standards, methods, materials, equipment, and environment. It should delineate the frequency and severity of generic risk factors (e.g., repeated and sustained static exertions, forces, postures, contact stresses, and exposures to vibration and low temperatures). It is desirable that the analysis also indicates the cause of major stresses-job-specific factors (e.g., flexing wrist six times per minute is caused by driving screws in a horizontal surface 1 m above the floor). Table 19-1 includes a list of job-specific factors associated with generic cumulative-trauma-disorder factors. This information will help plant personnel develop work interventions to accommodate the restricted worker.

In some cases it is not possible to visit the work site or even get a good analysis of the jobs. In those cases, the treating physician may obtain the information from a worker or someone at the plant. Table 19-2 lists some of the information that will be helpful for planning restrictions.

By focusing the restriction on a specific aspect of the job, it may make it possible for the employer to develop a workplace modification that would facilitate returning the worker to the same job and preventing future occurrences in other workers. For example, if the restriction focuses on torque associated with use of a hand tool, it may be possible for the employer to find an alternative tool with a lower torque reaction force to use as an articulating arm to eliminate the torque from the worker. A general list of factors associated with risk factors is summarized in Table 19-2. It is essential that all interventions be evaluated to ascertain their effectiveness.

**TABLE 19-1    WORK IMPROVEMENTS***

| | |
|---|---|
| Adjust production standards | R, S, D |
| Incentives | R, S, D |
| Rotations | R, S, D |
| Work enlargement | R, S, D |
| Mechanical aids | |
| Tools | R, S, D, F, P, C, V, T |
| Supports | S, F, P |
| Hoists and articulating arms | S, F, P |
| Motion economy | R, S, D |
| Weight of job work objects/materials | F |
| Friction | F |
| Gloves | F, V, T |
| Balance | F |
| Handles | F, C |
| Tool torque | F |
| Tool shape | F, P |
| Bits | F |
| Blades | F |
| Adjustable work surfaces | P |
| Isolation devices | V |
| Air temperature | T |
| Air leaks | T |
| Air line attachments | F, T |

\* R = Repetition
S = Static exertions
D = Work duration
F = Force
P = Posture
C = Contact stress
V = Vibration
T = Temperature

Several schemes have been proposed for analyzing jobs. These include checklists,[54,69] open-ended observational-based systems,[8,55] instrumental systems using goniometers and surface electromyography,[6,50,60,66,67] as well as a number of traditional interview and observational methods.[71] Descriptions of job analysis methods is beyond the scope of this discussion.

Control of cumulative trauma disorders entails participation and training of persons from many parts

**TABLE 19-2     JOB INFORMATION NEEDED FOR DEVELOPING WORK RESTRICTIONS. ANSWERING THE QUESTION 'WHY' WILL HELP DETERMINE THE FEASIBILITY OF INTERVENTIONS.**

---

**Documentation**

Job title? (including *all* jobs through which a worker may rotate)

What do you do?

Work standard?

Pay and incentive system.

List steps necessary to perform the job along with the work objects and locations.

List the work objects along with their size, weight, or other force information (e.g., torque, insertion force).

Describe the range of environments in which the job is performed (e.g., inside at room temperature, outside at ambient temperature).

List personal protective equipment (e.g., gloves).

**Assessment of Physical Stresses**

Does the worker have difficulty making production or keeping up with the line?

____Always?          ____Sometimes?          ____Why?

Does the worker work overtime?

____Always?          ____Sometimes?          ____Why?

Does the worker maintain the same position or hold a work object for prolonged periods?

____Always?          ____Sometimes?          ____Why?

Does the worker assume unnatural or awkward postures to perform the job?

____Always?          ____Sometimes?          ____Why?

Does the worker have difficulty exerting the force required to perform the job?

____Always?          ____Sometimes?          ____Why?

Do any work objects rub or create stress concentrations on the surface of the body?

____Always?          ____Sometimes?          ____Why?

Does the worker hold or touch anything that shakes or vibrates?

____Always?          ____Sometimes?          ____Why?

Does the worker hold or touch anything cold (less than 70° F)—tools, parts, air?

____Always?          ____Sometimes?          ____Why?

---

of the organization. A commitment is required from all levels of management to provide leadership and support for others in the organization. Commitment entails stating goals, assigning responsibilities, and maintaining accountabilities. It also entails allocating necessary time and monetary resources. Managers need training to understand the characteristics and causes of cumulative trauma disorders, their responsibility for providing workers with a safe and healthful workplace, the components of a control program, and the necessary resources.

Workers' participation is required to report possible health and job problems and to cooperate in implementing control measures. Workers need training about the characteristics and causes of cumulative trauma disorders, when and where they should report health and work problems, and the things they can do via work methods and work place adjustments to prevent cumulative trauma disorders.

Supervisors often are the first to hear of a worker's problem or to see a problem with equipment or materials. They must be vigilant for these problems and

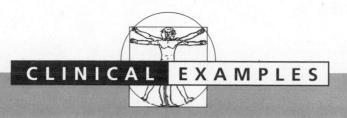

## CLINICAL EXAMPLES

## CUMULATIVE TRAUMA

EDITOR'S NOTE—Cumulative trauma is evaluated as a neurologic abnormality and is usually limited to the upper extremities (see Chapters 20 and 21). The history and physical examination are vital in this assessment because electrophysiological testing is not always confirmatory (87% sensitivity for carpal tunnel syndrome and 77% for ulnar neuropathy; see Chapter 40). Table 16 of the AMA *Guides* can be used to rate impairments caused by cumulative trauma, as can section 3.1k, which addresses the issues of impairment resulting from pain and sensory and motor deficits for afflictions of specific nerves.*

### EXAMPLE
#### History
A 48-year-old assembly line worker was evaluated for vague discomfort in the left elbow. This often awakened him from sleep. Other symptoms included intermittent paresthesias in the ring and little fingers and diminished strength in the left hand.

*All *tables* and *sections* referred to in this discussion are found in AMA *Guides to the evaluation of permanent impairment,* ed 4, Chapter 3—The Musculoskeletal System, American Medical Association, Chicago, 1993. All *chapter* citations are to chapters in this book.

#### Physical Examination
Light tapping over the ulnar nerve at the elbow reproduced the symptoms of paresthesias and discomfort (Tinel's sign).
#### Test Results
The elbow flexion test was positive (see Chapter 21). When radiographs were taken, an osteophyte was found on a cubital tunnel view. The NCV test was positive in the distribution of the ulnar nerve across the elbow.
#### Assessment Process
The history, physical examination, radiographs, and physiologic tests are consistent with a mild-to-moderate entrapment neuropathy involving the ulnar nerve and producing a 20% impairment of the upper extremity (Table 16). Using Table 3, this can be expressed as a 12% whole person impairment (WPI).
#### Evaluation
The diagnosis is entrapment neuropathy of the ulnar nerve or cubital tunnel syndrome. Recommendation is for job accommodation, nonsteroidal antiinflammatory medications, and a padded extension brace for use during sleep.

*Stephen L. Demeter*

must cooperate with the implementation of interventions. Supervisors need training about the characteristics and causes of cumulative trauma disorders, what they should do when workers report problems, and the need for work equipment to be set up and adjusted properly.

Engineering participation includes fixing equipment, identifying material and method problems as they are identified, and developing new designs that minimize physical work stresses. Engineers need training about the characteristics and causes of cumulative trauma disorders—especially with respect to the design of work equipment and methods. They need to be able to identify physical work stresses. They need to appreciate the range of physical and behavior differences in the working population and where to find work design information. Engineers need to appreciate the need to perform user trials on equipment before designs are finalized.[70]

The role of health-care providers in surveillance and medical management has already been described. They may need additional training to appreciate the unique properties of cumulative trauma disorders, and the use and limitations of surveillance methods, as well as to interpret job analysis information and develop recommendations.

Other health and safety personnel (such as the occupational safety expert) often participate through training and the analysis of data for injury and illness trends. Also, they may work with purchasing agents to be sure that new equipment and material acquisitions are reviewed for contributing avoidable stresses to workers. They need training about the characteristics and causes of cumulative trauma disorders, the organizational aspects of ergonomics programs, regulatory issues, and work analysis and design. The depth of their training will vary according to the role they play in plant program. Often, Safety and Health personnel set up, run, and evaluate preventive programs for workplaces. Other members of the organization may participate as necessary, and they should receive sufficient training regarding their role in the program.

Training should be tailored to each industry and setting. The training requirements of a large office facility will be different than those of a small manufacturing plant. Also, training should be an ongoing process. This often can be done in conjunction with a review of various program aspects or technical assistance needed for specific problems.

Because a control program for cumulative trauma disorders draws on a number of different skills, the assistance of one or more teams may facilitate preventive efforts. The team should be provided with training about the characteristics and causes of upper limb disorders. They also should be given training on how to analyze jobs. The team should meet at regular intervals to review new and existing cases. At that time the team may review the progress toward goals and recommend necessary program enhancements. Written records should be kept to document the team activities so that its progress can be evaluated. These records will also provide institutional memory of problems and solutions and will be useful in the future. Employers should be aware that some team activities may be a violation of the National Labor Relations Act of 1935.[16] They should consult with their personnel managers before setting up teams.

## SUMMARY

Cumulative trauma disorder refers to a group of muscle, tendon, and nerve disorders that can be caused, precipitated, or aggravated by repeated exertions of movements of the hand. Reports of these disorders dating back nearly 300 years demonstrate that they are a major cause of worker impairment and disability in some occupations. Causes of cumulative trauma disorders include personal and work-related factors. Contemporary regulations regarding worker safety and health, workers' compensation, and nondiscrimination obligate employers to identify and remedy hazardous work situations before disorders occur and to identify affected workers before they develop long-term consequences. This is best achieved by implementation of an on-going program that includes a written plan tailored to the needs of each organization, surveillance, analysis and design of jobs, management of affected workers, a team approach, and training for the team members.

## References

1. ADA: *The Americans with disabilities act of 1990,* Washington, DC, 1990, Public law: 110th Congress HR.
2. Amadio PC: Carpal tunnel syndrome, pyridoxine, and the workplace. *J Hand Surg* 12A5(part 2): 875-881, 1987.
3. ANSI Z-365: *Standards News* Jan. 1989.
4. Armstrong TJ, Chaffin DB: Some biological aspects of the carpal tunnel. *J Biomech* 12:567-570, 1979.
5. Armstrong TJ, et al: A conceptual model for work-related neck and upper-limb musculoskeletal disorders. *Scand J Work Environ Hlth* 19(2):73-84, 1993.
6. Armstrong T, Kochhar D: Work performance and handicapped persons. In Salvendy G, edi-

tor: *Handbook of industrial engineering,* New York, 1982, John Wiley & Sons.

7. Armstrong TJ: Some histological changes in carpal tunnel contents and their biomechanical implications. *JOM* 26(3):197-201, 1984.

8. Armstrong TJ: Ergonomics and cumulative trauma disorders. In Kasdan M, editor: *Hand clinics,* Philadelphia, 1986, WB Saunders.

9. Armstrong TJ: Mechanical considerations of skin in work. *Am J Ind Med* 8:463-472, 1985.

10. Armstrong TJ, et al: Ergonomic considerations in hand and wrist tendinitis. *J Hand Surg* 12A5(part 2):830-837, 1987.

11. Armstrong, TJ, et al: Investigation of cumulative trauma disorders in a poultry processing plant. *Am Ind Hyg Assoc J* 43(2):103-116,1982.

12. Barcroft H, Greenwood B, Whelan R: Blood flow and venous oxygen saturation during sustained contraction of the forearm. *J Physiol* 168:848-856, 1963.

13. Barnhart S, et al: Carpal tunnel syndrome among ski manufacturing. *Scand J Work Environ Health* 17:46-52, 1991.

14. Basmajian JV: Weight-bearing by ligaments and muscles. *Can J Surg* 4:166-170, 1961.

15. Basmajian JV, DeLuca CJ: *Muscles alive, their functions revealed by electromyography,* ed 5, Baltimore, 1985, Williams & Wilkins.

16. Bernstein A: Making teamwork work—and appeasing Uncle Sam, *Bus Week* p. 101, Jan. 1993.

17. Brain WR, Wright AD, Wilkinson M: Spontaneous compression of both median nerves in the carpal tunnel. *Lancet* 8:277-282, 1947.

18. Brand PW: *Clinical mechanics of the hand,* St. Louis, 1985, CV Mosby.

19. Bureau of Labor Statistics, USDOL *Occupational injuries and illnesses in the United States by industry,* Washington, DC, 1994, US Govt. Printing Office.

20. Bystrom, S, Sjogaard G: Potassium homeostasis during and following exhaustive submaximal static handgrip contractions. *Acta Physiol Scand* 142:59-66, 1991.

21. Cailliet R: *Soft tissue pain and disability,* Philadelphia, 1977, FA Davis.

22. Campbell CS: Gamekeeper's thumb. *J Bone Joint Surg* 37B(1):148-149, 1955.

23. Cannon LJ, Bernacki EJ, Walter SD: Personal and occupational factors associated with carpal tunnel syndrome. *JOM* 23(4):255-258, 1981.

24. Caplan A et al: Skeletal muscle. Chapter 6. In Woo SL, Buckwalter JE, editors: *Injury and repair of the musculoskeletal soft tissues,* Park Ridge, IL, 1988, American Academy of Orthopaedic Surgeons.

25. Chaffin DB: Localized muscle fatigue—definition and measurement. *JOM* 15(4):346-354, 1973.

26. Conn HR: Tenosynovitis. *Ohio State Med J* 27:713-716, 1931.

27. Corlett EN, Bishop RP: A technique for assessing postural discomfort. *Ergonomics* 19(2):175-182, 1976.

28. Courtney TK, Smith GD, Armstrong TJ: Ergonomics and OSHA: a chronological overview of enforcement and regulation development. In Kumar S, editor: *Advances in industrial ergonomics and safety—IV,* pp. 1313-1320, London, 1992, Taylor & Francis.

29. DeKrom MC, et al: Risk factors for carpal tunnel syndrome. *Am J Epidemiol* 132(6):1102-1110, 1990.

30. Duncan J, Ferguson D: Keyboard operating posture and symptoms in operating. *Ergonomics* 17(5):651-662, 1974.

31. Elkus R, Basmajian JV: Endurance in hanging by the hands. *Am J Phys Med* 52(3):124-127, 1973.

32. Fine LJ, Silverstein BA: Work-related disorders of the neck and upper extremity. In Levy B, Wegman D, editors: *Occupational health: recognizing and preventing work-related disease,* ed 3, Boston, 1995, Little, Brown.

33. Fine LJ, et al: The detection of cumulative trauma disorders of the upper extremities in the workplace. *JOM* 28(8):674-678, 1986.

34. Franklin GM, et al: Occupational carpal tunnel syndrome in Washington state—1984-88. *Am J Public Health* 81(6):741-746, 1991.

35. Franzblau A, et al: Workplace surveillance for carpal tunnel syndrome: a comparison of methods. *J Occup Rehab* 3(1):1-14, 1994.

36. Franzblau A, et al: Workplace surveillance for carpal tunnel syndrome using hand diagrams. *J Occup Rehab* 4(4):185-198, 1994.

37. Friden J, Sjostrom M, Ekblom B: A morphological study on delayed muscle soreness. *Experientia* 37:506-507, 1981.

38. Gelberman RH, et al: Tendon. In Woo SL, Buckwalter JE, editors: *Injury and repair of the musculoskeletal soft tissues,* Chapter 1, Park Ridge, IL, 1988, American Academy of Orthopaedic Surgeons.

39. Gelberman RH, et al: The carpal tunnel syndrome: a study of carpal tunnel pressures. *J Bone Joint Surg* 63A(3):380-383, 1981.

40. Gelberman RH, et al: Sensibility testing in peripheral-nerve compression syndromes. *J Bone Joint Surg* 65A(5):632-638, 1983.

41. Goldstein SA, et al: Analysis of cumulative

strain in tendons and tendon sheaths. *J Biomechanics* 20(1):1-6, 1987.

42. Hagberg M: Local shoulder muscular strain—symptoms and disorders. *J Human Ergology* 11:99-108, 1982.

43. Hagberg M: Occupational musculoskeletal stress and disorders of the neck and shoulder: a review of possible pathophysiology, *Int Arch Occup Environ Health* 53:269-278, 1984.

44. Hagberg M: Work load and fatigue in repetitive arm elevations. *Ergonomics* 24(7):543-555, 1981.

45. Hennekens CH, Buring JE: *Epidemiology in medicine,* Boston, 1987, Little, Brown.

46. Herberts P, et al: Shoulder pain in industry: an epidemiological study on welders. *Acta Orthop Scand* 52:299-306, 1981.

47. Herberts P, et al: Shoulder pain and heavy manual labor. *Clin Orthop* 191:166-178, 1984.

48. Hymovich L, Lindholm M: Hand, wrist and forearm injuries: the result of repetitive motions. *JOM* 8(11):573-577, 1966.

49. Jackson MJ, Jones DA, Edwards RHT: Experimental skeletal muscle damage: the nature of the calcium-activated degenerative processes. *Eur J Clin Invest* 14:369-374, 1984.

50. Jonsson B: The static load component in muscle work. *Eur J Appl Physiol* 57:305-310, 1988.

51. Katz JN, et al: The carpal tunnel syndrome: diagnostic utility of the history and physical examination findings. *Ann Intern Med* 112:321-327, 1990.

52. Katz JN: Validation of a surveillance case definition of carpal tunnel syndrome. *Am J Publ Hlth* 81(2):189-193, 1991.

53. Kenedi RM, Gibson T, Daly CH: Bioengineering studies of the human skin. In Kenedi RM, editor: *Symposium on biomechanics and related bio-engineering topics,* Proceedings, Glasgow, 1964, Pergamon Press, pp. II-147—II-158.

54. Keyserling WM, et al: A checklist for evaluating ergonomic risk factors associated with upper extremity cumulative trauma disorders. *Ergonomics* 36(7):807-831, 1993.

55. Keyserling WM, Armstrong TJ, Punnett L: Ergonomic job analysis: a structural approach for identifying risk factors associated with overexertion injuries and disorders. *Appl Occup Env Hyg* 6(5):353-363, 1991.

56. Kuorinka I, et al: Standardised Nordic health questionnaires for the analysis of musculoskeletal symptoms. *Appl Ergon* 18(3):233-237, 1987.

57. Kurppa K, Waris P, Rokkanen P: Peritendinitis and tenosynovitis: a review. *Scand J Work Environ Health* 5(suppl 3):19-24, 1979.

58. LeVeau B: In Williams and Lissner, editors: *Biomechanics of human motion,* Philadelphia, 1977, WB Saunders, pp. 151-1154.

59. Lind AR, McNicol GW, Donald KW: Circulatory adjustments to sustained (static) muscular activity, *Proc Symp Phys Activity Hlth Dis,* 1966, pp. 38-63.

60. Linderhed H: A new dimension to amplitude analysis of EMG. *Intl J Ind Ergonomics* 11:243-247, 1993.

61. Louis DS: The carpal tunnel syndrome. In Millender LH, Louis DS, Simmons BP, editors: *Occupational disorders of the upper extremity,* New York, 1992, Churchill Livingstone.

62. Lovlin R et al: Are indices of free radical damage related to exercise intensity? *Eur J Appl Physiol Occup Physiol* 56:313-316, 1987.

63. Lundborg G: *Nerve injury and repair,* New York, 1988, Churchill Livingstone.

64. Lundborg G, Rank F: Experimental intrinsic healing of flexor tendons based upon synovial fluid nutrition, *J Hand Surg* 3(1):21-31, 1978.

65. Luopajarvi R, et al: Prevalence of tenosynovitis and other injuries of the upper extremities in repetitive work. *Scand J Work Environ Health* 5(suppl 3)5:48-55, 1979.

66. Marras WS, Schoenmarklin RW: Wrist motions in industry. *Ergonomics* 36(4):341-351, 1993.

67. Mathiassen SE, Winkel J: Quantifying variation in physical load using exposure-vs-time data. *Ergonomics* 34(12):1455-1568, 1991.

68. Matte TD, Baker EL, Honchar PA: The selection and definition of targeted work-related conditions for surveillance under SENSOR. *Am J Publ Hlth* 79:21-25, 1989.

69. McAtamney L, Corlett EN: RULA: a survey method for the investigation of work-related upper limb disorders, *Appl Ergon* 24(2):91-99, 1993.

70. McClelland I: Product assessment and user trials. In Wilson JR, Corlett EN, editors: *Evaluation of human work: a practical ergonomics methodology,* New York, 1990, Taylor & Francis.

71. McCormick E: Job and task analysis. In Salvendy G, editor: *Handbook of industrial engineering,* New York, 1982, John Wiley & Sons.

72. McKenzie F, et al: A program for control of repetitive trauma disorders associated with hand tool operations in a telecommunications manufacturing facility. *Ind Hyg Assoc J* 46(11):674-678, 1985.

73. Moore JS: Function, structure, and responses of components of the muscle-tendon unit. *Occupational Medicine: State of the Art Reviews* 7(4):713-740, 1992.

74. Nathan PA, Meadows KD, Doyle LS: Occupation as a risk factor for impaired sensory conduction of the median nerve at the carpal tunnel. *J Hand Surg* 13B(2):167-170, 1988.

75. Nathan PA, et al: Obesity as a risk factor of sensory conduction of the median nerve in industry. *J Occup Med* 34(4):379-383, 1992.

76. Nathan PA, Meadows KD, Doyle LS: Relationship of age and sex to sensory conduction of the median nerve at the carpal tunnel and association of slowed conduction with symptoms. *Muscle Nerve* 11:1149-1153, 1988.

77. Newham DJ, Jones DA, Edwards RHT: Plasma creatine kinase changes after eccentric and concentric contractions. *Muscle Nerve* 9:59-63, 1986.

78. Obolenskaja AJ, Goljanitzki IA: Die serose tendovaginitis in der klinik und im experiment. *Dtsch z chir* 201:388-399, 1927.

79. Occupational Safety and Health Administration: Ergonomics safety and health management; proposed rule. *Federal Register* 57(149), 1992.

80. Occupational Safety and Health Administration: *Ergonomics program management guidelines for meatpacking plants*, OSHA-3121, Washington, DC, 1990, Bureau of National Affairs.

81. Occupational Safety and Health Administration: *Occupational safety and health act of 1970*, Public Law 91-596, Washington, DC, 1970, US Dept of Labor.

82. Occupational Safety and Health Administration: *Recordkeeping requirements under the occupational safety and health act of 1970*, Washington, DC, 1978, US Dept of Labor.

83. Occupational Safety and Health Administration: *Recordkeeping guidelines for occupational injuries and illnesses*, Washington, DC, 1986, US Dept of Labor.

84. Oxenburgh M: Musculoskeletal injuries occurring in word processor operators. In Adams A, Stevenson M, editors: *Proceedings of the 21st annual conference of the Ergonomics Society of Australia and New Zealand*, 1984, Sydney, Australia, pp. 137-143.

85. Ozkay A, Nordin M: *Fundamentals of biomechanics, equilibrium, motion and deformation*, New York, 1991, Van Nostrand Reinhold.

86. Phalen GS: The carpal-tunnel syndrome: seventeen years' experience in diagnosis and treatment of six hundred fifty-four hands. *J Bone Joint Surg* 48A(2):211-228, 1966.

87. Pipinich R, Getty R, Abbott W: Ergonomics: a high priority at Lockheed Fort Worth facility. *IE Magazine* 25(7):20-26, 1993.

88. Putz-Anderson V: *Cumulative trauma disorders—a manual for musculoskeletal diseases of the upper limbs*, New York, 1988, Taylor & Francis.

89. Ramazzini B: *Diseases of workers (de morbis artificum)*, Chicago, University of Chicago Press, originally published in 1713.

90. Reed JV, Harcourt AK: Tenosynovitis: an industrial disability. *Am J Surg* 62(3):392-396, 1943.

91. Saldana N, et al: A computerized method for assessment of musculoskeletal discomfort in the workforce: a tool for surveillance. *Ergonomics* 37(6):1097-1112, 1994.

92. Silverstein BA, Fine LJ, Armstrong TJ: Occupational factors and carpal tunnel syndrome. *Am J Indust Med* 11:343-358, 1987.

93. Smith EM, Sonstegard DA, Anderson WH: Carpal tunnel syndrome: contribution of flexor tendons. *Arch Phys Med Rehabil* 58:379-385, 1977.

94. Szabo RM, Chidgey LK: Stress carpal tunnel pressures in patients with carpal tunnel syndrome and normal patients. *J Hand Surg* 14A(4):624-627, 1989.

95. Taylor DC: Viscoelastic properties of muscle-tendon units: the biomechanical effects of stretching. *Am J Sports Med* 18(3):300-309, 1990.

96. Thompson AR, Plewes LW, Shaw EG: Peritendinitis crepitans and simple tenosynovitis: a clinical study of 544 cases in industry. *Brit J Industr Med* 8:150-160, 1951.

97. Waersted M, Bjorklund RA, Westgard RH: Shoulder muscle tension induced by two vdu-based tasks of different complexity. *Ergonomics* 34(2):137-150, 1991.

98. Wahl S, Renstrom P: Fibrosis in soft-tissue injuries. In Leadbetter WB, Buckwalter JA, Gordon SL, editors: *Sports induced inflammation: clinical and basic science concepts*, Park Ridge, IL, 1990, American Academy of Orthopaedic Surgeons.

99. Waris P, et al: Epidemiologic screening of occupational neck and upper limb disorders: methods and criteria. *Scand J Work Environ Health* 5(suppl 3):25-38, 1979.

100. WHO Expert Committee: Identification and control of work related diseases. *World Health Organization Technical Report Series*, 1985:3-11.

101. Winkel J, Mathiassen SE: Assessment of physical work load in epidemiologic studies: concepts, issues, and operation considerations. *Ergonomics* 37(6):979-988, 1994.

102. Yamaguchi DM: Carpal tunnel syndrome. *Minn Med* Jan. 1965, pp.-22-33.

103. Zollinger F: A few remarks on the question of tubercular tendovaginitis and bursitis after an accident. *Archiv fur Orthopadische und Unfall-Chirurgioe* 24:456-467, 1927.

# CHAPTER 20

# JOINT SYSTEMS: HAND AND WRIST

*Mark S. Cohen*

## ENTRAPMENT NEUROPATHIES

### Carpal Tunnel Syndrome

#### Anatomy/Pathophysiology

The median nerve passes through the wrist and palm through an unyielding fibroosseous canal termed the *carpal tunnel*. Compression of the median nerve within this canal is termed *carpal tunnel syndrome*. It occurs due to a mismatch between the volume of the canal and its contents, namely the median nerve and the flexor tendons of the digits (Fig. 20-1).

Carpal tunnel syndrome is associated with a variety of medical conditions such as diabetes, hypothyroidism, rheumatoid arthritis, and renal failure. In the workplace, carpal tunnel syndrome is associated with repetitive activities of the wrist and digits, prolonged or repetitive impact on the palm, and the use of vibratory tools.[17,38,39] Mechanically disadvantaged wrist positions such as the extremes of flexion and extension increase the pressure within the carpal canal.[20] Prolonged poor wrist posture may therefore add to compression of the median nerve.

#### Diagnosis

The diagnosis of carpal tunnel syndrome relies initially on the patient history. Symptoms consist of a combination of numbness (on the palmar surface of the radial 3½ digits innervated by the median nerve), tingling, burning pain, weakness, and decreased dexterity of the hand. They are often most pronounced during or after repetitive activity. Positions that increase carpal canal pressures such as wrist flexion during driving or sleep commonly aggravate the symptoms. Nocturnal paresthesia with awakening is thus a common complaint. Symptoms of advanced median nerve compression include loss of sensation (in the radial 3½ digits) and atrophy of the thenar eminence muscles at the base of the thumb that are supplied by the median nerve.

The physical examination is very important in establishing the diagnosis of carpal tunnel syndrome. Thenar muscle bulk and strength are evaluated and sensibility testing is performed. Two-point discrimination refers to the ability to distinguish two points on the pulp of the digit at decreasing distances.[40] Monofilaments are used as a quantitative sensory threshold test to assess light touch in the median nerve distribution.[22] Dryness or unusual texture of the radial digits signifies disruption of the sympathetic fibers carried by the median nerve.

A variety of provocative tests are used to reproduce/accentuate the symptoms of carpal tunnel syndrome. These tests have varying sensitivity and specificity (Table 20-1). Phalen's test refers to placing the wrist in fully flexed posture[46]; Tinel's test refers to percussion of the median nerve over the wrist.[56] The median nerve compression test involves direct pressure on the median nerve over the carpal canal.[13] These tests should reproduce the symptoms in patients with carpal tunnel syndrome.

Electrodiagnostic studies are often used to confirm the diagnosis of carpal tunnel syndrome. However, there is a documented 8 to 12% false-negative rate with the use of these tests (see Chapter 40).[26,36] Electromyograms and nerve conduction velocity studies thus help establish the diagnosis if it is in question, quantitate the degree of nerve injury, and rule out other pathologic nerve compression proximal to the wrist.

#### Treatment

Initial treatment for carpal tunnel syndrome without diminished sensation, atrophy, or denervation on the electromyogram involves splinting the wrist in a neutral, comfortable position. This rests the median nerve and keeps the carpal canal pressure at its lowest level. A cortisone injection into the carpal canal is often used in conjunction with splinting to decrease the inflammation of the canal contents. This injection

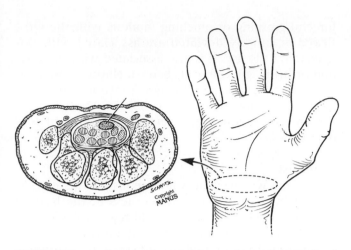

**FIGURE 20-1**    Cross-section of the carpal tunnel at the level of the wrist (carpal bones). The median nerve lies beneath the transverse carpal ligament with the flexor tendons of the digits. Compression of the median nerve within this canal leads to carpal tunnel syndrome. *(Courtesy of the Indiana Hand Center, Indianapolis, Indiana.)*

---

**TABLE 20-1    SENSITIVITY AND SPECIFICITY OF TESTS USED IN DIAGNOSING CARPAL TUNNEL SYNDROME***

|  | SENSITIVITY | SPECIFICITY |
|---|---|---|
| Two-point discrimination | 33% | 100% |
| Phalen's test | 71% | 80% |
| Tinel percussion | 44% | 94% |
| Semmes-Weinstein monofilaments | 91% | 80% |
| Monofilaments with Phalen's | 82% | 86% |
| Median nerve compression test | 87% | 90% |

*Sensitivity expresses the fraction of patients with carpal tunnel syndrome who are correctly identified by the test. Specificity expresses the fraction of normal patients (without carpal tunnel syndrome) who are correctly identified as normal (see Chapter 12). While expanded two-point discrimination in the median nerve distribution (≥ 6 mm) and the Tinel percussion test are the most specific findings in carpal tunnel syndrome, they are the least sensitive. The monofilament and median nerve compression tests appear to have the best combined sensitivity and specificity (see Chapter 40).[13,23,31]

is curative in a subset of patients with mild disease and is very helpful as a diagnostic tool. Patients who get temporary relief following injection are more apt to obtain similar relief from subsequent carpal tunnel release.[25] Job modification or rotation should be considered a part of initial treatment. Ergonomic evalua-tion with redesign of tools, work stations, and job requirements is helpful in this regard.

If patients have partial or only temporary relief following conservative measures and continue to have significant symptoms, surgical carpal canal decompression may be considered. Surgery is also indicated in the presence of thenar atrophy or diminished sensation. This may be performed under local or regional anesthesia as an outpatient procedure. Motion of the fingers is encouraged immediately after surgery to diminish tendon adhesions and digital stiffness. Newer approaches such as limited incision carpal tunnel releases[6,41] and releases done endoscopically have been developed to decrease the postoperative palm discomfort and quicken the return to activity and employment. The endoscopic technique has been shown to shorten the recovery period, but it has been associated with a higher incidence of complications including iatrogenic nerve injury.[1,8,10]

### Results

Splinting and injection provide dramatic short-term relief of symptoms in over 75% of patients when evaluated at six weeks.[19] It is curative in approximately 13 to 40% of patients followed for one year who had early diagnosis and milder disease. Conservative care may also diminish symptoms, obviating the need for carpal tunnel release in a much greater percentage. Good prognostic indicators of success with conservative treatment involve symptoms for less than one year, intermittent numbness, age over forty, male sex, and lack of advanced sensory changes and thenar atrophy.[19,60]

Operative release reliably improves pain and paresthesias. Improvement of numbness and weakness are less predictable. In patients with severe chronic nerve compression it is not unusual to have continued low-grade symptoms following a successful carpal tunnel release.[21] Individuals involved in strenuous labor may also have less complete relief of symptoms.[61] Palm and scar sensitivity, referred to as *pillar pain*, are quite common following median nerve release. Scar desensitization performed by an occupational therapist can be helpful in this regard when symptoms warrant. Scar tenderness characteristically resolves by 3 to 6 months but may take longer in some individuals. Returning to work with an anti-vibration glove to pad and protect the palm is often helpful. Activity restrictions are common for approximately six to eight weeks postoperatively. Grip strength improves predominantly over the first six months but can continue to improve for up to one year.[24,34] Most patients are able to return to their previous employment following successful carpal tunnel release.

## TENDINITIS/TENOSYNOVITIS

Tenosynovium functions as a low friction envelope around tendons, enhancing gliding through tendon sheaths or around bony prominences. Direct trauma, repetitive microtrauma, or repetitive shear forces can lead to inflammatory changes of this lining, termed *tenosynovitis*. This in turn leads to increased frictional forces with impaired tendon gliding. Pain, soft tissue swelling, and limited motion result. There is evidence that repetitive and forceful manual labor is associated with tendinitis of the hand and wrist.[4]

### DeQuervain's Tenosynovitis

#### Anatomy/Pathophysiology

The dorsal wrist contains six synovial-lined compartments that house the extensor tendons of the wrist and hand. The first compartment contains the abductor pollicis longus (APL) and the extensor pollicis brevis (EPB). It is located directly over the styloid process of the distal radius (Fig. 20-2). The compartment is an unyielding osteoligamentous tunnel approximately 1 to 2 cm in length with proximal and distal synovial extensions. Inflammation leads to tenosynovial proliferation, impeding excursion of the thumb tendons through this compartment. This is referred to as *DeQuervain's stenosing tenosynovitis.*

Repetitive microtrauma, an acute traumatic insult or more commonly repetitive activities requiring forceful grasping or pinching motions with the wrist flexed or ulnarly deviated are associated with De-Quervain's disease. It is also associated with rheumatoid arthritis, gout, and diabetes mellitus. A subdivision of the compartment by a septum appears to predispose individuals to the condition. In addition, it is seen more frequently in females by a ratio of 10:1 over males.

#### Diagnosis

Patients with DeQuervain's tenosynovitis experience pain, swelling, and tenderness at the base of the thumb over the radial styloid region. The pain is aggravated by thumb and wrist motion that are characteristically limited by the synovitis and fibrosis of the compartment. Crepitation with thumb flexion and extension is occasionally palpable as are small cysts (ganglia) over the diseased and inflamed compartment.

The Finkelstein test is the best objective tool in making the diagnosis of DeQuervain's tenosynovitis.[16] It consists in having the patient make a fist over the thumb, which is flexed into the palm, followed by ulnar deviation of the wrist (Fig. 20-3). This maneuver maximizes excursion of the tendons through the stenotic first dorsal compartment, producing significant discomfort if the condition is present. The differential diagnosis of DeQuervain's disease includes basilar thumb joint arthritis, trigger thumb, and other wrist tendonopathies that will be discussed below.

#### Treatment

Conservative treatment of DeQuervain's disease involves resting the inflamed tendons. Cortisone injections into the compartment are the mainstay of

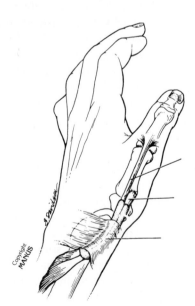

**FIGURE 20-2**    The first dorsal compartment of the wrist contains the abductor pollicis longus tendon and the short extensor of the thumb. These tendons pass through a fibroosseous tunnel that lies over the styloid process of the radius. Inflammation within this compartment leads to DeQuervain's stenosing tenosynovitis. *(Courtesy of the Indiana Hand Center, Indianapolis, Indiana.)*

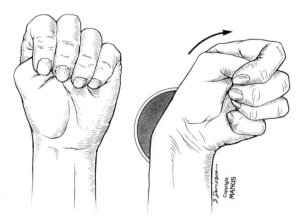

**FIGURE 20-3**    The Finkelstein test for DeQuervain's tenosynovitis involves ulnar deviation of the wrist with the thumb flexed into the palm. This increases the excursion of the first dorsal compartment tendons and leads to increased discomfort in individuals with this condition. *(Courtesy of the Indiana Hand Center, Indianapolis, Indiana.)*

treatment as is splint immobilization of the wrist and base of the thumb. The interphalangeal joint of the thumb can be left free, allowing use of the hand for writing or light activities. Nonsteroidal antiinflammatory medication may also be of benefit and job modification is required during initial treatment. Up to three cortisone injections are often performed over several weeks to months to diminish the inflammation and pain of the first dorsal compartment.

When conservative care fails to adequately relieve symptoms, surgical release of the compartment may be considered. This involves release of the fibrotic tendon sheath under local or regional anesthesia. Shortly after surgery, range of motion of the thumb and wrist is encouraged. Interval splinting is used if required for comfort and support initially.

## Results

First dorsal compartment release cures the vast majority of patients. Care must be made to adequately release all abnormal septa with the first compartment at surgery. Scar sensitivity is common following DeQuervain's release because branches of the dorsal radial sensory nerve lie directly over the compartment. Simple retraction of these nerves can cause hypersensitivity over the incision. A therapist can often help to desensitize the area and regain thumb and wrist motion and strength. Patients are generally able to return to unrestricted employment within four to eight weeks after surgery.

## Trigger Finger

### Anatomy/Pathophysiology

Stenosing tenosynovitis of the digital flexor tendons is referred to as trigger finger and trigger thumb. The digital flexor tendons enter an intricate set of pulleys that begin at the palmar metacarpophalangeal joint level (distal palmar flexion crease). The pulleys prevent bowstringing of the flexor tendons, thereby increasing the tendons' mechanical advantage during flexion. The first annular pulley acts as a fulcrum about which the flexor tendons bend. Inflammation in this region leads to tenosynovial proliferation with subsequent thickening of the tendon sheath and nodule development within the tendon (Fig. 20-4). Mechanical obstruction to tendon gliding follows with "catching or locking" of the digit. Once the trigger finger has developed, repeated attempts to pull the thickened tendon through the stenotic pulley aggravate the condition.

Trigger digits are associated with rheumatoid arthritis, gout, diabetes, amyloid deposition, and other metabolic conditions that cause changes within connective tissue and synovium. Repetitive resisted flexion of the digits is also associated with triggering. Repeated grasping with microtrauma to the palm produces high compressive and shear forces at the origin of the first annular pulley. This can contribute to the development of digital stenosing tenosynovitis.[5,47]

### Diagnosis

Symptoms of stenosing tenosynovitis can be present prior to the development of digital triggering. This involves tenderness along the palmar flexor tendon sheath over the first annular pulley in the distal palm with discomfort on repeated digital flexion. More commonly, patients have difficulty initiating extension of their fingers or thumb from a flexed position with accompanied pain. Examination reveals tenderness over the distal palmar flexion crease with a palpable nodule accentuated with active flexion and extension of the involved digit. Inability to completely extend the finger represents a "locked" or incarcerated trigger finger.

### Treatment

Conservative care of trigger digits involves activity modification along with cortisone injection into the digital flexor tendon sheath. Digital splinting of the metacarpophalangeal joint in extension for a short period may be added. In individuals whose trigger fingers are associated with the use of small narrow-handled tools, modification of these instruments to distribute forces over a greater area and require less digital flexion may be beneficial.[50]

If conservative management fails and symptoms warrant, surgical treatment may be considered.

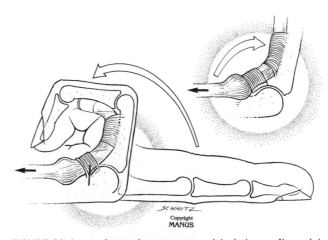

**FIGURE 20-4**    Stenosing tenosynovitis (trigger finger) involves the formation of a nodule on the flexor tendon that becomes restricted through a stenotic first annular pulley. Mechanical obstruction of the tendon ensues with "catching or locking" during digital motion. *(Courtesy of the Indiana Hand Center, Indianapolis, Indiana.)*

Surgery is also indicated in irreducibly locked digits. The operation consists of releasing the stenotic first annular pulley through a small palmar incision under local anesthesia. Patients are asked to actively flex and extend their fingers on the operating-room table to ensure adequate release. The postoperative dressing allows digital range of motion, which is encouraged.

### Results

Following injection, the majority of patients note a gradual decrease in triggering over the first one to two weeks. Reported cure rates following steroid injection range from 60 to 84%.[18,37,42] Recurrence of symptoms is often seen, especially if symptoms have been present for many months and the activity that led to the condition is not modified. Surgical release carries a 98% cure rate. Palmar incisional tenderness is quite common and often improves with occupational therapy scar programs. The therapist can also aid in regaining range of motion and strength of the involved digit. The majority of patients can return to unrestricted work activity between four and eight weeks postoperatively. Patients with diabetes or rheumatoid arthritis have a slower rehabilitation following surgical release.

### Other Tendonopathies of the Wrist/Hand

Tenosynovitis can occur in several less common tendons of the wrist and hand. *Intersection syndrome* refers to inflammation three to four fingerbreadths proximal to the wrist over the distal dorsoradial forearm. This is where the first dorsal compartment extensor tendons (APL/EPB) cross the second compartment tendons that radially extend the wrist (the extensor carpi radialis longus and brevis) (Fig. 20-5). This syndrome has been associated with repetitive use of the wrist in the workplace.[7] Patients exhibit inflammation and tenderness over this area often with palpable crepitation on wrist flexion and extension. Tenderness is well proximal and ulnar to the radial styloid process where it is seen in DeQuervain's disease.

Other wrist and digital tendons involved in tenosynovitis include the flexor carpi ulnaris (over the volar ulnar wrist flexion crease), the extensor carpi ulnaris (over the dorsal ulnar head), and the extensor pollicis longus (just ulnar to Lister's tubercle on the dorsal distal radius). Each of these is similar to DeQuervain's in its presentation with pain and limited range of motion. Treatment is also similar with splinting, activity modification, and steroid injection into the area of tenosynovitis. Surgical release is less

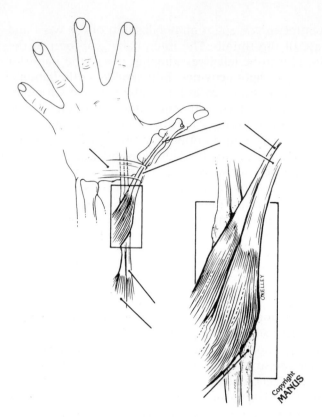

**FIGURE 20-5** Intersection syndrome involves inflammation at the intersection of the first and second dorsal wrist compartment tendons. Inflammation and discomfort occur several centimeters proximal to the radiocarpal joint. Crepitation is frequently palpable with wrist flexion and extension. *(Courtesy of the Indiana Hand Center, Indianapolis, Indiana.)*

commonly needed for these conditions, which usually respond to nonoperative measures.

### GANGLIA

Ganglia represent fluid-filled cavities that arise from a joint or tendon sheath. They contain lubricating fluid that is similar to the fluid within the sheath or tendon. Ganglia can arise from any joint capsule, interosseous ligament, or tendon sheath but occur in characteristic anatomical sites. The true cause of ganglia remains speculative, but most believe they represent the response of degenerative connective tissue to chronic stress. Direct or repetitive trauma is thought to lead to myxoid and mucinous degeneration of the normal capsular tissues or tendon sheath. This subsequently allows formation of an external cyst. Ganglion cysts communicate with the associated tendon or joint through a series of ducts that account for the intermittent enlargement and shrinking of the cyst seen clinically.[3,53]

## Carpal Ganglia

### Anatomy/Pathophysiology

Ganglia of the wrist occur most frequently over the dorsal radiocarpal joint near the midline of the dorsal wrist. They occur less commonly over the palmar radial carpus just radial to the flexor carpi radialis flexor tendon near the proximal palmar wrist flexion crease (Fig. 20-6). Dorsal ganglia predominantly arise from the scapholunate joint, whereas palmar ganglia most commonly originate from the scaphotrapezial region. The cysts may be multiloculated and far more extensive than clinically apparent. They can also exist quite far from their origin via a long stalk of ganglion tissue.

### Diagnosis

Patients with carpal ganglia complain of aching or vague discomfort of the wrist, which is exacerbated by activity. Loss of wrist motion secondary to pain may result. Occasionally an "occult" dorsal carpal ganglion will be too small to palpate. More commonly, a ganglion can be palpated as a firm mass or fullness in the aforementioned regions. Palmar flexion of the wrist will help accentuate the dorsally located cyst. If the diagnosis is in question, a needle aspiration will confirm the diagnosis of a cyst with the expression of clear jelly-like cyst material from the mass.

### Treatment

While wrist ganglia can lead to symptoms, they are often asymptomatic. Patients frequently request evaluation of a wrist lump that they noticed incidentally. These carpal ganglia may be tender to direct palpation, but they do not cause exertional discomfort or limit activities. No intervention is indicated for either asymptomatic or minimally symptomatic carpal ganglia.

For symptomatic dorsal carpal ganglia, aspiration and injection of cortisone into the cyst is successful in less than 50% of cases.[48] Injections are relatively contraindicated in volar wrist ganglia due to the close proximity of the radial artery. Temporary splinting of the wrist may lead to symptomatic improvement. Surgical excision of wrist ganglia is indicated only if symptoms warrant. This can be a rather extensive dissection to excise the entire ganglion down to the wrist capsule. As previously stated, the cysts can be quite loculated and extensive, originating far from the palpable mass. Volar wrist ganglia are usually intimate with the radial artery and are especially difficult in this regard.

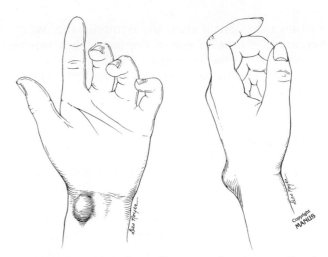

**FIGURE 20-6**    Carpal ganglia commonly arise over the dorsum of the wrist at the radiocarpal joint and at the palmar aspect of the wrist just radial to the flexor carpi radialis tendon. Ganglia can be multiloculated and thus more extensive than they appear on clinical examination. *(Courtesy of the Indiana Hand Center, Indianapolis, Indiana.)*

### Results

Surgical excision of carpal ganglia should offer a cure of the cyst in over 95% of cases. Failure to excise the deep capsular attachments of the cyst leads to a 30 to 50% recurrence rate.[2,3] The majority of recurrences occur within the first three months. Rehabilitation following cyst excision is very important. The majority of patients report continued low-grade aching for weeks to months following ganglion excision. Furthermore, wrist range of motion and strength returns slowly and usually requires a supervised occupational therapy program. Patients often lose a minor degree of terminal wrist motion postoperatively. This is more common in dorsal than palmar ganglia. Rapid rehabilitation of the wrist is important following surgery to decease the potential for wrist stiffness.

### Retinacular Ganglia

Ganglia arising from the flexor tendon digital sheath are termed *volar retinacular ganglia* or *retinacular cysts.* These show up as a small lump at the base of a digit adjacent to the digital flexor crease. The cyst is attached to the tendon sheath and thus does not move with the tendon like trigger finger nodules. Direct or repetitive microtrauma is implicated in their development.

Retinacular cysts are symptomatic due to their location on the palmar side of the digit. They commonly cause discomfort during activities that require gripping or holding objects in the palm. These ganglia need no treatment if they are asymptomatic. When they cause pain with use of the hand, they can be treated with needle aspiration and injection, with a higher rate of success than carpal cysts.[2,48] Alternatively, surgical excision performed under local anesthesia is usually successful.

## Mucous Cysts

Cysts that arise from degenerated distal interphalangeal joints are termed *mucous cysts*. These are invariably associated with osteoarthritis of the distal digital joint. Histologically they resemble ganglia and are believed to represent herniation of the synovial capsule with subsequent cyst formation.[29,30] Because of their location, mucous cysts can disrupt the germinal matrix of the nail and lead to longitudinal nail plate ridges or grooves (Fig. 20-7). Cysts can become quite tender when large and inflamed.

Aspiration and instillation of steroids may be attempted with mucous cysts, but they are rarely curative. Aspiration may also increase the likelihood of septic arthritis due to the poor soft-tissue cover of the distal interphalangeal joint. The cyst is related to joint degeneration and osteophytes, which must be removed to limit recurrence. Simple cyst excision carries a recurrence rate of 25% or greater.[29] Excision of the joint marginal osteophytes with the cyst is successful in over 95% of cases.[29,30] Recovery following mucous cyst excision is relatively rapid. Full and unrestricted use of the hand should be possible within three to six weeks.

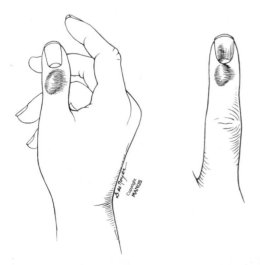

**FIGURE 20-7**   Mucous cysts are ganglia that arise from the distal interphalangeal joint. These cysts can compress the germinal nail matrix and lead to ridges or grooves in the nail plate. *(Courtesy of the Indiana Hand Center, Indianapolis, Indiana.)*

## Other Ganglia

Ganglion cysts can arise less commonly from any tendon sheath or joint in the hand. They can be found overlying the extensor tendons on the dorsum of the hand, the proximal interphalangeal joint of the fingers, or from a variety of carpal and carpometacarpal joints.[2] Treatment principles are similar to those discussed above.

## OSTEOARTHRITIS

Osteoarthritis is a slowly progressive disease of often unknown etiology. It appears to be part of the aging process, characteristically affecting the hands of middle-aged persons in a symmetrical distribution. The distal interphalangeal joint of the fingers is the most commonly affected joint in the hand, with the basilar thumb joint being the next most common. Osteoarthritis characteristically spares the metacarpophalangeal joints of the fingers. Hand involvement is more prevalent in females and there appears to be a hereditary component.[45] Several studies support overuse as having an influence on osteoarthritis of the hand.[43,45] The direct relationship of osteoarthritis to work, however, remains unclear.

### Wrist

#### Anatomy/Pathophysiology

Unlike the interphalangeal and basilar thumb joints, osteoarthritis of the wrist often occurs secondarily to a traumatic event or repetitive microtrauma. Intraarticular fractures of the distal radius, malunited or ununited scaphoid fractures, and ligamentous injuries all predispose the wrist to degeneration. Calcium pyrophosphate deposition disease has also been implicated in the development of wrist degenerative arthritis.[9,27] In many instances, however, a cause may not be readily identifiable.

An orderly sequence of joint deterioration has been described following ligamentous injury, scaphoid nonunion, and pyrophosphate deposition disease. This has been termed the *SLAC* (scapholunate advanced collapse) pattern of arthritis and is reportedly seen in over 70% of cases of osteoarthritis of the wrist.[59] Degeneration initially occurs at the distal radioscaphoid articulation, progressing to the proximal radioscaphoid joint and then to the capitolunate. The radiolunate joint is characteristically preserved. This degenerative pattern is occasionally associated with additional arthritis between the scaphoid, trapezium, and trapezoid.

### Diagnosis

Patients with wrist arthritis have pain, swelling over the dorsal carpus, loss of wrist mobility, and weakness. Crepitation during motion or loading activities is common in advanced disease. Examination reveals tenderness that is initially located at the tip of the radial styloid at its articulation with the scaphoid. Tenderness later becomes more global. Limitation of wrist motion is common as is weakness in grip strength. The diagnosis is confirmed on roentgenograms. Degeneration of the distal radioulnar joint is less common and manifests as pain and limitation of forearm rotation.

### Treatment

For early degenerative disease of the wrist, conservative measures are frequently successful. These include nonsteroidal antiinflammatory medication, wrist splints, activity modification, and steroid injection into the carpus. Once significant degenerative changes and pain have occurred, activity and job modification are usually required, as there is some degree of impairment. Intermittent wrist splint usage may be useful during more strenuous activities. Surgery is only indicated if conservative means fail and symptoms warrant. Options range from excision of the proximal row of carpal bones (proximal row carpectomy), various partial intercarpal fusions, and total wrist fusion. Surgical decision-making involves the type and degree of degenerative changes as well as the needs of the individual patient. Postoperative immobilization varies depending upon the surgical procedure and averages six to ten weeks for fusion procedures.

### Results

Like all degenerative joint disease, conservative therapy is more successful in less-advanced cases. Results of surgical treatment for wrist arthritis are favorable in terms of pain control. Motion retaining procedures such as partial wrist fusions and proximal row carpectomy require a considerable amount of therapy following cast removal. Grip strength and range of motion generally plateau by six months but can continue to improve for up to one year. Total wrist fusion is the most reliable in terms of pain relief and grip strength at the expense of wrist motion.

Impairment following partial or total wrist fusion involves primarily the loss of wrist motion. It may also include diminished grip strength and discomfort with heavy loading of the wrist. Potential restrictions following wrist reconstructive surgery must be determined on an individual basis, taking into account the degree of impairment and the specific job requirements.

## Thumb Basilar Joint

### Anatomy/Pathophysiology

The basilar joint of the thumb consists of the thumb metacarpal articulation with the trapezium. This is the most important joint of the hand as its unique saddle-shaped configuration affords the thumb exceptional mobility. It not only positions the thumb in space but provides a significant load-bearing function during pinch and grasp activities.[11] Arthritis of the basilar thumb joint is the second most common site for degenerative joint disease in the hand (following the distal interphalangeal joint). It is ten times more common in women than men.

### Diagnosis

Patients with basilar thumb joint arthritis have pain at the base of the thenar eminence with occasional proximal and distal radiation. The pain is exacerbated by pinching and gripping activities. It is characteristic for patients to have problems opening jars and turning door knobs. As the condition advances, pinch and grip strength are diminished and thumb range of motion becomes limited.

Examination often reveals a prominent carpometacarpal joint of the thumb as the metacarpal frequently subluxates in a radial and dorsal direction. Pain is reproduced when the joint is palpated on its radial and dorsal aspects. Stress applied to the joint through axial grinding and shearing of the base of the metacarpal radially exacerbates the pain (Fig. 20-8). This can be accompanied by palpable instability and crepitation. The Finkelstein test is

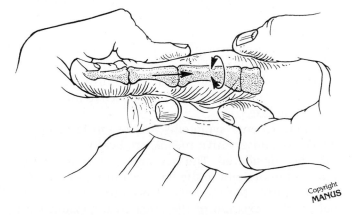

**FIGURE 20-8**    A thumb carpometacarpal joint "grind test" involves axial compression with rotation of the basilar thumb joint. This exacerbates the discomfort associated with basilar thumb joint degenerative arthritis. *(Courtesy of the Indiana Hand Center, Indianapolis, Indiana.)*

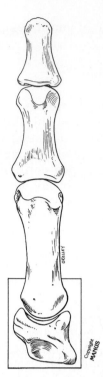

**FIGURE 20-9**     The Robert's view of the trapeziometacarpal (basilar thumb) joint is taken with the arm fully pronated, the shoulder internally rotated and the thumb abducted. This provides a true anteroposterior view of this saddle joint. *(Courtesy of the Indiana Hand Center, Indianapolis, Indiana.)*

negative, which helps distinguish basilar joint pain from DeQuervain's tenosynovitis. The diagnosis is confirmed by roentgenograms. These should include a hyperpronated anteroposterior Robert's view that readily projects the carpometacarpal joint (Fig. 20-9).[54]

### Treatment

Initial treatment of basilar thumb joint osteoarthritis includes activity modification, splint immobilization (leaving the interphalangeal joint free for writing and light activities), nonsteroidal antiinflammatory medication, and steroid injection into the joint. Splint wear is usually full-time for a period of three weeks. Conservative measures are more effective for less advanced disease.

When patients' symptoms are not satisfactorily relieved by conservative means, surgical intervention may be considered. The basilar thumb joint is the most common joint in the hand requiring surgery for osteoarthritis. Most surgical procedures require partial or total excision of the diseased trapezium with reconstruction or interposition using a wrist tendon.[15] These procedures require a short period of immobilization (three to four weeks) followed by a supervised rehabilitation program.

### Results

While pain relief is nearly universal, range-of-motion grip and pinch strength recover more slowly. Patients can continue to improve in these parameters for nine to twelve months postoperatively.[49] Work modification, therefore, may be required for many months following surgery.

Fusion of the basilar thumb joint is limited to younger individuals involved in manual labor. Arthrodesis provides excellent pain relief and strength at the expense of thumb mobility.[33] Fusion does lead to impairment secondary to the loss of thumb motion. However, individuals with a successful basilar thumb joint fusion should be able to return to heavy manual labor. Arthrodesis is contraindicated in the presence of scaphotrapezial degenerative changes.

### Proximal Interphalangeal Joints

#### Anatomy/Pathophysiology

Osteoarthritis of the proximal interphalangeal joint is relatively rare compared to the distal joint of the digit. Degeneration may be posttraumatic following an intraarticular fracture or joint dislocation. This is most likely the case in isolated arthritis of a single digit. Proximal interphalangeal joint degeneration occurs frequently in conjunction with distal joint degeneration, as solitary proximal interphalangeal joint involvement is highly unusual.[55]

#### Diagnosis

Swelling and stiffness is the first sign of early degenerative changes. Limited proximal interphalangeal joint motion follows with the development of marginal osteophytes (Bouchard's nodes.) Late joint degeneration leads to angular deformity and instability of the proximal interphalangeal joints (Fig. 20-10). A progressive loss of motion usually occurs although many severely involved joints will continue to function well with little discomfort. Roentgenograms confirm the diagnosis and document the degree of joint destruction (Fig. 20-11).

#### Treatment

Conservative measures of treatment include antiinflammatory medication, activity modification, and occasionally short-term splintage. Steroid injections can be used early in the degenerative process. If these fail and considerable symptoms remain, surgical intervention may be considered. Options include arthrodesis and Silastic replacement arthroplasty.[55,57] Arthrodesis is the most reliable method of eliminating pain and is superior in restoring pinch strength to the

Both procedures can be performed under a local or regional anesthetic block. Fusions are performed with pins, wires, or screws. Patients are protected postoperatively from heavy loading for approximately six to ten weeks or until fusion is documented on roentgenograms. Arthroplasties of the proximal interphalangeal joint should never be subjected to high stress or lateral shear forces to improve the longevity of the implant. They are thus preferred in lower demand individuals.

### Results

Fusion rates vary from 84 to 100% with excellent pain relief following successful arthrodesis.[35] Deformity is corrected and stability and strength are improved. Arthroplasties reliably preserve some motion and provide satisfactory pain relief.[55,57] Motion of the joint does, however, decrease over time. Arthroplasty carries the risk of implant failure, instability, and bone resorption around the implant.[44]

Impairment following fusion involves primarily the loss of joint motion. Grip strength may also be diminished, especially if the fusion involves the ulnar digits (which greatly contribute to grip strength). Impairment following arthroplasty may also include discomfort and instability.

### Distal Interphalangeal Joints

#### Anatomy/Pathophysiology

The distal interphalangeal joints of the fingers are the most frequently affected joints in the body in patients with osteoarthritis. Degeneration commonly involves multiple digits in a symmetrical distribution. In most cases, symptoms are mild and functional impairment is minimal. Isolated distal interphalangeal joint degeneration is usually the sequela of trauma to the joint. As previously stated, there is some evidence associating chronic overuse with degenerative disease in the small joints of the hand.[43,45]

#### Diagnosis

Swelling and stiffness are common in early joint degeneration. This typically occurs in the morning or after prolonged use of the digits. As the disease progresses, distal interphalangeal joint enlargement occurs secondary to osteophyte formation (Heberden's nodes) and painful limited motion results. Late in the disease joint deformity occurs with angular and rotational deformities of the digit tip. Roentgenograms again confirm the diagnosis and document the severity of involvement. Advanced disease is compatible with adequate function and minimal symptoms in many cases.

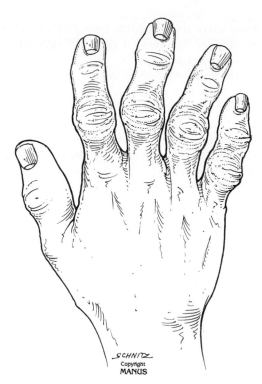

**FIGURE 20-10**    Late appearance of degenerative joint disease of the proximal interphalangeal joints. Osteophyte formation (Bouchard's nodes) leads to joint enlargement. Asymmetrical destruction leads to instability and angular deformity of the digits. *(Courtesy of the Indiana Hand Center, Indianapolis, Indiana.)*

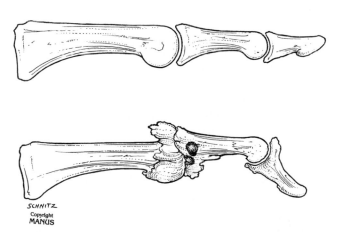

**FIGURE 20-11**    Proximal interphalangeal joint arthritis manifests as joint space narrowing and marginal osteophyte formation. Degenerative cysts and subchondral sclerosis are also prominent features of the degenerative process. *(Courtesy of the Indiana Hand Center, Indianapolis, Indiana.)*

index and middle digits. Fusion of the ulnar digits at the proximal interphalangeal level impairs grip strength and dexterity to a greater degree than the radial digits. Silicone arthroplasty preserves mobility but provides little stability to laterally directed forces.

## Treatment

Conservative care is successful in the majority of individuals. This includes nonsteroidal antiinflammatory medication with activity modification and occasional short-term splintage. Cortisone injections can also be of benefit. Surgery is reserved for late degenerative disease that does not respond to conservative measures and is causing significant pain, deformity, or instability. Distal interphalangeal joint arthrodesis is the procedure of choice, although Silastic arthroplasty can be considered for certain patients with special or limited needs.[12,52] Both procedures can be carried out under local anesthesia. Fusions are performed with screws or Kirschner wires. Postoperative protection from heavy loading is required for approximately six to ten weeks or until fusion is documented on roentgenograms.

## Results

Fusion reliably relieves pain, restores stability and strength, and improves the appearance of the involved digit. Successful distal interphalangeal joint fusion rates vary from 80 to 100%, with arthrodesis providing predictable long-lasting results.[28] Incisions placed at the pulp tip for screw insertion are frequently sensitive, requiring scar desensitization. Arthroplasty maintains some distal interphalangeal motion while providing adequate pain relief. Lateral instability and breakage of the implants are the potential complications.

Impairment following successful arthrodesis involves primarily the loss of motion and potential scar sensitivity. Impairment following arthroplasty may include additional discomfort and instability.

## REFLEX SYMPATHETIC DYSTROPHY

### Anatomy/Pathophysiology

Reflex sympathetic dystrophy (RSD) is a neurogenic disorder characterized by pain out of proportion to the level expected, swelling, vasomotor changes (autonomic dysfunction), and stiffness of the upper extremity. In the past it has been referred to by a variety of terms including *causalgia, Sudeck's atrophy,* and *shoulder-hand syndrome.* RSD can occur following a single traumatic event or a surgical procedure to the upper extremity. Alternatively, it can begin insidiously after the most trivial of injuries.

The pathogenesis of RSD remains poorly understood. Autonomic hyperactivity has been implicated in the syndrome. Nerve injuries are often linked to RSD. Psychological factors seem to play a role in many cases. Some clinicians believe in a diathesis or constitutional predisposition with dystrophy patients being more anxious, insecure, hysterical, passive-aggressive, or over-reactive to pain.[14,32] Whether patient personality characteristics predispose to the condition or are secondary is debatable. In either event, psychological factors clearly aggravate the symptom complex when present.

In many cases, full-blown reflex dystrophy progresses through a series of loosely defined stages. Initially pain, swelling, restricted motion, and vasomotor changes (hyperhidrosis, erythema and excessive warmth) predominate the symptom complex. Later, after several months, pain remains the dominant feature and swelling changes from a soft to a hard brawny edema. The hand becomes dry, stiff, and atrophied. Lastly, after many months to years, the skin assumes a shiny, glossy appearance and stiffness becomes marked with fixed contractures. It must be understood that all cases of RSD do not fit this temporal scheme. The condition represents a continuum with a variable presence and intensity of symptoms.

### Diagnosis

The diagnosis of RSD is made primarily on clinical findings but may be confirmed by a variety of objective tests. Diffuse pain out of proportion to the initial injury, diminished hand function secondary to stiffness or pain, and sympathetic dysfunction (edema, hyperhidrosis or anhidrosis, atrophy of skin, hair or nail changes, warmth or coolness, discoloration of skin) are present in varying degrees. The pain is frequently described as burning and intense and may be exacerbated with a light touch of the skin. Roentgenograms frequently reveal diffuse osteopenia secondary to demineralization within three to five weeks after the onset of symptoms. Three-phase bone scans show characteristic diffuse uptake in the involved areas.[14] Sympathetic blockade through stellate ganglion blockade or intravascular reserpine or guanethidine remains the most definitive means of establishing the diagnosis. Immediate relief following blockade confirms the presence of RSD.

### Treatment

The key to successful treatment of RSD is prompt diagnosis and intervention to break the pain cycle. Treatment should be initiated as soon as the diagnosis is suspected because prevention of the full-blown syndrome is the goal of therapy. The appearance and persistence of inordinate postoperative pain may be the first sign of early RSD. Care should be taken to eliminate any potential painful stimuli (wound hematoma, cast compression, etc).

Supervised active range of motion exercises, edema control, and interval splinting are initiated by an experienced therapist. A stress-loading program

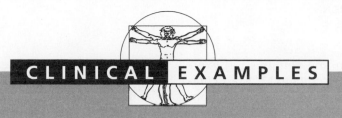

# CLINICAL EXAMPLES

## HAND AND WRIST

EDITOR'S NOTE—The assessment of the hand and wrist is complex because there are so many bones (19 in the hand and 8 in the wrist), joints, soft tissue structures, and planes of motion to be considered. Sections 3.1a to 3.1l of the AMA *Guides* clearly describe and illustrate these areas to facilitate the performance of the physical examination.* The guidelines set forth must be faithfully followed to avoid deriving nonequivalent figures.

Section 3.1m describes various clinical/pathological disorders. Exaggerated impairment percentages may be obtained following the methods outlined in Section 3.1m, so this section should only be used when the pathology can be more clearly described by the 3.1m subsections than by Sections 3.1a through 3.1l.

### EXAMPLE
#### History
A 29-year-old man injured his left index finger at work two years previously. He has no symptoms other than a minimal loss of strength.

#### Physical Examination
Range of motion (ROM) results are as follows:

| | |
|---|---|
| **DIP joint:** | Flexion (F), 20°; extension (E), 20° |
| **PIP joint:** | F, 70°; E, 20° |
| **MCP joint:** | F, 70°; E, 10° |

There is a slight loss of strength in the left index finger when compared to the right one. Two-point discrimination is intact at 7 mm except for the distal finger, where it is at 15 mm only.

*All *sections,* *figures,* and *tables* referred to in this discussion are found in the AMA *Guides to the evaluation of permanent impairment,* ed 4, Chapter 3—The Musculoskeletal System, American Medical Association, Chicago, 1993.

### Assessment Process
For the ROM abnormalities, the impairment percentages are as follows:

| | |
|---|---|
| **DIP:** | F (26%) + E (0%) = 26% |
| **PIP:** | F (18%) + E (0%) = 18% |
| **MCP:** | F (11%) + E (7%) = 18% |

(Note that F is added to E for each joint; see Figs. 12 to 14.) The Combined Values Chart (pp. 322–324) is used to derive the total ROM abnormalities. (Note that the impairments for each joint of the finger are *combined* rather than *added.*) Thus 26% is combined with 18% to yield a 39% value. The 39% is then combined with the remaining 18% for a total ROM value of 50%.

The sensory abnormality is 50% (p. 21) of 10% (Fig. 15), yielding a 5% sensory deficit. This is then combined with the 50% ROM impairment, yielding a 53% impairment of the right index finger (again note that these are combined rather than added).

Finally, Tables 1 to 3 are used to derive a whole person impairment (WPI) value. A 53% impairment of the index finger yields an 11% impairment of the hand, 11% of the hand yields a 10% of the upper extremity, and 10% of the upper extremity yields a 6% of the whole person. (Note that there is no distinction for "handedness," that is, whether the impairment exists in the dominant or nondominant hand. The *Guides* state: "Little evidence exists that there is a significant difference in grip strength between the dominant and nondominant hand. The *Guides* does not recognize such a difference" [p. 65].)

#### Evaluation
This individual with a well-healed, static impairment of the left index finger has a 6% WPI.

*Stephen L. Demeter*

consisting of active traction and compression exercises has also been shown to be helpful.[58] Transcutaneous electrical nerve stimulation (TENS) is occasionally useful in controlling pain in the early stages of RSD. Pharmacologic intervention involves the use of oral corticosteroids, alpha blockers, calcium channel blockers, and antidepressants. Stellate ganglion blocks provide immediate pain relief and are an integral component of treatment. They often must be repeated to break the cycle of RSD pain. Occasionally, a continuous stellate ganglion block is utilized.

Surgical intervention in RSD must be considered cautiously. Only if an identifiable pathological condition is present and thought to be contributing to the condition is this considered. Examples include a painful neuroma or compressive neuropathy that may have precipitated the condition. Surgery should not be performed if motion and function are improving. Perioperative stellate blockade is useful to thwart a possible flare-up of symptoms. Surgical sympathectomy is sometimes required in refractory cases.

## Results

The earlier intervention is instituted, the better the chance for a successful result. Once the chronic stages of RSD have occurred, results are much less favorable, with chronic stiffness and diminished function commonly resulting. In these patients, significant long-term impairment is the rule.

## References

1. Agee JM, McCarroll HR, Tortosa RD, et al: Endoscopic release of the carpal tunnel: a randomized prospective multicenter study. *J Hand Surg* 17A:987-995, 1992.
2. Angelides AC: Ganglions of the wrist and hand. In Green DP, editor: *Operative hand surgery*, ed 3, New York, 1993, Churchill Livingstone, pp 2157-2171.
3. Angelides AC, Wallace PF: The dorsal ganglion of the wrist: its pathogenesis, gross and microscopic anatomy, and surgical management. *J Hand Surg* 1:228-235, 1976.
4. Armstrong TJ, Fine LJ, Goldstein SA, et al: Ergonomic considerations in hand and wrist tendonitis. *J Hand Surg* 12A:830-837, 1987.
5. Bonnici AV, Spenser JD: A survey of "trigger finger" in adults. *J Hand Surg* 15:290-293, 1988.
6. Bromley GS: Minimal-incision open carpal tunnel decompression. *J Hand Surg* 19A:119-120, 1994.
7. Brooker AF: Extensor carpi radialis tenosynovitis: an occupational affliction. *Orthop Rev* 6:99-100, 1977.
8. Brown RA, Gelberman RH, Seiler JG, et al: Carpal tunnel release: a prospective randomized assessment of open and endoscopic methods. *J Bone Joint Surg* 75A:1265-1275, 1993.
9. Chen C, Chandnani VP, Kang HS, et al: Scapholunate advanced collapse: a common wrist abnormality in calcium pyrophosphate dihydrate crystal deposition disease. *Radiol* 177:459-461, 1990.
10. Chow JC: Endoscopic release of the carpal ligament for carpal tunnel syndrome: a 22-month clinical result. *Arthroscopy* 6:288-296, 1990.
11. Cooney WP, Chao EYS: Biomechanical analysis of static forces in the thumb during hand function. *J Bone Joint Surg* 59A:27, 1977.
12. Culver JE, Fleeger ES: Osteoarthritis of the distal interphalangeal joint. *Hand Clin* 3:385-402, 1987.
13. Durkam JA: A new diagnostic test for carpal tunnel syndrome. *J Bone Joint Surg* 73A:535-538, 1991.
14. Dzwierzynski WW, Sanger JR: Reflex sympathetic dystrophy. *Hand Clin* 10:29-43, 1994.
15. Eaton RG, Glickel SZ: Trapezial metacarpal osteoarthritis: staging as a rationale for treatment. *Hand Clin* 3:455-469, 1987.
16. Finkelstein H: Stenosing tenosynovitis of the radial styloid process. *J Bone Joint Surg* 30A:509, 1930.
17. Franklin GM, Haug J, et al: Occupational carpal tunnel syndrome in Washington State, 1984-1988. *Am J Public Health* 81(6):74, 1991.
18. Freiberg A, Mulholland RS, Levine R: Nonoperative treatment of trigger fingers and thumbs. *J Hand Surg* 14A:553-558, 1989.
19. Gelberman RH, Aronson D, Weisman MH: Carpal tunnel syndrome: results of a prospective trial of steroid injection and splinting. *J Bone Joint Surg* 62A:1181-1184, 1980.
20. Gelberman RH, Hergenroeder PT, Hargens AR, et al: The carpal tunnel syndrome: a study of carpal tunnel pressures. *J Bone Joint Surg* 63A:380, 1981.
21. Gelberman RH, Rydevik BL, Pess GM, et al: Carpal tunnel syndrome: a scientific basis for clinical care. *Orthop Clin North Am* 19:115-124, 1988.
22. Gelberman RH, Szabo RM, Williamson RV, et al: Sensitivity testing in peripheral-nerve compression syndromes. *J Bone Joint Surg* 65A:632-638, 1983.
23. Gellman H, Gelberman RH, Tan AM, et al: Carpal tunnel syndrome: an evaluation of the provocative diagnostic tests. *J Bone Joint Surg* 68A:735-737, 1986.
24. Gellman H, Kan D, Gee V, et al: Analysis of pinch and grip strength after carpal tunnel release. *J Hand Surg* 14A:863-864, 1989.
25. Green DP: Diagnostic and therapeutic value of

carpal tunnel injection. *J Hand Surg* 9A:850-854, 1984.

26. Grundberg AB: Carpal tunnel decompression in spite of normal electromyography. *J Hand Surg* 8:348-349, 1983.

27. Harrington RH, Lichtman DM, Brockmole DM: Common pathways of degenerative arthritis of the wrist. *Hand Clin* 3:507-525, 1987.

28. Jones BF, Stern PJ: Interphalangeal joint arthrodesis. *Hand Clin* 10:267-275, 1994.

29. Kasdan ML, Stallings SP, Leis VM, et al: Outcome of surgically treated mucous cysts of the hand. *J Hand Surg* 504-507, 1994.

30. Kleinert HE, Kutz JE, Fishman JH, et al: Etiology and treatment of the so-called mucous cyst of the finger. *J Bone Joint Surg* 54A:1455-1458, 1972.

31. Koris M, Gelberman RH, Duncan K, et al: Carpal tunnel syndrome: evaluation of a quantitative provocational diagnostic test. *Clin Orthop Rel Res* 251:157-161, 1990.

32. Lankford LL: Reflex sympathetic dystrophy. In Green DP, editor: *Operative hand surgery*, ed 3, New York, 1993, Churchill Livingstone, pp 627-660.

33. Leach RE, Bolton PE: Arthritis of the carpal metacarpal joint of the thumb: results of arthrodesis. *J Bone Joint Surg* 50A:1171, 1986.

34. Leach WJ, Esler C, Scott TD: Grip strength following carpal tunnel decompression. *J Hand Surg* 18B:750-752, 1993.

35. Leibovic SJ, Strickland JW: Arthrodesis of the proximal interphalangeal joint of the finger: comparison of the use of Herbert screw with other fixation methods. *J Hand Surg* 19A:181-188, 1994.

36. Louis DS, Hankin FM: Symptomatic relief following carpal tunnel decompression with normal electromyographic studies. *Orthop* 10:434-436, 1987.

37. Marks MR, Gunter SF: Efficacy of cortisone injection in treatment of trigger fingers and thumbs. *J Hand Surg* 14A:722-727, 1989.

38. Masear VR, Hayes JM, Hyde AG: An industrial cause of carpal tunnel syndrome. *J Hand Surg* 11A:222-227, 1986.

39. Miller RF, Lohman WH, Maldonado G, et al: An epidemiologic study of carpal tunnel syndrome and hand-arm vibration syndrome in relation to vibration exposure. *J Hand Surg* 19A:99-105, 1994.

40. Moberg E: Objective methods of determining functional value of sensibility in the hand. *J Bone Joint Surg* 44:454, 1958.

41. Nathan PA, Meadows KD, Keniston RC: Rehabilitation of carpal tunnel syndrome patients using a short surgical incision and an early program of physical therapy. *J Hand Surg* 18A:1044-1050, 1993.

42. Otto N, Wehbe MA: Steroid injections for tenosynovitis in the hand. *Orthop Rev* 15:290-293, 1986.

43. Palmieri TJ, Grand FM, Hay EL, et al: Treatment of osteoarthritis in the hand and wrist. *Hand Clin* 3:371-381, 1987.

44. Pelligrini VD, Burton RI: Osteoarthritis of the proximal interphalangeal joint of the hand: arthroplasty or fusion? *J Hand Surg* 15A:184-209, 1990.

45. Peyron JG: The epidemiology of osteoarthritis. In Moskowitz R, Howell D, Goldberg V, et al, editors: *Osteoarthritis: diagnosis and management*, Philadelphia, 1984, WB Saunders, pp 9-27.

46. Phalen GS: The carpal tunnel syndrome: seventeen years experience in diagnosis and treatment of 654 hands. *J Bone Joint Surg* 48A:211-228, 1966.

47. Pruzansky M: Stenosing tenosynovitis. In Chapman MW, editor: *Operative orthopaedics*, ed 2, Philadelphia, 1993, JB Lippincott, pp 1223-1235.

48. Richman JA, Gelberman RH, Engber WD, et al: Ganglions of the wrist and digits: results of treatment by aspiration and cyst wall puncture. *J Hand Surg* 12A:1041-1043, 1987.

49. Robinson D, Aghasi M, Halperin N: Abductor pollicis longus tendon arthroplasty of the trapezial-metacarpal joint: surgical technique and results. *J Hand Surg* 16A:504-509, 1991.

50. Rosenthal E: Tenosynovitis: tendon and nerve entrapment. *Hand Clin* 3:585-607, 1987.

51. Saunders WE: The occult dorsal carpal ganglion. *J Hand Surg* 10B:257-260, 1985.

52. Snow JW, Boyes JG, Greider JL: Implant arthroplasty of the proximal interphalangeal joint of the finger for osteoarthritis. *Plastic Recon Surg* 60:558-560, 1977.

53. Soren A: Pathogenesis and treatment of ganglions. *Clin Orthop* 48:173, 1966.

54. Steinberg DR: Management of the arthritic hand. In Chapman MW, editor: *Operative orthopaedics*, ed 2, Philadelphia, 1993, JB Lippincott, pp 1571-1578.

55. Stern PJ, Ho S: Osteoarthritis of the proximal interphalangeal joint. *Hand Clin* 3:405-412, 1987.

56. Stewart JD, Eisen A: Tinel's sign and the carpal tunnel syndrome. *Brit Med J* 2:1125-1126, 1978.

57. Swanson AB, Maupin BK, Gajjar NV, et al: Flexible implant arthroplasty in the proximal interphalangeal joint of the hand. *J Hand Surg* 10A:796-805, 1985.

58. Watson HK, Carlson L: Treatment of relex sympathetic dystrophy of the hand with an active

"stress loading" program. *J Hand Surg* 12A:779-785, 1987.

59. Watson HK, Vender MI: Wrist and intercarpal arthrodesis. In Chapman MW, editor: *Operative orthopaedics,* ed 2, Philadelphia, 1993, JB Lippincott, pp 1363-1377.

60. Weiss AP, Sachar K, Gendreau M: Conservative management of carpal tunnel syndrome: a re-examination of steroid injection and splinting. *J Hand Surg* 19A:410-415, 1994.

61. Yu GZ, Firrell JC, Tsai TM: Preoperative factors and treatment outcome following carpal tunnel release. *J Hand Surg* 17B:646-650, 1992.

# CHAPTER 21

# JOINT SYSTEMS: SHOULDER AND ELBOW

*Anthony A. Romeo*

## INTRODUCTION

Occupational disorders of the shoulder and elbow affect a substantial section of the workforce in the United States, with employment-related upper extremity and shoulder impairment occurring in more than 500,000 workers per year in the United States.[98] After back and knee conditions, the shoulder is the most common site of long-term impairment. Injuries to the shoulder area are usually related to overexertion, direct trauma, or a fall.[97]

Conditions of the shoulder and elbow resulting in impairment can be divided into two main categories: mechanical and nonmechanical. Nonmechanical problems are characteristically not related to specific activities or positions. They are difficult to localize, and are frequently accompanied by sensations of hot or cold, numbness, and intermittent swelling. Nonmechanical conditions are difficult to categorize into specific diagnostic groups and therefore make evaluation and treatment complex.

Mechanical conditions characteristically become symptomatic during certain activities and positions. They are reproducible, well-localized, and described by the patient in terms such as "weakness", "stiffness", "slipping" or "catching". For example, a muscle tear will be associated with weakness, whereas arthritis is generally associated with stiffness. Mechanical conditions often have typical signs and symptoms, leading to well-recognized diagnostic categories for which evaluation and management strategies have been developed.

## SHOULDER DISORDERS

Acute injuries to the shoulder include contusions, ligamentous sprains, muscular strains, and fractures. Treatment should be initiated within hours of the initial injury. The RICE concept of treatment includes rest, ice, compression, and elevation. This regimen provides relief of pain and limits inflammation and swelling. Physician evaluation should include a careful history with respect to the mechanism of injury, including the forces involved and the position of the arm at the time of injury. A thorough physical examination is followed by supporting radiographs.

If complaints such as pain and soreness are the patient's primary problem, the physician should initiate the RICE treatment protocol. Nonsteroidal antiinflammatory agents are often helpful in managing pain and inflammation. Physical therapy can be instituted early to maintain shoulder motion and gradually return the patient's shoulder to baseline strength. Most of these conditions improve within four to six weeks. If symptoms persist, particularly mechanical symptoms, then consideration of specific shoulder conditions should ensue.

### Impingement Syndrome

The most complex issue in the diagnosis of shoulder disorders relates to the diagnosis of "impingement syndrome".[73-75] The proposed pathophysiology is abutment of the proximal humerus and rotator cuff against the anterior acromion when the arm is in forward elevation (Fig. 21-1). The impingement syndrome is generally divided into three stages based on characteristic pathology and age. Stage I consists of reversible edema and hemorrhage in the rotator cuff tendon and subacromial bursa, usually seen in patients under the age of 25. Stage II consists of fibrosis and tendinitis of the rotator cuff (primarily the supraspinatus), typically in patients between 25 and 40 years of age. The pathology may not be reversible, and recurrence of pain with activity is common. Stage III includes acromion spur formation with associated rotator cuff tendon ruptures, usually in patients over the age of 40.

Unfortunately, the physical examination and radiographs are often insufficient to diagnose conclusively the impingement syndrome. Physical examina-

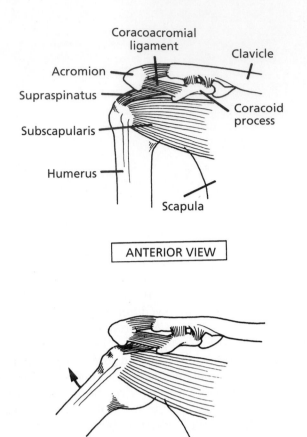

Coracoacromial
ligament

Clavicle

Acromion

Supraspinatus

Coracoid
process

Subscapularis

Humerus

Scapula

ANTERIOR VIEW

**FIGURE 21-1** Anatomy of the rotator cuff and acromion as it pertains to the impingement syndrome. Notice the potential abutment of the acromion on the rotator cuff when the arm is maximally elevated.

tion findings may include pain with forward elevation, posterior shoulder stiffness as evidenced by decreased cross-body adduction and internal rotation up the back, increased symptoms with rotation of the arm at 90° shoulder abduction, and a positive "impingement sign."[73] To demonstrate the impingement sign, the scapula is stabilized with the examiner's opposite hand, then the humerus is elevated in slight internal rotation so that the greater tuberosity progresses directly under the anterior acromion. These various findings are "sensitive" to shoulder conditions, but not "specific" to subacromial impingement. The accuracy of the physical examination may be improved by the impingement test. The subacromial space is injected with a local anesthetic such as 10 ml of 1% lidocaine. This injection ideally will eliminate the impingement sign, suggesting that the pathology does in fact exist in the subacromial space and rotator cuff region.

Additional useful information includes the clinical course of the symptoms and the response to treatment. This crucial information is often distorted when

issues of secondary gain are present. Nonoperative treatment primarily includes exercises that should be performed by the patient on a daily basis. The goal of therapy should be maximal shoulder flexibility, especially working on the posterior shoulder structures. Although circumduction motions, forward elevation, and external rotation are most frequently performed as part of the therapy, the presence of posterior tightness should encourage the use of internal rotation and cross-body adduction exercises as essential components of an effective stretching program. Once pain-free range of motion has improved, a strengthening program can be advanced. Strengthening is begun with isometric flexion, extension, abduction, and internal and external rotation with the elbow at the patient's side. Isometric exercise can then be advanced to include "theraband" exercises, then free-weights. Exercises that essentially reproduce the impingement sign (i.e., forward elevation of the arm with the patient's thumb directed toward the ground) should be strongly discouraged unless the patient has had more than three months of pain-free shoulder motion and is under the age of 40. Physical modalities such as ultrasonography are frequently used, but there is little objective evidence for their efficacy.[29] There is a paucity of literature on the natural history of impingement syndrome or the outcome of nonoperative management such as physical therapy, although most physicians believe that the majority of patients with this diagnosis improve without surgical management.[44,71]

Plain radiographic studies are obtained to rule out any contributing causes to impingement-like symptoms, such as calcific tendinitis. Standard radiographic evaluation of the shoulder should always include a true anteroposterior view of the glenohumeral joint and an axillary lateral view.[89] These two views will provide sufficient information for radiographic evaluation in the majority of patients with shoulder conditions. Supplementary views for impingement syndrome are directed toward better visualization of the acromion and include the supraspinatus outlet view[2] as well as the 30° caudal tilt view.[89] Radiographic studies are often noncontributory, especially in patients under the age of 40. Associated, nonspecific findings may include greater tuberosity sclerosis and cyst formation, acromial spurring, and degenerative changes of the acromioclavicular joint.

If a well-motivated patient does not respond to physical therapy after six to eight weeks of rehabilitation, a study to image the rotator cuff is indicated. Double-contrast arthrography of the glenohumeral joint is the gold standard for imaging the rotator cuff.[67] The accuracy of this test is greater than 95%.[40]

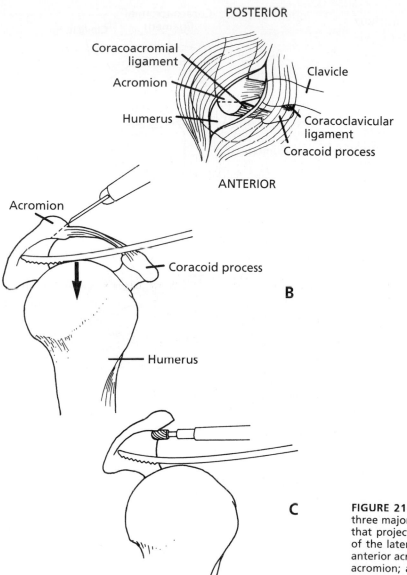

POSTERIOR

Coracoacromial ligament

Acromion

Humerus

Clavicle

Coracoclavicular ligament

Coracoid process

**A**

ANTERIOR

Acromion

Coracoid process

**B**

Humerus

**C**

**FIGURE 21-2** Technique of anterior acromioplasty. The three major steps include: (**A**) removal of the anterior acromion that projects beyond the plane parallel to the anterior surface of the lateral clavicle; (**B**) removal of the inferior aspect of the anterior acromion, parallel to the slope created by the posterior acromion; and (**C**) final smoothing of the undersurface of the acromion with a burr or rasp.

Ultrasonography has been proposed as an effective noninvasive method to image the rotator cuff,[62] but its use has not been widespread. Magnetic resonance imaging (MRI) has become the most frequently used imaging study of the shoulder after plain radiographs. MRI has replaced shoulder arthrograms in many centers after initial reports demonstrated sensitivity of 100% and specificity of 95% in the diagnosis of full-thickness rotator cuff tears.[6,47,48] However, MRI may not be able to discriminate between rotator cuff tendinitis, partial thickness tears of the rotator cuff, and small full-thickness tears of the rotator cuff. The studies are often overread, leading to a significant rate of false-positive results (i.e., full-thickness rotator cuff tear), especially in younger patients.[66] These false-positive reports encourage surgical intervention in a patient population that would be expected to have a high success rate with conservative management. MRI appears to have its greatest value at the two ends of the rotator cuff disease spectrum: no abnormalities or complete tears of the rotator cuff.

The timing of surgical management for impingement syndrome is not well defined. Surgical intervention appears to be indicated in patients with persistent impairment for one year despite adequate conservative treatment, including a well-motivated effort to eliminate stiffness.[3,31,37,42,44,46,60,64,73,74,83,90] Patients under the age of 40 must be carefully selected.[46,64]

Positive prognostic indicators of surgical success include well-motivated patients over the age of 40, the absence of posterior shoulder stiffness, the presence of reproducible subacromial crepitance, and pain relieved by the subacromial injection of lidocaine.[64,88] Poor prognostic factors include age under 40, stiffness, lack of relief by subacromial injection, attribution of the problem to occupation, concomitant evidence of glenohumeral instability, and neurogenic rotator cuff muscle weakness.

The surgical technique of subacromial decompression has been well-described, whether performed through an open shoulder incision or arthroscopically (Fig. 21-2).[3,37,42,44,46,64,73,74,83,90] Postoperative rehabilitation begins with an early range-of-motion program. During the first month, patients that have undergone an open procedure are started on a passive range of motion program, while patients that have undergone an arthroscopic procedure are advanced quickly to an active-assisted range-of-motion program. After one month, the two groups are rehabilitated at a similar pace. By eight weeks, a full range of motion should be achieved. The expected return to work is within three months, with maximum medical improvement achieved by three to six months in well-motivated patients. If favorable preoperative prognostic factors are present, the procedure is predictably effective; however, workers' compensation patients generally demonstrate results that are inferior to nonworkers' compensation patients.[44,46,83] In fact, approximately 25% of workers' compensation patients who are treated with an acromioplasty will demonstrate permanent impairment prohibiting return to their previous occupation. Furthermore, if a workers' compensation patient continues to have unresolving shoulder pain for nine months or more following an acromioplasty, the likelihood of their return to their previous occupation is less than 15%, even if a revision acromioplasty is performed.[45]

Three diagnoses that are often associated or labeled impingement syndrome include partial-thickness rotator cuff injury, full-thickness rotator cuff injury, and subacromial abrasion.

## Partial rotator cuff injury

The rotator cuff is defined by the coalescence of tendons from the subscapularis, supraspinatus, infraspinatus, and teres minor as they insert on the proximal humerus adjacent to the articular surface (Fig. 21-3). Its function is paramount to normal shoulder function, although other muscles may compensate remarkably in the absence of the rotator cuff. The rotator cuff is highly resistant to injury in people under the age of 40; however, increasing age and disuse are associated with its failure. Symptomatic partial tears of the rotator cuff usually occur in younger patients between the ages of 30 and 50.[65] They are almost always associated with tearing of the supraspinatus tendon, most commonly on the undersurface of the tendon.[17] Patients commonly report an injury where an unexpected or overwhelming eccentric load was

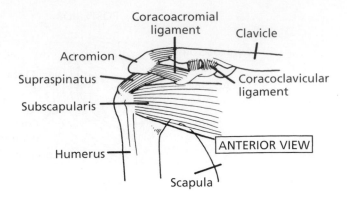

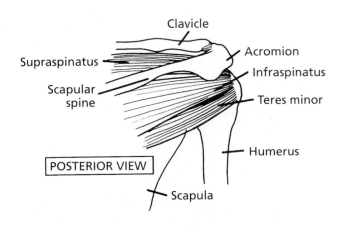

**FIGURE 21-3**    Rotator cuff anatomy. The rotator cuff is formed by the coalescence of the tendons from the supraspinatus, infraspinatus, teres minor, and subscapularis as they insert on the tuberosities of the humerus. The supraspinatus is most commonly involved in pathologic processes that affect the rotator cuff. Note its position in relationship to the anterior acromion.

applied to the arm, resulting in shoulder pain. Mechanical symptoms include difficulty in active elevation, especially against resistance.

The physical examination must be effective in eliminating other diagnoses, while focusing on the rotator cuff. The most sensitive provocative test is the impingement sign, which is frequently positive in various shoulder conditions.[74,76] The most specific sign of rotator cuff pathology is weakness of the rotator cuff.[11,63,75] The strength of the cuff muscles can be tested by resisted elevation of the arm at 90° and resisted external rotation with the elbow at the patient's side. External rotation weakness may be directly related to cuff deficiency.[11] Patients are generally able to move the shoulder through a substantial arc of motion, but resisted external rotation and abduction results in increased pain and is consistent with rotator cuff pathology (positive cuff signs).[65] Associated findings with partial rotator cuff tears include mild atrophy of the supraspinatus muscle belly (located in the supraspinatus fossa of the scapula), and crepitation emanating from the subacromial space when the arm is internally and externally rotated in abduction. Also, stiffness of the posterior shoulder is frequently demonstrated. The patient will have limited internal rotation and cross-body adduction, signifying posterior shoulder stiffness.

Although the diagnosis of partial-thickness rotator cuff tears may be strongly suspected from the history and physical examination, it must be differentiated from small full-thickness tears. This distinction is important as the management of the two conditions differs. Plain radiographs are of little benefit in differentiating partial-thickness tears from small full-thickness tears. Double-contrast arthrography of the glenohumeral joint has the ability to distinguish partial thickness from full thickness tears, and is considered the gold standard for imaging the rotator cuff.[67] The value of MRI in the determination of partial-thickness tears appears to be inferior to double-contrast arthrography at this time. The integrity of the rotator cuff should be evaluated with an advanced imaging study if there is a poor response to treatment after six weeks. Additionally, if 80% of preinjury level of function has not been achieved by three months, an imaging study is recommended.

The management of partial-thickness rotator cuff tear begins with the RICE protocol. Nonsteroidal anti-inflammatory medication is useful for decreasing symptoms of pain and inflammation. Physical therapy is essential due to the associated stiffness that frequently accompanies this condition. The therapist needs to specifically instruct the patient to work on flexibility of the posterior aspect of the shoulder. Internal rotation and cross-body adduction, as well as the traditional motions of forward elevation and external rotation, must be stressed.[63,65] Most patients experience a substantial reduction in their shoulder symptoms within six weeks.[71] Return to one-handed work can begin after the acute symptoms have improved (one to two weeks), with a gradual advance of work responsibilities using the involved limb. If the patient is well-motivated and responds to physical therapy, maximum medical improvement should be achieved by three months.

Despite appropriate management and a motivated patient, symptoms may persist well beyond the three months. These symptomatic, partial-thickness rotator cuff tears pose a dilemma for the patient, the physician, and the workers' compensation system. There is good evidence that these conditions continue to improve beyond three months, and that very few patients need surgery if appropriate management continues for up to one year.[44,46,64,71,73,74,83] However, employers and insurance companies are generally not willing to accept limitations for up to one year. Six months of nonoperative management is generally accepted. If a patient has a partial-thickness cuff tear, or if the patient does not improve by six months, surgery can be considered. If a full-thickness tear is demonstrated on the imaging studies, repair is indicated.

Surgical treatment of partial-thickness rotator cuff tears includes acromioplasty, with or without a repair of the torn section of the rotator cuff. The gold standard is an acromioplasty performed through an open incision as previously discussed. Recent reports have suggested that arthroscopic acromioplasties may return the patient's function sooner than open acromioplasties.[3,37] However, the arthroscopic procedure remains technically demanding, and three to six month comparisons of patient results even in the hands of experienced arthroscopists have not demonstrated a clear advantage. For the majority of orthopaedic surgeons, an open acromioplasty may provide better results.[44,60,71,83] One potential advantage of arthroscopic surgery is the ability to visualize carefully the rotator cuff, from both the articular side and the bursal side. Repair of partial-thickness tears of the rotator cuff still remains controversial, but when more than 50% of the rotator cuff tendon thickness is involved, surgical repair is recommended.[104] When the tear involves less than 50% of the rotator cuff thickness, debridement of the partial-thickness tears combined with an acromioplasty yields a satisfactory result in the majority of patients.[3,37]

Following surgery, range-of-motion exercises are started immediately. Some patients benefit from continuous passive motion devices following surgery, but the final outcome may not be improved with patients who exercise consistently.[20,35,51,78] Patients progress from passive to active range-of-motion exercises over the first four to six weeks. Strengthening of the deltoid and rotator cuff is started between four and six weeks. Light manual labor work can begin between eight and twelve weeks, with gradual advancement of work status after three months. Maximum medical improvement is usually achieved by six months, although patients may continue to improve in strength for more than a year.

### Full-thickness cuff tear

Full-thickness tears of the rotator cuff are potentially labor-ending injuries, even when appropriate management is provided. Although full-thickness cuff tears are often treated as the end-stage impingement, acute work-related injuries are responsible for a substantial number of full-thickness tears. The diagnosis should be achieved within the first six weeks following the injury as the outcome of chronic tears (greater than three months) is less successful than acute tears.[5]

In the general population, the typical age of patients with full-thickness rotator cuff tears is between 48 and 75 years.[65] Patients under the age of 60 are more likely to suffer a full-thickness rotator cuff tear after a major eccentric load occurs to the arm, such as in a fall or with a sudden forceful above-shoulder movement or lift. Work-related full-thickness rotator cuff tears are associated commonly with these injury mechanisms. Patients older than 60 often have the insidious onset of shoulder pain with a gradual decrease in shoulder function, particularly in overhead activities. In these older patients, the tear of the rotator cuff tendon may be relatively atraumatic, occurring secondarily to the attrition of cuff tissue, either by disuse or from the progression of the impingement disease.

Physical examination findings include atrophy of the rotator cuff musculature and tenderness at the greater tuberosity. The most common site of a rotator cuff tear is at the supraspinatus tendon insertion,[17] which can be palpated on examination by locating the proximal aspect of the bicipital groove, then advancing 1 cm laterally. More specific findings on examination include deficit in active motion when compared to passive motion, weakness of elevation of the arm, weakness of external rotation, and frequently painful crepitation in the subacromial region with internal and external rotation in abduction. Weakness of external rotation with the elbow by the patient's side appears to be the most sensitive indicator of the extent of rotator cuff disease.[11]

Specialized imaging studies are recommended if the history, physical examination, and radiographs are consistent with a substantial injury to the rotator cuff, or when patients do not respond to six to eight weeks of rehabilitation exercises. The gold standard for specialized evaluation of the rotator cuff integrity is the double-contrast arthrogram. However, many physicians have replaced shoulder arthrograms with MRI. MRI is very accurate in determining whether a full-thickness rotator cuff tear is present. However, partial-thickness tears challenge the interpretative skills of radiologists, as the images of tendinitis, partial-thickness rotator cuff tears, and small full-thickness rotator cuff tears can be similar. MRI findings other than "complete full-thickness rotator cuff tear" should be interpreted with caution. Surgical management should be strongly supported by the history and physical examination, or by an arthrogram.

Patients seen with chronic symptoms of rotator cuff disease are initially treated in the same way as patients with partial-thickness cuff tears: RICE, anti-inflammatory medications, occasionally a subacromial injection of cortisone, and physical therapy focused on improving shoulder motion. Special attention is directed towards the posterior shoulder stiffness that frequently accompanies rotator cuff conditions. Chronic, symptomatic tears that do not respond to therapy should be treated with the primary goal of pain relief. Improvement in strength is less predictable.

Acute full-thickness tears of the rotator cuff are repaired soon after the diagnosis is confirmed. Repair within six weeks of the initial injury is recommended.[5] Preoperative factors suggestive of good postoperative prognosis include the acute onset of symptoms, specific injury to the shoulder, younger age, good maintenance of external rotation strength (Grade 3 or 4), and normal radiographs.[5,32,63] Poor postoperative function is associated with long duration of pain, older patients, severe weakness (< Grade 3) of abduction and external rotation, decreased acromiohumeral interval on plain radiographs, and revision rotator cuff repairs.[23,32,42] Functional results of nonoperative management of full-thickness tears of the rotator cuff are inferior to open rotator cuff repair.[8]

Following rotator cuff repair, the shoulder is protected with a sling during the first four to six weeks. The rehabilitation program begins either on the day of surgery or the following morning. Although patients will experience substantial discomfort that requires appropriate pain management, the benefit of early mobilization has been documented.[7,49,63,65] For the first eight weeks, the primary goal of therapy is to reestablish a full range of shoulder motion. Strengthening exercises, beginning with active-assisted range of motion and isometric exercises controlled by the patient, are started between six and twelve weeks depending on intraoperative findings. If the rotator cuff tear is small and repair is easily accomplished, strengthening begins at six weeks; if the rotator cuff tear is large or attrition of the tissues provides a precarious repair, strengthening begins at twelve weeks. At three months, the strengthening program is advanced as tolerated, while continuing to improve on pain-free range of motion. Adequate rehabilitation of full-thickness rotator cuff repair requires a minimum of six months and may need up to twelve months following the surgery. The strength of the shoulder muscles and therefore the shoulder function substantially increases from six to twelve months following rotator cuff repair, supporting continued rehabilitation during this postoperative period.[101] If there is no further injury and the cuff remains intact, the results do not appear to deteriorate within the first five years.[41,43] The determination of maximal medical improvement is thus best performed at one year following surgery.

In terms of return to work, no significant use of the extremity is allowed for the first three months, as even writing or simple sedentary responsibilities that require the hand to be positioned slightly away from the person's side will aggravate the symptoms. At three months sedentary office-type work is allowed with gradual advancement to light physical activities. Medium-to-heavy physical labor may be initiated at approximately six months. Often, a work-hardening program helps bridge the gap from relatively short, intense exercise to the more long-term activities of a normal workday. Maximum heavy physical labor (such as a construction worker using a jackhammer) is not suggested until at least one year after surgery has been performed.

With these guidelines, one should consider job modifications or vocational rehabilitation in certain situations. The 55-year-old male who does heavy manual labor and develops the insidious onset of shoulder pain with confirmation of a rotator cuff tear is highly unlikely to return to his previous occupation without substantial restrictions, even after an extended rehabilitation. The employer and employee often benefit from an early decision to change occupational responsibilities to a lighter physical activity with no above-shoulder responsibilities. The employee will have the potential to return to work at an earlier date, substantially decreasing the risk of long-term disability.

### Subacromial abrasion

Subacromial abrasion is another subset of the frequently-used diagnosis of impingement. The shoulder function is compromised due to roughness or a "catching" sensation experienced by the patient, usually in the intermediate positions of shoulder elevation.[65] The symptoms are generally localized to the anterior shoulder region. There may be a history of a previous injury or strain to shoulder area, without evidence of substantial weakness.

The examination is pathognomonic of this disorder. With the arm abducted 90°, internal and external rotation of the humerus demonstrates crepitation that the patient recognizes as the etiology of the shoulder's dysfunction. This finding is termed the *abrasion sign*.[65] Patients may also demonstrate *tendon signs* as seen with rotator cuff injuries. Posterior shoulder stiffness with decreased internal rotation and cross-body adduction is often present. Radiographs demonstrate a normal glenohumeral relationship. Special imaging of

the rotator cuff is indicated if tendon signs are clearly evident on examination.

The initial management is similar to the management for partial-thickness cuff tears, including the RICE protocol, nonsteroidal antiinflammatory medications, and occasionally a subacromial cortisone injection. However, if patients have reproducible crepitation or catching that is directly related to their initial symptoms, an acromioplasty may be recommended earlier than six months.

Postoperative rehabilitation is similar to surgery for partial-thickness cuff tears that do not require a repair of the tendon. Full use of the extremity for activities of daily living should be achieved by three months, with light physical labor allowed at three months, advancing as tolerated to heavy physical labor by six months.

### Biceps Tendon Disorders

Proximal biceps tendon disorders can be divided into three categories: biceps tendinitis, biceps instability, and biceps/superior labrum lesions. The vast majority of biceps pathology is related to conditions of the rotator cuff.[75] Biceps tendinitis is seen rarely as a primary condition with thickening of the tendon and stenosis at the bicipital groove.[26] Biceps instability occurs when the normal restraining mechanism, the transverse humeral ligament, is incompetent.[16] This is frequently associated with large rotator cuff tears that involve the subscapularis.[63] The treatment of these conditions is related to the primary pathology as discussed.

Lesions involving the superior labrum and biceps attachment site can be a source of persistent shoulder pain, although an actual reproducible functional deficit directly attributable to this lesion remains to be defined.[95] The superior labral injury generally involves the labrum from the anterior bicep attachment to the posterior superior aspect, hence the term *SLAP lesion*. Most commonly, the patient will have discomfort with overhead activities.[4,87,95] Occasionally, a click or snap will be present with activities at shoulder level or above. This condition is often found coexisting with the other conditions such as partial-thickness rotator cuff tears, and its significance remains unclear. However, when found on arthroscopic examination, this lesion should be stabilized because increasing evidence exists that patients respond favorably to arthroscopic stabilization of this condition.[87] Postoperatively, lifting is restricted for at least six weeks, although passive and active-assisted range-of-motion exercises are encouraged after the first few days. Most patients have good function but continued pain at three months. This dull, aching pain usually resolves by six months. Some patients will demonstrate objective findings of permanent impairment, primarily related to strenuous lifting and overhead activities. Maximum medical improvement is achieved at six months when this is an isolated condition.

## Acromioclavicular Joint Disease

Acromioclavicular joint pathology generally occurs secondary to trauma.[92] The traumatic event is frequently an injury to the stabilizing structures of the joint as well as to the intraarticular meniscus or fibrocartilage. Acute injuries to the acromioclavicular joint with compromise of the supporting ligaments and joint capsule represent the majority of acromioclavicular pathology in the nonphysical labor population. However, early degenerative joint disease and distal clavicular osteolysis represent two conditions that commonly occur in the worker with heavy physical demands or frequent above-shoulder-level responsibilities.

The acromioclavicular joint is a diarthrodial joint formed by the acromion and lateral clavicle, with the articular surfaces covered with fibrocartilage (Fig. 21-4). A fibrocartilaginous interarticular disc, meniscoid in shape, exists between the two articular surfaces. This tissue undergoes degeneration with age and is no longer functional by the fifth decade.[25] The acromioclavicular joint motion is limited to only 5 to 8°.[54,92]

The most common mechanism of injury to the acromioclavicular joint is a direct blow to the top of the shoulder. Indirect mechanisms of injury include a fall on the elbow, particularly with the arm extended. In more severe cases, there is an obvious deformity of the lateral aspect of the shoulder, because the acromion and upper extremity are displaced downward, while the lateral end of the clavicle remains in its anatomic position. Acromioclavicular joint separations have been classified into six different types,[91] based on the anatomical structures injured and the radiographic appearance of the clavicle and acromion relationship (Fig. 21-5). Type I is a sprain of the acromioclavicular joint without displacement. Type II involves a sprain with displacement, but the acromion and clavicle remain in a close relationship. Type III involves a complete separation of the acromion and clavicle, which occurs when the injury involves not only the acromioclavicular joint, but also the coracoclavicular ligaments. Types IV, V, and VI are indicative of severe displacement of the relationship between the acromion and clavicle, with complete disruption of the ligamentous attachments from the clavicle to the scapula.

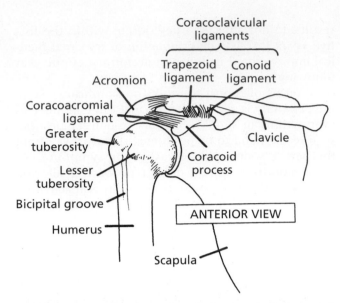

**FIGURE 21-4**   Normal anatomy of the acromioclavicular (ac) joint. The acromioclavicular ligaments are the primary horizontal stabilizers of the ac joint and they are more frequently involved in ac joint injuries. The coracoacromial ligaments are the primary vertical stabilizers of the ac joint. Substantial forces are required to rupture both the acromioclavicular ligaments as well as the coracoclavicular ligaments.

Types I, II, and III are generally treated nonoperatively with good results.[57,61,99] Treatment includes the RICE protocol, with immobilization in a sling to support the upper extremity. With Grade I injuries, range of motion can be started within one to two weeks following the injury, advancing to a strengthening program when a full range of pain-free motion has been achieved (four to six weeks). With Grade II and III injuries, the extremity is supported for one to two weeks to allow the pain and swelling to subside. Range-of-motion activities are then initiated. A full range of pain-free motion is usually achieved by six weeks. At six weeks, strengthening exercises are added to the rehabilitation regimen. Recovery from this injury is approximately three months, although Grade I injuries heal more rapidly, while Grade II and III injuries may take longer.

While most patients with Grade III acromioclavicular joint separations are appropriately treated nonoperatively, one exception may be the laborer who is constantly required to lift heavy objects (i.e., wheelbarrow work). These workers have symptoms of fatigue and/or paresthesias with repetitive heavy lifting. This is because the upper extremity work is being supported by soft tissues, without the usual support of the acromioclavicular structures and coracoclavicular ligaments. On examination, the only objective findings may be the displacement of the acromioclavicular joint. Objective testing of the strength of the

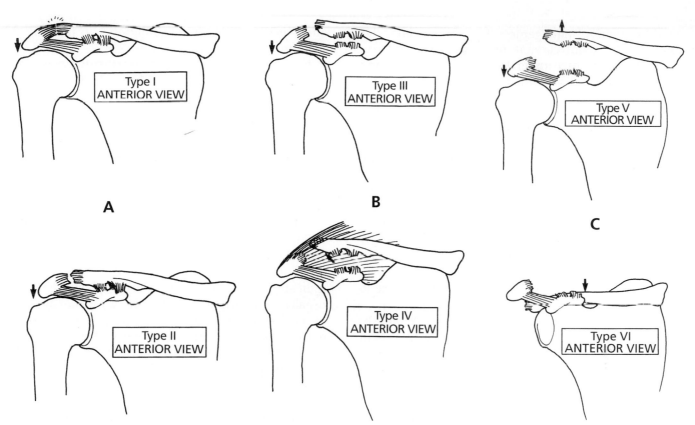

**FIGURE 21-5**    Classification of acromioclavicular joint injuries. **A,** Types I and II. **B,** Types III and IV. **C,** Types V and VI. Clinically, the most important differentiation is between Type III and Type V dislocations, because Type III dislocations are generally treated nonoperatively, while Type V dislocations are treated with stabilization. Type IV and VI are easily diagnosed with appropriate radiographs, and are also treated with surgical stabilization.

shoulder is usually noncontributory because the worker is able to demonstrate good strength during strenuous activities of short duration.[102] The surgical management, when indicated, involves reduction of the acromion back to the level of the clavicle, stabilization of the coracoclavicular junction, and commonly a resection of the distal clavicle.[91]

Types IV, V, and VI are best managed operatively.[91,92,103] In these injuries, there is a disruption of the acromioclavicular joint as well as the coracoclavicular ligaments, with substantial injury to the remaining soft tissues. In essence, the supporting structures of the upper extremity and scapula are separated from the remainder of the torso. Weakness, paresthesias, and chronic discomfort are common. Stabilizing the scapula to the clavicle by reconstruction of the coracoclavicular ligaments is successful in relieving the symptoms and providing excellent functional results.[54,91,92,103]

Chronic discomfort of the acromioclavicular joint secondary to degenerative arthritis may be related to occupational activities. However, the causal relationship is circumstantial. There is no study that docu-

ments a direct relationship between specific occupational activities and an increased risk of osteoarthritis of the acromioclavicular joint compared with the normal population. The acromioclavicular joint begins to deteriorate in the second decade with gradual loss of the fibrocartilaginous disc; by age 50, substantial narrowing of the joint space exists in the general population.[25,81,82]

An associated condition is osteolysis of the distal clavicle. This may be seen in workers who have occupational demands that include frequent strenuous use of their upper extremities.[13,92] It is also common in weight lifters. The proposed etiology is repetitive trauma across the acromioclavicular joint. Usually, pain begins insidiously, directly in the area of the acromioclavicular joint. On occasion, the worker remarks that a distinct pull or strain to the upper shoulder occurred. Examination demonstrates point tenderness at the acromioclavicular joint, which can be exacerbated by cross-body (horizontal) adduction. Glenohumeral joint motion is unaffected. Radiographs demonstrate osteopenia of the distal clavicle, often with tapering and cystic changes.[72]

Conservative management for acromioclavicular arthritis or distal clavicle osteolysis includes ice, avoiding strenuous upper-extremity activities, and nonsteroidal antiinflammatory medication. An intraarticular injection of cortisone is often very helpful if there is no response to initial management after four to six weeks. The physician should be confident that the cortisone is actually in the acromioclavicular joint. Using a 20-gauge needle, a gentle "pop" is felt as the joint is entered, and only a small volume of fluid (usually less than 2 cc, with a 1:1 ratio of cortisone and anesthetic agent) is accepted. Patients have an acute worsening of their presenting symptoms from the pressure in the joint, followed by complete relief of their symptoms within 5 min. This injection can be repeated in two to three months, ideally in those patients who demonstrated a good response to the initial injection.

Patients who have had symptoms for six months or more despite appropriate conservative treatment can be considered for distal clavicle resection. Distal clavicle resection is an effective treatment for both osteoarthritis of the acromioclavicular joint as well as distal clavicle osteolysis, resulting in decreased pain and return to precondition levels of function.[13,38,80,92] However, the return of normal strength takes much longer than three to six months. Even in well-motivated athletes, objective strength testing noted a >10% deficit in side-to-side testing at one year following a distal clavicle resection.[18] Therefore, the postsurgical return-to-work guidelines must be modified based on the worker's upper-extremity (especially overhead) occupational demands. Light use of the extremity with the elbow by the side is possible at six to twelve weeks. Full use of the extremity for activities of daily living and light manual labor can be expected around three months. Medium labor activities will be possible between four to six months, and heavy labor, particularly overhead lifting, will be restricted for six to twelve months. Maximum medical improvement is achieved between six to twelve months, although strength may continue to improve beyond one year.

### Degenerative Arthritis of the Glenohumeral Joint

As with osteoarthritis of the acromioclavicular joint, the relationship between osteoarthritis of the glenohumeral joint and occupation remains vague. Occupations that require heavy labor with large forces occurring across the shoulder have been associated with a higher incidence of degenerative arthritis of the glenohumeral joint.[9,53,58] Typically, patients with osteoarthritis of the glenohumeral joint are between 54 and 74 years of age.[65] Functional problems often include difficulty sleeping and an inability to perform activities of daily living.

Patients with glenohumeral arthritis have pain, worsened by motion, and stiffness. Reduced glenohumeral motion is present in all planes, but is particularly evident with rotation of the humerus with the arm by the patient's side. Glenohumeral crepitance may be demonstrated with shoulder motion. Plain radiographs are diagnostic, eliminating the need for advanced imaging studies. The required diagnostic views include a true anteroposterior view of the glenohumeral joint and an axillary lateral view.[89]

Initially, management includes avoidance of aggravating activities, antiinflammatory medication, and occasionally an injection of cortisone. With increasing pain and decreasing function, shoulder arthroplasty is indicated.[105] After shoulder arthroplasty, patients usually have little or no pain and a functional range of motion. Lifetime restrictions for patients who require a glenoid resurfacing along with the proximal humeral articular surface replacement include no lifting of more than 10 lb on a regular basis, no impact-loading tasks such as shoveling, and no repetitive overhead activities. Light use of the extremity for occupational demands can begin between six and twelve weeks. Activities of daily living are successfully achieved between two to four months, and patients achieve full use of their extremity with the above mentioned restrictions at four to six months.

## ELBOW DISORDERS

Acute injuries to the elbow primarily include contusions, muscular strains, and fractures. Early intervention is recommended, with the RICE protocol. The initial evaluation should include a careful history and physical examination, with supporting radiographs as indicated. Fractures involving the elbow are treated with techniques that allow early range of motion. Loss of elbow motion, especially terminal extension, is common with most elbow pathology. Fortunately, loss of some elbow motion is well-tolerated because the vast majority of daily and occupational activities are possible with an extension-flexion arc of 30 to 130°.[70] Supervised therapy must be instituted early to maintain elbow motion. Most minor injuries resolve within four to six weeks. If symptoms persist, particularly mechanical symptoms, then consideration of specific elbow conditions should ensue.

### Tendinitis: Lateral and Medial Epicondylitis

The elbow is susceptible to injury when substantial forces generated by the shoulder overwhelm the

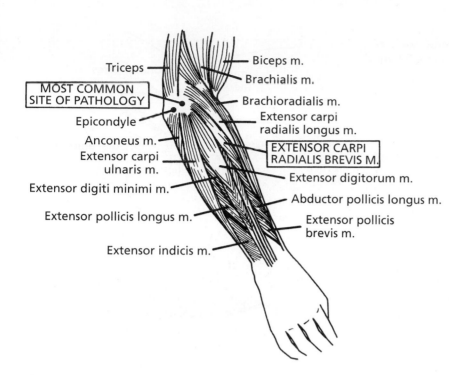

Triceps

MOST COMMON
SITE OF PATHOLOGY

Epicondyle

Anconeus m.

Extensor carpi
ulnaris m.

Extensor digiti minimi m.

Extensor pollicis longus m.

Extensor indicis m.

Biceps m.

Brachialis m.

Brachioradialis m.

Extensor carpi
radialis longus m.

EXTENSOR CARPI
RADIALIS BREVIS M.

Extensor digitorum m.

Abductor pollicis longus m.

Extensor pollicis
brevis m.

**FIGURE 21-6**    Anatomy of lateral epicondylitis. The extensor muscles of the forearm originate at the lateral epicondyle of the distal humerus. The structure most frequently involved in the condition of lateral epicondylitis is the origin of the extensor carpi radialis brevis, which originates at the lateral epicondyle and inserts at the base of the third metacarpal.

muscles of the elbow region, or alternatively, when the wrist and elbow are used in a chronic and repetitive manner. Frequently, the lateral aspect of the elbow is involved, and the term *lateral epicondylitis* (*tennis elbow*) is used to describe this condition. When the medial aspect of the elbow is involved, medial epicondylitis (golfer's elbow) is used. Lateral epicondylitis occurs at the origin of the extensor muscles of the forearm, primarily the extensor carpi radialis brevis (Fig. 21-6). Medial epicondylitis occurs at the origin of the flexor-pronator mass on the medial epicondyle of the distal humerus. Although the use of epicondylitis implies an inflammatory process, the histology of these conditions is more consistent with a chronic degenerative process,[14,52,86] suggesting that epicondylosis may be the appropriate diagnostic term.

Typically, epicondylitis of the elbow occurs in patients between the ages of 30 and 50, with a mean of 41 years.[79] Younger patients frequently report its association with sports participation such as tennis. Usually, the dominant arm is affected, and there does not appear to be any correlation with gender. The condition is commonly associated with repetitive eccentric wrist use, such as the activities of carpenters or welders. In addition, repetitive low-level activities such as typing or data entry may cause microtrauma to the involved tissues, resulting in epicondylitis.[15,28,79]

Although epicondylitis appears to be associated with work-related activities, the fact that this is a degenerative process histologically implies that work related tendon degeneration may be superimposed on the normal aging process. The incidence of lateral epicondylitis is significantly correlated with increasing age.[28] It is also occupation dependent, with estimated elbow stress directly proportional to the prevalence of epicondylitis.[28] The overall prevalence in a study of industrial workers was less than 10%, with one-third of the cases directly work-related, one-third due to sports or recreation, and one-third without a specific cause. Analyzing the reports of patients with lateral epicondylitis who were seen by the company physician shows that 50% of the patients claimed work-related causes.[27]

The diagnosis of epicondylitis is suspected after a careful history, implicating an eccentric load or repetitive activity involving the wrist and elbow. Pain may be diffuse, but is commonly localized to a very specific area at the anterolateral (lateral epicondylitis) or anteromedial (medial epicondylitis) aspect of the distal humerus. Often, the worker will complain of pain radiating down the forearm, and decreased grip strength and dexterity. Resisted wrist extension may intensify the pain. Radiographs are usually normal, but up to 25% of patients may have soft-tissue calcifications involving the tendon origins, which have no prognostic value.[79]

The initial management of elbow epicondylitis is directed toward decreasing the stresses across the elbow and decreasing pain. The inciting activity must be avoided, or ideally, stopped until the acute phase has resolved. Cryotherapy is useful to decrease the discomfort. The benefits of nonsteroidal antiinflammatory medication are primarily pain relief; their role in the reparative process remains vague. The healing process may be facilitated by other modalities such as electrical stimulation or iontophoresis, but their efficacy is unproven.[10,19,56] A crucial component of rehabilitation is a consistent effort by the worker to stretch the affected area. Wrist extension with medial epicondylitis or wrist flexion with lateral epicondylitis should be performed three to five times per day. As the end-range of motion increases with decreasing pain, from two to four weeks, then strengthening exercises can be initiated.

Counterforce bracing has been shown to improve wrist and grip strength, as well as decrease pain.[100] Bracing may be particularly useful in workers who continue with their occupational responsibilities. A controlled, prospective study evaluating the effects of various modalities and medications has not been done.

If the worker does not respond to initial management, an injection of cortisone may be considered. In some patients, a single injection may permanently relieve their problem, while in many patients, the pain relief is only transient.[84] The detrimental effects of cortisone on the normal healing process of collagen and other tissues leads to the recommendation that corticosteroid injections should be used sparingly.[33]

Workers who are well-motivated, exercise (stretch) daily, avoid aggravating activities, and yet continue to suffer the effects of elbow epicondylitis after six to twelve months are considered for surgical intervention. This should represent less than 10% of all patients who have symptoms of lateral epicondylitis.[15,79] If surgery is not performed for a minimum of 12 months following the onset of symptoms, then less than 5% of all patients with lateral or medial epicondylitis would require surgery. Numerous surgical techniques have been described for the treatment of elbow epicondylitis.[10,19,50,77,79] As with any surgical procedure, the guiding principle should be determination of the exact pathology preoperatively, with an anatomical restoration of the tissues. However, with elbow epicondylitis, the technique most commonly used is an excision of pathologic tissue and release of any remaining affected tendon origin. The overlying fascia of the extensor communis (lateral epicondylitis) or flexor-pronator group (medial epicondylitis) is usually repaired when closing the wound (Fig. 21-7). The success rate is 90% or better. Success is primarily described in terms of pain relief, because other parameters such as objective measurements may demonstrate substantial deficits despite complete relief of pain.[50]

Postoperatively, the elbow may be splinted briefly, but an early range-of-motion program should be instituted. After four weeks, a gradual strengthening program is started, initially with light resisted isometrics. This is advanced, as tolerated, at six weeks fol-

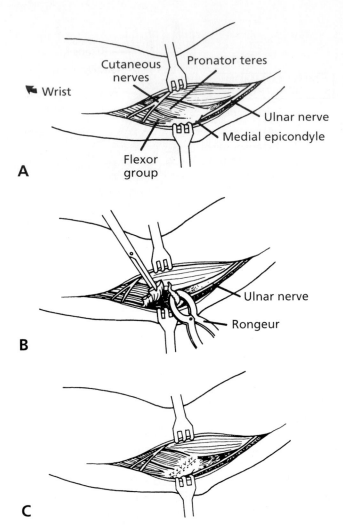

**FIGURE 21-7**    Surgical management of medial epicondylitis. The stages include: **(A)** exposure of the fascia of the common flexor-pronator group originating at the medial epicondyle; **(B)** reflection of the common flexor-pronator group origin and debridement of the involved tissue; and **(C)** repair of the fascia of the common flexor-pronator group.

lowing surgery. Grip strengthening is gradually advanced. Stretching remains an essential component of the rehabilitation, with the patient instructed to stretch three to five times per day, beginning with the elbow slightly flexed and advancing to stretching activities with the elbow fully extended. At three months following surgery, lifting activities and more athletic work responsibilities are permitted. For occupations that include high levels of elbow and wrist stress, full return to duty should occur between four and six months. If progress remains slow at four to five months, an intensive work-hardening program may be beneficial. Symptoms persisting beyond six months may indicate failure of the surgical procedure, often requiring advanced evaluation techniques to determine the cause of surgical failure.[68]

## Olecranon Bursitis

Olecranon bursitis generally has a traumatic origin, although occasionally it may be related to an overuse or repetitive stress phenomenon, such as miner's elbow. Olecranon bursitis may also herald a systemic process such as gout or inflammatory arthropathies. A succinct history should determine the etiology. The differential diagnosis between nonseptic and septic bursitis can be challenging.[69] Septic bursitis predominantly affects young and middle-aged men involved in manual labor (e.g., plumbers, truck drivers, and automechanics).[85] Predisposing medical conditions are evident in more than 70% of patients with septic olecranon bursitis.

Physical examination findings include a visible enlargement of the posterior aspect of the olecranon with a mobile, usually soft mass. Traumatic olecranon bursitis is painful at the time of injury, but the pain quickly resolves. Septic bursitis is associated with a persistence or worsening of pain. Patients with septic bursitis have pain 80% of the time, whereas patients with aseptic bursitis have pain less than 20% of the time after resolution of acute symptoms.[93] The skin temperature over a septic olecranon bursa is approximately 4°C warmer than the nonaffected side. Loss of motion, particularly flexion, may be present and more likely suggests a septic process.[85]

Radiographs demonstrate an olecranon spur in less than 25% of patients.[69] Bursal fluid aspiration contents depend on the underlying etiology. Remarkably, a Gram stain may be positive in only 50% of patients with septic bursitis, although a high leukocyte count would suggest an infectious process.[69]

Treatment for acute olecranon bursitis without an associated systemic disease includes the avoidance of the inciting activity and protection of the posterior elbow from recurrent trauma with a protective elbow sleeve. Antiinflammatory medications usually provide pain relief. Aspiration may be indicated when the swollen bursa is painful and interferes with daily activities. However, a simple aspiration and then application of a compressive dressing is associated with a high rate of recurrence. Repeat aspirations can not be recommended. Aspiration of the bursal fluid, instillation of methylprednisolone, and application of a compressive dressing may result in the lowest recurrence rate,[94] but the use of corticosteroids has been associated with a prohibitive risk of infection that may be as high as 12%, and a 20% risk of subdermal atrophy.[105] If the bursa persists despite conservative management, resection of the entire bursa through a midline incision is recommended. The patient is started on range-of-motion exercises after immobilizing the elbow in flexion for one to two weeks. Return to full activities is generally accomplished within six weeks.

For septic olecranon bursitis, the bursa must be drained. Drainage can be adequately accomplished through a small incision. A small suction drain or Penrose drain allows adequate decompression of the septic bursa. Antibiotic therapy effective against Gram-positive organisms (e.g., staphylococci, streptococci) is started. Initially, antibiotics are adjusted according to the Gram stain, while definitive treatment is based on culture results at 48 hours. Recovery is generally complete within two to three weeks. Surgical removal of the bursa is rarely indicated in the acute phase of either septic or nonseptic olecranon bursitis.[69]

Surgical removal is considered if symptoms interfere with activities of daily living or occupational responsibilities. The entire bursa is removed through a longitudinal incision, a compressive dressing is applied, and the elbow is splinted for 10-14 days. After the wound has healed, an olecranon pad is used to protect this area and return to work is accomplished within two to four weeks.

## Entrapment of the Ulnar Nerve at the Elbow: Cubital Tunnel Syndrome

Ulnar neuropathy at the elbow level is not uncommon, although the vast majority of compressive neuropathies involving the upper extremity are related to compression of the median nerve in the carpal tunnel. The ulnar nerve travels in a specific path, descending from the brachial plexus in the anterior compartment of the arm, passing through the intramuscular septum at the arcade of Struthers approximately 6 to 8 cm above the medial epicondyle, then continuing posterior to the medial epicondyle (Fig. 21-8). After passing the medial epicondyle, it enters into the flexor carpi ulnaris, underneath a connecting fibrous band. Compression or irritation of the nerve can occur at any of these three relatively fixed points. The term *cubital tunnel syndrome* initially referred to constriction of the nerve by the tunnel formed from the band crossing the ulnar nerve between the two heads of the flexor carpi ulnaris;[34] however, the term is now commonly used to describe most ulnar nerve conditions around the elbow.

Most commonly, symptoms begin with an insidious onset of intermittent paresthesias involving the ulnar nerve distribution into the little finger and ring finger. A vague discomfort at the posteromedial aspect of the elbow may be present. Symptoms are aggravated by repetitive or prolonged elbow flexion. Gradually, the paresthesias become more persistent, and loss of sensation, particularly in the ulnar aspect

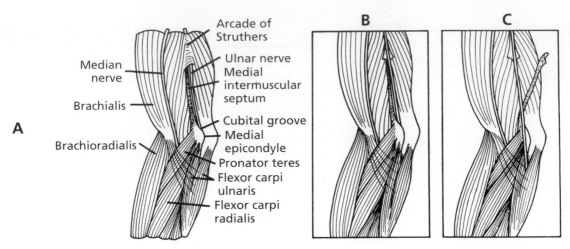

**FIGURE 21-8**    Cubital tunnel syndrome. Anatomy of the ulnar nerve. The normal dimensions of the ulnar nerve can be encroached upon at three important levels: **(A)** proximally, at the arcade of Struthers; **(B)** in the ulnar nerve groove at the posterior aspect of the medial epicondyle; and **(C)** distally by a fibrous band across the two heads of the flexor carpi ulnaris as the nerve enters into this muscle. Anterior transposition of the ulnar nerve requires release of the arcade and fibrous band at the flexor carpi ulnaris.

of the hand, can occur. Other complaints include loss of grip strength and decreased hand dexterity. Cubital tunnel syndrome can also begin with a single traumatic event from which the patient does not completely recover, although this mechanism is uncommon. Other disorders that may have similar associated symptoms include cervical radiculopathy and thoracic outlet syndrome.

On examination, light tapping with the index finger over the ulnar nerve distribution may elicit pain and paresthesias (positive Tinel's sign). Another useful test is the elbow flexion test.[12] The elbow is held in flexion with the wrist in extension for up to 3 min. A positive test results in reproduction or worsening of the initial symptoms. Late findings include atrophy of the hypothenar eminence and the flexor carpi ulnaris, weakness of the intrinsic muscles of the hand, and gradual clawing of the small and ring fingers. Instability of the ulnar nerve (subluxation of the nerve out of the medial epicondylar groove with elbow flexion) is present in approximately 16% of the general population and therefore is not directly related to the development of ulnar neuropathy at the elbow level.[23] However, ulnar nerve instability may predispose patients to ulnar neuropathy if their occupation or recreation is associated with frequent flexion of the elbow beyond 90°.

Radiographs and electromyographic studies contribute to the evaluation of patients with cubital tunnel syndrome. The cubital tunnel is visualized on plain radiographs with the cubital tunnel view.[96] The elbow is fully flexed, placed on the radiographic plate, and the humerus is externally rotated 20°. The radiographic beam is directed perpendicular to the plate. This radiograph is particularly useful when the patient

has a prior history of trauma. Osteophytes or a malunion in this area may encroach on the usual ulnar nerve pathway as it traverses along the medial edge of the trochlea. Electromyographic (EMG) studies can confirm the suspected clinical diagnosis, but occasionally they may be normal despite clinical findings.[21] Conduction velocities are tested across the elbow with the intrinsic muscles of the hand used to determine the motor velocity. The little finger is tested for sensory deficits. The electromyographer must be skilled, the region to be tested should be clearly described, and the patient must be cooperative. The EMG may be unable to demonstrate the exact site of the ulnar nerve pathology in up to one-third of all cases.[30] Electromyographic studies are particularly useful when the diagnosis of this condition remains uncertain based on clinical findings, because the results can assist in differentiating other conditions such as cervical radiculopathy or thoracic outlet syndrome.

Management includes avoiding the inciting activity. If a source of external trauma is evident, padding of the elbow is helpful. Modification of the work area, such as changing the height of the keyboard, may be helpful. Repetitive flexion activities can also be decreased by job restrictions or job rotation. A padded extension brace can be fabricated to prevent the elbow from flexing more than 30° during sleep. If an inflammatory component is recognized, an antiinflammatory medication is prescribed. Treatment may last three to nine months and is often successful. When only mild paresthesias are present, the likelihood of surgery over the following six years is 21%; however, if muscle atrophy is present on examination, the likelihood of surgery over the following three years is 62% despite conservative treatment.[23]

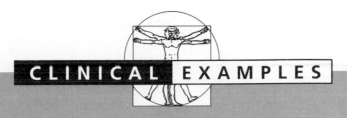

# CLINICAL EXAMPLES

## SHOULDER AND ELBOW

EDITOR's NOTE—Apart from the miscellaneous categories of joint assessment (section 3.1m), neurological abnormalities, and vascular problems, impairment evaluation of the shoulder and elbow involves essentially measurement of active range of motion (ROM).* Abnormalities of strength are assessed only when they result from a neurologic disorder; then assessment of those abnormalities supersedes the ROM evaluation. Any other cause of diminished strength is considered part of the pathologic condition associated with the diminished ROM, and these impairment values reflect the contribution of diminished strength. Pain is similarly evaluated.

### EXAMPLE

#### History

While at work, a 55-year-old self-employed female had a penetrating injury of the left elbow. She had had osteoarthritis involving many joints for several years. Five days after the injury, she saw her physician because of pain, swelling, and redness over the elbow. A soft, fluctuant mass was visible over the posterior aspect of the olecranon. Aspiration revealed a white blood cell count of 18,000/mm³, all neutrophils. A Gram stain was negative. Treatment consisted of RICE and nonsteroidal antiinflammatory medication. Follow-up examination at 5 days revealed worsening of her symptoms and a fever (38.2° Celsius). A repeat aspiration revealed increasing white blood cell counts and gram-positive cocci. She was admitted to the hospital for surgical therapy. Six months later, she sees a physician for an impairment evaluation.

#### Physical Examination

There is a well-healed scar over the elbow. Strength and sensation are normal. Crepitation is noted with both active and passive ROM. Flexion (F) is 110°, extension (E) is 30°, pronation (P) is 50°, and supination (S) is 50°.

#### Assessment Process

Based on the diminished ROM, the patient has 12% impairment of the upper extremity (F = 4%, E = 3%, P = 2%, S = 1%) and a 6% whole person impairment (WPI) (Figs. 12 and 13, Table 3, p. 20). Using Tables 18 and 19 (p. 59), an impairment rating could be based on joint crepitation. The percentage would be 30% ("severe: constant during passive range of motion") × 42 (entire elbow) = 13% WPI. This represents an additional 7% impairment rating. However, caution must be exercised. Joint crepitation as a source of impairment reflects synovial or cartilage degeneration. The question must be asked: Could her septic joint have caused this problem? This pathologic condition could have caused the diminished ROM and attendant stiffness but, as a discrete pathologic entity, could it have caused her joint tissue degeneration? The history of osteoarthritis must also be considered.

On examination of the right elbow, crepitation is found constantly during active ROM, although the ROM is normal. Based on the crepitation alone, an 8% WPI (20% × 42) is found for the opposite, unaffected joint, with the source of the crepitation being osteoarthritis. The 8% should be subtracted from the 13% in the left elbow to reflect the contribution of the independent pathologic condition, yielding a 5% impairment based solely on the contribution of the injury.

#### Evaluation

Since the right elbow ROM is normal, the 5% WPI of the left elbow, reflecting the diminished ROM caused by the injury, is considered an appropriate value.

*All *sections,* *tables,* and *figures* referred to in this discussion are found in AMA *Guides to the evaluation of permanent impairment,* ed 4, Chapter 3—The Musculoskeletal System, American Medical Association, Chicago, 1993.

*Stephen L. Demeter*

Surgery is reserved for those patients with a clear clinical picture of cubital syndrome who do not respond to conservative management with six months. Subcutaneous, submuscular, or intramuscular transposition is recommended.[1,21,22,55,59] Other techniques, such as medial epicondylectomy, may also achieve good results.[1,36,39,55] After transposition of the nerve, the arm is rested with a splint for up to two weeks. Active range of motion can be started after removal of the splint. At four to six weeks, a strengthening program is instituted. Most patients will be able to resume full activities without restrictions by eight to twelve weeks.

## References

1. Adson AW: The surgical treatment of progressive ulnar paralysis. *Minn Med* 1:455-460, 1918.
2. Alexander OM: Radiography of the acromioclavicular articulation. *Med Radiogr Photogr* 30:34-39, 1954.
3. Altchek DW, Warren RF, Wickiewicz TL, et al: Arthroscopic acromioplasty: technique and results. *J Bone Joint Surg* 72-A:1198-1207, 1990.
4. Andrews RJ, Carson WG, McLeod WD: Glenoid labrum tears related to long head of the biceps. *Am J Sports Med* 13:337-341, 1985.
5. Bassett RW, Cofield RH: Acute tears of the rotator cuff: the timing of surgical repair. *Clin Orthop* 175:18-24, 1983.
6. Beltran J: The use of magnetic resonance imaging about the shoulder. *J Shoulder Elbow Surg* 1:321-332, 1993.
7. Bigliani L, Cordasco F, McIlveen S, et al: Operative treatment of failed repairs of the rotator cuff. *J Bone Joint Surg* 74-A:1505-1515, 1992.
8. Bokor DJ, Hawkins RJ, Huckell GH, et al: Results of nonoperative management of full-thickness tears of the rotator cuff. *Clin Orthop* 294:103-110, 1993.
9. Bovenzi M, Fiorito A, Volpe C: Bone and joint disorders in the upper extremities of chipping and grinding operators. *Int Arch Occup Environ Health* 59:189-198, 1987.
10. Boyd HB, McLeod AC: Tennis elbow. *J Bone Joint Surg* 55-A:1183, 1973.
11. Brems JJ: Digital muscle strength measurement in rotator cuff tears. Paper presented to American Shoulder and Elbow Surgeons, 3rd Open Meeting, San Francisco, 1987.
12. Buerhler MJ, Thayer DT: The elbow flexion test: a clinical test for the cubital tunnel syndrome. *Clin Orthop* 233:213-216, 1988.
13. Cahill BR: Osteolysis of the distal part of the clavicle in athletes. *J Bone Joint Surg* 64-A:1053-1058, 1982.
14. Chard MD, Cawston TE, Riley GP, et al: Rotator cuff degeneration and lateral epicondylitis: a comparative histological study. *Ann Rheum Dis* 53:30-34, 1994.
15. Ciccotti MG, Lombardo SJ: Medial and lateral epicondylitis. In Jobe FW: *Upper extremity injuries in sports*, St. Louis, 1994, CV Mosby.
16. Clark JM, Harryman DT II: Tendons, ligaments, and capsule of the rotator cuff. *J Bone Joint Surg* 74-A:713-725, 1992.
17. Codman EA: *The shoulder: rupture of the supraspinatus tendon and other lesions in or about the subacromial bursa.* Boston, 1934, Thomas Todd.
18. Cook FF, Tibone JE: The Mumford procedure in athletes: an objective analysis of function. *Am J Sports Med* 16:97-100, 1988.
19. Coonrad RW, Hooper WR: Tennis elbow: its course, natural history, conservative and surgical management. *J Bone Joint Surg* 55-A:1177, 1973.
20. Craig EV: Continuous passive motion in the rehabilitation of the surgically reconstructed shoulder: a preliminary report. *Orthop Trans* 219, 1986.
21. Dawson DM: Entrapment neuropathies of the upper extremities. *N Eng J Med* 329:2013-2018, 1993.
22. Dellon, AL: Review of treatment results for ulnar nerve compression at the elbow. *J Hand Surg* 14:688-699, 1989.
23. Dellon AL, Hament W, Gittelshon A: Nonoperative management of cubital tunnel syndrome: an 8-year prospective study. *Neurology* 43:1673-1677, 1993.
24. DeOrio JK, Cofield RH: Results of a second attempt at surgical repair of a failed initial rotator cuff repair. *J Bone Joint Surg* 66-A:563-567, 1984.
25. DePalma AF: The role of the disks of the sternoclavicular and acromioclavicular joints. *Clin Orthop* 13:7-12, 1959.
26. DePalma AF, Callery GE: Bicipital tenosynovitis. *Clin Orthop* 3:69-85, 1954.
27. Dimberg L: Lateral humeral epicondylitis (tennis elbow) among industrial workers. Swedish Work Environment Fund, 1983.
28. Dimberg L: The prevalence and causation of tennis elbow (lateral humeral epicondylitis) in a population of workers in an engineering industry. *Ergonomics* 30:573-580, 1987.
29. Downing DS, Weinstein A: Ultrasound therapy of subacromial bursitis: a double-blind trial. *Phys Ther* 66:194-199, 1986.
30. Eisen A: Early diagnosis of ulnar nerve palsy:

an electrophysiologic study. *Neurology* 24:256-262, 1974.

31. Ellman H: Diagnosis and treatment of incomplete rotator cuff tears. *Clin Orthop* 254:64-74, 1990.

32. Ellman H, Hanker G, Bayer M: Repair of the rotator cuff: end-result study of factors influencing reconstruction. *J Bone Joint Surg* 68-A:1136-1144, 1986.

33. Fadale PD, Wiggins ME: Corticosteroid injections: their use and abuse. *J Am Acad Orthop Surg* 2:133-140, 1994.

34. Feindel W, Stratford J: The role of the cubital tunnel in tardy ulnar palsy. *Can J Surg* 38:287-300, 1958.

35. Flowers K: CPM for postop rotator cuff repair: a case history. *Contin Care* 1990.

36. Froimson AI, Zahrawi F: Treatment of compression neuropathy of the ulnar nerve at the elbow by epicondylectomy and neurolysis. *J Hand Surg* 5:391-395, 1980.

37. Gartsman GM: Arthroscopic acromioplasty for lesions of the rotator cuff. *J Bone Joint Surg* 72-A:169-180, 1990.

38. Gartsman GM: Arthroscopic resection of the acromioclavicular joint. *Am J Sports Med* 21:71-77, 1993.

39. Goldberg BJ, Light TR, Blair SJ: Ulnar neuropathy at the elbow: results of medial epicondylectomy. *J Hand Surg* 14A:182-188, 1989.

40. Goldman AB, Ghelman B: The double-contrast shoulder arthrogram. *Radiology* 127:655-663, 1978.

41. Gore DR, Murray MP, Sepic SB, et al: Shoulder-muscle strength and range of motion following surgical repair of full-thickness rotator cuff tears. *J Bone Joint Surg* 68-A:266-272, 1986.

42. Ha'eri GB, Wiley AM: Shoulder impingement syndrome: results of operative release. *Clin Orthop* 168:128-134, 1982.

43. Harryman D II, Mack L, Wang K, et al: Repairs of the rotator cuff. *J Bone Joint Surg* 73-A:982-989, 1991.

44. Hawkins RJ, Abrams JS: Impingement syndrome in the absence of rotator cuff tear (Stages 1 and 2). *Orthop Clin North Am* 18:373-382, 1987.

45. Hawkins RJ, Chris T, Bokor MB, Kiefer G: Failed anterior acromioplasty. *Clin Orthop Rel Res* 243:106-111, 1989.

46. Hawkins RJ, Kennedy JC: Impingement syndrome in athletes. *Am J Sports Med* 8:151-158, 1980.

47. Holt R, Helms C, Steinbach L, et al: Magnetic resonance imaging of the shoulder: rationale

and current applications. *Skeletal Radiol* 19:5-14, 1990.

48. Iannotti J, Zlatkin M, Esterhai J, et al: Magnetic resonance imaging of the shoulder: sensitivity, specificity, and predictive value. *J Bone Joint Surg* 73-A:17-29, 1991.

49. Iannotti JP: Full-thickness rotator cuff tears: factors affecting surgical outcome. *J Am Acad Orthop Surg* 2:87-95, 1994.

50. Jobe FW, Ciccotti MG: Lateral and medial epicondylitis of the elbow. *J Am Acad Orthop Surg* 2:1-8, 1994.

51. Johnson DP: The effect of continuous passive motion on wound healing and joint mobility after knee arthroplasty. *J Bone Joint Surg* 72:1353-1358, 1990.

52. Kannus P, Jozsa L: Histopathological changes preceding spontaneous rupture of a tendon. *J Bone Joint Surg* 73-A:1507-1525, 1991.

53. Katevuo K, Aitasalo K, Lehtinen R, et al: Skeletal changes in dentists and farmers in Finland. *Commun Dent Oral Epidemiol* 13:23-25, 1985.

54. Kennedy JC, Cameron H: Complete dislocation of the acromioclavicular joint. *J Bone Joint Surg* 36-B:202-208, 1954.

55. Kleinman WB, Bishop AT: Anterior intramuscular transposition of the ulnar nerve. *J Hand Surg* 14A:972-979, 1989.

56. Labelle H, Guibert R, Joncas J, et al: Lack of scientific evidence for the treatment of lateral epicondylitis of the elbow. *J Bone Joint Surg* 74-B:646-651, 1992.

57. Larsen E, Bjerg-Nielsen A, Christensen P: Conservative or surgical treatment of acromioclavicular dislocation. *J Bone Joint Surg* 68-A:552-555, 1986.

58. Lawrence JS: Rheumatism in coal miners: Part III—Occupational factors. *Br J Indust Med* 12:249-261, 1955.

59. Leffert RD: Anterior submuscular transposition of the ulnar nerve by the Learmonth technique. *J Hand Surg* 7:147-152, 1982.

60. Lirette R, Morin F, Kinnard P: The difficulties in assessment of results of anterior acromioplasty. *Clin Orthop* 278:14-16, 1992.

61. MacDonald PB, Alexander MJ, Frejuk J, et al: Comprehensive functional analysis of shoulders following complete acromioclavicular separation. *Am J Sports Med* 16:475-480, 1988.

62. Mack LA, Matsen FA III, Kilcoyne JF, et al: Sonographic evaluation of the rotator cuff: accuracy in patients without prior surgery. *Clin Orthop* 234:21-28, 1988.

63. Matsen FA III, Arntz C: Rotator cuff tendon failure. In Rockwood CA, Matsen FA III: *The*

*shoulder*. Philadelphia, 1990, WB Saunders, pp 647-677.

64. Matsen FA III: Subacromial impingement. In Rockwood CA, Matsen III FA: *The shoulder*. Philadelphia, 1990, WB Saunders, p 638.

65. Matsen FA III, Lippitt SB, Sidles JA, et al: *Practical evaluation and management of the shoulder*. Philadelphia, 1994, WB Saunders.

66. Miniaci A, Willits K, Vellet AD: Magnetic resonance imaging evaluation of the asymptomatic shoulder. Paper presented to American Academy of Orthopaedic Surgeons, 61st Annual Meeting, New Orleans, 1994.

67. Mink JH, Harris E, Rappaport M: Rotator cuff tears: evaluation using double-contrast shoulder arthrography. *Radiology* 153:621-623, 1985.

68. Morrey B: Reoperation for failed surgical treatment of refractory lateral epicondylitis. *J Shoulder Elbow Surg* 1:47-55, 1992.

69. Morrey BF: *The elbow and its disorders*. ed 2, Philadelphia, 1993, WB Saunders, pp 872-880.

70. Morrey BF, Askew LJ, An KN, et al: A biomechanical study of normal elbow motion. *J Bone Joint Surg* 63-A:872, 1981.

71. Morrison DS, Frogameni A, Woodworth P: Conservative management for subacromial impingement of the shoulder. Paper presented to American Shoulder and Elbow Surgeons, Ninth Open Meeting, San Francisco, 1993.

72. Murphy OB, Bellamy R, Wheeler W, et al: Post-traumatic osteolysis of the distal clavicle. *Clin Orthop* 109:108-114, 1975.

73. Neer CI: Anterior acromioplasty for the chronic impingement syndrome in the shoulder. *J Bone Joint Surg* 54-A:41, 1972.

74. Neer CS II: Impingement lesions. *Clin Orthop* 173:70-77, 1983.

75. Neer CS II: *Shoulder reconstruction*. Philadelphia, 1990, WB Saunders.

76. Nelson M, Leather G, Nirschl R, et al: Evaluation of the painful shoulder. *J Bone Joint Surg* 73-A:707-716, 1991.

77. Neviaser TJ, Neviaser RJ, Neviaser JS, et al: Lateral epicondylitis: results of outpatient surgery and immediate motion. *Contemp Orthop* 11:43, 1985.

78. Nicholson GG: The effects of passive joint mobilization on pain and hypomobility associated with adhesive capsulitis of the shoulder. *J Orthop Sports Phys Ther* 6: 1985.

79. Nirschl RP, Pettrone F: Tennis elbow: the surgical treatment of lateral epicondylitis. *J Bone Joint Surg* 61-A:832, 1979.

80. Novak P, Romeo AA, Hager CA, et al: Open distal clavicle resection: an objective and subjec-tive analysis of results. *J Shoulder Elbow Surg* 1994.

81. Peterson CJ: Degeneration of the acromioclavicular joint: a morphological study. *Acta Orthop Scand* 54:434-438, 1983.

82. Peterson CJ, Redlund-Johnell I: Radiographic joint space in normal acromioclavicular joints. *Acta Orthop Scand* 54:431-433, 1983.

83. Post M, Cohen J: Impingement syndrome: a review of late stage II and early stage III lesions. *Clin Orthop* 207:126-132, 1986.

84. Price R, Sinclair H, Heinrich I, et al: Local injection treatment of tennis elbow: hydrocortisone, triamcinolone, and lidocaine compared. *Br J Rheumatol* 30:39-44, 1991.

85. Raddatz DA, Hoffman GS, Franck WA: Septic bursitis: presentation, treatment, and prognosis. *J Rheumatol* 14:1160-1163, 1987.

86. Regan W, Wold L, Coonrad R, et al: Microscopic histopathology of chronic refractory lateral epicondylitis. *Am J Sports Med* 20:746-749, 1992.

87. Resch H, Golser K, Thoeni H, et al: Arthroscopic repair of superior glenoid labral detachment. *J Shoulder Elbow Surg* 2:147-155, 1993.

88. Rockwood CAJ, Matsen FA III: *The shoulder*. Philadelphia, 1990, WB Saunders.

89. Rockwood CAJ, Szalay EA, Curtis RJ, et al: X-ray evaluation of shoulder problems. In Rockwood CAJ, Matsen FA III: *The shoulder*. Philadelphia, 1990, WB Saunders.

90. Rockwood CAJ, Lyons FR: Shoulder impingement syndrome: diagnosis, radiographic evaluation and treatment with a modified Neer acromioplasty. *J Bone Joint Surg* 75-A:409-424, 1993.

91. Rockwood, CAJ, Williams GR, Young DC: Injuries to the acromioclavicular joint. In Rockwood CAJ, Green DP, Bucholz RW: *Fractures in adults*. Philadelphia, 1984, JB Lippincott, pp 1181-1251.

92. Rockwood CAJ, Young DC: Disorders of the acromioclavicular joint. In Rockwood CAJ, Matsen FA III: *The shoulder*. Philadelphia, 1990, WB Saunders pp 413-476.

93. Smith DL, McAfee JH, Lucas LM, et al: Septic and nonseptic olecranon bursitis: utility of the surface temperature probe in the early differentiation of septic and nonseptic cases. *Arch Intern Med* 149:1581-1588, 1989.

94. Smith DL, McAfee JH, Lucas LM, et al: Treatment of nonseptic olecranon bursitis: a controlled, blinded prospective trial. *Arch Intern Med* 149:2527-2530, 1989.

95. Snyder, SJ, Karzel RP, Del Pizzo W, et al: SLAP

lesions of the shoulder. *Arthroscopy* 6:274-279, 1990.

96. St John JN, Palmaz JC: The cubital tunnel in ulnar entrapment neuropathy. *Radiology* 158:119-121, 1986.

97. Injury and illness data from 1987 workers' compensation records. US Department of Labor, 1990.

98. National Health Interview Survey, Data tapes, 1988.

99. Taft TN, Wilson FC, Oglesby JW, Dislocation of the acromioclavicular joint. *J Bone Joint Surg* 69-A:1045-1051, 1987.

100. Wadsworth CT, Nielsen DH, Burns LT, et al: The effect of the counterforce armband on wrist extension and grip strength and pain in subjects with tennis elbow. *J Orthop Sports Phys Ther* 11:192-195, 1989.

101. Walker SW, Couch WH, Boester GA, et al: Isokinetic strength of the shoulder after repair of a torn rotator cuff. *J Bone Joint Surg* 69-A:1041-1044, 1987.

102. Walsh WM, Peterson DA, Shelton G, et al: Shoulder strength following acromioclavicular injury. *Am J Sports Med* 13:153-158, 1985.

103. Weaver JK, Dunn HK: Treatment of acromioclavicular injuries, especially complete acromioclavicular separation. *J Bone Joint Surg* 54-A:1187-1197, 1972.

104. Weber SC: Arthroscopic versus open treatment of significant partial thickness rotator cuff tears. Paper presented to 13th Annual Meeting, Orlando, Fla., 1994.

105. Weinstein PS, Canoso JJ, Wohlgethan JR: Long-term follow-up of corticosteroid injection for traumatic olecranon bursitis. *Ann Rheum Dis* 43:44-49, 1984.

106. Wilde AH: Shoulder arthroplasty: what is it good for and how good is it? In Matsen FA III, Fu FH, Hawkins RJ: *The shoulder: a balance of mobility and stability*, Rosemont, Ill., 1992, American Academy of Orthopaedic Surgeons, pp 459-481.

# CHAPTER 22

## JOINT SYSTEMS: KNEE AND HIP

*James V. Luck, Jr.*

Early musculoskeletal impairment evaluation systems were strictly anatomic and focused only on range of motion and amputation.[10,26] They were simple and reproducible but failed to cover most clinical situations adequately. A more comprehensive system is, of necessity, more complex, requiring more judgement and expertise. The fourth edition of the AMA *Guides to the Evaluation of Permanent Impairment (Guides)* embodies major changes in the lower extremity section enabling the evaluator to assess accurately many more clinical situations.[2] This chapter applies this system to a broad range of pathology in the lower extremity and is intended to be used in conjunction with the fourth edition of the *Guides*.

More than in the upper extremity or spine, the evaluation of lower-extremity impairment lends itself to the utilization of all three general rating methodologies: anatomic, diagnostic, and functional (see Chapter 13). The upper extremity utilizes all three but is primarily anatomic, based on range of motion (ROM). The spine is predominately diagnostic but is anatomic under certain entities. Although most scholars agree that functional assessment, such as strength and endurance measurement, is the ultimate method for impairment rating, its application will only progress when assessment techniques and equipment become more objective, valid, and reproducible. By including some of the simpler and more reproducible functional assessment methodologies, this section takes another step forward in that progression.

The principal advantage of utilizing all three methodologies is the flexibility that it gives the physician to match more closely the methodology to each patient's physical impairment and thus to more accurately and appropriately rate each patient. Some physical impairments are more accurately rated by alterations in the range of motion, whereas others fit best under diagnostic categories or functional assessment. In some cases, a combination of two or three methodologies will be required. However, using more than one rating methodology for a single anatomic lesion is only allowed under certain circumstances as described in this chapter and the AMA *Guides*. Careful adherence to these principles will make it easier for the evaluating physician to select the best methodology and also ensure the highest degree of consistency between evaluators of the same patient and between patients with the same physical impairment. Combining the three methodologies requires medical knowledge, experience, and judgement as well as careful and thoughtful evaluation. It should only be undertaken by physicians who are adequately trained and experienced in examination techniques of the musculoskeletal system.

## LOWER EXTREMITY EVALUATION AND RATING METHODOLOGIES

In the fourth edition of the AMA *Guides*, lower extremity impairment includes nine separate methodologies each with its own rating scale (Table 22-1).[2] Arriving at the correct impairment for a specific clinical situation requires a thorough history, careful physical examination, musculoskeletal specialty expertise, and a thoughtful selection of the optimal methodology or combination of methodologies. Where a choice exists between methodologies, the one with the greatest objectivity, specificity, and reliability should be selected.

Objectivity relates to the successful elimination of confounding factors such as motivation that might influence the resulting impairment rating. Active range-of-motion (AROM) and manual muscle testing for strength are dependent on patient cooperation and motivation. Electromyographic (EMG) and radiographic findings are highly objective. Reflex changes are much more objective than sensory changes.

Reliability refers to the consistency of results between two or more medical evaluators. Limb girth measurements may have a high variance between observers because of differences in technique, varia-

**TABLE 22-1    LOWER EXTREMITY IMPAIRMENT METHODOLOGIES***

| METHODOLOGY | OBJECTIVITY | RELIABILITY | SPECIFICITY |
| --- | --- | --- | --- |
| Limb length discrepancy | 1 | 1 | 1 |
| Gait derangement | 3 | 1 | 3 |
| Muscle atrophy | 1 | 3 | 2 |
| Manual muscle testing | 2 | 2 | 2 |
| Range of motion | 2 | 2 | 2 |
| Arthritic degeneration | 1 | 1 | 1 |
| Diagnosis-related estimates | 1 | 2 | 1 |
| Amputations | 1 | 1 | 1 |
| Peripheral nerve deficits | 1 | 2 | 1 |

*SCALE: 1 = good; 2 = fair; 3 = poor.

tions in local edema, and presence or absence of joint effusion. Limb-length measurement by tele-roentgenograms is much more reliable than by tape measure. For musculoskeletal disorders of the lower extremity, diagnostic-based methodologies should be highly reliable.

Specificity refers to the accuracy with which a given methodology or combination of methodologies describes a specific clinical situation. Amputation rating scales are highly specific. Radiographically-measured arthritic degeneration of a joint is moderately specific. Muscle-girth measurement, as an indicator of muscle strength and endurance, is objective but not specific. Manual muscle testing is less objective but much more specific. In a cooperative and reliable patient who is able to make a maximal effort, manual muscle testing should be utilized over girth measurements.

Few tests score high marks in all three areas (objectivity, reliability, and specificity), but in making decisions between choices, all of these factors must be considered.

The gait derangement scale is based on the use of assistive devices for ambulation. It is highly dependent on patient integrity, reliability, and motivation and should rarely be used as a primary rating scale. Its greatest value is in serving as a general guide

against which other lower extremity impairment values may be compared. The use of a cane or crutch for low-back pain is generally inappropriate and would be a poor example of the use of this scale. However, a patient with superior gluteal nerve injury and no hip abductor function should use a cane on the opposite side and would be an appropriate use of this scale as a check against the other rating variables such as manual muscle testing or peripheral nerve deficit. Of these, the peripheral nerve deficit scale is the most objective, reliable, and specific. Under no circumstances should the gait disturbance scale be added to other impairment values for the same extremity.

Diagnosis-related estimates are objective and specific. However, reliability is only fair because of occasional physician disagreement over the appropriate diagnostic value especially when it relates to the outcome of surgery. For example, the operating surgeon may rate the result of an anterior cruciate ligament repair as good with no residual laxity (0% impairment), where an independent evaluating physician rates the same patient as fair with moderate residual laxity (17% lower extremity impairment).[2] This scale is designed to stand alone except where specifically instructed to be used in combination with another method. A femoral neck fracture malunion, for example, is rated at 30% lower extremity impairment plus the value produced by ROM abnormalities.[2] These patients will generally have significant restriction of motion. Those values would be added to the diagnostic values using the combined values chart.

In a patient with moderate-to-advanced degenerative arthritis, either ROM or radiographic measurement of cartilage interval can be utilized. In a patient where the ROM was deemed reliable, the method giving the greatest value should be selected.

## THE PELVIS

Work-related pelvic fractures are usually the consequence of motor vehicle-related injuries, falls, or crush injuries and are relatively uncommon. Subsequent musculoskeletal impairment evaluation and rating may be divided into three areas: sacroiliac joint injuries, acetabular fractures, and nonarticular fractures.

### Sacroiliac Joint Injuries

Fractures that appear undisplaced on plain radiography may result in significant impairment if there is joint surface derangement or neuroforaminal encroachment on sacral roots. Computed tomography (CT) is essential to define these problems (Fig. 22-1). Isotopic bone scans will also identify an occult sacral

A

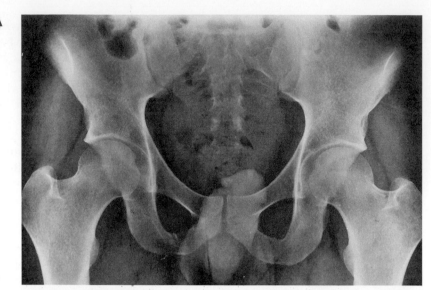

B

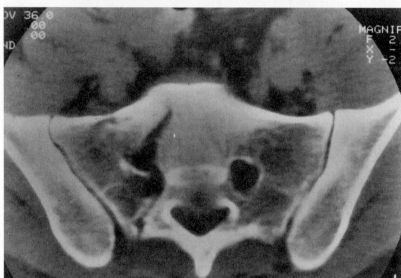

**FIGURE 22-1** **A,** AP pelvis x-ray of a 29-year-old male who fell from a ladder. The x-ray shows some loss of definition of the right S1 foramen but, because of overlying bowel gas, fails to define the presence or absence of a fracture. In reality, this x-ray would usually be interpreted as normal. **B,** CT scan of the pelvis clearly demonstrating a displaced comminuted sacral fracture with significant involvement of the second sacral foramen. Other CT views demonstrated involvement of the first, second, and third sacral foramina. The patient clinically had weakness of plantar flexion of his right foot and ankle, which gradually recovered over a 6-month period.

fracture, but CT scans will still be necessary to define it clearly.[5,31] In most instance, CT alone is more cost-effective. Posttraumatic radiculopathy is associated with objective clinical findings and a positive EMG for the upper two sacral roots, but may only be manifested by perianal anesthesia for the lower roots. As long as the injury is unilateral, it is unlikely to result in loss of bowel or bladder control. Radiculopathy caused by undisplaced fractures often improves, and it is important not to rate the patient until a permanent and stationary status is reached, which may take 12 to 18 months. According to the AMA *Guides,* fourth edition, radiculopathy of the lower sacral roots does not result in impairment.[2] However, residual pain that follows the appropriate anatomic dermatome(s) should be rated the same as residual pain from a sacroiliac (SI) joint fracture (1-3% whole person).[2] Rarely, spinal root injuries from neuroforaminal fractures may result in residual causalgia that is impossible to measure and difficult to document. Rating musculoskeletal impairment on the basis of pain is highly controversial. The reader is referred to the AMA *Guides,* fourth edition, section 3.1k, page 46, and Chapter 15.[2]

Sacroiliac joint derangement from intraarticular fractures often results in some residual pain and limited ambulatory capacity warranting an impairment rating. Objective findings include a positive FABER or Patrick's test and a CT scan clearly indicative of joint surface abnormalities, although the plain x-ray may be deceptively negative. Undisplaced fractures with severe joint space narrowing produce a 3% whole person impairment rating.[2] Rarely, a degenerative SI joint is symptomatic enough to warrant arthrodesis. A fused SI joint would not rate any permanent impairment unless there were associated physical findings such as loss of hip range of motion or neurological deficit.

Displaced SI joint fractures, such as a Malgaigne fracture that is associated with an anterior ring disruption, can rate as high as 10%.[2,33,35,40] Malgaigne fractures result in significant shortening of the lower extremity. In this case the pelvic fracture rating would be combined with the limb length discrepancy rating using the combined values table.[2] Furthermore, these injuries are frequently associated with sciatic nerve injury for which the nerve rating would be combined with the others, again using the combined values table. Patients with severe pelvic fractures often have associated lower extremity trauma such as femur fractures with which any pelvic impairment values would be combined. An estimate for loss of motion as a consequence of prolonged immobilization would also be combined if it were deemed substantial by the evaluating physician.

## Acetabular Fractures

Truly undisplaced acetabular fractures are actually quite rare. All acetabular fractures should be evaluated with a CT scan to determine offset, separation, the presence of intra-articular fragments, and associated femoral head injury.[5,9,33,36,38,42] Many that appear undisplaced on plain radiographs will show separation or offset of a few millimeters (Fig. 22-2). Minor separation has a better prognosis than offset. Fractures that have only minor displacement should heal rapidly, within six to twelve weeks. When CT confirms union, muscle strengthening and activities can begin. Once permanent and stationary, the patient and impairment can be rated by whichever scale is the most objective and best describes the impairment. The options include diagnostic values, range of motion, radiographic cartilage interval, or manual muscle testing. The latter is difficult to perform objectivity and may vary between evaluators. A minimally displaced fracture should not change the cartilage interval until many years later, so the most appropriate rating methods are diagnostic or range of motion. The fourth edition of the AMA *Guides* does not have a diagnostic value for acetabular fractures, per se, and suggests that range of motion be utilized.[2] If the range is not significantly abnormal, the Trendelenburg test is clearly normal with no demonstrable abductor weakness, and if no narrowing of the cartilage interval is present, then there is no ratable permanent impairment. Potential future arthritic changes are not ratable. The forces necessary to cause an acetabular fracture can crush the articular cartilage, resulting in progressive posttraumatic degenerative arthritis over time, but, in this group of patients with "undisplaced" acetabular fractures, it is difficult to predict in which cases this will occur. It is essential

that the evaluating physician indicate that this possibility exists, so that if and when it does occur the patient can be reassessed.

## Nonarticular Pelvic Fractures

Minimally-displaced pubic ramus fractures heal rapidly. Residual symptoms are often related to associated soft tissue trauma. Minimally displaced ramus fractures warrant no rating. Displaced ramus fractures may be assessed on the basis of limb-length discrepancy, associated nerve deficit, or loss of hip motion in the case of significant periarticular soft tissue injury with residual contracture. Fractures involving the sciatic nerve and the sciatic notch may injure the superior and/or the inferior gluteal nerves. If permanent and complete, impairment from these nerve injuries is a very significant (superior gluteal = 25%, inferior gluteal = 15%, and sciatic = 30% impairment of the whole person).[2] The superior and inferior gluteal nerves are pure motor nerves and the muscles they supply (hip abductors and hip extensors, respectively) should be checked very carefully. Residual weakness due to partial denervation may be difficult to determine on a routine office examination, but with extended walking the muscle fatigues, which results in an abnormal gait and limited ambulatory capacity. If this is suspected, an EMG can clarify the issue. If the EMG confirms partial denervation, rating can be on the basis of manual muscle testing by a physician or trained physical therapist.

## THE HIP JOINT

Degenerative arthritis of the hip is rarely work-related unless it is the consequence of trauma either on the basis of intraarticular fracture or avascular necrosis of the femoral head. The latter condition may pose a difficult dilemma for the evaluating physician.[25] The relationship between avascular necrosis and a femoral neck fracture is clear. However, the more common situation is that of the patient with avascular necrosis of nontraumatic etiology who claims the hip became symptomatic as a consequence of work-related activities, "repetitive trauma", or a minor injury. These patients present with Ficat stage IIb or III radiographic changes showing fracture of the subchondral cortex (Fig. 22-3).[11,34] While the hip may have become symptomatic at work, the etiology of the avascular necrosis is, with rare exception, not work related. The evaluating physician is often asked to determine if the subchondral fracture and onset of symptoms is in any way work-related. This is an impossible question to answer with any certainty, but

A

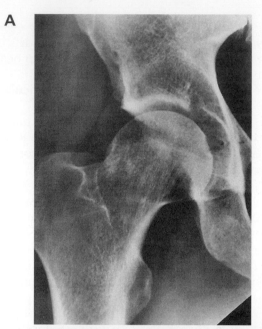

B

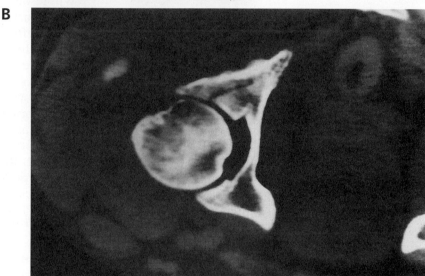

C

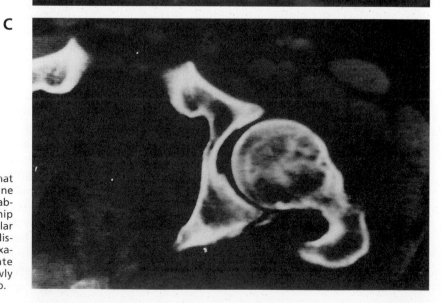

**FIGURE 22-2**    **A,** AP x-ray of the right hip that shows a pelvic fracture involving the ischial spine but does not define the involvement of the acetabular articular surface. **B,** CT scan of the right hip demonstrates a 2 mm displacement of the articular surface. **C,** A more distal CT scan view shows displacement of the posterior rim and slight subluxation of the femoral head. There is a moderate probability that this patient will develop slowly progressive degenerative arthritis of the right hip.

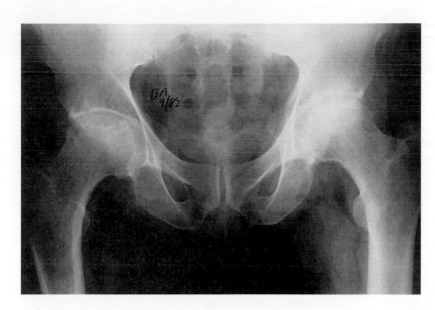

**FIGURE 22-3**    AP pelvis x-ray of a 52-year-old worker who complained of right-hip pain after a twisting injury at work. The x-ray shows avascular necrosis of both hips, grade 2b with collapse of the subchondral cortex on the right and grade 2a on the left.

medical probability is the legal benchmark. If the patient is involved in heavy lifting or carrying, or if there was a specific injury, a partial relationship to work is usually established based on aggravation of a preexisting condition. Lacking a specific injury, and given work activities that are no more strenuous than routine activities of daily living, the progression of the avascular necrosis is probably unrelated to work. In most states, if the condition is even partially work-related, the workers' compensation system is responsible for covering medical expenses to correct the problem. Two critical issues remain to be addressed by the evaluating physician: future medical coverage of the diseased hip and potential secondary disease in the opposite hip. Treatment of the avascular necrosis will depend on the stage, but in cases with fracture and collapse of the subchondral cortex, hip replacement is usually needed. Avascular necrosis is bilateral in up to 80% of cases depending on etiology and clinical series. It is essential that the opposite hip be carefully evaluated by MRI and isotope scan at the initial examination and that the evaluator comment on the likelihood of opposite-side involvement. If opposite-side involvement later occurs, the patient and representing attorney will commonly question whether the increased load borne during the convalescence of the first hip accelerated the progression of disease in the other hip. Medically this seems quite unlikely. However, commentary on this issue will often prevent a controversy later.

Degenerative arthritis that is not severe enough to warrant surgical intervention is best rated using either range of motion or radiographically measured cartilage interval. The method of choice is the one that awards the highest value consistent with objec-

tivity. If range of motion is difficult to assess due to subjective factors, such as excessive pain behavior, measured cartilage interval may be the preferred procedure. The cartilage interval, commonly referred to as *joint space*, must be assessed by taking a radiograph directly over the involved joint with the source 36 inches from the cassette and the hip in as close to neutral position as possible. Because the hip is a ball-and-socket joint, position is not as critical as it is in the knee and weight bearing is not required.

Patients will often have remarkable function with only 1 mm of cartilage interval, but when the last remnant of cartilage wears down, symptoms become severe and unrelenting, and require total hip replacement. Until the fourth edition of the AMA *Guides,* hip replacement was rated using a single, diagnostic value recommended by the American Academy of Orthopedic Surgeons (AAOS) in its 1962 edition of the *Manual for Orthopaedic Surgeons in Evaluating Permanent Physical Impairment.*[1] This value was based on prophylactic work restrictions to protect the prosthetic joint. In this system all hip replacement patients would be rated the same. For many years, clinical research studies have utilized various scales to evaluate the results of hip replacement.[4,6] In the fourth edition of the AMA *Guides,* a modified Harris rating scale was utilized.[14] This allows the impairment rating to reflect the result of the hip replacement as measured by multiple parameters including pain, gait, activities of daily living, deformity, and range of motion, and follows a widely-used and widely accepted research instrument (Table 22-2).

Management of occupational injuries includes future medical care for the specific area involved. Joint replacements in a working-age population are likely

**TABLE 22-2    RATING HIP REPLACEMENT RESULTS***

| | NO. OF POINTS | | NO. OF POINTS |
|---|---|---|---|
| **a. Pain** | | Public transportation | |
| None | 44 | Able to use | 1 |
| Slight | 40 | Unable to use | 0 |
| Moderate, occasional | 30 | **d. Deformity** | |
| Moderate | 20 | Fixed adduction | |
| Marked | 10 | <10° | 1 |
| **b. Function** | | ≥10° | 0 |
| Limp | | Fixed internal rotation | |
| None | 11 | <10° | 1 |
| Slight | 8 | ≥10° | 0 |
| Moderate | 5 | Fixed external rotation | |
| Severe | 0 | <10° | 1 |
| Supportive device | | ≥10° | 0 |
| None | 11 | Flexion contracture | |
| Cane for long walks | 7 | <15° | 1 |
| Cane | 5 | ≥15° | 0 |
| One crutch | 3 | Leg length discrepancy | |
| Two canes | 2 | <1.5 cm | 1 |
| Two crutches | 0 | ≥1.5 cm | 0 |
| Distance walked | | **e. Range of motion** | |
| Unlimited | 11 | Flexion | |
| Six blocks | 8 | >90° | 1 |
| Three blocks | 5 | ≤90° | 0 |
| Indoors | 2 | Abduction | |
| In bed or chair | 0 | >15° | 1 |
| **c. Activities** | | ≤15° | 0 |
| Stair climbing | | Adduction | |
| Normal | 4 | >15° | 1 |
| Using railing | 2 | ≤15° | 0 |
| Cannot climb readily | 1 | External rotation | |
| Unable to climb | 0 | >30° | 1 |
| Putting on shoes and socks | | ≤30° | 0 |
| With ease | 4 | Internal rotation | |
| With difficulty | 2 | >15° | 1 |
| Unable to do | 0 | ≤15° | 0 |
| Sitting | | | |
| Any chair, 1 hour | 4 | | |
| High chair | 2 | | |
| Unable to sit comfortably | 0 | | |

*Add the points from categories *a, b, c, d,* and *e* to determine the total and characterize the result of replacement. (From *AMA Guides to the evaluation of permanent impairment,* ed 4, American Medical Association, Chicago, 1993.)

to include the need for surgical revision. This raises significant apportionment issues in cases where the origin of the degenerative arthritis is nonindustrial but the condition was aggravated by occupational factors, and is often a source of controversy in patients with avascular necrosis. If the occupational injury was only an aggravating factor and the joint replacement would have been needed in the relatively near future anyway, future medical care, after the patient's condition is permanent and stationary, would seem to be nonindustrial.

## THE THIGH AND FEMUR

Work-related injuries to the thigh may be divided into soft-tissue trauma, fractures, or combined injuries. Lacerations to muscle often heal without impairment. Manual muscle testing is fairly accurate and reproducible for grades I to III if performed by a physical therapist or physician trained in these techniques.[37] Accuracy is also very dependent on patient cooperation and the ability to make a maximal effort, which may be inhibited by pain, fear of pain, or motivational problems. For this reason, two evaluators' results should be consistent to use this methodology for impairment rating.

Grades IV and V are difficult to differentiate on manual muscle testing. In the case of the quadriceps and hamstring muscle groups, isokinetic testing is well developed and can accurately differentiate between grade IV and V when the opposite side is normal for comparison.[22] Associated nerve injury, if complete, should be rated using peripheral nerve impairment scales.[2] Partial motor deficits should be rated using manual muscle testing. Sensory or dysesthesia components may be added from the table.

## Proximal Femoral Fractures

Femoral neck fractures may heal without impairment but are subject to a variety of potential complications resulting in significant permanent impairment. Malunion and nonunion are rated under the diagnostic section, and a loss-of-motion impairment estimate would be combined with either impairment. Trochanteric bursitis, if chronic and associated with a positive Trendelenburg gait or abductor lurch, is rated in the diagnostic section of the AMA *Guides* at 3% whole person.[2]

Intertrochanteric fractures rarely result in nonunion or avascular necrosis. Residual impairment estimates for these and femoral shaft fractures are based on examination findings, principally loss of motion and weakness, with a few exceptions. Malunion with angular deformity would be rated using specific values in Table 64 of the AMA *Guides* to which examination findings such as loss of motion or shortening are additive.[2] Tape measurement is highly variable due to imprecise landmarks, especially in obese or edematous patients. Any hip or knee flexion will also invalidate the result. Standing measurements, using the iliac crest, are dependent on hip and knee position as well as the ability of the examiner to measure accurately the difference between the two sides in spite of the overlying soft tissues. The range of error with these two methods is 1 to 2 cm, whereas teleroentgenograms are accurate to within less than 1 cm.[18]

## Distal Femur Fractures

Values for angular deformity of supracondylar fractures are in the knee section of Table 64 in the AMA *Guides,* because that is the joint where the effect is manifest.[2] Loss of motion will be at this site as well. More severe angular deformities may result in gradually progressive degenerative arthritis of the adjacent joint. This effect will be accelerated if the joint has as-

sociated or pre-existing damage. As in acetabular fractures, the evaluating physician should comment on potential future problems and apportion those problems between pre-existing and work-related etiologies. Physicians appropriately view this task as onerous because there is no scientific basis that would allow quantification. Many figuratively "throw their hands up in the air" and decline to comment on these issues. Insurance administrators and legal representatives are equally frustrated and explain to the physicians that, even though a definitive scientific answer is impossible, a musculoskeletal specialist physician by virtue of his training and experience can give a far better estimate than they. "Medical probability" is a legal construct that falls in the realm of opinion not to be confused with medical science. Like it or not, these determinations are best made by physicians. To decline to comment is to relegate the responsibility to others less qualified.

## THE KNEE JOINT

### Intra-articular Fractures

Intra-articular fractures involving the knee may be divided into four categories (intercondylar, osteochondral, tibial plateau, patellar), which have quite different prognoses and anticipated impairments. All of these fractures require a high level of patient cooperation to obtain an optimal result.

Intercondylar fractures may heal with minimal impairment if the weight bearing articular surfaces are minimally involved. If the fracture is through the trochlea and is anatomically reduced with enough stability to allow early range of motion, the end result may be excellent. At the opposite end of this spectrum is the comminuted, displaced, intraarticular fracture of the distal femur that, even if optimally reduced, will lead to progressive degenerative arthritis. The rate of progression is dependent on many factors but mostly on accuracy of reduction and the ability to initiate early range of motion.

Isolated osteochondral fractures, involving weight bearing surfaces, have a guarded prognosis. If repaired early and anatomically, they may heal without significant impairment. However, the articular segment is avascular and may collapse at a later time, giving rise to degenerative arthritis.

Tibial plateau fractures are frequently comminuted and displaced, and analogous to the displaced intercondylar femur fractures in their prognosis. Open reduction and some form of stabilization that will allow early range of motion are required for any displaced tibial plateau fracture. Unlike intercondylar femoral fractures, these fractures are often associated with meniscal and/or ligament injury, which increases the degree of permanent impairment.

Patellar fractures, if minimally displaced and stable, may be treated nonoperatively. As in all intraarticular fractures, surface reduction is critical and offset adversely affects the prognosis. Unstable fractures, even if reducible, require internal fixation, which allows earlier range of motion than casting alone, and minimizes loss of motion and maximizes muscle function.

Arthrofibrosis refers to the development of dense adhesions, fibrous pannus, and capsular hypertrophy.[24] It is common following intraarticular fractures that are immobilized and may result in severe loss of motion. Early motion will help prevent this complication as well as maintain the health of the articular cartilage and muscle function.

Permanent impairment may be evaluated once the fracture is healed and the patient has achieved maximum benefit from rehabilitation. Deformities including varus, valgus, or malrotation are rated using numerical values in the diagnostic section.[2] Loss of motion, loss of cartilage interval on standing x-ray, and shortening are combined. The examining physician must carefully evaluate ligament integrity because ligament injury may be associated with any intraarticular or periarticular fracture and may be overlooked due to the more obvious fracture.

## Ligament Injuries

Injuries of the collateral or cruciate knee ligaments are common and serious injuries of the lower extremity, and they often result in permanent impairment. This is especially true of the anterior cruciate ligament, which because of its intraarticular location, is difficult to repair with a durable long-term result. These repairs may stretch out over two years, with recurrent problems of instability with twisting and pivoting activities. This results in joint subluxation and severe damage to the lateral meniscus and articular surface. Because of uncertain results and a prolonged rehabilitation following anterior cruciate repair, patients who do not engage in pivoting activities are often treated nonoperatively with quadriceps and hamstring strengthening and the use of an orthosis for sports. Some of these patients will require a late reconstruction because of significant instability and progressive joint surface damage. In those patients, an early repair might have prevented the joint damage and the result of repair before joint surface damage is better.

Posterior cruciate ligament (PCL) injuries are much less frequent and repairs, when indicated, are more predictable and successful. The principal impairment resulting from PCL instability is difficulty descending stairs and kneeling.

Isolated collateral sprains require repair only if they are associated with significant laxity. Mild-to-moderate sprains will often heal without problems, and mild laxity of the medial collateral ligament will usually diminish over six month.[15] All acute ligament injuries require an MRI or arthroscopy for evaluation because of the high incidence of associated injuries to menisci and the articular surfaces. Mild ligament sprains may be isolated but severe ones almost never are.

Impairment evaluation in patients with ligament injuries requires the physician's ability to determine the degree of laxity (mild, moderate, or severe) on physical examination.[7] These examination techniques require significant experience and should only be performed by physicians who are trained to do this. Instrumentation, a knee arthrometer, has been developed to quantify the amount of force used in the anterior drawer or Lochman tests, so that the amount of anterior tibial displacement will be more consistent among examiners.[27] This equipment was developed for clinical research but might be useful in impairment evaluation. Muscle atrophy is common following these injuries and is included in the *Guides* impairment rating. Loss-of-motion impairment would be combined as would arthritic degeneration impairment demonstrated on standing radiographs. Discussion in the impairment report about prognosis and future medical care with special reference to arthritic degeneration is critical for patients with ligament and articular surface injury.

## Meniscal Injuries

Small acute meniscal tears that are adequately symptomatic require arthroscopic debridement but usually result in no permanent impairment.[20] Large acute tears, if simple, are best treated with repair, and this may result in some permanent loss of motion. Chronic tears are often associated with articular degeneration, especially in middle-aged and older patients.[16] This raises the issue of causation. Since the advent of MRI, it has become apparent that most individuals have degenerative changes in the posterior horn of their medial menisci by early middle age if not sooner. In fact, the vast majority of tears are the result of minor trauma superimposed on meniscal degeneration.[41] This degeneration is slowly progressive and can eventually result in a full-thickness degenerative tear or horizontal cleavage lesion without specific trauma. Arthroscopy in the individuals with degenerative tears usually reveals fairly extensive chondromalacia not limited to the area of the meniscal tear.

If patients associate the onset of symptoms in their knee with work activity or a minor injury, the evaluating physician is asked to determine causation as well as to rate impairment. Often there is no clear answer, and each case must be decided on its specific merits. The need for future medical care and apportionment must also be determined. In the absence of a specific injury, the type of work is critical. If the patient is involved in frequent squatting, twisting, carrying heavy objects, or climbing, his work probably played a role in the acceleration of the degenerative disorder. In this case, the need for acute care is work related. However, the degenerative arthritis will continue to progress. Eventually the patient may require further work restrictions and even a knee replacement.

The evaluator must determine if and how these further problems relate to work activities. Once the initial meniscal tear is accepted as work related, the future degenerative changes also are related, in part, because excision of a meniscus is believed to accelerate degenerative arthritis.

As mentioned above, a degenerative tear of the lateral meniscus may follow anterior cruciate instability. For example, a worker with anterior cruciate laxity from a high school football injury later develops lateral meniscal pathology that he relates to his work as a plumber. The evaluating physician must decide if the lateral meniscal degeneration would have occurred within the same time frame, absent this patient's work activities. If it is decided that the work played some role, then the same situation as described above for degenerative tear of the posterior horn of the medial meniscus exists here with all of its ramifications for future medical care and apportionment issues.

With the substantial concurrent and future costs involved, the reader can readily appreciate why these cases result in the need for multiple expert opinions and may be highly contested. Under these circumstances, treatment is often delayed until financial responsibility can be resolved. Much of this may be avoided if these issues are addressed comprehensively and authoritatively by the initial physician.

Impairment rating of meniscal injuries under the diagnostic section is divided into partial and complete lesions. Involvement of both menisci is rated greater than double that for a single meniscus because of the significant decrease in function with both sides of the knee involved. Loss of motion, which is usually only present in meniscal lesions if there is associated degenerative arthritis, is combined using the combined values chart. Loss of cartilage interval on standing x-ray, if significant, is also combined using the combined values chart.[2]

## Chondromalacia

Tibiofemoral chondromalacia in weight-bearing zones is progressive at a variable rate and has been discussed in the sections on fractures, ligament, and meniscal injuries. Patellofemoral chondromalacia is quite another issue.

Patellofemoral crepitation with active range of motion is common in the general population from adolescence on and usually asymptomatic. Patients commonly have a complaint of anterior knee pain that follows a minor contusion to the patella or state that the pain came on spontaneously after repetitive squatting or prolonged use of stairs. Physical examination reveals mild patellofemoral crepitation on the symptomatic side. Diagnostic studies, including MRI, are usually negative except for degenerative changes within the meniscus without a tear. The physician is posed with a dilemma, again, in which it must be determined if the symptoms are related to the mild patellofemoral chondromalacia and whether there is a significant work-related injury. Examination of the opposite, asymptomatic knee may help resolve this issue if there is similar mild patellofemoral crepitation. Often this is the case. Although it does not rule out an industrial aggravation of a preexisting problem, it certainly adds credence to the assertion that some patellofemoral chondromalacia existed before the industrial "injury". Furthermore, the presence of patellofemoral crepitation does not mean the latter is the source of symptoms.[21] Anterior knee pain has many causes including patellar tendinitis, inflammation of the iliotibial band insertion at Gerty's tubercle, inflammation of the insertion of the anterior knee capsule or menisci, and fat pad syndrome. All of these should be self-limited and not result in permanent impairment. For all of these reasons, mild patellofemoral chondromalacia is not a ratable disorder. However, it is ratable if it is associated with narrowed cartilage interval on lateral radiographs, which indicates moderate-to-severe degeneration, or if there is associated loss of motion or measurable muscle atrophy.

## Extensor Mechanism Injuries

These injuries may result from trauma to the quadriceps, fracture of the patella, or rupture or avulsion of the quadriceps (patellar) tendon. Quadriceps lacerations or crush injuries will heal but often with some residual loss of function. This is best measured by manual muscle testing for strength grades I-III and by isokinetic testing for grades IV and V. There may also be significant residual fibrosis, contracture, and loss of motion; if the latter is significant, an impairment estimate for it may be combined. There is also atrophy, which is difficult to measure because of scar tissue and local swelling. Furthermore, if strength is used as the parameter, atrophy is not combined because it would be duplicative.

Patellar tendon ruptures, lacerations, and avulsions, if complete, require repair followed by immobilization for three to six weeks. If the tendon becomes infected as a consequence of severe open trauma and part of the substance is lost from necrosis, reconstruction is very difficult and may require several procedures. The permanent impairment is significantly more than with closed injuries and simple primary repair.

Complete loss of knee extension is valued at 10% whole person in addition to any loss of passive knee motion such as a fixed flexion contracture or loss of flexion range. An individual with complete loss of the extensor mechanism can walk normally on level surfaces by using the gluteus maximus and gastrocsoleus muscle groups to lock the knee. This is contingent upon having full hip and knee extension. Only very strong patients with loss of the extensor mechanism can climb stairs, alternating in a normal fashion. Descending hills or stairs is quite difficult.

### Degenerative Arthritis

Many causes of posttraumatic degenerative arthritis and the possible relationships to occupational factors have been described above. According to the Framingham Study, the incidence of degenerative arthritis of the knee is clearly higher in certain occupations.[12] Rate of progression is variable, but ultimately knee replacement may be required. Avascular necrosis of the knee is rare and is mostly seen in patients with systemic diseases such as sickle cell disease, systemic lupus erythematosus, or patients on high-dose steroids. Bilaterality is much less common than with avascular necrosis of the hip.

For younger patients with predominately unicompartmental degenerative arthritis, distal femoral or high tibial osteotomy may be performed to shift the weight to the healthier compartment, which may avoid the need for knee replacement for several years. The outcome of this procedure is less predictable than knee replacement. Poor results are rated using examination criteria including loss of motion and arthritic degeneration.

Knee replacements may be unicondylar or total condylar. They have various degrees of built-in constraint to compensate for loss of cruciate or collateral stability. The need and indications for patellar resurfacing are currently debated and it may or may not be included when the joint is replaced. The results of knee replacement, once permanent and stationary,

are rated using the Knee Society rating system that is analogous to the methodology used for hip replacements (Table 22-3).[19] Longevity of knee replacements appears to exceed that of hip replacements, but future revisions may need to be addressed.

**TABLE 22-3     RATING KNEE REPLACEMENT RESULTS***

|  | **NO. OF POINTS** |
|---|---|
| **a. Pain** | |
| None | 50 |
| Mild or occasional | 45 |
| Stairs only | 40 |
| Walking and stairs | 30 |
| Moderate | |
| Occasional | 20 |
| Continual | 10 |
| Severe | 0 |
| **b. Range of motion** | |
| Add 1 point per 5° | 25 |
| **c. Stability** | |
| (maximum movement in any position) | |
| Anteroposterior | |
| <5 mm | 10 |
| 5-9 mm | 5 |
| >9 mm | 0 |
| Mediolateral | |
| 5° | 15 |
| 6°-9° | 10 |
| 10°-14° | 5 |
| ≥15° | 0 |
| Subtotal | |
| **d. Deductions (minus)** | |
| **Flexion contracture** | |
| 5°-9° | 2 |
| 10°-15° | 5 |
| 16°-20° | 10 |
| >20° | 20 |
| **e. Extension lag** | |
| <10° | 5 |
| 10°-20° | 10 |
| >20° | 15 |
| **f. Alignment** | |
| 0°-4° | 0 |
| 5°-10° | 3 points per degree |
| 11°-15° | 3 points per degree |
| >15° | 20 |
| Deductions subtotal | — |

*The point total for estimating knee replacement results is the sum of the points in categories *a*, *b*, and *c* minus the sum of the points in categories *d*, *e*, and *f*. (From AMA Guides to the evaluation of permanent impairment, ed 4, American Medical Association, Chicago, 1993.)

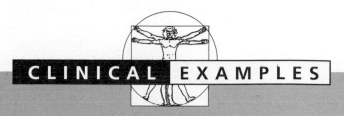

# CLINICAL EXAMPLES

## HIP, THIGH, KNEE, AND LEG

EDITOR'S NOTE—Using the AMA *Guides* for the assessment of lower extremity impairment requires an awareness of the three methods of diagnosis—anatomic, diagnostic, and functional—as well as superb diagnostic skills and appropriate radiographs. In general, the highest award possible, based on the most appropriate of the three methods, is the preferred rating. Difficulties may arise when adequate medical records or radiographs are unavailable or when the physician is not skilled in musculoskeletal examination.

Assessment of the lower extremities using the third edition of the *Guides* was based principally on evaluation of range of motion (ROM), that is, a functional method. The 1993 guidelines (ed 4) are more complex, so evaluators must be thoroughly familiar with the three methods of assessment and study section 3.2 of the *Guides*.*

### EXAMPLE
#### History

A 45-year-old man had a comminuted fracture of his right femur after an industrial accident. He had appropriate surgical care, including debridement of the wound and rod insertion with cerclage cables. His postoperative course was complicated by a wound infection, which resulted in two further surgeries for debridement, bone removal followed by grafting, revision of the fixation, and skin grafting. Two years later, after the patient has had extensive physical therapy, he needs an assessment.

#### Physical Examination

The patient's symptoms include mild discomfort with ambulation, diminished strength, mild problems with balance, and anesthesia in the area of the skin graft. He uses only one cane but has an orthotic shoe device. The right thigh is 3.5 cm smaller than the left, and the right calf is 2.6 cm smaller than the left when measured at similar levels. There is grade 4 motor strength when hip flexion and extension are examined and grade 4 in knee flexion and extension. Hip abduction and adduction, ankle strength, and great toe strength are all rated grade 5. The right side is weaker than the left side. There is a 3.1 cm limb length discrepancy when measured clinically; no radiographs are available for limb length assessment. The radiographs that are available show the results of the surgical intervention. The cartilage interval of the hip is 2 mm, the knee 2 mm, and the patellofemoral joint 3 mm. There is no angulation or malrotation of the femur.

ROM testing of the right hip shows the following results:

| | |
|---|---|
| **Flexion (F):** | 85° |
| **Extension (E):** | 0° |
| **Internal rotation (IR):** | 20° |
| **External rotation (ER):** | 25° |
| **Abduction (AB):** | 20° |
| **Adduction (AD):** | 10° |
| **Abduction contracture:** | None |

The ROM of the knee is F 110° and E 0°. The knee alignment is within normal limits at 8° valgus.

#### Assessment Process

To assess this complicated situation, it is best to divide the process according to the subsections of section 3.2 and use the appropriate subcomponents.

*Limb length discrepancy (3.2a)*—The limb length discrepancy is best measured with x-ray or CT scanograms in patients with pelvic angulation, knee flexion contractures, or significant ankle edema. None of these are present in this case. Therefore the results of the clinical examination are deemed appropriate. A 3.1 cm limb length discrepancy yields a 4% to 5% whole person impairment (WPI) (Table 35). The 4% figure is used based on the

---

*All *sections*, *tables*, and *figures* referred to in this discussion are found in AMA *Guides to the evaluation of permanant impairment*, ed 4, Chapter 3—The Musculoskeletal System, American Medical Association, Chicago, 1993.

*Continued.*

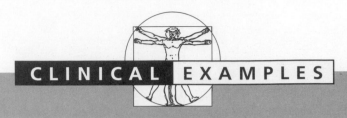

spread of 4% to 5% for a discrepancy of 3.0 to 3.9 cm and the patient's value of 3.1 cm.

*Gait derangement (3.2b)*—A cane is used for walking and an orthotic shoe appliance is used. A leg brace is not used. This yields a 15% WPI (mild "C," Table 36).

*Muscle atrophy (3.2c)*—The muscle atrophy found in this example is assumed to be measured correctly; that is, 10 cm above the patella with the knee fully extended and the muscles relaxed for the thigh and the maximal calf circumference. The 3.5 cm discrepancy for the thigh yields a 5% WPI and the 2.6 cm for the calf yields a 3% to 4% WPI, with the 4% value chosen (Table 37). These values, 5% and 4%, are combined using the Combined Values Chart (pp. 322-324), giving a 9% WPI.

*Manual muscle testing (3.2d)*—The motor examination is relatively normal, except for flexion and extension of the hip and knee. All four areas are graded at level 4, yielding WPI values of 2%, 7%, 5%, and 5% (Tables 38 and 39). Using the Combined Values Chart (pp. 322-324), an 18% WPI is determined.

*Range of motion (3.2e)*—The results of the ROM examination yield the following impairment values (Tables 40 and 41):

**Hip:** F 2%, E 0%, IR 0%, ER 2%, AB 2%, AD 0%
**Knee:** F 0%, varus 0%, valgus 0%

Using the Combined Values Chart, this yields a 6% WPI.

*Joint ankylosis (3.2f)*—No joint ankylosis is found.

*Arthritis (3.2g)*—The cartilage intervals are diminished to 2 mm in both the knee and the hip. This yields values of 8% and 8% (Table 61), resulting in a 15% WPI using the Combined Values Chart. It assumes that the radiographs were taken appropriately, as described in section 3.2g. Additionally, there is no direct trauma to the patellofemoral joint, complaints of patellofemoral pain, or joint crepitation to produce an award for this joint independent of a diminished cartilage interval.

*Amputations (3.2h)*—This section is not applicable.

*Diagnosis-based estimates (3.2i)*—No angulation of the femur is present nor are any of the diagnoses listed for the knee in Table 64. Therefore this section is not applicable. The same applies for Tables 65 and 66, addressing joint replacement.

*Skin loss (3.2j)*—The skin graft anesthesia issues are not adequately addressed by Table 67 nor are they adequately addressed under a sensory deficit caused by the peripheral nerve injury (section 3.2k, Table 68). Therefore this impairment is assessed using Table 2 in Chapter 13 (Skin). Because of the potential abnormalities created by the appearance possible perturbations in thermoregulation and wound repair, and the alteration in sensory perception (Table 1), a 4% WPI is appropriate.

*Whole person impairment calculation*—To derive a proper WPI for this injury, a combination of the function and anatomic abnormalities with the skin impairment is needed. The leg length discrepancy award (3.2a) of 4% stands alone and is combined with other values. The gait derangement (3.2b) is rated at 15% but can also be assessed by measurements found in sections 3.2c, d, e, and g. The muscle atrophy (3.2c) yields a value of 9%, the manual muscle testing (3.2d) 6%, and the peripheral nerve section (3.2k) was not used. Only one of these values is to be used, generally the highest. Accordingly, the 15% WPI is used for sections 3.2b, c, d, and k.

The impaired ROM (3.2g) yields a 6% WPI rating. This impairment is felt to be a contributory factor in the gait abnormality and is therefore discarded.

Arthritis (3.2g) is assessed based on diminished cartilage intervals. Since this injury would not be expected to produce this type of radiologic abnormality, the 15% WPI rating is discarded. However, if it is decided that

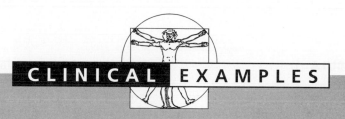

## HIP, THIGH, KNEE, AND LEG—cont'd

these abnormalities result from the injury (and radiographs of the unaffected side would strengthen this argument), then the 15% WPI for arthritic degeneration is used in preference to manual muscle testing and ROM, assuming those values are within the range expected for the degree of arthritic change in this case. Since the gait disturbance results from arthritic degeneration and associated stiffness and weakness, only the higher of these two ratings is used. In this case they are identical at 15% WPI. The gait derangement section is designed to test the validity of the other sections. In general, the summation of the other appropriate sections should equal the gait derangement section, as it does in this case. Because the other sections are more specific and objective than gait derangement, they should be used in preference when there is a difference in values.

**Evaluation**

The final WPI is a combination of the limb-length discrepancy (4%) and the gait abnormality (15%) or the arthritic degeneration (15%), and the skin impairment (4%). When combined, the final value is a 21% WPI.

*Stephen L. Demeter*

## LEG, UPPER TIBIA, AND FIBULA

Work-related injuries to the proximal and mid-shaft tibia and fibula and surrounding soft tissues are relatively common as a result of motor vehicle accidents, falls, and direct trauma from heavy equipment such as forklifts. Isolated fractures of the fibula are rare. Fractures of the tibia frequently require internal fixation except in the case of compound fractures, which may be stabilized with an external fixator, at least until the wound is healed. Tibial fractures, especially those associated with soft-tissue trauma, have a significant risk of anterior compartment syndrome that results in muscle ischemia. If uncorrected by fasciotomy, this ischemia may result in permanent weakness of foot and ankle dorsiflexion. Less commonly, the posterior compartment may be involved as well.

Intramuscular and peritendinous scarring following these high-energy injuries frequently results in contractures of the ankle, foot, and toes. The earlier motion can be restored, the less severe these contractures will be. At the time of impairment evaluation following leg injuries, attention must be focused on the foot and ankle to assess and identify carefully any fixed contractures, loss of motion, or weakness. These findings are in addition to the diagnostic ratings for the fractures that are based on malalignment including rotation, varus, or valgus. A shortening impairment would be combined, as would one related to peripheral nerve deficit.

Chronic osteomyelitis of the tibia is much less common today, but it can still follow major (type IV) tibial fractures with severe associated soft tissue trauma. If present when the patient's impairment is declared permanent and stationary, it warrants an additional impairment percent that is listed in the diagnostic section. All the combined values may not exceed that for below-knee amputation.

## AMPUTATION

Amputations are rated using Table 63 of the AMA *Guides*. Estimates for additional factors that limit prosthesis use would be combined. These would include significant phantom pain, symptomatic neuromas, loss of protective sensation, chronic wound drainage, or recurrent skin breakdown. Skin breakdown can occur as a result of vascular insufficiency, loss of protective sensation, and scarring or split-thickness skin graft with limited durability. As indicated in the table, stump length in the thigh or leg must be greater than three inches to have adequate function, and a distal-thigh amputation is more favorable for the patient than a mid-thigh amputation. Posttraumatic amputation patients often have significant psychological problems and, as a group, do not function as well as patients in other amputation categories.[23]

## CONCLUSION

The evaluation of musculoskeletal impairment has evolved from earlier systems that used amputation and ankylosis as their primary assessment models. Diagnostic accuracy and rating flexibility are the hallmarks of present models.

Methodologies vary in objectivity, reliability, and specificity. As the rating system and diagnostic and therapeutic technology continue to evolve, these factors will improve, resulting in increased accuracy that will make the job of the evaluating physician less judgemental and the ultimate awards more fair. The number of contested cases and the length of the contests will decrease, which will have a positive economic and rehabilitive impact. Furthermore, by reducing adversity, more injured workers will successfully return to work sooner. This evolution is not automatic but will require extensive research and diligence. Fortunately, there is an increasing interest in orthopaedic and other musculoskeletal academic programs that are studying and improving these systems.

### References

1. American Academy of Orthopaedic Surgeons: *Manual for orthopaedic surgeons in evaluating permanent physical impairment*, Chicago, 1962, American Academy of Orthopaedic Surgeons.
2. American Medical Association: *Guides to the evaluation of permanent impairment*, ed 4, 3/75-3/93, Chicago, 1993, American Medical Association.
3. American Medical Association: *Guides to the evaluation of permanent impairment*, ed 4, 3/85-3/86, Chicago, 1993, American Medical Association.
4. Andersson G: Hip assessment: A comparison of nine different methods. *J Bone Joint Surg* 54B: 621, 1972.
5. Burgess AR: Fractures of the pelvis. In Rockwood CA, Green DP, Bucholz RW, editors: *Fractures*, vol 2, pp. 1399-1441, New York, 1991, JB Lippincott.
6. Callaghan JJ, Dysart SH, Savory CF, et al: Assessing the results of hip replacement. *J Bone Joint Surg* 72B:1008, 1990.
7. Daniel DM, Stone ML: Diagnosis of knee ligament injuries: tests and measurement of knee motion limits. Feagin JA Jr, editor, In *The crucial ligaments*, New York, 1994, Churchill Livingston.
8. DeLee JC: Fractures and dislocations of the hip.

In Rockwood CA, Green DP, Bucholz RW, editors, *Fractures,* vol 2, pp. 1481-1652, New York, 1991, JB Lippincott.

9. Dunn EL, Berry PH, Connally JD: Computed tomography of the pelvis in patients with multiple injuries. *J Trauma* 23:378, 1983.

10. Esquemeling J: *The Buchaners of America,* New York, 1967, Dover.

11. Ficat RP: Ideopathic bone necrosis of the femoral head. *JBJS* 67B:3-9, 1985.

12. Felson DT, Hannan MT, Naimark A, et al: Occupational physical demands, knee bending, and knee osteoarthritis: results from the Framingham Study. *J Rheumatol* 18:10, 1587, 1991.

13. Garth WP: Current concepts regarding the anterior cruciate ligament. *Orthop Rev* 5:565, 1992.

14. Harris WH: Traumatic arthritis of the hip after dislocation and acetabular fractures: treatment by mold arthroplasty. *J Bone Joint Surg* 51A:737, 1969.

15. Hastings DE: The non-operative management of collateral ligament injuries of the knee joint. *Clin Orthop* 147:22, 1980.

16. Helfet AJ: Mechanism of derangements of the medial semilunar cartilage and their management. *JBJS* 41B:319-336, 1959.

17. Henning CE, Lynch MA, Glick KR Jr: Physical examination of the knee. In Nicholas JA, Hershman EB, editors, *The lower extremity and the spine in sports medicine,* vol 1, pp. 765-800, St Louis, 1986, Mosby.

18. Hoikka V, Ylikoski M, Tallroth K: Leg-length inequality has poor correlation with lumbar scoliosis. *Arch Orthop Trauma Surg* 108:173, 1989.

19. Insall JN, Dorr LD, Scott RD, et al: Rationale of The Knee Society clinical rating system. *Clin Orthop* 248:13, 1989.

20. Katz JN, Harris TM, Larson MG, et al: Predictors of functional outcomes after arthroscopic partial meniscectomy. *J Rheumatol* 19:1938, 1992.

21. LaBrier K, O'Neill DB: Patellofemoral stress syndrome: current concepts. *Sports Med* 16(6):449, 1993.

22. Lord JP, Aitkins SG, McCrory MA, et al: Isometric and isokinetic measurement of hamstring and quadriceps strength. *Arch Phys Med Rehabil* 73:324-330, 1992.

23. Livingston DH, Keenan D, Kim D, et al: Extent of disability following traumatic extremity amputation. *J Trauma* 37:495, 1994.

24. Luck JV: Traumatic arthrofibrosis. *Bull Hosp Joint Dis* 12:394-403, 1951.

25. Luck JV Jr, Beardmore TD, Kaufman R: Disability evaluation in arthritis patients. *Clin Orthop* 221:59-67, 1987.

26. Luck JV Jr, Florence DW: A Brief history and comparative analysis of disability systems and impairment rating guides. *Orthop Clin North Am* 19:839-844, 1988.

27. Markolf KL, Graff-Radford A, Amstutz HC: In vivo knee stability. *JBJS* 60A:664-674, 1978.

28. Matsen FA: Compartmental syndrome. *CORR* 113:8-13, 1975.

29. Mitchell DG, Steinberg ME, Dalinka MK, et al: Magnetic resonance imaging of the ischemic hip. *CORR* 244:60-77, 1989.

30. Mubarak SJ, Owen CA, Hargens AR, et al: Acute compartment syndrome: Diagnosis and treatment with the aid of the Wick catheter. *JBJS* 60A:1091-1095, 1978.

31. Nutton RW, Pinder IM, Williams D: Detection of sacroiliac injury by bone scanning in fractures of the pelvis and its clinical significance. *Injury* 13(6):473, 1982.

32. Olson SA, Matta JM: The computed tomography subchondral arc: a new method of assessing acetabular articular continuity after fracture (a preliminary report). *J Orthop Trauma* 7:402, 1993.

33. Peltier L: Joseph Malgaigne and Malgaigne's fracture. *Surgery* 44:777-784, 1958.

34. Schroer WC: Current concepts on the pathogenesis of osteonecrosis of the femoral head. *Orthop Rev* June 1994, p 487.

35. Semba RT, Yasukawa K, Gustilo RB: Critical analysis of results of 53 Malgaigne fractures of the pelvis. *J Trauma* 23:535, 1983.

36. Tile M: Fractures of the acetabulum. In Rockwood CA, Green DP, Bucholz RW, editors, *Fractures,* vol 2, pp. 1442-1479, New York, 1991, JB Lippincott.

37. Tobis JS, Chang-Zern H: Muscle testing. In Kottke FJ, Lehman JF, editors, *Krusen's handbook of physical medicine and rehabilitation,* ed 4, pp. 33-60, Philadelphia, 1990, WB Saunders.

38. Walker RH, Burton DS: Computerized tomography in assessment of acetabular fractures. *J Trauma* 22:227, 1982.

39. Ward EGW, Bodiwala GG, Thomas PD: The importance of lower limb injuries in car crashes when cost and disability are considered. *Accid Anal Prev* 24:613, 1992.

40. Webb LX, Caldwell K: Disruption of the posterior pelvic ring caused by vertical shear. *South Med J* 81:1217, 1988.

41. Weber M: Die Beurteilung des Unfallzusammenhangs von Meniskusschaden. *Orthopade* 23:171, 1994.

42. White MSI: Three-dimensional computed tomography in the assessment of fractures of the acetabulum. *Injury* 22:13, 1991.

# CHAPTER 23

# JOINT SYSTEMS: FOOT AND ANKLE

*George B. Holmes, Jr.*
*Lee C. Woods*

Impairment and disability evaluations of the foot and ankle are performed most frequently for work-related injuries. According to a recent survey, injuries to the foot and ankle account for approximately 7.5% of all occupational injuries.[6] Statistics from state Labor Departments in 1993 indicate that injuries of the foot and toes were responsible for 5% of work-related injuries and 3% of those that received compensation.[8] Injuries to the foot and ankle accounted for $3.4 to $8.7 billion of the estimated $115.9 billion in work accident costs in 1992.[6,8]

The worker with an injury to the foot or ankle is most typically a male, aged 30 to 40 years, who works in jobs of manual labor or vehicular operations.[6] Most such work-related injuries (58.4%) are caused by a blow to the foot or ankle. In a study from the Rush-Presbyterian-St. Luke's Occupational Health Clinic (RPSLOHC), 22% of the foot and ankle injuries were fractures, sprains, or strains,[6] and 5% of these injuries were caused by vehicles. The peak incidence of these injuries occurred in the summer months.

An appreciation of the nature of the injury and a description of the injury's cause and circumstance are helpful in the overall determination of the diagnosis, rehabilitation, time for recovery, temporary disability, permanent disability, and return-to-work status. Table 23-1, from a 1981 publication of the U.S. Department of Labor, categorizes foot injuries according to the description of the accident and the involved part of the foot.[10] The most common occurrence was when the foot was struck by a falling object. Injuries to the toes and metatarsal bones accounted for the vast majority of foot and ankle injuries. The most common specific injuries were contusions, lacerations (or punctures), fractures, and sprains.

## CONTUSIONS, CRUSH INJURIES, AND BRUISES

The impact of contusion and crush injuries to the foot, as it relates to temporary or permanent impair-

ment, is in large part based upon the location and degree of soft tissue injury. The degree of injury can in part be assessed by the size and weight of the object striking the foot. However, in many instances the initial estimation of soft-tissue damage is incorrect or misleading.

Significant crush injury can result in local or regional necrosis of skin and muscle. Large defects may require split thickness skin grafts or the grafting of one of several types of flaps. The possibility of compartment syndrome must always be considered in the presence of moderate-to-severe crush injury. Failure to appreciate the magnitude of the injury can lead to an inadequate awareness of a permanent sensory loss or loss of motor function. A lack of early intervention can lead to contractures or, possibly, the need for wider amputation. Regardless of the type of treatment, patients with severe crush injuries to the foot and ankle may be left with chronic pain and a limb that is unable to bear weight repetitively, a major disability particularly in an environment of manual labor and vehicular operation. Physical therapy and occupational therapy should stress the re-establishment of normal or near-normal range of motion, soft-tissue mobilization, strengthening, and proprioception training. A return to normal function is predicated on the achievement of these goals. Recovery from minor bruises and contusions can be expected to occur within 3 to 6 weeks of the time of injury. Maximal medical improvement from more severe injuries can take 12 to 24 months. Not unexpectedly even following this period some patients may continue to have chronic pain, swelling, and functional deficits.

Contusions to the toes are common, especially if the worker is not wearing safety-tipped shoes at the time of the injury. Because of the lack of significant soft-tissue protection, the toes are particularly susceptible to chronic swelling after such injuries. This may result in chronic pain that is exacerbated by cold weather and constricting footwear. Adequate warmth and a shoe with an enlarged toebox are measures

**TABLE 23-1**     FOOT INJURIES BY DESCRIPTION OF ACCIDENT, SELECTED STATES, JULY-AUGUST, 1979[10]

| ITEM | ALL WORKERS | | WORKERS WEARING SAFETY SHOES | |
|---|---|---|---|---|
| | NUMBER | PERCENT | NUMBER | PERCENT |
| **How did the accident occur?** | | | | |
| Total | 1,251 | 100 | 283 | 100 |
| Stepped on sharp object | 194 | 16 | 24 | 8 |
| Struck by falling object | 721 | 58 | 191 | 67 |
| Object rolled onto or over foot | 168 | 13 | 36 | 13 |
| Squeezed between two surfaces | 59 | 5 | 13 | 5 |
| Struck foot against object | 28 | 2 | 3 | 1 |
| Occurred in another way | 81 | 6 | 16 | 6 |
| **What part of your foot was injured?** | | | | |
| Total* | 1,251 | * | 283 | * |
| Toes | 719 | 57 | 118 | 42 |
| Toes only | 557 | 45 | 69 | 24 |
| Toes and other part(s) of foot | 162 | 13 | 49 | 17 |
| Metatarsal | 475 | 38 | 179 | 63 |
| Metatarsal only | 291 | 23 | 124 | 44 |
| Metatarsal and other part(s) of foot | 184 | 15 | 55 | 19 |
| Sole | 241 | 19 | 45 | 16 |
| Sole only | 153 | 12 | 19 | 7 |
| Sole and other part(s) of foot | 88 | 7 | 26 | 9 |
| Heel | 69 | 6 | 19 | 7 |
| Heel only | 28 | 2 | 4 | 1 |
| Heel and other part(s) of foot | 41 | 3 | 15 | 5 |
| Ankle and other part(s) of foot | 59 | 5 | 19 | 7 |
| **Were both feet injured?** | | | | |
| Total | 1,195 | 100 | 269 | 100 |
| No | 1,176 | 98 | 266 | 99 |
| Yes | 19 | 2 | 3 | 1 |

*Because the categories listed are not mutually exclusive, the sum of the parts will exceed the total.

NOTE—Due to rounding, percentages may not add to 100. Because incomplete questionnaires were used, the total number of responses may vary by question.

SOURCE—Survey questionnaire.

that will decrease symptoms and prolong weight bearing tolerance. In nondiabetic patients partial- and multiple-toe amputations are usually well-tolerated without significant compromise of stability, balance, and energy expenditure. Multiple amputations and amputations of the great toe in diabetic patients will necessitate a significant reduction in the weight bearing status or a significant modification in footwear. These modifications include (1) use of an extra-depth shoe with a plastizoate liner and rocker bottom, and

(2) change to a semi-sedentary status with lifting, climbing, and walking restrictions.

A common complication after direct impact trauma to the toes or metatarsals is the development of one or more interdigital (Morton's) neuromas. Neuromas cause pain that increases with weight bearing, stair climbing, or the use of tight shoes. If metatarsal pads, a rigid shoe, or a wider shoe do not decrease the pain, the injured worker may require excision of the interdigital nerve. This will result in a satisfactory response in 80% of the cases.[2,7] The remaining 20% may require a reduction in weight bearing status along with various shoe modifications.

## FRACTURES AND DISLOCATIONS

A specific discussion of every fracture and dislocation of the foot and ankle along with its treatment, rehabilitation, and impairment is beyond the scope of this text. A framework for the evaluation of fractures and their outcomes will be presented within the context of impairment rating. In general, the treatment for a fracture or dislocation of the foot and ankle is appropriate reduction and immobilization followed by rehabilitation and mobilization in order to achieve a return to optimal functioning. In specific instances, such as with intraarticular fractures treated with rigid internal fixation, early range of motion is initiated to enhance a more rapid and complete return to normal motion and function.

Permanent impairment is manifested by pain, loss of motion, decreased strength, or swelling. Loss of motion and pain occurs in the presence of arthritis, malunion, and soft-tissue scarring along with associated nerve and muscle injury. Pain can be secondary to the presence of avascular necrosis, delayed union, nonunion, or chronic infection. These possibilities must be assessed thoroughly, because the status of temporary impairment versus permanent impairment depends in large part on the establishment of the correct diagnosis. Obviously, in the absence of an early accurate diagnosis and treatment, the chances are increased for the development of a more protracted temporary disability and permanent impairment.

Lisfranc fracture-dislocations and fractures of the calcaneus are common workplace injuries. A Lisfranc fracture-dislocation can easily be overlooked, especially in a worker with multiple injuries. This is in sharp contrast to a calcaneus fracture that usually exhibits a dramatic clinical and radiographic picture. The diagnosis and treatment of these two differing injuries is quite instructive in evaluation of temporary and permanent disability of the injured worker.

Prompt treatment of a Lisfranc fracture-dislocation via open or closed reduction and internal fixation of the tarsometatarsal joints provides the injured worker with the greatest opportunity to return to pain-free weight bearing (Fig. 23-1). The recovery time is usually between 3 and 6 months. Commonly, when the fracture is subtle, the initial radiographs are normal. After a brief period on crutches, the worker attempts to return to regular duties and develops pain and/or swelling in the area of the midfoot. If this situation persists, arthritis can develop, which will later be ob-

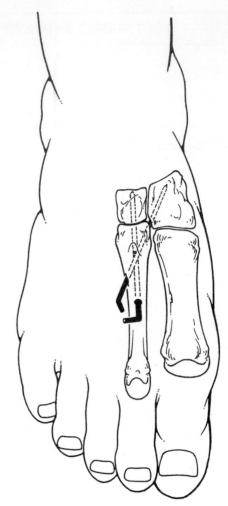

**FIGURE 23-1**    Internal fixation using smooth K-wires. (From Holmes GB: *Surgical approaches to the foot and ankle*, New York, McGraw-Hill.)

served on radiographs. The treatment becomes one of selective midfoot arthrodesis, which has a low rate of success in terms of relieving pain.[1] These patients may require the long-term use of a steel-shank rocker-bottom type of shoe and are often unable to return to an unrestricted level of activity. However, if diagnosed early and treated appropriately most patients will be able to return to an unrestricted or minimally restricted weight-bearing status.

A fracture of the calcaneus is frequently a devastating, career-ending injury for the manual laborer. This is especially true when the fracture involves the posterior facet, when associated with a loss of the heel height, when there is comminution, and when the heel has undergone significant widening (Fig. 23-2). There is also a high association of injury to the posterior tibial nerve and its branches due to direct injury or concomitant swelling. The initial prognosis for return to unrestricted weight bearing is poor. However,

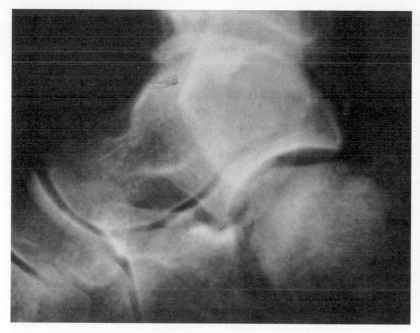
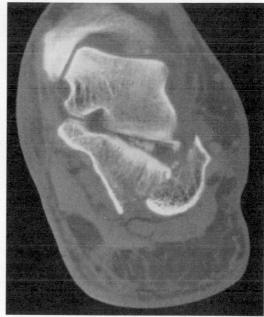

**FIGURE 23-2**    Fracture of the calcaneus.

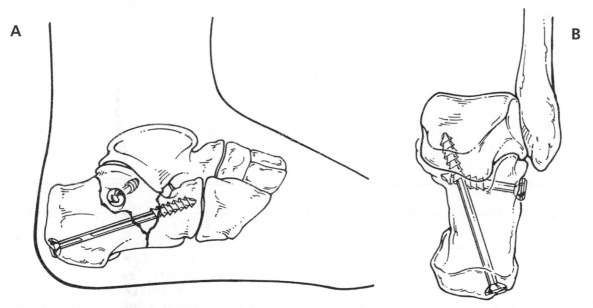

**FIGURE 23-3**    **A,** Lateral view after insertion of screws. **B,** Harris view: fixation for facet split and joint depression. (From Holmes GB: *Surgical approaches to the foot and ankle,* New York, McGraw-Hill.)

several options can significantly improve the likelihood of return to a level of weight bearing that may allow the worker to return to his or her former employment. The prompt reduction of soft-tissue swelling, accurate anatomic reconstruction of the posterior facet, narrowing of the heel, and restoration of heel height can improve the overall prognosis (Fig. 23-3). Maximal medical improvement is usually seen in 12 to 18 months. If the patient continues to have significant pain related to the subtalar joint of the hindfoot (as opposed to nerve injury), a subtalar fusion or triple arthrodesis offers an excellent chance for the elimination of pain. However, if significant subtalar motion and flexibility are required to perform the worker's job (e.g., in the case of a roofer), significant activity restrictions may be essential even though there has been a reduction or elimination of pain. Workers over the age of 50 will have a greater likelihood of developing chronic post-injury pain after a calcaneus fracture regardless of the initial treatment.[9] Therefore, the overall prognosis for return to pain-free weight-bearing function is worst for the middle-aged or older worker.

## CUTS, LACERATIONS, AND PUNCTURES

Simple cuts, lacerations, and punctures of the foot are usually easy to treat and carry a low propensity of long-term permanent impairment. However, since most structures of the foot and ankle are relatively superficial, careful assessment is necessary to ensure that vital structures have not been compromised by a seemingly minor injury.

A cut of the foot can result in injury to vessels, tendons, or ligaments. It may also penetrate a joint and lead to sepsis or an abscess. Cuts and lacerations associated with an adjacent fracture convert the injury to an open fracture that will require irrigation, exploration, and debridement.

Tendon injuries most frequently result from a worker stepping on, kicking, or dropping a sharp object on the foot or ankle. About 75% of these injuries occur in the forefoot.[4] Injuries to the lesser extensor and flexor tendons of the foot generally do not require surgical repair. These injuries lead to very little functional deficit. However, acute complete lacerations of the flexor hallucis longus, extensor hallucis longus, anterior tibial tendon, posterior tibial tendon, and peroneal tendons demand surgical repair. In most instances significant functional losses can be expected if there is no repair.

A laceration of the arteries and veins of the foot and ankle will cause injury in proportion to the importance of the vessel and the area supplied or drained by that vessel. If viability of the foot or even a portion of the foot is compromised, long-term functional losses may be anticipated.

Puncture wounds of the plantar aspect of the foot can be quite serious. Puncture wounds through a shoe or sneaker have a significant risk for the development of *Pseudomonas* infection of the soft tissue and adjacent bone. Prevention of complications calls for prompt irrigation, debridement, and appropriate antibiotic coverage.[3,5] Development of a chronic infection can lead to post-infection scarring, chronic pain, and chronic swelling.

## SPRAINS AND STRAINS

Strains and sprains of the foot and ankle are quite common. They are frequently graded on a scale of 1 to 3, with the latter representing complete ligamentous disruption along with instability. In the most common instances of Grade 1 and Grade 2 injuries, early range of motion and rehabilitation will significantly reduce the period of total temporary impairment. The techniques of soft-tissue mobilization, contrast baths, proprioception training, electrical stimulation, and dynamic support are crucial in the achievement of an early recovery. Slower recovery can be anticipated in middle-aged or older workers, workers with prior ligamentous injuries in the same location, or patients with associated injuries such as fractures or nerve damage.

The primary problem in the recovery from strains and sprains lies in the underdiagnosis of more serious problems. A seemingly simple strain or sprain may actually represent a posterior tibial tendon rupture, spring ligament injury, subluxation or rupture of a peroneal tendon, formation of an intra-articular loose body, turf toe, reflex sympathetic dystrophy, or Lisfranc fracture-dislocation. This list could be expanded further, but the main point is to eliminate other diagnostic possibilities associated with strains and sprains, especially when the patient's recovery is unexpectedly prolonged.

## NEUROLOGIC INJURIES

Neurologic injuries can be broadly categorized as being either local or diffuse. Local neurologic injuries of the foot and ankle usually result in one of several characteristic patterns of injury. There may be very discrete pain at the site of injury to a somatic nerve. This may or may not be associated with a positive Tinel's test over the proximal, and occasionally the distal, aspect of the nerve. With disruption of the nerve fibers there is also the possibility of a loss of sensation distal to the distribution of the nerve. This pattern of injury is typical of neuromas. In general, treatment options consist of desensitization techniques, relative immobilization (stiff shoe or orthosis), TENS, local anesthetic injection (diagnostic purposes), lysis of adhesions, or surgical excision. It may take several months for the injured worker to experience decrease in symptoms with the initial use of conservative and nonoperative techniques, but these techniques are generally successful.

Diffuse injuries will affect a wider area of the foot. The most common forms of injury include tarsal tunnel syndrome, the sequela of compartment syndrome, and reflex sympathetic dystrophy. The long-term prognosis for recovery, the success of nonoperative and operative modalities, and the avoidance of permanent impairment are less than

**TABLE 23-2      TEMPORARY AND PERMANENT IMPAIRMENT**

| INJURY | PROJECTED TEMPORARY IMPAIRMENT | RISK OF LONG-TERM PERMANENT IMPAIRMENT |
|---|---|---|
| **Minor/Mild Contusions** | | |
| Toe(s) | 3–6 wks | Low |
| Dorsum foot | 3–6 wks | Low |
| **Severe Contusions** | | |
| Toe(s) | 6–12 wks | Low |
| Dorsum foot | 6–12 wks | Mild–Moderate |
| **Ankle** | | |
| Avulsion | 1–3 months | Low |
| Lat. malleolar | 3–5 months | Low-Mild |
| Bimalleolar | 3–5 months | Low-Mild |
| Trimalleolar | 3–5 months | Low-Mild |
| Plafond | 3–6 months | Moderate |
| **Hindfoot** | | |
| Extra-articular calc. | 3–6 months | Low-Mild |
| Intra-articular calc. | 6–18 months | Moderate-High |
| Talus | 6–18 months | Mild-High |
| **Mid-Foot** | | |
| Navicular | 3–4 months | Mild-Moderate |
| Cuboid | 2–3 months | Low |
| Cuneiforms | 2–3 months | Low |
| Lisfranc | 3–6 months | Mild-Moderate |
| **Forefoot** | | |
| Metatarsals | 1–3 months | Low-Mild |
| Phalanges | 1–2 months | Low |
| Sesamoids | 2–6 months | Mild-Moderate |
| Compartment syndrome | 6–12 months | Moderate-High |
| Tarsal tunnel syndrome | 3–6 months | Moderate-High |
| Sinus tarsi syndrome | 3–6 months | Mild-Moderate |
| Reflex sympathetic dystrophy | 6–30 months | Moderate-High |

would be expected for more discrete injuries such as neuromas. Injuries such as tarsal tunnel syndrome or reflex sympathetic dystrophy may require several months of examinations and tests before the diagnosis can be established by objective measures, such as an EMG, NCV, or bone scan.

Early diagnosis and intervention are important in reducing the short-term impairment and the probability of progression to long-term impairment associated with tarsal tunnel syndrome or reflex sympathetic dystrophy. From a rating standpoint these injuries pose a special problem in that patients may initially be seen with relatively well-maintained range of motion and normal motor function. However, they will have significant functional problems based on the presence of significant pain exacerbated by weight bearing.

## CONCLUSION

The approach to determining temporary and permanent impairment (see Table 23-2) with respect to the foot and ankle is more efficient than those of other regions of the body such as the spine. Unlike other areas of the trunk, the anatomy of the foot and ankle is quite visible, which enhances its assessment by physical examination. Ancillary studies such as radiographs, bone scan, tomography, and magnetic resonance imaging are also enhanced by the relatively superficial nature of the anatomy. The key to a successful outcome of treatment and rehabilitation is the early, accurate assessment of the problem, with the anatomy of the foot lending itself to the correct diagnosis.

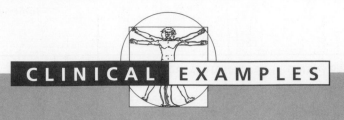

## FOOT AND ANKLE

EDITOR'S NOTE—Impairment assessment of the foot and ankle presents the same challenges as assessment of the rest of the lower extremity and for the same reasons. Chapter 22 of this text reviews these challenges and offers an example of a complex situation involving impairment of the lower extremity. As with the remainder of the lower extremity, the evaluation of the foot and ankle is more complex in the fourth edition of the *Guides* than in the third edition, where impairment was primarily assessed by measuring range of motion (ROM).

### EXAMPLE

#### History

A 22-year-old man suffered traumatic amputation of the left great toe nine months previously. The amputation is well healed, but he states that he has difficulty walking because of the injury and any weight bearing causes pain. A neuroma has been diagnosed at the site of amputation.

#### Assessment Process

This individual can be assessed in one of two ways: (1) based on his gait abnormality (Table 36) or (2) using a combination of the amputation plus the dysesthesia (Tables 63 and 68).* Using the former method of analysis, this individual would have a 7% whole person impairment (WPI) based on an antalgic limp. The pain could not be adequately assessed, however, using this method.

Using the second method (Tables 63 and 68), there is a 5% WPI for amputation of the great toe at the MTP joint. Furthermore, the neuroma in the distribution of the medial plantar nerve is associated with a 2% whole person impairment. When combined, this yields a 7% WPI.

#### Evaluation

The impairment percentages are identical with these two methods. Note that the first method of analysis did not specifically include pain, but Table 36 was constructed so that issues such as pain or arthritic changes are included as factors causing the gait derangement. Therefore either assessment method would yield a 7% WPI.

*Stephen L. Demeter*

*All *tables* referred to in this discussion are found in AMA *Guides to the evaluation of permanent impairment,* ed 4, Chapter 3—The Musculoskeletal System, American Medical Association, Chicago, 1993.

## References

1. Arntz CT, Veith RG, Hansen ST: Fractures and fracture-dislocations of the tarsometatarsal joint. *J Bone Joint Surg* 70A:173, 1988.
2. Bradley N, Miller WA, Evans JP: Plantar neuroma analysis of results following surgical excision in 145 patients. *South Med J* 69:853, 1976.
3. Fitzgerald RH, Cowan JDE: Puncture wounds of the foot. *Orthop Clin North Am* 6:965, 1975.
4. Floyd DW, Heckman JD, Rockwood CA Jr: Tendon lacerations in the foot. *Foot Ankle* 4:8, 1983.
5. Johnson JE, Hall RL: Management of foot infections. In Gould JS, editor: *Operative foot surgery,* 1982, Philadelphia, WB Saunders, p. 274.
6. Oleski DM, Hahn JJ, Leibold M: Work-related injuries to the foot. *J Occupation Med* 34(6):650, June 1992.
7. Mann RA, Reynolds JD: Interdigital neuroma: a critical clinical analysis. *Foot Ankle* 3(4):238, 1983.
8. National Safety Council: *Accident facts,* ed 3, Itasca, Ill., 1993, National Safety Council.
9. Paley D, Hall H: Intra-articular fractures of the calcaneus: a critical analysis of results and prognostic factors. *J Bone Joint Surg* 75A:342, 1993.
10. U.S. Dept of Labor: Accidents involving foot injuries (Report 626). Washington, D.C., 1981.

# JOINT SYSTEMS: CERVICAL SPINE

*Jeffrey D. Klein*
*Steven R. Garfin*

The clinical evaluation of patients with suspected cervical spine disorders can be divided into a discussion of patients with neck pain, patients with arm pain, and patients who have signs and symptoms of myelopathy. The physician must then distinguish between the many causes of neck and arm pain based on the history, physical examination, and radiographic findings.

## NECK PAIN

### Cervical Spondylosis

The process of aging and degenerative change in the cervical spine involves all elements of the motion segment. Disc degeneration is accompanied by osteophyte formation around the degenerate disc and neurocentral joints, facet arthritis, and ligamentous thickening. Subluxation and disc herniation may also be present. Taken together, these changes are referred to as *cervical spondylosis.*

Cervical spondylosis is very common in patients older than 40 years, and generally is asymptomatic or causes mild neck pain.[3] Patients may initially be seen, however, with significant neck pain, symptoms associated with nerve root compression (cervical spondylotic radiculopathy), symptoms associated with spinal cord compression (cervical spondylotic myelopathy), or a combination of the above.

The neck pain associated with cervical spondylosis is generally gradual in onset, though it can be exacerbated by superimposed trauma. The pain varies in severity, is generally activity related, and is often accompanied by stiffness. The pain is commonly posterior in the mid-cervical spine, but referred pain to the shoulders and upper arms may be present. Headaches are not unusual and may be due to prolonged paraspinal muscle spasm secondary to nerve irritation or to specific compression of the greater occipital nerve.

The physical examination of patients with painful cervical spondylosis is notable for a limited range of motion. Extension is usually lost first, and passive extension by the examiner may be painful.[11] The neurological examination is generally normal. Paraspinal muscle spasm may be present, and tenderness may be elicited in the midsubstance of the trapezius muscle.

Radiographs are useful and are generally obtained early in the evaluation of cervical spondylosis. The later view may reveal disc space narrowing, loss of normal cervical lordosis, ankylosis, osteophytosis, and subluxation (Fig. 24-1, *A*). Disease may be seen at one level, or at many levels. The most mobile segments (C5-6, C6-7, and C4-5) are most commonly involved (in that order). Dynamic lateral (flexion and extension) films may demonstrate instability. The oblique views demonstrate the intervertebral foramen and may show osteophytes from the neurocentral joints projecting into the neuroforamen. These latter views, however, do not offer significant, clinically useful information.

Compressive lesions of the nerve roots or spinal cord require neurodiagnostic evaluation with computed tomography (with or without myelography) or magnetic resonance imaging (Fig. 24-1, *B*). It is important to note that the correlation of radiographic changes with neck pain and degenerative joint disease is extremely poor. Patients with radiographic findings of severe cervical spondylosis may be asymptomatic, whereas patients with minimal radiographic findings may have severe pain. Boden et al reported that MRI evidence of disc degeneration, disc space narrowing, and nerve compression was seen in 25% of asymptomatic patients younger than 40 years, and 60% of asymptomatic patients older than 40 years.[23]

### Pathoanatomy

Progressive dehydration and fibrosis of the intervertebral disc results in loss of the normal disc architecture, and ultimately loss of the demarcation between the nucleus pulposus and the annulus fibrosus.

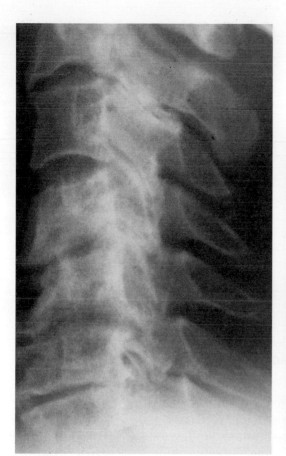

A

**FIGURE 24-1**    Cervical spondylosis.

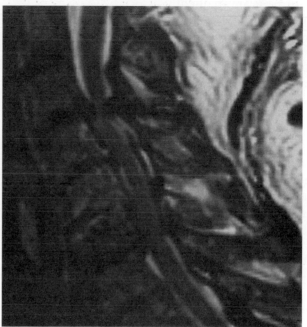

B

There is a gradual loss of the gelatinous nucleus pulposus, coarsening of the annular lamellae, and later fissuring of the annulus.[20,24]

Histologically, there is loss of the normal fibrillar structure of the nucleus accompanied by progressive cavitation, desiccation, fibroblastic proliferation, and calcium deposition.[6] A decrease in overall proteoglycan content is also observed.[4] Proteoglycans are responsible for disc hydration by virtue of their osmotic properties.

### Natural history

The morphologic changes of cervical spondylosis are progressive and not reversible. There is no correlation, however, between the structural changes of disc degeneration and the clinical syndrome of pain without neurologic involvement.[31]

Cervical spondylosis with isolated neck pain exhibits a variable course. Symptoms generally wax and wane. Short-term relief is quite common. DePalma et al reported that 21% had complete relief, 49% had partial relief, and 22% had no relief after three months of conventional nonoperative care.[9] Gore et al reported that, at a ten-year follow-up, 79% of patients improved, with 43% pain-free; 32%, however, had severe residual symptoms.[14]

### Treatment

A number of nonoperative modalities are available in the treatment of cervical spondylosis and are usually used in combination. Rest and immobilization are used to reduce irritation of inflamed supporting structures. A soft cervical collar can be used to maintain the neck in a neutral or slightly flexed position. Hyperextension of the neck may aggravate the patient's symptoms.[12]

Nonsteroidal antiinflammatory drugs play a useful role in the treatment of these patients. Muscle relaxants can be used as well in patients with definite muscle spasm. They should be used, however, for brief periods only.

Physical therapy is used routinely in the treatment of cervical spondylosis. During acute episodes, exercise may make the pain worse, but should be performed as tolerated. Aerobic exercise should be encouraged. Other modalities, such as heat, cold, ultrasonography, and transcutaneous electrical stimulation, may be helpful in the acute setting. Patients should be instructed in isometric neck-strengthening activities and to avoid positions that provoke symptoms. Modifications at the workplace, such as telephone headsets and elevated work stations, are sometimes helpful. After the acute episode has resolved, exercises are used to strengthen the cervical musculature and decrease the frequency of future episodes.

The neck pain of cervical spondylosis is generally cyclical. The initial episode usually responds to simple conservative measures within two to three weeks. Episodes of pain are frequently associated with periods of increased physical activity and generally respond to modification of these activities. More chronic conditions require prolonged therapy with less certain results.

Surgical treatment is rarely indicated for neck pain in the absence of radiculopathy or myelopathy. Cervical spine fusion may be considered in very select patients with incapacitating mechanical neck pain, and preferably, one-level involvement in patients younger than 40 years. Provocative discograms may help to identify the symptomatic level. Such surgery, however, is controversial. Evidence of focal cervical "instability" in the setting of limited cervical spondylosis may also be an indication for a one-level fusion.

## Differential Diagnosis

### Tumor

Although cervical spondylosis is the most common cause of neck pain, other diseases must be considered in the differential diagnosis. Neck pain is the most common complaint of patients with tumors causing significant bony destruction. The pain is classically constant and often worse at night. Destruction of structures that render the spine unstable may cause the pain to be worse with neck motion and activity. Direct nerve-root compression may result in typical radicular findings. Compression of the spinal cord may result in signs and symptoms of myelopathy. Neural deficits may be due to collapse of bony structures or extension of the tumor mass.

Metastatic lesions constitute, by far, the largest group of malignant bone tumors. Common primary sites include the breast, prostate, lungs, thyroid, kidney, and parathyroid (Fig. 24-2). Primary bone tumors are rare in the cervical spine, accounting for only 1% of primary bone tumors. Primary malignant neoplasms of the cervical spine are extremely rare. Malignant tumors are frequently associated with large soft-tissue masses and significant destruction. These often result in major neurologic deficits.

Apical carcinomas of the lung (Pancoast tumors) may encroach upon the brachial plexus or subclavian vessels. These lesions commonly present with shoulder pain, upper-extremity weakness, and Horner's syndrome. The classic sensory deficit is along the ulnar nerve distribution. These tumors are difficult to

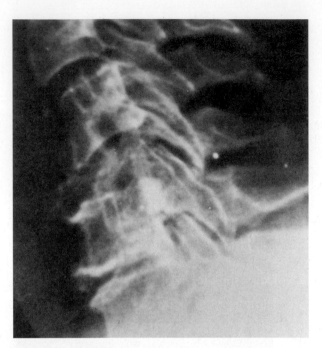

**FIGURE 24-2**    Metastatic lesion.

detect on routine chest film and frequently require apical lordotic views.

Primary benign neoplasms include osteoid osteoma, osteoblastoma, and osteochondroma, all of which predilect the posterior elements. Benign tumors of bone that occur in the vertebral body include hemangioma, fibrous dysplasia, eosinophilic granuloma, giant cell tumor, and aneurysmal bone cyst. Giant cell tumors and aneurysmal bone cysts may be associated with large soft tissue masses and significant lytic destruction.

Most symptomatic tumors of the cervical spine will be seen on plain radiographs, although bone scans may be positive earlier. Fifty to 60% of bone mineral must be lost before a significant change is noted on plain films. Bone scans are particularly useful in the patient with unremitting, axial neck pain and normal plain films. The remainder of the skeleton can also be evaluated for metastatic lesions. It should be remembered that multiple myeloma is frequently cold on bone scan.

CT and MRI scans are useful for further delineation of the lesions. CT is particularly helpful in the evaluation of the bony architecture. MRI best demonstrates an associated soft-tissue mass as well as the neural elements.

### Infection

Patients with infection of the cervical spine are seen most commonly with neck pain. As with tumors, the pain is generally not relieved by rest. Often,

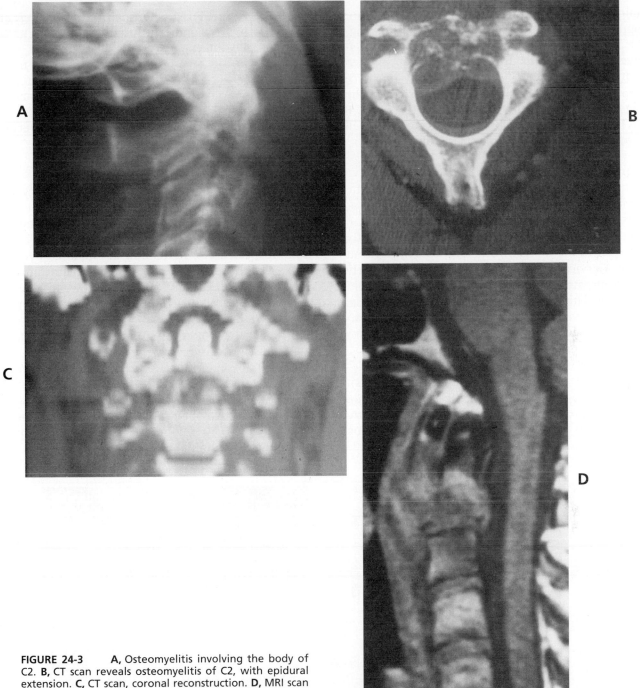

**FIGURE 24-3**    **A,** Osteomyelitis involving the body of C2. **B,** CT scan reveals osteomyelitis of C2, with epidural extension. **C,** CT scan, coronal reconstruction. **D,** MRI scan reveals osteomyelitis of C2, with epidural extension.

the symptoms have persisted for several months or more. This is significant because 90% of patients with benign mechanical pain have resolution of their symptoms within two months.[10]

Concurrent symptoms may include fever, malaise, and weight loss. Vertebral osteomyelitis is seen more often in older, debilitated patients and intravenous drug users. A history of antecedent infection or immunologic compromise is common. The erythrocyte sedimentation rate (ESR) and C-reactive protein (CRP) are usually elevated, although the white blood cell count (WBC) is often normal. Approximately 50% of the patients are clinically malnourished at presentation (albumin <3.5 g/dl, total lymphocyte count <1500/mm³).[28]

Plain films are usually normal early in the course of the disease. Later, lytic lesions may be seen (Fig. 24-3, *A*). These may span across the disc space, a finding that helps distinguish infection from tumor radiographically. This contributes to the delay in diagnosis, which is unfortunately common in osteomyelitis. Bone scans are positive early. Although CT scans are useful, MRI is now the study of choice in the evaluation of spinal infection, especially in the setting of concurrent neurologic findings (Fig. 24-3, *B* to *D*). Bony, as well as epidural, involvement is well seen, and the neural structures clearly identified.

## Systemic disorders

Inflammatory arthritides commonly involve the cervical spine and may lead to pain complaints as well as focal or generalized stiffness. The pain and stiffness of the spondyloarthropathies is typically most severe in the morning and improves throughout the day. Cervical spine involvement is particularly common in patients with rheumatoid arthritis, especially those with long-standing polyarticular disease. Neck pain and occipital headaches are common complaints. These patients must be followed carefully for the development of myeloradiculopathy.

The bony changes in rheumatoid arthritis are destructive, rather than productive (as in osteoarthritis). Common radiographic findings include osteopenia and instability, both in the upper cervical spine and, to a lesser extent, in the subaxial cervical spine (Fig. 24-4, *A*). Neurodiagnostic studies (CT myelography, MRI) are required when neurologic findings are present, or when significant instability is noted in the neurologically intact patient (Fig. 24-4, *B*).

Neck pain can be a prominent symptom in metabolic diseases such as gout and renal osteodystrophy. Cervical spine involvement varies from minimal-to-severe destructive lesions. Treatment must be directed toward the cervical spine as well as correction of the underlying metabolic abnormality.

## Fractures and instabilities

The patient with acute cervical spine injury will have neck pain and tenderness, with or without associated neurologic deficit. Plain films should be obtained initially. Fractures are further defined by CT scan. Suspected disc herniation is evaluated by MRI. Patients with neck pain and negative plain films require lateral flexion and extension views to rule out ligamentous instability. If flexion/extension views are negative, a hard collar is worn for seven to ten days and repeat dynamic evaluation performed after the acute muscle spasm has resolved.

Patients experiencing neck pain after the time of the injury also require plain films, including lateral flexion/extension views to assess for chronic instability (Fig. 24-5). An open-mouth odontoid view should be obtained, because nondisplaced odontoid fractures can be missed on initial evaluation.

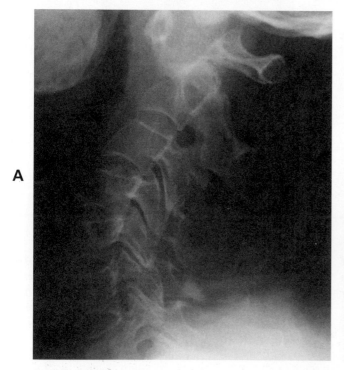

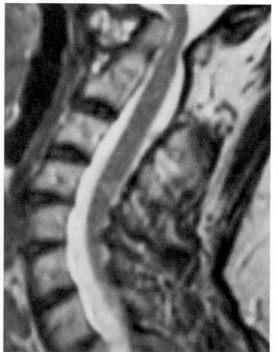

**FIGURE 24-4**    **A,** Rheumatoid arthritis, C1-2 instability. **B,** Rheumatoid pannus in the atlantodens interval; decreased space available for the cord at C1-2.

## ARM PAIN

The patient with cervical spondylosis may initially complain of arm pain. This can be referred pain secondary to degenerative joint disease, without evidence of nerve root involvement. It is, however, more commonly described as a shooting, radicular pain associated with numbness and paresthesias in a dermatomal distribution. Focal neurologic findings referrable to a specific nerve root may be identified. Nerve root compression may be due to uncovertebral osteophyte (hard disc), herniation of degenerative disc (soft disc), spondylotic bars, or a combination of these. In cervical spondylosis, multiple nerve root involvement may occur.

Acute, isolated cervical disc herniation is a separate entity. This is usually a posterolateral herniation in patients younger than 50 years. There is usually a specific onset of the symptoms, regardless of whether a traumatic event is noted. In acute cervical disc herniation, single nerve root deficits are common.

### Associated Tests

The **cervical compression** test is a provocative maneuver performed by applying axial pressure on the top of the patient's head. A positive response includes neck, and more importantly, arm pain (note a

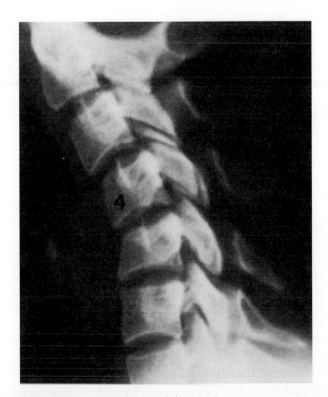

**FIGURE 24-5**    Posterior instability, C4-5.

radicular pattern if present). This is generally seen in the setting of disc herniation or neuroforaminal encroachment of the nerve root. **Spurling's** test includes compression of the patient's head with the neck extended and rotated to the side of the radicular pain. A positive test includes complaints of reproduction of the radiating arm pain, and again suggests spinal nerve root entrapment in the neuroforamen. The **cervical distraction** test is performed by gradually distracting the patient's head. Patients with nerve root compression from herniated discs or neuroforaminal narrowing may note diminution of pain, because the distraction maneuver tends to enlarge the neuroforamen and decrease the load across the facet joints. The **shoulder abduction** test is performed by passively abducting the patient's involved arm. This reduces nerve root tension and relieves arm pain in many patients with cervical radiculopathy due to extradural compression.

### Neurologic Evaluation

The examination of the upper extremity by neurologic levels is directly related to the physical examination of the cervical spine. Motor, sensory, and reflex activity, if appropriate, should be assessed at each root level. The critical importance of this examination warrants a review of these levels (Fig. 24-6).

The C5 nerve root innervates the deltoid muscle and, along with C6, the biceps muscle. It supplies sensation to the lateral arm (over the shoulder) and is primarily responsible for the biceps reflex. Patients with C5 radiculopathy may complain of shoulder pain and weakness. Loss of shoulder function creates a significant functional deficit. Some physicians recommend early (6 weeks) decompression for C5 radiculopathy with significant neurologic findings.

The C6 root innervates the wrist extensors and, along with C5, the biceps muscle. The C6 sensory distribution includes the lateral forearm, the thumb, the index finger, and occasionally part of the middle finger. The posterior ramus of C6, as well as those of C7 and C8, supply sensation to the region overlying the scapula. The associated reflex at this level is the brachioradialis. The C7 motor distribution includes the triceps muscle, the wrist flexors, and the finger extensors. C7 provides sensation to the middle finger and is primarily responsible for the triceps reflex.

The C8 neurologic level includes motor innervation of the middle finger flexors and the interossei. The sensory supply is to the ulnar side of the hand and the distal half of the ulnar aspect of the forearm. There is no reflex test for the C8 level. The T1 level includes motor innervation of the interossei. Sensory

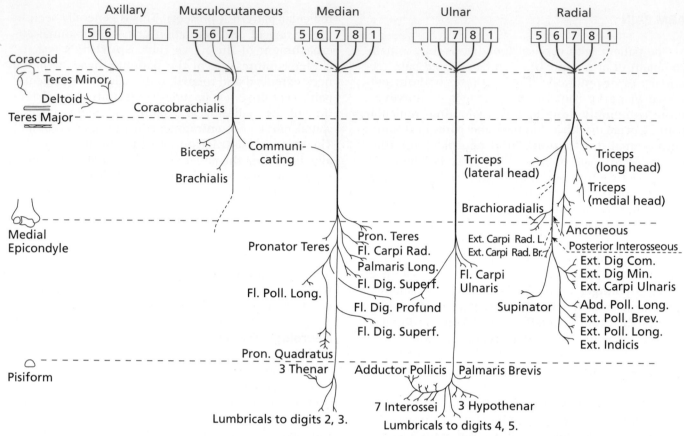

**FIGURE 24-6** Motor innervation of the upper extremity. (Courtesy American Medical Association.)

supply is to the ulnar side of the proximal forearm and distal arm. There is no associated deep tendon reflex. Loss of intrinsic hand function creates a significant functional deficit, and many surgeons recommend early (6 weeks) decompression if marked neurologic deficit is present.

### Natural History

DePalma and Subin reported a five-year study of nonoperative management for cervical spondylosis and disc herniation. Sixty-nine percent of patients had neck and radicular pain and 31% had neck pain only. Overall, 45% of patients had resolution of symptoms. Of those whose symptoms did not resolve, 23% were significantly impaired.[5] Another series that reviewed nonoperatively treated athletes with acute cervical radiculopathy showed that 17 of 20 returned to full activity at an average of 17 weeks. Neurologic deficits took up to five months to improve.[27]

### Diagnosis

Plain films are obtained initially. These are followed by either MRI or CT myelography, if surgery is being considered (Fig. 24-7, *A*). MRI is superior for evaluating soft-tissue structures, such as discs and the neural elements, and provides information on the intrinsic status of the spinal cord as well (Fig. 24-7, *B*). The CT myelogram adds a dynamic quality, because the passage of dye can be followed. The CT scan also provides the best evaluation of the bony anatomy. Carefully performed electromyography (EMG) and nerve conduction velocity (NCV) studies can be useful to confirm radiculopathy and rule out peripheral neuropathy.

### Treatment

The nonoperative modalities used are the same as described for cervical spondylosis, namely rest and immobilization, physical therapy after the acute episode has abated, anti-inflammatory medication, and time. Natural history studies have shown that neck and arm pain usually improve spontaneously within a few weeks.[1,29]

The primary indication for the surgical management of cervical spondylotic radiculopathy and cervical disc disease is nerve root compression with persistent radicular signs and symptoms, not responsive to

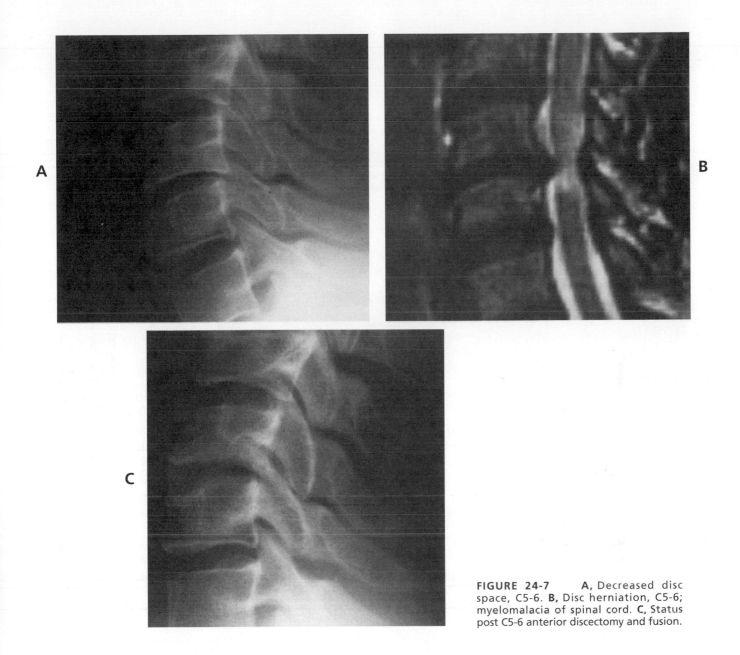

**FIGURE 24-7**    **A,** Decreased disc space, C5-6. **B,** Disc herniation, C5-6; myelomalacia of spinal cord. **C,** Status post C5-6 anterior discectomy and fusion.

nonoperative measures. The findings on physical examination should correspond to the findings on the neurodiagnostic studies. Early surgical intervention should be considered for more severe neurologic deficits, and certainly with progression of the neurologic deficit. Some recommend intervention at six weeks if the C5 and C8 nerve roots are involved, because of the significant loss of function associated with neurologic compromise at these levels.[15]

The surgical approaches for cervical radiculopathy include anterior discectomy and fusion, and numerous posterior procedures. These include foraminotomy with or without lateral, free fragment discectomy for single level disease, and multilevel foraminotomy, laminectomy, and laminoplasty for multilevel involvement. Both approaches achieve excellent results when properly performed. To a certain extent, the choice depends on the preference of the surgeon. If there is one level, unilateral involvement, with radiculopathy alone, and no associated neck pain or instability, the posterior foraminotomy approach may be desirable. The anterior approach is preferred if there is concurrent instability at the involved level that requires decompression and stabilization, associated neck pain, midline pathology, or bilateral involvement. The anterior approach has the added benefit of opening the neuroforamen by widening the disc space with a well-fashioned bone graft (Figs. 24-7, *C,* and 24-8).

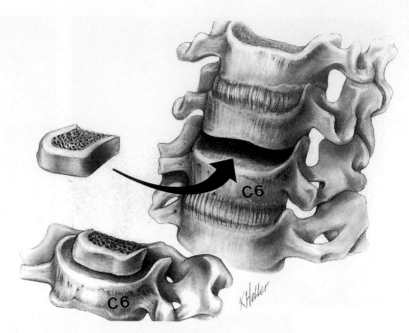

**FIGURE 24-8**   Anterior cervical discectomy and fusion. (From Abitol JJ, Garfin SG: *Semin Spine Surg* 1(4):233, 1989.)

## Differential Diagnosis

### Tumor and infection

Cervical disc disease is the most common cause of cervical radiculopathy. Nonetheless, many other conditions can have similar findings.

The spectrum of cervical spine tumors was reviewed in the discussion on neck pain. Bony collapse, extension of the tumor mass, and local inflammatory reaction can all cause nerve root compression, with subsequent radicular pain and neurologic findings.

Schwannomas and meningiomas are rarely seen in the cervical region, but when present, frequently occur with radicular symptoms. Schwannomas arise from the spinal nerve root and thus tend to compress the root at the level of the neuroforamen. Meningiomas, too, arise in the region of the dorsal root, and thus can be compressive in the neuroforamen. Both may cause foraminal enlargement seen on oblique radiographs, CT scan, or MRI.

Infection, like tumor, can cause nerve-root compression on the basis of bony collapse, or extension of disease into the epidural space. Primary epidural abscess can also result in radicular findings. Clinical suspicion must be very high with any patient who has constant, unremitting neck pain associated with neurologic deficits.

### Entrapment syndromes

The peripheral nerves of the upper extremity may be compressed at specific sites along their course. This can produce sensory and motor findings in characteristic patterns. The median, ulnar, and radial nerves, and their branches, may all be involved at various levels. These syndromes can mimic cervical radiculopathy, but careful examination will reveal deficits referable to peripheral nerves and not nerve roots. The other peripheral nerves innervated by the nerve roots in question will be entirely normal. Electromyography and nerve conduction velocity studies help distinguish between radiculopathy and peripheral compressive neuropathies.

### Thoracic outlet syndrome

Thoracic outlet syndrome is an entity characterized by intermittent vascular or neurologic compromise in the upper extremity due to compression of the subclavian vessels, or the lower two nerve roots (C8, T1) of the brachial plexus. Occasionally, a cervical rib may be palpable in the supraclavicular fossa. Compression of these neurovascular structures as they pass between the scalenus anticus and scalenus medius muscles can also cause this syndrome. Vasomotor symptoms usually affect the radial side of the hand, whereas neurologic symptoms usually involve the ulnar side of the hand. One maneuver to assess this compression is **Adson's test.** For this, the patient's radial pulse is palpated and noted before and after the arm is passively abducted, extended, and externally rotated. The patient is then told to turn his head towards the arm in question. Diminution or loss of the pulse suggests compression of the subclavian artery and a possible diagnosis of thoracic outlet syndrome.

### Brachial neuritis

Patients with idiopathic brachial neuritis generally have unilateral neck and shoulder pain that within two weeks is followed by significant upper-extremity weakness. The axillary, long thoracic, and suprascapular nerves are most often involved. Shoulder abductor weakness is common and often the brachial plexus is tender, in either the supraclavicular fossa or axilla. Electrodiagnostic studies are very helpful in establishing the diagnosis. The etiology is unknown (possibly viral). It often follows a systemic illness or a period of stress (e.g., surgery). The disease process is frequently self-limited over weeks to months. Anti-inflammatory medication may be helpful in reducing the symptoms.

### Shoulder disease

Numerous disorders of the shoulder girdle cause local pain and weakness. These symptoms may mimic proximal cervical radiculopathy. The physical examination can usually help distinguish between shoulder and spine pathology, but it may be confusing, particularly if there are concurrent processes. Tenderness is usually present with rotator cuff tears, subacromial bursitis, impingement syndrome, and degenerative disease of the acromioclavicular and glenohumeral joints. Shoulder weakness is generally due to pain, spasm, or in the proper clinical setting, a large rotator cuff tear. Once again, electrodiagnostic studies may help distinguish cervical spine radiculopathy from primary shoulder pathology (see Chapter 21).

## MYELOPATHY

The degenerative changes seen with advanced cervical spondylosis may be associated with compression of the spinal cord, causing cervical spondylotic myelopathy (CSM). Cervical spondylotic myelopathy is the most common cause of spinal cord dysfunction in patients older than 55 years.[26]

The spinal canal may be narrowed by degenerative disc bulges with or without herniation, transverse bony bars adjacent to the disc, osteophytes, and/or facet and ligamentum flavum hypertrophy. Subluxation also decreases the space available for the spinal cord. This pathology may occur at single or multiple levels.

Cervical spondylotic myelopathy exhibits a protracted course with episodic progression.[29] There can be long periods without progression, and even regression. Conversely, mild trauma, such as a minimal hyperextension injury, can produce an acute neurologic deterioration. Clarke and Robinson reported that 75% of patients had episodic symptoms, 20% had slow progression, and 5% had rapid deterioration.[13] Early diagnosis may be important because the results of treatment are related to the severity of the condition and the duration of findings.[16]

Generalized upper and lower extremity weakness, especially in concert with gait disturbance and bladder dysfunction, suggests myelopathy. Early findings may include neck pain; numb, cold, or painful hands; decreased fine motor skills; and subtle gait disturbances (broad-based). Some patients may exhibit a mild scissoring gait or describe a perceived loss of control. Others describe a foot drop, or slapping, when they walk, or an inability to rotate internally or externally a lower extremity smoothly. Radiculopathy and myelopathy may also coexist.

The findings of physical examination are those of cervical spondylosis in general, with the addition of pathologic upper motor neuron reflexes in both the upper and lower extremities. Neck range-of-motion is generally decreased, particularly in extension. Weakness may be present in the upper and/or lower extremities. Decreased vibratory sense and proprioception are subtle signs seen early in the course of myelopathy. **L'hermitte's sign** is characterized by shock-like pains radiating down the arms or legs with passive flexion and compression of the neck. **Babinski's test** involves firmly stroking the plantar surface of the foot with a sharp instrument, starting from the heel and proceeding distally along the lateral aspect of the sole and then medially across the forefoot. The normal, or negative, response consists of no movement or downward motion of the toes. A positive response consists of extension of the great toe and spreading (fanning) of the lesser toes.

Generalized hyperreflexia is also associated with myelopathy, especially when in conjunction with a positive Babinski sign. **Clonus** is a rhythmic, repetitive oscillation of the foot at the ankle in response to sudden, maintained dorsiflexion of the foot and stretching of the Achilles tendon. The presence of clonus also suggests myelopathy. **Hoffman's sign** is a pathologic reflex that is elicited in the upper extremity. The hand is held in a comfortable resting position, and the nail of the middle finger is "flicked." A positive reaction consists of flexion of the terminal phalanx of the thumb and index finger. If one elicits pathologic reflexes in the lower extremity, and Hoffman's sign is negative, this may suggest that the problem lies below the level of the cervical spinal cord. This would be further supported by hyperreflexia limited to the lower extremities.

"Myelopathy hand" refers to the loss of power of adduction and extension of the ulnar two or three fingers due to weak intrinsics.[17] These fingers may spontaneously abduct, giving rise to the "finger escape sign." These findings, together with hyperreflexia, are suggestive of cervical myelopathy, usually above the C6-7 level.

Plain films, including flexion/extension views, are obtained initially (Fig. 24-9, A). In the setting of

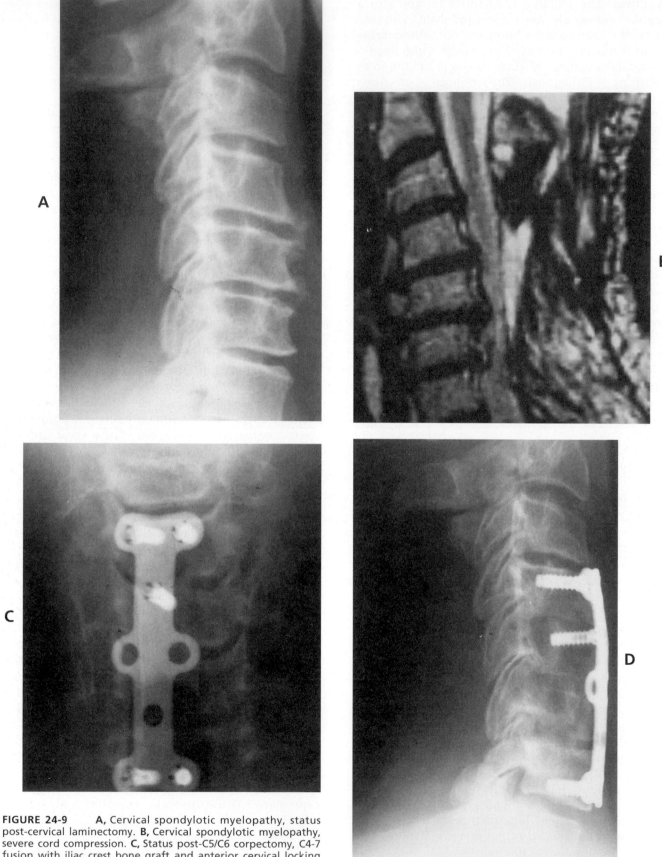

**FIGURE 24-9**    **A,** Cervical spondylotic myelopathy, status post-cervical laminectomy. **B,** Cervical spondylotic myelopathy, severe cord compression. **C,** Status post-C5/C6 corpectomy, C4-7 fusion with iliac crest bone graft and anterior cervical locking plate. **D,** Postoperative lateral view.

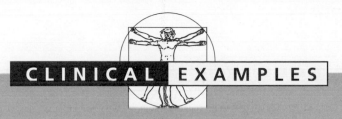

# CLINICAL EXAMPLES

## CERVICAL SPINE

EDITOR'S NOTE—The fourth edition of the AMA *Guides* represents a major departure from previous editions with respect to spinal examination. Deficiencies noted in prior examination models included (1) "other clinical data and diagnostic information tended to be ignored;" (2) there was concern about "the accuracy and reproducibility of mobility measurements;" and (3) this method of examination failed to "account for the effects of aging" (p. 94). Accordingly, an entirely new approach to the evaluation of spinal impairment was created, called the injury model or the diagnosis-related estimates (DRE) model; the older, range of motion (ROM) model is also referred to as the functional model. The DRE model is the presently preferred model of analysis. However, if disagreement exists between physicians over which category in the DRE model fits the patient's impairment, then the ROM model should be used (p. 101).

The DRE system appears to be on a trial basis. The authors freely acknowledge that "the approach is different from that of previous *Guides* editions, and that future developments may lead to refinement or to a different recommendation altogether" (p. 94).*

Two other problems make the spine one of the most difficult areas to assess for impairment. First, according to the *Guides,* section 3.3, "it is emphasized that if an impairment evaluation is to be accepted as valid under the *Guides* criteria, the impairment being evaluated should be a *permanent* one, that is, one that is stable, unlikely to change within the next year, and not amenable to further medical or surgical therapy . . ." (p. 94).* But neck and back symptoms seem to fluctuate over time, and supervening and intervening injuries often occur, so that an evaluation at any given time is unlikely to be performed in

*All *sections* and *tables* referred to in this discussion are found in AMA *Guides to the evaluation of permanent impairment,* ed 4, Chapter 3—The Musculoskeletal System, American Medical Association, Chicago, 1993.

an individual with a "permanent" impairment. Since evaluations cannot be deferred indefinitely, they are done when the injury is not necessarily permanent.

Second, since individuals limit their ROM based on their symptoms and there is no "healthy" limb available for comparison with the spine, the ROM examination is not always reliable. ROM can vary from day to day and from observer to observer. To address this concern, other elements of the physical examination can be used to affirm the limitations found in ROM testing. For example, the straight leg raising test is supposed to be an independent check of limited ROM. However, as seen in Chapter 25, limitations can be found in this examination as well as various other types of examinations used to "double-check" straight leg raising. Thorough familiarity with all the alternative examinations is needed to provide the most accurate examination possible.

**EXAMPLE**
### History
A 54-year-old, right-hand-dominant painter came to his physician with neck pain. Symptoms had developed gradually over the previous two years. He had pain and stiffness in the posterior cervical spine and shoulders and occasionally had headaches. His symptoms have been stable for 18 months.
### Physical Examination
On examination, there is mild rigidity of the cervical spine muscles and in the trapezius muscles bilaterally. His head is held semi-erect. There is diminished sensation to pain and light touch in the distribution of C6 on the left side. The musculature about the left shoulder appears atrophic compared to the right shoulder, and there is a 2 cm difference in the size of the left upper arm and a 2 cm difference in the left lower arm when compared with measurements taken at similar lo-

*Continued.*

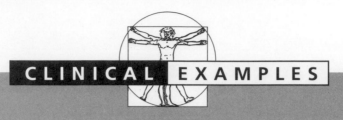

cations on the right side. Strength in the shoulder and left upper arm is graded at 5/6; it is 6/6 in the right shoulder, right arm, and left lower arm.

### Test Results

An EMG demonstrates evidence of radiculopathy in the C6 distribution on the left side. Other distributions of the left side and all the areas of the right side are normal. Neck x-rays reveal osteophytes on multiple levels throughout the cervical spine. An MRI shows compression of the nerve root on the right side at the C5-6 level as well as on both sides at the C6-7 level. Because of suspected radiculopathy, failure of nonoperative management in relieving his arm symptoms, and confirmatory imaging studies, a surgical referral is made. However, he declines any surgical intervention.

### Assessment Process

The preferred method of assessment is the DRE method. This individual falls into Category III (Tables 70, 71, and 73), yielding a 15% whole person impairment (WPI). No long tract signs were found by history or physical examination, radiculopathy is present, and no loss of segment integrity or multilevel neurologic compromise has occurred. A 15% WPI is determined.

If the functional (ROM) model is used, assessment starts with Table 75. This individual has had no operation, has a stable condition, and has medically documented injury, pain, and rigidity. Moderate-to-severe degenerative changes are found on the structural tests, and he has a radiculopathy. Therefore he has a 6% WPI based on cervical level of abnormality. In addition, he has an extra 1% because he has degenerative changes found on x-rays taken at multiple levels. Thus he has a 7% WPI based on a specific spine disorder.

Next, radiculopathy is evaluated using Table 13. He has minor motor deficits and some sensory deficits, both in the region of C6 on the left. The maximum upper extremity impairment caused by combined motor and sensory deficits is 40%, and the majority of this is related to the motor deficit. Since the motor deficit is minor, a 10% to 15% upper extremity impairment is probably appropriate. (This reflects the examiner's previous experience.) A 10% impairment of the upper extremity, using Table 3, yields a 6% WPI.

Finally, the ROM of the cervical spine is examined. After three separate sets of measurements of all six ROM areas, with all measurements falling within 10% of each other, the following were observed:

| | |
|---|---|
| **Flexion (F):** | 30° |
| **Extension (E):** | 50° |
| **Right lateral flexion (RLF):** | 30° |
| **Left lateral flexion (LLF):** | 10° |
| **Right rotation (RR):** | 40° |
| **Left rotation (LR):** | 20° |

Using Tables 76 to 78, this yields a 2% WPI for F, 1% for E, 1% for RLF, 3% for LLF, 2% for RR, and 4% for LR. The range-of-motion abnormalities are added, yielding a 13% WPI. This impairment is combined with the specific spine disorder (7%) and the unilateral spinal nerve impairment (6%) to produce a 24% WPI.

### Evaluation

As already indicated, the DRE method is preferred and produced a 15% WPI as opposed to the functional (ROM) model, which produced a 24% impairment.

*Stephen L. Demeter*

myelopathy, neurodiagnostic evaluation with CT myelography or MRI is needed to search for sites of cord compression. MRI also provides information on the intrinsic status of the spinal cord (Fig. 24-9, *B*).

## Treatment

All of the nonoperative modalities discussed for cervical spondylosis can be used in these patients. Improvement of sensory and motor deficits has been reported in 33 to 50% of patients with cervical spondylotic myelopathy treated conservatively.[2,8] Such improvement, however, is generally mild to moderate. Furthermore, it is difficult to predict the pattern and timing of progression. Since the results of surgical treatment are related to the duration of myelopathic findings, there is general agreement that early surgical intervention is indicated for myelopathy, especially with documented neurologic progression.[16,21,22]

The decompression of cervical spondylotic myelopathy (CSM) can be performed from the anterior or posterior approaches. Anterior procedures include decompressive discectomy and corpectomy, followed by fusion (Fig. 24-9, *C* and *D*). Posterior procedures include laminectomy (with or without fusion) and laminoplasty. The side of maximal compression (anterior or posterior) should be determined on preoperative imaging studies. Generally, if the impingement is anterior, as it often is, an anterior approach should be utilized. If the impingement is posterior, as with hypertrophied ligamentum flavum or ossification of the posterior longitudinal ligament, posterior approaches should be used.

The posterior approach should be avoided, if possible, in the patient with a kyphotic cervical spine. In this situation, the spinal cord is draped over the spondylotic discs and vertebrae anteriorly, resulting in direct spinal cord compression, and possibly ischemic compromise as well. Posterior decompression cannot address this pathoanatomy. Additionally, with loss of the posterior elements, further progression of the deformity, as well as symptoms and signs, may occur. Some authors reserve the posterior approach for patients with three or more involved levels, particularly in stiff spines, and with elderly patients.[25]

The results of surgical decompression for CSM are generally good. Numerous recent reports document improvement in 70 to 80% of patients.[7,18,19] Neurologic return may be seen as late as one to two years after surgery. Anterior surgery tends to provide greater long-term relief than posterior decompression.[30] The primary goal, however, is to arrest the progressive myelopathic process.

## Differential Diagnosis

As discussed in previous sections, tumor and infection, particularly epidural abscess, can cause acute or progressive myelopathy. These entities, however, are generally easily distinguished from CSM on imaging studies. One should always be alert to the possibility of concurrent tumor or infection in the patient with CSM, especially in the setting of an acute episode of pain and neurologic deficit in a previously stable patient.

The involvement of the cervical spine in rheumatoid arthritis was also discussed earlier. Due to the instability that may develop in either the upper or subaxial cervical spine, myelopathy, with or without radiculopathy, is not an uncommon presentation. These patients are generally severely involved with polyarticular disease. Deformity of the extremities makes neurologic assessment difficult and unreliable. Nonetheless, distinguishing them from CSM is generally not difficult, based on clinical examination and diagnostic features on imaging studies.

Multiple sclerosis can present with acute sensory and motor loss in the extremities and can mimic cervical myelopathy. These patients are generally younger, with the average age of onset of 32 years. Frequent findings include central vision loss, diplopia, incoordination, and chronic fatigue.

## SUMMARY

Cervical disc disease and cervical spondylosis are the most common causes of neck and arm pain, as well as upper extremity radiculopathy and myelopathy. Poor correlation between the clinical examination and radiographic findings makes it difficult to prognosticate for any given patient. Evaluation and treatment must be individualized. Reasonable outcomes can be expected generally, though certainly not uniformly. Early diagnosis of myelopathy is critical because early surgical treatment (i.e., decompression) enhances the likelihood of obtaining a good result.

## References

1. Boden S, McCowin PR, Davis DO, et al: Abnormal magnetic resonance scans of the cervical spine in asymptomatic subjects. *J Bone Joint Surg* 72A:1178-1184, 1990.
2. Boden SD, Wiesel W: Conservative treatment for cervical disc disease. *Semin Spine Surg* 1:229, 1989.
3. Bradshaw P: Some aspects of cervical spondylosis. *Q J Med* 2:177, 1957.

4. Campbell AM, Phillips DG: Cervical disc lesions with neurological disorder: differential diagnosis, treatment, and prognosis. *Br Med J* 2:481, 1960.

5. Clarke E, Robinson P: Cervical myelopathy: a complication of cervical spondylosis. *Brain* 79:483-510, 1956.

6. Coventry MB, Ghornley RK, Kernohan JW: The intervertebral disc: its microscopic anatomy and pathology: Part II—Changes in the intervertebral disc concomitant with age. *J Bone Joint Surg* 27A:233-247, 1945.

7. Coventry MB, Ghormley RK, Kernohan JW: The intervertebral disc: its microscopic anatomy and pathology: Part III—Pathologic changes in the intervertebral disc. *J Bone Joint Surg* 27A:460-474, 1945.

8. Crandall PH, Batsdorf U: Cervical spondylotic myelopathy. *J Neurosurg* 25:57-66, 1966.

9. DePalma A, Rothman R, Lewinnek G, et al: Anterior interbody fusion for severe cervical disc degeneration. *Surg Gynecol Obstet* 134:755-758, 1972.

10. DePalma AF, Subin DK: Study of the cervical syndrome. *Clin Orthop* 38:135-141, 1965.

11. Dillane JB, Fry J, Kaiton G: Acute back syndrome: a study from general practice. *Br Med J* 3:82, 1966.

12. Gore DR, Sepic SB, Garner GM, et al: Neck pain: a long-term follow-up study of 205 patients. *Spine* 12:1-5, 1987.

13. Hanai K, Fujiyoshi F, Kamei K: Subtotal vertebrectomy and spine fusion for cervical spondylotic myelopathy. *Spine* 11:310, 1986.

14. Harris RI, Macnab I: Structural changes in the lumbar intervertebral discs: their relationship to low-back pain and sciatica. *J Bone Joint Surg* 36B:304-322, 1954.

15. Herkowitz HN: Surgical management of cervical disc disease: "open-door" laminoplasty. *Semin Spine Surg* 1:245, 1989.

16. Irvine DH, Foster JB, Newell DJ, et al: Prevalence of cervical spondylosis in general practice. *Lancet* 1:1089, 1965.

17. Ishida Y, Suzuki K, Ohmori K, et al: Critical analysis of extensive cervical laminectomy. *Neurosurgery* 24:215, 1989.

18. Kamano K, Umeyama T: Cervical disc injuries in athletes. *Arch Orthop Trauma Surg* 105:223-226, 1986.

19. Klein JD, Hey LA, Lipson SJ: Arthrodesis of the subaxial cervical spine in rheumatoid arthritis. Presented at the Annual Meeting of The Cervical Spine Research Society, New York, 1993.

20. Klein JD, Young EP, Klein BB, et al: Perioperative nutritional status and postoperative complications in the treatment of vertebral osteomyelitis. Presented at the Annual Meeting of The North American Spine Society, Minneapolis, 1994.

21. Lawrence JS: Disc degeneration: its frequency in relationship to symptoms. *Am Rheum Dis* 28:121, 1969.

22. Lees F, Turner JW: Natural history and prognosis of cervical spondylosis. *Br Med J* 11:1607, 1963.

23. Lipson SJ: Cervical disc disease: pathogenesis and natural history. *Semin Spine Surg* 1:190, 1989.

24. MacNab I: Symptoms in cervical disc degeneration. In Cervical Spine Research Society: *The cervical spine*, ed 2, Philadelphia, 1989, JB Lippincott.

25. Nurick S: The natural history and the results of surgical treatment of the spinal cord disorder associated with cervical spondylosis. *Brain* 95:101, 1972.

26. Ono K, Ebara S, Fiji T, et al: Myelopathy hand. *J Bone Joint Surg* 69B:215-219, 1987.

27. Phillips DG: Surgical treatment of myelopathy with cervical spondylosis. *J Neurol Neurosurg Psychiatr* 36:879, 1973.

28. Simeone FA: Surgical management of cervical disc disease: posterior approach. *Semin Spine Surg* 1:239, 1989.

29. Urban JPG, McMullin JF: Swelling pressure of the lumbar intervertebral discs: influence of age, spinal level, composition, and degeneration. *Spine* 13:179-187, 1988.

30. White A, Southwick W, DePonte R, et al: Relief of pain by anterior cervical spine fusion for spondylosis. *J Bone Joint Surg* 55A:525, 1973.

31. Whitecloud T: Anterior surgery for cervical spondylotic myelopathy: Smith-Robinson, Cloward, and vertebrectomy. *Spine* 13:861, 1988.

# CHAPTER 25

# JOINT SYSTEMS: LUMBAR AND THORACIC SPINE

*Gunnar B. J. Andersson*
*John W. Frymoyer*

Determining impairment in patients with painful conditions of the lumbar and thoracic spine is difficult not only because the actual impairment is difficult to assess, but also because there is no single universally-accepted diagnostic classification system. It is the purpose of this chapter to describe the two major classification approaches currently used, which can serve as a basis upon which impairment and disability can be rated. The first approach is based on symptoms, the second on pathoanatomic causation. Before describing these classification approaches, however, a brief review of how to evaluate patients with back pain is presented. This evaluation process is the foundation on which any classification system is based.

## PATIENT EVALUATION

The evaluation of a patient with low-back pain must always start with history and physical examination. Most patients with acute symptoms rapidly recover and do not require further tests. Others with recurrent or chronic symptoms, more severe, unrelenting pain, or with neurological deficits, may require imaging, electrodiagnostic, or laboratory studies. These tests should be based on specific indications derived from the history and physical examination, and the results must be correlated to the history and physical examination. Patients with chronic symptoms sometimes need a psychologic evaluation as well, and attention also may be diverted to psychosocial issues sometimes accompanying a work-related "injury".

### Clinical Examination

#### History

A complete history should contain information about present and previous symptoms, other significant medical diseases, and use of medications. The onset of the symptoms should be explored in detail, including the specific events when trauma is reported. Pain is the most important symptom. It should be evaluated in terms of its intensity, localization, distribution, pattern, and factors that accentuate and relieve pain. Pain intensity is impossible to quantify, but it is useful to use verbal descriptors: slight, moderate, severe, etc., or to use visual analogue scales, usually calibrated from no pain to the worst possible pain. The quality of pain (sharp, stabbing, burning, or aching,) is also helpful to determine. Localization and distribution of pain can conveniently be recorded on a "pain drawing" (Fig. 25-1) and serves as a major determinant in the symptom classification systems. A pain drawing can also be used to screen for inappropriate pain distribution, and thus can serve as one indicator of the need for further psychological evaluation. The duration of the painful episode is also important, and is part of some classification systems. The natural history for recovery of most back conditions is excellent, but the chance of recovery lessens the longer the duration of a pain complaint (Fig. 25-2). The time of day when pain is most severe is valuable information. Worsening throughout the day suggests a mechanical etiology and is the most common pattern. Pain when the patient first arises in the morning with improvement during the day suggests the possibility of an inflammatory condition. Pain that is most severe at night and awakens the patient is unusual, and a sign of possible malignancy or infection. Factors that accentuate or relieve pain are also important indicators of its etiology (mechanical vs. nonmechanical). Most types of back pain are aggravated by mechanical loading, such as lifting and bending, and are relieved by rest. Function is greatly influenced by pain and should therefore be analyzed, including ability to walk, sit, stand, lift, bend, drive, and work.

Neurologic symptoms should be sought by specific questions regarding sensory changes (numbness and

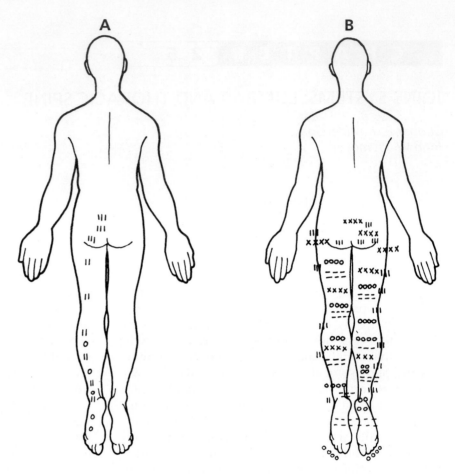

**FIGURE 25-1** Example of a pain drawing from a patients with **(A)** an S1 root lesion and **(B)** a nonspecific nonorganic pain distribution. (After Pope MH, et al: *Occupational low-back pain.* St. Louis, 1991, Mosby–Year Book.)

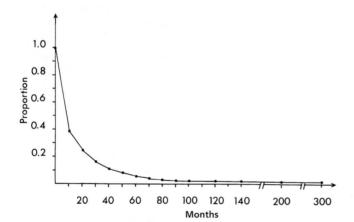

**FIGURE 25-2** Proportion of subjects still absent from work as a function of time (in months). Based on 1588 sickness absence periods. (From Andersson GBJ, et al: The intensity of work recovery in low-back pain. *Spine* 8:880–884, 1983.)

tingling), subjective sense of lower extremity weakness, and changes in bladder and bowel control or sexual function. Loss of ability to initiate voiding and loss of urinary and/or fecal control are symptoms of a cauda equina syndrome, which requires urgent evaluation. Progressive weakness and "foot drop" are other symptoms requiring further evaluation.

Information about previous painful episodes should include possible causative factors, as complete a pain description as possible, and associated disability. The success or failure of treatment, including surgery, is also important information. Significant other medical diseases such as diabetes or vascular disease, previous surgery, and previous or current use of medication should also be determined. Smoking and alcohol habits should be explored as well as any drug abuse.

A careful history will lead to plausible differential diagnoses that can be further evaluated during the physical examination. Serious conditions, such as tumors, infections, fractures, and cauda equina syndrome, are often indicated by the patient's history (Table 25-1).

### Physical examination

The physical examination includes inspection, palpation, range-of-motion measurements, and neurologic tests. It is useful to develop a system for the examination because it reduces the time involved and ensures completeness (Table 25-2).

Inspection provides information about postural abnormalities such as kyphosis, lordosis, scoliosis, list-

**TABLE 25-1** PERFORMANCE CHARACTERISTICS OF THE MEDICAL HISTORY IN THE DIAGNOSIS OF SPINE DISEASES CAUSING LOW BACK PAIN

| DISEASE TO BE DETECTED | MEDICAL HISTORY | SENSITIVITY | SPECIFICITY | SAMPLE |
|---|---|---|---|---|
| Cancer | Age ≥ 50 years | 0.77 | 0.71 | Unselected primary care |
| | Previous history of cancer | 0.31 | 0.98 | Unselected primary care |
| | Unexplained weight loss | 0.15 | 0.94 | Unselected primary care |
| | Failure to improve with a month of therapy | 0.31 | 0.90 | Unselected primary care |
| | No relief with bed rest | >0.90 | 0.46 | Unselected primary care |
| | Duration of pain >1 month | 0.50 | 0.81 | Unselected primary care |
| Spinal Stenosis | Pseudoclaudication | 0.60-0.90 | ? | Surgical case series |
| | Age ≥ 50 years | 0.90 ? | 0.70 | Surgical case series |
| Spinal Osteomyelitis | IV drug abuse, urinary tract infection, skin infection | 0.40 | ? | Multiple case series |
| Herniated Disc | Sciatica | 0.98 | 0.88 | Surgical cases series (sens.); population survey of patients with back pain (spec.) |
| Compression Fracture* | Age ≥ 50 years | 0.84 | 0.61 | Primary care patients having x-ray |
| | Age ≥ 70 years | 0.22 | 0.96 | Primary care patients having x-ray |
| | Trauma | 0.30 | 0.85 | Unselected primary care |
| | Corticosteroid use | 0.06 | 0.995 | Unselected primary care |

*Previously unpublished data from 833 patients with back pain at a walk-in clinic, all of whom received plain lumbar roentgenograms. (From Andersson GBJ, Deyo RA: Sensitivity, specificity, and predictive value: a general issue in screening for disease and in the interpretation of diagnostic studies in spinal disorders. In Frymoyer JF, editor: *The adult spine,* ed 2, in press.)

ing, asymmetry, and skin abnormalities. Body movements, gait, and posture provide information about the severity of symptoms and indicate functional limitations. Ability to walk on heels and toes suggests intact function of the L5 and S1 nerve roots. Quadriceps function, which tests the L2, 3, and 4 roots, can be assessed by asking the individual to squat and rise. The range of flexion-extension, lateral bending, and axial rotation are observed and measured. [2] The pattern of motion (rhythm) is important as is any pain resulting from it. Although range of motion (ROM) is sometimes considered an objective test, it is greatly influenced by the patient.

The lower extremities are examined to determine the presence of significant joint deformities and to assess neurologic function. Hip motion should also be evaluated, because hip conditions can sometimes pro-

duce leg pain that is difficult to distinguish from lumbar radiculopathies.

The evaluation of nerve root tension signs is one of the most important parts of the examination. The straight leg raising test (SLR) is easiest to perform with the patient supine. The leg is elevated with the knee extended. The examining hand is placed on the pelvis to gauge against pelvic motion. The test is positive when sciatica (posterior leg pain) is reproduced. The degree of elevation at which pain occurs is recorded. Often, the patient will complain of low-back pain rather than sciatica. In this circumstance, the degree of elevation should be recorded, but the test is not positive for nerve-root tension. The SLR test should also be performed with the patient sitting, for reasons of consistency. Straight leg raising may be restricted by tightness of the hamstring muscles.

**TABLE 25-2    PHYSICAL EXAMINATION**

| | | |
|---|---|---|
| Patient Standing | Posture | Scoliosis |
| | | Lordosis-kyphosis |
| | Gait | |
| | Range of motion | Flexion |
| | | Extension |
| | | Lateral bend |
| | | Axial rotation |
| | Screening muscle strength test | Heel-toe walk |
| | | Squatting |
| Seated | Observation | Seated posture |
| | Neurologic | Reflexes (ankle, knee) |
| | | Straight leg raising |
| Patient Recumbent (supine) | Measurements | Circumferences |
| | | Leg length |
| | Neurologic exam | Reflexes (ankle, knee) |
| | Nerve tension sign | Posterior tibial |
| | | Sensation |
| | | Muscle strength |
| | Nerve tension sign | Straight leg raising |
| | Other tests | Abdominal exam |
| | | Peripheral pulses |
| | | Hip range of motion |
| Recumbent (prone) | Neurologic | Sensation |
| | | Femoral stretch test |
| | Palpation | Muscle spasm |
| | | Spinous process |
| | | Interspinous spaces |

Again, this should also be recorded but is not a positive SLR test. Sometimes sciatic pain will occur in the opposite leg as the test is being performed. This finding, referred to as the *contralateral or crossed positive SLR test*, is highly specific for lumbar disk herniation.[20] A variety of other root tension tests have been described. They include the Lasegue test, where the hip and knee joints are flexed 90° and the knee extended to the point where sciatica is reproduced. The test can be further refined by dorsiflexing the foot.

The minimum testing of neurologic function of the lower extremities in patients with radicular symptoms includes the knee and ankle reflexes, the strength of the extensor hallucis longus, and the sensory function. Figure 25-3 illustrates the typical L4, L5, and S1 neurologic findings. About 98% of all herniations occur at those levels. Knee (quadriceps) and ankle (Achilles) reflexes should be obtained in the sitting and/or supine positions. The knee reflex is primarily a test of L4 nerve root function, while the ankle reflex is primarily mediated by the S1 nerve root. Sensation can be grossly evaluated by touch but,

when indicated, is more precisely determined by means of a sterile, sharp object (pin prick), light touch, a vibrating tuning fork and the ability of the patient to feel position. Nonspecific loss of sensation must be differentiated from well-defined dermatomal loss. Strength of the extensor hallucis longus is typically affected by an L5 nerve root compression. The testing of muscle may also include ankle and toe dorsiflexors and ankle invertors (L4, L5 roots), ankle plantar flexors and evertors (S1, S2 roots), knee extensors and hip adductors (L2, L3, L4) and hip flexors (T12, L1, L2, L3). The Babinski sign and the presence of clonus are measures of upper-motor neuron involvement. A summary of common lumbar radicular syndromes is provided in Table 25-3.

With the patient in the prone position, palpation of the spinous processes, interspinous spaces, paraspinal muscles, sacroiliac joint, and sciatic nerve is performed. Palpation should include the thoracic spine. A femoral stretch test is sometimes performed to detect radicular pain from the L2-4 nerve roots. A complete examination should include ab-

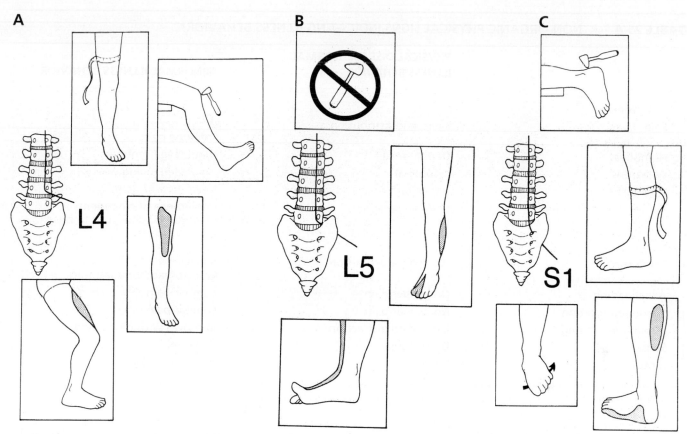

**FIGURE 25-3**    Typical findings in L4, L5, and S1 syndromes. L4 lesions are characterized by a loss of the knee reflex **(A)**, L5 by a weakness of the extensor hallucis longus **(B)**, and S1 by a loss of the ankle reflex **(C)**. (After Pope MH, et al.: *Occupational low-back pain.* St. Louis, 1991, Mosby–Year Book.)

**TABLE 25-3    LUMBAR RADICULAR SYNDROMES***

| DISC LEVEL | ANY CENTRAL DISC HERNIATION | L5/S1 | L4/5 | L3/4 |
|---|---|---|---|---|
| Nerve root involved | Cauda equina (L4/5 > L5/S1 | S1 | L5 | L4 |
| Pain referral pattern | Perineum | Unilateral | Unilateral | Unilateral |
| | Low back | Low back | Low back | Low back |
| | Buttocks | Buttocks | Buttocks | Buttocks |
| | Either or both legs | Posterior leg | Lateral leg and thigh | Posterolateral leg |
| Motor deficit | Unilateral or bilateral leg weakness | Unilateral weakness; plantar flexion of foot; difficulty with toe walking | Unilateral weakness; dorsiflexion of foot; difficulty with heel walking | Unilateral quadriceps weakness |
| Sensory deficit | Perineum/buttocks, low back, thighs, legs, feet | Lateral foot, postero-lateral calf | Lateral calf; between 1st and 2nd toes | Knee distal, anterior thigh |
| Reflexes compromised | Ankle jerk | Ankle jerk | 0 | Knee jerk |

*After Andersson GBJ, McNeill TW: *Lumbar spine syndromes: evaluation and treatment,* Vienna, 1989, Springer-Verlag.

**TABLE 25-4   NON-ORGANIC PHYSICAL SIGNS INDICATING ILLNESS BEHAVIOR***

| | PHYSICAL DISEASE/NORMAL ILLNESS BEHAVIOR | ABNORMAL ILLNESS BEHAVIOR |
|---|---|---|
| **Symptoms** | | |
| Pain | Anatomic distribution | Whole leg pain<br>Tailbone pain |
| Numbness | Dermatomal | Whole leg numbness |
| Weakness | Myotomal | Whole leg giving way |
| Time pattern | Varies with time and activity | Never free of pain |
| Response to treatment | Variable benefit | Intolerance of treatments<br>Emergency admissions to hospital |
| **Signs** | | |
| Tenderness | Anatomic distribution | Superficial<br>Widespread nonanatomic |
| Axial loading | No lumber pain | Lumbar pain |
| Simulated rotation | No lumbar pain | Lumbar pain |
| Straight leg raising | Limited on distraction | Improves with distraction |
| Sensory | Dermatomal | Regional |
| Motor | Myotomal | Regional, jerky, giving way |

*After Waddell G, Bircher M, Finlayson D, et al: Symptoms and signs: physical disease or illness behavior? *Br Med J* 289:739, 1984.

dominal palpation and evaluation of the peripheral pulses. If ankylosing spondylitis is suspected, chest expansion should be measured. Normally there is a difference greater than 1.5 cm between expiration and inspiration.

A variety of tests have been developed to determine the reproducibility and consistency of patient responses. The best researched are those described by Waddell et al[47] (Table 25-4). These tests should alert the examiner to the possibility of psychologic distress and/or malingering, and may signify the need for psychological testing.

In addition to the tests included in the standard examination described above, there are a number of other tests that are sometimes used. They include the *Patric test,* in which the hip is flexed, abducted and externally rotated, and the *pelvic rock test,* where the pelvis is forcefully compressed by the examiner exerting force on both iliac tubercles. Both of these tests are done to determine sacroiliac joint involvement. Another test to the same purpose is the *Gaenslen test.* With the patient supine and the buttock over the edge of the table, the unsupported leg is allowed to drop down while the other leg is flexed and held to the chest. None of these tests have a high degree of specificity.

Other tests are the *Milgram test,* where the patient simultaneously lifts both legs off the table and holds for 30 seconds. This increases the intrathecal pressure and is used to rule out intrathecal pathology. The *Naffziger test* is another test aimed at increasing the intrathecal pressure. In this test, both jugular veins are compressed until the patient's face begins to flush, at which point the patient is asked to cough. The test is positive if radicular pain occurs. A large number of additional tests, some with eponyms, are being used. In general, their contribution to a specific diagnosis is small.

At the completion of the history and physical examination, a general formulation can be made of the patient's low-back problem, including decisions regarding the need for any further diagnostic tests. An initial therapeutic plan can usually be initiated at this time as well.

### Diagnostic Studies

For the majority of patients, further diagnostic studies are not required. If additional tests are indicated, two general categories are considered: those performed to detect physiologic abnormalities, and those to detect anatomic abnormality and provide anatomic definition. Physiologic tests include serologic studies, bone scans, and electrodiagnostic studies. Anatomic tests include x-rays and other imaging studies such a computed tomography (CT) and magnetic resonance imaging (MRI). In select cases a psychological evaluation may also be required.

## Serologic studies

Serologic tests have limited value in the evaluation of patients with back pain but are indicated when there is clinical suspicion of systemic disease including infection, inflammation, and malignancy.

## Spinal radiography

Radiographs are commonly used and can reveal a variety of bony and structural abnormalities of which only a few are associated with back pain. For general diagnostic screening, spinal radiographs have limited value and findings correlate poorly with the presence of back pain.[12] Degenerative changes are common in patients with and without back problems, and are typically unrelated to the patients' pain. Spondylolisthesis, severe deformity, and severe degenerative changes are the main findings of clinical importance. Fractures, osseous tumors, and some infections can also be detected, but are rare. Thus plain film radiographs are indicated primarily in patients with recent trauma, suspicion of osteoporosis, a history of malignancy or recent infection, and when the clinical symptoms are suggestive of malignancy, infection, or fracture.

Flexion/extension radiographs are taken to detect abnormal motion between vertebrae (i.e., instability). However, this type of radiographic study is difficult to evaluate because of the inability to accurately identify bony landmarks. A positive test of instability requires a minimum of 4 to 5 mm translation.[42] Flexion/extension views are also used to assess the integrity of a previously performed spinal fusion. Again, caution must be exerted in interpreting results. When instrumentation is used, flexion/extension films may show absence of movement even when the fusion has not healed.

## Other imaging techniques

A variety of other imaging techniques are available to assess patients with back pain and sciatica including CT scanning, MRI scanning, myelography, and discography, the uses of which are described in Chapter 15). These tests allow assessment of the anatomy of the spinal canal and its contents. Estimates of the sensitivity and specificity of these tests are provided in Table 25-5, and further discussed in Chapter 12. They should be used only when there is a clear indi-

### TABLE 25-5 SENSITIVITY AND SPECIFICITY OF IMAGING TESTS USED FOR THE DIAGNOSIS OF HERNIATED DISCS (HNP) AND SPINAL STENOSIS (SS)*

| | TEST | SENSITIVITY | SPECIFICITY |
|---|---|---|---|
| HNP | CT | 0.90 | 0.70 |
| | MRI | 0.90 | 0.70 |
| | CT myelography | 0.90 | 0.70 |
| SS | CT | 0.90 | 0.80-0.95 |
| | MRI | 0.90 | 0.75-0.95 |
| | Myelography | 0.77 | 0.70 |

*After Andersson GBJ, McNeill TW: *Lumbar spine syndromes: evaluation and treatment,* Vienna, 1989, Springer-Verlag.

cation based on the patient's history and physical examination. These studies are only valid when correlated with the clinical signs and symptoms. Imaging abnormalities are common in individuals who have never had low-back symptoms ar sciatica, occurring in about 25% of asymptomatic people with larger percentages in older populations.[9, 22, 23, 27, 49, 50] Further, a number of other findings of questionable or unknown importance are commonly observed. These include disc bulging and disc degeneration, which are both nonspecific and present in the majority of the adult population.

Four imaging tests, CT, MRI, myelography and myelo-CT, are used in similar clinical situations and often provide similar types of information.[24, 25] Significant technologic advances in these imaging modalities are currently taking place. As a result, there has been a gradual shift from myelography towards CT and, more recently, from CT towards MRI. Discography and Disc-CT are other tests used more specifically by some to determine severe degenerative changes of the disc (see Chapter 15).

## Electrodiagnostic studies

Electrodiagnostic studies are used to evaluate the physiologic function of the spinal cord, nerve roots, and peripheral nerves.[1] They include electromyography, reflex studies, somatosensory-evoked potentials, and nerve conduction velocity studies. The use and value of these tests are further described in Chapters 38 through 40. They should only be used to confirm specific clinical suspicions.

## Psychological Assessment

Patients with chronic back pain occasionally require a psychological assessment. A variety of tests and techniques have been developed for that purpose.[28] They include personality and psychological test instruments, behavioral assessment methods, cognitive-behavioral assessment methods, and psychophysiological measures. Some of these tests are the Minnesota Multiphasic Personality Inventory (MMPI) and the Million Behavioral Health Inventory (see Chapters 43 and 45).

## CLASSIFICATION

As discussed earlier, there is a lack of agreement on the classification of patients with back disorders. The two currently used approaches are briefly discussed here.

## Symptom Diagnosis

The most comprehensive system based on symptoms was developed by the Quebec Study Group.[44] Table 25-6 outlines the system, which is applicable to all anatomic regions of the spine. Broadly, it contains four symptom categories with diagnostic specificity, four categories based on pathoanatomic cause, two postsurgical categories, and one category that is unspecified.

Category 1 represents the majority of patients with low-back disorders. These patients have pain that is typically aggravated by mechanical factors such as activity, worsens during the day, and is relieved by rest. Acute low-back pain of this type can develop following single or repetitive loading events and can also develop from minor postural changes such as bending or twisting, from simple coughing, or, in the majority of cases, is triggered by an unknown event. Examination typically reveals loss of lumbar lordosis, varying

---

**TABLE 25-6      THE QUEBEC CLASSIFICATION SYSTEM**

| CLASSIFICATION | SYMPTOMS | DURATION OF SYMPTOMS FROM ONSET | WORKING STATUS AT TIME OF EVALUATION |
|---|---|---|---|
| 1 | Pain without radiation | | |
| 2 | Pain + radiation to extremity, proximally | a (<7 days) | W (working) |
| 3 | Pain + radiation to extremity, distally | b (7 days-7 weeks) | I (idle) |
| 4 | Pain + radiation to upper/lower limb neurologic signs | c (>7 weeks) | |
| 5 | Presumptive compression of a spinal nerve root on a simple roentgenogram (ie, spinal instability or fracture) | | |
| 6 | Compression of a spinal nerve root confirmed by (1) specific imaging techniques (i.e., computed axial tomography, myelography, or magnetic resonance imaging) or (2) other diagnostic techniques (e.g., electromyography, venography) | | |
| 7 | Spinal stenosis | | |
| 8 | Postsurgical status, 1-6 months after intervention | | |
| 9 | Postsurgical status, >6 months after intervention<br>9.1 Asymptomatic<br>9.2 Symptomatic | | |
| 10 | Chronic pain syndrome | | W (working) |
| 11 | Other diagnoses | | I (idle) |

From Spitzer WO, LeBlanc FE, Dupuis M, et al: Scientific approach to the assessment and management of activity-related spinal disorders: a monograph for clinicians. Report of the Quebec Task Force on Spinal Disorders. *Spine* 12(Suppl 7):S1-S59, 1987.

degrees of back-muscle tightness and spasm, and restriction of spinal motion. None of these signs have particular diagnostic significance. Neurologic signs and symptoms are absent. Commonly-used diagnoses for this patient group include low-back strain or sprain, implying a muscular or ligamentous injury. Unfortunately these suspected diagnoses are almost never verifiable; thus these are nonspecific terms. Imaging studies are *not* required to classify patients into this group, or indeed to develop an initial treatment plan, but if done, should be negative with respect to a specific diagnosis. Disc degeneration is often present in patients of Category 1.

Category 2 is characterized by a proximal leg pain distribution. That pain distribution can be induced experimentally by mechanical stimuli or injection of noxious substances, such as hypertonic saline, into back muscles, facet joints, ligaments and bone.[21, 29, 35, 37] Referred pain caused by stimulation of connective tissue structures is frequently referred to as *sclerotomal*. All of the structures that produce this type of pain derive their innervation from the posterior primary rami.

Category 3 represents pain that radiates distally into the legs. This pain may arise from three sources: by irritation of structures innervated by the posterior primary rami;[38] by increased tension, compression, or inflammation of an anterior primary rami; or by a reduction in the space available for the cauda and/or nerve roots. Mono- or poly-radiculopathies are both included in this group, but are better defined in Categories 4, 6, and 7. Monoradiculopathies in Category 3 are typically called *sciatica*. Category 3 does not present with specific neurologic signs.

Category 4 increases the diagnostic specificity of mono-or poly-radiculopathies by requiring neurologic signs, such as a positive nerve root tension sign (SLR), loss (or reduction) of reflexes, sensation, or motor power. In the instance of a monoradiculopathy, the presence of these signs will accurately identify a lumbar disc herniation in a high proportion of patients affected.[20] When root tension signs such as a contralaterally positive straight leg raising test are present, the probability of lumbar disc herniation approaches 98%.[41] Confirmation of cause of root involvement by an imaging study transfers a patient in Category 4 to Category 6.

Category 5 includes spinal fractures that compromise the bony spinal canal, as well as the more subtle and controversial problem of segmental instability, which will be discussed later in this chapter. In these patients the presence or absence of nerve root compromise is evaluated from clinical and radiographic presentation.

Category 6 is an extension of Category 4 and requires confirmation of nerve root compression by imaging techniques such as myelography, CT scans, and MRI, as well as physiologic techniques such as electromyography.

Category 7 includes the most common cause of polyradiculopathy and neurogenic claudication—spinal stenosis. If the patient has significant or advancing neurologic dysfunction, the diagnosis should be confirmed by the imaging techniques discussed above.

Categories 8 and 9 include patients who have undergone a surgical intervention for a spinal disorder. Dividing the postoperative period into 1 to 6 months, and greater than 6 months, is meaningful, because most patients with simple disc excisions should have recovered and returned to work within 6 months of the intervention. The separation of Category 9 into two classifications (9.1 asymptomatic, 9.2 symptomatic) is important for impairment evaluation purposes and long-term prognosis.

Category 10, chronic pain syndrome, signifies a situation where acute pain has been transferred into a chronic pain syndrome and psychological and psychosocial factors gradually have become most important. Physical findings are inconclusive and often nonorganic, and "pain behavior" is common. There is no direct relationship between an identifiable physical pathology and the patients' initial symptoms and disability. Determination of impairment in these patients should ideally not be made without psychological or psychiatric consultation.

A special group of patients who may belong in this last category have the so-called deconditioning syndrome. The deconditioning syndrome develops after injuries of unknown etiology suspected to involve the soft tissues. In these conditions the physiologic measurements of motion, strength, cardiovascular fitness, and lifting capacity are all significantly below normal. Determination of impairment should not be made until correction of this decondition state has been attempted.

Category 11 contains all other types of back pain not included in the 10 other categories. Although this list is extensive, including tumors, infections, metabolic, and inflammatory causes, it comprises only a small minority of patients with back disorders.

The Quebec classification introduces two other important parameters: duration of symptoms and working status. Based on duration, symptoms are generally divided into acute, subacute, or chronic. The Quebec Study Group suggests acute symptoms are 7 days or less in duration; subacute, 7 day to 7 weeks; and chronic, more than 7 weeks. Others use somewhat different time sequences: acute, less than 1 month; subacute, 1 to 3 months; and chronic, greater than 3 months.[18, 39] Figure 25-2 demonstrates the normal recovery curve after an acute low-back episode. About 90% of patients are recovered within 3 months.[6] Failure to recover during that time increases the probability that a chronic pain syndrome will develop.

Another subset of patients not discussed in the Quebec classification system are those who have recurrent pain complaints. It is estimated that 60% of patients who have an acute low-back episode and recover will have a recurrence, usually within the first two years.[8, 45] Patients with sciatica have an increased risk of recurrence.

Subclassification by work status also has major implications to prognosis. As time passes, there is rapidly diminishing likelihood that the individual will ever return to work (see Fig. 25-2).

An alternative classification system was developed by the Back Strategy Committee of the Australian Work Cover Corporation and has been endorsed by a variety of Australian medical associations and colleges (Table 25-7). It combines symptom diagnoses and anatomical diagnoses.[52] It is presented here to illustrate an even more simplified approach than the Quebec System. The Australian system has only three groups: two based on the patient's descriptions and one based on known etiology. It is anticipated that over 90% of work-related back pain will fall into Groups one and two. It is also anticipated that classifications for a particular injury will change as more sophisticated diagnostic techniques become available. Interestingly, the classification system does not accept a diagnosis of back strain after eight weeks, because of the normal healing time of muscle. After this, a different classification must be selected.

The American Medical Association has also included a classification system in the fourth edition of its *Guides to the Evaluation of Permanent Impairment.*[2] This system, which applies particularly to patients with traumatic injuries, is referred to as the "injury model", and assigns the patient to one of eight categories called *Diagnosis-Related Estimates (DREs).* These estimates, which are listed in Table 25-8 for lumbosacral injuries, are differentiated based on clinical findings: guarding, loss of reflexes, decreased muscle circumference (atrophy), diagnostic tests (electrodiagnostics, lateral motion roentgenograms, cystometrograms), and neurologic deficits (cauda equina-like syndromes and paraplegia). Further, structural changes (such as fractures and dislocations) are included. The injury model "attempts to document physiologic and structural impairments relating to insults other than common developmental findings, such as (1) spondylolysis, (2) spondylolisthesis, (3) herniated discs without radiculopathy, and (4) aging changes".[2] The injury model is applicable to only a small percentage of patients with spinal conditions.

**TABLE 25-7    AUSTRALIAN WORK COVER CLASSIFICATION SYSTEM***

| | |
|---|---|
| Group One | Back pain (non-specific) |
| Group Two | Back strain (diagnosis is not appropriate if 8 weeks or more have passed since the injury) |
| Group Three | Back pain with specific diagnosis. For all diagnoses in Group Three, it is stressed that the symptoms, signs, and investigatory findings must be in concordance. |

1. Disc prolapse
2. Symptomatic disc or facet degeneration
3. Stenosis -
    Central
    Subarticular
    Foraminal
4. Spondylolisthesis
5. Fracture and/or dislocation

*Relevant intercurrent medical conditions affecting the lumbosacral spine should be noted, for example, inflammatory arthritides.

Also included in the AMA *Guides* is a listing of specific spine disorders that are combined with range of motion impairment estimates and impairment estimates involving sensation, weakness and other conditions. They fall into four categories; (1) fractures, (2) intervertebral discs or other soft tissue lesions, (3) spondylolysis and spondylolisthesis, not operated on, and (4) spinal stenosis, segmental instability, spondylolisthesis, fracture, or dislocation operated on and will be discussed.

### Pathoanatomic Classification

The second main classification method is by pathoanatomic etiology. This system is presently applicable to only a few percent of all patients with low-back pain, if degenerative changes are excluded, but has major significance in the treatment and prognosis of this small subset. The majority of patients with specific pathoanatomic causes for pain will fall into Quebec Categories 4 through 7. A small, but very important, minority will be classified as belonging in Category 11.

### Degenerative spinal disorders

Degenerative spinal disorders are the bases for the most common pathoanatomic causes of low-back pain, mono- and poly-radiculopathies, and claudica-

**TABLE 25-8**     LUMBOSACRAL SPINE IMPAIRMENTS DESCRIBED AS DIAGNOSIS-RELATED ESTIMATES (DRES) AND CLASSIFIED INTO EIGHT CATEGORIES

| DRE-CATEGORY | COMPLAINTS OR SYMPTOMS | STRUCTURAL INCLUSION |
|---|---|---|
| I | No Impairment | None |
| II | Minor Impairment | Vertebral Fx |
| III | Radiculopathy | Vertebral Fx |
| IV | Loss of Motor Segment Integrity (MSI) | Vertebral Fx or Dislocation |
| V | Radiculopathy and Loss of MSI | Structural Compromise |
| VI | Cauda Equina-Like Syndrome (Without Bowel or Bladder Paralysis) | None |
| VII | Cauda Equina Syndrome with Bowel or Bladder Paralysis | None |
| VIII | Paraplegia, Total Loss of Lumbosacral Spinal Cord Function | None |

From American Medical Association: *Guides to the evaluation of permanent impairment,* ed 4, Chicago, 1993.

tion. While this is true, it is very important not to assume that degeneration is synonymous with back pain and, indeed, is the cause of pain in an individual patient. Currently we cannot, with certainty, determine the difference between a disc that is degenerated and symptoms producing and one that is degenerated and asymptomatic.

It is critical to place the normal, age-related, spinal degeneration in perspective as a background for considering clinically significant degenerative syndromes, and to recognize that disc degeneration, as such, is usually not clinically significant. All human spines degenerate with time. Most autopsy specimens, and MRI studies in normal subjects, show the onset of gross and microscopic evidence of intervertebral disc degeneration by the third decade of life. These morphologic changes are accompanied by alterations in the biochemical composition of the disc, such as a decrease in water and proteoglycan content, and an increase in collagen.[15] The onset of changes occurs earlier in life in the male and affects more commonly the L4/5 and L5/S1 discs.

Radiographic changes such a disc-space narrowing, endplate sclerosis, and spinal osteophytes lag behind the histologic and chemical events. However, the prevalence of these degenerative changes is equivalent in patients with and without low-back pain. The presence of a narrowed intervertebral disc is not correlated with the risk for, or the presence of, a disc herniation. In fact, disc space narrowing in one study

was a negative predictor for lumbar disc herniation at that level.[20] Based on radiographs, disc degeneration has sometimes been divided into minimal, moderate, and severe. This division has no particular value to the determination of impairment.

The advent of MRI scanning allows earlier detection of disc degeneration, as discussed in Chapter 15, and has revealed that disc degeneration is present in many people in their twenties. Again, the presence of these so-called "black discs" on the T2 weighted MRI images does not imply clinical significance or impairment.

**Herniated nucleus pulposus**

Clinically, the syndrome of a herniated nucleus pulposus (HNP) is characterized by sciatica, usually accompanied or preceded by low-back pain. Physical examination reveals the presence of one or more objective neurologic changes such as reflex asymmetry, sensory change in the distribution of a nerve root, or muscle weakness (Fig. 25-3). The diagnosis of disc herniation requires a combination of appropriate radicular pain distribution, positive nerve root tension sign, objective neurologic abnormality, and a positive confirmatory structural examination (CT, Myelo, Myelo-CT, MRI, Discogram, Disco-CT). For the straight leg raising test to be positive, sciatic pain should develop below the knee. Neurologic signs can be absent. It is important to remember that reflex abnormalities, when present, can be a residual from a previous herniation, since the reflex usually does not reappear even after successful treatment. Although a positive structural examination is a requirement, the presence of a disc abnormality is not sufficient for diagnosis in the absence of clinical symptoms and signs, since more than 25% of healthy individuals have an abnormal imaging test (see Chaper 15). The structural examination should show a clear expansion of disc material posteriorly or posterolaterally, and displacement or indentation on the spinal cord if the lesion is above L1, the thecal sac if below L1 or one or both nerve roots at the affected level. An extraforamenal (far lateral) disc herniation can be present without obvious nerve root displacement. Diffuse disc bulging is not sufficient for diagnosis nor is an abnormal EMG where there are no clinical and structural correlates (see Chapters 38 and 40).

It is important to emphasize that the majority of patients who fit the clinical criteria of HNP will recover from acute symptoms with conservative treatment and have minimal residual functional or work capacity impairment. However, patients who have had a known disc herniation are more likely to have a recurrent herniation. Surgical treatment is indicated in patients who do not respond to conservative treatment, or who develop progressive motor deficit. Between 0.3 and 1% of patients who have lumbar disc herniations will have a massive extrusion of nuclear material sufficient to interfere with nerve control of bladder and bowel function.[34, 43] This so-called cauda equina syndrome is a true surgical emergency, since failure to decompress the lesion may result in permanent loss of bladder and bowel control.

### Spinal stenosis

Spinal stenosis is defined as a narrowing of the vertebral canal, lateral recesses, or vertebral foraminae.[4] Narrowing of the central lumbar spinal canal in its sagittal or coronal dimensions (central spinal stenosis) may occur at a single level or at many levels of the spine (Fig. 25-4). When multiple levels are involved, typical symptoms include recurrent or continued low-back pain aggravated by specific body postures and/or physical exertion. As stenosis increases, extension of the spine often becomes more painful while flexion provides relief. Neurogenic claudication is a common symptom, but reflex, motor, and sensory changes are often confusing because of the involvement of multiple nerve roots. Neurologic findings also can be completely absent despite substantial neural encroachment. Unlike lumbar disc herniations, positive nerve root tension signs such as the straight leg raising test are usually absent. Diffuse narrowing of the spinal canal may be due to many

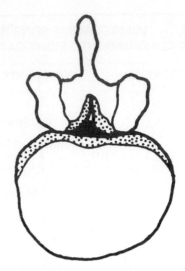

**FIGURE 25-4**    In central spinal stenosis, the spinal canal is narrowed. As seen on the figure, ligamentous tissue often contributes to this narrowing. (After Andersson GBJ, McNeill TW: *Lumbar spinal stenosis*, St. Louis, 1992, Mosby–Year Book.)

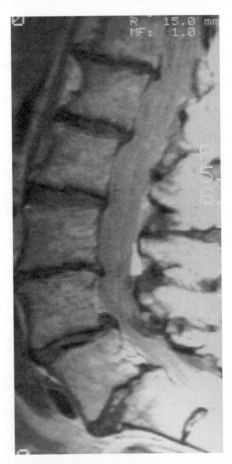

**FIGURE 25-5**    Magnetic resonance scan of a patient with degenerative lumbar spine changes and a degenerative spondylolisthesis at L4/L5.

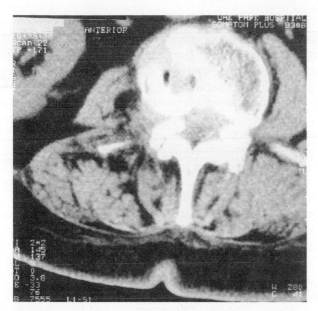

**FIGURE 25-6** CT scan of a patient with lateral spinal stenosis. Note the large osteophytes at the facet joints.

---

**TABLE 25-9**  CLASSIFICATION OF SPINAL STENOSIS

**Etiologic Classification***

I. Congenital—Developmental Stenosis
  (a) Idiopathic (hereditary)
  (b) Achondroplastic

II. Acquired Stenosis
  (a) Degenerative
  (b) Combined congenital and degenerative stenosis
  (c) Spondylolytic/Spondylolisthetic
  (d) Iatrogenic
    (i) Post-laminectomy
    (ii) Post-fusion
    (iii) Post-chemonucleolysis
  (e) Post-traumatic
  (f) Metabolic
    (i) Paget's disease
    (ii) Fluorosis

**Anatomic Classification**

I. *Central Stenosis*—The central canal is narrowed in the sagittal or coronal plane or in both planes.

II. *Lateral Stenosis*—The nerve root canal is narrowed in the lateral recess or nerve root canal or both.

*Etiologic classification after Arnoldi CC, Brodsky AE, Cauchoix J, et al: Lumbar spinal stenosis and nerve root entrapment syndromes: definition and classification. *Clin Orthop* 115:4, 1976.

---

causes, but most commonly the stenosis results from degeneration with posterior osteophytes projecting into the spinal canal, hypertrophy of the articular facets, and buckling of the ligamentum flavum.

A second group of stenotic lesions are associated with more focal degenerative disease. Degenerative spondylolisthesis is the most common of these and typically affects females during the fifth and sixth decades of life (Fig. 25-5). It occurs most commonly at the L4/L5 level. Radiographic surveys have shown that as many as 9.1% of females and 5.8% of males have this deformity, although many have no symptoms.[46] In other patients, disc space collapse leads to backward displacement (retrospondylolisthesis), which may lead to compromise of the nerve root canals or central spinal stenosis.

Another group of patients is characterized as having predominantly lateral (nerve root canal) stenosis (Fig. 25-6). In this situation, a combination of facet hypertrophy and varying degrees of disc bulge reduces the space available at the affected disc level(s) and compromises the nerve root(s). Lateral spinal stenosis may present as a mono- or poly-radiculopathy, but the characteristic complaints of neurogenic claudication are less likely to be present. Yong-Hing and Kirkaldy-Willis[30] have emphasized the interrelationships between spinal stenosis and disc herniations. When the spinal canal and lateral nerve root canal are narrowed, a relatively small disc herniation can produce clinically significant symptoms such as sciatica, which would not have occurred if the canal

had been of adequate dimensions. This exemplifies how a pre-existing condition can contribute to the development of symptoms.

Spinal stenosis can be classified etiologically as well as anatomically (Table 25-9). Impairment evaluation, however, is based on symptoms, not on classification. Diagnosis is not purely clinical but requires a positive imaging test.

**Other degenerative changes**

Two peculiar types of degenerative changes of minor clinical importance are idiopathic vertebrogenic sclerosis and diffuse idiopathic spinal hyperostosis (DISH). The former is characterized by severe low-back pain, focal severe disc space narrowing, and diffuse sclerosis of the vertebral body adjacent to the disc. Most commonly the L4 vertebral body is affected. Women are affected four to five times more often than men. In contrast, DISH affects multiple vertebrae, is most common in men, and is characterized radiographically by diffuse flowing osteophytes, which bridge over a minimum of three vertebral levels. Patients commonly have associated metabolic conditions such as diabetes and gout, and may also have other joints affected.

## Degenerative conditions of less certain significance

Three diagnoses are commonly considered causes of low-back pain, with or without radiculopathies: segmental instability, facet syndrome, and disc disruption syndrome.

### SEGMENTAL INSTABILITY

Many patients with low-back pain have recurring episodes of increasing severity, sometimes transiently associated with nerve root irritation and usually triggered by minor mechanical overloads.[18, 32] Radiographic criteria associated with this diagnosis have included the presence of disc space narrowing and spinal osteophytes projecting away from the disc space, the so-called traction spur.[36] The most important criterion is abnormal shifts in the alignment of vertebrae observed on lateral spinal radiographs taken with the patient in a flexed and extended position.[14, 33] Friberg[17] proposed a different method whereby the spine is overloaded by a back pack and then placed in traction (traction/compression films). Attempts to classify segmental instability associated with spinal degeneration have not been uniformly accepted.[19] Despite the absence of certain clinical and radiographic criteria, segmental instability remains one of the most commonly used indications for lumbar spinal fusion. The diagnosis should require translation of at least 4 mm as measured from the dynamic radiographs.

### FACET SYNDROME

Sixty years ago, it was proposed that many causes of low back pain originated from the facet joints. Mooney and Robertson[38] repopularized this diagnosis. They described a patient group who had pain mainly in spinal extension or rotation, often accompanied by referred pain to the upper buttocks, posterolateral thigh, and sometimes even into the calf. Spinal radiographs were often normal. Provocative injections with saline into the facet joints resulted in referred pain, while relief of pain followed injection of the facet with local anesthetic. In other patients, radiographic evidence of degeneration of the facets was present, and this group was given the diagnosis of facet arthritis. Treatment with antiinflammatory medication, and in some instances local cortisone injection into the affected joint, was associated with symptom relief. Denervation has also been attempted. Since this original description, there have been a number of attempts to characterize precisely

the clinical syndrome and develop rational therapy. A comprehensive analysis of over 400 patients led to the conclusion that facet syndrome cannot be classified with any certainty.[26] A small subset of patients can have facet pathology associated with a degenerative cyst. If this projects into the nerve root, it can produce symptoms indistinguishable from lumbar disc herniation.

### DISC DISRUPTION SYNDROME

Crock[10] described the disc disruption syndrome as characterized by severe, unrelenting, mechanical low-back pain, following a suspected compression injury. He reported that spinal radiographs were usually normal and the diagnosis was dependent on discography whereby injection of the radiopaque contrast media into the disc must faithfully reproduce the patient's pain, and also demonstrate disruption of the normal disc architecture. Disc disruption syndrome is a source of controversy and uncertainty, as is the use of discography (see Chapter 15).

## Congenital abnormalities

In the normal development of the spine, defects in the formation of spinal structures may occur. The majority of these abnormalities have minimal significance but are often erroneously believed to cause low-back pain. Most of the common congenital abnormalities occur equally in populations with and without back pain. The most common are spina bifida occulta and segmentation abnormalities such as lumbarization and sacralization.

### SPINA BIFIDA OCCULTA

As the neural arch forms, incomplete closure may occur, accompanied by partial or complete absence of the spinous process. In a small subgroup (1/100,000), the bony defect is accompanied by a herniation of the neural elements through the defect. This condition is termed meningomyelocele and is associated with a variety of neurologic defects usually apparent at birth. For the vast majority of patients, spina bifida occulta is a finding of no significance.

### SEGMENTATION ABNORMALITIES

There are wide variations in the number and shape of lumbar vertebrae. Lumbarization is where the first sacral segment has the appearance of a lumbar vertebra and, thus, there are six rather than five lumbar segments. Conversely, the fifth lumbar vertebra may be incorporated into the sacrum (sacralization), resulting in only four mobile lumbar vertebrae (Fig. 25-7). Sometimes the incorporation occurs only on one side (hemisacralization), and in a small patient group may be associated with the development of a false joint between the ilium and the elongated transverse process of the fifth lumbar vertebrae. In general, segmentation abnormalities are not associated with an in-

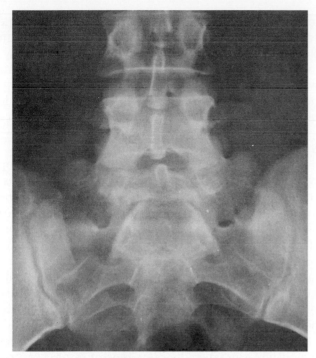

**FIGURE 25-7**   Sacralization of the fifth lumbar vertebrae (L5).

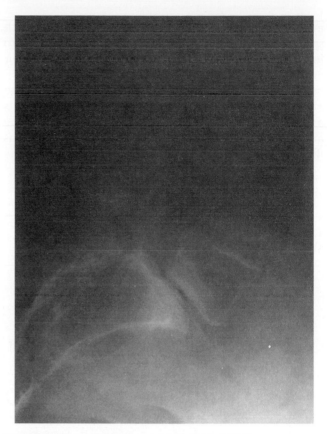

**FIGURE 25-8**   Grade 2 spondylolisthesis (L5/S1).

creased risk of back pain and are not the cause of back pain *per se*. A few patients with hemisacralization may have pain arising from the false joint, and also there is some evidence of increased susceptibility to L4/5 disc herniations in this group, the so-called Bertelocci syndrome. Segmentation abnormalities are important sources of confusion in determining the level of a herniated disc or stenosis.

### CONJOINED NERVE ROOTS

Anatomic variants may also occur in neural structures. For example, nerve roots may be conjoined. This condition has minimal significance excepted as a possible cause of sciatica, but may pose technical problems in surgical interventions. It can also confuse the interpretation of an imaging examination, particularly myelograms, since the conjoint root can produce a picture resembling a disc herniation.

## Spondylolysis and spondylolisthesis

Spondylolisthesis is broadly defined as forward displacment of one vertebra relative to the next lower vertebra (Fig. 25-8). This condition can arise from numerous causes.[51] The most common form is isthmic spondylolisthesis, which involves an acquired or, more rarely, congenital defect in the neural arch at the pars interarticularis. The defect is termed *spondylolysis* and may be unilateral or bilateral. The presence of the defect varies widely in the population and ranges from 1 to 10%. Isthmic spondylolisthesis is less common, affecting 1 to 4% of populations. The

most common site of isthmic spondylolisthesis is at L5, slipping forward on S1, and the lesion is far more common in males than females. Importantly, continuation of forward slippage ceases with adulthood and, thus, adult patients with the common L5/S1 lesion do not have an unstable spine.[16] When the isthmic lesion occurs at L4/5, there is evidence slippage may continue in adulthood, unlike the L5/S1 lesion.

The development of spondylolysis and subsequent isthmic spondylolisthesis is thought to be due to a fatigue failure of the neural arch in many patients rather than being a congenital abnormality. Typically, this occurs in childhood or adolescence and when recognized on radiographs later in life have no appearance or signs of an overt fracture. In a few patients, the fracture is recent but can only be identified by the presence of increased radioisotope uptake within the neural arch, and no bony defect is observed on routine spinal radiographs. In these patients, bracing may resolve the symptoms and the actual defect may never develop (i.e., the fracture heals). Because spondylolysis is more common in certain athletes such as football linemen and female gymnasts, repetitive flexion-extension forces have been thought to be the mechanism of injury. Spondylolysis is equally common in populations with and without pack pain. However, workers with spondylolisthesis are somewhat more susceptible to low back pain, particularly if the slip is Grade 2 or greater.

The type of spondylolisthesis should be described etiologically and anatomically. Table 25-10 presents an etiologic classification of spondylolysis.[7] The anatomic classification describes the degree of slip as illustrated in Figure 25-9. In Grades 3 and 4 spondy-

lolisthesis, additional measures may have prognostic value. The level at which spondylolisthesis is present should be specified, since patients with L4/5 spondylolisthesis have more clinical symptoms than patients with an equivalent spondylolisthesis at L5/S1. Diagnosis should be based on radiographs, and the grade of slip measured on true lateral views (Chapter 15).

### Spine trauma

Acute fractures and fracture dislocations develop when an external load exceeds the strength of the tissues. The resulting type of injury is a function of the magnitude and velocity and direction of the applied loads. A variety of classifications have been devised (Fig. 25-10).[11] The most common fracture is the result of a fall landing on the buttocks and is termed a *compression fracture*. Compression fractures are usually quantified by the degree of vertebral body collapse that has occurred. Because of the structure of the trabecular network, the anterior part of the body is usually more compressed than the posterior. If the force magnitude is greater, the same type of trauma can result in a burst fracture of the vertebral body where bony fragments may be displaced into the spinal canal, sometimes resulting in neurologic compromise.

With the exception of very severe (greater than 50% of vertebral body height) compression fractures, burst fractures, and fracture-dislocations, the majority

---

**TABLE 25-10    ETIOLOGIC CLASSIFICATION OF SPONDYLOLISTHESIS**

I. Dysplastic (congenital)

II. Isthmic (pars lesion)
   (a) Lytic (fatigue fracture)
   (b) Elongated (but intact pars)
   (c) Acute fracture

III. Degenerative

IV. Traumatic

V. Pathologic (bone disease)

After Wiltse LL, Newman PH, Macnab I: Classification of spondylolysis and spondylolisthesis. *Clin Orthop* 117:23, 1976.

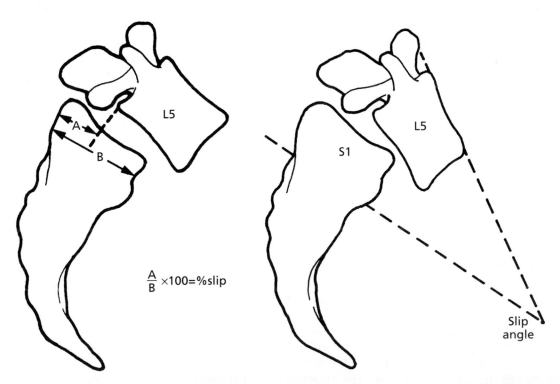

$$\frac{A}{B} \times 100 = \% slip$$

**FIGURE 25-9**    Measurements in spondylolisthesis. The degree of slip is measured as a percentage obtained by dividing the amount of displacement *(A)* by the A-P diameter of the inferior vertebra (here sacrum) *(B)* and multiplying by 100. Commonly, the olisthesis is classified as grade 1 (0-25%), 2 (25-50%), 3 (50-75%), and 4 (75-100%). The slip angle is a measure of the angular relationship of L5 and S1. A higher slip angle is associated with a greater potential for progressive slip.

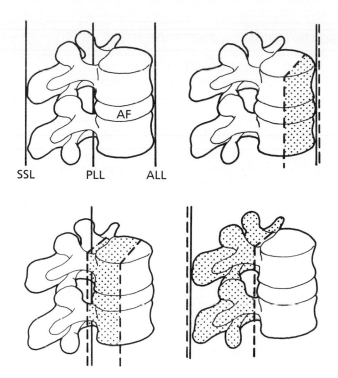

**FIGURE 25-10**    The three-column concept divides the spine into an anterior column (the anterior longitudinal ligament, anterior disc, and anterior vertebral body), a middle column (the posterior disc, posterior vertebral body, and posterior longitudinal ligament), and a posterior column (posterior bony complex and ligamentous complex). Failure of two columns results in an unstable spine. (After Denis F: The three-column spine and its significance in the classification of acute thoraco-lumbar spinal injuries. *Spine* 8:817, 1983.)

of these injuries do not require operative treatment, heal uneventfully, and are compatible with the resumption of normal activities after healing is complete. Neurologic dysfunction associated with more severe injuries has major functional implications, including paraplegia.

### Spinal infections

Acute or chronic bacterial infections of the spine are uncommon. Acute infections are the result of hematogenous spread of bacteria to the vertebrae and are rare in individuals who are otherwise healthy. Predispositions include diabetes, the use of corticosteroids or other immunosuppressive drugs, and recent genitourinary surgery. Intravenous drug abusers and patients with AIDS are also at risk. Staphylococci are the most commonly cultured bacteria, but a variety of other organisms are becoming more common. Tuberculosis infections are common in underdeveloped countries, still exist in the United States, and are increasing in the drug-abusing populations. Postoperative infections occur after disc surgery in about 0.25% of patients, almost always in the form of discitis.

The history of these patients is variable, ranging from very acute, severe systemic illness with pain and fever to an insidious onset with minimal, if any, systemic symptoms. An acute onset is most common with blood-borne bacterial infections, whereas insidious onset is typical of tuberculosis. A distinctive characteristic is the complaint of pain at night. Physical examination varies widely, ranging from restricted spinal motion and muscle spasm, to excruciating pain. In the small subset of patients with epidural abscesses, neurologic dysfunction may be rapidly progressive and constitute a surgical emergency.

Early in the course of these infections the spinal radiographs may be normal. Radioisotope scans and magnetic resonance imaging are often necessary for diagnosis. Later, destruction of the vertebral bodies with collapse and obliteration of the disc space may occur. The outcome of these patients and their ability to return to their occupation depends on the underlying disease that may have predisposed to the condition, and the successful eradication of the infection by appropriate antibiotics. The need for surgical intervention depends on the infecting organism, the response to antibiotics, and the development of neurologic symptoms and signs. Many of the patients ultimately resume fairly normal activities, particularly those with postoperative disc space infections.

### Inflammatory spinal conditions

Inflammatory lesions affecting the lumbar spine are termed *spondyloarthropathies*, of which ankylosing spondylitis is most prevalent, affecting 2% of the population. The patient is typically a male less than 40 years of age. The onset of back pain is insidious. The patients often describe early awakening and spinal stiffness, particularly in the morning. These symptoms often improve as the day progresses. Physical examination reveals decreased chest expansion and reduced spinal mobility. Early radiographic studies are often normal but eventually demonstrate erosive changes at the sacroiliac joints. In severe cases, complete ankylosis (fusion) of the spine may occur. Laboratory studies can be normal, but more commonly there are mild elevations of the erythrocyte sedimentation rate, and in 95% of patients a specific serum antigen, the HLA-27B antigen, is present. However, a positive HLA-27B test alone is not diagnostic because 5 to 12% of the population has this finding, most of whom do not have the disease.

Other types of spondyloarthropathy include Reiter's syndrome (a disease characterized by the triad of genitourinary inflammation [urethritis], eye inflammation [uveitis], and sacroiliitis) and spondylitides associated with psoriasis or inflammatory bowel disease such as ulcerative colitis (Table 25-11).

**TABLE 25-11** DIFFERENTIAL DIAGNOSES OF SERO-NEGATIVE SPONDYLOARTHROPATHIES

| | ANKYLOSING SPONDYLITIS | REITER'S SYNDROME | INFLAMMATORY BOWEL DISEASE | PSORIASIS |
|---|---|---|---|---|
| Sacroiilitis | 100% early Symmetric | 20% late Symmetric | 20% Symmetric | 20% late Asymmetric |
| Peripheral arthritis | Hips and shoulders | Lower extremity | Hips and shoulders | Upper extremity |
| Calcaneous periostitis | Frequent | Very frequent | Occurs | No |
| Extraarticular | Occurs | Frequent (eye/skin) | Occurs | Frequent (skin) |
| Sex | M > F | M > F | F = M | F > M |
| Age at onset | ≥20 | >20 | Any | Any spine |
| Onset | Gradual | Sudden | Variable | Gradual |

After Andersson GBJ, McNeill TW: *Lumbar spine syndrome: evaluation and treatment*, Vienna, 1989, Springer-Verlag.

The majority of patients with inflammatory spinal conditions are able to carry on normal physical activities. In the most severely affected individuals, limitation of spinal mobility or involvement of other joints, such as the hips, may preclude all but sedentary occupations.

### Fibromyalgia

Fibromyalgia or myofascial pain syndrome are conditions that are thought to be caused by muscle inflammation. These controversial diagnoses are characterized by the symptom of nonspecific and chronic low-back pain, sometimes radiating into the upper parts of the lower legs. There are three major criteria, which the proponents feel are required for diagnosis (Table 25-12). With the exception of trigger points, these major criteria are similar to those symptoms reported by patients with nonspecific chronic low back pain. A number of minor criteria strengthen the diagnosis but are not absolutely required. The important diagnostic criterion is the presence of trigger points, which are localized tender areas of tissue within the muscle and the fascia. Relief of symptoms by anesthetic injections into these trigger points is thought to be diagnostic. Sleep disturbances are common. Almost half of the patients report that they are awakened during the night and fatigue is often a significant functional problem. While some physicians are strong proponents of fibromyalgia and myofascial pain as distinct disease entities, others believe they are simply variants of idiopathic chronic low-back pain.

**TABLE 25-12** CRITERIA FOR THE DIAGNOSIS OF FIBROMYALGIA

**Major Criteria (required)**
1. Chronic generalized aches, pains, or stiffness (involving at least three musculoskeletal regions for at least three months)
2. Absence of other systemic conditions to account for these symptoms
3. Multiple tender points at characteristic locations (trigger points)

**Minor Criteria**
1. Disturbed sleep
2. Generalized fatigue
3. Subjective swelling or numbness of extremities
4. Pain in neck or shoulders
5. Chronic headache
6. Irritable bowel symptoms

Treatment of fibromyalgia is nonspecific and includes muscle relaxants, heat, stretching, aerobic exercises, and education. Prognosis is generally good but symptoms may persist for a long period. These patients are sometimes unnecessarily subjected to expensive and sometimes invasive diagnostic tests. Fibromyalgia does not by itself result in permanent impairment.

### Metabolic disorders

The most important spinal metabolic disorder is osteoporosis. It most commonly affects women after the

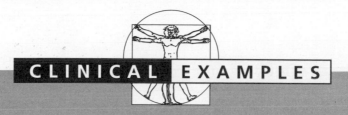

# CLINICAL EXAMPLES

## LUMBAR AND THORACIC SPINE

EDITOR'S NOTE—Please refer to comments made in the Clinical Example in Chapter 24, Cervical Spine.

### EXAMPLE

#### History

A 42-year-old female assembly-line worker is to be evaluated for "low-back sprain/strain." She was first injured five years previously. At that time she was bending, twisting, and lifting when she felt a sudden "popping" in her back. She consulted her physician who made a diagnosis of low-back sprain. She was treated with rest, analgesics, and muscle relaxants, remaining off work for three months. Physical therapy was started at that time, but, dissatisfied with the results, the patient went to a chiropractor. She was treated with spinal manipulations, electrical stimulation of the back, ice packs, and thermal massage, which she felt improved her symptoms.

Since her first injury, she has reinjured her back on three separate occasions. One occurred while she was at work and, as determined after a very careful and detailed history, two occurred in the home setting, both while she was playing badminton with her children. On all these occasions, she consulted her chiropractor, who kept her off work for 6 to 24 weeks while intensive therapy was given.

She continues to have low-back discomfort for an average of three to four hours at a time, five of seven days per week. She awakens two nights out of seven with pain in her back, and she is limited with regard to many activities. She states that she is no longer capable of enjoying sexual intercourse because it increases her back discomfort. She walks into the office grimacing with discomfort. Her gait is stiff, and she holds her body very erect.

#### Physical Examination

No muscle spasm is elicited, although she is tender throughout the back region, especially in the sacroiliac joint areas. Range of motion (ROM) examination reveals the following:

| | |
|---|---|
| T12 inclination angle in extension | 10° |
| Sacral inclination angle in extension | 10° |
| True lumbar extension | 0° |
| Total hip motion (flexion + extension) | 30° |

The straight leg raising test is performed and found to be 50° in each leg. Right lateral flexion is 15° and left lateral flexion 20°.

The deep tendon reflexes in the lower extremities are normal. The sensory examination (pain, light touch, and temperature) in the lower extremity is normal. The motor examination reveals loss of strength in the flexion and extension of the upper and lower aspects of both legs.

#### Test Results

She has never had a CT scan, MRI, or orthopedic consultation. Multiple back x-rays all attest to malalignment and slippage of the vertebral bodies. Two thermograms are reported to be positive.

#### Assessment Process

This individual's problem would not be considered permanent because she is receiving ongoing treatment. In addition, intervening injuries have caused further problems. Evaluation of the initial injury, which occurred five years ago, cannot be accomplished without considering the impact of the three subsequent injuries. Finally, total hip motion is 30° and straight leg raising 50°; therefore, following any edition of the AMA *Guides*, this would be an invalid test because the *Guides* state that "if the tighter SLR angle exceeds the sum of the sacral flexion and extension angles by more than 15°, the lumbosacral flexion test is invalid. The examiner should either repeat the test or disallow impairment for lumbosacral spine flexion or extension" (p. 127).* Regardless of these issues, an evaluation has been requested, a situation frequently found in practice.

*All *sections* and *tables* referred to in this discussion are found in AMA *Guides to the evaluation of permanent impairment*, ed 4, Chapter 3—The Musculoskeletal System, American Medical Association, Chicago, 1993.

*Continued.*

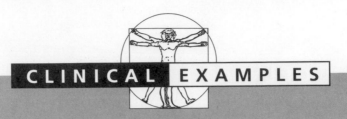

# CLINICAL EXAMPLES

## LUMBAR AND THORACIC SPINE—cont'd

Assuming that a real pathologic condition is present, assuming that this is a permanent problem, assuming that it is static and well-stabilized, and assuming that the test is valid, assessment using the ROM model could be performed.

Sacral (hip) flexion angle is 20°, so, using Table 81, the sacral (hip) flexion angle category of 0-29 is used. Three true lumbar spine flexion angles are provided: 0, 15, and 30+°; the true lumbar flexion of 20° falls between 15 and 30+. Based on all of this, 7% whole person impairment (WPI) for flexion is found. The true lumbar spine extension is 0°. Therefore a 7% WPI for extension is chosen. Right lateral flexion is 15°, which, using Table 82, yields a 2% WPI. Left lateral flexion is 20°, yielding a 1% WPI. The total impairment caused by ROM abnormalities of the lumbar spine is 17% (7% combined with 7% combined with 2% combined with 1%).

Nothing has been added for impairment based on the specific spine disorder, as exemplified in Table 75, because of the lack of radiographic confirmation. Nothing is added for diminished muscle strength because this is believed to reflect back pathology and the rest of the neurologic examination is normal.

**Evaluation**

This case exemplifies the problems associated with the ROM or functional model, showing why the diagnosis-related estimates (DRE) model was developed. The DRE model concentrates on the historical symptoms, physical examination, radiographic abnormalities, and results of previous surgeries. Using Tables 70 to 72, this individual would most likely be classified in Category I or II. Radiographs help differentiate between these two. A 0% to 5% WPI would be considered appropriate for this particular individual based on the DRE model. Because this is the preferred method of examination, this value would be reported, rather than the 17% found with the ROM evaluation.

*Stephen L. Demeter*

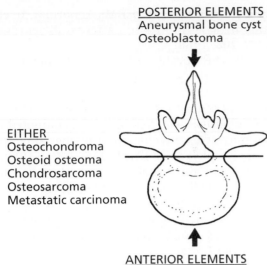

POSTERIOR ELEMENTS
Aneurysmal bone cyst
Osteoblastoma

EITHER
Osteochondroma
Osteoid osteoma
Chondrosarcoma
Osteosarcoma
Metastatic carcinoma

ANTERIOR ELEMENTS
Round cell tumors
   Ewing's
   Multiple myeloma
   Reticulum cell sarcoma
Hemangioma
Giant cell tumor
Eosinophilic granuloma
Hemangioendothelioma
Chordoma

**FIGURE 25-11**    Frequent location of spinal tumors. (After Andersson GBJ, McNeill TW: *Lumbar spine syndromes: evaluation and treatment*, Vienna, 1989, Springer-Verlag.)

age of 50. Other risk factors include northern European descent, small stature, early menopause, positive family history on the female side, smoking, and chronic treatment with corticosteroids. The major consequence of osteoporosis is weakening of the bone, which makes the individual more susceptible to compression fractures. Awareness of this problem in older individuals is important and it may be necessary to reduce the affected individual's lifting and bending requirements.

## Neoplasms

Tumors can involve osseous or neural structures, producing pain or neurologic dysfunction. They are rare in patients before age 50. The most common tumors are the result of metastatic spread from some other primary site, most commonly breast cancer in the female, prostatic cancer in the male, and lung, kidney, and thyroid cancer in both sexes (Fig. 25-11). Multiple myeloma is the most common primary malignant bone tumor, but a variety of other, rarer primary bone or neural tumors may cause low-back pain or sciatica. Bony malignant tumors often present with the insidious onset of pain, although acute pain may occur if structural weakening causes a compression fracture. The characteristic pain complaint is night pain, awakening the patient. The spinal radio-

graph is often diagnostic, but early in the development of a tumor, bone scan, CT scan, or MRI may be required for definitive diagnosis.

## SUMMARY

The lumbar spine is susceptible to a variety of pathologic conditions, but the majority of patients do not have a definable pathoanatomic causation for their pain, if strict diagnostic criteria are used. The Quebec Classification overcomes the reliance on the more classic, pathoanatomic classification systems and has the important attributes that not only is the pain pattern characterized, but the duration and effect on work status are incorporated. These factors are more important in defining treatment and employability than is the actual diagnosis in the majority of patients. However, the examiner must remember that there is a smaller subgroup of patients who have a clear diagnosis for their symptoms, which is more likely when sciatica or claudication accompany the complaint. The patient's complaint of pain must be carefully evaluated and may give important clues to the causation. Because radiographic abnormalities are so common in asymptomatic individuals, the most important lesson in clinical diagnosis is to correlate the radiographic studies with the patient's clinical complaint, rather than define or rate impairment solely upon a radiographic diagnosis of "spinal degeneration or disk degeneration."

*ACKNOWLEDGEMENT*

Parts of this chaper are based on previously published material by the authors, which appeared in Pope MH, Andersson GBJ, Frymoyer JW et al: *Occupational Low Back Pain: Prevention, Diagnosis and Treatment*, St. Louis, 1991, Mosby–Year Book.

## References

1. Aiello I, Serra G, Tugnoli V, et al: Electrophysiological findings in patients with lumbar prolapse. *Electromyogr Clin Neurophysiol* 24(4):313-20, May 1984.
2. American Medical Association: *Guides to the evaluation of permanent impairment*, ed 4, Chicago, 1993.
3. Andersson GBJ, Deyo RA: Sensitivity, specificity, and predictive value: a general issue in screening for disease and in the interpretation of diagnostic studies in spinal disorders. In Frymoyer JF, editor: *The adult spine*, ed 2, in press.
4. Andersson GBJ, McNeill TW: *Lumbar spinal stenosis*, St. Louis, 1992, Mosby–Year Book.
5. Andersson GBJ, McNeill TW: *Lumbar spine syndromes: evaluation and treatment*, Vienna, 1989, Springer-Verlag.

6. Andersson GBJ, Svensson H-O, Oden A: The intensity of work recovery in low-back pain. *Spine* 8:880-884, 1983.

7. Arnoldi CC, Brodsky AE, Cauchoix J, et al: Lumbar spinal stenosis and nerve root entrapment syndromes: definition and classification. *Clin Orthop* 115:4, 1976.

8. Bergquist-Ullman M, Larsson U: Acute low back pain in industry. *Acta Orthop Scand (suppl)* 170:1, 1977.

9. Boden S, Davis DO, Dina TS, et al: Abnormal magnetic resonance scans of the lumbar spine in asymptomatic subjects. *J Bone Joint Surg (Am)* 72(3):403-408, 1990.

10. Crock HV: Internal disc disruption: a challenge to disc prolapse fifty years on. *Spine* 11:650, 1986.

11. Denis F: The three-column spine and its significance in the classification of acute thoraco-lumbar spinal injuries. *Spine* 8:817, 1983.

12. Deyo RA, Diehl AK: Lumbar spine films in primary care: current use and effects of selective ordering criteria. *J Gen Intern Med* 1(1):20-25, Jan-Feb, 1986.

13. Deyo RA, Rainville J, Dent DL: What can the history and physical examination tell us about low-back pain? *JAMA* 268(6): 760-765, Aug 12, 1992.

14. Dupuis PR, Yong-Hing K, Cassidy JD, et al: Radiologic diagnosis of degenerative lumbar spinal instability. *Spine* 10:262, 1985

15. Eyre D, Buckwalter J, et al: The intervertebral disk: Part B—Basic science perspective. In Frymoyer JW, Gordon SL, editors: *New perspectives on low-back pain.* American Academy of Orthopaedic Surgeons, Park Ridge, Ill., pp. 147-207, 1989.

16. Fredrickson BE, Baker D, McHolick WJ, et al: The natural history of spondylolysis and spondylolisthesis. *J Bone Joint Surg* 66A:699, 1984.

17. Friberg O: Lumbar instability: a dynamic approach by traction-compression radiography. *Spine* 12:119, 1987.

18. Frymoyer JW: Back pain and sciatica. *N Engl J Med* 318:291, 1988.

19. Frymoyer JW, Selby DK: Segmental instability: rationale for treatment. *Spine* 10:280, 1985.

20. Hakelius A, Hindmarsh J: The significance of neurological signs and myelographic findings in the diagnosis of lumbar root compression, *Acta Orthop Scand* 43:239, 1972.

21. Hirsch C, Inglemark B-E, Miller M: The anatomical basis for low back pain: studies on the presence of sensory nerve endings in ligamentous, capsular and intervertebral disc structures in the human lumbar spine. *Acta Orthop Scand* 33:1, 1963.

22. Hitselberger WE, Witten RM: Abnormal myelograms in asymptomatic patients. *J Neurosurg* 28:204-208, 1968.

23. Holt EP: The question of lumbar discography. *J Bone Joint Surg (Am)* 50(4):720-6, June 1968.

24. Jackson RP, Cain JE, Jacobs RR, et al: The neuroradiographic diagnosis of lumbar herniated nucleus pulposus: I—A comparison of computed tomography (CT), myelography discography, and CT-discography. *Spine* 14(12):1356-1360, 1989.

25. Jackson RP, Cain JE, Jacobs RR, et al: Neuroradiographic diagnosis of lumbar herniated nucleus pulposus: II—A comparison of computed tomography (CT), myelography, CT-myelography, and magnetic resonance imaging. *Spine* 14(12):1362-1367, 1989.

26. Jackson RP, Jacobs RR, Montesano PX: Facet joint injection in low-back pain, a prospective statistical study. *Spine* 13:966, 1988.

27. Jensen MC, Brant-Zawdzki MN, Obuchowski N et al: Magnetic resonance imaging of the lumbar spine in people without back pain. *N Engl J Med* 331:69-73, 1994.

28. Keefe FJ, Beckham JC, Fillingim RB: The psychology of chronic back pain. In Frymoyer JW, editor: *The adult spine: principles and practice.* New York, 1991, Raven Press, pp 185-197.

29. Kellgren JH: The anatomical source of back pain. *Rheumatol Rehabil* 16:3, 1977.

30. Yong-Hing K, Kirkaldy-Willis WH: The pathophysiology of degenerative disease of the lumbar spine. *Orthop Clin North Am* 14:491, 1983.

31. Kent DL, Haynor DR, Larson EB, et al: Diagnosis of lumbar spinal stenosis in adults: a meta-analysis of the accuracy of CT, MR, and myelography. *Am J Roentgenol* 158:1135-1144, May 1992.

32. Kirkaldy-Willis WH, Farfan HF: Instability of the lumbar spine. *Clin Orthop* 165:110, 1982.

33. Knutsson F: The instability associated with disk degeneration in the lumbar spine. *Acta Radiol* 25:593, 1944.

34. Kostuik JP, Harrington I, Alexander D, et al: Cauda equina syndrome and lumbar disc herniation. *J Bone Joint Surg* 68A:386, 1986.

35. Lewis T, Kellgren JH: Observations relating to referred pain, visceromotor reflexes, and other associated phenomena. *Clin Sci* 4:47, 1939.

36. Macnab I: The traction spur: an indicator of segmental instability. *J Bone Joint Surg* 53A:663, 1971.

37. McCall IW, Park WM, O'Brien JP: Induced pain referral from posterior lumbar elements in normal subjects. *Spine* 4:441. 1979.

38. Mooney V, Robertson J: The facet syndrome. *Clin Orthop* 115:149, 1976.

39. Nachemson AL, Andersson GBJ: Classification of low-back pain. *Scand J Work Environ Health* 8:134, 1982.

40. Pope MH, Andersson GBJ, Frymoyer JW, et al: *Occupational low-back pain.* St. Louis, 1991, Mosby–Year Book.

41. Scham SM, Taylor TKF: Tension signs in lumbar disc prolapse. *Clin Orthop* 75:195, 1971.

42. Shaffer W, Spratt K, Weinstein J, et al: The consistency and accuracy of roentgenograms for measuring sagittal translation in the lumbar vertebral motion segment. *Spine* 15:741-750, 1990.

43. Spangfort EV: The lumbar disc herniation: a computer aided analysis of 2504 operations. *Acta Orthop Scand (Suppl)* 142:1, 1972.

44. Spitzer WO, LeBlanc FE, Dupuis M, et al: Scientific approach to the assessment and management of activity-related spinal disorders: a monograph for clinicians. Report of the Quebec Task Force on Spinal Disorders. *Spine* 12(Suppl 7):S1-S59, 1987.

45. Troup JDG, Martin JW, Lloyd DCEF: Back pain in industry: a prospective survey. *Spine* 6:61, 1981.

46. Valkenburg HA, Haanen HCM: The epidemiology of low-back pain. In White AA, Gordon SL, editors: *American Academy of Orthopaedic Surgeons symposium on idiopathic low-back pain.* St. Louis, 1982, CV Mosby.

47. Waddell G, McCulloch JA, Kummel E, et al: Nonorganic physical signs in low-back pain. *Spine* 5:117, 1979.

48. Waddell G, Bircher M, Finlayson D, et al: Symptoms and signs: physical disease or illness behavior? *Br Med J* 289:739, 1984.

49. Walsh TR, Weinstein JN, Spratt KF, et al: Lumbar discography in normal subjects: a controlled, prospective study. *J Bone Joint Surg (Am)* 72(7):1081-1088, Aug. 1990.

50. Wiesel SW, Tsourmas N, Feffer HL, et al: A study of computer-assisted tomography: I—The incidence of positive CAT scans in an asymptomatic group of patients. *Spine* 9(6):549-51, Sept. 1984.

51. Wiltse LL, Newman PH, Macnab I: Classification of spondylolysis and spondylolisthesis. *Clin Orthop* 117:23, 1976.

52. Work Cover Guidelines for the management of back-injured employees. Adelaide, South Australia, Work Cover Corporation. 1993.

# SECTION B
# Internal Medicine Assessment

# DISABILITY ISSUES IN INTERNAL MEDICINE EVALUATIONS

*Stephen L. Demeter*

## PHYSIOLOGIC FACTORS IN DETERMINING DISABILITY

Internal medicine is the branch of medicine that deals with the diagnosis and treatment of diseases and disorders of the internal structures of the human body. Disparate organ systems are involved, each having its own peculiar anatomy and physiologic function. They share a purpose—maintenance of the supporting systems vital to the body's function. The broad categories of functions are energy substrate acquisition, waste product removal, and protection from the external environment. In addition, these organ systems interact to regulate each other. For example, the primary functions of the pulmonary system are to acquire oxygen and release carbon dioxide (the energy substrate and the waste product). No conversion is necessary in terms of this energy substrate. The pulmonary system also assists the kidneys in regulating pH balance and protects against potentially harmful substances in the inhaled air (for example, particulates, microorganisms, or toxic gases) via mechanical, cellular, and humoral defense mechanisms. The digestive system is another example. Its principal functions are energy substrate acquisition, substrate conversion, and waste elimination. However, the digestive system also provides environmental protection via cellular and mechanical defense mechanisms throughout the gastrointestinal tract. Even the skin functions in ways other than environmental protection by regulating waste heat and fluid balance as well as by manufacturing vitamin D.

Not all of the functions of the internal organs fit neatly into the conceptual framework just described. For example, the reproductive system functions in species continuation as well as pleasure, neither of which conform to the functions listed for internal organs.

Deviation from normal physiological function defines impairment as it affects internal medicine. Deviations sufficient to create abnormalities in energy substrate acquisition, substrate conversion, waste elimination, regulation or protective functions can potentially produce a disability. For example, how do the multiple fistulas of Crohn's disease alter the physiological function of the gastrointestinal tract? Is there a problem with energy substrate acquisition or conversion (for example, malabsorption leading to diarrhea resulting in electrolyte and protein depletion resulting in weight loss?) or protection from the environment (repeated infection?). Does a person with a ureterosigmoidostomy (for urinary diversion after bladder removal from cancer) have a physiological alteration? Does a person with a pneumonectomy have impairment? Physiological alterations are the key to understanding all system impairments.

The following chapters will describe the physiological basis for impairment specific to internal medicine concerns. The functions of each organ system and the tests used to evaluate these functions are mentioned only in passing; the reader is referred to medical and physiology textbooks. It is assumed that the reader possesses sufficient background so that derangements of physiological function need not be explained. The tests detailed are those used by the various rating systems to determine impairment.

Two chapters focus more specifically on tests. Pulmonary function testing is described in detail because the pulmonary system is frequently involved in impairments evaluated by internal medicine specialists and because this parameter, while frequently evaluated, remains poorly understood.

The other chapter detailing a discrete test (Chapter 29) focuses on the cardiopulmonary exercise stress test. This test represents an important assessment currently and potentially will grow in importance. In evaluating disability, one defines the capability, from a physiological standpoint, of an individual to perform sustained work. The cardiopulmonary stress test measures this ability to work by testing the soundness of the combined pulmonary-cardiac-vascular systems, as well as the blood, as energy substrates are acquired and carried to the tissues, and wastes are eliminated.

Looking at the broad concepts of physiological function alterations seen in internal medicine practice, one would hope for a test that addresses the body as a whole, not merely a collection of organ systems. This field is too large, complex, and diverse for any one test to assume that role. However, the cardiopulmonary stress test does provide evidence of ability to work by assessing the physiologic functions of various organ systems. Currently, the test is performed on a treadmill or bicycle and measures the person's peak capabilities in terms of watts or metabolic equivalents (mets). By extrapolation, these measurements are fitted to job requirements and an estimate of sustained ability is derived by multiplying the peak ability by 40%. For example, if a person is capable of performing to 10 mets before the anaerobic threshold is achieved (assuming a normal level is 12 mets for an individual of that age), then the individual is assumed to be able to sustain work for 8 hours at 4 mets. If the job in question is that of a logger and requires 8 mets of sustained capacity, then the individual is disabled for that particular job.

For this test to become more universally applicable, research is required to determine what is normal and what a particular job requires. In addition, the test would ideally be performed under a real or simulated job situation, similar to the functional capacity assessment performed by orthopedists. Lastly, this type of test would be ideal, in a manual labor occupation, to test an individual's fitness for duty, return to work, or capacity to perform the essential job tasks (under the Americans with Disabilities Act) (see Chapters 17, 50, and 51).

## MOTIVATIONAL FACTORS

### Effects on Testing

Motivation can exert a powerful influence on the level of work one can perform. Tests to evaluate impairment are ideally sufficiently sensitive so that issues of motivation are controlled and physiological capacities are accurately assessed. Tests of serum blood urea nitrogen, creatinine measurements, and the free thyroxine index are largely objective. However, bulimia may produce abnormalities in serum albumin content, or patients with alcoholic hepatitis who "binge" before liver function testing may be able to create "motivational" abnormalities even in blood tests.

It is the examining physician's responsibility to assess as accurately as possible the health status of the examinee. Often the results of the history, physical, and laboratory tests must be balanced against the physician's clinical experience to arrive at an accurate evaluation.

### Effects on Health Choices

Information concerning healthy behaviors such as refraining from smoking, avoiding alcohol excess, watching caloric intake, exercising regularly, consulting a physician regularly, and avoiding diets rich in saturated fats abounds. Motivation clearly plays a vital role in how avidly we adopt these health-seeking behaviors. It is possible that the individual may adopt disease-seeking behaviors, which will profoundly influence or even constitute the sole factor in producing impairment and possibly disability. Such behaviors can produce impairment or influence assessment. For example, among Black Lung Act awardees, cigarette smoking has been designated "the primary variable associated with pulmonary impairment severe enough to warrant a financial award under present legislation."[1] How many cases of impairment due to hepatitis or cirrhosis result from occupational or environmental exposures and how many from alcohol excess? Will the pulmonary testing of a smoker be affected? The answers are obvious.

Another issue involves medications. Is a patient following the prescribed dosage? Is he or she taking the medication at all? Clearly, motivational factors underpin, first, seeking out a physician regarding alterations in health, and, second, following the recommendations given by that physician.

## SUMMARY

Each of these issues must be addressed in an impairment and disability evaluation. Further information is given in the following chapters as specific systems are evaluated.

### Reference

1. U.S. Department of Health and Human Services. *Disability evaluation under Social Security*, U.S. Government Printing Office, 1992.

# CHAPTER 27

## PULMONARY FUNCTION TESTING

*Stephen L. Demeter*
*Edward M. Corsasco*
*Timothy Wolfe*

In the investigation of the pulmonary system as part of an impairment evaluation leading to a disability rating, greater reliance is given to pulmonary function tests than on the history and physical examination. Reasons for this include the following:

1. These tests provide quantifiable discriminations between degrees of impairment.
2. Pulmonary function tests are reliable and historically valid.
3. Compared to the history and physical examination, these tests are generally more accurate, more reliable, and more readily reproduced.

Specific to impairment evaluation, the goal of pulmonary function testing is to determine the degree of an impairment or deviation from normal in a person with a breathing disorder. The various rating systems specify different tests and different endpoints that reflect the function of that particular system. In addition, the American Thoracic Society has published criteria for the machine used,[1] the selection of reference values for normal,[3] testing for asthma,[3,10] tests of diffusing capacity,[2] use of computers,[15] quality assurance in the pulmonary function laboratory,[16] and persons performing the test.[17,18,20] In addition, NIOSH provides both guidelines and training seminars for the personnel who provide these tests.[20]

Tests of lung function address lung volumes, expiratory flow rates, and gas exchange. In impairment evaluations, tests of lung volumes are rarely used, but these measurements do provide important background information regarding disease states and abnormalities found when other areas are tested. Impairment rating systems emphasize tests of flow rates and gas exchange. Flow rates relate to the ability to breathe and, therefore, to perform work on a sustained basis; they are also used for asthma testing. Gas exchange testing includes the diffusing capacity and arterial blood gas levels, culminating in the cardiopulmonary exercise stress test (see Chapter 28), which combines the elements of breathing ability and gas exchange both in the lungs and in the various organs of the body.

Many variables can influence pulmonary function testing, including the following: height, age, weight, sex, race, posture, altitude at which the test is done, the ambient environment on the day of testing, presence of disease, presence of training (for example, a wind instrument player), presence of disease, recent exposure to inhaled irritants, diurnal rhythms (including time of day or year or time in menstrual cycle for women), motivation, choice of "normal" values, and prior testing.[4,9]

### TESTS OF FLOW RATES

A flow-volume loop is the standard measurement performed in most pulmonary function laboratories. It measures flow (liters per second) versus volume and requires a computer for the resulting calculations. These measurements, once limited to expensive and comprehensive laboratories, are now done with simpler machines and are performed frequently in private offices.

The flow-volume loop (Fig. 27-1) graphically represents flow rates, makes the peak expiratory flow easily discerned, and produces a shape that yields important information (see Fig. 27-2, in which the erratic flow-volume loops clearly convey information regarding consistency of effort).

Spirometers can also produce a volume-time curve from which forced vital capacity is measured and various flow rates calculated. Volume-time curves are required by the Social Security Administration (SSA) for pulmonary function testing.

The classic flow rates measured include the forced expiratory volume in one second ($FEV_1$), which is the total volume exhaled in the first second of exhala-

Name: 000                          ID:                    08-03-1994      12:32:48
Age:  44      Height: 66.0 in.      Sex: M      Ethnic: C      Normal: Knudson/IMTS
Medications:
**Test** #1 lasted 5.4 s
Last calibration: 08-03-1994

| Expiratory | Actual | Pred. | %Pred. | Inspiratory | | |
|---|---|---|---|---|---|---|
| FVC | 4.19 L | 4.47 L | 93.8% | IVC | 4.17 L | 4.17 L |
| $FEV_{0.5}$ | 3.08 L | 2.90 L | 106.1% | $FIV_1$ | 3.78 L | 3.78 L |
| $FEV_1$ | 3.68 L | 3.68 L | 100.1% | PIF | 4.34 L/s | |
| $FEV_3$ | 4.19 L | 4.27 L | 98.2% | FIF 50% | 3.84 L/s | |
| $FEV_{0.5}/FVC$ | 73.5% | 65.0% | 113.1% | $FEF_{50}/FEF_{50}$ | 1.49 | |
| $FEV_1/FVC$ | 87.9% | 82.4% | 106.7% | | | |
| $FEV_3/FVC$ | 100.0% | 95.5% | 104.7% | | Analysis | |
| | | | | | Test is within | |
| PEF | 13.05 L/s | 8.24 L/s | 158.3% | | NORMAL limits | |
| FEF 25-75% | 4.65 L/s | 3.59 L/s | 129.5% | | | |
| FEF 75-85% | 1.40 L/s | 1.06 L/s | 132.2% | | Current BEST test | |
| FEF 50% | 5.73 L/s | 4.44 L/s | 128.9% | | | |
| FEF 75% | 1.88 L/s | 1.70 L/s | 110.6% | | | |
| $FEF_{0.2-1.2}$ | 12.50 L/s | 7.14 L/s | 175.2% | | | |

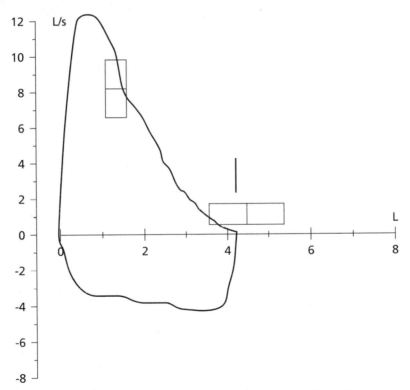

**FIGURE 27-1**    Flow volume loop with subdivisions. See text for explanation. Note the calibrations made for age, height, sex, and race. Also, note the date of the last calibration of the spirometer.

tion; the forced expiratory flow between 200 and 1200 cc ($FEF_{200-1200}$), which reflects the rate of airflow between the points on the volume axis representing the first 200 cc and the next 1 L of air exhaled; and the forced expiratory flow between 25% and 75% of the total exhaled volume ($FEF_{25-75}$, see Fig. 27-1).

## $FEV_1$

A low $FEV_1$ value can result from airway obstruction, air trapping, poor effort, or restrictive lung discases. Since the $FEV_1$ actually represents a volume (and not a flow rate), any disease that seriously impairs the total volume will have a parallel change in the $FEV_1$.

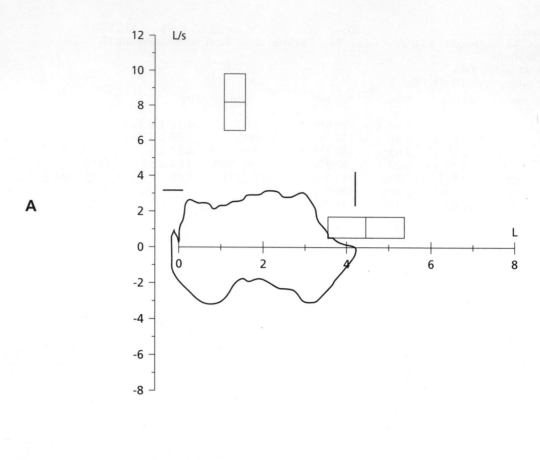

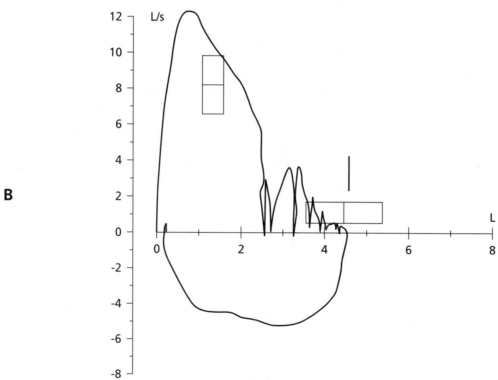

**FIGURE 27-2**    Examples of poor flow-volume curves. **A,** Poor effort resulting in a low peak flow. **B,** Inconsistent effort resulting in an erratic curve.

## FEV₁/FVC

The $FEV_1/FVC$ is believed to be a more sensitive measurement of airflow than the $FEV_1$ alone in determining the presence of true obstructive phenomena. Generally the $FEV_1/FVC$ is about 75% to 80%, meaning that the normal individual exhales 75% to 80% of the total exhaled volume in the first second when done as a forceful maneuver. If the FEV is 4.0 L, then the $FEV_1$ is expected to be approximately 3.0 L. If the forced vital capacity (FVC) diminishes (for whatever reason), then the $FEV_1$ must also decrease.

## FEF₂₅₋₇₅

The $FEF_{25-75}$ (also termed the *mid-maximal expiratory flow* [MMEF]) is considered an excellent test of small airway flow rates. In small airflow obstruction (the earliest physiological abnormality in smokers who are developing emphysema), it is abnormal (decreased).

## Other Flow Rate Tests

### Peak expiratory flow

The peak expiratory flow (PEF) represents the greatest flow rate achievable during a forceful exhalation, thus it is highly effort-dependent. In contrast, small airflow rates, such as the $FEF_{25-75}$, are considered effort-independent. The PEF represents the highest point on the flow-volume curve.

The four major differential diagnoses with a decreased PEF are (1) moderate or severe airflow obstruction, (2) neuromuscular disease, (3) poor effort, and (4) upper airway obstruction (for example, tracheal stenosis, endobronchial foreign bodies or tumors, or laryngeal obstructions). The PEF is not used as a criterion of impairment; it is a factor in asthma testing, where variable amounts of airflow obstruction can be found when measured over time. This simple test can provide evidence for obstructive phenomena occurring at variable times, providing the effects of variable effort are eliminated.

MVV test lasted 12.2 s at 153 breaths/min

MVV = 195 L/min or 154% of predicted 126 L/min

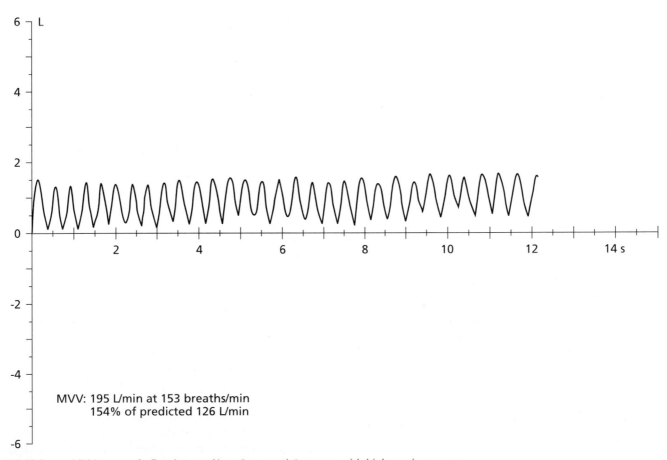

MVV: 195 L/min at 153 breaths/min
154% of predicted 126 L/min

**FIGURE 27-3**    MVV curves. **A,** Good curve. Note "sawtooth" pattern with high respiratory rate.

*Continued.*

MVV test lasted 12.0 s at 35 breaths/min

MVV = 106 L/min or 84% of predicted 126 L/min

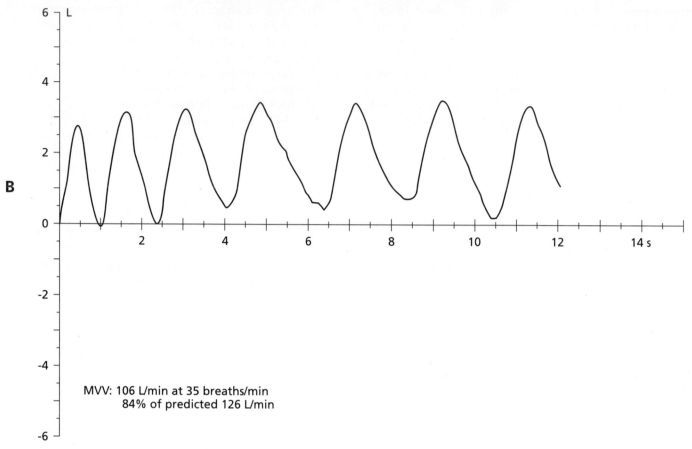

FIGURE 27-3, cont'd.    B, Unacceptable curve. Note good "sawtooth" but low rate.

### Maximum voluntary ventilation

The maximum voluntary ventilation (MVV) is a special test measuring the individual's maximal ability to breathe in and out during a 60-second period. The test is conducted over 12 to 15 seconds and extrapolated to a full 60-second period. The waveforms during a "good" test are uniform and give a classic "sawtooth" appearance (Fig. 27-3).

Presently, this test is applied during cardiopulmonary exercise testing to determine breathing reserve (see Chapter 28) and for Social Security disability determinations.

### Application in Impairment Evaluations

For impairment evaluations, the only flow rate determinations considered in any of the rating systems are the $FEV_1$, the $FEV_1/FVC$, and the $FEF_{25-75}$. In special circumstances the PEF and MVV may be mea-sured. These values are all easily derived from volume-time curves.

### TESTS OF GAS EXCHANGE

The primary function of the lungs is gas exchange, specifically oxygen acquisition and carbon dioxide release. The one alveolus-one capillary model shown in Figure 27-4 illustrates the basic elements necessary for gas exchange: an intact airway, a functional alveolus, a normal interstitial compartment, a normal capillary, and hemoglobin. If any of these elements are abnormal or missing, gas exchange will be abnormal. However, the lungs are not made up of a single alveolus/single capillary, but many such units, about 350 million. Because many units do not participate in respiration on a normal basis, there exists a large reserve under resting conditions. Thus tests of gas ex-

MVV test lasted 12.0 s at 60 breaths/min

MVV = 106 L/min or 84% of predicted 126 L/min

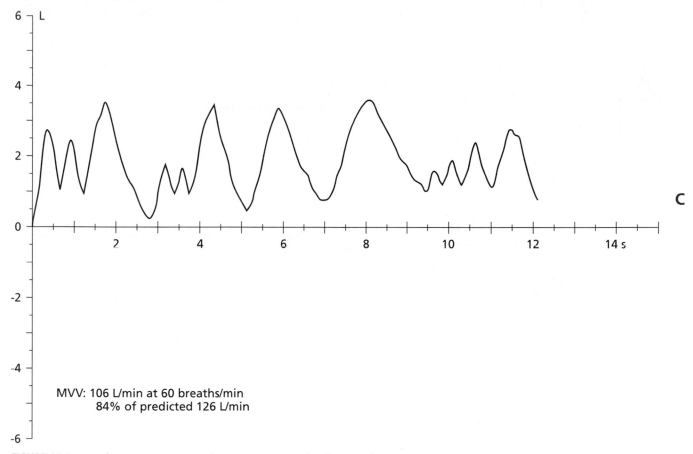

MVV: 106 L/min at 60 breaths/min
      84% of predicted 126 L/min

**FIGURE 27-3, cont'd.    C,** Unacceptable curve. Note erratic effort, moderate rate.

change under resting conditions rarely show abnormalities until severe disease is present. Diseases of the airways, alveoli, interstitium, or blood supply only become detectable if they are severe or are tested during exercise. (Exercise testing is discussed in Chapter 28.)

The gas exchange tests to be discussed here are the diffusing capacity and arterial blood gases.

### Diffusing Capacity

The diffusing capacity ($D_{LCO}$) measures gas transfer from the alveolus to the capillary. Carbon monoxide (CO) represents the best gas for testing the diffusing capacity because it is readily diffusible, is normally not present either in the inhaled air or in the blood, and readily attaches to the hemoglobin molecule so that as soon as it transfers across the membrane, it is immediately removed, thereby maintaining a zero

level in the blood presented to the alveolar-capillary interface. Any existing CO in the blood creates problems with diffusion measurements (as is seen in cigarette smokers).

Figure 27-5 serves as an example of how the $D_{LCO}$ is measured. The reservoir for inhaled air contains 100 molecules of CO. All molecules are drawn into the lungs, and the number of molecules in the exhaled air are counted. If only 80 are present, the amount of residual air in the lungs would be expected to contain 10 molecules (after complete mixing of the gases). The 10 missing molecules are assumed to diffuse across the alveolar-capillary membrane, yielding a $D_{LCO}$ of 10%. If the blood to the alveoli already contains CO, extra CO is found in the exhaled air as a result of back-diffusion (blood to alveolus to airway). This would result in a drop in the measured $D_{LCO}$.

Factors influencing the $D_{LCO}$ include elevated lev-

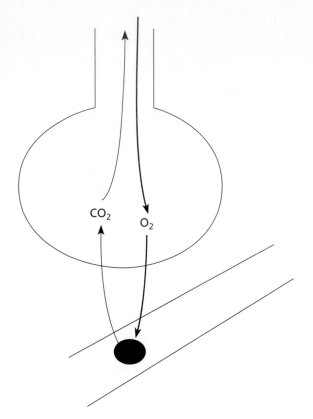

**FIGURE 27-4** One alveolus/one capillary model.

els of carbon monoxide pre-existent in the blood (HgCO), reduced hemoglobin content, and abnormal lung volumes. These confounding factors can be addressed during complete pulmonary function testing in sophisticated laboratories. It should be noted that the AMA *Guides* recommend that "the patient should be instructed not to smoke for at least 8 hours before the test" (p. 161).[13]

### Arterial Blood Gas Levels

Arterial blood gas levels (ABGs) are rarely used alone in impairment evaluations for determination of disability. The $FEV_1$ is preferred in the AMA *Guides;*[13] the Social Security System uses ABGs, but it cites three important qualifiers with respect to the oxygen level:

1. The altitude must be specified. Since the amount of oxygen presented to the alveolus is a function of the number of oxygen molecules in the air (the partial pressure of oxygen [$Po_2$]) and, since this is a function of altitude, or barometric pressure, the expected $Pao_2$ should be adjusted for altitude.
2. The arterial partial pressure of carbon dioxide ($Paco_2$) must be known. Hyperventilation increases $Pao_2$.

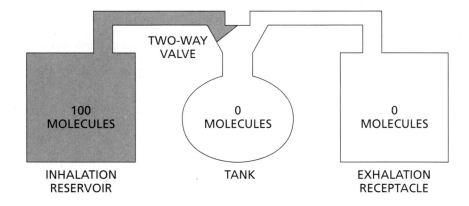

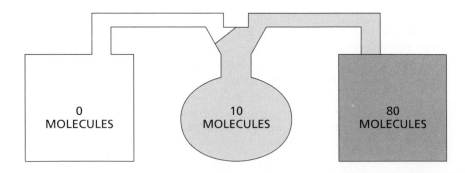

**FIGURE 27-5** Gas diffusion model.

3. The $Pao_2$ must be tested after exercise, not in the resting state. This depicts the condition of the lungs more accurately.

In addition, the Social Security System provides tables of expected $Pao_2$ levels in obese individuals. The Black Lung Benefits Law uses the $Pao_2/Paco_2$ levels at rest or at exercise.[12]

## LUNG VOLUMES

*Total lung capacity* (TLC) is defined as the total amount of air the lung can hold at the end of a full inhalation (Fig. 27-6). TLC can be considered to comprise the "respirable" air of the lung as well as the "structural" air (some air must remain within the lungs, or the work of breathing would become excessive, so that the body would spend a disproportionate amount of its energy simply breathing). This volume of air remaining in the lungs is the *residual volume* (RV). The difference between the TLC and the RV is called the *vital capacity* (VC).

Other lung volumes are expressed as follows:
1. Tidal volume (TV): the volume of a normal resting breath.
2. Functional residual capacity (FRC): FRC = ERV + RV. (ERV = expiratory reserve volume)
3. Inspiratory capacity (IC): IC = TLC − FRC.
4. Inspiratory reserve volume (IRV): IRV = TLC − (FRC + TV).

Except for TV, these are rarely used in impairment evaluations. TV is usually small (approximately 250 to 350 cc). During exercise, however, it increases as the demands for oxygen acquisition and carbon dioxide removal increase.

## RV

The RV reflects the size of the lungs, which itself reflects the size of the body. Prediction formulas for the RV include the variables of height, sex, age, and race.

If the size of the alveoli could increase, the RV would increase. While this does not happen, it is mimicked by four conditions: aging, emphysema, air trapping, and cysts or blebs. During the aging process, the integrity of the elastic tissue of the lung diminishes. In emphysema, lung tissue is destroyed. Thus, where alveoli, respiratory bronchioles, and connecting tissue surrounding these alveoli once existed, a large "mega-alveolus" exists. In air-trapping states (such as mucous plugs or asthma), the air is not allowed to escape, so the individual cannot exhale completely. Therefore the air at the end of a forceful exhalation (the definition of RV) increases. Finally air-occupying abnormalities such as cysts, blebs, or bronchopleural fistulas can increase the RV by a similar mechanism.

## VC

The VC may be measured either as a long, slow breath from TLC to RV (also called the *slow vital capacity* [SVC]) or as a quick, forceful breath from TLC to RV (known as *forced vital capacity* [FVC]). Diseases causing air trapping can cause a discrepancy between these two values, and the FVC is the value cited in the various rating systems of pulmonary impairment. The advantages of FVCs are ease of measurement, low cost, and reproducibility of findings. Depending on the skill of the technician, spirometric machines produce accurate and reproducible FVCs using a quick test, usually less than 3 to 5 minutes, and costing less than $45.

The four major differential diagnoses of a low FVC are emphysema, interstitial lung disease, severe airflow obstruction with or without air trapping, and poor effort. Emphysema can decrease the FVC by producing a reciprocal increase in the RV (Fig. 27-7). Restrictive or interstitial lung diseases decreases the air-occupying spaces of the lungs and replace or collapse them by increasing the solid tissue of the lungs with inflammatory cells, collagen, or tumor cells. Obliteration or filling of the air spaces can cause a similar physiologic change and occurs in pneumonias, pulmonary edema, and alveolar proteinosis, among other diseases. If air trapping exists (for example, involving a mucous plug or an endobronchial tumor), less total air is expelled during a complete

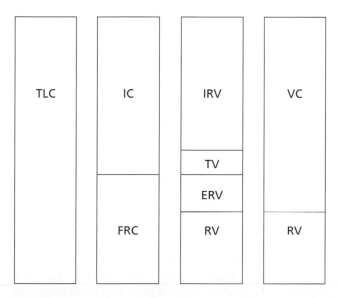

**FIGURE 27-6**    Lung compartments.

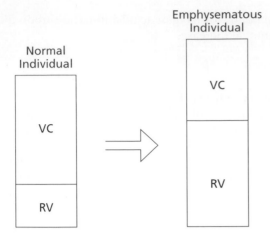

**FIGURE 27-7**     Changes with emphysema.

exhalation. Severe airway obstructive states also diminish total exhaled volume. Finally, poor effort (either voluntarily or nonvoluntarily as in a patient with a fractured rib or neuromuscular disorder) diminishes the FVC. Repeated testing helps discriminate between these two conditions; the individual giving less than optimal effort voluntarily will have erratic flow-volume loops and variable volumes in the FVC. The individual with nonvoluntary, incomplete effort-induced reductions in the FVC often has characteristic flow-volume loops and a relatively constant volume of air.

### Application in Impairment Evaluations

As shown in Figure 27-6, if the TLC remains constant, a reciprocal relationship exists between the RV and the VC. Disease states increasing the RV diminish the VC. This is a major reason why the VC is an integral component of many rating systems. In addition, the VC is much easier and cheaper to obtain than the RV and the TLC. Individuals with severe emphysema can be adequately assessed using a relatively simple test.

Disease states such as emphysema often increase the TLC (Fig. 27-7), as can be seen in the "barrel-chest" of emphysema patients or the "low diaphragms" on chest x-rays of patients with emphysema or status asthmaticus (an example of air trapping). Emphysematous and air-trapping diseases often have co-existent abnormalities in either airflow rates or gas exchange systems. These latter two areas have proven sensitive in determining ability to work and, hence, disability.

The FVC can provide most of the information needed to properly assess most patients with structural lung abnormalities.

## ASTHMA TESTING

Asthma is characterized by reversible airflow rates. This factor and the need to test the individual in the absence of wheezing make it difficult to assess impairment due to asthma using the FVC, the $FEV_1$, the $FEV_1$/FVC, the $FEF_{25-75}$, and the MVV alone. This difficult issue will be addressed at length in Chapter 29. The various tests used in asthma testing, however, are presented briefly here.

Two principal tests address the issue of variable airflow rates: bronchodilation studies and bronchoconstriction studies. A simple spirometric test is done and the FVC or the flow rates are contrasted after a dilator or constrictor agent is inhaled. Many controversies exist concerning which test is better, how much change is needed, and the sensitivity and specificity of each in diagnosing asthma.[5,26]

When wheezing is heard or when the flow rates on the screening spirometry are low, an asthma test using a bronchodilator substance is generally chosen. The expected result is increased flow rates. When flow rates are normal and wheezing is not heard, a constrictor agent is used. The expected result is decreased airflow rates. When wheezing is heard or airflow rates are low, constrictor agents may precipitate an asthmatic attack that can be severe, delayed, and possibly require hospitalization (rarely death results).

The PEF is used principally in asthma testing where serial testing can often provide useful information about specific events possibly responsible for diminished airflow rates or where there is concern regarding the timing of asthma (for example, a bronchospastic event can be delayed several hours after the exposure has occurred). The peak flow meter assesses the severity of airflow obstruction as well as the response to treatment. Since it is portable, small, and inexpensive, it can also be given to patients for home use. Its greatest value lies in the diagnosis of asthmatic reactions following specific exposures, as in occupational asthma (see Chapter 29). Its greatest disadvantage is its dependence on effort and the patient's full cooperation for reliable results. For litigation purposes a bronchoprovocative test would appear to be more reliable than the PEF.[6,11,14]

### Bronchoprovocative Testing

Because constrictor agents provoke an asthmatic or bronchospastic response, they are also called bronchoprovocative agents and the test may be termed a bronchoprovocative test or maneuver. It can be performed with a variety of agents, each with its own sensitivity and specificity (see Table 27-1). Included are

**TABLE 27-1**    INHALATION CHALLENGE TESTS

|  | METHACHOLINE | HISTAMINE | ANTIGEN | EXERCISE | COLD AIR | OSMOTIC |
|---|---|---|---|---|---|---|
| Clinical usefulness | High | High | Low | Moderate | High | High |
| Sensitivity | High | High | Moderate | Moderate | High | High |
| Specificity | Moderate | Moderate | High | High | High | High |
| Reproducibility | High | High | Moderate | Moderate | High | High |
| Adverse effects | Low | Low | Potent; high | Potent; high | Low | — |
| Cost | High | High | High to very high | Moderate | High | — |

histamine, acetylcholine (acetylcholine is liberated from nerve endings in the lungs, causing bronchospasm), methacholine, cold air, dry air, exercise, hyperventilation, inhaled hypo-osmolar substances, and even ice cubes applied to the face. Theoretically, however, the most sensitive test would use a substance to which an individual has a suspected reaction. Table 27-1 and the accompanying boxes at right and at top left on page 314 provide examples of diseases and environmental factors associated with hyperresponsiveness (that is, can give false-positive values) and the sensitivity and specificity of some common bronchoprovocative tests.[5]

Inhalation challenges have been used to determine the extent of airway reactivity for three decades.[22] Challenge procedures are incorporated into research projects as well as clinical medicine and are used to document occupational asthma or other work-related disorders.

Bronchoprovocation has been validated in many separate studies as a useful tool in the diagnosis of occupational asthma.[7,8,23,24] Provocation testing is particularly helpful in patients with normal or borderline lung function as defined by standard pulmonary function testing (normal $FEV_1$ and maximal midexpiratory flow rates).[8]

Nonspecific inhalation challenge testing using methacholine or histamine is often needed to establish the presence and degree of bronchial hyperactivity. These nonspecific procedures provide evidence of sensitization to occupational inhalants when performed before and after work resumption or as a return-to-work challenge.[21]

The measurement of bronchial hyperactivity after inhaling specific occupational agents, such as formaldehyde, isocyanates, drugs, or wood dusts, has

## INFLUENCES ON AIRWAY RESPONSIVENESS

### FACTORS THAT ENHANCE HYPERRESPONSIVENESS

Aeroallergens (late phase response)
Chemical sensitizers (toluene diisocyanate, western red cedar dust)
Noxious gases (ozone, $SO_3$, $NO_2$)
Cigarette smoke (chronic exposure)
Viral respiratory infections

### FACTORS THAT DO NOT ENHANCE HYPERRESPONSIVENESS

Aeroallergens (early phase response)
Pharmacologic agents (histamine, methacholine)
Cold air
Exercise and hyperventilation
Cigarette smoke (acute exposure)

been defined as chemical bronchoprovocation or specific inhalation challenge.[8] Indications and contraindications are listed in the box at top right on page 314. Chemical inhalation challenge is used in investigating distinct or unusual exposure to airborne dusts, gases, vapors, or fumes. These tests are time consuming and complex, and therefore are not considered practical or beneficial in most cases of possible occupational-environmental asthma or hypersensitiv-

## SUBSTANCES ASSOCIATED WITH OCCUPATIONAL ASTHMA

Animal in origin
    Allergens from hair, scales, urine, serum, and remains of arthropods
Vegetable in origin
    Wood, roots, leaves, flowers, cereals, grains, green coffee beans, castor beans, vegetable gums (arabic, adragante, karaya)
Textiles
    Cotton, jute, flax, hemp
Chemical products
    Pharmaceuticals (penicillin, ampicillin, cephalosporin powder, macrolides, tetracyclines)
Metals
    Chromium, nickel, platinum, vanadium, mercury
Plastic materials
    Isocyanates (toluene diisocyanate, diphenyl methane diisocyanate, hexamethylene diisocyanate), phthalic anhydrides, trimellitic anhydride, formaldehyde

## MAJOR INDICATIONS AND CONTRAINDICATIONS FOR SPECIFIC INHALATION CHALLENGE

### INDICATIONS

- New chemical exposures related to occupational asthma.
- Assessment of specific and unusual agents in complex industrial environments (multiple chemical exposures).
- Medicolegal purposes (rarely).
- Research studies including epidemiologic and air pollution investigations.[19]

### CONTRAINDICATIONS

- Lack of experienced personnel who can recognize and assess the occurrence of clinical changes that will require therapeutic intervention.
- Lack of emergency facilities (must be done in a hospital where facilities for emergency respiratory care are immediately available).
- Medication interference, including sustained-release theophyllines, beta-adrenergic agents, antihistamines, and mast cell stabilizers. Mast cell stabilizers should be avoided for 24 hours, antihistamines for 48 hours, and beta-adrenergic agents and short-term theophylline compounds for 8 hours. All these agents will inhibit or totally block the response to chemical challenge.
- Moderately to markedly abnormal baseline pulmonary function tests. Since severe reductions in pulmonary function can occur with bronchoprovocation testing (especially if baseline values are less than 65% to 70% of predicted), it is best to avoid this procedure in these circumstances. However, if an intermediate-type reaction is expected, the test can usually be performed, since treatment with a beta-antagonist reverses the constrictive effect quickly. Late-type responses usually require corticosteroids.[25]

ity pneumonitis.[21] These studies are potentially dangerous and involve risk for both the patient and the investigator. Therefore, they should be performed in a hospital setting and a physician should always be present.

The methods used to challenge individuals have been published by many authors.[8,16] Some investigators have devised whole body chambers to quantify accurately chemical reactions in a dose-responsive relationship.[7,21] These chambers and their accompanying apparatus control the complete sample environment, including temperature, relative humidity, airflow rate, air quality, aerosol generation, and exposure level. It may even be possible to reproduce conditions in the laboratory that can approximate or equal those found in the industrial environment. Once the appropriate conditions are reproduced, detailed studies can be done to evaluate human response to individual chemical compounds.

By combining the occupational history, time course of symptoms, industrial hygiene data, and evaluation of the appropriate Material Safety Data Sheets (MSDS), a specific chemical can be identified or be strongly suspected of a causal relationship. Under such circumstances, a controlled inhalation challenge in the pulmonary laboratory is probably the best course to follow. Table 27-2 and Figure 27-8 illustrate the short-term effects of polyisocyanate during a chemical challenge test.

**TABLE 27-2**     POLYISOCYANATE CHALLENGE*

| | FVC | FEV₁ | FEF₂₅₋₇₅% | PEF | RAW | SGAW |
|---|---|---|---|---|---|---|
| Predicted | 5.52 | 4.57 | 288 | 592 | 1.10 | 0.23 |
| Baseline | 6.49 | 4.38 | 158 | 594 | 1.13 | 0.20 |
| Saline control | 6.34 | 4.30 | 159 | 569 | 1.11 | 0.21 |
| 0.00091 cc/ml | 6.29 | 4.20 | 151 | 541 | 1.38 | 0.16 |
| 0.00182 cc/ml | 5.94 | 3.65 | 106 | 431 | 2.14 | 0.11 |
| 30 min | 6.23 | 4.27 | 166 | 531 | 1.81 | 0.15 |
| 1 hour | 6.15 | 4.19 | 157 | 531 | 1.49 | 0.17 |
| 2 hours | 6.20 | 4.16 | 151 | 527 | 1.47 | 0.18 |
| 3 hours | 6.24 | 4.15 | 144 | 500 | 1.37 | 0.19 |
| 4 hours | 6.28 | 4.17 | 142 | 529 | 1.37 | 0.20 |
| 5 hours | 6.10 | 4.18 | 161 | 493 | 1.29 | 0.21 |
| 6 hours | 6.11 | 4.19 | 159 | 549 | 1.15 | 0.23 |

*31-year-old male caucasian (180 cm and 77 kg). RAW = airway resistance, SGAW = specific conductance.

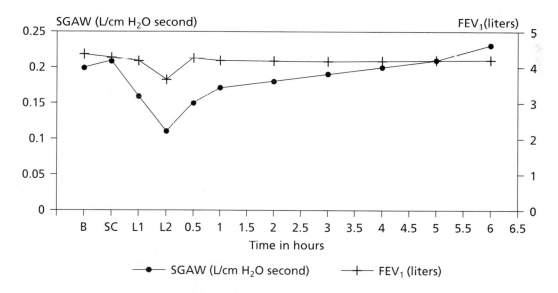

B = baseline; SC = saline control
L1 = 0.00091 cc/ml polyisocyanate
L2 = 0.00182cc/ml polyisocyanate

**FIGURE 27-8**     Polyisocyanate challenge.

## Application in Impairment Evaluations

Asthma testing is more difficult than tests of lung volumes, airflow rates, or gas exchange. As shown in Chapter 29, asthma is also the most difficult pulmonary disease to which to apply disability criteria. The establishment of a diagnosis of asthma is usually insufficient to warrant impairment or disability. Supporting evidence of disability in an asthmatic has traditionally rested on documentation of hospitalizations and/or emergency room visitations. But frequent and repeated emergency room or hospital stays have become less reliable indicators of functional impairment and thus disability because (1) more medications are available and effective in the treatment or prophylaxis of asthma; (2) newer theories have emerged regarding asthmagenesis and the crucial role of preventing airway inflammation; and (3) more specialists have entered the field of pulmonary and allergic diseases. The use of specific bronchoprovocative tests and the testing of serial lung functions with a peak-flow meter will probably, in the near future, become the criteria of choice in disability evaluations.

## References

1. American Thoracic Society: Standardization of spirometry—1987 update. *Am Rev Respir Dis* 136:1285-1298, 1987.
2. American Thoracic Society: Single-breath carbon monoxide diffusing capacity (transfer factor): recommendations for a standard technique. *Am Rev Respir Dis* 136:1299-1307, 1987.
3. American Thoracic Society: Lung function testing: selection of reference values and interpretative strategies. *Am Rev Respir Dis* 144:1202-1218, 1991.
4. Becklake MR, White N: Sources of variation in spirometric measurement: identifying the signal and dealing with noise. In Eisen EA, editor: *Occupational medicine: state of the art reviews*, Vol. 8, No. 2, Philadelphia, 1993, pp. 241-264, Hanley & Belfus.
5. Braman SS, Corrao WM: Bronchoprovocation testing. In Mahler DA, editor: *Clinics in chest medicine*, Vol. 10, No. 2, Philadelphia, 1989, pp. 165-176, WB Saunders.
6. Burge PS: Use of serial measurements of peak flow in the diagnosis of occupational asthma. In Eisen EA, editor, *Occupational medicine: state of the art reviews*, Vol. 8, No. 2, Philadelphia, 1993, pp. 279-302, Hanley & Belfus.
7. Butcher BT: Inhalation challenge testing with toluene diisocyanate. *J Aller Clin Immunol* 64:655-657, 1979.
8. Chan-Yeung M, Lam S: State of art: occupational asthma. *Am Rev Respir Dis* 133:686-703, 1986.
9. Clausen JL: Prediction of normal values in pulmonary function testing. In Mahler DA, editor: *Clinics in chest medicine*, Vol. 10, No. 2, Philadelphia, 1989, pp. 135-143, WB Saunders.
10. Cropp GJA, Bernstein IL, Boushey HA, et al: Guidelines for bronchial inhalation challenges with pharmacologic and antigenic agents. *Am Thorac Soc News* Spring:11-19, 1980.
11. Dahlqvist M, Eisen EA, Wegman DH, Kriebel D: Reproducibility of peak expiratory flow measurements. In Eisen EA (ed). *Occupational medicine: state of the art reviews*, Vol. 8, No. 2, Philadelphia, 1993, pp. 295-302, Hanley & Belfus.
12. Department of Labor, Employment Standards Administration. Standards for determining coal miners' total disability or death due to pneumoconiosis. *Fed Reg* 45:13678-13712, 1980.
13. Doege TC, Houston TP, editors: *Guides to the evaluation of permanent impairment*, ed 4, Chicago, 1993, American Medical Association.
14. Eisen EA, Wegman DH, Kriebel D: Application of peak expiratory flow in epidemiologic studies of occupation. In Eisen EA, editor: *Occupational medicine: state of the art reviews*, Vol. 8, No. 2, Philadelphia, 1993, pp. 265-277, Hanley & Belfus.
15. Gardner RM, Clausen JL, Cotton DJ, et al: Computer guidelines for pulmonary laboratories. *Am Rev Respir Dis* 134:628-629, 1986.
16. Gardner RM, Clausen JL, Crapo RO, et al: Quality assurance in pulmonary function laboratories. *Am Rev Respir Dis* 134:625-627, 1986.
17. Gardner RM, Clausen JL, Epler G, et al: Pulmonary function laboratory personnel qualifications. *Am Rev Respir Dis* 134:623-624, 1986.
18. Gardner RM, Crapo RO, Nelson SB: Spirometry and flow-volume curves. In Mahler DA, editor: *Clinics in chest medicine*, Philadelphia, 1989, pp. 145-154, WB Saunders.
19. Hackney JD, Linn WS, Avol EL: Acid fog: effects on respiratory function and symptoms in healthy and asthmatic volunteers. *Environ Health Perspect* 79:159-162, 1989.
20. Hankinson JL: Instrumentation for spirometry. In Eisen EA, editor: *Occupational medicine: state of the art reviews*. Philadelphia, 1993, pp. 397-407 Hanley & Belfus.
21. Hendrick DJ: Bronchopulmonary disease in the workplace: challenge testing with occupational agents. *Ann Allergy* 51:179-184, 1983.
22. Parker CD, Bilbo RE, Reed CE: Methacholine aerosol as test for bronchial asthma. *Arch Intern Med* 115:452-458, 1965.
23. Pepys J, Hutchcroft BJ: State of the art: bronchial provocation tests in etiologic diagnosis and analy-

sis of asthma. *Am Rev Respir Dis* 112:829-859, 1975.

24. Rosenthal RR: Inhalation challenge—procedures, indications, and techniques: the emerging role of bronchoprovocation. *J Allergy Clin Immunol* 64:564-568, 1979.

25. Schlueter DP: Environmental challenge. *Allergy Proc* 10:339-344, 1989.

26. Shin C. Response to bronchodilators. In Mahler DA, editor: *Clinics in chest medicine*, Vol. 10, No. 2, Philadelphia, 1989, pp. 155-164, WB Saunders.

# CHAPTER 28

# INTEGRATED CARDIOPULMONARY EXERCISE TESTING

*James E. Hansen*
*Karlman Wasserman*

The objective of this chapter is to inform physicians who evaluate individuals for impairment about the importance, value, indications, economy, and safety of integrated cardiopulmonary exercise testing using gas exchange measurements. The authors briefly review the basic physiology of exercise to show why measures of $O_2$ uptake ($\dot{V}_{O_2}$) and $CO_2$ output ($\dot{V}_{CO_2}$) provide important data for an informed assessment of work capacity. The authors also review how exercise-testing equipment, methods, measures, and protocols can be used to understand how they discriminate between diseases involving the respiratory, circulatory, and musculoskeletal systems. Such testing assists in identifying the dominant disorder when multiple disorders coexist, and helps exclude or quantitate impairment. Further reading[3,54,60] and training are required before testing patients. The box on page 319 lists and defines the abbreviations used in this chapter.

## ESSENTIALS OF EXERCISE PHYSIOLOGY

### Bioenergetics of Muscle Contraction

In brief, muscle contraction and relaxation depend upon the immediate availability of high-energy phosphates in the form of adenosine triphosphate (ATP) and creatine phosphate (CP).[37] At the start of exercise there are ample stores of ATP, CP, and $O_2$ in the muscle. In the muscle cell mitochondria, $O_2$ is utilized to regenerate ATP in the energy-yielding electron-transport process, keeping the level of ATP relatively constant while the CP decreases in proportion to the work rate, and $CO_2$ and water are produced predominantly in the tricarboxylic acid cycle.[35] If exercise continues, cellular respiration ($CO_2$ production and $O_2$ consumption) continues at a rate proportional to the power output and substrate respiratory quotient (RQ).[54]

## Coupling of External Exchange with the Atmosphere to Cellular Respiration

As depicted in Figure 28-1, the delivery of $O_2$ to the muscle and removal of $CO_2$ from the muscle depends on several processes: the effectiveness of the heart and blood in transporting $O_2$ and $CO_2$, the ability of the peripheral and pulmonary circulations to exchange $O_2$ and $CO_2$ at the muscle and pulmonary capillaries, respectively, and the effectiveness of the lungs and ventilatory apparatus in transporting $O_2$ and $CO_2$ from and to the atmosphere.[50]

## The Mechanism and Consequences of Exercise Lactic Acidosis

If $O_2$ delivery to the exercising muscles is adequate, the catabolism of glycogen or glucose, fatty acid, ethanol, or (rarely) amino acids through the tricarboxylic acid cycle and $O_2$ transport chain results in the production of $H_2O$ and $CO_2$ plus large amounts of ATP (36 ATP from 6 molecules of $O_2$ and 1 molecule of glucose).[35] When adequate $O_2$ is not delivered to the cell, there is a major decrease in the efficiency of production of ATP (i.e., 1 molecule of glucose produces only 2 ATP molecules). This is accompanied by the obligate conversion of 2 molecules of pyruvate to 2 molecules of lactate with 2 accompanying hydrogen ions.[35]

When metabolism is partially anaerobic, the lactic acid produced must be immediately buffered in the cells because its pK is 3.9 while the cell pH is about 7.0. The hydrogen ion reacts immediately with the bicarbonate, resulting in the immediate production of carbonic acid which dissociates into water and $CO_2$.[51] This $CO_2$ can be considred "excess" since it did not come directly from aerobic metabolism. On a molar basis, the decrease in bicarbonate approximately equals the increase in lactate; 22 ml of $CO_2$ are produced for each mEq of lactate formed (Fig. 28-2).[54] With mild anaerobiasis, the normal respiratory tract

## ABBREVIATIONS

| Symbol | Meaning |
|--------|---------|
| AT | Anaerobic threshold |
| ATP | Adenosine triphosphate |
| BTPS | Body temperature, pressure, saturated |
| $C(a-v)_{O_2}$ | Difference in $O_2$ content between arterial and mixed venous blood |
| $Ca_{O_2}$ | $O_2$ content in arterial blood |
| $Cv_{O_2}$ | $O_2$ content in mixed-venous blood |
| COHb | Carboxyhemoglobin |
| CP | Creatine phosphate |
| $D_{LCO}$ | Diffusing capacity for carbon monoxide |
| $f$ | Frequency of ventilation |
| $FEV_1$ | Forced expiratory volume in one second |
| FVC | Forced vital capacity |
| HR | Heart rate |
| IC | Inspiratory capacity |
| LAT | Lactic acidosis threshold |
| MRT | Mean response time |
| MVV | Maximal voluntary ventilation |
| Peak HR | Highest heart rate |
| Peak $\dot{V}_{O_2}$ | Highest $O_2$ uptake |
| $P(A-a)_{O_2}$ | Alveolar-arterial $O_2$ pressure difference |

| Symbol | Meaning |
|--------|---------|
| $P(a-ET)_{CO_2}$ | Arterial-end tidal $CO_2$ pressure difference |
| $Pa_{CO_2}$ | Arterial $CO_2$ pressure |
| $PA_{CO_2}$ | Alveolar $CO_2$ pressure |
| $Pa_{O_2}$ | Arterial $O_2$ pressure |
| $PET_{CO_2}$ | End tidal $CO_2$ pressure |
| $PET_{O_2}$ | End tidal $O_2$ pressure |
| $R$ | Respiratory exchange ratio |
| RQ | Respiratory quotient |
| $Sa_{O_2}$ | Arterial $O_2$ saturation |
| STPD | Standard temperature, pressure, dry |
| $S\bar{v}_{O_2}$ | Mixed venous $O_2$ saturation |
| $\dot{V}_{CO_2}$ | $CO_2$ output |
| VD | Dead space |
| VD/VT | Dead space/tidal volume ratio |
| $\dot{V}E$ | Expired ventilation |
| $\dot{V}E/\dot{V}_{O_2}$ | Ventilatory equivalent for $O_2$ |
| $\dot{V}E/\dot{V}_{CO_2}$ | Ventilatory equivalent for $CO_2$ |
| $\dot{V}E_{max}$ | Maximum exercise ventilation |
| $\dot{V}_{O_2}$ | $O_2$ uptake |
| VT | Tidal volume |
| $\Delta\dot{V}_{O_2}/\Delta WR$ | Change in $O_2$ uptake per change in work rate |
| $\Delta\dot{V}_{O_2}(6-3)$ | Change in $O_2$ uptake from 3 to 6 min |

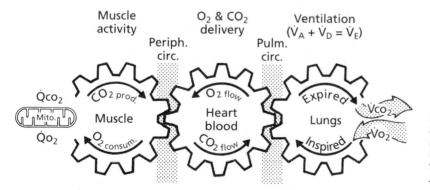

**FIGURE 28-1**    Schematic representation of $O_2$ and $CO_2$ transport between atmospheric air and muscle mitochondria during exercise. External and internal (cellular) respiration are linked through the circulatory system. (From Wasserman K: *N Engl J Med* 298:780, 1978. Used by permission.)

eliminates this excess $CO_2$ promptly. With increasing anaerobiasis and lactic acid production, the blood becomes more acid and ventilation is further stimulated, thereby enhancing $CO_2$ output. This decreases the alveolar $P_{CO_2}$ ($PA_{CO_2}$) and arterial $P_{CO_2}$ ($Pa_{CO_2}$) in those who are not limited in ventilatory capability.[58] While anaerobiasis in some muscular sites produces lactate from pyruvate, lactate can be concurrently re-

converted to pyruvate in other body sites where oxygenation is adequate.[56]

### Fuel Utilization and the Respiratory Quotient (RQ)

The ratio of $CO_2$ production to the $O_2$ consumption at the cellular level is identified as the respiratory quotient (RQ) and is partially dependent on the sub-

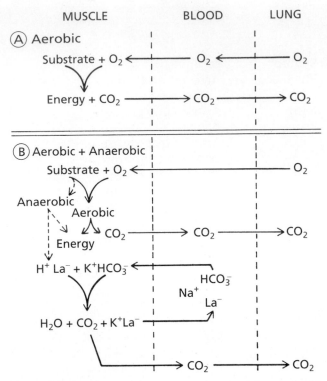

**FIGURE 28-2**    Gas exchange during aerobic **(A)** and aerobic plus anaerobic **(B)** exercise. In the former situation, $O_2$ is used and $CO_2$ is produced in approximately equal volumes. In the latter situation, cell lactic acid is produced, which must be immediately buffered at the pH of cell water, primarily by bicarbonate. The buffering reaction increases $CO_2$ production by 22 ml for each mEq of bicarbonate buffering lactic acid. This excess $CO_2$ must be eliminated through the lungs. (From Wasserman K, et al: *Principles of exercise testing and interpretation*, ed 2, Philadelphia, 1994, Lea & Febiger. Used by permission.)

strate metabolized.[18] The metabolism of 1 gram of fatty acid yields 9 kcal of energy: for each 4.7 kcal of energy, approximately 1.0 L of $O_2$ is used and 0.7 L of $CO_2$ is produced ($\dot{V}CO_2/\dot{V}O_2$ or RQ = 0.7 for fat). The metabolism of 1 gram of carbohydrate yields 4 kcal of energy: for each 5.1 kcal of energy, approximately 1 L of $O_2$ is used and 1 L of $CO_2$ is produced ($\dot{V}CO_2/\dot{V}O_2$ or RQ = 1.0 for carbohydrate). Because of the small differences in $O_2$ requirements per liter of $O_2$ (4.7 kcal versus 5.1 kcal) and the fact that a mixture of substrates is usually utilized, energy requirements expressed as kcal/L $O_2$ are relatively insensitive to the dietary source. Thus $\dot{V}O_2$ has a high correlation with power output during aerobic work.

## Metabolic Requirements to Perform Work: Effects of Body Size, Work Efficiency, and Work Intensity

Total metabolic requirements depend on body size and the external work performed, which are directly related to kcal or $\dot{V}O_2$ measurements. Resting metabolism increases with body size, fever, and many ill-nesses. Although the ease or difficulty of performing an external task depends in part on the intelligence, skill, and agility of the worker, its metabolic requirement is primarily based on the action of the musculoskeletal system in overcoming resistance and gravity.[3]

Work efficiency, however, is reasonably similar for all persons. It is defined as the $\dot{V}O_2$ required to perform external work above the $\dot{V}O_2$ cost of moving the body without external load.[62] Several studies have shown that the $\dot{V}O_2$ requirement to perform 1 W of external cycling work (after subtracting the $\dot{V}O_2$ of unloaded cycling at the same frequency) is 10 ± 1 ml of $O_2$ per minute, regardless of age, gender, or body size.[26,27,57]

The ability of the musculoskeletal system to perform work depends on the ability of the circulatory and respiratory systems to transport $O_2$ from the atmosphere to the working muscles and remove $CO_2$ and lactic acid from them, since work is rarely limited by the availability of water, carbohydrate, or fatty acids.[54] The ability to increase $\dot{V}O_2$ also depends on the quantity of muscle involved in the task performed; the more muscle involved the higher the possible $\dot{V}O_2$. For example, the peak $\dot{V}O_2$ is less for arm cycling than for leg cycling because of the greater muscle mass in the legs than in the arms. It is still higher for treadmill walking or running or other exercise that combines the use of both arms and legs.[54] The ambulatory peak $\dot{V}O_2$ of normal, sedentary, middle-aged adults is about ten times that at rest.

The intensity of work depends on the relative ease of increasing $\dot{V}O_2$ compared to the $\dot{V}O_2$ required to perform that task and the task duration.

For the approximate relationships between activity, metabolic rate (expressed as $\dot{V}O_2$ in L/min), and work intensity (from minimal to extreme) in several individuals differing in body size and health,[1,3,8,18] the key points are as follows: (1) For a given age, gender, and height, the peak $\dot{V}O_2$ usually depends on the adaptation of the weakest link in the cardiovascular, respiratory, and musculoskeletal systems of the individual. (2) Individuals differ little in work efficiency, once we account for the differences between individual metabolic requirements to perform activity without an external load and the learned ability to perform motor skills. (3) Despite similar work efficiency, the energy (and $\dot{V}O_2$) requirements for a given task are higher in larger individuals, especially when movement of the body or large body parts are involved, because they must use more energy to move a larger mass. Tasks that require lifting the person's body weight as in climbing (rather than just moving the legs as in cycling) cause even greater differences in the $\dot{V}O_2$ requirements between smaller and larger

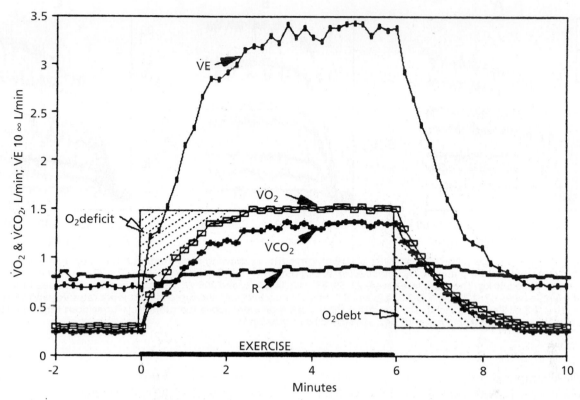

**FIGURE 28-3**     Gas exchange values for 6 min of exercise on a cycle ergometer at 100 W in a healthy subject. $O_2$ uptake ($\dot{V}O_2$), $CO_2$ output ($\dot{V}CO_2$), minute ventilation ($\dot{V}E$), and respiratory exchange ratio (R) values are plotted. The exercise is preceded by 2 min of rest and followed by 4 min of recovery. Note the more rapid rise in $\dot{V}O_2$ than in $\dot{V}CO_2$ or $\dot{V}E$, the decline in R immediately after the onset of exercise (due to the increasing stores of $CO_2$ in the body), and the plateau of these values after 3 min of exercise. The latter indicates that the work rate is below the lactic acidosis threshold of the subject and that a steady state has been reached. The $O_2$ deficit and $O_2$ debt (crosshatched areas) are equal in size. (From Hansen JE, Tierney DF, editors: *Current pulmonology*, Vol. 14, St. Louis, 1993, Mosby-Year Book, p 43. Used by permission.)

individuals. (4) The intensity of a task increases as the ratio of the task $\dot{V}O_2$ to the individual's peak $\dot{V}O_2$ approaches 1.0. (5) Tasks of very heavy intensity can be performed for only brief periods.

## The Steady State, Gas Exchange Kinetics, $O_2$ Deficit, and $O_2$ Debt

A person can be considered to be in a "steady state" when metabolism is constant. In such a state variables such as heart rate (HR), blood pressure, $\dot{V}E$ (expired ventilation), $\dot{V}O_2$, $\dot{V}CO_2$, and blood chemistry also remain constant, and the metabolic rate ($\dot{V}O_2$) can be maintained indefinitely. During this state the work task is being performed without anaerobic metabolism or increasing $O_2$ debt, and there is no lactic acidosis (i.e., the work rate is below the subject's lactic acidosis threshold [LAT]).[54] Commonly, work tasks fluctuate, so the above variables change with time delays related to changes in the body stores of $O_2$, $CO_2$, ATP, and CP. Figure 28-3 shows the changes in $\dot{V}O_2$, $\dot{V}CO_2$, R (respiratory exchange ratio or $\dot{V}CO_2/\dot{V}O_2$), and $\dot{V}E$ in a normal person during a 12 min test: rest for 2 min, loaded cycling at a work rate of 100 W,

and a recovery period of 4 min. During exercise a steady state is reached well before 6 min with a $\dot{V}O_2$ of 1.50 L/min. After the onset of exercise, $\dot{V}O_2$, $\dot{V}CO_2$, $\dot{V}E$, and HR abruptly rise, $\dot{V}O_2$ increasing more rapidly than $\dot{V}CO_2$, which in turn increases more rapidly than $\dot{V}E$.[13,16] $\dot{V}O_2$ reaches a plateau by 3 min and $\dot{V}CO_2$ and $\dot{V}E$ reach a plateau by 4 min.

The mean response time (MRT) (the time to reach 63% of the way between the original and new steady state) is used as a measure of the response kinetics for each variable. It assumes a first order (single exponential) response from the start of exercise despite the fact that the response may have several components that distort the response curve from that of a single exponential function.[54]

The terms *$O_2$ deficit* and *$O_2$ debt* (Fig. 28-3) identify the differences in $O_2$ volume consumed and $O_2$ volume required at the *onset* and *offset* of exercise, respectively.[3] The $O_2$ deficit is the difference between $\dot{V}O_2$ metabolically required to perform the work rate and the actual $\dot{V}O_2$ during this time. The $O_2$ debt is the quantity or volume of $\dot{V}O_2$ during recovery in excess of that required during rest (i.e., the amount that was repaid to replete body $O_2$ stores and regenerate ATP and

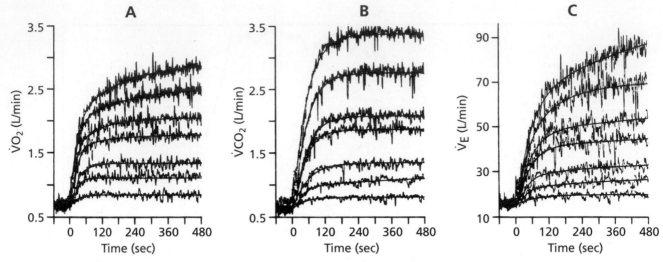

**FIGURE 28-4**     Gas exchange values, second-by-second, with curve fitting, showing the transition from unloaded pedalling to seven levels of work rate sustained for 6 min. **A,** $O_2$ uptake ($\dot{V}O_2$). **B,** $CO_2$ output ($\dot{V}CO_2$). **C,** Ventilation ($\dot{V}E$). The 32-year-old male subject was 180 cm tall and weighed 80 kg. The work levels were 29, 59, 88, 117, 146, 176, and 205 W. Venous blood lactate values 1 min after the cessation of exercise were 1.2, 1.4, 1.4, 1.7, 3.2, 4.3, and 8.7 mEq/L, respectively. At the three-highest work rates $\dot{V}O_2$ and $\dot{V}E$ continued to rise, indicating the absence of a steady state and that these work rates were above the subject's lactic acidosis threshold for leg cycling. (From Casaburi R, et al: *J Appl Physiol* 67:547, 1989. Used by permission.)

CP). In the example shown, both $O_2$ deficit and $O_2$ debt approximate 1 L. With exercise of mild-to-moderate intensity, the $O_2$ deficit and $O_2$ debt are similar in quantity. With heavy or higher-intensity exercise, $O_2$ deficit may not be quantified accurately because the true $O_2$ requirement is unknown (a plateau in $\dot{V}O_2$ is not reached); the $O_2$ debt also may not be accurately quantified when the $\dot{V}O_2$ remains elevated above resting levels for a long period (even hours).[3]

## Responses to Constant Work of Differing Intensities

Figure 28-4 shows the changes in $\dot{V}O_2$, $\dot{V}CO_2$, and $\dot{V}E$ from unloaded cycling to loaded cycling at seven exercise levels from mild to very heavy.[13] At the four lower work rates (29, 59, 88, and 117 W) this person could work for several hours without resting, if needed, because the work is supported completely by atmospheric $O_2$. At the three higher work rates (146, 176, and 205 W) this person cannot support the work rate totally by aerobic sources. This exercise is above the anaerobic threshold (AT) or lactic acidosis threshold (LAT).* Blood lactate levels, VE, HR, and blood pressure also continue to rise during work levels above the LAT. Work rates higher than 205 W cannot be sustained for even 6 min.

*Lactic acidosis develops at the $\dot{V}O_2$ above which metabolism cannot be fully supported aerobically for a long period of time. This is referred to as the *lactic acidosis threshold* (LAT). It is also referred to as the *anaerobic threshold* (AT), since the lactic acidosis develops when anaerobic energy-producing mechanisms supplement the aerobic energy-producing mechanisms. These terms, therefore, identify the same $\dot{V}O_2$ (i.e., they are equivalent).

At work rates above the LAT, many variables demonstrate characteristic changes. The $\dot{V}CO_2$ exceeds the $\dot{V}O_2$ due to the production of excess $CO_2$ resulting from the dissociation of bicarbonate as it buffers the intracellularly accumulating lactic acid.[52] Initially the ventilatory response is isocapnic (i.e., the $PaCO_2$ remains relatively constant) as $\dot{V}E$ is tightly linked to $\dot{V}CO_2$.[59] As exercise continues so that lactic acid accumulation increases, the arterial bicarbonate and pH decrease. The latter stimulates the carotid body chemoreceptors to increase ventilation even more than that predicted from the $CO_2$ load to the lung. The disproportionate decrease in $PACO_2$ and $PaCO_2$ minimizes the decrease in blood pH. The disproportionate increase in $\dot{V}E$ to $\dot{V}O_2$ raises the alveolar $PO_2$ ($PAO_2$).[38] Thus, despite an increase in the difference between $PAO_2$ and $PaO_2$ ($[P(A-a)O_2]$) commonly found with very heavy exercise in normal persons, the $PaO_2$ does not usually decrease below resting levels.[28] Except for occasional elite athletes with high cardiac outputs and high tolerance for discomfort, the arterial oxygen saturation ($SaO_2$) rarely declines with exercise in normal persons.[20]

## WHAT IS INTEGRATED CARDIOPULMONARY EXERCISE TESTING?

### Definition

Integrated cardiopulmonary exercise testing assesses the physiologic mechanisms that couple external to cellular respiration.[54] As such it measures not only the electrocardiogram (ECG), but also evaluates the functional status of the heart, peripheral and pulmonary circulations, the lungs, and matching of ventilation to pulmonary blood flow as they relate to changing metabolic rate. Exercise testing can be performed using a cycle or treadmill ergometer. The collected data should be accurately measured and displayed in such a manner that an informed decision can be made with regard to the subject's functional capacity (including that for all daily activities) and the components limiting gas transport. The latter often reduces the need for further, more costly or invasive investigations.[54]

## How Measurements are Made

After a preliminary history, physical, and laboratory examination (including chest roentgenogram, resting ECG, and spirometry), multiple noninvasive measures of cardiopulmonary variables are obtained in 20 minutes or less (i.e., during rest, constant low-intensity exercise, incremental exercise to tolerance, and recovery.) After preliminary evaluations, the patient is introduced to the general laboratory environment and ergometer (cycle or treadmill) and familiarized with the mouthpiece, breathing valve and instrumentation (flow or volume meters and rapidly-responding $CO_2$ and $O_2$ analyzers).[7,31,45,60] Informed consent is obtained and electrodes are placed for recording of a 12-lead ECG, from which HR and ECG pattern can be determined. Together, the simultaneous gas exchange and ECG recordings allow repetitive measurement of HR, $\dot{V}E$, breathing frequency ($f$), tidal volume (VT), $\dot{V}CO_2$, $\dot{V}O_2$, end-tidal $CO_2$ pressure (PET$CO_2$) and end-tidal $O_2$ pressure (PET$O_2$). With appropriate analyzers and computer software, gas exchange data can be measured breath-by-breath and displayed breath-by-breath or averaged over any interval. Additionally, the external work rate can be computer-controlled and estimated in the case of treadmill or quite accurately measured in the case of a cycle. If an arterial line is used, samples can be taken for measurement of $PaO_2$, $PaCO_2$, pH, and lactate values and arterial blood pressure tracings can be recorded. If not, blood pressure is measured by auscultation, arterial blood can be sampled once or twice during exercise, and ear or finger oximetry values can be obtained. Either an incremental or constant work rate protocol may be used. A dedicated microcomputer is commonly used to calculate, tabulate, and display the results graphically. The latter is particularly important, in order to interrelate the multiple ventilatory, circulatory, blood, and work rate variables. A nine-panel plot (Fig. 28-5) of these variables displays the most information,[54] but a four-panel plot, as shown in Figure 28-6, illustrates the major findings.[24]

## Ergometry Methods

For impairment and clinical evaluations, leg cycling or treadmill exercise are most commonly used. The cycle can be used for upper-extremity exercise if leg exercises on the cycle or treadmill are unsuitable. Table 28-1 lists some of the advantages and disadvantages of each of these ergometers. Because persons on the treadmill can be "dragged along" without actually climbing or propelling themselves, any connection other than that between the exercising person's feet and the treadmill belt can reduce the external work performed. The opportunity to accurately quantitate the relationship of $\dot{V}O_2$ to work rate (e.g., panel 3 of Fig. 28-5) is a major advantage of cycle ergometry.[54]

## Exercise Protocols

### Incremental work

Usually, a progressively increasing work-rate protocol to tolerance gives all the necessary information for impairment evaluation with the least effort on the part of the patient. On the cycle ergometer, a useful protocol includes data collection during (a) 2 to 3 min of rest, (b) 3 to 4 min of unloaded pedalling at a rate of 60 rpm, (c) 7 to 10 min of continued pedalling while work rate is increased in equal increments to tolerance, and (d) 2 min of recovery. Work can be increased in ramp fashion or in one-minute steps. If a treadmill is used, the unloaded cycling is replaced by walking at an easy pace for 3 to 4 min at zero grade, followed by increasing the grade the same amount (1 to 3%) every minute to tolerance.

Usually a work rate increment can be selected (considering the evaluee's age, gender, body size, usual activity level, and known illnesses) so that the incremental work rate period lasts 6 to 14 min. Too short a period (under 6 min) may prevent the investigator from obtaining enough data for an accurate interpretation. Too long a period (over 14 min) leads to boredom or physical discomfort at a submaximal work rate.[10,54]

As evaluees cannot speak while on the mouthpiece during the exercise test, they are taught to signal discomfort by pointing to the site of discomfort and to quantitate severity by extending one, two, or three digits or pointing to a scale (Borg or visual analog) displaying the degree of distress.

The evaluee and the monitors are closely observed during exercise. Exercise is not stopped because the evaluee reaches some predetermined percentage of the predicted peak HR or maximal voluntary ventilation (MVV), but is continued as long as safely tolerated. The development of a significant arrhythmia, substernal pressure or discomfort of more than mild severity, hypotension, hypertension greater than 260

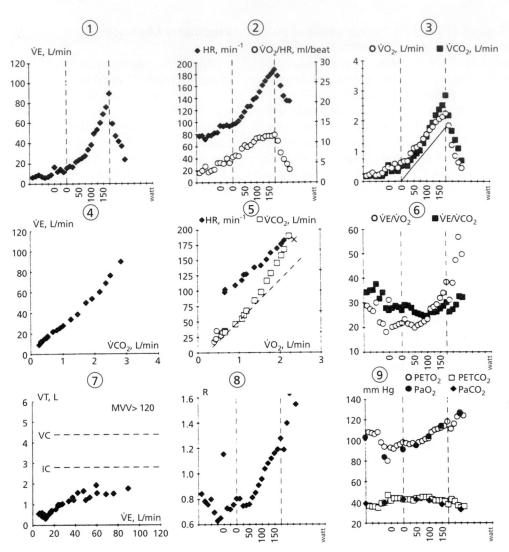

**FIGURE 28-5**    A nine-panel plot of a cycle exercise study in a 37-year-old shipyard machinist complaining of dyspnea. After 3 min of rest, the evaluee pedalled at 60 rpm for 3 min. The work load was then increased 25 W/min to his symptom-limited tolerance. Intra-arterial blood was obtained from a brachial catheter. He stopped exercise because of fatigue. Resting and exercise ECGs were normal. Values are measured breath-by-breath and plotted every 30 sec. Abbreviations are: ventilation ($\dot{V}E$), heart rate (HR) $O_2$ pulse ($\dot{V}o_2$/HR), $O_2$ uptake ($\dot{V}o_2$), $CO_2$ output ($\dot{V}co_2$), ventilatory equivalents for $O_2$ and $CO_2$ ($\dot{V}E/\dot{V}o_2$ and $\dot{V}E/\dot{V}co_2$), tidal volume (VT), vital capacity ($\dot{V}C$), inspiratory capacity (IC), maximal voluntary ventilation (MVV), respiratory exchange ratio (R), arterial and end-tidal $Po_2$ ($Pao_2$ and $PETo_2$), and arterial and end-tidal $Pco_2$ ($Paco_2$ and $PETco_2$). The vertical dashed lines in several panels indicate the beginning and end of the incremental work period. The solid line in the right upper panel indicates a $\dot{V}o_2$/work rate relationship ($\Delta\dot{V}o_2/\Delta WR$) of 10 ml/min of $O_2$/W. The "X" in the center panel indicates the predicted peak $\dot{V}o_2$ and peak HR; the diagonal dashed line has a slope of 1.0. The exercise findings shown in this figure are normal. (From Wasserman K, et al: *Principles of exercise testing and interpretation*, ed 2, Philadelphia, 1994, Lea & Febiger. Used by permission.)

mm Hg systolic or 130 mm Hg diastolic, pallor, or lightheadedness is sufficient to stop the study. After the mouthpiece has been removed, patients should be asked in a nonleading fashion to explain exactly why they stopped exercise. If, after the exercise test, the investigator considers that the evaluee stopped prematurely, the study can be repeated after a short rest period.[54]

**Constant work**

Occasionally evaluees are so infirm that they can perform only unloaded pedalling or walking at a slow pace. For that reason it would be impractical to use an increasing work rate protocol. At other times, constant work protocols can be used to evaluate the efficacy of $O_2$ breathing or drug therapy in relieving symptoms or for an accurate measure of the LAT or $\dot{V}o_2$ kinetics.[40]

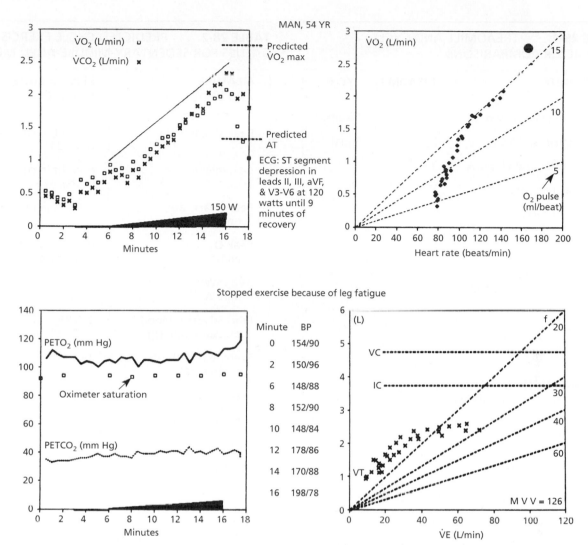

**FIGURE 28-6** A four-panel plot of a cycle exercise study in a 54-year-old asbestos-exposed worker (191 cm and 98 kg) referred by a government agency for disability evaluation because of 15 years of work exposure to asbestos. He was an ex-smoker. He noted leg numbness after walking 20 min. Crackles were heard at the left lung base and linear scarring was seen on roentgenograms. Heart sounds and resting ECG were normal. The vital capacity ($\dot{V}C$) and diffusing capacity for carbon monoxide ($D_{LCO}$) were normal, but the $FEV_1/\dot{V}C$ of 64% was reduced. The exercise protocol included 3 min of rest, 3 min of unloaded pedalling at 60 rpm and work increments of 15 W/min until the patient stopped at 16 min (150 W) with leg fatigue. Values of $O_2$ uptake ($\dot{V}O_2$), $CO_2$ output ($\dot{V}CO_2$), ventilation ($\dot{V}E$), and heart rate (HR) were measured breath-by-breath but plotted every 30 seconds. The black circle in the upper right panel indicates the predicted peak HR, peak $\dot{V}O_2$, and peak $O_2$ pulse. The solid line in the left upper panel slope is a $\Delta\dot{V}O_2/\Delta WR$ of 10 ml/W. Significant downsloping ST-segment depressions were noted in the inferior and lateral ECG leads from 14 min of exercise until they resolved completely by 9 min of recovery. The evaluee denied chest pain or pressure or shortness of breath during or after exercise. The peak $\dot{V}O_2$ and peak HR were reduced. The anaerobic threshold (AT) and the $\Delta\dot{V}O_2/\Delta WR$ were normal, but the $O_2$ pulse did not increase for the last 3 min of exercise. The abnormal exercise ECG and the concurrent failure of the $O_2$ pulse and diastolic pressure to increase during late exercise indicate the likelihood of significant cardiovascular problem as the cause of the abnormal $O_2$ transport. Breathing reserve was ample. The ventilatory equivalents for $O_2$ and $CO_2$ (not graphed) and ear oximeter values were normal, all indicating that significant ventilation/perfusion mismatching was unlikely. Other abbreviations are: end-tidal $P_{O_2}$ and $P_{CO_2}$ ($PET_{O_2}$ and $PET_{CO_2}$), inspiratory capacity (IC), and maximum voluntary ventilation (MVV). Although this evaluee had evidence for obstructive and interstitial lung disease at rest, he was limited in his exercise tolerance by a cardiovascular problem, likely previously unsuspected coronary artery disease. Further workup was recommended.

**TABLE 28-1    TREADMILL AND CYCLE ERGOMETER COMPARISONS**

| ATTRIBUTE | TREADMILL | CYCLE |
|---|---|---|
| Quantify external work | Fair | Excellent |
| Highest HR and $\dot{V}E$ | Equal | Equal |
| Highest $\dot{V}O_2$ and $O_2$ pulse | Yes | |
| Familiarity of exercise | Yes | |
| Fewer artifacts in physiologic measurement | | Yes |
| Can be used supine | | Yes |
| Ease of obtaining arterial blood specimens | | Yes |

## MEASUREMENTS DESCRIBING PHYSIOLOGICAL IMPAIRMENTS

### Presentation of Data

Because of the large number of important variables that can be measured and displayed during incremental exercise and later can be graphed or tabulated, it is easy to overwhelm the interpreter or viewer with information. For over a decade, a group at the Harbor-UCLA Medical Center have reported the results of exercise testing using a format that includes (1) a brief history of the patient and description of the protocol, (2) a figure of 9-panels displaying key variables plotted either versus time and work rate or versus each other (Fig. 28-5), (3) a large table listing 10 to 20 variables every half minute, (4) a small table listing key predicted and measured parameters, and (5) an interpretation of the study with recommendations.[54] Table 28-2 lists the more important predicted values for sedentary adult men; Table 28-3 gives exercise data for a typical adult man.

A simpler, but less complete, graphical method of visual presentation of exercise data in another impairment evaluee is shown in Figure 28-6.[24] The two panels on the left illustrate the patterns of $\dot{V}O_2$ and $\dot{V}CO_2$ (upper left) and $PETO_2$, $PETCO_2$, and related blood values (lower left) during rest, three minutes of unloaded cycling exercise, incremental cycling exercise, and recovery. The two panels on the right show the relationships of $\dot{V}O_2$, HR and $O_2$ pulse (upper

**TABLE 28-2    PREDICTED CYCLE EXERCISE VALUES FOR SEDENTARY MIDDLE-AGED MEN**

| MEASURE AND UNITS | APPROXIMATE MEAN VALUE |
|---|---|
| Peak $\dot{V}O_2$, ml/min | (Height in cm – Age in yrs) $\times$ 21 |
| LAT, ml/min | (Height in cm – Age in yrs) $\times$ 11 |
| Peak heart rate, beats/min | 220 – Age in yrs |
| Peak $O_2$ pulse, ml/beat | Peak $\dot{V}O_2$/Peak heart rate |
| $\Delta\dot{V}O_2/\Delta WR$, ml/min/W | 10 |
| Brachial artery blood pressure, mm Hg | 205/95 |
| Exercise breathing reserve, L/min | 35 |
| Breathing frequency, end-exercise, breaths/min | 40 |
| VT/IC, end-exercise | 0.6 |
| $\dot{V}E/\dot{V}CO_2$ at LAT | 29 |
| $\dot{V}E/\dot{V}O_2$ at LAT | 27 |
| $PaO_2$, end-exercise, mm Hg | 90 |
| $P(A–a)O_2$, end-exercise, mm Hg | 20 |
| $P(a–ET)CO_2$, end-exercise, mm Hg | –3 |
| VD/VT, end-exercise | 0.20 |
| Bicarbonate, arterial, end-exercise, mEq/L | 20 |
| pH, arterial, end-exercise | 7.35 |
| Respiratory exchange ratio (R), end-exercise | 1.2 |

right) and the interrelationships of exercise $\dot{V}E$, VT, and $f$ to the preliminary measures of $\dot{V}C$, IC, and MVV (lower right). The center space gives additional information.

## TABLE 28-3  CYCLE EXERCISE VALUES FOR A TYPICAL SEDENTARY 50-YEAR-OLD MAN (170 CM AND 70 KG)

| MEASURE AND UNITS | RESTING | PEAK |
|---|---|---|
| $\dot{V}O_2$, ml/min | 300 | 2300 |
| Heart rate, beats/min | 74 | 170 |
| $O_2$ pulse, ml/beat | 4.2 | 15 |
| Brachial artery blood pressure, mm Hg | 120/72 | 206/95 |
| $\dot{V}E$, L/min | 8 | 102 |
| Breathing frequency, breaths/min | 14 | 42 |
| VT, L | 0.5 | 1.8 |
| $\dot{V}E/\dot{V}CO_2$ | 35 | 29* |
| $\dot{V}E/\dot{V}O_2$ | 30 | 27* |
| $PaO_2$, mm Hg | 88 | 96 |
| $P(A-a)O_2$, mm Hg | 14 | 24 |
| $P(a-ET)CO_2$, mm Hg | 3 | -3 |
| VD/VT | 0.40 | 0.20 |
| Bicarbonate, arterial, mEq/L | 24 | 17 |
| pH, arterial | 7.40 | 7.34 |
| Respiratory exchange (R) | 0.85 | 1.15 |

*At LAT rather than at peak exercise.

Note—Resting values: $\dot{V}C$ = 4.3 L; IC = 2.8 L; $FEV_1$ = 3.3 L; MVV = 135 L/min.

Other values: LAT = 1.2 L/min; breathing reserve = 33 L/min.

Heart rate reserve = 0 beats/min; $\Delta\dot{V}O_2/\Delta WR$ = 10 ml/W.

## Cardiovascular

### Peak $\dot{V}O_2$

A person's ability to increase $\dot{V}O_2$ (measured in L/min or ml/min/kg) to its highest values depends not only on the circulatory system, but also on the quantity of muscle involved in the task being performed: the more muscle involved, the higher the possible $\dot{V}O_2$. For example, in untrained individuals, the peak $\dot{V}O_2$ reached will be least for arm cycling (approximately 50 to 60% of treadmill exercise), much greater for upright leg cycling (approximately 90% of treadmill exercise), and highest for treadmill walking or running (uphill rather than on the level) or tasks that include arm and leg exercise (such as cross-country skiing or combined arm and leg cycling).

Multiple studies have shown that an individual's peak $\dot{V}O_2$ for a given task is similar whether determined by (a) a series of constant work rate tasks repeated at progressively higher intensities (the classical approach, which takes one or more days), or (b) continuous incremental exercise to exhaustion (the practical approach), as long as the incremental work period lasts for a reasonable period of time (e.g., 6 to 14 min).[23,54]

Predicted or "normal" peak $\dot{V}O_2$ values for a given age, weight, gender, and degree of fitness differ slightly between reported series, primarily because of the different attributes of the population selected to be tested.[9,28,30,32] Values derived primarily from nonobese athletes, faculty, graduate students, or military personnel may be inappropriate to use for impairment evaluation. Additionally, peak $\dot{V}O_2$ values derived from Japanese and European populations tend to be higher than values from Canadian or American populations. This is probably due to a lower level of physical activity and physical fitness in North American inhabitants.[30] For disability testing, the authors usually select peak $\dot{V}O_2$ reference values from a sedentary, working, blue-collar population rather than a population oriented to regular leisure sports.[28,54] Readers should refer to Table 28-2 for predicted values and to references for more complete information.[31,54]

Peak $\dot{V}O_2$ values are usually expressed in units of ml/min/kg of body weight for athletes and competitors, with predicted values based on gender, age, and fitness. It is reasonable to express cardiovascular performance this way in nonobese individuals, as peak $\dot{V}O_2$ has a high correlation with lean body mass (which is primarily muscle). Peak $\dot{V}O_2$ values (in L/min) tend to be higher in early adult life, in larger and taller individuals, in men than women of the same age and size, and most importantly, in those engaged in endurance training and more-active lifestyles.

On the other hand, peak $\dot{V}O_2$ values for patients or impairment evaluees should (nearly always) be related to predicted values based primarily on age, gender, and body height rather than age, gender, and body weight.[54] This is not a minor distinction considering the high percentage of overweight evaluees and patients that are referred for exercise testing. Figure 28-7 shows the high incidence of obesity in men and women sent to the authors for exercise testing. On average, 60% of the referred men were 19% overweight, whereas 63% of the referred women were

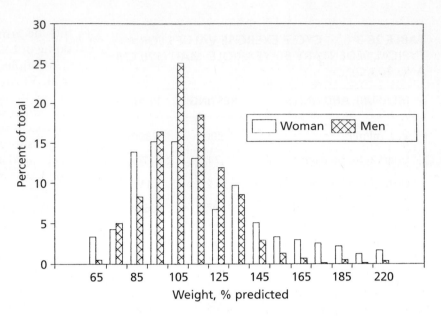

**FIGURE 28-7.** Relationship of actual to predicted weight in approximately one thousand men and women evaluated at the authors' exercise laboratory. Predicted weight for men is 0.79 kg, height is 60.7 cm. Predicted weight for women is 0.65 kg, height is 42.8 cm. Each column indicates the percentage of the total of each gender by decile of predicted weight (e.g., 65 = 60–69.9% of predicted weight), continuing until the last column that indicates those with a mean value of 220% of predicted weight. Values are skewed to the right, indicating more corpulence than a normal population. Less than 1% of the men are less than 70% of their predicted weights, while 14.6% exceed 130% of their predicted weights; 3.4% of the women are less than 70% of their predicted weights, while 28.7% exceed 130% of their predicted weights.

33% overweight. If predicted values for peak $\dot{V}_{O_2}$ (and consequently peak $O_2$ pulse and LAT) in these overweight patients had been based on weight and age rather than height and age, about two-thirds of the healthy men would have had a reduced peak $\dot{V}_{O_2}$, peak $O_2$ pulse, and LAT (81% or less of predicted) and about two-thirds of the healthy women would have had a measured peak $\dot{V}_{O_2}$, peak $O_2$ pulse, and LAT of 67% or less than predicted solely on the basis of excess body weight.

In nonathletes, we conclude that changes in body weight are much more often due to increased body fat than muscle. Consequently, in comparing two individuals of the same height, age, and gender, we should not expect an otherwise healthy individual with 40% body fat to have a peak $\dot{V}_{O_2}$ 20% higher than another person with 20% body fat.

When predicted values for $\dot{V}_{O_2}$, $O_2$ pulse, and LAT are based on weight rather than height (as is done in some laboratories), the obese person with normal cardiovascular function and normal peak $\dot{V}_{O_2}$, $O_2$ pulse, and LAT for height, gender, and age may be deemed to have abnormal cardiovascular function because their measured values will be below the predicted values for peak $\dot{V}_{O_2}$, $O_2$ pulse, and LAT. Indeed, such a person likely has a decreased ability to perform external work, but this decreased work ability is due to obesity rather than cardiovascular disease. Thus, it is of great importance to select appropriate predicted values in impairment evaluation.[54]

### Lactic acidosis threshold (LAT)

Tasks that require an energy expenditure above the LAT require rest periods for recovery. Energy expenditure requiring $\dot{V}_{O_2}$ below the LAT should be considered as moderate or of lesser intensity, whereas $\dot{V}_{O_2}$ above the LAT is considered as heavy, very heavy, or extreme-intensity exercise.[52,55]

In the average young person, the LAT occurs at a $\dot{V}_{O_2}$ value that is approximately 45 to 60% of the peak $\dot{V}_{O_2}$.[54] The LAT does not necessarily occur synchronously with the respiratory compensation point (ventilatory threshold) or when the respiratory exchange ratio exceeds 1.0. It can be detected with repeated arterial blood lactate measurements. It is easiest, however, to recognize the LAT using noninvasive gas exchange measurements with a graphical display of $\dot{V}_{CO_2}$ versus $\dot{V}_{O_2}$ values (center panel of Fig. 28-5) during a progressively increasing work rate test of less than 12 min duration.[6,47] The LAT value should be expressed in units of $\dot{V}_{O_2}$ rather than work rate. Regardless of age, gender, or body size, a LAT that is less than 40% of the predicted (not the measured) peak $\dot{V}_{O_2}$ is abnormal (below the 95% confidence limits) and is indicative of circulatory dysfunction.[54] With physical training, both the LAT and the peak $\dot{V}_{O_2}$ increase. Generally the LAT/peak $\dot{V}_{O_2}$ ratio also increases, to as high as 0.85 in some highly-trained endurance athletes. With maintenance of good health, the LAT/peak $\dot{V}_{O_2}$ ratio also increases with age, probably more in women than men.[54]

### Oxygen uptake/work rate ($\Delta\dot{V}_{O_2}/\Delta WR$) relationships

The opportunity to quantify the $\Delta\dot{V}_{O_2}/\Delta WR$ is an important advantage of cycle ergometry.[26,27] When a steady state is reached during multiple constant work-rate-cycle ergometry tests below the LAT, the steady state $\dot{V}_{O_2}$ increases by approximately 10 ml/min/W, regardless of age, gender, or body size.[13]

Similarly during incremental cycle ergometry to exhaustion of reasonable duration (5 to 20 min), the $\dot{V}_{O_2}$ also increases in healthy persons (after a delay of about ¾ min) by approximately 10 ml/min/W.[26] A smaller increase in $\dot{V}_{O_2}$ per watt increase in work rate (low $\Delta\dot{V}_{O_2}/\Delta WR$) during an incremental test reflects a reduced rate of aerobic metabolism and an increased rate of anaerobic metabolism. Possible causes include failure of the lung to oxygenate the pulmonary blood at an appropriate rate, an inability of the circulatory system effectively to transport $O_2$, a high resistance to diffusion at the capillary level, or a defect in aerobic enzymes or the electron transport chain in muscle mitochondria.[27] Although not everyone with these disorders has a statistically significant decrease in $\Delta\dot{V}_{O_2}/\Delta WR$, the finding of a low $\Delta\dot{V}_{O_2}/\Delta WR$ indicates a reduced use of atmospheric $O_2$ and a higher-than-normal use of anaerobic metabolism to support muscle bioenergetics.

### Oxygen pulse ($\dot{V}_{O_2}/HR$)

Regardless of age, gender, or body size, a near-linear relationship between $\dot{V}_{O_2}$ and HR from rest to exhaustive exercise is noted in every healthy person.[54] The $\dot{V}_{O_2}$ in ml/min divided by the HR in beats/min equals the $\dot{V}_{O_2}/HR$ in ml/beat and is identified as the *$O_2$ pulse*. Graphically, these relationships can be observed in Figures 28-5 and 28-6. Note that the linear intercept of HR versus $\dot{V}_{O_2}$ intersects the HR axis well above zero.

The predicted peak $O_2$ pulse for normal individuals can be calculated by dividing their predicted peak $\dot{V}_{O_2}$ (based on age, gender, and height) by their predicted peak HR (220 minus age). From the Fick principle, which relates cardiac output to $\dot{V}_{O_2}$, it can be shown that the $O_2$ pulse is the product of *(a)* effective ventricular stroke volume and *(b)* the difference between the arterial and mixed-venous $O_2$ contents. Any process that *(a)* decreases maximal stroke volume (e.g., valvular heart disease, cardiomyopathy, coronary artery disease, pulmonary vascular disease, or peripheral vascular disease), *(b)* decreases arterial $O_2$ content (anemia, hypoxemia, or carboxyhemoglobinemia), or *(c)* increases mixed-venous $O_2$ content (poor peripheral $O_2$ extraction or inability to increase exercise to higher levels because of the presence of other systemic disease) will reduce the peak $O_2$ pulse.[54]

During incremental exercise the $O_2$ pulse normally increases in a curvilinear fashion from rest to exhaustion (Fig. 28-5, top center panel). A change from this pattern during an incremental exercise test indicates dysfunction in $O_2$ transport. A smaller than appropriate increase of the $O_2$ pulse during increasing exertion indicates that the product of stroke volume and $O_2$ extraction has prematurely reached its maximal

value. In many persons with coronary artery disease who have myocardial ischemia with exercise without angina, the $O_2$ pulse abruptly stops increasing concurrent with the development of significant ST segment or T wave abnormalities, indicating ventricular dysfunction.[54] (See the reference for case examples of this functional impairment of cardiac output detected non-invasively when ECG changes consistent with myocardial ischemia develop.) This finding is important because the ECG changes alone may be difficult to interpret. (See also Fig. 28-6.)

### $\dot{V}_{O_2}$ kinetics: mean response time (MRT) and change in $\dot{V}_{O_2}$ from 3 to 6 min [$\Delta\dot{V}_{O_2}(6-3)$]

In the transition from a low metabolic steady state (sitting or cycle exercise with unloaded pedalling at 60 cycles per minute) to a moderate-intensity exercise in normal persons, it takes two to three minutes for the $\dot{V}_{O_2}$ to reach a steady state. The normal $\dot{V}_{O_2}$ MRT (63% of the steady-state response) is approximately ½ min. Longer values indicate $O_2$ delivery or utilization problems, such as primary cardiac disease, pulmonary vascular disease, or peripheral vascular disease.[41] In the latter illness, the MRT is much improved following surgical correction of the vascular obstructions and reestablishment of better $O_2$ delivery to the exercising leg muscles.[4]

During exercise at a constant work rate above the LAT, the $\dot{V}_{O_2}$ does not reach a constant value in 3 min but continues to rise. The higher the intensity of the exercise, the more obvious is the lack of a steady state. In such constant work tests, the difference in the $\dot{V}_{O_2}$ between 3 and 6 min can be quantitated.[13,40] The finding of a positive $\Delta\dot{V}_{O_2}(6-3)$ identifies exercise above the LAT. The $\Delta\dot{V}_{O_2}(6-3)$ is proportional to lactate in normal subjects and patients with heart disease.[54]

### Blood pressure

Both systolic and diastolic pressures continue to rise as work rate increases with the systolic rising much more than the diastolic. Commonly systolic pressure reaches values over 200 mm Hg while intra-arterial recorded diastolic pressure reaches about 100 mm Hg. By auscultation, fifth phase diastolic pressures may rise, but usually remain stable or decline minimally.[39]

### Electrocardiogram

The development of downsloping ST segment depression is suggestive, but not diagnostic, of myocardial ischemia. The development or increase in the number of premature ventricular contractions or a significant atrial arrhythmia during exercise also suggests myocardial ischemia.

## Respiratory Mechanics

When resting respiratory function testing does not reveal severe abnormalities in respiratory mechanics, exercise tests are needed to determine impairment. In evaluees with moderate airway obstruction or restriction, exercise studies are needed to evaluate ventilation/perfusion mismatching and whether hypoxemia develops. For example, the comparison of integrated cardiopulmonary exercise tests with resting respiratory function tests is helpful in deciding whether a person is limited in ventilatory ability during exercise. Preliminarily, it is preferable to measure the maximal voluntary ventilation (MVV) directly; if this is not done, it should be estimated by multiplying the $FEV_1$ times 40.[11] Initially, as exercise begins, $\dot{V}E$ rises primarily by increasing VT; as the work rate increases, ventilatory frequency (f) also increases. Ventilation is likely to be limiting exercise if (a) the maximum exercise ventilation ($\dot{V}E_{max}$) closely approaches (i.e., within 10 to 15 L/min) the maximal voluntary ventilation (MVV) measured prior to exercise (identified as a low exercise breathing reserve); (b) the exercise VT approaches to within 10% the resting inspiratory capacity (IC); or (c) the f exceeds 50 per minute.[54]

There are two other findings suggestive of ventilatory limitation. One is a rise in $Pa_{CO_2}$ during heavy exercise. With normal ventilatory control, the development of a lactic acidosis during heavy exercise stimulates ventilation causing $PA_{CO_2}$ and $Pa_{CO_2}$ to decline, which in turn, tends to minimize the acidemia. If ventilation is mechanically limited, it fails to increase appropriately in response to the exercise lactic acidosis. The resulting increase in $Pa_{CO_2}$ late in the exercise test aggravates the metabolically induced acidemia so that arterial pH decreases more than normal. Such a respiratory acidosis is sometimes seen in patients with severe obstructive or (less commonly) restrictive lung disease who are limited in ventilatory ability. A mild respiratory acidosis is also tolerated by some elite athletes who have learned to reduce their ventilatory requirements at very high work levels.[54]

The other evidence for ventilatory limitation, which can be recognized without blood gas measures, is a lack of the normal prompt decrease in $\dot{V}E$ early during recovery accompanying the prompt decrease in HR early in recovery.

## Ventilation/Perfusion Mismatching

### Ventilatory equivalents for $O_2$ ($\dot{V}E/\dot{V}O_2$) and $CO_2$ ($\dot{V}E/\dot{V}CO_2$)

Ventilatory equivalents express the efficiency of ventilation related to metabolism. They are defined as the liters of $\dot{V}E$, BTPS (body temperature and pressure, saturated) required per liter of $\dot{V}O_2$ or $\dot{V}CO_2$, STPD (standard temperature and pressure, dry). Normally, the $\dot{V}E/\dot{V}CO_2$ and the $\dot{V}E/\dot{V}O_2$ decline from resting values of 35 to 60 to values of 30 or less near the LAT for $\dot{V}E/\dot{V}CO_2$, and 27 or less for $\dot{V}E/\dot{V}O_2$. They then increase considerably as metabolic acidosis develops. If the $\dot{V}E/\dot{V}O_2$ and $\dot{V}E/\dot{V}CO_2$ do not decline appropriately at the LAT, a high VD/VT (dead space volume/tidal volume ratio) is likely to be the cause. However, elevated ventilatory equivalents can also be due to an unusually low $Pa_{CO_2}$ (as with acute hyperventilation, chronic respiratory alkalosis, or chronic metabolic acidosis).[54] In evaluees with elevated ventilatory equivalents at the LAT, the authors recommend that arterial blood gas measurements be made and matched to concurrent expired gas measurements during high intensity exercise. These simultaneous measurements should clarify the cause of the high $\dot{V}E/\dot{V}O_2$.

End-tidal pressures of $O_2$ and $CO_2$ ($PET_{O_2}$ and $PET_{CO_2}$), which are easy to obtain noninvasively, give indications of mean alveolar values of $O_2$ and $CO_2$ and their trends only in normal persons but cannot reliably predict alveolar or arterial $p_{CO_2}$ or $p_{O_2}$ values in patients or evaluees.

### Dead space/tidal volume ratio (VD/VT)

The evaluee's physiologic VD/VT is calculated from knowing mixed expired $CO_2$, $Pa_{CO_2}$, VT, and the dead space of the breathing valve and mouthpiece or face mask. Physiologic VD/VT cannot be validly measured noninvasively without measures of $Pa_{CO_2}$ (in contrast to that purported by some commercial exercise systems). Normally the VD/VT decreases from rest to exercise as the VT increases and perfusion of the airspaces with high $CO_2$-laden blood increases. In normal older men, the VD/VT falls to 0.30 or less at maximal exercise; in younger men the decrease is even greater.[28,33,44,54,56] In persons with primary or secondary pulmonary vascular disease or severe maldistribution of ventilation to perfusion, the VD/VT does not decline appropriately and may be increased at rest and markedly increased with exercise.

### Arterial-end tidal carbon dioxide pressure difference [P(a-ET)$_{CO_2}$]

The $Pa_{CO_2}$ at rest, which reflects the ideal $PA_{CO_2}$, is slightly higher than the $PET_{CO_2}$.[33] As exercise progresses, the $PET_{CO_2}$ normally becomes higher than the $Pa_{CO_2}$. This finding is so consistent that a positive P(a-ET)$_{CO_2}$ at the end of exercise is equivalent to a pathologic increase in physiologic VD/VT (over 0.30) (i.e., evidence for uneven ventilation/perfusion relationships due to lung or pulmonary vascular disease).[44,54]

## Alveolar-arterial $O_2$ pressure difference [$P(A-a)o_2$]

The $P(A-a)o_2$ may remain constant but usually increases during exercise, even to as high as 30 to 35 mm Hg.[54] Greater increases are usually due to ventilation/perfusion mismatching but may also be due to diffusion abnormalities or blood shunting through a patent foramen ovale.

## Other Measures

Normally there is a few percentage increase in hematocrit and hemoglobin during incremental exercise. With heavy exercise, the $Sao_2$ remains relatively constant despite a decrease in pH (rightward shift in oxyhemoglobin dissociation curve) due to a small increase in $Pao_2$. Values found with ear or finger oximetry during exercise often, but not invariably, parallel simultaneously directly measured arterial oxyhemoglobin saturation.[17] The discrepancies between directly measured and peripherally estimated blood saturations are likely to be greater during intense exercise, when perfusion of the ear or finger may be compromised.[25]

With high-intensity exercise not limited by ventilatory disorders, arterial bicarbonate decreases approximately equimolar to the increase in blood lactate concentration.[5] Concurrently, mixed-venous $po_2$ oxyhemoglobin saturation, $O_2$ content, and pH decline precipitously, while mixed-venous $pco_2$ and actual bicarbonate levels rise strikingly.[14,42]

The respiratory exchange ratio (R) rises with the production and elimination of excess $CO_2$ during exercise. During early recovery, R increases further, reflecting the abrupt decrease in $\dot{V}o_2$ and elimination of tissue $CO_2$ stores that had increased during exercise and further hyperventilation secondary to arterial acidemia. If R does not increase to over 1.05 during recovery, it is likely that the maximal exercise level was below the LAT.[28,44,54]

## PATHOPHYSIOLOGY OF WORK INTOLERANCE AND DISEASE

For a comprehensive presentation of pathophysiology, readers should refer to Reference 54 for actual case reports, partially illustrated here in the form of 9-panel plots (Fig. 28-5). The box on this page lists some case examples from the reference. Limited comments on pathophysiology follow.

## CASE REPORT EXAMPLES AVAILABLE FOR REVIEW AND STUDY*

Normal men and women
Normal athlete
Cycle and treadmill compared
Air and $O_2$ breathing compared
Effect of acute cigarette smoking
Pre-β and post-β adrenergic blockade
Poor effort
Acute hyperventilation
Coronary artery disease
Cardiomyopathy
Valvular heart disease
Congestive heart failure
Heart disease with oscillatory gas exchange
Congenital heart disease
Vasoregulatory asthenia
Patent ductus arteriosus
Pulmonary arterio-venous fistulae
Peripheral vascular disease
Anemia
Carboxyhemoglobinemia
Pulmonary hypertension with patent foramen ovale
Thromboembolic pulmonary vascular disease
Pulmonary vasculitis
Mica pneumoconiosis
Pulmonary microlithiasis
Idiopathic interstitial lung disease, before and after corticosteroids
Alveolar proteinosis, before and after lavage
Sarcoidosis
Asbestosis
Mixed connective tissue disease
Lung cancer with preoperative evaluation
Bullous emphysema
Emphysema
Chronic bronchitis
Asthma
Obstructive lung disease, before and after rehabilitation
Obstructive lung disease, room air and oxygen
Extreme obesity

*Many of the 70+ cases have more than one disorder. (From Wasserman K, Hansen JE, Sue DY, et al: *Principles of exercise testing and interpretation*, ed 2, Philadelphia, 1994, Lea & Febiger.)

## Obesity

Obesity is an important factor in work intolerance for many reasons. Obese persons have higher $\dot{V}_{O_2}$ requirements at all work rates than their leaner counterparts.[49] The effect of obesity on the $\dot{V}_{O_2}$ requirement for work depends on how overweight the subject is and whether the body is supported or ambulatory when performing the work tasks. Ambulatory work, especially, has higher $\dot{V}_{O_2}$ requirements in the obese. It should be stressed that the $\dot{V}_{O_2}$ requirement for unloaded cycling (no external work accomplished) is primarily dependent on the weight of the legs. The efficiency in performing external work while cycling in normal obese subjects is normal (i.e., $\Delta\dot{V}_{O_2}/\Delta WR = 10$ ml/min/W.

It is preferable to discriminate between cardiovascular disease and obesity by basing predicted peak $\dot{V}_{O_2}$ values on height rather than on weight.[28,54] Resting hypoxemia is common in obese persons and may suggest that an evaluee has primary lung disease. The relief of hypoxemia during mild-to-moderate exercise, however, indicates that the resting hypoxemia was due to obesity-induced atelectasis at the lung bases, which cleared as tidal volume increased.[54] Thus obesity is a significant disadvantage, even without considering accompanying complicating illnesses such as atherosclerosis, hypertension, and diabetes mellitus.

## Heart, Pulmonary Vascular, and Peripheral Vascular Disease

Many persons with cardiovascular disorders have normal electrocardiographic, hemodynamic, and gas exchange findings at rest but have distinctly abnormal findings during integrative cardiopulmonary exercise testing. Any of these disorders may manifest a reduced ability to transport $O_2$ from the lungs to the cells, as evidenced by a low peak $\dot{V}_{O_2}$, low LAT, low or abnormal $O_2$ pulse, or low $\Delta\dot{V}_{O_2}/\Delta WR$. In the case of coronary artery disease, these abnormalities plus electrocardiographic abnormalities may be evident only at high-work intensities. Patients with cardiomyopathy or valvular heart disease often evidence dysfunction at lower work rates.[54]

Cardiac output increase in response to exercise may also be severely limited by pulmonary vascular disease, whether embolic, secondary to destruction of the pulmonary vascular bed (e.g., interstitial lung disease or emphysema) or idiopathic (e.g., primary pulmonary hypertension). An increase in pulmonary vascular resistance impedes blood flow from the right ventricle to the left ventricle. The low cardiac output response causes a low work rate lactic acidosis that stimulates ventilation. Additionally, with pulmonary vascular disease, the VD/VT is increased (which increases the ventilatory requirement) while hypoxemia (a potent ventilatory stimulus) commonly develops during exercise. Thus dyspnea is a common feature of pulmonary vascular disease.

With peripheral vascular disease, sclerotic vessels may restrict blood flow to the exercising extremities. In addition to low peak $\dot{V}_{O_2}$, LAT, $O_2$ pulse and $\Delta\dot{V}_{O_2}/\Delta WR$, the MRT is elevated and systemic blood pressure usually rises more than expected for the level of exercise performed. Commonly, pain in the affected lower leg or legs is given as the reason for stopping exercise.

## Obstructive Lung Disease

Resting pulmonary function tests are usually abnormal in persons with asthma, chronic bronchitis, or emphysema, except for those with only exercise-induced asthma. Exercise limitation may be due to airway obstruction (with reduced ability to increase ventilation) and/or ventilation/perfusion mismatching (which increases the ventilatory requirement). When ventilation is limiting, the exercise breathing reserve (resting MVV - $\dot{V}_{E_{max}}$) is low (usually in the range of -5 to +15 L/min). Patients with predominant obstructive disease rarely have exercise ventilatory frequencies higher than 45/min. When exercise is ventilatory limited, it is common for the peak $\dot{V}_{O_2}$ to be reduced, the HR reserve to be high, and the subject to complain of dyspnea as the limiting factor during the exercise test. With well-motivated persons with obstructive lung disease, the $Pa_{CO_2}$ may rise near the end of incremental exercise, indicating that a respiratory acidosis is accompanying the exercise-induced metabolic acidosis. If exercise is chronically limited by obstructive lung disease, then the LAT may be also reduced because of the inactivity of the patient.[54]

## Restrictive Lung Disease

Some interstitial diseases are subtle and difficult to diagnose even after thorough laboratory and radiologic investigation at rest. In such individuals, exercise testing may be critically important because hypoxemia during heavy exercise may be the only conclusive evidence short of open lung biopsy of otherwise latent interstitial lung disease.[22] Other patients with restrictive disease have obvious abnormalities at rest and exercise. In patients with severe interstitial lung disease, the breathing reserve tends to be low, breathing frequency high, and VT/IC approaches 1.0, while blood gases, P(a–ET)$_{CO_2}$ and VD/VT may be clearly abnormal.[54]

With either obstructive or restrictive lung disease, an accompanying pulmonary vascular disease (which may be evidenced by a low gas transfer index or diffusing capacity for carbon monoxide [$D_{LCO}$] at rest) commonly causes a reduction in maximal stroke volume and maximal cardiac output so that the peak $\dot{V}_{O_2}$, LAT, $O_2$ pulse, and $\Delta\dot{V}_{O_2}/\Delta WR$ may also be abnormal, causing more impairment than is evident from resting pulmonary function studies.[54]

Similarly, measurements of VD/VT, P(a–ET)$_{CO_2}$, Pa$_{O_2}$, and P(A–a)$_{O_2}$ during exercise are often more useful than resting measurements for the purpose of defining ventilation-perfusion mismatching.

## Anemia, Carboxyhemoglobinemia, and Cigarette Smoking

Any mechanism that reduces the capacity of blood to take up $O_2$ in the lungs also reduces the ability of the circulatory system to deliver $O_2$.[34] Even if the Pa$_{O_2}$ and Sa$_{O_2}$ are normal, the $O_2$ content of arterial blood (Ca$_{O_2}$) is reduced in proportion to the reduction in available hemoglobin. At rest and at low activity levels, such a reduction in Ca$_{O_2}$ may be compensated for by increased extraction of $O_2$ from the peripheral blood (a lower mixed-venous $O_2$ content) and/or by an increase in cardiac output. Because of reduced $O_2$ transport, lactic acidosis develops at a reduced work rate, and the LAT and peak $\dot{V}_{O_2}$ are reduced in proportion to the reduction in available hemoglobin.[34] The same work rate, consequently, is less-well tolerated than in an individual not so affected. A reduction in available hemoglobin due to carboxyhemoglobinemia increases the work of the heart more than a reduction due to anemia because the carboxyhemoglobin must be circulated. Acute cigarette, cigar, or pipe smoking not only cause carboxyhemoglobinemia, but also increase HR and blood pressure and may decrease ventilation/perfusion matching.[29] The adverse effects of chronic tobacco abuse on the respiratory and circulatory systems are too numerous to enumerate here.

## β-Adrenergic Blockade

Patients on β-adrenergic blocking drugs are frequently referred for disability evaluation. The practice is to evaluate and exercise such persons without modifying their drug intake. If the β-blockade is high, the likely changes from predicted exercise values (in persons with otherwise normal cardiovascular systems) are likely to be a large reduction in peak HR, a mild-to-moderate reduction in peak $\dot{V}_{O_2}$, and a moderate increase in the peak $O_2$ pulse.[54] The high $O_2$ pulse reflects an increase in time of ventricular filling

and a resultant increase in effective stroke volume. Whether the patient should be retested after reducing β-blockade depends on whether β-blockade can be safely decreased, and the desire to increase the patient's exercise tolerance.

## Defects in Bioenergetics

Rarely persons are found to have deficiencies in $O_2$ utilization by the exercising muscle due to enzymatic or metabolic disorders, usually genetic. Because $O_2$ is not extracted from the capillary blood and metabolized normally by patients with these disorders, the muscle end-capillary and mixed-venous $O_2$ contents do not decline to low levels during intense exercise, as they do in normal subjects and patients with the usual circulatory disorders.[36,54] Patients with these defects usually demonstrate a high peak HR, low peak $\dot{V}_{O_2}$, and low $O_2$ pulse during exercise testing. In patients with McArdle's syndrome, for example, there is considerable muscle pain during maximal exercise without elevation of blood lactate values.[36] The HR response is high and $O_2$ extraction is low, indicating the failure of the muscles to utilize $O_2$ normally. In other patients, muscle biopsy and enzymatic analysis or measurements of mixed-venous blood may be necessary to establish a diagnosis.

## Secondary Gain and Anxiety

In some individuals, the secondary gain associated with disability evaluation makes testing more difficult. All evaluees are encouraged to perform as well as possible during all preexercise and exercise tests so that the evaluation will provide a conclusive diagnosis to which the evaluees' symptoms can be attributed. When behavior and test results are erratic, the evaluees are told that such findings are not advantageous for them. If an exercise test shows a low peak $\dot{V}_{O_2}$, a high HR reserve, a high breathing reserve, no suggestion of gas exchange abnormality, a normal LAT, a low recovery $R$, no local musculoskeletal cause for cessation of exercise, and the reason the evaluee stopped exercise is not clear and logical, there is no choice but to attribute the limited performance to poor effort. The evaluee is encouraged to repeat the exercise test. If the ventilatory equivalents are high or if oximetry is not entirely normal, a second test with an arterial line is helpful.[54]

Evidences for high anxiety are a bizarre or irregular ventilatory pattern with intermittent and episodic breathing, especially at rest and early in exercise; a high $R$ during rest and early exercise (hyperventilation) and a high resting HR. Ordinarily, the physiologic requirements of increasing work rate soon override the manifestations of anxiety, and the circulatory and ventilatory response approach normal.[54]

## APPLICATIONS OF CARDIOPULMONARY EXERCISE TESTING FOR DISABILITY EVALUATION AND FOLLOW-UP

### The Risk in Relying on Resting Studies Alone

In a 1971 study of 14 patients with extremely severe obstructive lung disease (mean $FEV_1$ 29% of predicted), Vyas et al[48] found that 80% of the variance of peak $\dot{V}O_2$ was explained by the $FEV_1$. Thus it is tempting to rely on the American Thoracic Society statement[2] hypothesis that exercise limitation and peak $\dot{V}O_2$ can be correctly predicted by regression analysis using resting respiratory function tests alone in impairment evaluees with a diversity of lung diseases.

Sue has recently summarized and pointed out several problems in the use of this hypothesis.[43] First, in individuals with demonstrated reduced ventilatory capacity at rest ($FEV_1$ or MVV), ventilatory requirements during exercise are dependent not only on ventilatory capacity but on the ventilatory requirement. The latter depends on the efficiency of gas exchange (ventilation/perfusion matching or mismatching), the ventilatory set point ($PaCO_2$), ventilatory drive (lung receptors, hypoxemia, metabolically induced acidemia), and the respiratory exchange ratio. Second, data from a recent larger study did not validate the hypothesis that exercise limitation can be quantified by resting pulmonary function testing. Cotes and coworkers,[19] in examining 157 referred men with a variety of lung diseases and abnormal resting studies (low $FEV_1$, FVC, $FEV_1$/FVC, or $D_{LCO}$) who stopped exercise because of dyspnea (rather than other causes), found that the best combination of resting pulmonary function tests could account for only 29% of the variance of peak $\dot{V}O_2$ and 14% of the peak $\dot{V}O_2$ in % predicted. As might be expected, both Cotes[19] and Carlson,[12] with 110 patients, found that adding values obtained during exercise appreciably improved their ability to predict peak $\dot{V}O_2$ or peak work rate using multiple regression analysis, but that the high variability of the prediction limited its usefulness in individual patients. Dillard[21] points out the difficulty in transferring such predicting formulas from one laboratory to the other. Third, ventilatory limitation is frequently not the factor limiting exercise in patients with known lung disease.[54] Lastly, the finding of abnormal blood gases during exercise is poorly predicted from resting studies.[46]

### Differential Diagnosis

Many potential evaluees have symptoms and findings at rest that are suggestive of either or both heart and lung disease. Exercise testing with has exchange measurements is a logical early step in deciding which organ system is most limiting to evaluees in their work. An example will be given.

Consider an obese 53-year-old, cigarette-smoking, male foundry worker who has dyspnea, a daily cough, infrequent wheezing, and complains of vague epigastric discomfort with exertion or emotional upset. Routine examination discloses systemic hypertension, normal heart and breath sounds, normal 12-lead ECG, and chest roentgenograms suggestive of interstitial lung disease. Respiratory function studies show a mildly reduced VC, a moderately reduced $FEV_1$, MVV, and $D_{LCO}$. Resting arterial blood shows mild hypoxemia, mild hypercarbia, and a carboxyhemoglobin of 6%. It is unclear whether the evaluee's dyspnea is due primarily to obesity, obstructive or interstitial lung disease, or to coronary artery disease. On incremental cycle ergometry with gas exchange, arterial blood, and ECG measurements, one of the following scenarios might occur:

1. At a moderate work rate the ECG shows 2 mm ST segment depression in the lateral chest leads, while the $\dot{V}O_2$ increases more slowly and the $O_2$ pulse does not increase appropriately as exercise is continued beyond this work rate. This strongly suggests that coronary artery disease is limiting cardiac output and $O_2$ transport increase when the ECG changes. Thus coronary artery disease is likely the dominant disorder.

2. The evaluee's exercise ventilation reaches his MVV with a ventilatory frequency of 55. The evaluee's peak $\dot{V}O_2$ nearly reaches his predicted peak $\dot{V}O_2$. However, he also becomes progressively hypoxemic and has an elevated VD/VT. The ECG remains normal. The finding of progressive hypoxemia, increased VD/VT, and tachypnea during exercise suggests that he has interstitial lung disease and not coronary artery disease.

3. The resting hypoxemia resolves with exercise and the ECG remains normal. This indicates that the resting hypoxemia is due to obesity atelectasis rather than intrinsic lung disease.

4. The evaluee remains minimally hypoxemic and stops exercise close to his MVV with a ventilatory frequency of 35, a peak HR of 140, and a normal ECG. This indicates that the disorder limiting the evaluee's exercise tolerance is obstructive lung disease.

In patients with known obstructive or restrictive lung disease, exercise testing may clarify not only whether impairment exists but also whether the limitation is primarily ventilatory or whether the impairment is secondary to accompanying pulmonary vascular disease and its effect on cardiac output.

## Severity of Impairment

Exercise testing also assists in quantitating the severity of the impairment. This is one of the many sources of data that helps the examiners, both medical and nonmedical, in deciding the extent of impairment and whether a person is disabled. In the example given above, the exercise findings would assist not only in establishing a diagnosis, but also in planning the most effective therapy and follow-up.

## Assessment of Therapy

Exercise studies are often more useful than resting measures in assessing the results of therapy, whether it be pharmacotherapy (e.g., β-blockers for heart disease or β-agonists for obstructive lung disease); vessel repair of coronary artery or peripheral vascular disease; physical therapy for rehabilitation of patients with ventilatory limitation,[15] obesity, or coronary artery disease; $O_2$ therapy for interstitial, obstructive, or pulmonary vascular disease; or adjustment of cardiac pacemakers.

## References

1. Ainsworth BE, Haskell WL, Leon AS, et al: Compendium of physical activities: classification of energy costs of human physical activities. *Med Sci Sports Exerc* 25:71, 1993.
2. American Thoracic Society: Evaluation of impairment/disability secondary to respiratory disorders. *Am Rev Respir Dis* 133:1205, 1986.
3. Astrand P-O, Rodahl K: *Textbook of work physiology: physiological bases of exercise*, ed 3, New York, 1986, McGraw-Hill.
4. Auchincloss JH Jr, Ashoutosh K, Rana S, et al: Effect of cardiac, pulmonary, and vascular disease on one-minute oxygen uptake. *Chest* 70:486, 1976.
5. Beaver WL, Wasserman K, Whipp BJ: Bicarbonate buffering of lactic acid generated during exercise. *J Appl Physiol* 60:472, 1986.
6. Beaver WL, Wasserman K, Whipp BJ: A new method for detecting the anaerobic threshold by gas exchange. *J Appl Physiol* 60:2020, 1986.
7. Beaver WL, Wasserman K, Whipp BJ: On-line computer analysis and breath-by-breath graphical display of exercise function tests. *J Appl Physiol* 34:128, 1973.
8. Brooks GA, Fahey TD: *Exercise physiology: human bioenergetics and its applications*. New York, 1984, Wiley.
9. Bruce RA, Kusimi F, Hosmer D: Maximal oxygen uptake and nomographic assessment of functional aerobic impairment in cardiovascular disease. *Am Heart J* 85:546, 1973.
10. Buchfuhrer MJ, Hansen JE, Robinson TE, et al: Optimizing the exercise protocol for cardiopulmonary assessment. *J Appl Physiol* 55:1558, 1983.
11. Campbell SC: A comparison of the maximal voluntary ventilation with forced expiratory volume in one second: an assessment of patient cooperation. *J Occup Med* 24:531, 1982.
12. Carlson TA: Exercise capacity in patients with chronic obstructive lung disease. *Chest* 100:297, 1991.
13. Casaburi R, Barstow TJ, Robinson T, et al: Influence of work rate on ventilatory and gas exchange kinetics. *J Appl Physiol* 67:547, 1989.
14. Casaburi R, Daly J, Hansen JE, et al: Abrupt changes in mixed venous blood gas composition after the onset of exercise. *J Appl Physiol* 67:1106, 1989.
15. Casaburi R, Patessio A, Ioli F, et al: Reduction in exercise lactic acidosis and ventilation as a result of exercise training in patients with obstructive lung disease. *Am Rev Respir Dis* 143:9, 1991.
16. Casaburi R, Weissman ML, Huntsman DJ, et al: Determinants of gas exchange kinetics during exercise in the dog. *J Appl Physiol* 46:1054, 1979.
17. Clark JS, Votteri B, Ariagno RL, et al: Noninvasive assessment of blood gases. *Am Rev Respir Dis* 145:220, 1992.
18. Consolazio CF, Johnson RE, Pecora LJ: *Physiological measurements of metabolic functions in man*, New York, 1963, McGraw-Hill.
19. Cotes JE, Zejda J, King B: Lung function impairment as a guide to exercise limitation in work-related lung disorders. *Am Rev Respir Dis* 137:1089, 1988.
20. Dempsey JA, Hansen PG, Henderson, KS: Exercise-induced arterial hypoxemia in healthy persons at sea level. *J Physiol* (London) 355:161, 1984.
21. Dillard TA: Exercise capacity in patients with chronic obstructive pulmonary disease. *Chest* 100:297, 1991.

22. Epler GR, McLoud TC, Gaensler EA, et al: Normal chest roentgenograms in chronic diffuse infiltrative lung disease. *N Engl J Med* 298:934, 1978.

23. Hansen JE: Exercise instruments, schemes, and protocols for evaluating the dyspneic patient. *Am Rev Respir Dis* 129:S25, 1984.

24. Hansen JE: Exercise testing for the pulmonologist. In DF Tierney, editor: *Current pulmonology,* 14:43-72, St Louis, 1993, Mosby-Year Book.

25. Hansen JE, Casaburi R: Validity of ear oximetry in clinical exercise testing. *Chest* 91:333, 1987.

26. Hansen JE, Casaburi R, Cooper DM, et al: Oxygen uptake as related to work rate increment during cycle ergometer exercise. *Eur J Appl Physiol* 57:140, 1988.

27. Hansen JE, Sue DY, Oren A, et al: Relation of oxygen uptake to work rate in normal men and men with circulatory disorders. *Am J Cardiol* 59:669, 1987.

28. Hansen JE, Sue DY, Wasserman K: Predicted values for clinical exercise testing. *Am Rev Respir Dis* 129:S49-S55, 1984.

29. Hirsch GL, Sue DY, Wasserman K, et al: Immediate effects of cigarette smoking on cardiorespiratory responses to exercise. *J Appl Physiol* 58:1975, 1985.

30. Itoh H, Tanaguchi K, Koike A, et al: Evaluation of severity of heart failure using ventilatory gas analysis. *Circulation* 81(Suppl 2):31, 1990.

31. Jones NL, Campbell EJM: *Clinical exercise testing,* ed 3, Philadelphia, 1988, WB Saunders.

32. Jones NL, Makrides l, Hitchcock C, et al: Normal standards for an incremental progressive cycle ergometer test. *Am Rev Respir Dis* 131:700, 1985.

33. Jones NL, McHardy GJR, Naimark A, et al: Physiological dead space and alveolar-arterial gas pressure differences during exercise. *Clin Sci* 31:19, 1966.

34. Koike A, Weiler-Ravell D, McKenzie DK, et al: Evidence that the metabolic acidosis threshold is the anaerobic threshold. *J Appl Physiol* 68:2521, 1990.

35. Lehninger AL: *Biochemistry,* New York, 1971, Worth.

36. Lewis SF, Haller RG: The pathophysiology of McArdle's disease: clues to regulation in exercise and fatigue. *J Appl Physiol* 61:391, 1986.

37. McGilvery RW: *Biochemistry: a functional approach,* Philadelphia, 1970, WB Saunders.

38. Rahn H, Fenn WO: A graphical analysis of the respiratory gas exchange: the $O_2$-$CO_2$ diagram. Washington, DC, 1955, American Physiological Society.

39. Robinson TE, Sue DY, Huszczuk A, et al: Intra-arterial and cuff blood pressure responses during incremental cycle ergometry. *Med Sci Sports Exerc* 20:142, 1988.

40. Roston WL, Whipp BJ, Davis JA, et al: Oxygen uptake kinetics and lactate concentration during exercise in man. *Am Rev Respir Dis* 135:1080, 1987.

41. Sietsema KE: Oxygen uptake kinetics in response to exercise in patients with pulmonary vascular disease. *Am Rev Respir Dis* 145:1052, 1992.

42. Stringer WL: Personal communication.

43. Sue DY: Exercise testing in the evaluation of impairment and disability. *Clin Chest Med* (in press).

44. Sue DY, Hansen JE: Normal values in adults during exercise testing. *Clin Chest Med* 5:89, 1984.

45. Sue DY, Hansen JE, Blais M, et al: Measurement and analysis of gas exchange during exercise using a programmable calculator. *J Appl Physiol* 49:456, 1980.

46. Sue DY, Oren A, Hansen JE, et al: Single breath diffusing capacity for carbon monoxide as a predictor of lung function and exercise gas exchange. *N Engl J Med* 316:1301, 1987.

47. Sue DY, Wasserman K, Moricca RB, et al: Metabolic acidosis during exercise in chronic obstructive pulmonary disease. *Chest* 94:931, 1988.

48. Vyas MN, Banister EW, Morton JW, et al: Response to exercise in patients with airways obstruction. *Am Rev Respir Dis* 103:410, 1971.

49. Wasserman K: Dyspnea on exertion. *JAMA* 248:2093, 1982.

50. Wasserman K: Breathing during exercise. *N Engl J Med* 298:780, 1978.

51. Wasserman K: The anaerobic threshold measurement to evaluate exercise performance. *Am Rev Respir Dis* 129(Suppl):35, 1984.

52. Wasserman K, Beaver WL, Whipp BJ: Gas exchange theory and the lactic acidosis (anaerobic) threshold. *Circulation* 81(Suppl 2):4, 1990.

53. Wasserman K, Hansen JE, Sue DY: Facilitation of oxygen consumption by lactic acidosis during exercise. *News Physiol Sci* 6:29, 1991.

54. Wasserman K, Hansen JE, Sue DY, et al: *Principles of exercise testing and interpretation,* ed 2, Philadelphia, 1994, Lea & Febiger.

55. Wasserman K, McIlroy MB: Detecting the threshold of anaerobic metabolism in cardiac patients during exercise. *Am J Cardiol* 14:844, 1964.

56. Wasserman K, Van Kessel Al, Burton GG: Interaction of physiological mechanisms during exercise. *J Appl Physiol* 22:71, 1967.

57. Wasserman K, Whipp BJ: Exercise physiology in health and disease. *Am Rev Respir Dis* 112:219, 1975.

58. Wasserman K, Whipp BJ, Koyal SN, et al: Anaerobic threshold and respiratory gas exchange during exercise. *J Appl Physiol* 35:236, 1973.

59. Wasserman K, Whipp BJ, Koyal SN, et al: Effect of carotid body resection on ventilatory and acid-base control during exercise. *J Appl Physiol* 39:354, 1975.

60. Weber KT, Janicki JS, editors: *Cardiopulmonary exercise testing: physiologic principles and clinical applications,* Philadelphia, 1986, WB Saunders.

61. Whipp BJ, Seard C, Wasserman K: Oxygen deficit-oxygen debt relationships and efficiency of anaerobic work. *J Appl Physiol* 28:452, 1970.

62. Whipp BJ, Wasserman K: Efficiency of muscular work. *J Appl Physiol* 26:644, 1969.

# CHAPTER 29

# ASSESSMENT OF RESPIRATORY IMPAIRMENT AND DISABILITY

*Philip Harber*
*Moira Chan-Yeung*

Respiratory disability assessment is greatly facilitated by the availability of excellent objective tests of physiologic function. Thus, it differs from disability assessment for many other organ systems (e.g., musculoskeletal system) for which subjective data are often more important. This chapter will describe general principles of disability assessment. Generic, rather than job-specific, disability will be described.

## GENERAL PRINCIPLES

Several concepts underlie the process of respiratory disability assessment. *Impairment* is the actual loss of physiologic function. On the other hand, *disability* is the impact of the physiologic loss.* As a result, disability may be viewed from several perspectives: general disability and job-specific disability. Disability for everyday life describes the impact on common life activities. Occupational disability may be described as *general occupational disability* or as *job specific disability*. That is, the effect of the impairment on the general ability to earn a living may be described, or for job-specific disability, the ability to perform a very specific job with its attending tasks and exposures may be the relevant perspective in some instances. A final concept is that of *residual ability*. This represents "what the patient can do," rather than being based upon loss of function or activities/jobs which the individual cannot do. This chapter will view disability from a more general perspective.

Disability assessment for the pulmonary system differs from the establishment of a clinical diagnosis or an impairment assessment. Because disability assessment is functionally rather then diagnostically oriented, testing to establish a highly specific clinical diagnosis may not always be requisite. Conversely, adequate testing to describe accurately the functional impact may occasionally extend beyond that which is typically done for diagnostic purposes, therapeutic purposes, or an impairment assessment in other systems.

There are several published and widely accepted general guidelines for assessment of respiratory impairment. In the United States, the American Medical Association (AMA) *Guidelines for the Evaluation of Permanent Impairment*[3] are widely employed. In addition, the American Thoracic Society (ATS) has prepared general guidelines for permanent total impairment[4] and an updated version including recommendations for less than total impairment.[5] The American Thoracic Society has also promulgated recommendations specific for assessment of impairment due to asthma.[6] Government agencies have also prepared guidelines that may be advisory or mandatory. The Social Security Disability Insurance system[7] and the United States Railroad Retirement Board have established specific criteria for impairment. Notably, these criteria are based solely on the functional characteristics of the individual without regard to the cause of the respiratory illness. Other guidelines, however, require that the cause be specifically delineated (at least in theory); for example, the United States Black Lung compensation laws and many state workers' compensation systems are predicated upon the assumption that the underlying illness arises out of employment and in the course of employment.

Notably, all these guidelines or regulations are based upon "expert opinion" rather than empirical data. Thus, they have been largely established by committees of designated "experts" rather than by actually determining the functional characteristics of individuals on an empirical basis. Fortunately, many of these guidelines (e.g., the ATS) were carefully developed by committees intentionally to provide a balance of expertise and viewpoints.

---

*In Europe, slightly different definitions are used. Impairment is the loss of lung function (e.g., decreased $FEV_1$); disability is the consequent decrease in exercise ability; and handicap is the impact on life.[1,2]

This chapter includes four parts:
1. Description of categories of respiratory disease
2. Discussion of test procedures
3. Special considerations for asthma assessment
4. Practical step-by-step approaches

## RESPIRATORY SYSTEM DISORDERS

The respiratory system is complex and is composed of several functional and anatomic components. Some tests are effective in providing an integrated view of the functioning of several systems, whereas in other instances, specific tests are particularly effective for certain functions. Hence, some tests will be useful in nearly all impairment assessment cases; however, some cases must require careful selection depending upon the specific clinical condition and the specific question being asked.

The *upper airway* includes structures ranging from the nose and mouth through the oropharynx, nasopharynx, and larynx. Anatomic or functional disorders can produce significant symptoms. Functional assessment tests, unfortunately, are not well standardized. For example, nasal airflow and resistance can be evaluated by rhinomanometry, but this is rarely used for impairment assessment because it is a complicated technique and because there is considerable short-term variability within individuals.

The *airways* represent a second functional unit. These are composed of the large airways such as the trachea and bronchi, and the small airway region, which is composed of the terminal airways with diameters less than 0.3 mm. Abnormalities may be present within the small airways without being clinically evident due to the very large cross-sectional area in total (typically, there are 23 branches of the airway). Abnormalities in the small airways may be considered to be a early indicator of many disorders; however, from the functional standpoint, small-airway abnormality may have only limited impact in itself in terms of limiting exercise ability.

*Airway abnormalities* fall into three general functional categories: structural, fixed, and reversible. Structural abnormalities are composed of physical obstructions and similar abnormalities (e.g., tumors). Fixed airflow obstruction occurs when the barrier to airflow is not easily reversible (e.g., this is termed "fixed" or "irreversible"). However, variable airflow reduction occurs in disorders such as asthma, in which there may be considerable variability in the magnitude of obstruction that is present. This may occur because of compression of the airway by contraction of muscles (brochoconstriction) or due to airway inflammation. Since both these phenomena are

reversible, testing performed at one time may not directly indicate the permanent condition of the subject.

The *alveolar region and supporting tissues* are the areas where gas exchange occurs. In addition, there are numerous other immunologic and related responses that occur here. This area is significantly affected by alveolar inflammatory processes such as hypersensitivity pneumonitis and by pulmonary fibrotic processes. Such disorders are often termed "interstitial" (because of location) or "restrictive" (because of associated spirometric abnormality).

Disease of the alveolar and interstitial regions can lead to acute inflammatory responses, granuloma formation, or pulmonary fibrosis. The same disease may show different manifestations. For example, sarcoidosis may be primarily a granulomatous disorder or it may be manifested mainly as interstitial fibrosis.

*Hypersensitivity pneumonitis* (IIP) includes a spectrum of disorders caused by repeated inhalation of organic antigens with subsequent allergic sensitization. HP can present as an acute alveolar filling or granulomatous process or, alternatively, it may be seen as an insidiously developing pulmonary fibrotic process.

The *pulmonary vasculature* has the function of transporting nearly the entire cardiac output through the lungs. Unlike the systemic circulation, the pulmonary vascular circulation is a low pressure, high capacitance circulation. Therefore, it has considerable vascular reserve and can recruit new vascular areas as blood flow increases (e.g., due to exercise). Because of this large reserve, there can be considerable disease present without being evident when studies are made at rest (unstressed) conditions. Furthermore, destruction of pulmonary vasculature can lead to indirect effects on the heart, as the right ventricle progressively fails working to overcome the markedly-increased pulmonary vascular resistance. Thus, heart failure (cor pulmonale) may be a major manifestation of lung disease.

Disorders of *respiratory control* may occur in conjunction with other respiratory disorders or may occur as independent phenomena. Disordered breathing during sleep (sleep apnea) with consequent daytime somnolence and possible heart failure is an example of a functional disorder of this category. Other disorders such as chronic obstructive pulmonary disease may be frequently accompanied by a significant component of abnormal respiratory control, decreasing the tendency of the patient to compensate appropriately for the other physiologic changes. For example, carbon dioxide retention and respiratory acidosis may occur.

Finally, the respiratory system also has components that function as a *sense organ*. Such functions range from obvious aspects such as olfaction to sensation produced by the stretch receptors in the lung. Specific sensations associated with breathing may be consciously sensed or may produce more subtle discomfort (e.g., mild dyspnea due to the disproportion between work expended and airflow achieved).

In evaluating patients with possible respiratory impairment, the physician must select the appropriate test procedures. In addition, the modality of the impairment and/or disability should be clearly delineated. The impact of severe mechanical derangement of ventilatory function is quite different from a sensation of upper airway irritation. Not all tests are appropriate for all settings. Often, a provisional clinical diagnosis or an initial estimate of the severity of disease can guide the choice of test. When a disorder of airway responsiveness such as asthma is suspected, it can be both diagnostically and functionally assessed with tests such as methacholine challenge testing (see below). On the other hand, the full assessment of functional impact of interstitial lung disease may be better evaluated with tests of diffusing capacity of the lung for carbon monoxide and occasionally by pulmonary exercise testing.

## TEST PROCEDURES

### Spirometry

Spirometry is a well-standardized and simple test, and it should be employed in nearly all respiratory impairment evaluations. Spirometry is useful only if it is properly performed. The subject must be adequately motivated and receive proper instruction before test performance. The technician performing the test must be qualified to calibrate the equipment and conduct various aspects of the testing. The existence of an automated spirometer does not eliminate the need for a well-qualified technician. In some patients, particularly those who cannot or will not cooperate, adequate spirometry cannot be achieved. The technician must be comfortable in reporting that testing was not adequate.

Published guidelines exist for both equipment and test performance.[8,9] Factors to consider include adequacy of equipment, training of technicians, regular calibration of equipment, and method of performance.

Properly administered spirometry requires that the patient perform the test procedure at least three times. The two best values must be within 5% of each other. For this reason, in some instances, the test must be repeated as many as eight times. If adequate consistency cannot be achieved, the test data

should still be considered, although its significance must be carefully evaluated. The inability to achieve adequate consistency may itself be an indicator of the presence of disease; alternatively, it simply may represent inadequate technician or patient effort. A large number of parameters may be calculated from spirometry. However, for impairment assessment purposes, only two are of primary importance: the forced expiratory volume in one second ($FEV_1$) and forced vital capacity (FVC).

$FEV_1$ is the volume of air that can be expelled in the first second of a maximal effort. A slow start to maximal expiratory effort can lead to a falsely low measurement, and such tests (with a large extrapolated volume) should be discarded. FVC is the total amount that can be exhaled. When interpreting these results, one must remember that the $FEV_1$ and the FVC represent the amount of air exhaled and do not in themselves represent the actual lung volume. The ratio between the $FEV_1$ and FVC ($FEV_1$/FVC) is a good index of the presence of obstructive lung abnormality.

Other parameters that may be derived from the spirogram include the forced expiratory flow in the mid-portion of the vital capacity, currently termed the forced expiratory flow from 25–75% ($FEF_{25-75\%}$). Many feel that this is an indicator of small airway function. It is often a sensitive test for the presence of early abnormality, but in itself it does not appear to lead to symptoms or significant functional limitations. For this reason, it is not considered in many formal rating schemes such as that of the AMA.

The maximal voluntary ventilation (MVV) test has a long historical tradition but has very little utility in pulmonary assessments. It is highly effort-dependent and generally adds little information to that which is otherwise obtained. Therefore, it should be used only if it is specifically mandated by the referring agency.

### Post-Bronchodilator Spirometry

The spirogram may be repeated after administration of an inhaled bronchodilator. A significant increase is defined as a greater than 15% increase in the $FEV_1$ from the best prebronchodilator result. The ATS recommends that a positive response be defined by the presence of both a 12% increase in either the FVC or $FEV_1$ and a 200 ml or greater increase in either.[10] This presupposes that the prior baseline result was accurately performed and that the improvement is not simply a "learning effect." A significant bronchodilator response may have two implications. First, such a response, if valid, indicates the presence of airway variability, a marker of asthma. Second, the post-bronchodilator result is indicative of the level of function that can be obtained with proper treatment; therefore, assessing functional capacity based solely on the pre-bronchodilator result would underestimate ability. This is discussed further in the Asthma section.

## Diffusing Capacity of the Lung for Carbon Monoxide ($D_{LCO}$)

The diffusing capacity of the lung for carbon monoxide is a useful test in many impairment evaluations, but it may not be essential in every case. It is less useful when the spirometry demonstrates variable airflow obstruction (e.g., asthma) than in other situations.

The test name ("diffusing capacity") is actually a misnomer. This test procedure is a highly integrative test and is dependent upon distribution of airflow, lung volumes, pulmonary vasculature, hemoglobin concentration, and vascular volumes as well as diffusion *per se*. Hence, the British term, *transfer factor*, may be more appropriate.

The $D_{LCO}$ is highly nonspecific since it incorporates so many different functions. However, the $D_{LCO}$ is useful in pulmonary evaluations because of its excellent integrative capacity. As a result, it is sensitive but nonspecific.

Performance of the diffusing capacity test requires careful attention to detail. Recommendations for standardization are available.[11] Unlike spirometry, test results are less subject to external validation of accuracy, and it is therefore particularly important that the test be performed in a credible fashion.

The test result is highly dependent upon the hemoglobin concentration. For this reason, most experts suggest that the result should be adjusted for hemoglobin concentration if anemia is present.[11] There are several equations available for adjusting the observed $D_{LCO}$ for hemoglobin concentration.[12-14] The ATS recommends use of the equation:

Adjusted $D_{LCO}$ – Observed $D_{LCO}$ ([10.22 + Hb]/1.7 Hb)

where Hb = hemoglobin concentration.[11] Otherwise, impairment may be ascribed to respiratory disease when it is actually hematologic in origin.

In individuals who smoke, the blood may contain a significant back diffusion pressure of carbon monoxide. Some authorities recommend that the blood carboxyhemoglobin (from a venous sample) be measured in order to allow the diffusing capacity test to be adjusted for such back diffusion.[15] There is controversy about the necessity of this; in marginal cases, it may have sufficient effect to change the impairment assessment. At the very least, subjects should not smoke overnight prior to the test.

## Arterial Blood Gas Analysis

Arterial blood gas analysis describes the oxygen and carbon dioxide tension in the sample of arterial blood, generally obtained while at rest. In addition, the pH level is measured. Most impairment assessment systems consider the arterial blood gas analysis to be only an adjunctive procedure, only occasionally useful. The AMA guidelines, for example, do not incorporate it as a primary test and consider it to be "invasive." Several systems, however, do place greater emphasis upon this.

The major limitation to arterial blood gas analysis is the lack of validated relationships between changes in arterial oxygen tension and actual functional limitation. In addition, results are variable within individuals.[16] Severe abnormalities of arterial blood gas analysis, however, are likely to be significant.

## Pulmonary Exercise Testing

Pulmonary exercise testing is a quantitative measure of integrated exercise ability. Detailed discussion of the methodology and interpretation protocols are presented in Chapter 27.

Pulmonary exercise testing can provide the answers to the following questions:

1. Is any physiologic abnormality present? Studies have shown that exercise testing may reveal abnormalities when other tests are normal.[17]
2. What is the maximal exercise level that the subject has attained for a short time?
3. What is the estimated sustainable exercise capacity?

There is some controversy about how frequently exercise testing is needed in respiratory impairment assessments. Some consider frequent exercise testing necessary because the maximum oxygen consumption cannot be well predicted by resting pulmonary function data.[18,19] However, the ATS[5] notes that functional impact can generally be assessed from the basic pulmonary function tests and that exercise testing will be needed only in unusual cases. It may be particularly useful when evaluating ability to do a specific job with a heavy, sustained workload.[5]

Exercise testing must be performed properly. In general, maximal, rather than submaximal, exercise tests should be employed if the technique is utilized at all. Oxygen consumption must be directly measured and should not be estimated on the basis of the external workload (e.g., treadmill speed and grade).

In selected cases, exercise testing can be an extremely valuable technique. When the statement of dyspnea by the patient is disproportionate to the results of more simple function tests, and the evaluating physician feels that the patient's statement of symptoms has a high likelihood of being accurate, then exercise testing should be strongly considered. A completely normal exercise test serves as strong evidence that significant disabling pulmonary physiologic abnormalities of the interstitium, vasculature, or fixed obstructive types are unlikely to be present. Conversely, in some instances, this will be the indication that significant abnormalities are present.

If properly interpreted, exercise testing can yield considerable information about the physiologic origin. For example, it may suggest that ventilatory limitation is present, or alternatively, may point to gas exchange as the limiting factor. Such testing may also show that physical deconditioning (e.g., due to voluntary lack of exercise) accounts for the inability to achieve expected levels of work. It may also point to cardiac disease as the origin of symptoms. One study found that 78% of cases of unexpectedly-low exercise tolerance in the course of pulmonary impairment evaluations were actually due to cardiac disease.[17]

Exercise testing may also be useful for quantifying the degree of abnormality present. It is widely held that oxygen consumption is the best single measure of work ability, and exercise testing measures this directly. As generally practiced, pulmonary exercise testing measures the maximal (peak) exercise attainable. This directly indicates the maximal exercise that could be performed at work for short periods. The exercise level that the patient could be reasonably expected to sustain for more prolonged periods is estimated as a proportion of the actually-measured maximal exercise. Typically, it is assumed that an individual could maintain between 40% and 60% of the maximal. This is based upon limited empirical data, drawn largely from individuals with obstructive lung disease.

In some instances, subjects may not exercise maximally because of intentionally malingering or for psychological reasons. When this occurs, the subject terminates exercise at a time that the physiologic parameters do not show a physiologic basis for the limitations. Unfortunately, it is difficult to differentiate deconditioning from lack of maximal effort, although a high heart rate in the absence of other evidence of cardiac disease may suggest deconditioning rather than voluntary premature exercise termination.

The major rating schemes do not mandate that exercise testing be performed, but most will utilize the data if it is collected. As a result, there is some flexibility in the frequency with which evaluating physicians will order such testing as part of the evaluation process.

The complete set of data are utilized in determining the presence and type of physiologic abnormalities. However, for categorizing the degree of impairment, measurement of the maximum-attained oxygen consumption is the focus. The AMA system relies upon the measured oxygen consumption, based upon the weight-adjusted peak-attainable oxygen consumption, commonly expressed in units of milliliters of oxygen uptake per kilogram per minute. Another commonly used measure is METS. One MET corresponds to an oxygen consumption of 3.7 ml/kg/min. In theory, one MET is the baseline oxygen consumption for performing no activity. Unlike the method commonly used in cardiac exercise testing, in which exercise levels are expressed in METS although this is not actually measured, pulmonary-exercise testing requires actual measurement.

The significance of the weight adjustment must be recognized for obese subjects. In such persons, the oxygen consumption to weight ratio may appear disproportionately low because the denominator is so significantly increased. Therefore, obesity alone without the presence of actual lung disease may diminish the weight-adjusted oxygen consumption measurements.

## Chest Radiography

Chest radiographs generally do not play a major role in assessing respiratory disability. However, they are often needed when interstitial lung disease, such as asbestosis, is being considered.

A standard method for interpreting chest radiographs for pneumoconiosis (dust disease of the lung) has been developed. It is known as the ILO (International Labor Organization) system.[20] Although it was developed for epidemiologic rather than clinical purposes, it has been used widely in such settings. In the United States, physicians may be certified for competency in the standardized reading method by the National Institute for Occupational Safety and Health (NIOSH). Physicians who are certified for this purpose are known as B-readers.

There is nothing absolute about results of the ILO reading system. Specifically, the interpretations are for findings "consistent with" rather than "diagnostic of" pneumoconiosis. In essence, it is a descriptive rather than a diagnostic method.

In this system, a series of letters and numbers rather than prose descriptions are used for reporting purposes. Interpretation by B-readers does not guarantee accuracy and objectivity of interpretation, but it does provide a standardized communication modality. Interpretation is done by comparing the patient's radiograph to a standard series of radiographs. The reference radiographs are graded 0, 1, 2, or 3. The best match to the patient's radiograph is used to describe it. However, because a patient's radiograph may be intermediate between two reference categories, two numbers are often assigned. For example, "1/0" means the patient's film is intermediate between reference film "1" and reference film "0" but is "closer" to "1". On the other hand, "0/1" means it is intermediate but closer to "0". These terms describe the "profusion" or amount of opacities.

The size and shape are described with letters. Small opacities (<1 cm) are classified as "p, q, r" if they are rounded and as "s, t, u" if linear. Large opacities are described by the capital letters "A, B, or C" depending on their extent. "C" implies extensive replacement of lung tissue.

The ILO system is also used to describe pleural plaques that occur in asbestos-exposed persons. However, the precision and accuracy of such descriptions of plaque and pleural thickening is generally considered to be less than for profusion.

Technically, interpretation is limited to the PA (posteroanterior) view only, although other views (e.g., lateral) may be employed.

## EVALUATION OF IMPAIRMENT IN PATIENTS WITH ASTHMA AND OCCUPATIONAL ASTHMA

Occupational asthma has become the most prevalent occupational lung disease in developed countries. In Canada, the number of compensated cases of occupational asthma exceeded the total number of cases of pneumoconiosis in both Quebec and British Columbia.[21,22] In Finland and in the United Kingdom, occupational asthma has also become the most frequently-reported occupational lung disease.[23,24] Many follow-up studies have shown that the majority of patients with occupational asthma had not recovered several years after the removal from exposure. Since these patients did not have asthma before they entered the industry and they were shown by objective testing to have sensitivity to an agent present in the workplace, the persistence of symptoms is likely to be due to previous exposure.[25] Compensation for these patients has become an important issue.

For many years, the assessment of impairment in patients with asthma or occupational asthma has been based on the same guidelines as those used in patients with any other respiratory disorders, such as those recommended by the ATS.[4,5] The 1986 ATS guidelines for evaluation of impairment and disability secondary to respiratory disorders attempted to address the issue of asthma in some of the recommendations,[5] but they were quite inadequate.[26] The most recent *Guidelines to the Evaluation of Permanent Impairment,* published by the American Medical As-

sociation in 1993,[3] states that "asthma represents a difficult problem in impairment evaluation because results of pulmonary function studies may be normal or near normal between attacks" (p. 164). The *Guides* addresses asthma's treatment, testing, and specific occupationally-acquired precipitating factors, but does not discuss the issue of how to provide an impairment rating.

## Rationale for Separate Guidelines for Patients with Asthma

Asthma has unique features that distinguish it from all other respiratory diseases. First, asthma is characterized by variable airflow obstruction. The results found on one day may not reflect the subject's true status. This is different from pneumoconiosis in which subjects show little variation in lung function. Second, unlike pneumoconiosis, asthma is amenable to therapy. The lung function ($FEV_1$) of subjects with asthma can be improved to within normal limits with appropriate therapy sometimes including the use of systemic corticosteroid therapy. Third, in contrast to pneumoconiosis, there are no radiologic changes in asthma. Fourth, subjects with asthma have evidence of bronchial hyperresponsiveness that may render them less able to work in an environment with continued exposure to irritants or cold air even though they are not exposed to the initial causative agent. The use of guidelines designed for evaluation of patients with irreversible lung damage in patients with asthma is inappropriate.

## Approach to Impairment Assessment in Asthma Patients[6,27]

The process of asthmatic impairment evaluation includes establishing or confirming the diagnosis of asthma and assessing the impairment. It is recommended that assessment should take place at least on two occasions: (1) temporary impairment assessment is to be carried out immediately after the diagnosis; (2) permanent impairment assessment is to be carried out two years after the subject has been removed from exposure. The details of these assessments have been published,[6] and the following is a brief description of the recommendations.

### Diagnosis of asthma
The diagnosis of asthma requires both relevant symptoms and the presence of airflow limitation that is partially or completely reversible either spontaneously or after treatment, or the presence of airway hyperresponsiveness.

## Temporary impairment

Once the diagnosis of asthma is made, a temporary rating for impairment can be given based on the results of the tests for establishing the diagnosis of asthma.

## Permanent impairment

1. *Timing of Evaluation*—Evaluation for permanent impairment should be done after the patient's asthma is under optimal control and the objectives of treatment of asthma have been attained. Optimal control means that additional treatment is unlikely to improve further functional status. The objectives of treatment of asthma include achieving and maintaining control of asthma to prevent acute exacerbations. To achieve these objectives, avoidance of exposure to the offending agent and other nonspecific irritants is essential, together with judicious use of medications. Treatment should be given to maintain the best result for each subject with minimal side effects.

2. *Clinical and Physiological Parameters*—As no one clinical or physiologic parameter has been validated as a measure of impairment in asthma, a combination of parameters is recommended.

(*a*) *Clinical parameters*—The amount and type of medication required to maintain asthma under optimal control have the merit of being semiquantitative compared with other clinical measures such as frequency of wheeze, hospitalization, and emergency department visits, which may reflect poor control of asthma. A hierarchy of asthmatic severity, based on treatment, has been constructed as follows (Table 29–4, p. 349):

(*i*) No medications
(*ii*) Occasional bronchodilators, not daily and/or occasional cromolyn
(*iii*) Daily bronchodilator and/or daily cromolyn sodium and/or daily low dose (< 1000 μg beclomethasone or equivalent) inhaled steroids
(*iv*) Daily high dose (> 1000 μg beclomethasone or equivalent) inhaled and/or occasional course (1–3/yr) systemic corticosteroids and bronchodilator on demand
(*v*) Daily high dose inhaled steroid (> 1000 μg beclomethasone or equivalent) and daily systemic steroid and bronchodilator on demand

Since physicians tend to vary in their prescribing habits, reliability of the treatment scale depends upon the treatment of asthma in a uniform manner according to published guidelines.[28-31] It should be pointed out that none of the above clinical parameters has been validated; investigating this constitutes an important subject area for research.

(*b*) *Physiological parameters*—In addition to spirometry, it is recommended that the test for reversibility of air flow obstruction or measurement of nonspecific bronchial hyperresponsiveness should be done.[16]

- *Spirometry* should be done using standardized methods.[9] Inhaled β2-adrenergic agents should be withheld for 8 hours and theophylline preparations for 24 hours before the test. Withdrawal of inhaled and systemic corticosteroids is not advisable because of the potential risk to the subject.

- *Testing for reversibility of airflow obstruction* should be carried out whenever the baseline $FEV_1$ is below the lower limit of normal.[10]

- *Measurement of nonspecific bronchial responsiveness (NSBH)* to histamine or methacholine using standardized protocols[32-35] should be done only when the baseline $FEV_1$ is above the lower limit of normal[10] because the degree of NSBH is highly correlated with the baseline airway calibre. Conditions such as chronic bronchitis with airflow obstruction may be associated with NSBH.

*Exercise testing* is not recommended routinely in the investigation of asthma. As in pneumoconiosis, an exercise test is indicated in subjects in whom dyspnea cannot be explained by lung function tests. Another indication for exercise testing is to induce exercise-induced bronchospasm for grading of impairment in jobs requiring physical exertion. The precise role of the exercise test in impairment assessment in subjects with asthma has yet to be clearly established.

*Measurement of diffusing capacity and measurement of lung volumes* are not required for the impairment assessment in subjects with asthma once the diagnosis is clearly established.

3. *Grading of Impairment*—The grading of impairment should be based on both clinical and physiologic parameters in accordance with Tables 29-2 to 29-5 (pages 348 and 349). The degree of impairment is calculated as the sum of scores for postbronchodilator $FEV_1$, reversibility of $FEV_1$ or $PC_{20}$ and medication need. The class of impairment is expressed as Class 0 to V. Class V or total impairment in a subject with asthma is defined as asthma that cannot be controlled adequately despite maximal treatment,

including >20 mg prednisone per day on a regular basis, and the $FEV_1$ remains below 50% predicted despite aggressive medicine usage (Table 29–5). In addition, the evaluating physicians should indicate the effects asthma has on the subject's quality of life, including the impact on the subject's ability to perform his or her normal job.

4. *Periodic Examination*—There should be provision for reassessment. Subjects with persistent asthma after removal from exposure seldom deteriorate with good ongoing medical care. If there is a significant change in the clinical course, reassessment should be carried out.

## Special Considerations for Subjects with Occupational Asthma

Assessment of subjects with occupational asthma should be done by physicians with expertise in this area. The subject should be considered 100% permanently disabled for the job that caused the illness and for other jobs entailing exposure to the same causative agent. Several alternatives should be considered for the subject: relocation to a new job either in the same plant or in a different plant where there is no exposure; rehabilitation into a new job; or early retirement. Financial compensation should be offered in every instance where there is a loss of earning. In some situations, modifications in the job, such as improved ventilation or process substitution, may enable the worker to remain. It is important to remember that if the agent induces immunologic asthma, the subject may respond to levels of exposure well below those considered safe for subjects without prior sensitization.

The subjects should be assessed for permanent impairment two years after removal from exposure to the offending agent since improvement in symptoms, lung function, and bronchial hyperresponsiveness appears to plateau after this period of time.[36] Although the study that documented this effect was conducted specifically in workers with occupational asthma due to high molecular weight compounds and in those who were intermittently exposed to the offending agent, there is no reason to believe that occupational asthma due to low molecular weight compounds would behave differently. It is important to assess the subjects when their asthmatic conditions are under reasonable control. If medication is required, they should be on maintenance doses. Recent acute exacerbation of asthma or severe upper-respiratory infection precludes impairment evaluation (generally within two months).

## PRACTICAL APPROACH TO RESPIRATORY DISABILITY ASSESSMENT

This section will provide a practical, step-by-step approach to respiratory impairment assessment. In general, it is consistent with the recommendations of the AMA and several of the ATS guidelines. Steps are summarized in the box below.

1. *Determine the administrative nature of the evaluation.* This includes answering the following questions:
   —What is the purpose of the disability assessment?
   —Does the scope of the evaluation include determination of specific diagnosis or simply assessment of functional level?
   —Must the individual be assessed for ability to do a specific job or is the evaluation generic?
   —Are there specific tests that are required by the referring agency, and is there a specific report format?

2. *Review records.* Perform a preliminary record review of available medical records. If necessary, request additional information.

3. *Obtain respiratory and medical history.* Obtain a medical history from the patient that focuses on the respiratory system. Major elements of the history are

### PRACTICAL STEPS IN ASSESSING RESPIRATORY DISABILITY

1. Determine the administrative nature of the evaluation.
2. Review records.
3. Obtain respiratory and medical history.
4. Physical examination, focusing on the respiratory system.
5. Perform basic lung function tests.
6. Radiography (if indicated).
7. Determine if there is sufficient information to determine impairment and assess the magnitude of disability.
8. Determine if any additional testing or additional records are needed.
9. After all data have been acquired, determine if impairment and disability have been demonstrated to be present.
10. Classify the magnitude of impairment and consequence of disability.
11. Identify any modifiers.
12. Assess occupational disability (optional).
13. Prepare report.

## ELEMENTS OF HISTORY

### RESPIRATORY SYMPTOMS

Dyspnea
Cough
Sputum
Wheeze
Nasal and sinus symptoms

### RESPIRATORY MEDICAL HISTORY

Current medications
Prior medications
Physician visits
Frequency of respiratory infections
Any history of treatment for respiratory disease
Prior hospitalizations for respiratory disease
Prior surgical treatment/bronchoscopic evaluation of respiratory disease

### ALLERGIC HISTORY

Allergies
History of allergic reactions
Hay fever, childhood asthma, and related history
Family history of allergies

### FUNCTIONAL STATUS

Exercise ability
Typical exercise at home and work
Any limitations due to respiratory symptoms
Hobbies

### OCCUPATIONAL AND ENVIRONMENTAL HISTORY

List all jobs held in lifetime, including duration and use of protective equipment:
Industry
Job title
Employer
Chemical exposures
Any effects on respiratory symptoms
Hobbies
Possible home allergens (e.g., pets)

### FAMILY HISTORY OF RESPIRATORY DISORDERS

### TOBACCO EXPOSURE HISTORY

Active smoking
Environmental tobacco smoke exposure

---

shown in the box above. This should be obtained directly by the evaluating physician. While questionnaires or information may be collected by less experienced and trained individuals, they do not substitute for the carefully-obtained history. The physician must consider not only the "facts" about symptoms reported by the patient but must also in many cases of impairment assessment consider whether there is a tendency to understate or overstate symptoms. Such an assessment cannot be achieved without talking to the patient in detail.

Such subjective information is essential for guiding the choice of tests, and in some instances, it affects the overall interpretation. However, for respiratory impairment assessment, symptoms *per se* do not play a major role in determining the presence or extent of respiratory impairment or disability. Fortunately, there are objective tests that avoid reliance upon subjective data.

It is important to emphasize functional impact as well as simply obtaining information about symptoms.

In addition, the evaluating physician should ask about how these symptoms limit the patient's activities.

4. *Perform a physical examination, focusing on the respiratory system*—An adequate physical examination should be conducted. Special focus upon the respiratory system is important. In addition to evaluating the presence of physical signs (e.g., rubs, crackles, wheezes), the patient should be carefully observed to determine if actions are consistent with symptoms. The patient who complains of severe continuous dyspnea yet is observed to walk very quickly down the hall following examination is suspect.

While the pulmonary focus of the examination is intuitively obvious, other areas should be carefully assessed. In particular, symptoms related to upper-airway problems are often interpreted by patients as causing "shortness of breath." Therefore, careful examination for evidence of nasal congestion, turbinate enlargement, or polyps is advisable. In addition, because of the high frequency of the coexistence of upper-airway and lower-airway diseases, valuable information may be obtained by assessing the upper airway. Dyspnea may also have other causes, and a careful cardiac examination is important. Furthermore, functional observations in the course of the examination (e.g., getting on or off the examining table and walking in the hall) may be an essential component of the physical examination. The clinician should also evaluate if any specific factors are present that would make the day of the examination atypical (e.g., a current upper or lower respiratory tract infection may temporarily affect lung function).

5. *Perform basic lung function tests*—In most instances, this will include determination of spirometry and diffusing capacity of the lung for carbon monoxide. However, if it is clear from the preliminary assessment that asthma is the relevant clinical diagnosis, then the diffusing capacity determination may not be necessary.

Spirometry should be repeated after administration of a short-acting aerosolized bronchodilator if the baseline results are abnormal (as described above). In general, the baseline spirogram is considered to be abnormal if the $FEV_1$ or FVC is less than 80% of predicted.

6. *Obtain radiograph (if necessary)*—A chest radiograph is not usually essential, but for "tradition sake" many referring agencies request a chest radiograph. Methods have been discussed earlier. CT scans are generally not needed. While they are highly sensitive for emphysema and interstitial lung disease, they have only limited value in reflecting physiologic impact.

7. *Determine if information is sufficient*—Based upon the available information from the examination, the interview, and the basic laboratory tests, the physician should determine if there is sufficient information to determine the presence of absence of any significant impairment and for assessing the magnitude of disability. In many instances, good clinical sense can guide this, but in other cases, reference to specific tables provided by published guidelines (e.g., AMA, ATS) or the referring agency should be utilized.

8. *Obtain additional information (if needed)*—From the preliminary assessment, determine if any additional testing or additional records are needed. If asthma is seriously considered as a likely cause of the symptoms reported, then specific evaluation methods should be employed.

Exercise testing should be considered under the following circumstances:

(*a*) When it is specifically required by the referring agency and there is no medical contraindication.

(*b*) When necessary to determine precisely the level of physiologic impairment.

(*c*) When the physician's evaluation of symptoms suggest that significant dyspnea may be present, yet other functional tests do not adequately reflect the degree of abnormality felt to be clinically present.

(*d*) When exercise-induced bronchospasm is considered likely. (For this purpose, a different form of exercise testing is necessary.)

9. *Determine if impairment and disability are present*—After all data have been acquired, determine if impairment and disability have been demonstrated to be present. Furthermore, if the referring agency requires that the organ system leading to the disability be specifically identified, determine if there is a specific clinically diagnosable condition of the respiratory system.

Specifically, the evaluator must answer two questions: (1) Is there any *significant* impairment with consequent disability present? (2) If such impairment is present, is there sufficient information to rate (scale) its magnitude?

In some instances, a "permanent" assessment may not be possible at the time the evaluation is performed. For example, for asthmatics, the current treatment may be perceived to be inadequate; therefore the physiologic tests may underestimate the actual functional capacity of the individual. In other instances, the underlying medical condition may be temporary (such as the consequences of an infection) or the pulmonary condition may be otherwise amenable to a therapeutic trial.

Notably, the AMA *Guides* are specifically designed only for *permanent* impairment, and they therefore cannot (theoretically) be used in all instances. However, many physicians have found it convenient to apply them to the current data; however, in the written discussion, they note that this should not be misconstrued as permanent.

10. *Classify the magnitude of impairment and consequence of disability*—The next step is performed in most disability assessments. If there is any impairment present, an expression of its magnitude is made. In most instances, a standard classification scheme is utilized as a default. Such schemes employ lung function data to place the individual into one of an ordered series of categories. These are generally based upon specified combinations of test results. For example, the classification schemes recommended by the AMA and ATS are shown in Table 29-1. As shown in Table 29-1, the classification schemes of the AMA and ATS are similar. They differ in the cutpoints for $D_{LCO}$. In addition, the ATS system places greater emphasis on the $FEV_1/FVC$ ratio than does the AMA system.

As shown in Table 29-1, subjective data are not incorporated for the purpose of classifying the extent of

**TABLE 29-1    RATING SCHEMES OF AMA AND ATS***

| | FVC | FEV$_1$ | FEV$_1$/FVC | D$_{LCO}$ | V̇$_{O2}$ | COMMENT |
|---|---|---|---|---|---|---|
| Class 1 (None) | ≥80% Pr (≥80% Pr) | ≥80% Pr (≥80% Pr) | ≥0.70 (≥0.75) | ≥70% Pr (≥80% Pr) | >25 (—) | Must meet *all* the criteria |
| Class 2 (Mild) | 60–79% Pr (60–79% Pr) | 60–79% Pr (60–79% Pr) | — (0.60–0.74) | 60–69% Pr (60–79%) | 20–25 (—) | Must meet *only one* criterion |
| Class 3 (Moderate) | 51–59% Pr (51–59% Pr) | 41–59% Pr (41–59% Pr) | — (0.41–0.59) | 41–59% Pr (41–59% Pr) | 15–20 (—) | Must meet *only one* criterion |
| Class 4 (Severe) | ≤50% Pr (≤50% Pr) | ≤40% Pr (≤40% Pr) | — (≤0.40) | ≤40% Pr (≤40% Pr) | ≤15 (—) | Must meet *only one* criterion |
| Prediction Equation | Crapo 1980 | | | Crapo 1981 | Units: ml O$_2$/min/kg weight | |

*Classification schemes recommended by the AMA and ATS (in parentheses). %Pr = percent of predicted value. The ratio FEV$_1$/FVC is expressed as an *absolute* number, not as percentage of predicted; to emphasize this and to avoid confusion, the ratio is expressed as a decimal in this table.

the impairment and disability. Furthermore, these tables are primarily for fixed obstructive disease (e.g., COPD) or restrictive lung disease. For asthma, the current edition of the AMA *Guides* suggests using the rating tables shown but then reconsidering based upon the severity of the manifestations of the asthma. Recognizing the unique aspects of disability assessment in asthma, the American Thoracic Society has developed a specific set of guidelines. The ATS *Guidelines* established a classification by adding together "points" from each of three distinct categories: severity of airflow obstruction (e.g., FEV$_1$), airway responsiveness (as determined by methacholine challenge testing or variability of lung function), and bona fide need for medication (see Tables 29-2 to 29-5).

11. *Identify any modifiers*—The use of tables and similar techniques can only provide an approximate default classification of severity. In most instances, this will be accurate (albeit occasionally arbitrary). However, in some cases, information collected in the course of the medical evaluation will suggest that the classification described in Step 10 above may either overestimate or underestimate the actual impairment. For example, the tables may overestimate impairment if the patient is not receiving good therapy or continues to smoke. Similarly, tables may underestimate disability significantly under several circumstances:

(a) To achieve a level of lung function measured, very large doses of drugs (such as high dose systemic corticosteroid therapy) are utilized, which in themselves may lead to significant disabling effects.

**TABLE 29-2    POSTBRONCHODILATOR FEV$_1$**

| SCORE | FEV$_1$ (% PREDICTED) |
|---|---|
| 0 | > lower limit of normal |
| 1 | 70–lower limit of normal |
| 2 | 60–69 |
| 3 | 50–59 |
| 4 | < 50 |

From American Thoracic Society: Guidelines for the evaluation of impairment/disability in patients with asthma. *Am Rev Respir Dis* 147:1056-1061, 1993.

(b) The medical condition is likely to rapidly deteriorate (e.g., with active inflammatory alveolitis or progressive pulmonary fibrosis).

(c) The patient has a respiratory condition that is not reflected physiologically in tests such as spirometry or diffusing capacity. For example, respiratory control disorders will produce very significant impairment and disability in many individuals without affecting these tests.

(d) There are reasons to believe that the testing was inaccurate or otherwise is misleading.

12. *Assess occupational disability (optional)*—In some evaluations, it is necessary specifically to evaluate occupational disability, either for all jobs or for specific jobs. This is not necessary in all cases but may be required in certain instances. Doing so requires knowl-

**TABLE 29-3    REVERSIBILITY OF FEV$_1$ OR DEGREE OF AIRWAY HYPERRESPONSIVENESS***

| SCORE | FEV$_1$ CHANGE | OR | PC$_{20}$ MG/ML OR EQUIVALENT |
|---|---|---|---|
| 0 | <10 | | >8 |
| 1 | 10–19 | | 8– >0.5 |
| 2 | 20–29 | | 0.5– >0.125 |
| 3 | ≥30 | | ≤0.125 |
| 4 | — | | — |

*When FEV$_1$ is above the lower limit of normal, PC$_{20}$ should be determined and used for rating of impairment; when FEV$_1$ is < 70% predicted, the degree of reversibility should be used; when FEV$_1$ is between 70% predicted and the lower limit of normal, either reversibility or PC$_{20}$ can be used.

Reversibility with bronchodilator is calculated as:

$$\frac{\text{FEV}_1 \text{ post-bronchodilator} - \text{FEV}_1 \text{ pre-bronchodilator}}{\text{FEV}_1 \text{ pre-bronchodilator}} \times 100\%$$

Airway responsiveness is expressed as that concentration of agent that will provoke a fall in FEV$_1$ of 20% from the lowest post-saline value. Plot the concentration of methacholine/histamine against the fall in FEV$_1$ using a logarithm scale for the doubling concentrations. The PC$_{20}$ is obtained by interpolation between the last two points. The formula for linear interpolation of the PC$_{20}$ from the log dose response curve is as follows:

$$\text{PC}_{20} = \text{antilog } C1 + \frac{(\log C2 - \log C1)(20 - R1)}{(R2 - R1)}$$

where C1 = second last concentration (< 20% FEV$_1$ fall)
C2 = last concentration (> 20% FEV$_1$ fall)
R1 = % fall FEV$_1$ after C1
R2 = % fall FEV$_1$ after C2
(From American Thoracic Society: Guidelines for the evaluation of impairment/disability in patients with asthma. *Am Rev Respir Dis* 147:1056-1061, 1993.)

**TABLE 29-4    MINIMUM MEDICATION NEED***

| SCORE | MEDICATION |
|---|---|
| 0 | No medication |
| 1 | Occasional bronchodilator, not daily and/or occasional cromolyn, not daily |
| 2 | Daily bronchodilator and/or daily cromolyn and/or daily low-dose inhaled steroid (< 800 μg beclomethasone or equivalent) |
| 3 | Bronchodilator on demand and daily high-dose inhaled steroid (> 800 μg beclomethasone or equivalent) or occasional course (1–3/yr) systemic steroid |
| 4 | Bronchodilator on demand and daily high-dose inhaled steroid (> 1000 μg beclomethasone or equivalent) and daily systemic steroid |

*The need for minimum medication should be demonstrated by the treating physician (e.g., previous records of exacerbation when medications have been reduced). (From American Thoracic Society: Guidelines for the evaluation of impairment/disability in patients with asthma. *Am Rev Respir Dis* 147:1056-1061, 1993.)

**TABLE 29-5    SUMMARY IMPAIRMENT RATING CLASSES***

| IMPAIRMENT CLASS | TOTAL SCORE |
|---|---|
| 0 | 0 |
| I | 1–3 |
| II | 4–6 |
| III | 7–9 |
| IV | 10–11 |
| V | Asthma not controlled despite maximal treatment (i.e., FEV$_1$ remaining <50% despite use of ≥20 mg prednisone/day) |

*The impairment rating is calculated as the sum of the patient's scores from Tables 29-2, 29-3, and 29-4. (From American Thoracic Society: Guidelines for the evaluation of impairment/disability in patients with asthma. *Am Rev Respir Dis* 147:1056-1061, 1993.)

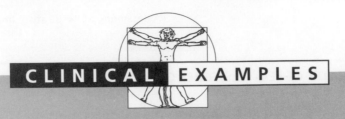

## RESPIRATORY SYSTEM

### EXAMPLE I

EDITOR'S NOTE—The concept of asthma in the AMA *Guides* is not clearly defined. Since its publication, the American Thoracic Society has published its own recommendations with respect to asthma (see discussion in the text and in Reference 6).

#### History

A 34-year-old man works in a factory involved in making various paints and dealing extensively with chemicals. He has worked in this factory for six years. He is exposed to isocyanates. He is Caucasian and 187 cm tall. He was diagnosed as having asthma five years ago. His symptoms can be initiated by work exposures and by environmental factors such as dust, fumes, second-hand cigarette smoke, and cold air. He has three to four respiratory infections per year and has been hospitalized twice in the past five years for asthma. In addition, he has been seen in the emergency room on two other occasions. He has been followed very closely by his physician for this condition. He has come for an evaluation based on shortness of breath associated with wheezing, coughing, and mucus production. On the day of evaluation, he is taking his usual medications, which include theophylline, 900 mg per day; cromolyn sodium, 2 puffs four times a day; ipratropium bromide, 2 puffs four times a day; beclomethasone dipropionate, 3 puffs four times a day; and albuterol, 2 puffs every 4 hours on an as-needed basis. He indicates that he needs to take oral steroids an average of 5 days each month because of shortness of breath. He has been off work (on vacation) for approximately 2 weeks and wheezes are absent. He reports no shortness of breath on the day of evaluation.

#### Physical Examination

His chest auscultation is normal.

#### Test Results

A chest x-ray is normal. Pulmonary function tests show the following values: forced vital capacity (FVC), 5.48 L; $FEV_1$, 4.39 L; and $D_{LCO}$, 40.2 ml/min/mm Hg. These values reflect 101%, 99%, and 100% respectively of predicted values.

#### Assessment Process

You note that this individual has been off work for two weeks and away from his occupational exposures. He states that he has improved and is presently asymptomatic. You feel that his assessment is probably not representive of his usual state of health so you request old records.

In a review of old records, you note that this individual has had wheezing on almost every occasion when seen by a physician. There have been a number of screen spirometries obtained. These have shown variable values. However, in most circumstances, the FVC has ranged between 40 and 68% of predicted and the $FEV_1$ has ranged between 20% and 54% of predicted.

He has had a methacholine challenge test performed in the past. You carefully assess his records to find out if the criteria discussed in this chapter and in Chapter 27 with respect to medications, timing, and clinical symptomatology were met. They were. The methacholine challenge test was also done when he was on another vacation. He was found to have a $PC_{20}$ of 0.11 mg/ml. On another occasion, while he was actively involved in the work force, his $FEV_1$ was noted to change, on a post-bronchodilator spirometric examination, by 38%, to a value to 72%.

Using Table 29–1,* he would be placed in a Class 1 impairment level if only the results of the present examination and testing were used. Thus, he would have a 0% impairment rating, one which hardly represents the impact of his disease on his life and workability. Using Table 29–2 and his prior test results, he would have a score of 1, reflecting the post-bronchodilator value of 72%. Using Table 29–3, he has a score of 4 based upon a $PC_{20}$ of 0.11 mg/ml. Using Table 29-4, he has a score of 3 based upon his medication requirements. Adding up the total scores, he has a total of 8 points, placing him into a Class III impairment.

---

*All *tables* cited in this paragraph refer to tables in this chapter.

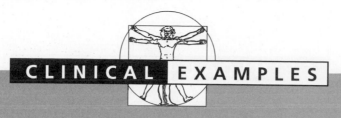
## RESPIRATORY SYSTEM—cont'd

Using Table 8, found on page 162 of the AMA *Guides,*[†] this individual would have a 25% to 50% impairment of the whole person based upon his asthma. The exact number would be at the discretion of the examining physician. The variables that would have to be considered would include his symptoms while away from work, the number of hospitalizations that he has had, the number of emergency room visits that he has had, the frequency of respiratory infections, and the frequency of systematic steroid usage. A 35% value might be appropriate in this particular individual.

Lastly, it should be appreciated that he is 100% impaired for his present occupation. Asthma is a disorder that can be life-threatening on occasion. He is working in a factory that produces chemicals known to not only create asthma but to exacerbate asthma. More definitive testing (for example, a RAST test to determine the presence of antibodies to isocyanates in her serum) would be appropriate to determine his status. This would also help from a legal standpoint.

### Addendum

It is two years later. He has changed jobs. His medication usage has dropped dramatically, and he is no longer using the steroids except during exacerbations caused by infections. He has not been seen in the hospital or emergency room, and his physician visits have diminished by 70%.

## EXAMPLE II

EDITOR'S NOTE—There are times when the evaluator has questions about the "fairness" of an evaluation. For example, in a person who is an active smoker and takes no medications for his breathing disorder, are the values measured truly representative of what this person is capable of doing? Is this individual truly comparable to another individual who,

for example, may have had similar symptoms yet took various medications and quit smoking ten years before examination?

The official stance of the AMA *Guides* is that "a patient may decline treatment of an impairment with a surgical procedure, a pharmacological agent, or other therapeutic approach. The view of the *Guides* contributors is that if a patient declines therapy for a permanent impairment, that decision should neither decrease nor increase the estimated percentage of the patient's impairment. However, the physician may wish to make a written comment in the medical evaluation report about the suitability of the therapeutic approach and describe the basis of the patient's refusal" (page 9).

Finally, a permanent impairment is defined as "one that has become static or stabilized during a period of time sufficient to allow optimal tissue repair, and one that is unlikely to change in spite of further medical or surgical therapy" (page 1). Clearly, an individual who smokes does not meet this definition. An active smoker is not in a "static or stabilized" condition. Even if he were to quit, a "period of time sufficient to allow opitmal tissue repair" may not have elapsed. Generally, the inflammatory changes, in the smoker, resolve over a period of six to twelve months. The emphysematous changes, of course, do not disappear. Further, this condition is likely to change with further medical therapy. Therefore, an individual who smokes and takes no medications could be considered non-evaluable based upon the concept and definition of "permanent impairment."

### History

A 55-year-old black man comes for an evaluation. He has smoked two packs of cigarettes per day for the last 37 years of his life. He works in a foundry and wears no respiratory protection. He states that the environment is constantly dirty, dusty, and smoky. His symptoms are predominantly those of shortness of breath. He has dyspnea on exertion when he walks at his own pace on the level.

---

[†]All *tables, figures,* and *sections* referred to in this discussion, unless indicated otherwise, are found in AMA *Guides to the evaluation of permanent impairment,* ed 4, Chapter 5—The Respiratory System, American Medical Association, Chicago, 1993.

*Continued.*

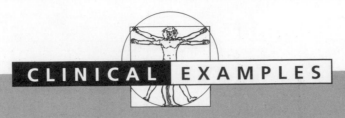
His daily cough is productive of a tan/brown sputum. The remainder of his medical history is negative. He takes no medications at the present time. He is 180 cm tall.

### Physical Examination

On examination, he has mild wheezing throughout the lungs. The expiratory phase of respiration is prolonged, but no other abnormalities are found.

### Test Results

A chest x-ray shows emphysematous changes in the lungs. The results of pulmonary function testing are FVC, 2.82 L; $FEV_1$, 2.02 L; and $D_{LCO}$, 32.10 ml/min/mm Hg. The spirometry is done in accordance with the requirements listed in section 5.2.

Since this individual is wheezing, a repeat study is performed using bronchodilators. The results are FVC, 3.41 L; $FEV_1$, 2.91 L; and $D_{LCO}$, 28.12 ml/min/mm Hg. These values represent 78%, 84%, and 84% of normal predicted for an individual of this height, age, sex, and race. (Please note that for North American blacks, there is a reduction factor necessary for the spirometric values. These factors are 0.88, 0.88, and 0.93, respectively, for the FVC, $FEV_1$, and $D_{LCO}$. Also, this individual required a spirometry *after* bronchodilator treatment.)

### Assessment Process

Tables 2, 4, and 6 are used to derive the predicted values for this individual. First, the values between 54 and 56 years of age are extrapolated. Based on his height, the FVC is predicted to be 4.97 L, which, when multiplied by 0.88, yields a value of 4.37 L. This is divided into 3.41, producing the 78% value already noted.

Using Table 1 (page 154), this individual has moderate dyspnea, specifically shortness of breath "when walking at your own pace on the level." Using Table 8, he has mild whole person impairment (WPI) based on the post-bronchodilator study. Thus the FVC is between 60% and 79% of predicted. The $FEV_1$ and $D_{LCO}$ are larger than in a Class II impairment and would place him into a Class I impairment. However, such a determination indicates that all three levels must be larger than the predicted formula. Class II, however, indicates that the FVC, *or* FEV, *or* the $D_{LCO}$ is lower than predicted. Therefore the Class II category would be more appropriate.

### Evaluation

Using the Class II impairment found in Table 8, this individual has a 10% to 25% WPI. Since the $FEV_1$ and $D_{LCO}$ are above predicted values and FVC is 78% with a spread of 60% to 79%, this individual would be ranked closer to the 10% value.

*Stephen L. Demeter*

edge of the job, its physical demands, and associated exposures.

When causation, particularly occupational causation, is an issue to be examined, it is essential to obtain an adequate evaluation of workplace exposures. This information can be obtained from a variety of sources. The patient, for example, can provide information including names and chemical descriptions of workplace exposures (MSDS Sheets). In many instances, industrial hygiene surveys of the workplace (e.g., measurement of air levels of toxins) may be obtainable from previous assessments. In particularly complex cases, it may be necessary to conduct a new exposure assessment to examine the specific and unique issues pertinent to the case. Another source of information may be standard textbooks of occupational lung disease.[37-41] Of course, such information is relevant only if determination of occupational causation is a significant component.

Additional specific considerations occur when there has been sensitization to a particular workplace agent (for example, isocyanates). Under such circumstances, even extremely small exposures can be hazardous. Usually, it is possible to establish the diagnosis by carefully conducting history and exposure assessment. In rare instances, specific bronchoprovocation testing with the suspected agent may be needed. Such testing is complex, costly, and entails risk for the patient. Therefore, it should only be performed by qualified laboratories.

*13. Prepare report*—The final step is the preparation of the summary report. The format should be appropriate for the "customer," which is often the agency who referred the patient for evaluation. Unlike therapeutic patient care, in impairment assessment, the quality of the written report may be just as important as the clinical assessment. Inadequately communicated information will not achieve the original intent of the evaluation. Therefore, the report should be prepared carefully.

The written report often provides the opportunity to add relevant information to that which is collected on a mandatory basis. For example, many administrative systems mandate that spirometry and diffusing capacity determination should be performed, but additional information about the patient's history or other available information may be added here. General principles of report preparation as well as ethical and legal considerations are discussed further in Chapters 10 and 11.

## SUMMARY

Assessment of respiratory disability and impairment can be accomplished with accuracy and objectivity. Judicious use of lung-functioning testing is particularly useful in documenting the presence or absence of respiratory disease and for scaling its severity.

## References

1. World Health Organization: *International classification of impairments, disabilities, and handicaps,* Geneva, 1980, WHO.
2. Cotes J, Zejda J, King B: Lung function impairment as a guide to exercise limitation in work-related lung disorders. *Am Rev Respir Dis* 137:1089-1093, 1988.
3. American Medical Association: *Guides to the evaluation of permanent impairment,* ed 4, Chicago, 1993, American Medical Association.
4. American Thoracic Society: Evaluation of impairment/disability secondary to respiratory disease. *Am Rev Respir Dis* 126:945-951, 1982.
5. American Thoracic Society: Evaluation of impairment/disability secondary to respiratory disorders. *Am Rev Respir Dis* 133:1205-1209, 1986.
6. American Thoracic Society: Guidelines for the evaluation of impairment/disability in patients with asthma. *Am Rev Respir Dis* 147:1056-1061, 1993.
7. Social Security Administration: *Disability evaluation under Social Security: a handbook for physicians,* DHEW Publication No. (SSA)79-10089, Washington D.C., 1979, Department of Health, Education, and Welfare.
8. Ferris BG: Recommended standardized procedures for pulmonary function testing. *Am Rev Respir Dis* 118(Part 2):55-88, 1978.
9. American Thoracic Society: Standardization of spirometry—1987 update. *Am Rev Respir Dis* 136:1285-1298, 1987.
10. American Thoracic Society: Lung function testing: selection of reference values and interpretative strategies. *Am Rev Respir Dis* 144:1202-1218, 1991.
11. American Thoracic Society: Single breath carbon monoxide diffusing capacity (transfer factor): recommendations for a standard technique. *Am Rev Respir Dis* 136:1299-1307, 1987.
12. Cotes JE, Dabbs JM, Elwood PC, et al: Iron-deficiency anaemia: its effects on transfer factor for the lung (diffusing capacity) and ventilation and cardiac frequency during sub-maximal exercise. *Clin Sci* 42:325-335, 1972.
13. Dinakara P, Blumental WS, Johnston RF, et al: The effect of anemia on pulmonary diffusing capacity with derivation of a corrected equation, *Am Rev Respir Dis* 102:965-969, 1970.
14. Mohsenifar Z, Brown HV, Schnitzer B, et al: The effect of abnormal levels of hematocrit on the

single breath diffusing capacity. *Lung* 160:325-330, 1982.

15. Mohsenifar Z, Tashkin DP: Effect of carboxyhemoglobin on the single breath diffusing capacity: derivation of an empirical correction factor. *Respiration* 37:185-191, 1979.

16. Morgan WKC, Zaldivar GL: Blood gas analysis as a determinant of occupationally related disability. *J Occup Med* 32(5):440-443, 1990.

17. Oren A, Sue DY, Hansen JE, et al: The role of exercise testing in impairment evaluation. *Am Rev Respir Dis* 135:230-235, 1987.

18. Cotes JE, Zejda J, King B: Lung function impairment as a guide to exercise limitation in work-related lung disorders. *Am Rev Respir Dis* 137:1089-1093, 1988.

19. Sue DY, Oren A, Hansen JE, Wasserman K: Diffusing capacity for carbon monoxide as a predictor of gas exchange during exercise. *N Engl J Med* 316:301-306, 1987.

20. International Labor Office: *Guidelines for the use of the ILO International Classification of radiographs of pneumoconioses,* Geneva, 1980, International Labor Office.

21. Malo J-L: Compensation for occupational asthma in Quebec. *Chest* 98(suppl):236S-239S, 1990.

22. Contreras G, Chan-Yeung M: Short report: a voluntary occupational lung disease registry in British Columbia. (submitted)

23. Keskinen H: Registers for occupational diseases. *Br Med J* 303:597-598, 1991.

24. Meredith S, Taylor V, McDonald J: Occupational respiratory disease in the United Kingdom 1989: a report to the British Thoracic Society and the Society of Occupational Medicine by the SWORD project group. *Br J Ind Med* 48:292-298, 1991.

25. Chan-Yeung M: State of the art: occupational asthma. *Chest* 98:148S-161S, 1990.

26. Chan-Yeung M: Pulmonary perspective: evaluation of impairment/disability in patients with occupational asthma. *Am Rev Respir Dis* 135:950-951, 1987.

27. Report of the working groups: Workshop on environmental and occupational asthma. *Chest* 98:240S-250S, 1990.

28. *Guidelines for the diagnosis and management of asthma,* Expert Panel Report of National Asthma Education Program, National Institute of Health Publication No. 91-3042A, 1991, National Heart, Lung and Blood Institute.

29. British Thoracic Society: Guidelines for management of asthma in adults: I—Chronic persistent asthma. *Br Med J* 301:651-653, 1990.

30. Woolcock A, Rubinfeld AR, Seale JP, et al: Asthma management plan—1989. *Med J Aust* 151:650-653, 1989.

31. Hargreave FE, Dolovich J, Newhouse M: The assessment and treatment of asthma: a conference report. *J Allergy Clin Immunol* 85:1097-1111, 1990.

32. Ramsdale EH, Morris MM, Roberts RS, Hargreave FE: Bronchial responsiveness to methacholine in chronic bronchitis: relationship to airflow obstruction and cold air responsiveness. Thorax 39:912-918, 1984.

33. Juniper EF, Cockcroft DW, Hargreave FE: *Histamine and methacholine inhalation tests: tidal breathing method: laboratory procedure and standardization,* Canadian Thoracic Society, 1991.

34. Yan K, Salome C, Woolcock AJ: Rapid method for measurement of bronchial responsiveness. *Thorax* 38:55-61, 1983.

35. Fabbri LM, Mapp CE, Hardick DJ: Standardization of the dosimeter method for the measurement of airway responsiveness in man. In Hargreave FE, Woolcock AJ, editors: *Airway responsiveness, measurement, and interpretation,* 1985, pp. 29-34, Astra Pharmaceuticals Canada Ltd.

36. Malo J-L, Cartier A, Ghezzo H, et al: Patterns of improvement on spirometry, bronchial hyperresponsiveness, and specific IgE antibody levels after cessation of exposure in occupational asthma caused by snow crab processing. *Am Rev Respir Dis* 138:807-812, 1988.

37. Parkes WR: *Occupational lung disorders,* ed 2, London, 1991, Butterworth.

38. Morgan WKC, Seaton A, editors: *Occupational lung diseases,* ed 2, Philadelphia, 1984, WB Saunders.

39. Merchant JA, editor: *Occupational respiratory diseases,* Appalachian Laboratory for Occupational Safety and Health (NIOSH), US Department of Health and Human Services, NIOSH Publication No. 86-102, 1986.

40. Harber P, Schenker M, Balmes J: *Occupational and environmental respiratory disease,* St. Louis, 1995, Mosby-Year Book.

41. Cotes JE, Steel W: *Work-related lung disorders,* Oxford, 1987, Blackwell Scientific.

# CHAPTER 30

# CARDIAC DISABILITY

*Harvey L. Alpern*

Cardiac impairment evaluation is challenging since it involves an often difficult assessment of subjective complaints. Of the array of objective diagnostic modalities that can be utilized in support of an evaluation, many are expensive and some more sensitive than others. An examiner must rely most significantly on his or her judgment in making a final assessment of impairment, in light of all the subjective and objective facts of a given case.

Impairment ratings will be based on objective measurements and use of various scales, including those adapted from AMA *Guides to the Evaluation of Permanent Impairment.*[3] Estimating the degree of the patient's *impairment* is the physicians' responsibility. In general, physicians do not judge *disability.*[3]

## CORONARY ARTERY DISEASE

Numerous risk factors are associated with coronary artery disease. Impairment examinations should include a careful history of the patient to determine all that are applicable. Gender, age, and a family history of coronary artery disease are factors that cannot be controlled; however, hypertension, hyperlipidemia, cigarette smoking, diabetes mellitus, obesity, sedentary lifestyle, and psychological stress are risk factors that can be modified to prevent coronary artery disease.

A history should provide details as to the duration and severity of risk factors identified with a given case. How long has the hypertension been present? When did treatment commence? Describe the degree and type of hyperlipidemia. Report the length of time of cigarette smoking and the number of cigarettes per day. If smoking has stopped, when did this occur? This is an important detail given the direct relationship between the number of cigarettes smoked and the incidence of cardiac events, and that this risk returns to near-normal approximately one year after smoking is discontinued. Diabetes mellitus must be noted because it contributes to an increased incidence

of atherosclerosis and small vessel disease. Obesity greater than 30% of ideal body weight is a notable risk factor. Lesser degrees of obesity do not contribute to coronary artery disease and need not be reported. Exercise abstinence is a risk factor to document.

Psychological stress, a potent risk factor, can precipitate a cardiac event. Studies have focused on chronic stress as it contributes to the development of coronary artery disease; some are now attempting to identify the toxic sub-components of Type A behavior that may lead to coronary disease. An association has been suggested between hostility and anger, and cardiac morbidity and mortality.[9,19,23] High levels of chronic stress, social isolation, and an inability to control, alter, or avoid stress are all associated with the risk of a cardiac event.[18,22,25]

Damage to the epithelium of the coronary vessel due to the effects of associated risk factors provides the catalyst for the gradual development of coronary artery disease and myocardial infarction. In response to the damage, macrophages in the form of foam cells enter the area to promote healing of the epithelium, and bring with them lipid particles from the bloodstream. Platelets accumulate, and calcification begins to occur. The foam cells and platelets release a substance that stimulates the growth of fibrous tissues in the area. The cumulative effect is a progressive development of atherosclerotic plaque. Myocardial infarction occurs when, with increased platelet stickiness, a thrombus results and occludes the vessel. Emotional and physical stresses are additionally linked to myocardial infarction because such stresses tend to increase the coagulability of blood and platelet aggregation.

### Diagnosis of Coronary Artery Disease

A careful history and a physical examination are crucial to any diagnostic procedure. All applicable risk factors should be documented. Note the initial onset of symptoms, the frequency of their occurrence, and their relationship to any physical or emotional activity. The notation of angina symptoms should include a detailed description of the patient's personal perception of the angina, and a description of any precipitating activity. In case of heart attack, include a detailed account of the precipitating event.

The physical examination should include vital signs, a description of the eyegrounds, jugular venous pressure, carotid pulse with a description of duration and upstroke, and evidence of bruits. Pulmonary findings should be noted. The heart examination should include a description of cardiac impulse felt for in the left lateral decubitus position. Heart tones, extra heart sounds, and murmurs may be reported according to standard procedure. The abdominal examination should include the presence or absence of bruits. Describe venous abnormalities and the quality of arterial supply as found during an examination of the extremities.

Diagnostic studies are not indicated if these have been done recently and the results are available, unless their accuracy is in question. A complete blood cell count, renal function studies, liver function studies, and lipid concentrations are usually appropriate laboratory studies. Thyroid function studies are indicated when there are findings in the history or on examination.

A resting electrocardiogram and chest x-rays are appropriate if these have not been recently done. An echocardiogram, most likely a stress echocardiogram, would be of help in diagnosing cardiac enlargement secondary to hypertension, or in attempting to assess areas of dyskinesia due to coronary disease. Based upon the extent of information needed for a thorough diagnosis, a standard stress test, a pharmacologic stress test, or one associated with an echocardiogram or radionuclide material might be indicated. If coronary artery disease is suspected and there is a history of hypertension, a stress echocardiogram, to determine the level of cardiac impairment from heart disease and simultaneously diagnose any enlargement from hypertension, is a cost-effective test. If the diagnosis of coronary artery disease is at issue, and there is an equivocal standard treadmill test available, then a radionuclear stress test using thallium, or a combination of thallium and technetium-99 sestamibi, would provide information about wall motion function and the area of ischemia to the heart.

In patients with intermittent chest pain or palpitations, a Holter monitor worn during a twenty-four hour period of normal activity may provide information useful to an evaluation of arrhythmias. Patients with chest pain may have ST-segment changes indicating evidence of spasm or ischemic heart disease. A Holter monitor used for this purpose should have a high frequency response to ensure that the ST-segment evaluation is reliable.

Treadmill exercise time can be used to predict the $\dot{V}o_2$max (maximum oxygen consumption). If oxygen consumption can be directly measured during the treadmill test, this is ideal; but if not logistically feasible, one may estimate $\dot{V}o_2$max by the time of exercise on the treadmill.[21] Tables and nomograms are available for this purpose.[14] A variance in the results up to 30% has been suggested when direct oxygen consumption cannot be measured.[16] The results of treadmill testing should be expressed in metabolic units called *METs* (Table 30-1).[13] Each MET represents 3.5 cc of oxygen consumption per kilogram per minute. One MET equals oxygen uptake at rest. Since protocols vary with regard to exercise testing, this method of reporting provides common ground for physicians in communicating the degree of exercise accomplished. The peak level in METS should always be stated. When exercise is stopped, note the reason, including any symptoms and signs that occurred. Note any arrhythmias, describe the degree of ST-segment depression, horizontal or downsloping, and report the blood pressure response to exercise.

Discontinue exercise testing if the individual is limited by chest pain, dyspnea, or orthopaedic problems. Testing should be stopped subsequent to the onset of supraventricular tachycardia or runs of three or more ventricular ectopics. Unifocal ectopic beats generally are not a reason to stop exercise. Blood pressure changes with systolic greater than 250 mm Hg signal the need to stop exercise, but lesser levels do not. Diastolic blood pressure normally increases mildly with exercise. A 10 mm Hg drop in systolic blood pressure with exercise may indicate ventricular dysfunction and is an indication to stop exercise.

Thallium, once the standard radionuclide used to measure areas of death of tissue of the myocardium and reversible ischemia, has been generally replaced by SPECT thallium-201 or SPECT technetium-99 sestamibi. SPECT (single-photon tomography) increases quantification of the extent of left ventricular dysfunction. Use of Tc-99 sestamibi, one of several newer radioactive agents, allows for better imaging and simultaneous assessment of first-pass ejection fraction and wall motion.

Pharmacologic stress testing is indicated when debility or musculoskeletal problems preclude exercise. Dipyridamole or adenosine is commonly used. Dobutamine is frequently used with stress echocardiogram studies.

Echocardiography with stress testing, either pharmacologic with dobutamine or treadmill, gives comparable results to radionuclear studies. The relative

**TABLE 30-1    RELATIONSHIPS OF METS AND FUNCTIONAL CLASS ACCORDING TO FIVE TREADMILL PROTOCOLS**

| METS | 1.6 | 2 | 3 | 4 | 5 | 6 | 7 | 8 | 9 | 10 | 11 | 12 | 13 | 14 | 15 | 16 |
|---|---|---|---|---|---|---|---|---|---|---|---|---|---|---|---|---|
| **Treadmill tests** | | | | | | | | | | | | | | | | |
| **Ellestad** | | | | | | | | | | | | | | | | |
| Miles per hour | | | | | 1.7 | 3.0 | | | 4.0 | | | | | | 5.0 | |
| % grade | | | | | 10 | 10 | | | 10 | | | | | | 10 | |
| **Bruce** | | | | | | | | | | | | | | | | |
| Miles per hour | | | | | 1.7 | | 2.5 | | 3.4 | | | | 4.2 | | | |
| % grade | | | | | 10 | | 12 | | 14 | | | | 16 | | | |
| **Balke** | | | | | | | | | | | | | | | | |
| Miles per hour | | | | 3.4 | 3.4 | 3.4 | 3.4 | 3.4 | 3.4 | 3.4 | 3.4 | 3.4 | 3.4 | 3.4 | 3.4 | 3.4 |
| % grade | | | | 2 | 4 | 6 | 8 | 10 | 12 | 14 | 16 | 18 | 20 | 22 | 24 | 26 |
| **Balke** | | | | | | | | | | | | | | | | |
| Miles per hour | | | 3.0 | 3.0 | 3.0 | 3.0 | 3.0 | 3.0 | 3.0 | 3.0 | 3.0 | 3.0 | | | | |
| % grade | | | 0 | 2.5 | 5 | 7.5 | 10 | 12.5 | 15 | 17.5 | 20 | 22.5 | | | | |
| **Naughton** | | | | | | | | | | | | | | | | |
| Miles per hour | 1.0 | 2.0 | 2.0 | 2.0 | 2.0 | 2.0 | 2.0 | | | | | | | | | |
| % grade | 0 | 0 | 3.5 | 7 | 10.5 | 14 | 17.5 | | | | | | | | | |
| METS | 1.6 | 2 | 3 | 4 | 5 | 6 | 7 | 8 | 9 | 10 | 11 | 12 | 13 | 14 | 15 | 16 |
| **Clinical status** | | | | | | | | | | | | | | | | |
| Symptomatic patients | ←————————————→ | | | | | | | | | | | | | | | |
| Diseased, recovered | | | ←————————→ | | | | | | | | | | | | | |
| Sedentary healthy | | | | | ←————————————→ | | | | | | | | | | | |
| Physically active | | | | | | ←——————————————————————————→ | | | | | | | | | | |
| **Functional class** | IV | ←— III —→ | | ←II→ | | ←———————— I and Normal ————————→ | | | | | | | | | | |

Adapted from AMA *Guides to the evaluation of permanent impairment*, ed 4, Chicago, 1993, American Medical Association.

sensitivity and specificity of these modalities are shown in Table 30-2.[7]

Positron emission tomography (PET) gives information about metabolic viability of the myocardium. There are usually fewer artifacts with this technique and the sensitivity and specificity is >90%. The test is infrequently used due to its expense, although now is becoming cheaper due to less expensive radionuclides.

Ejection fraction, obtained from echocardiograms, multigated radionuclide studies, or cardiac catheterization, is a useful figure since a reduced value of less than 50% is associated with a risk of higher mortality over five years.

When exercise is discontinued due to dyspnea, one should consider a cardiopulmonary exercise test where oxygen consumption is measured and one can collect data to differentiate between cardiac causes of dyspnea and pulmonary causes of dyspnea (see Chapter 28).[28]

Cardiac catheterization provides valuable information, although this study is seldom ordered in conjunction with impairment evaluation. Data regarding ventricular function, wall motion, pressures in the ventricle, valvular abnormalities, and the anatomy of the coronary arteries is obtained through coronary angiography and catheterization; coronary artery vasospasm can be seen.

Coronary artery vasospasm is frequently implicated as a cause of chest pain at rest; however, most

**TABLE 30-2    SENSITIVITY AND SPECIFICITY OF EXERCISE TESTS[7]**

|  | SENSITIVITY | SPECIFICITY |
|---|---|---|
| Stress ECG | 68% | 77% |
| Thallium-201 | 84% | 87% |
| Quantified thallium | 89% | 89% |
| SPECT thallium | 90% | 89% |
| Tc-99 sestamibi | 89% | 90% |
| SPECT Tc-99 sestamibi | 90% | 93% |
| Dipyridamole thallium-201 | 85% | 87% |
| Stress echo | 80% | 90% |
| During exercise | 93% | 86% |
| Dobutamine | 89% | 85% |
| PET scan | 95% | 95% |
| History and physical examination | 79% | 83% |

of these chest pains are not of cardiac etiology. Coronary artery vasospasm of the Prinzmetal variant type occurs in a normal coronary artery during the nocturnal hours generally, and is usually associated with ST-segment elevation. Fixed coronary artery lesions are also associated with coronary artery spasm. These lesions may be seen on angiography if ergonovine is given, or if a mental stress test is given simultaneously. Lesions of this type are often responsive to a stimulus of emotional stress.

A mental stress test can be administered during a standard electrocardiogram, Holter monitor testing, or studies measuring cardiac ischemia through other methods. Public speaking is a potent stimulus for mental stress testing. Engaging the individual in word recognition games, arithmetic, or computer games is another technique.[23]

The choice of the appropriate diagnostic test requires matching the best test to a particular patient. Many patients will require no testing since all studies have been done in the recent past. If tests were done in the past six months and there were no historical clinical changes, no further testing would likely be needed. If the question is not diagnosis but only detection of symptoms at a measured exercise level, then a simple stress test would be reasonable. If diagnosis of chest pain is required and past studies have

not been done or were not diagnostic, then a radionuclear stress study or stress echocardiogram would be the better choice. If both evaluation of wall thickness due to hypertension and diagnosis of coronary artery disease is the goal, then a stress echocardiogram would be the cost-effective choice. If risk stratification for future mortality were needed, an ejection fraction could be estimated from a Tc-99 sestamibi or echocardiogram study.

If no diagnostic studies were available and only the history and physical examination were done, the diagnosis of coronary artery disease could be made with about the same sensitivity and specificity as the standard treadmill test, but less than that of a radionuclear exercise study or stress echocardiogram. Regardless of the quoted sensitivity and specificity of the history and physical examination, standard treadmill tests are usually ordered and performed to accommodate the requirements of various impairment schemes including the AMA *Guides* and the Social Security System.[3,30]

**Impairment Ratings**

In the past, occupational tables were used to categorize impairment. The energy used to accomplish a particular job was calculated in METS.[15] If during testing an individual could achieve a level of METS greater than the number on the work table associated with a particular occupation, that individual was deemed able to do the job. The problem with categories is that they are based on averages of energy needed, and peak energies are often much higher. Also, healthy individuals, not those with coronary artery disease, participated in the studies that determined the categories.

Haskell has devised a simple classification of work based upon MET level achieved that ranges from very heavy work to sedentary work (Table 30-3).[15] Individuals who can do more than 7 METS of work, or greater than a $\dot{V}O_2max$ of 25, are said to have no impairment; those with a $\dot{V}O_2max$ of less than 15 are totally impaired (Table 30-4). Graphs that correlate exercise capacity for normal individuals, both active and inactive men and women, can be used as a reference.

Another method of expressing cardiac impairment is to take the current measurement of work or exercise capability in METS in comparison with preinjury or preillness level of METS (either previously measured or estimated) and then calculate the percentage of impairment as a result of the injury or illness:[17]

Percentage Impairment =
    (1 – current MET level/ prior MET level) × 100%

The New York Heart Association Functional Classi-

**TABLE 30-3**    HASKELL WORK CLASSIFICATION[15]

|  | PEAK METS | ACTIVITY |
|---|---|---|
| Very Heavy | >6 | Climb stairs |
| Medium | 4-6 | Carry 50 lbs |
| Light | 2-4 | Carry 20 lbs |
| Sedentary | <2 | Sit/carry 10 lbs |

Adapted from Haskell, W, et al: Task Force II: determination of occupational working capacity in patients with ischemic heart disease. *JACC* 1989; 14:1027.

**TABLE 30-4**    IMPAIRMENT RATING

| $\dot{V}_{O_2}$MAX | PEAK METS | ACTIVITY |
|---|---|---|
| >25 | >7 | None |
| 20-25 | 5-7 | Mild to moderate |
| 15-20 | 2.5-5 | Severe |
| <15 | <2.5 | Total |

Adapted from AMA *Guides to the evaluation of permanent impairment,* ed 4, Chicago, 1993, American Medical Association.

**TABLE 30-5**    NEW YORK HEART ASSOCIATION FUNCTIONAL CLASSIFICATION OF CARDIAC DISEASE

| CLASS | DESCRIPTION |
|---|---|
| 1 | Ordinary activity does not cause symptoms of undue fatigue, palpitations, dyspnea, or anginal pain |
| 2 | Greater than ordinary physical activity results in symptoms |
| 3 | Ordinary physical activity results in symptoms |
| 4 | Symptoms at rest, and worse with any physical activity |

Adapted from AMA *Guides to the evaluation of permanent impairment,* ed 4, Chicago, 1993, American Medical Association.

fication has been in use since 1964 (Table 30-5). This classification is based entirely upon subjective evaluation. The AMA Impairment Classification of classes one through four is based upon subjective and objective evaluations,[3] where impairment is measured objectively in METS as described above (Table 30-6).

Disability is determined by evaluating how this impairment limits the individual in the work place as well as in everyday activities. When chest pain is thought to be noncardiac, an opinion as to the etiology, and the reason for this opinion, should be stated. A description of precipitating or aggravating factors and a rating of the severity of the pain should be given.

Individuals with cardiac disease should be advised as to whether they can maintain an eight-hour workday, based on a figure of approximately 40% of the maximum MET level achieved during testing. Assuming that usual breaks are taken, the individual can perform sustained work at this level for 8 hours. Concerning maximal short-term work—less than 15 min once a day—an individual who does not have current symptoms can accomplish 80% of maximum MET level, assuming that the end-point of exercise is physical fitness. The figure does not apply to an individual who is posttreatment, for example, from coronary artery bypass graft surgery and symptomatic. If cardiac symptoms are the end-point of exercise, 70% of the tested MET level should be considered the level of maximum short-term work the patient can achieve.[4,5,29]

## HYPERTENSIVE HEART DISEASE

The most common form of hypertension is essential hypertension. An evaluation for hypertension must address a history of any factors that may reveal a primary cause for hypertension other than essential. Questions should focus on past history of renal infections or other renal disease, and symptoms suggestive of paroxysmal elevations such as those associated with pheochromocytoma. The history should expose any secondary effects of the hypertension on other organ systems including neurologic symptoms and visual changes. The complete physical examination, in addition to determining the blood pressure in both upper extremities in the supine and standing positions, allows the physician to look for evidence of neurologic abnormalities, cardiac enlargement, a fourth heart sound, and abdominal bruits.

Hypertension has been defined and categorized in The Fifth Report of the Joint National Committee on Detection, Evaluation, and Treatment of High Blood Pressure. According to this classification, a blood pressure of less than 130 mm Hg systolic and less than 85 mm Hg diastolic is considered normal; a blood pressure of 130-139 mm Hg systolic and 85-90 mm Hg diastolic is high normal. Hypertension occurs when blood pres-

**TABLE 30-6**     IMPAIRMENT CLASSIFICATION FOR CORONARY HEART DISEASE

| CLASS 1<br>(0%-9% IMPAIRMENT<br>OF THE WHOLE PERSON) | CLASS 2<br>(10%-29% IMPAIRMENT<br>OF THE WHOLE PERSON) | CLASS 3<br>(30%-49% IMPAIRMENT<br>OF THE WHOLE PERSON) | CLASS 4<br>(50%-100% IMPAIRMENT<br>OF THE WHOLE PERSON) |
|---|---|---|---|
| Because of serious implications of reduced coronary blood flow, it is not reasonable to classify degree of impairment as 0 through 9 in any patient who has symptoms of coronary heart disease corroborated by physical examination or laboratory tests; this class of impairment should be reserved for patients with equivocal histories of angina pectoris on whom coronary angiography is performed, or for patients on whom coronary angiography is performed for other reasons and in whom less than 50% reduction in cross sectional area of coronary artery is found; METS determination is not applicable. | Patient has a history of myocardial infarction or angina pectoris documented by appropriate laboratory studies, but at time of evaluation, patient has no symptoms while performing ordinary daily activities or even moderately heavy physical exertion (functional class 1);<br><br>**and**<br><br>Patient may require moderate dietary adjustment or medication to prevent angina or to remain free of signs and symptoms of congestive heart failure;<br><br>**and**<br><br>Patient is able to walk on the treadmill or bicycle ergometer and obtain heart rate of 90% of predicted maximum heart rate without developing significant ST-segment shift, ventricular tachycardia, or hypotension; if patient is uncooperative or unable to exercise because of disease affecting another organ system, this requirement may be omitted; METS >7;<br><br>**or**<br><br>Patient has recovered from coronary artery surgery or angioplasty, remains asymptomatic during ordinary daily activities, and is able to exercise as outlined above; if patient is taking a beta-adrenergic blocking agent, he or she should be able to walk on treadmill to level estimated to cause energy expenditure of at least 7 METS as substitute for heart rate target. | Patient has history of myocardial function documented by appropriate laboratory studies, and/or angina pectoris documented by changes on resting or exercise ECG or radioisotope study suggestive of ischemia;<br><br>**or**<br><br>Patient has either fixed or dynamic focal obstruction of at least 50% of coronary artery, angiography, and function testing;<br><br>**and**<br><br>Patient requires moderate dietary adjustment or drugs to prevent frequent angina or to remain free of symptoms and signs of congestive heart failure but may develop angina pectoris after moderately heavy physical exertion (functional class 2); METS >5 but <7;<br><br>**or**<br><br>Patient has recovered from coronary artery surgery or angioplasty, continues to require treatment, and has symptoms described above. | Patient has history of myocardial infarction that is documented by appropriate laboratory studies, or angina pectoris documented by changes on resting ECG or radioisotope study highly suggestive of myocardial ischemia;<br><br>**or**<br><br>Patient has either fixed or dynamic focal obstruction of at least 50% of one or more coronary arteries, demonstrated by angiography and function testing;<br><br>**and**<br><br>Patient requires moderate dietary adjustments or drugs to prevent angina or to remain free of symptoms and signs of congestive heart failure, but continues to develop symptoms of angina pectoris or congestive heart failure during ordinary daily activities (functional class 3 or 4), or there are signs or laboratory evidence of cardiac enlargement and abnormal ventricular function; METS <5;<br><br>**or**<br><br>Patient has recovered from coronary artery bypass surgery or angioplasty and continues to require treatment and have symptoms as described above. |

Adapted from AMA *Guides to the evaluation of permanent impairment,* ed 4, Chicago, 1993, American Medical Association.

sure exceeds 140/90. Mild hypertension is 140-159/90-99; moderate hypertension is 160-179/100-109; and severe hypertension is 180-209/110-119. Critical hypertension is higher than this.[24]

Hypertension is not a simple disease. Research by Eliot has concluded that stress is a major and often overlooked component of the illness.[10-12] Studies by Schnall et al show that job strain is a potential risk factor for hypertension and for structural changes in the heart, leading to an increased left ventricular mass index.[6] Impairment evaluations must include a careful history of stress, if stress is relevant to the case.[26] Of particular concern is any pattern of continuous, unrelenting stress where the individual is in a trapped position with no options for avoiding or altering the stress.[20,25] Evaluate the possible presence of a "hot reactor"—an individual who has a normal blood pressure at rest and may appear calm, but with mental stress has marked increase in blood pressure. This increase in blood pressure may be due to increased cardiac contraction or increased peripheral resistance or both. Eliot has described a method for identifying a hot reactor by determining blood pressure and, through noninvasive techniques, peripheral vascular resistance, so as to individualize therapy (pharmacologic and non-pharmacologic). When a cerebrovascular accident (CVA) occurs in a hypertensive individual, and the CVA is not felt to be embolic, a history of any stress that might have elevated blood pressure immediately proximal to the event should be noted.

## Classification of Hypertension

The AMA *Guides* define as Class I those individuals who are normotensive with medication and have no end-organ damage (Table 30-7). A Class II individual shows abnormalities of urine without evidence of renal impairment or a history of a cerebrovascular episode or retinal changes. There may be no symptoms. Class III individuals have renal insufficiency, a history of stroke, left ventricular hypertrophy, or retinopathy. An individual whose high blood pressure cannot be controlled belongs in this category. Individuals who have more than one of the Class III complications or have cardiac decompensation belong in the Class IV category.[3] In essence, impairment as a result of hypertension is related to end-organ damage. An individual should be considered temporarily impaired until the hypertension is controlled with medication, then rated as to his or her level of impairment to brain, eye, heart and kidneys. Progressive doses or additions of medication are considered an additional impairment.

## VALVULAR HEART DISEASE

Any history suggestive of rheumatic fever should be noted. The progression of symptoms of shortness of breath should be documented by an estimation of prior and current tolerance to exercise. Obtain a history of the number of stairs the individual could climb in past years as compared to present time, for example, and any history of treadmill testing. Slowly progressive cardiac decompensation is seen most often in conditions such as mitral stenosis or aortic stenosis. Aortic regurgitation may not be symptomatic until there is relatively rapid decompensation. These conditions are not known to be related to work phenomena; however, an impairment evaluation and the rating for such an impairment is necessary to determine a feasible work assignment for the individual.

Rating the level of impairment for an individual with valvular heart disease is especially important when there are co-existing conditions, such as coronary artery disease. Co-existing conditions may also impair the individual. An attempt must be made to distinguish the level of impairment for all existing conditions so that the impairment classification may be appropriately judged (Table 30-8).

Testing for valvular heart disease when the diagnosis is known may only require a history to determine activity level or a treadmill study to document this level in METS. Chest X-ray for evaluation of heart size and pulmonary vasculature is another objective measure of the effect of valvular heart disease. An echocardiogram to determine chamber size and estimate valve area is usually required. Valve area is usually estimated from echocardiographic measurement, but the information may also be derived from catheterization data if available. Cardiac catheterization is usually not required for an impairment rating but would usually be done before surgery to determine if coronary or other cardiac abnormalities are present. If coronary artery disease and valvular disease are present the physician should indicate whether the exercise test was terminated due to angina. Fatigue or dyspnea could result from either coronary or valvular disease.

Existing tables that measure the severity of valve disease are based upon valve diameter and exercise tolerance (Table 30-9). The AMA guidelines are dependent on the number of METS achieved and the necessity of therapy for heart failure.

## CARDIAC ARRHYTHMIAS

A complete physical examination is necessary for the impairment evaluation and should focus on

**TABLE 30-7** IMPAIRMENT CLASSIFICATION FOR HYPERTENSIVE CARDIOVASCULAR DISEASE

| CLASS 1 (0%-9% IMPAIRMENT OF THE WHOLE PERSON) | CLASS 2 (10%-29% IMPAIRMENT OF THE WHOLE PERSON) | CLASS 3 (30%-49% IMPAIRMENT OF THE WHOLE PERSON) | CLASS 4 (50%-100% IMPAIRMENT OF THE WHOLE PERSON) |
|---|---|---|---|
| Patient has no symptoms but diastolic pressures are repeatedly > 90 mm Hg; **and** Patient is normotensive with antihypertensive medications and has *none* of the following abnormalities: (1) abnormal urinalysis or renal function tests; (2) history of hypertensive cerebrovascular disease; (3) evidence of left ventricular hypertrophy; (4) hypertensive vascular abnormalities of optic fundus, except minimal narrowing of arterioles. | Patient has no symptoms but diastolic pressures are repeatedly > 90 mm Hg; **and** Patient is taking antihypertensive medication and has *any* of the following abnormalities: (1) proteinuria and abnormalities of the urinary sediment, but no impairment of renal function as measured by serum urea nitrogen (SUN) and serum creatinine determinations; (2) history of hypertensive cerebrovascular damage; (3) definite hypertensive changes in retinal arterioles, including crossing defects and old exudates. | Patient has no symptoms but diastolic pressure readings are consistently > 90 mm Hg; **and** Patient is taking antihypertensive medication and has *any* of the following abnormalities: (1) diastolic pressure readings usually > 120 mm Hg; (2) proteinuria or abnormalities in urinary sediment, with evidence of impaired renal function as measured by elevated SUN and serum creatinine, or by creatinine clearance below 50%; (3) hypertensive cerebrovascular damage with permanent neurologic residual; (4) left ventricular hypertrophy according to findings of physical examination, echocardiography, ECG, or chest roentgenogram, but no symptoms, signs, or evidence by chest roentgenogram of congestive heart failure; (5) retinopathy, with definite hypertensive changes in arterioles, such as "copper" or "silver wiring," or arteriovenous crossing changes, with or without hemorrhages and exudates. | Patient has a diastolic pressure consistently > 90 mm Hg; **and** Patient is taking antihypertensive and has *any* 2 of the following abnormalities: (1) diastolic pressure readings usually > 120 mm Hg; (2) proteinuria and abnormalities in urinary sediment, with impaired renal function and evidence of nitrogen retention as measured by elevated SUN and serum creatinine or by creatinine clearance below 50%; (3) hypertensive cerebrovascular damage with permanent neurologic deficits; (4) left ventricular hypertrophy; (5) retinopathy as manifested by hypertensive changes in arterioles, retina, or optic nerve; (6) history of congestive heart failure; **or** Patient has left ventricular hypertrophy with persistence of congestive heart failure despite digitalis and diuretics. |

Adapted from AMA *Guides to the evaluation of permanent impairment,* ed 4, Chicago, 1993, American Medical Association.

symptoms and signs of cardiac abnormality. The history of an individual with cardiac arrhythmias should include the onset of symptoms of palpitations, whether they start or stop suddenly, and whether they are associated with any neurologic symptoms. Any factors that may have caused the onset of arrhythmia should be explored in the history. Questions should be asked concerning the history of a possible thyroid condition and symptoms of hyperthyroidism. If the patient is taking thyroid medication, note the dosage.

Impairments in patients with arrhythmias are the result of decreased blood flow during the arrhythmia, resulting in dizziness or syncope. There are other subjective complaints in addition to dizziness such as palpitations, dyspnea, and chest pain. Objective findings are the recording of the arrhythmia, such as on a Holter monitor recording, and associating this finding with ischemic ST change, syncope, or seizure. Emboli from the left atrium in atrial fibrillation may result in dysfunction in a variety of different organs (e.g., brain, gut, extremities) and, hence, impairment of any target body part.

In situations of cardiac arrhythmia, laboratory studies are a reasonable part of the impairment evaluation in order to diagnose anemia, check levels of potassium and electrolytes, and assess thyroid function.

Sometimes a simple electrocardiogram and rhythm

**TABLE 30-8**    IMPAIRMENT CLASSIFICATION FOR VALVULAR HEART DISEASE

| CLASS 1 (0%-9% IMPAIRMENT OF THE WHOLE PERSON) | CLASS 2 (10%-29% IMPAIRMENT OF THE WHOLE PERSON) | CLASS 3 (30%-49% IMPAIRMENT OF THE WHOLE PERSON) | CLASS 4 (50%-100% IMPAIRMENT OF THE WHOLE PERSON) |
|---|---|---|---|
| Patient has evidence by physical examination or laboratory studies of valvular heart disease, but no symptoms in the performance of ordinary daily activities or even on moderately heavy exertion (functional class 1); **and** Patient does not require continuous treatment, although prophylactic antibiotics may be recommended at time of surgical procedure to reduce risk of bacterial endocarditis; **and** Patient remains free of signs of congestive heart failure; **and** There are no signs of ventricular dysfunction or dilation, and severity of stenosis or regurgitation is estimated to be mild; METS >7; TMET (Bruce protocol) >6 min; **and** In patient who has recovered from valvular heart surgery, all of above criteria are met. | Patient has evidence by physical examination or laboratory studies of valvular heart disease, and there are no symptoms in performance of daily activities, but symptoms develop on moderately heavy physical exertion (functional class 2); **or** Patient requires moderate dietary adjustment or drugs to prevent symptoms or to remain free of signs of congestive heart failure or other consequences of valvular heart disease, such as syncope, chest pain, and emboli; **or** Patient has signs or laboratory evidence of cardiac chamber dysfunction and/or dilation, severity of stenosis or regurgitation is estimated to be moderate, and surgical correction is not feasible or advisable; METS >5 but <7; TMET (Bruce protocol) >3 min; **or** Patient has recovered from valvular heart surgery and meets above criteria. | Patient has signs of valvular heart disease and has slight to moderate symptomatic discomfort during performance of ordinary daily activities (functional class 3); **and** Dietary therapy or drugs do not completely control symptoms or prevent congestive heart failure; **and** Patient has signs or laboratory evidence of cardiac chamber dysfunction or dilation, severity of stenosis or regurgitation is estimated to be moderate or severe, and surgical correction is not feasible; METS >2 but <5; TMET (Bruce protocol) >1 min; **or** Patient has recovered from heart valve surgery but continues to have symptoms and signs of congestive heart failure including cardiomegaly. | Patient has signs by physical examination of valvular heart disease, and symptoms at rest or in performance of less than ordinary daily activities (functional class 4); **and** Dietary therapy and drugs cannot control symptoms or prevent signs of congestive heart failure; **and** Patient has signs or laboratory evidence of cardiac chamber dysfunction or dilation, severity of stenosis or regurgitation is estimated to be moderate or severe, and surgical correction is not feasible; METS <1; TMET <1 min; **or** Patient has recovered from valvular heart surgery but continues to have symptoms or signs of congestive heart failure. |

strip will suffice as an analysis of cardiac arrhythmias; however, a 24-hour Holter monitor may be necessary at least once. If symptoms recur less frequently, an event monitor recording is indicated. The Holter monitor records every heart beat over 24 hours and is analyzed both visually and by computer to determine the frequency of ectopic beats and the type. If symptoms are rare, an event monitor with fixed leads or a chest contact box monitor may be used. The usual event monitor records when an individual puts the box on the chest and presses a button to activate the recording when symptoms occur. This device can be carried for weeks at a time.

An attempt should be made to uncover and document in the history any emotional stress that may relate to the onset of the arrhythmias.[1]

AMA *Guides to Permanent Impairment Evaluation* are clear in delineating the four classes of arrhythmias. Class 1 distinguishes an individual who is asymptomatic, does not have a complex arrhythmia, and has no evidence of organic heart disease. A Class 2 individual may be symptomatic. A person in this category is undergoing treatment for symptoms, or has been diagnosed with organic disease. A Class 3 individual is one under treatment whose symptoms from arrhythmia continue infrequently. A Class 4 type is

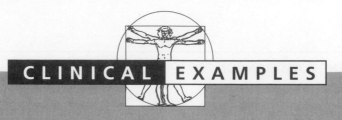

## CLINICAL EXAMPLES

## CARDIAC DISEASE

### EXAMPLE

#### History

A 54-year-old Caucasian firefighter has come for an evaluation. He is 180 cm tall and has a history of coronary artery disease, diagnosed by signs, symptoms, and an angiogram performed previously. Angiographic findings showed an 80% lesion of the circumflex artery, 75% lesion of the left anterior descending artery, and 60% lesion in the right coronary artery. He has symptoms of angina approximately three times per month. He has difficulty performing his work and is now on medical leave.

Further evaluation reveals a history of high cholesterol levels; his total cholesterol level currently is 302, and the HDL fraction is diminished. There is also a family history of hypercholesterolemia. Additionally, he has shortness of breath with exertion. He is presently taking nitroglycerin on an as-needed basis, and a calcium channel blocker; he has a nitroglycerin patch. He was also taking a theophylline product, but discontinued it due to stomach upset.

#### Physical Examination

He has no wheezing. A pulmonary function test is obtained. His forced vital capacity (FVC) is 4.85 L; FEV$_1$, 3.02 L; and D$_{LCO}$, 34.1 ml/min/mm Hg. An S4 gallup is identified, the blood pressure is normal, and no other abnormalities are found.

#### Assessment Process

With respect to coronary artery disease, this individual would fall into Class III impairment using Table 6 (p. 178).* However, an exercise stress test was not performed. To be completely compliant with the Table 6 classification scheme, this test would be needed to determine the individual's METS achievable. With the information available, however, he best fits Class III. The spread for the cardiac impairment is 30% to 49%. Based on all the facts presented, the lower value would be more appropriate, leading to a 35% impairment considering the relative infrequency of nitroglycerin use. Additionally, his spirometric values indicate a mild respiratory impairment using Table 8 (p. 162). A 10% impairment would be considered appropriate based on his pulmonary impairment.

#### Evaluation

The 10% pulmonary impairment is combined with the 35% cardiovascular impairment, producing a 42% whole person impairment (WPI).

*Stephen L. Demeter*

---

*All *tables* referred to in this discussion are found in AMA *Guides to the evaluation of permanent impairment,* ed 4, Chapter 5—The Respiratory System, and Chapter 6—The Cardiovascular System, American Medical Association, Chicago, 1993.

**TABLE 30-9    SEVERITY OF VALVE STENOSIS**

| SEVERITY OF STENOSIS | MEAN VALVE GRADIENT (MM HG) | VALVE AREA (CM$^2$) |
|---|---|---|
| Aortic valve | | |
| Mild | <25 | >1.2 |
| Moderate | 25-50 | 0.7-1.2 |
| Severe | >50 | <0.7 |
| Mitral valve | | |
| Mild | <5 | >1.5 |
| Moderate | 5-10 | 1.0-1.5 |
| Severe | >10 | <1.0 |

Adapted from AMA *Guides to the evaluation of permanent impairment,* ed 4, Chicago, 1993, American Medical Association.

functionally a NYHA Class 3 or 4 and has palpitations or syncope even though under treatment.[3]

If arrhythmias occur during exercise, the MET level attained would establish the impairment level. Supraventricular arrhythmias may result in impairment related to the extent of subjective symptoms. It should be noted that ventricular arrhythmias in the presence of ventricular dysfunction are associated with increased mortality.[8]

## CARDIOMYOPATHY

Cardiomyopathy is frequently the result of an unknown condition. Congenital or hereditary factors may lead to cardiomyopathy, or it may be secondary to infections of many types, usually viral. Amyloid or thyroid disease or parasitic conditions can result in cardiomyopathy. There is no evidence that the illness is in any way related to emotional stress. A history and physical examination is similar to that indicated for patients with coronary and valvular disease. Myocardial biopsy may be done for diagnosis or research, but is unnecessary for an impairment evaluation. Treadmill exercise testing would give the level of impairment by noting the MET level where exercise is stopped due to fatigue or dyspnea. A stress echocardiogram would also give this information along with an ejection fraction. Given that the diagnosis was previously made, radionuclear exercise testing would not be needed.

The impairment rating for cardiomyopathy is a function of the patient's ability to exercise as determined by a treadmill test. When symptoms are present, the impairment rating is also based on the New York Heart Association Guidelines. Arrhythmia may add to the impairment by causing dizziness and palpi-

tations. Guidelines similar to those for coronary artery disease are applicable. Some patients will need surgery for hypertrophic cardiomyopathy or transplant therapy, but overall ratings would depend upon measured impairment on an exercise study after recovery from surgery.

## CONGESTIVE HEART FAILURE

When congestive heart failure (CHF) complicates any cardiac condition, treatment is undertaken; only when maximal medical therapy has been given is an impairment rating considered. The impairment rating guides outlined for coronary heart disease may be used to determine the impairment rating for CHF (Table 30-6). It would be expected that the limiting factor on exercise testing would be dyspnea or fatigue rather than angina. If exercise cannot be done, an ejection fraction measured by echocardiogram or by angiogram—either radionuclear or at catheterization—may be used to estimate impairment. An ejection fraction of greater than 50% is generally considered as normal or no impairment. However, a normal ejection fraction at rest may be seen when there is significant coronary or other heart disease and may be lower with exercise. An ejection fraction of less than 25% indicates severe impairment, with moderate impairment for ejection fractions between 25% and 50%.

## OTHER CARDIAC DISEASE

Congenital heart abnormalities may be rated by exercise capability as outlined in the sections on coronary disease and congestive heart failure. Pericardial disease usually is an acute problem with temporary total impairment. When there is a chronic pericardial disease, such as when tuberculosis or carcinoma involve the pericardium and no further medical or surgical intervention is planned, an impairment rating would be based on exercise tolerance as outlined previously.

Heart block or any slow arrhythmia resulting in symptoms is generally treated with a pacemaker implantation. Impairment rating would be as described in the section on cardiac arrhythmias if further arrhythmias or symptoms were present after pacemaker insertion.

## References
1. Allen R, et al: Is coronary heart disease a lifestyle disorder? A review of psychologic and behavioral factors. *CVR&R*, Dec. 1992.

2. Alpern HL: Cardiac disability: an overview. *J Disabil* 1:2 April 1990.

3. American Medical Association: *Guides to the evaluation of permanent impairment,* ed 4, Chicago, 1993.

4. Astrand I: Aerobic work capacity in men and women with special reference to age. *Acta Physiol Scand* 49 (Suppl 169), 1960.

5. Astrand I: Degree of strain during building work as related to individual aerobic work capacity. *Ergonomics* 10:293-303, 1967.

6. Barker S: High-strain jobs' role in hypertension. *Cardiology World News,* March 1993.

7. Beller GA: *New stress testing methods.* Presented at the ACC Lake Louise Cardiologists' Conference, March 1994.

8. Clark WL, Alpern HL, et al: Suggested guidelines for rating cardiac disability on workers' compensation. *West J Med* 158:263-267, March 1993.

9. Denollet J, et al: Coping subtypes for men with coronary heart disease: relationship to well-being, stress, and Type-A behaviour. *Biol Psychol* 34(1):1-4, Oct. 1992.

10. Eliot RS: *Stress and the heart,* New York, 1988, Futura.

11. Eliot RS: The dynamics of hypertension—an overview: present practices, new possibilities, and new approaches. *Am Heart J* 116:2, Aug. 1988.

12. Eliot RS: Psychophysiologic stress testing as a predictor of mean daily blood pressure. *Am Heart J* 116:2, Aug. 1988.

13. Fletcher GF, et al: Exercise standards. *Circulation* 82:6, Dec. 1990.

14. Froelicher VF, et al: Nomogram for exercise capacity using METs and age. *Highlights* 8:2, Winter 1992.

15. Haskell et al: Task Force II: determination of occupational working capacity in patients with ischemic heart disease. *J Am Coll Cardiol* 14:1016-1042, Oct. 1989.

16. Higginbotham MB, editor: *Cardiopulmonary exercise testing,* St. Paul, 1993, Medical Graphics Corporation.

17. Industrial Medical Council, *State of California guidelines for evaluation of cardiac disability,* March 1994.

18. Johnson JV, et al: Combined effects of job strain and social isolation on cardiovascular disease, morbidity and mortality in a random sample of the Swedish male working population. *Scan J Work Environ Health* 15(4):271-279, Aug. 1989.

19. Lachar BL: Coronary-prone behavior: type A behavior revisited. *Tex Heart Inst J* 20:3, 1993.

20. Markovitz JH, et al: Psychological predictors of hypertension in the Framingham study: is there tension in hypertension? *JAMA* 270:20, Nov. 24, 1993.

21. McConnell TR, et al: Prediction of maximal oxygen consumption during handrail-supported treadmill exercise. *J Cardio Rehab* 7:324-331, 1987.

22. McEwen BS, et al: Stress and the individual. *Arch Intern Med* 153, Sept. 27, 1993.

23. Merz CNB, et al: Mental stress and myocardial ischemia: correlates and potential interventions. *Tex Heart Inst J* 20:3, 1993.

24. NIH National Heart, Lung, and Blood Institute, *The Fifth Report of the Joint National Committee on Detection, Evaluation, and Treatment of High Blood Pressure,* March 1994.

25. Rosengren A, et al: Self-perceived psychological stress and incidence of coronary artery disease in middle-aged men. *Am J Cardiol* 68, Nov. 1, 1991.

26. Schnall, et al: The relationship between "job strain," workplace diastolic blood pressure, and left ventricular mass index. *JAMA* 263:14, April 11, 1990.

27. Shaw LK, Pryor DB, et al: Sensitivity and specificity of the history and physical examination for coronary artery disease. *Ann Intern Med* 118:81-90; 120:344-345, 1993.

28. Wasserman K: Dyspnea on exertion: is it the heart of the lungs? *JAMA* 248:2039-2043, 1982.

29. *Work practices guides for manual lifting,* NIOSH Publication No. PB82-178948.

30. USDHHS Social Security Administration: Disability evaluation under Social Security, Washington, DC, 1990, Dept. of Health and Human Services.

# CHAPTER 31

# EVALUATION OF THE PATIENT WITH PERIPHERAL VASCULAR DISEASE

*Dennis J. Wright*

Evaluation of the patient with peripheral vascular disease may be considered according to location of the disease (upper vs. lower extremity) and the nature of the disease (arterial vs. venous). When the evaluation is being performed for disability purposes, a third characteristic, the degree of impairment caused by the disease, also exists. Arterial disease of the lower extremity will be considered first, followed by upper extremity arterial occlusive disease. Finally venous disease of both the upper and lower extremities will be considered together.

## LOWER EXTREMITY ARTERIAL DISEASE

### History

An impairment evaluation of the vascular patient is dependent on the history obtained regarding the patient's symptoms. This history should be taken in a systematic and complete fashion. A sample worksheet for the vascular history is shown in Figure 31-1. This type of checklist can be helpful to ensure the completeness of the history.

Coexistent medical conditions are very important in the vascular history. Associated cardiovascular disease is typified by angina, myocardial infarction, congestive heart failure, and cardiac arrhythmias. Diabetes, regardless of its severity, duration, or insulin dependence, is a cause of significant vascular comorbidity. Any history of hypertension should also be sought. Because patients may deny having hypertension if their blood pressure is controlled on medication, the physician should ask if the patient is taking medication and, if so, ascertain the type and the reason. Hyperlipidemia and hypercholesterolemia, treated or untreated, should be identified. Tobacco use is one of the most serious contributors to progressive arterial occlusive disease and its use should be documented. Other important aspects of the history include a history of stroke, renal vascular disease, collagen vascular disease, arthritis, degenerative back disease, and back injury. A history of any previous vascular operations must be complete.

Once these points of general history are obtained, specific questioning regarding the lower extremity should be performed. Claudication is the hallmark symptom of chronic peripheral arterial occlusive disease. This symptom may be identified by a series of terms used by patients to describe the discomfort associated with ambulation. "Cramping", "aching", "weakness", "tightness," and "giving out," are all commonly used to describe the feeling in the legs while ambulating. The classic description of claudication is one of cramping, usually beginning in the calves, that extends proximally as ambulation continues. This pain is consistently reproduced with ambulation and is relieved with several minutes of rest.[1]

The distribution of claudicatory symptoms may vary depending on the anatomic level of arterial occlusion. Aortoiliac occlusions are often accompanied by hip, thigh, and buttock claudication. Superficial femoral occlusive disease is associated with calf claudication. Foot claudication alone is rare but may indicate severe disease of the infrapopliteal vessels (e.g., thromboangiitis obliterans, Buerger's disease). In all cases symptoms may be unilateral or bilateral depending on the site and involvement of the disease.[1-3]

A detailed description of the claudication itself must also be sought. Attention should be paid to symptoms that occur while the patient is standing still or that cannot be relieved unless the patient sits or lies down. Spinal stenosis and other neurospinal compressions of the low back may have claudicatory symptoms. The pain in these conditions is often a numbing weakness and may well be associated with paresthesia (see Chapter 25). Lateral and/or anterior distribution of the leg pain is unusual with vascular claudication but may be seen more frequently with neurospinal claudicatory syndromes.[2]

Arthritis may be exacerbated by exercise and may be confused with vascular claudication. In this situa-

VASCULAR HISTORY/PHYSICAL INTAKE EXAMINATION

Name _____    Age _____    Sex _____

General History

Medications _____

_____

Allergies _____

Diabetes _____        Hypercholesterolemia _____

Tobacco _____        Duration _____        Currently Smoking? _____

Cardiac History _____    MI _____    Angina _____    CHF _____    Arrhythmia _____

Hypertension _____        Duration _____

CVA _____        COPD _____        Renal Insufficiency _____

Arthritis _____        Collagen Vascular Disease _____

Back Injury/Surgery _____

Other Injury _____

Previous Operations _____

Prior Vascular Operations _____

Description of Symptoms

_____

_____

_____

_____

_____

EXAMINATION

Height _____        Weight _____        Pulse _____        BP    R _____        L _____

Upper Extremity

Swelling    R _____    L _____        Bilateral _____        Measurements    R _____        L _____

Ulceration    R _____    L _____        Description _____

| Pulses | Right | Left | Comments (Bruit/Aneurysm) |
|---|---|---|---|
| Carotid | | | |
| Subclavian | | | |
| Axillary | | | |
| Brachial | | | |
| Radial | | | |
| Ulnar | | | |

FIGURE 31-1    Sample worksheet for obtaining vascular history.

Lower Extremity

Swelling    R _____    L _____    Bilateral _____    Measurements    R _____    L _____

Ulceration    R _____    L _____    Description _____

| Pulses | Right | Left | Comments (Bruit/Aneurysm) |
|---|---|---|---|
| Aortic | | | |
| Iliac | | | |
| Femoral | | | |
| Popliteal | | | |
| D. Pedal | | | |
| P. Tibial | | | |

**FIGURE 31-1, cont'd**    For legend see opposite page.

tion, as with neurospinal problems, careful questioning may delineate subtle differences. While vascular claudication is consistent and reproducible, arthritic pain is often variable and changes with regard to degree of exercise needed to induce the symptoms. Often, pain will not be noted until exercise is stopped and a period of rest occurs. Also, arthritic pain may vary with time of day and with changes in the weather, neither of which will alter the severity of vascular claudication. Finally, if pain does occur with exercise, it will often not subside on the cessation of ambulation.[2]

Other signs and symptoms should be sought in the patient who complains of claudication. Temperature changes in the involved extremity and any history of color changes such as blanching, bluish discoloration, or persistent rubor should be recorded. Persistent numbness in a patient with otherwise classic vascular claudication may be a symptom of ischemic neuropathy. Loss of muscle mass may be a complaint in long-standing cases. In the patient with hip, thigh, and buttock claudication an associated history of impotence may suggest severe aortoiliac occlusive disease (Leriche syndrome).

However, of all other associated symptoms, the two that mark the most severe disease in a patient with claudication are rest pain and tissue loss. Ischemic rest pain usually involves the foot distal to the midfoot and may be associated with an ischemic ulcer or early gangrene of the toes. This pain is often unrelenting and may not be relieved with pain medication. The only relief for this type of pain is often maintaining the foot in a dependent position, thus recruiting extra perfusion by means of gravity. The pa-

tient may have a history of a red, swollen foot due to continuous dependent positioning. Although some arthritic conditions may have pain in the same anatomic distribution, they tend not to have this classic picture of vascular rest pain, and an irregular waxing and waning course is more common. Rest pain implies severe impairment of function and is a precursor to ischemic tissue loss.[1-3]

The presence of ischemic ulceration or obviously gangrenous tissue is a sign of far-advanced arterial occlusive disease. The history as to how the ulcer or necrosis developed is often vague and it is blamed on a myriad of other problems including work-associated injuries. It is imperative that if tissue loss is the presenting complaint, other historical indicators of ischemic vascular disease, such as claudication and rest pain, should be sought. The patient with tissue loss as the presenting complaint often will be headed for amputation if revascularization cannot be performed.

## Physical Examination

The physical examination of the lower extremity begins with good general examination principles. The apical pulse should be checked for regularity and the heart auscultated for murmurs. Blood pressure should be assessed for the presence of hypertension. The abdomen should be palpated for aneurysms and auscultated for bruits. Atrial fibrillation, valvular heart disease, and aneurysms may not only identify vascular comorbidities, but also may serve as the source for emboli in the patient with a vascular abnormality. Abdominal bruits may suggest significant stenoses of the aorta and its branches.

Pulses must be examined carefully and completely. Femoral pulses should be evaluated just below the inguinal ligament. This may be difficult in the patient who is obese or quite muscular. Popliteal pulses may be quite difficult to assess even when a great deal of care and time is given to this examination. The dorsal pedal pulse, on the dorsum of the foot, should be assessed along with the posterior tibial pulse at the ankle level. It is important to check for both of these pulses because the dorsal pedal pulse may be absent as a normal variant in about 5% of the population. Each pulse should be assessed for its presence or absence, the presence of a bruit (where appropriate), and any evidence of aneurysm.

Other indicators of vascular disease on the examination are hair loss, decreased skin temperature, and poor capillary refill. Muscles and joints should be inspected for signs of muscle atrophy or joint swelling. The skin should be examined for its color in both the dependent and elevated positions. Marked dependent rubor that disappears with elevation is often seen with severe occlusive disease. Less severe disease may be associated with normal appearing legs that blanch on elevation. Any ischemic ulcer or necrotic tissue must be thoroughly documented with regard to its extent and its location.

In addition to these routine examinations, an examination with a pocket Doppler should be performed. This is an excellent adjunct test in documenting the presence or absence of blood flow in the areas where pulses have been assessed. The presence of Doppler flow does not exclude vascular disease even when good flow is noted, nor does this exam take the place of more extensive noninvasive testing. However it does serve to confirm what findings are made on palpation. In addition, the complete absence of Doppler flow in a patient with complaints of rest pain or tissue loss should prompt referral to a vascular specialist.

### Noninvasive Testing

The standard noninvasive test for lower extremity arterial occlusive disease is segmental Doppler pressures with plethysmographic arterial waveform analysis. This testing must be performed both at rest and after the patient has exercised on a treadmill.[4] While the methods of any qualified, competent facility are acceptable, recommendations for Social Security disability are that the test be performed for 5 min on a 2 mph treadmill adjusted to a 10% or greater grade.[5] Certain patients with cardiac and respiratory problems may not be able to perform treadmill testing, and no patient in whom treadmill testing is contraindicated should perform this. Resting pressures may be performed in all circumstances and when

significant disease is present, color duplex scanning or arteriography may indicate the severity of disease in patients who cannot perform treadmill testing.

Normal ankle/arm ratio (blood pressure measured at the ankle/blood pressure measured at the arm) is considered to be greater than 0.8. At any level below this claudicatory symptoms begin to appear. Disabling claudication usually occurs with resting ankle/arm ratios of less than 0.5 or when the ankle blood pressure falls to less than 50% of pre-exercise levels, and if it requires 10 min to return to baseline.[5] Again it is very important in evaluating the patient for impairment that the results of this exercise testing include the level of exercise (i.e., treadmill settings), the duration of exercise, any symptoms that develop, reasons for stopping the testing if desired level of exercise is not obtained, the post-exercise ankle blood pressure, and finally the amount of time required to return the ankle pressure to its preexercise levels. This is perhaps the single most important examination for determining impairment because it recreates the physiologic conditions that cause the patient's symptoms.

Once the patient is placed on the treadmill, subclinical disease may become evident. Physiologic stresses induced by exercise cause peripheral vasodilation in the vascular beds of the muscles. The patient with fixed occlusive disease cannot compensate for this increased demand for flow, and pressure decreases. Even patients with good collateral circulation and relatively good ankle/arm ratios (>0.5) at rest may show significant decreases in ankle pressure after physiologic stress of the leg. Conversely, just because a fixed obstruction is present, one will not necessarily see significant drops in pressure with exercise if extensive collateralization has occurred with longstanding obstruction.[4] It is especially important to note if a patient has symptoms without significantly decreased pressures either at rest or after exercise. Two significant situations where this occurs are in patients with neurologic and musculoskeletal etiologies for their symptoms.

A third situation may also cause this finding, and is one of the primary reasons for obtaining plethysmographic waveform analysis. This is the case where pressures are falsely elevated due to incompressibility of the vessels under the blood pressure cuffs. Diabetics will often have incompressible vessels due to calcific sclerosis. Because there is still Doppler flow even when the cuffs may be inflated to greater than 200 mm Hg, pressure testing alone may be inaccurate in assessing the degree of disease in this group of patients. Normal plethysmographic waveforms show sharp upstroke, prompt sharp downstroke, and the presence of a dicrotic notch. As vascular disease progresses, the waveforms become progressively blunted with loss of amplitude as well as loss of the normal waveform appearance. In the most severe circumstances, the waveform will become flat. These changes in waveform are not dependent on vessel compressibility and therefore will be present in patients with occlusive disease and incompressible vessels. Thus a diabetic patient who has ankle/arm ratios of greater than 1.0 but has significant alterations in waveform analysis probably has significant occlusive disease and should be considered for more invasive diagnostic procedures.[2,4]

## Invasive Testing

Arteriography is the gold standard for anatomic evaluation of arterial occlusion. Patients who are referred for arteriography should have symptoms that would warrant intervention if occlusion is identified. These include life-style limiting claudication, ischemic rest pain, or ischemic tissue loss. The information provided by arteriography includes the exact location of the arterial occlusion, the overall extent of occlusive disease in the other patent vessels of the extremity, and identification of possible therapeutic interventions.

This information cannot and does not replace the physiologic information provided by the noninvasive testing already discussed. However, when evaluating a patient for disability there are several situations where arteriography is required to assess the extent of disease. As previously mentioned, certain patients with severe cardiac or pulmonary conditions cannot undergo exercise testing on a treadmill. In these patients arteriography may be the only way to determine the extent of occlusive disease especially if resting ankle/arm ratios are not normal but do not fall below 0.5. Another group of patients where arteriography is important are diabetics with incompressible vessels and significant disturbance in waveform analysis. Here the arteriogram may be the only reliable method to assess the vascularity of the affected extremity.

Arteriography is not without risk. Renal insufficiency and failure occur due to exposure to the contrast agents in a small but significant number of patients. Other risks such as anaphylaxis, embolization, and puncture site complications are also present. For these reasons alternatives to arteriography are constantly being sought. Both color duplex imaging and magnetic resonance angiography have shown promise in certain settings. At this time and in most institutions, standard contrast arteriography must still be considered the diagnostic procedure of choice if intervention appears warranted.

## Intervention for Lower Extremity Occlusive Disease

There are a number of therapeutic interventions available for patients with peripheral arterial occlusive disease. Endovascular procedures range from recanalization procedures such as angioplasty and atherectomy to endovascular stents and grafts. Standard operative procedures are also quite successful and are most appropriate in a large number of patients. Any of these procedures may improve a previously impaired extremity to a normal physiological status.

## Assessing the Degree of Impairment

Patients with severe claudication and rest pain will often be seen for an impairment evaluation. This determination should be made on the basis of the patient's symptomatology, physical examination findings, and noninvasive tests with or without associated arteriography. It is important that attention be paid to the other possible causes that have been mentioned for these problems, especially in the patient who has convincing symptomatology but does not have identifiable vascular disease on examination or testing.

The Social Security Administration requires one of four circumstances be present for disability. The first is amputation at or above the tarsal level. The second is resting ankle/arm ratio of less than 0.5. In patients with ankle/arm ratios greater than 0.5 disability may still be determined if there is a decrease in ankle pressure 50% or more below resting levels and it is determined that the pressure takes 10 minutes or more to return to preexercise levels. A final circumstance is that of severe claudication with failure to visualize the common femoral or deep femoral artery on arteriogram.[5]

A different approach is outlined in the American Medical Association's *Guides to the Evaluation of Permanent Impairment*. The information is summarized in Table 31-1.[6] It combines the information obtained from the symptom history, physical examination findings, surgical history, response to treatment, and diagnostic tests.

A final mention should be made of the fact that no evaluation of a vascular patient can be considered simple. Vascular disease in the lower extremities is a dynamic problem that can progress rapidly or slowly. The symptoms may change drastically or they may only gradually deteriorate. Noninvasive testing may serve as a tool at both initial evaluation and later to document changes that occur over time. This may be of significant help in determining when a patient has crossed over from well-compensated disease to one

**TABLE 31-1**     IMPAIRMENT OF THE LOWER EXTREMITY DUE TO PERIPHERAL VASCULAR DISEASE

| CLASS 1 (0%–9% IMPAIRMENT) | CLASS 2 (10%–39% IMPAIRMENT) | CLASS 3 (40%–69% IMPAIRMENT) | CLASS 4 (70%–89% IMPAIRMENT) | CLASS 5 (90%–100% IMPAIRMENT) |
|---|---|---|---|---|
| The patient experiences neither claudication nor pain at rest; | The patient experiences intermittent claudication on walking at least 100 yards at an average pace; | The patient experiences intermittent claudication on walking as few as 25 yards and no more than 100 yards at average pace; | The patient experiences intermittent claudication on walking less than 25 yards, or the patient experiences intermittent pain at rest; | The patient experiences severe and constant pain at rest; |
| **and** | **or** | **or** | **or** | **or** |
| The patient experiences only transient edema; | There is persistent edema of a moderate degree, incompletely controlled by elastic supports; | There is marked edema that is only partially controlled by elastic supports; | The patient has marked edema that cannot be controlled by elastic supports; | There is vascular damage as evidenced by signs such as amputations at or above the ankles of two extremities, or amputation of all digits of two or more extremities, with evidence of persistent vascular disease or of persistent, widespread, or deep ulceration involving two or more extremities |
| **and** | **or** | **or** | **or** | |
| On physical examination, not more than the following findings are present: loss of pulses; minimal loss of sub-cutaneous tissue; calci-fication of arteries as detected by roentgeno-graphic examination; asymptomatic dilation of arteries or of veins, not requiring surgery and not resulting in curtailment of activity | There is vascular damage as evidenced by a sign such as a healed, painless stump of an amputated digit showing evidence of persistent vascular disease, or a healed ulcer | There is vascular damage as evidenced by a sign such as healed amputation of two or more digits of one extremity, with evidence of persisting vascular disease or superficial ulceration | There is vascular damage as evidenced by signs such as an amputation at or above an ankle, or amputation of two or more digits of two extremities with evidence of persistent vascular disease, or persistent widespread or deep ulceration involving one extremity | |

From American Medical Association: *Guides to the evaluation of permanent impairment,* ed 4, Chicago, 1993.

that will no longer allow the performance of normal daily activities.

## UPPER EXTREMITY ARTERIAL DISEASE

### History

Upper extremity arterial disease is much more complex in the etiologies of its vascular occlusive disease. Thus a much more detailed history must be obtained. While lower extremity occlusive disease is al-

most solely due to atherosclerotic disease, occlusive disease of the upper extremity is more commonly due to other disorders such as vasculitis, vasospastic disease, and thoracic outlet problems. Atherosclerotic disease occurs but is unusual and often confined to the elderly. Because of this diversity in etiologies, the history needs to address each of the possible causes. However, before investigating any particular etiology a good general history similar to that described for lower extremity disease should be the first priority.

Once this is accomplished, the individual's presenting complaints often direct the initial questioning. A patient with painful digits and a history of color changes associated with temperature changes should be considered for the possibility of vasospastic disorders. Careful questioning should be first given to the classic white, then blue, then red color changes that occur on exposure to cold or strong emotional stimuli. This history should prompt a careful questioning with regard to any type of connective tissue disease. Inquiries should be made with regard to arthralgia, rashes, myalgia, hair loss, arthritis, telangiectasia, dysphagia, sclerodactyly, and mouth ulcers. If these are present, an evaluation for connective tissue disorder should be considered as part of the evaluation of the upper extremity vascular disease.[1]

Arterial occlusions that occur with thoracic outlet syndrome are relatively unusual. They may present with digital ischemia or with upper extremity pain on exertion. A common occupational complaint in patients with thoracic outlet syndrome is pain when working with the arms abducted or over the head. Here it is very important to determine the distribution of the symptoms to help differentiate symptoms related to nerve compression as opposed to those associated with arterial insufficiency. Pain with exertion that involves the entire arm or forearm is more likely to be vascular in origin as opposed to pain in the distribution of a branch of the brachial plexus. Digital ischemia in this setting often is of sudden onset because it may be related to embolic phenomena. Other etiologies of digital ischemia must also be considered both here and in the setting of vasospastic disease. These include hypothenar hammer syndrome, frostbite, intraarterial drug injection, heavy metal poisoning, ergot intoxification, and other sources for proximal emboli (e.g., valvular heart disease).[1-3]

Arteritis may also be the cause of significant upper extremity symptoms. Takayasu's arteritis, giant cell arteritis, and Buerger's disease all have been associated with upper extremity symptoms such as exertional pain and digital ulceration. When considering Takayasu's arteritis the physician should ask for symptoms associated with other great vessel involvement. A history of cerebrovascular events or vertebrobasilar insufficiency should suggest the possibility of this problem, especially if the patient fits the epidemiologic pattern of a female in the second or third decade of life. Giant cell arteritis affects a much-older population group and is an unusual cause of upper extremity disease as well. It should be suspected, however, in patients that complain of significant jaw pain with chewing, dysphagia, headache and visual disturbance along with their extremity pain. Lastly, Buerger's disease is associated with a young male having digital ulcerations, a history of tobacco use, and a history of superficial phlebitis.[1]

In addition to these causes of upper extremity vascular disorders, about 10% of patients will have atherosclerotic disease as the cause of their upper extremity pain. The pain occurs with exertion and often is associated with activities that require significant overhead arm motion such as hair combing. Digital ischemia due to atherosclerotic disease is rare, and its presence should suggest (at least initially) another cause for the patient's symptoms such as the ones previously discussed.

## Physical Examination

The examination of the upper extremity begins with the blood pressure in both arms, making note of any significant discrepancies. Each arm should then be checked for pulses at the subclavian, axillary, brachial, radial, and ulnar areas. The presence or absence of pulsation, bruit, or aneurysm should be documented. Fingers should be examined for the presence of acute or remote ulceration. Muscle-wasting in the hand should be documented and its distribution noted: this can occur with both the thoracic outlet and carpal tunnel syndromes. Any associated signs of connective tissue disorders should also be noted. Finally, as in the lower extremity, the examination of the arterial system should be confirmed with pocket Doppler examination. In contrast to the foot, the palmar arch and digital arteries can be assessed with respect to the presence or absence of flow. Any alterations in Doppler flow should be documented and prompt noninvasive laboratory evaluation.

## Noninvasive and Invasive Testing

Evaluation of the upper extremity for vascular insufficiency is accomplished by both noninvasive and invasive means. Doppler pressures can be measured with cuffs on the upper arm and forearm and at the digital levels. Pressures are compared from arm to arm as well as between upper and lower arm. Waveform analysis should also be performed simultaneously. Significant decrements in either pressure (>20 mm Hg) or waveform amplitudes are recorded. For patients with Raynaud's disease, stress testing with ice water may be performed. In this test, submersion of the extremity in ice water reproduces the symptoms of the condition and causes decreased pressure and loss of waveform amplitude.

Arteriography is performed for two reasons in patients with upper extremity vascular disease. The first is to confirm the presence of digital arterial occlusion and examine the arterial disease pattern associated with it. The second is to identify proximal arterial etiologies for distal symptoms such as pain and ulceration. Confirmation of the anatomic causes for these problems may assist in treatment strategies and provide documentation needed in impairment evaluation.

### Assessing the Degree of Impairment

The impairment assessment for upper extremity vascular disease is more complex than that for lower extremity disease. While certain situations such as those that have resulted in amputation may be assessed as to their musculoskeletal impairment, vascular problems with pain (either claudicatory or at rest) as their primary symptom have not been as well-defined. The degree of impairment has been outlined in the AMA *Guides*. Table 31-2 summarizes the recommendations made in this publication.[6]

Care must be taken to avoid minimizing symptoms in patients with upper extremity vascular disease. Failure to assess and counsel patients with vasospastic

**TABLE 31-2**     IMPAIRMENT OF THE UPPER EXTREMITY DUE TO PERIPHERAL VASCULAR DISEASE

| CLASS 1 (0%–9% IMPAIRMENT OF THE WHOLE PERSON) | CLASS 2 (10%–39% IMPAIRMENT OF THE WHOLE PERSON) | CLASS 3 (40%–69% IMPAIRMENT OF THE WHOLE PERSON) | CLASS 4 (70%–89% IMPAIRMENT OF THE WHOLE PERSON) | CLASS 5 (90%–100% IMPAIRMENT OF THE WHOLE PERSON) |
|---|---|---|---|---|
| Patient experiences neither intermittent claudication nor pain at rest; | Patient experiences intermittent claudication on severe usage of the upper extremity; | Patient experiences intermittent claudication on mild upper extremity usage; | Patient experiences intermittent claudication on mild upper extremity usage; | Patient experiences severe and constant pain at rest; |
| or | or | or | or | or |
| Patient experiences only transient edema; | There is persistent edema of a moderate degree, controlled by elastic supports; | There is marked edema that is only partially controlled by elastic supports; | There is marked edema that cannot be controlled by elastic supports; | There is vascular damage evidenced by signs such as amputation at or above the wrists of both extremities, or amputation of all digits of both extremities with evidence of persistent, widespread, or deep ulceration involving both upper extremities; |
| and | or | and | or | |
| On physical examination not more than the following findings are present: loss of pulses; minimal loss of subcutaneous tissue of fingertips; calcification of arteries as detected by radiographic examination; asymptomatic dilation of arteries or of veins, not requiring surgery and not resulting in curtailment of activity; | There is vascular damage evidenced by a sign such as a healed, painless stump of an amputated digit showing evidence of persistent vascular disease, or a healed ulcer; | There is vascular damage evidenced by a healed amputation of 2 or more digits of 1 extremity, with evidence of persisting vascular disease or superficial ulceration; | There is vascular damage as evidenced by signs such as an amputation at or above a wrist, or amputation of 2 or more digits of both extremities with evidence of persistent vascular disease; or persistent widespread or deep ulceration involving 1 extremity; | or |
| or | or | or | or | Raynaud's phenomenon occurs on exposure to temperatures lower than 20° C (68° F) and is poorly controlled by medication. |
| Raynaud's phenomenon that occurs with exposure to temperatures lower than 0° C (32° F) but is readily controlled by medication. | Raynaud's phenomenon occurs on exposure to temperatures lower than 4° C (39° F) but is controlled by medication. | Raynaud's phenomenon occurs on exposure to temperatures lower than 10° C (50° F), and it is only partially controlled by medication. | Raynaud's phenomenon occurs on exposure to temperatures lower than 15° C (59° F), and it is only partially controlled by medication. | |

From American Medical Association: *Guides to the evaluation of permanent impairment,* ed 4, Chicago, 1993.

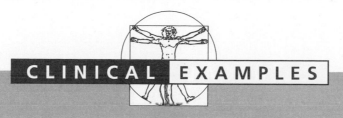

## PERIPHERAL VASCULAR DISEASE

### EXAMPLE

#### History

A physician is asked to perform a specialist impairment evaluation of the lower extremities for a 42-year-old man who has a history of juvenile-onset diabetes. His condition has been "brittle" for the last 22 years, and he now has an insulin pump inserted into the abdomen. He has had multiple manifestations of "small vessel" disease associated with diabetic vascular changes, including diminished vision in the right eye, partial blindness in the left eye, renal insufficiency (he has not been placed on dialysis yet), myocardial infarction, mild congestive heart failure, and a lesion on the lower left leg that required skin grafting two years previously. He has a below-the-knee amputation on the right. He cannot walk because of pain in the stump when he uses his prosthesis.

#### Physical Examination

He has no symptoms of claudication. The pulses in the left foot (dorsalis pedis and posterior tibial) are normal. There are two superficial ulcerations above the ankle. Delayed capillary refilling time is seen when the nails are pressed. Vibratory sensation is absent in the left foot. The deep tendon reflex is normal. Motor strength is considered to be normal, but there is diminished sensation below the knee on the left. However, the patient gives inconsistent responses with respect to anatomic landmarks on repeated examination using cold, light touch, and pain. No edema is present in the lower left extremity.

#### Assessment Process

As indicated, the impairments caused by the visual system, cardiac system, and renal system are not considered in the evaluation. At some point in the future, they can be evaluated independently and the results combined with the impairment results provided for the lower extremity.

The amputation is not addressed per se, as covered in Table 14. Similarly, the skin and peripheral nervous system abnormalities are not evaluated separately. Only the vascular changes responsible for these problems are considered in this section.

Using Table 14 (p. 198), this individual would be considered to have an impairment between Classes IV and V.* This individual cannot walk without pain in the stump; the pain is not caused by claudication. Thus the part of the evaluation dealing with claudication is not performed. There is no evidence for edema, but marked vascular damage is indicated by poor capillary refilling time, amputation, neurologic abnormality, and skin ulceration. Therefore, from a peripheral vascular disease standpoint, the whole person impairment (WPI) caused by the lower extremity abnormalities would be considered to be between 85% and 90%, which is also reflected in Table 69 (p. 89). Section 3.2 (p. 75) states that the lower extremity impairment is multiplied by 0.4 to yield WPI. Therefore 85% times 0.4 yields a 34% WPI based on peripheral vascular disease of the lower extremities.

If the impairment were evaluated using a combination of the amputation, skin changes, and neurologic deficits, the resulting impairment value would be much greater. Using Table 63 (p. 83), there is a 32% WPI based on the amputation below the knee on the right side. This individual would fall into a Class III impairment based on the signs of skin disorder, and there are limitations of many of the activities of daily living because of the fear of trauma and infection created by the vascular abnormality; intermittent-to-constant treatment may be required. The rating would be 35%. The neurologic deficit is more difficult to assess. Loss is sensory only and does not follow the distribution of any single peripheral nerve or dermatome. However, for the purposes of this example, there would be sensory impairment in the saphenous, lateral

---

*All *tables, figures,* and *sections* referred to in this discussion are found in AMA *Guides to the evaluation of permanent impairment,* ed 4, Chapter 3—The Musculoskeletal System, American Medical Association, Chicago, 1993.

*Continued.*

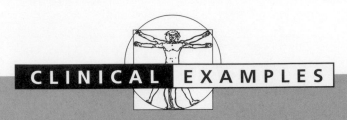

## PERIPHERAL VASCULAR DISEASE—cont'd

sural cutaneous, superficial peroneal, sural, deep peroneal, medial plantar, lateral plantar, and medial calcaneal nerves based on Figure 59 (p. 93). Table 68 rates impairment from a sensory standpoint only for five of these nerves. When combined, these yield a value of 5%. When the 32%, 35%, and 5% impairments are combined using the Combined Values Chart (pp. 322-324), a 58% WPI is found. For this reason, the peripheral vascular system is regarded as a whole, with the consequences of the vascular disorder combined in the appropriate tables. Otherwise, lengthy impairment assessments could be required when there are signs of peripheral vascular disease in various areas of the extremities. Overestimates would result.

**Evaluation**

As already stated, the preferred procedure would yield a 34% WPI.

*Stephen L. Demeter*

disorders when evaluated at an early stage may result in those same patients' becoming permanently disabled due to ongoing unsafe cold exposure. Also patients with tissue loss must be warned against unnecessary risks of trauma to the hands, which may cause further loss of digits.

## VENOUS DISEASE

Venous disease of the upper and lower extremities will be considered here along with lymphedema. However, from the standpoint of impairment evaluation, the problems have a relatively common ground. These are diseases of swelling, pain, and ulceration and it is on the basis of how severe each of these is that judgement is made about severity of the impairment. The most important findings are those in the history and those identified on physical examination. While invasive and noninvasive evaluations are helpful in acute venous problems, they are best ordered by vascular specialists when evaluating the patient with chronic disease. Specific tests may be required for each individual circumstance, but these are beyond the scope of this chapter.

### History

As in the case of patients with arterial disease, a thorough general health history should be obtained. Patients should be questioned with regard to cardiac and pulmonary problems. Specific questions must be asked with regard to the problems of swelling and pain. The duration and pattern of the swelling should be determined. The presence or absence of varicosities should be determined. Dermatitis or ulceration either current or healed must also be appraised.[1]

Pain may be present in one of several patterns. Pain associated with an ulcer is often quite severe and localized. The generalized aching that occurs after long periods of standing is much more insidious in nature, but is often relieved once legs are elevated. Venous claudication, felt as a bursting or throbbing in the calf and thigh with walking, can be seen in severe cases of venous insufficiency. Painless swelling may occur in venous disease, but its presence without other signs of venous disease may indicate a lymphatic etiology.

Other notes of import in the history are prior occurrences of deep vein thrombosis (including site, date, treatment, and complications). A history of recurring superficial phlebitis may also be obtained. One should also question the patient as to the use of support stockings. These may have been prescribed or instituted by the patient to alleviate symptoms. Response to stocking therapy should be noted.

### Physical Examination

The hallmark of longstanding venous insufficiency is swelling. This edema is often firm and may or may not pit on palpation. It is often associated with brawny induration, a brownish-purple discoloration of the skin that does not blanch. Varicosities may be present or absent, and evidence of venous "spiders" and actual varicosity rupture may be present. Venous eczema as evidenced by dry, cracked, poorly nourished skin is present as the duration of the disease increases.

Venous ulcers occur in the so-called gaiter distribution of the lower third of the leg. Their most common location is just posterior and just superior to the medial malleolus of the ankle. The ulcers tend to be ill-defined and without sharply demarcated edges. They may be multiple, but usually they show good granulation tissue in the base of the wound. Rarely do venous ulcers appear on the foot. Distal ulcers, a sharply punched out margin or poorly vascularized tissue in the base of the ulcer should raise the question of arterial insufficiency.[1] The presence of combined arterial and venous disease is not uncommon and may well be suggested by the associated risk factors in the history.

### Assessing the Degree of Impairment

Venous disease and lymphedema create impairment by their inability to be controlled. Stocking therapy with graduated compression stockings may well control venous disease so that minimal impairment is experienced. However, disease that cannot be controlled or that is associated with uncontrolled, non-healing ulcers may require the patient to restrict their activity severely, at least until healing has occurred. Recurring problems may be a cause for permanent impairment. Tables 31-1 and 31-2 outline the guidelines for impairment due to venous disease as it affects the lower and upper extremities, respectively.[6]

### References

1. Veith FJ, Hobson RW, Williams RA, et al: *Vascular surgery: principles and practice*, New York, 1994, McGraw-Hill.
2. Rutherford RB: *Vascular surgery*, Philadelphia, 1989, WB Saunders.
3. Moore WS: *Vascular surgery: a comprehensive review*, 1994, Grune and Stratton.
4. Zwiebel WJ: *Introduction to vascular ultrasonography*, San Diego, 1986, Grune and Stratton.
5. U.S. Department of Health and Human Services: *Disability evaluation under social security*, Social Security Administration, SSA Publication No. 64-039, 1992.
6. American Medical Association: *Guides to the evaluation of permanent impairment*, ed 4, Chicago, 1993.

# CHAPTER 32

# THE GASTROINTESTINAL TRACT AND LIVER

*Thomas A. LoIudice*
*Stephen L. Demeter*

Impairments due to disease or abnormalities in the gastrointestinal (GI) tract are similar to other organ-specific causes of impairment. They are produced as a direct result of aberrations in the normal physiologic functions of the various organs in the GI tract, or as a result of anatomical alterations. A good case could be made that diseases of the GI tract cause impairments in a person's lifestyle (for example, an individual with a stoma and external bag-collecting system or an individual whose disease expresses itself in a need to seek a bathroom for bowel evacuation 10-15 times a day), but this type of discussion centers more upon disability rather than impairment *per se* (see Chapter 1). The impairment examiner must be cognizant of this discrimination and be able to accommodate this distinction when assessing for impairment in the GI tract.

Perhaps no other organ system of the body (except the endocrine system) encompasses so many different organs as does the GI tract. While the overall functions of the GI tract can be summarized as nutrition acquisition, assimilation, and excretion, the variety of anatomical forms, physiological functions, biochemical processes, and disease alterations makes the GI tract a formidable organ system for assessing impairment. This is most clearly expressed in the variety of hormones produced within the various organs, most of which are organ-specific and function-specific although some overlap is seen. Fortunately, impairments due to GI abnormalities are uncommon and can generally be lumped together by addressing the principal activity of the GI tract—namely, nutrition acquisition—and assessing this indirectly by measuring the loss in total caloric or specific nutrient acquisition. Thus, this chapter is not as detailed as textbooks encompassing thousands of pages. This chapter primarily considers the overall effect of inadequate caloric or nutrient acquisition upon the body as a whole or upon other organ systems in impairment evaluation.

This chapter will separate the six organs of the GI tract (upper tract, stomach, small intestine, colon, liver, and pancreas) and discuss various diseases, anatomical alterations, and tests designed to measure abnormalities.

## UPPER TRACT (MOUTH, THROAT, ESOPHAGUS)

The functions of the upper GI tract include debulking of food, enzyme secretion, and transportation. These functions can be divided into the following steps: (1) chewing the food (requiring teeth and proper functioning of the jaws), (2) admixture with the saliva (for moisture, for ease of swallowing, and for initial enzymatic degradation), (3) transport to the pharynx (action of the tongue), and (4) swallowing (esophageal transport). None of these steps are critical for survival and all can be bypassed. The edentulous person will voluntarily switch to soft or liquid foods. The person without a tongue learns to accommodate this loss by alterations in swallowing. The individual with salivary gland disease (e.g., Sjögren's syndrome) sips water with food to facilitate swallowing. The person with esophageal disease can accommodate with extra chewing, using liquid foods, or by bypassing the esophagus by having tubes directly implanted into the stomach either surgically or endoscopically (percutaneous endoscopic gastrostomy [PEG]), which convey liquid foodstuffs directly to the stomach, thereby bypassing the entire upper tract.

Nevertheless, upper tract diseases, especially diseases of the esophagus, can and do produce impairment when the individual is unable or unwilling to make the above (occasionally drastic) alterations in normal lifestyle. This is especially prominent in the mid-course of some of the diseases of these organs.

Certain symptoms, such as dysphagia, pyrosis or heartburn, retrosternal pain, bleeding, weight loss, and vomiting may be important clues to esophageal dysfunction. Evaluations of these symptoms should include history, physical examination, laboratory studies, radiography with contrast materials, endoscopy with or without biopsy, and manometric studies. Medical or surgical treatment is based on these evaluations and the treatment itself is then evaluated. Based upon the data obtained, one can determine the degree and character of the patient's impairment.

Important tests to assess esophageal function include liquid or solid (barium cookie) swallowing tests assessed fluoroscopically, and manometry (pressure wave testing). Tests of esophageal anatomy include barium swallows and esophagoscopy. These tests are capable of reasonably good discriminations in the alteration of physiological or anatomical abnormalities. However, the sensitivity, specificity, or degree of abnormality is rarely an issue in an impairment evaluation. Impairment estimates involving esophageal abnormalities are principally based upon the degree of symptomatology, the establishment of an appropriate diagnosis, the impact upon the total nutritional status of the patient (usually expressed as deviations in weight since the only concern here is with calorie acquisition), and degree of remediation capable, based upon the pathological diagnosis. Therefore, an individual with diffuse esophageal spasm whose symptoms are reflected in weight loss due to an inability to swallow comfortably will have impairment regardless of the degree of alteration seen on a barium swallow or a manometric study. These studies are thus used to confirm the diagnosis and provide clues to prognosis and response to therapy, not as impairment discriminators.

## Swallowing Disorders

Diseases affecting swallowing, both neurologic and neuromuscular, have a particular propensity for permanence. Add this to secondary causes, most notably cerebrovascular disease due to hemorrhage or infarction, and a significant modifier of impairment to the whole person is established.[5] Attempted treatment for these conditions rarely, if ever, works and patients usually survive in a debilitated state with feeding tubes (see Chapter 39). Obstructions that are permanent and not treatable by dilation or surgery occasionally occur and are treated in a similar fashion.

## Stomach and Duodenum

Once considered merely a holding organ, the stomach is now held to be the principal site for early enzymatic breakdown of foodstuffs, due to enzyme or acid secretion and churning (calorie acquisition) or enzyme secretion for micronutrient absorption (intrinsic factor for vitamin $B_{12}$ absorption).

The task of calorie and nutrient acquisition is completed in the small intestine (duodenum, ileum, and jejunum) and requires either intrinsic enzymes or extrinsic enzymes (e.g., from the pancreas or the liver), as well as anatomical constituents that allow the absorption from these organs into the bloodstream.

When performing an impairment evaluation in patients with diseases of the stomach and duodenum, the history more than the physical examination may provide the important clues. Nausea and vomiting, particularly soon after eating, early satiety, and weight loss with or without bleeding may be important clues to gastric carcinoma but may also be seen with peptic ulcer disease that is present long enough to narrow the gastric outlet secondary to scar formation or edema. In some cases, severe gastritis may produce similar symptoms. Feeding generally makes the duodenal ulcer patient symptomatically better while worsening the symptoms of the patient with gastric inflammation. Deficiencies of vitamin $B_{12}$, iron, and folate may be sequelae of these illnesses. Physical examination usually shows epigastric tenderness, but in some cases may be negative even though significant disease exists.

Radiography with a contrast medium, endoscopy with biopsy, blood laboratory studies such as a complete blood cell count (CBC), electrolytes and vitamin levels, and Schilling's test for pernicious anemia may be valuable in confirming the initial diagnostic impression.

Medical treatment with a variety of agents including H-2 blockers, cisapride, omeprazole, antacids, and anticholinergics in a specifically designed regimen for a particular individual has been proven highly effective for those with an inflammatory condition. Tumors must be surgically removed and obstructions surgically corrected.

## Small Intestine

Diseases of the small intestine mostly manifest themselves with diarrhea or pain and nausea and vomiting secondary to obstruction. Bleeding may be a less-common initial sign but may occur with ulcer disease, arteriovenous malformations, and tumors. Weight loss is seen when malabsorption or maldigestion is present, and steatorrhea is seen in both these circumstances (stool fat >7 g/24 hr). Additionally, $d$-xylose absorption studies are abnormal (5-hr urine xylose <4 g).

Radiography of the small bowel with barium, endoscopy with biopsy, a Schilling's test, and routine lab screens including a biochemical profile, and CBC may also aid in the diagnosis.

Treatment for diarrhea, steatorrhea, and malabsorption ranges from dietary measures to anti-inflammatory medication including steroids. Obstruction is treated surgically.

As with the rest of the upper tract, diagnostic studies are meant to provide pathologic diagnoses, evidence for causes of specific nutrient malabsorption, or anatomical alteration. Usually, the degree of impairment is based upon evidence of nonabsorption (weight loss reflecting total calorie malabsorption) or specific micronutrient malabsorption (e.g., iron, vitamins, fats). Diagnostic studies will also provide clues for prognosis and results of therapeutic success.

Two additional topics need to be amplified under discussions of the stomach and small intestine because they represent specific disease states or situations commonly encountered in GI impairment: inflammatory bowel disease and post-surgical states.

### Inflammatory bowel disease

Three entities are considered a part of inflammatory bowel disease: (1) Crohn's disease or regional enteritis, (2) ulcerative colitis, and (3) radiation enteritis. These three diseases share the common features of debilitating diarrhea and anemia. Only ulcerative colitis has frequent rectal bleeding. Malabsorption, and hence debilitating weight loss, is more common in Crohn's disease and radiation enteritis, but may be seen also with ulcerative colitis in severe cases. It is the malabsorption and anemia that account for the impairment in severe forms of these diseases. The mechanisms by which this occurs, however, are different for the three entities.

In Crohn's disease, anemia may be the result of terminal ileal disease with impairment of vitamin $B_{12}$ absorption, anemia of chronic disease, and/or iron deficiency in those cases with duodenal and/or jejunal involvement. Malabsorption may be related to steatorrhea, brush border problems, fistulas, or rapid transit of food substances depending on the location and extent of the small bowel disease. Involvement of the colon primarily produces fluid and electrolyte problems.

In ulcerative colitis, malabsorption of fluids and electrolytes is the main problem, and the resulting debility relates to the denuding of colonic mucosa and the additional losses of protein. Bleeding results in an iron-deficiency anemia. Anemia of chronic disease may also be superimposed.

In radiation enteritis, anemia is usually due to chronic disease factors. With small bowel involvement, anemia may also be the result of malabsorption of iron, vitamin $B_{12}$, and folate. Depending on the location of the radiation injury, magnesium, fluid, and electrolyte abnormalities may play roles in producing impairment.

Treatment of regional enteritis, ulcerative colitis, and radiation enteritis may at one time or another involve the use of total parenteral nutrition for life support plus corticosteroids to reduce inflammation. Advanced cases with complications lasting over one year may be causes of total impairment because of the chronic debilitating nature of these diseases in many cases, even with sound treatment.

### Post-surgical states

Three postsurgical problems that commonly produce prolonged disability are (1) anal incontinence, (2) gastric surgery, and (3) extensive small bowel resection. Anal incontinence is discussed elsewhere in this chapter. Although most cases result from aging and weakening of the anorectal musculature, anal incontinence may be produced as an adverse event at anorectal surgery for fistulas, fissures, and internal hemorrhoids. Such a circumstance may result in significant debility of the whole person.[3]

Gastric surgery may lead to prolonged impairment or disability. The worst scenario is one that may follow total gastrectomy, which is most commonly done as part of gastric cancer therapy. Problems from this type of surgery include malnutrition, malabsorption, failure of upper gastrointestinal tract emptying, "dumping syndrome," and anemia.[8] Lesser degrees of resection may produce similar results but usually the severity of impairment is lower.[8]

Extensive surgery to the small bowel may have even greater consequences. Although the small bowel has a unique ability to compensate by adaptation to losses in its length and absorptive surface, there is a limit to this adaptation beyond which absorption of usual food substances cannot occur. Although there is some variability, it is generally expected that loss of greater than 100 cm of ileum or more than 45% of total small bowel absorptive surface will result in severe consequences, even to the extent of requiring total parenteral nutrition for the remainder of the patient's life. Circumstances that lead to such a state include ischemic bowel disease with infarction, Crohn's disease with numerous operations, and radiation injury to the small bowel with extensive resection. These patients tend to be severely impaired because of frequent diarrhea, vitamin deficiencies, fluid and electrolyte abnormalities (including sodium, potassium, calcium, iron, magnesium, and zinc) which are difficult to replace orally, and hyperacidity secondary to the increased production of gastrin.[10]

## LOWER GASTROINTESTINAL TRACT

Impairment due to lower GI tract disease can be caused by distention from ileus, constipation, or obstruction or overfunction (resulting in diarrhea). Pain is the universal manifestation of all of these diseases. Other causes include anorectal problems resulting in rectal pain, fever, tenesmus, or bleeding from abscesses, fistulas, fissures, or hemorrhoids. Anal incontinence is a particularly distressing and difficult impairment that may be due to neurologic or muscular disease, or may originate after surgery.

Commonly used diagnostic studies used for colonic disorders include stool cultures; stool examinations; digital examinations or endoscopic examinations including proctoscopy, sigmoidoscopy and colonoscopy, any of which may include biopsy; and barium enema examinations. Medical treatment is available for treatment of colitis, diverticulitis, and infections; local therapy is used for hemorrhoids and fissures. Abscesses require drainage and antibiotics. Tumors require resection although polyps may be removed endoscopically. Anal incontinence, evaluated with anal manometry, may be helped with anal exercises or surgery. However, this disorder remains extremely difficult to treat and is extremely distressing for patients who must learn to live with fecal soiling. Obstruction requires surgery.

### Pancreas

The two principal functions of the pancreas are its enzyme production for the GI tract and its hormonal role in the endocrine system. The latter will be discussed in Chapter 37.

Diagnostic tests of the pancreas are designed to provide information about either loss of function (enzyme production and transport) or alterations in anatomy; loss of normal anatomy is usually reflective of prognosis as opposed to functional alterations. Anatomical tests include an upper GI series, CT scans, ultrasonography, and endoscopic retrograde cholangiopancreatography (ERCP) and pathological entities are confirmed with appropriate biopsies. Functional tests include secretin stimulation studies, glucose tolerance tests, direct measurements of bicarbonate and enzyme levels in duodenal secretions, and calcium infusion studies. These tests of function and anatomy give important information on diagnosis and prognosis. The impact upon the person, however, is best assessed by more indirect means, such as how is nutrient (calorie or specific micronutrient) absorption impaired? Some of these tests include caloric adequacy as judged by body weight, serum cholesterol, serum protein, albumin, and pre-albumin levels. These deviations are the principal cause of medical impairments.

## LIVER AND BILIARY TRACT

Impairment of the liver may result from intrinsic disease or extrinsic compression or obstruction of the biliary tree. Signs and symptoms include nausea, vomiting, anorexia, loss of strength and stamina, decreased resistance to infection, jaundice, and pruritus. When primary liver disease becomes chronic and advanced, ascites, anasarca, esophageal varices with or without bleeding because of portal hypertension, hepatic encephalopathy, and renal impairment may be seen.

Commonly used studies for liver dysfunction include obtaining serum bilirubin and hepatic enzyme levels, prothrombin time, serum protein measurements, as well as performing nuclide scintography, CT scan, angiography, and liver biopsy. Post-hepatic obstructive disorders and primary biliary tract disease are usually diagnosed with ultrasonography, CT scan, and percutaneous or endoscopic cholangiography. The treatment for post-hepatic obstructive disease is surgery. Primary liver disease can occasionally be treated with medication depending on the disease entity.

Advanced liver disease leading to cirrhosis is the final common pathway for a host of exposures and toxicities, including those involving chemicals and drugs, especially alcohol.[4,6,11] Chemicals that can cause cirrhosis include 1,1,1–trichloroethane, trichloroethylene, styrene, chlorinated and nonchlorinated organic solvents, vinyl chloride (which also causes angiosarcoma), ionizing radiation, and beryllium.[2] Medications may also be associated with cholestatic liver injury and may lead to cirrhosis.[7]

The major site of transformation of foreign chemicals is the liver. In the process of detoxifying chemicals, permanent hepatic injury may occur. Typically, chemicals such as those listed above are transformed into more polar and excretable forms. Usually this occurs in the endoplasmic reticulum of the hepatocyte in the cytochrome P450 system. The process of detoxification itself, in many cases, may lead to the formation of toxic intermediates, which trigger destructive cytotoxic reactions.[12]

The liver may also become compromised by chronic viral hepatitis (A, B, C, D, and E), Wilson's disease, alpha-1-antitrypsin deficiency, primary biliary cirrhosis, and other chronic liver ailments, all of which may lead to cirrhosis.

The treatment of cirrhosis revolves around treatment of its complications, principally ascites. This

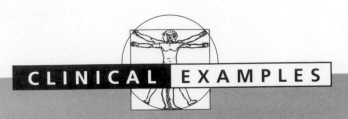

## CLINICAL EXAMPLES

## GASTROINTESTINAL TRACT

### EXAMPLE

#### History

A 32-year-old woman has asked for an impairment evaluation based on her history of ulcerative colitis. This disease started when she was 15 years old. From previous endoscopic examination reports, the physician finds that the disease involved the entire colon. By age 28 years, she developed infrequent rectal bleeding. Over the next 3 years, the rectal bleeding became more frequent and signs of malabsorption syndrome developed. Because of this progression and the fear of cancer, she had a complete colectomy. She now has an ileostomy.

#### Physical Examination

Other than the ileostomy, her physical examination is relatively normal. She appears thin, though not cachectic. However, when asked, she states that she has increased her body weight since the time of her surgery and now weighs 15 lb over that level. She feels well and has had no blood in her stool.

#### Test Results

Biochemical evaluations over the past 6 months have been normal. Her complete blood count is also normal.

### Assessment Process

Previously she would have been determined to have a disability based on colonic impairment, falling into Class III or perhaps even Class IV range. This would have been based on her symptoms of pain, frequent diarrhea, hematochezia, and biochemical manifestations of malabsorption. Restrictions on her activities of daily life would have required documentation. However, currently she is in a stable state. The surgical treatment corrected her original disease, so she no longer has disability based on the ulcerative colitis. Her body weight is normal, and no adverse sequelae followed the surgical procedure. Therefore, any impairment would be based solely on the presence of the ileostomy.

### Evaluation

Using Table 5 (page 243), a 15% to 20% whole person impairment would be assigned, with the actual number left to the discretion of the examiner.*

*Stephen L. Demeter*

*All *tables* referred to in this discussion are found in AMA *Guides to the evaluation of permanent impairment*, ed 4, Chapter 10—The Digestive System, American Medical Association, Chicago, 1993.

treatment consists of sodium and fluid restriction and diuretics. Cirrhosis may also lead to hepatic encephalopathy due to the inability to detoxify various substances in the blood. Lactulose and/or neomycin are hallmarks of medical treatment for this condition. Portacaval shunts for intractable encephalopathy, ascites or bleeding may be needed. Acute bleeding from esophageal varices may be managed using combination medical therapy and endoscopy. Since cirrhosis is not reversible, the impairment it causes, when complicated, is permanent.[4]

## MISCELLANEOUS DISORDERS

### Anal Disease and Hernias

Under this category are two conditions that are included in the AMA *Guides:* anal impairment and impairment due to hernias.[1] Both of these problems relate to anatomical alterations, but the functional implications are primarily related to lifestyle and are more appropriately regarded as a disability rather than an impairment. Nevertheless, restrictions in daily life, not just in work-related activities, can be caused by related problems (especially incontinence) or hernias (pain), which have the potential for requiring emergency surgery.

### Stoma

Another anatomical alteration giving rise to an impairment rating in the AMA *Guides* is the presence of a surgically created stoma.[1] The mechanism of impairment caused by stomas is similar to that caused by anal abnormalities and hernias.

### Fistulas

Lastly, fistulas are mentioned in the AMA *Guides* as creating impairment due to dysfunction in the organ of origin. These are listed as supporting points under inflammatory bowel disorders by the Social Security System.[9] These items were covered under the section on Inflammatory Bowel Diseases in this chapter.

### SUMMARY

Except for liver diseases, the role of diagnostic testing in GI diseases is to provide a pathological diagnosis, a rationale for malabsorption, and a clue to prognosis and treatment. In the liver, diagnostic tests are used in these roles as well but also to determine the severity of the abnormality. Except in the instance of the liver and some miscellaneous categories, diseases of the GI tract create impairment due to alterations in the principal role of the GI tract, namely nutrient acquisition, and are measured, as a rule, by indirect means of measuring the effects of malabsorption upon body weight and other measures (protein or vitamin levels).

## References

1. American Medical Association: *Guides to the Evaluation of permanent impairment,* ed 4, Chicago, 1993, pp 235-248.
2. Fleming LE: Unusual occupational gastrointestinal and hepatic disorders. In Shusterman DJ, Blanc PD, editors. *State of the art reviews: occupational medicine,* Philadelphia, 1992, pp 434-439, Hanley and Belfus.
3. Greenberger NJ: *Gastrointestinal disorders: a pathophysiologic approach,* Chicago, 1986, pp 184-190, Year Book Medical Publishers.
4. Lieber CS: Alcoholic liver disease. In Wright R, Alberti KGMM, Karran S, Millward-Sadler GH, editors: *Liver and biliary disease,* Philadelphia, 1979, pp 735-773, WB Saunders.
5. Pope CE: Motor disorders of the esophagus. In Sleisenger MH, Fortran JS, editors: *Gastrointestinal disease,* Philadelphia, 1988, pp 424-446, WB Saunders.
6. Read AE: The liver and drugs. In Wright R, Alberti KGMM, Karran S, et al, editors: *Liver and biliary disease,* Philadelphia, 1979, pp 822-847, WB Saunders.
7. Sherlock S: *Diseases of the liver and biliary system,* London, 1981, pp 295-322, Blackwell Scientific Publications.
8. Stabile BE, Passaro E: Sequelae of surgery for peptic ulcer. In Berk JE, editor: *Gastroenterology,* Philadelphia, 1985, pp 1225-1254, WB Saunders.
9. USDHHS Social Security Administration: *Disability evaluation under Social Security,* Washington, DC, 1990, pp 8-9, Department of Health and Human Services.
10. Weser E, Urban E: The short bowel syndrome. In Berk JE, editor: *Gastroenterology,* Philadelphia, 1985, pp 1792-1802, WB Saunders.
11. Zimmerman HJ: *Hepatoxicity,* New York, 1978, pp 349-369, Appleton-Century-Crofts.
12. James RC: Hepatoxicity: toxic effects in the liver. In Williams PL, Burson JL, editors: *Industrial toxicology,* New York, 1985, pp 78-105, Van Nostrand Reinhold.

# CHAPTER 33

## HEMATOLOGIC AND ONCOLOGIC CAUSES OF DISABILITY

*Ralph O. Wallerstein, Sr.*
*Stephen L. Demeter*

### HEMATOLOGIC CONSIDERATIONS

The three major hematologic cell types are erythrocytes (red blood cells), leukocytes (white blood cells), and platelets. Impairment resulting from low levels of these cells involves alterations in either physiologic or cellular function and place the body at risk for major disruptive events, such as uncontrolled infection or bleeding. High levels of these cells can produce vascular occlusive events (either systemic or pulmonary). These latter events are covered more completely in chapters addressing the specific organ functions. Other hematologic disorders include abnormalities of clotting proteins, immune globulins, and the spleen. These disorders and HIV disease are discussed later in this chapter.

When assessing hematologic disease as a potential cause of impairment, it must be fully appreciated that the three blood cell components only support the organism. Thus the manifestations of disease are measured primarily as dysfunctions in other organ systems and are expressed in terms of how they disturb the performance of activities of daily life (ADL). A useful paradigm for assessing such disturbances is given in the box on this page. This table is nonspecific with regard to cell type and provides no quantification of "whole person impairment." Reliance on clinical experience is vital in developing a meaningful and justifiable estimate of long- or short-term impairment.

### Red Blood Cells

The primary function of red blood cells is to transport oxygen and carbon dioxide. Through several biochemical reactions, oxygen is attached to the hemoglobin molecule until, with lowered oxygen tensions, the oxygen molecules are passed on to tissues. Carbon dioxide is a waste by-product of tissue metabolism and must be eliminated. While some carbon dioxide dissolves in plasma, the majority is removed by conversion to bicarbonate, which occurs primarily in the erythrocytes. In addition, some carbon dioxide is carried directly in carbamino compounds. Thus, with decreased levels of erythrocytes carbon dioxide transport is impaired.

Other erythrocyte functions include transport of gases other than oxygen and carbon dioxide and metabolism. Impairment may also be produced in these areas if erythrocyte levels decline; one example would be the methemoglobinemias.

### Criteria for impairment

Erythrocyte abnormalities can be either quantitative (for example, anemia) or qualitative (for example, hemoglobinopathies). Oxygen transport disturbances can be measured using the cardiopulmonary exercise stress test (Chapter 28), although this is rarely needed for impairment evaluations other than with the hemoglobinopathies. Usually, combining physiologic complaints, hemoglobin level, and transfusion requirements suffices to depict the disorder. Both the AMA *Guides* and the Social Security *Handbook* stress the importance of these three components.

> ## PARADIGM FOR ASSESSING IMPAIRMENT FOR HEMATOLOGICAL AND ONCOLOGICAL DISEASES
>
> Disturbances in global physiological function
> Disturbances in activities of daily life
> Acute vs. chronic
> Ability to respond to and degree of response to therapy
> Ability to cause other organ system impairment that is independently assessed
> Frequency and duration of above dysfunctions
> Prognosis

PHYSIOLOGIC COMPLAINTS

Anemia *per se* can cause alterations in physiology as a result of its role in gas transport. The signs and symptoms of anemia are listed in the box below.

HEMOGLOBIN LEVELS

The AMA *Guides* list three hemoglobin levels and grade them according to symptoms and transfusion requirements, producing four levels of impairment (Table 33-1).[2] The Social Security *Handbook* defines impairment as a reduction in erythrocytes of 30% or more.[3]

Impairment in oxygen transport can be quantitatively tested by the cardiopulmonary stress test. However, while this test reveals tissue delivery of oxygen and is abnormal when alterations are present (such as anemia, hemoglobinopathies, vascular obstruction, carbon monoxide poisoning, and cyanide poisoning), no formal studies have used this test in this manner.[4] Thus oxygen delivery reductions are related empirically to reductions in erythrocyte mass.

Two major problems attend this approach to erythrocyte dysfunction:

1. Acute anemia has a far greater impact on the body than chronic anemia because in chronic states the body adapts. For example, patients with malaria may tolerate hemoglobin levels as low as 2 to 5 g well with little physiologic dysfunction.

2. Subtle abnormalities may exist in some adaptive mechanisms. For example, with chronic anemia, the respiratory and cardiovascular systems increase their performance to compensate for the diminished oxygen-carrying capacity. While mild abnormalities in one or several systems may be insufficient to produce impairment alone, the combination with the anemia may produce physiologic problems. Yet careful quantification of each element, or the combined quantification, may produce no impairment rating.

The cardiopulmonary exercise stress test may compensate for the latter problem.

TRANSFUSION REQUIREMENTS

Patients with disorders where the erythrocyte count is reduced (such as bleeding or destruction of red blood cells by immunologic or mechanical processes coupled with a relative inability to replenish erythrocyte numbers) are often given transfusions at a predetermined point in their disorder. These arbitrary levels are based on laboratory tests. Transfusion may also be employed when the patient develops signs or symptoms of inadequate oxygen-carrying capacity.

Transfusion requirements (1) reflect the rapidity of loss related to the bone marrow's inability to replace the loss, which is an index of the disease's severity, and (2) serve as a useful paradigm for im-

---

**TABLE 33-1    IMPAIRMENT BASED UPON ANEMIA**

| SYMPTOMS | HEMOGLOBIN LEVEL (G/L) | TRANSFUSION REQUIREMENT | IMPAIRMENT (%) |
|---|---|---|---|
| None | 100–120 | None | 0 |
| Minimal | 80–100 | None | 10–29 |
| Moderate to marked | 50–80* | 2–3 U every 4–6 wks[†] | 30–69 |
| Moderate to marked | 50–80* | 2–3 U every 2 wks[†] | 70–100 |

*Level before transfusion.
[†]Implies hemolysis of transfused blood.
From AMA *Guides to the evaluation of permanent impairment,* ed 4, Chicago, 1993, American Medical Association.

---

## SIGNS AND SYMPTOMS OF ANEMIA

### SYMPTOMS

1. Dyspnea on exertion
2. Dizziness
3. Throbbing headaches
4. Palpitations
5. Easy fatigability
6. Increased symptoms of pre-existent vascular disease
   a. Angina pectoris
   b. Claudication
   c. CNS

### SIGNS

1. Skin pallor
2. Tachycardia
3. Systolic ejection murmur
4. (Possible) peripheral edema

pairment classification. Both the AMA *Guides* and the Social Security *Handbook* rely on transfusion requirements to discriminate among the various levels of impairment. The AMA *Guides* lists values as follows: (1) no transfusion requirements, (2) two to three units per 4 to 6 weeks, and (3) two to three units per 2 weeks.[2] The Social Security *Handbook* cites a level of "one or more transfusions on an average of at least once every 2 months."[3]

## Hemoglobinopathies

Hemoglobinopathies are diseases associated with and caused by alterations in the erythrocyte itself. The expressions of these abnormalities, for impairment purposes, can be divided into those causing alterations in oxygen transport and those causing chronic anemia.

Oxygen transport hemoglobinopathies are characterized by alterations in the resting $Pao_2$ or the uncoupling of oxygen at the tissue level. $Pao_2$ levels (ideally determined using the cardiopulmonary exercise stress test) are assessed according to the respiratory guidelines of the disability rating system.

Abnormalities causing chronic anemia are assessed as already outlined, using physiologic complaints, hemoglobin levels, and transfusion requirements. It should be noted that a few diseases have manifestations expressed in organ systems other than the hematologic system, including sickle cell disease and thalassemia. The impairments in the hematologic system must be coupled with the extra-hematologic manifestations to yield an accurate impairment rating. For example, a young adult man may have sickle cell disease, recurrent painful arthroses, mild renal insufficiency, and suffered a previous, although mild, stroke. The combined impairment ratings for these disease manifestations may not reflect his global disability. Mild organ-specific diseases usually yield minimal impairment percentages in the AMA system and none under the Social Security system. Yet the totality of disease is so profound as to make this individual totally nonemployable.

### SICKLE CELL ANEMIA

Patients with sickle cell anemia usually have moderately severe anemia. More important than the anemia are the various manifestations in other organ systems, including recurrent acute painful episodes or "crises" due to vasoocclusive disease especially involving the back, long bones, and abdomen, and leading to strokes. Repeated episodes may lead to extensive organ damage involving the heart, lungs, liver, and kidneys. Cardiomegaly, recurrent pneumonia, and chronic jaundice are frequent findings. Sickle cell anemia is often fatal before the individual reaches 40 years of age. Sickle cell-thalassemia and

sickle cell-hemoglobin C disease present clinical pictures similar to the picture typical of sickle cell anemia, although somewhat less severe.

### THALASSEMIA

Thalassemia minor, which is the most common hemoglobinopathy, causes only minimal anemia, no abnormal physical findings, and no symptoms. Thalassemia major and its variants usually produce profound anemia, require transfusion maintenance, and result in total impairment.

### POLYCYTHEMIA

Polycythemia is usually easily controlled with serial phlebotomies, and patients will rarely be impaired. Even when a marked elevation in erythrocyte count (that is, an erythrocyte count approaching 7 million/$mm^3$) requires the addition of a myelosuppressive agent such as hydroxyurea, patients remain relatively symptom-free.

### MYELOFIBROSIS

Most patients can continue full activity during the early phases of myelofibrosis when phlebotomies are no longer needed and the hemoglobin level declines, although a few patients experience excessive fatigue, perspire, or have low-grade fevers. Objective assessment of these largely subjective symptoms may be difficult. Most patients will be unable to carry on with normal activities when the hemoglobin level falls below 7 gm/dl. Transfusions do not restore these patients' strength, and complications, such as massive splenomegaly, add to the patients' problems.

## White Blood Cells

White blood cells primarily protect the body against substances that are considered abnormal or foreign. This protection encompasses such activities as fighting infections (foreign micro-organisms), participating in graft versus host disease (foreign tissue), and functioning in cancer (abnormal material). Diseases resulting from leukocyte abnormalities are generally described as either quantitative abnormalities (the -penias or -cytoses of the various elements, reflecting either too few or too many leukocytes) or qualitative abnormalities (rare diseases where the total leukocyte counts are normal but function is diminished, thus yielding the same results as quantitative abnormalities). An example of the latter is chronic granulomatous disease, wherein leukocytes cannot provide the "respiratory burst" needed for destruction of certain microorganisms.

Causes for these disorders relate to bone marrow dysfunction, the effects of drugs or radiation, and infections (HIV is the prototype). Proper disease categorization yields important information relating to prognosis and effect of treatment.

## Leukemias

The leukemias—acute, chronic, lymphatic, and nonlymphatic—vary considerably with regard to course, prognosis, management, and degree of impairment. Patients with acute leukemia are usually unable to perform ADL during their courses of chemotherapy and/or marrow transplantation, but can undergo complete remissions and return to full-time activity. Unless there is complete hematologic remission from acute leukemia, patients usually remain totally impaired because of fatigue, infection, or side effects of chemotherapy.

Patients who have chronic lymphatic leukemia may remain free of symptoms for years and may continue to work even during those times when oral therapy is needed. Limitations to activity result primarily from anemia; enlargement of lymph nodes, liver, and spleen; recurrent infections; and possibly bleeding.

Chronic myelocytic leukemia can usually be controlled for several years using hydroxyurea, which has virtually no side effects, or alpha-interferon, which may cause disabling symptoms in some patients such as acute interstitial nephritis and bronchiolitis obliterans.[5] Since neither of these agents can prevent the eventual progression to blast crisis, marrow transplant has become the preferred treatment, but it also carries the potential for impairment, because of rejection, infection, or the side effects of immune-modulating medications.

Hairy cell leukemia, a lymphocyte variant, frequently responds to alpha-interferon or 2-chlorodeoxyadenosine. The side effects of these agents, such as nausea and vomiting, myalgias, arthralgias, headaches, and "flu-like" symptoms, are transient, and most patients are able to resume normal activities when these effects subside.

## Multiple myeloma and macroglobulinemia

Patients with multiple myeloma may remain symptom-free for several years, but anemia, bone pain, and sometimes renal failure can lead to total impairment. This condition is usually permanent, but a few relatively symptom-free years may be salvaged for patients whose disease responds to Alkeran and prednisone treatment.

Those patients with macroglobulinemia may also be asymptomatic initially, with the disease manifested only by certain laboratory abnormalities. When symptoms occur, they generally result from anemia, which may be treated with oral chemotherapy, and/or transfusion or hyperviscosity of the serum, for which plasmapheresis is usually used successfully.

## Hodgkin's disease and non-Hodgkin's lymphoma

All patients with Hodgkin's disease require therapy with radiation, chemotherapy, or a combination of these treatments, depending on the stage and location of the disease. During therapy patients are usually unable to complete ADL because of the rigors or the logistics of therapy, but once the disease is in remission, patients may exhibit no impairment or subsequent disability. In a few cases, clinically noteworthy fibrosis may occur after radiation therapy.

Some patients with low-grade non-Hodgkin's lymphoma remain relatively symptom-free for a number of years, require no treatment, and thus are not considered disabled. All others require chemotherapy or, rarely, radiation. The impairments noted are similar to those seen in Hodgkin's disease.

## Inflammatory cells

Exciting research into the various proteins and cells involved in inflammation has taken place over the last two decades. However, specific quantitative or qualitative disease states are yet to be diagnosed, so impairment assessment remains many years away. An extensive review of this field is provided elsewhere.[1]

## Platelets and Clotting Disorders

Platelets help to form thrombi and stop hemorrhage. A platelet thrombus is formed through a series of events involving various proteins, termed a clotting cascade. It was initially believed that these cascades could be separated into intrinsic and extrinsic pathways and there were twelve "clotting factors." We now know that innumerable proteins participate in these pathways. Research has explored the various proteins associated with the inflammatory process, the effects of prostaglandin or leukotriene chemicals, the protein deficiencies associated with spontaneous clotting or hemorrhagic episodes, and the natural mechanisms for clot dissolution.

Evaluation of impairment resulting from thrombotic or hemorrhagic manifestations of defects in platelets or clotting proteins requires that the physician have an appropriate clinical background and the ability to make sound "educated guesses." Although these abnormalities can be quantified, the overall impact on a person's life, meaning impairment and disability, can rarely be measured, except in thrombocytopenia. For example, two patients may have a protein S deficiency, both with levels of 30% of normal. The first patient may have a past history of two pulmonary emboli, a spontaneous abortion, and now, at 28 years of age, an embolic occlusion of her left popliteal artery. The second patient is in his mid-sixties and is suffering from deep venous thrombophlebitis. Thus, even though both patients have the same defect at the same quantifiable level, the differences in their physiologic functioning, the impact on their ADL, and their prognosis are significant.

### Platelet disorders

Thrombocytopenia does not constitute an impairment unless it is severe enough to cause bleeding, either spontaneously or after slight trauma. Purpura rarely occurs with platelet counts above 40,000 and may not develop at counts of 20,000 to 40,000. In general, it is not worthwhile to treat patients who have immune thrombocytopenic purpura (ITP) with platelet counts above 40,000. Thrombocytopenia associated with a malignancy or aplastic anemia reflects the impairment attending those diseases.

Functional platelet disorders are most frequently secondary to other disturbances, such as azotemia or renal failure. Primary functional defects are uncommon and rarely cause serious clinical difficulties.

Thrombocytosis is generally a reactive abnormality, but even when it is primary, the platelets function poorly. Hence, bleeding is a more common problem and thrombosis is generally not seen.

### Hemophilia

Recurrent, painful hemarthroses constitute the major source of impairment in patients with hemophilia. Infusion of factor VIII or IX concentrate is usually given as home therapy, but during an acute, painful bleeding episode, patients may be completely disabled for a few days. The frequency of these episodes varies considerably; hemarthroses occur weekly, monthly, or less often. Damage to the joints, despite infusion therapy, causes permanent impairments; these are evaluated in accordance with the criteria used for musculoskeletal disorders (see Part A, Musculoskeletal System). Experience shows that patients with severe hemophilia may have an impairment rating of 15% to 50%, depending on the frequency of bleeding episodes and the severity of the joint damage.

HIV infection, which can be acquired through infusion therapy, has become an important source of impairment in patients with hemophilia. Evaluation of impairment in these cases is carried out as in other patients with HIV disease (see below).

### Von Willebrand's disease

Although von Willebrand's disease is the most common hereditary hemorrhagic disorder, bleeding is frequently mild, occurring only after trauma or surgery. Therefore the condition does not generally lead to disability. However, some patients may be severely impaired by recurrent gastrointestinal bleeding.

### HIV Disease

Infection with the human immunodeficiency virus (HIV-1) is manifested primarily by alterations in the immune system. The progression of disease from virus acquisition to disease expression varies and is best reflected by following the decline in the CD-4 subset of the T-lymphocyte. Most patients are generally healthy until these lymphocytes fall below 200 to 400/mm$^3$; normal levels are 800 to 1200/mm$^3$. The primary disease manifestations result from immunologic interference and consist of infectious illnesses and tumors.

Determination of medical impairment for patients with HIV infection is probably best addressed using the methods for assessing oncology (see later discussion). Being HIV-positive can be compared to being in remission with cancer. HIV disease (or AIDS complex) corresponds to metastatic carcinoma, and the side effects of drugs used to treat the various organ system infections or cancers are compared with antineoplastic drug effects.

### Disorders of the Spleen

The spleen is the largest single collection of lymph tissue in the body and a secondary site of blood cell manufacture. Splenic disorders rarely cause significant impairment. Splenectomy is usually performed after trauma to the abdomen significantly injures this organ. Splenectomy generally produces only subtle erythrocyte abnormalities and slight elevation of the platelet count. Medical conditions for which splenectomy may be performed include idiopathic thrombocytopenic purpura, some hemolytic anemias, and very large spleens in polycythemia and myelofibrosis. In fewer than 2% of these patients, the failure to clear certain encapsulated bacteria, such as pneumococcus, from the blood may lead to sudden overwhelming infection. Pneumovax offers considerable, but not complete, protection.

## ONCOLOGIC CONSIDERATIONS

Impairment assessment for oncologic disorders depends on various factors. The paradigm listed in the box on page 390 can be of value in this assessment.

Impairment in patients with cancer results from pain, weakness, emotional factors, convalescence from surgery, side effects from radiation or chemotherapy, and site-specific involvement. Evalua-

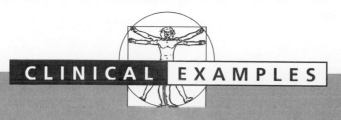

## CLINICAL EXAMPLES

## HEMATOPOIETIC SYSTEM

EDITOR'S NOTE—Most of the abnormalities associated with the hematopoietic system and/or cancer are associated with involvement of a specific organ (see appropriate chapters and the AMA *Guides*). For example, an individual with a history of carcinoma of the colon who may now have a permanent colostomy but is otherwise stable would be evaluated using the colostomy section found in Table 5 (p. 243).* An individual who has carcinoma of the thyroid, who has had a total thyroidectomy, and who is now taking replacement thyroid hormone would be evaluated under section 12.2. An individual who has sickle cell anemia with frequent sickle cell crises would be evaluated under the appropriate organ sections, including those involving the eye, central nervous system, peripheral nervous system, joints, spleen, and peripheral nervous disease. The following is an example of a purely hematopoietic problem.

### EXAMPLE
#### History

A 38-year-old man has shortness of breath with exertion. This condition has existed all

*All *tables* referred to in this discussion are found in AMA *Guides to the evaluation of permanent impairment,* ed 4, Chapter 5—The Respiratory System, and Chapter 7—The Hematopoietic System, American Medical Association, Chicago, 1993.

his life, so that he is not even aware of it, but he does state that he has difficulty keeping up with other individuals, cannot climb more than one flight of stairs without having a problem breathing, and could not keep up with other children when he was in school. There is a family history of thalassemia.
#### Test Results

This individual's hemoglobin level is 9.2 g/dl with a hematocrit of 32.5%. The MCV is 65 fl/RBC. A cardiopulmonary exercise stress test reveals maximum $\dot{V}_{O_2}$ of 21.3 ml/kg/min; he achieved 6.8 METS. The RBC is 5.0 mil/µl of blood.
#### Assessment Process

This individual has thalassemia minor. Based on Table 1 (p. 202), he has minimal symptoms, a moderate to marked deficiency of hemoglobin, no transfusion requirement, and a confusing impairment percentage. Oxygen is transported by red blood cells, and this chronic condition is not considered a disorder that needs and/or responds to treatment. Using Table 8 (p. 162), this individual would fall into a mild whole person impairment (WPI). The spread is 10% to 25%.
#### Evaluation

Considering the physiologic abnormalities, a 20% WPI is considered appropriate.

*Stephen L. Demeter*

## FACTORS CAUSING IMPAIRMENT IN ONCOLOGIC DISEASE

Primary organ (system) involved
Secondary organ(s) (system(s)) involved
Response to therapy
Prognosis
Presence of ongoing therapy
    A. Type
    B. Frequency
    C. Dosage
    D. Disturbance in physiological function
        1. Global
        2. Site specific
Psychological factors

tion findings are mostly subjective, although weight loss, anemia, low-grade fever, and low serum albumin levels provide objective measurements. Most side effects from chemotherapy dissipate over time, but residual neuropathies, such as loss of reflexes, foot drop, or ataxia, may be permanent after the use of vinca alkaloids; cardiomyopathy may be permanent after the use of anthracyclines; and renal damage may be irreversible after the use of cisplatin.

From 25% to 33% of all patients with cancer receive radiation therapy during the course of their disease. When used to achieve a cure, as in prostatic cancer or after lumpectomy in breast cancer, ill effects such as fatigue or local discomfort last only a short time. However, reactions to head and neck radiation may be severe.

Cancers that do not cause impairment include most skin cancers (except melanoma), some prostate cancers, and most successfully-resected cancers.

Incurable cancers and those that become resistant to therapy eventually produce permanent disability. Examples are cancer of the pancreas, kidney, and esophagus, most lung cancers, and many brain tumors.

Most cancers that become metastatic render patients permanently disabled; examples include metastatic melanoma, adenocarcinomas, and sarcoma. Patients with radiologically demonstrable bone metastases to the breast or those with prostate cancer sometimes remain relatively asymptomatic over a period of a few months to two years.

In addition to the general symptoms listed, some cancers have more specific symptoms. Site-specific involvement depends on the natural history of certain types of cancer. Spreading ovarian cancer causes recurrent bowel obstruction, and lung cancer produces severe dyspnea. These can be evaluated objectively by radiologic studies and pulmonary function tests, respectively.

## References

1. Demeter SL, Koo PH, Pipoly DJ: Lung defense mechanisms. In Cordasco EM, Demeter SL, Zenz C, editors: *Environmental respiratory disease,* New York, 1994, Van Nostrand Reinhold.
2. Doege TC, Houston TP, editors: *Guides to the evaluation of permanent impairment,* ed 4, Chicago, 1993, American Medical Association.
3. U.S. Department of Health and Human Services: *Disability evaluation under Social Security,* 1992, U.S. Government Printing Office.
4. Wasserman K, Hansen JE, Sue DY, Whipp BJ, editors: *Principles of exercise testing and interpretation,* Philadelphia, 1987, Lea & Febiger.
5. Ogata K, Koga T, Yagawa K: Interferon-related bronchiolitis obliterans organizing pneumonia. *Chest* 106:612-613, 1994.

# CHAPTER 34

# ASSESSMENT OF RENAL IMPAIRMENT AND DISABILITY

*Donald F. Eipper*

Chronic renal disease tends to be progressive and may not be manifested until renal excretory function is severely reduced. The accumulation of uremic toxins leads to progressive dysfunction and damage of body organ systems and, ultimately, the uremic syndrome of irreversible, or end-stage, renal disease. Organ system dysfunction and damage in early stages may be reversible by renal replacement therapy (dialysis or transplantation). In late stages the damage may be reversible by specific therapy (such as parathyroidectomy for uremic hyperparathyroidism and osteodystrophy) or may be irreversible (as in advanced peripheral neuropathy).

Because renal failure has such widespread deleterious effects and may also be part of a systemic disease, such as diabetes mellitus, which directly causes organ system damage, impairment and disability assessment in a patient with renal disease can be complex. Furthermore, there may be considerable disparity between the severity of impairment and the severity of disability depending on the physical and mental demands of the daily activities or work activities of the individual. For example, individuals with no systemic problems other than end-stage renal disease may require three four-hour dialysis sessions each week. These sessions may significantly impair their ability to attend work or perform work-related and recreational activities.

## CATEGORIES OF RENAL DISEASE

Chronic renal disease may cause permanent impairment and disability. Acute renal disease, such as acute glomerulonephritis, is usually reversible, although, in some cases, progression to renal failure may occur. The degree of renal impairment can be measured by laboratory testing. However, disability must be determined on an individual basis because no predictable correlation between these two issues exists.

For purposes of devising an approach to assessing impairment of the whole person and disability, grouping patients into appropriate categories of renal disease and treatment can be helpful.

## Chronic Renal Disease (CRD)

1. Evidence of renal disease persisting more than 3 months and expected to last 12 months or more.
2. Usually progressive and often results in end-stage renal disease (ESRD).
3. The degree of renal impairment may be modified by treatment.
4. With some chronic renal disorders, acute events or morbidity from chronic symptomatology may increase impairment independent of severity of loss of renal function:
   *(a)* Recurrent urinary tract infections
   *(b)* Recurrent nephrolithiasis
   *(c)* Nephrotic syndrome—edema, serum albumin less than 3.5 g/dl, urinary protein excretion greater than 3.5 g/24 hr

## End-Stage Renal Disease (ESRD)

1. Dialysis
2. Renal transplantation

## DETERMINATION OF THE PRESENCE OF CRD AND EXTENT OF IMPAIRMENT

Through examination of the patient with suspected or known renal disease, the physician must determine not only the nature and severity of the renal disease but the extent and severity of organ system complications caused by renal failure and/or comorbid conditions, such as diabetes mellitus. The history and physical examination must cover all organ systems. Interpretation and weighing of the findings must take into account the interacting effects of impairment of several organ systems.

The history focuses on documentation of renal abnormalities. Information should be elicited pertaining to systemic diseases, such as diabetes mellitus or lupus erythematosus, that might have renal involvement. Also, the history should address voiding problems, the appearance of urine, the amount and location of peripheral edema, and hypertension. Finally, a thorough review of systems should be recorded, as well as a complete review of social, occupational, recreational, and past medical histories.

The physical examination findings the physician must look for include the general appearance, nutritional status, and blood pressure. The skin should be examined for excoriations and ecchymosis. The lungs should be auscultated for rales, pleural friction rubs, or pleural effusions. The heart should be examined for the presence of pericardial friction rubs, pericardial effusions, or gallops. The abdomen should be examined for organomegaly, including the possibility of palpable kidneys and ascites. The extremities should be examined for edema, joint swelling, and limitation of motion. The nervous system should be evaluated for mental status impairment, muscle weakness, blunted or absent sensation, and diminished or absent reflexes.

Laboratory abnormalities to look for include high levels of blood urea nitrogen (BUN), serum creatinine, phosphorus, uric acid, potassium, glucose (with or without underlying diabetes), and parathyroid hormone. Low values of bicarbonate, albumin, hemoglobin, and hematocrit can be expected. Physicians examining the results of urinalysis tests should look for protein, blood, white blood cells, and glucose. A urinary protein excretion greater than 3.5 grams per 24 hours is consistent with nephrotic syndrome. Creatinine clearance less than 50 ml per minute is indicative of renal failure.

A renal ultrasound may reveal small kidneys (indicative of chronic renal disease), hydronephrosis (indicative of obstruction), or polycystic kidneys. Chest x-rays may reveal a large heart, pleural effusion, or uremic pneumonitis. Cardiac ultrasound is more sensitive when diagnosing pericardial effusion or impaired ventricular contractility. X-rays of bones, particularly those of hands and clavicles, may reveal subperiosteal resorption, bone dissolution, osteomalacia, or fractures.

Nerve conduction velocity studies in patients with renal failure show slowed sensory and motor conduction.

## PROGRESSION OF CHRONIC RENAL DISEASE (CRD)

As CRD progresses, physiological derangements and organ system impairments begin to appear, and persist, as the loss of renal function passes through successively more severe stages. These stages are not sharply demarcated and there is considerable overlap, but they do provide compass points to guide the examiner in the evaluation process.

### Loss of Renal Reserve (Creatinine Clearance: 75–50)

1. Usually asymptomatic
2. BUN and serum creatinine usually normal
3. Serum calcium and phosphorus normal; parathyroid hormone (PTH) may be elevated (early uremic hyperparathyroidism)

### Renal Insufficiency (Creatinine Clearance: 50–25)

Add:
1. Azotemia—BUN, creatinine and uric acid elevated
2. Elevated PTH
3. Impaired urinary concentration and dilution
4. Depressed erythropoietin (EPO) production

### Renal Failure (Creatinine Clearance: 25–10)

Add:
1. Isosthenuria (urine with the same osmolality as the serum) and fluid retention
2. Hypocalcemia
3. Hyperphosphatemia
4. Hyperkalemia
5. Depressed vitamin D (1,25–dihydroxy D3) production
6. Anemia

### ESRD (Creatinine Clearance < 10)

Add:
1. Uremic signs and symptoms
2. Multiple organ system dysfunction
3. Death if there is no renal replacement therapy

## ORGAN SYSTEM COMPLICATIONS OF CRD CAUSING IMPAIRMENT AND DISABILITY

Uremia is a systemic disorder causing impairment of all body organ systems. While the renal disease causing renal failure may be irreversible, conservative management and renal replacement therapy may ameliorate or even reverse the impairments. However, some impairments persist or even progress. This is particularly true of diabetics, who make up about one third of the dialysis population, and who become disabled from vision loss, neuropathy, and cardiovascular complications.

Cardiovascular complications include hypertension, accelerated atherosclerosis, congestive heart failure, or uremic pericarditis (with or without effusion). Accelerated atherosclerosis may present as coronary artery disease (CAD), with manifestations of angina pectoris, myocardial infarction, stroke, or peripheral vascular occlusive disease. Congestive heart failure may be due to hypertension, fluid overload, CAD, uremia (reversible) or ischemia (not reversible), and cardiomyopathy.

Neuropsychiatric abnormalities can include encephalopathy, peripheral sensory and motor neuropathy, autonomic neuropathy, carpal tunnel syndrome, and depression.

Musculoskeletal abnormalities can include myopathy, tendonitis, arthritis, and hyperparathyroidism (presenting as osteodystrophy or osteomalacia).

Endocrinologic and metabolic manifestations include uremic hyperparathyroidism, impaired glucose metabolism, hypothyroidism, impotence, protein and energy malnutrition, and salt and water retention. This retention can present as peripheral edema, pulmonary edema, and hypertension.

Respiratory manifestations include uremic pneumonitis, uremic pleuritis (with or without effusion), and pulmonary fibrosis.

Gastrointestinal abnormalities may include anorexia, peptic ulceration or gastritis, gastroparesis (especially in diabetics), and chronic HBV or HCV hepatitis (caused by blood transfusions).

Hematologic abnormalities include anemia (normochromic or normocytic), bleeding due to platelet dysfunction, or impaired immunity.

Dermatologic manifestations may involve intractable itching (with excoriations due to hyperparathyroidism), ecchymosis, painful hematomas, and various rashes.

## DISABILITY ASSESSMENT IN THE PATIENT WITH CRD OR ESRD

Assessment of the disability in a patient with CRD or ESRD must take the following into account:

1. Severity of loss of renal function
2. Extent of organ system impairment and damage
3. The composite effects of impairment of multiple organ systems (e.g., by using the AMA combined values chart[2])
4. The impact of the impairments on activities of daily living and ability to carry out occupational demands (e.g., by using the Sickness Impact Profile [SIP][3])

While it may make sense that the impact upon various organ systems should be evaluated by assessing those organ systems as if they have primary diseases, the AMA *Guides,* when rating impairment caused by renal disease, takes this into account. The *Guides* contain a table that categorizes renal disfunction according to the creatinine clearance and symptoms of renal disease.

Data from several reports[4-9] allow some general statements to be made:

1. Disability as measured by the SIP in patients with renal insufficiency and renal failure can be serious and perhaps worse than in ESRD patients who are getting renal replacement therapy with dialysis.[6]
2. Disability rates are lower, and rehabilitation rates are higher, in transplanted patients than in dialysis patients.[4,5]
3. Disability rates are higher, and rehabilitation rates are lower, in diabetic patients than in nondiabetic transplanted patients.[9]
4. More dialysis and transplant patients are able to work than are actually working.[8,9]

The same study reports provide useful information about disability and rehabilitation in patients in the renal disease categories as well as comparisons between dialysis and transplant patients and between diabetic and nondiabetic patients. The chronic renal disease group has been less studied than the dialysis and transplantation groups. Harris et al[6] measured SIP in 360 patients with calculated creatinine clearance less than 50 cc/min of more than six months duration. These patients had a higher mean SIP score (greater disability) than patients on dialysis. Independent correlates with higher SIP scores were lower educational level and income, prior diagnosis of coronary artery disease or stroke, and lower serum albumin. A plausible explanation for the relatively poor quality of life in these patients with renal insufficiency and failure is that they received less than optimal care, since they were not subject to the intense medical management and support afforded dialysis and transplant patients. Studies of ESRD patients[4,5] show that 59% stopped working because of physical limitation or disability. Transplanted patients did better than dialysis patients.

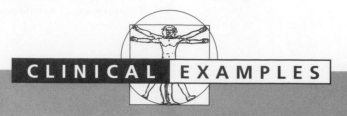

## RENAL SYSTEM

EDITOR'S NOTE—The following example illustrates the ongoing nature of impairment evaluation in renal disease.

### EXAMPLE

#### History

At 18, this woman was diagnosed with slowly progressive chronic glomerulonephritis based on a biopsy. No cause was found. At 21 years of age, she graduated from college with a teaching degree.

#### Test Results

She was mildly anemic with a hemoglobin level of 10.2 g/dl (normal for her age and sex is 12.0 to 16.0 g/dl). A 24-hour urine sample was obtained, revealing a creatinine clearance of 31 ml/min (normal, 62 to 145 ml/min/1.73 m$^2$). Her serum calcium, potassium, and sodium levels were all normal. Her blood urea nitrogen (BUN) was 28 mg/dl (normal, 6 to 20 mg/dl), and her creatinine level was 1.3 mg/dl (normal, 0.7 to 1.5 mg/dl).

#### Assessment Process

Based on altered creatinine clearance, this person would belong in a Class III whole person impairment (WPI) category. However, she can still perform most activities of daily life, including her job as a schoolteacher. Therefore, she would have a 40% WPI. Further alterations of the BUN, creatinine, or electrolytes would merit a higher impairment percentage. Using Table 1 (page 202) of the American Medical Association *Guides,* her anemia would, while present, not produce an impairment rating, although it could be assessed by a cardiopulmonary exercise stress test.*

#### Evaluation

A 40% WPI would be assigned at this point in the patient's course.

*All *tables* referred to in this discussion are found in AMA *Guides to the evaluation of permanent impairment,* ed 4, Chapter 11—The Urinary and Reproductive Systems, American Medical Association, Chicago, 1993.

#### Repeat History and Test Results

Two years later the patient developed a progressive decline in health. Her creatinine clearance was 21 ml/min and hemoglobin was 8.2 mg/dl. The creatinine level increased to 2.4 mg/dl, and the BUN increased to 48 mg/dl. Her physician recommended that she be carefully watched for the need for dialysis and/or transplantation.

One year later, her creatinine clearance fell to 12 ml/min. The creatinine level was 3.1 mg/dl, and the BUN was 58 mg/dl. Her hemoglobin remained at 8.2 mg/dl.

#### Assessment Process

She now merits a Class IV impairment. In addition, she now has impairment caused by the anemia that would be rated as 10% to 29%. Since the renal abnormality places her in Class IV, the 10% value may be more appropriate. A Class IV renal impairment produces a 60% to 95% WPI, and 70% would probably be appropriate.

#### Evaluation

Combining the 70% with the 10% yields a WPI value of 73%.

#### Repeat History and Test Results

Two years later she had clearly deteriorated, receiving dialysis 3 days each week. Her hemoglobin remained at 8.2 mg/dl, but creatinine level fell to 1.2 mg/dl and BUN to 38 mg/dl. The creatinine clearance was measured at 5 ml/min. Her serum calcium level diminished as did her serum protein levels. Phosphorus concentration was elevated, although her other electrolytes remained relatively stable.

#### Assessment Process

As before, she would be found to have a Class IV impairment, but the level would have increased to 90%.

#### Evaluation

Combining the 90% with the 10% impairment caused by the anemia produces a 91% WPI.

#### Final History

One year later, she had a successful renal transplantation. She comes now, one year

*Continued.*

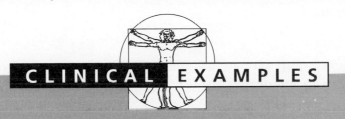
after transplantation, for an impairment evaluation. She is being maintained on cyclosporin and prednisone. She has developed no significant complications from the use of either of these medications, with the exception of two episodes of pneumonia and the presence of diabetes mellitus. The diabetes is being controlled with diet and oral hypoglycemic medications. Her weight has increased by 35 kg. However, she has had no vascular complications from the diabetes, osteoporosis with fractures, or chronic infections.

### Test Results

Creatinine clearance is 85 ml/min, hemoglobin value is 10.1 mg/dl, and electrolytes are normal.

### Assessment Process

This individual now exhibits a Class I WPI. The causes of her impairment are independent of the renal disorder, due instead to diabetes, Cushing's syndrome, and anemia. None of these produce independent impairment presently. However, she should be followed closely to determine if impairment may develop in the future.

### Evaluation

Presently this patient has a 0% to 14% WPI based on her classification in Category I. A 10% to 14% value would probably be appropriate for her at this point.

*Stephen L. Demeter*

One year prior to ESRD 67% of all patients were working full- or part-time, while afterward 46% of transplanted patients were working compared with 30% of dialysis patients. Over 80% of the dialysis patients reported limitations of vigorous physical activity. Over 50% of dialysis patients and 35% to 40% of transplanted patients reported trouble walking several blocks, climbing stairs, lifting or carrying weights, or bending or stooping. Complaints common to both groups were fatigue, lack of energy, trouble sleeping, nervousness, anxiety, or depression.

With respect to those patients whose livelihood and social functioning depends on manual dexterity, Chazot et al[10] reported that many of the 66 patients hemodialyzed for over ten years demonstrated hand dysfunction. Arthropathies, carpal tunnel syndrome, ulnar neuropathy, and tendinous lesions and nerve entrapment due to amyloidosis were the abnormalities commonly responsible for the impairments.

The changing scene in home dialysis no longer allows general statements to be made regarding disability and rehabilitation. Home hemodialysis (HHD) has consistently shown better rates of rehabilitation than center hemodialysis (CHD). Since the introduction of home peritoneal dialysis (CAPD or CCPD), HHD, by comparison, showed better results early[4,5] and about the same results more recently.[11] At the present time there are no good reasons to believe that disability and rehabilitation rates differ significantly between the different dialysis modalities.

A recent study of transplanted patients done by the Battelle-Seattle Research Center[9] revealed that transplantation does not allow as many patients to work as might be expected from a treatment that reverses all of the pathophysiology of CRD and uremia. Functional impairments and work-related limitations were common, especially in diabetics who had impairments due to retinopathy and neuropathy. Of concern was the discrepancy between how many patients were able to work (62%) and how many were actually working (43%), especially when health problems prevented working in only 39%. Social, economic, and motivational factors appear to be playing a big role in blocking rehabilitation.

While significant impairment may ensue from CRD or ESRD, the degree of disability reported appears excessive for the severity of the physical limitations. The crushing of motivation and interest by the weight of chronic illness discourages many from even trying to pursue a vocation. Some patients who want to work may find their jobs too physically demanding. In some cases economic disincentives or employer discrimination inhibit an attempt to reenter the workforce.[9] Avoidance of disability requires early intervention to avert job loss or vigorous vocational rehabilitation for those dialysis and transplant patients who stopped work. Most importantly, the attitude of patients, physicians, and employers must change from a grim expectation that disability is inevitable in CRD or ESRD to an optimistic willingness to strive for adequate functioning in the home or in the workplace. Providing realistic and valid impairment ratings, rather than deciding that all patients with renal failure are permanently and totally impaired and therefore disabled, would be an important first step in achieving this attitude change.

The passage of the Americans with Disabilities Act (see Chapter 50) may further address this change.

## References

1. Social Security Administration: *Disability evaluation under social security*, USD, HHS, SSA, SSA Pub. No. 64-039, Oct. 1992.
2. American Medical Association: *Guides to evaluation of permanent impairment*, ed 4, Chicago, 1993.
3. Bergner M: Development, testing and use of the sickness impact profile. In: Walker SR, Rosser RM, editors: *Quality of life: assessment and application*, Boston, 1988:79, MPT Press.
4. Health Care Financing: *Special report on findings from the national kidney dialysis and kidney transplantation study*, U.S. Dept of HHS, HCFA, Office of Research and Demonstrations, Oct. 1987.
5. Evans RW, et al: *Procedures manual: National Kidney Dialysis and Kidney Transplantation Study*, Seattle, 1982, Health and Population Study Center, Battelle Human Affairs Research Centers.
6. Harris LE, Luft FC, Rudy DW, Tierney WM: Clinical correlates of functional status in patients with chronic renal insufficiency, *Am J Kidney Dis* 21(2): 161-166, 1993.
7. Gorlen, T, Abdelnoor M, Enger E, et al: Quality of life after kidney transplantation: A 10-22 years follow-up, *Scan J Urol Nephrol* 27(1):89-92, 1993.
8. Kirtner NG, Brogan D, Fielding B: Employment status and ability to work among working-age chronic dialysis patients, *Am J Nephrol* 11(4):334-340, 1991.
9. Manninen DL, Evans RW, Dugan MK: Work disability, functional limitations and the health status of kidney transplantation recipients posttransplant, *Clin Transpl* 193-203, 1991.
10. Chagot C, et al: Functional study of hands among patients dialyzed for more than ten years, *Nephrol Dial Transplant* 8(4):347-351, 1993.
11. Rubin J, Case G, Bower J: Comparison of rehabilitation in patients undergoing home dialysis, *Arch Int Med* 150(7):1429-1431, 1990.

# CHAPTER 35

# ASSESSMENT OF UROGENITAL IMPAIRMENT AND DISABILITY

*Martin Fritzhand*
*Eric L. Jenison*

This chapter will focus on the lower urinary tract, as well as the male and female reproductive systems. There are specific sections discussing the bladder, urethra, and the specific anatomical components of the male and female reproductive systems. The sections are oriented in a manner similar to the AMA *Guides,* and the classification schemes are adapted from this source. There is little in the literature addressing impairment and disability of the urogenital system, and many examples are provided incorporating the classification scheme to demonstrate the principles of the grading system.

## I. LOWER URINARY TRACT

## BLADDER

### Definitions and Functions

The bladder is well-suited for its two functions: the storage (filling) and the expulsion (micturition) of urine. It is a hollow organ lying deep in the pelvic cavity in both males and females and is covered with smooth (detrusor) muscle. This viscus distends as it fills with urine, and the fundus gradually expands and rises in the pelvis, exposing itself more readily to injury. Urine is stored in the bladder under minimal pressure. In normal circumstances, the bladder can hold 400 to 700 cc of urine with little rise in intravesical pressure during filling. The distention of the bladder by urine does not trigger muscular (detrusor) contractions; this is termed *stability* (i.e, voluntary control of micturition). A neurogenic bladder is an unstable bladder where there is poor control of bladder activity. The end result of an unstable bladder is urinary incontinence with the unwanted premature expulsion of urine from the bladder (involuntary micturition).

### Disorders Resulting in Impairment

Bladder function can be compromised intrinsically by injury and disease directly involving the bladder tissue or extrinsically by similar kinds of lesions affecting bladder innervation. Intrinsic vesical lesions adversely affect the bladder's function as a reservoir, causing the bladder to be incapable of holding the usual quantity of urine and resulting in urinary frequency. Painful micturition may be an end result of a diseased bladder. Extrinsic lesions affecting the cerebrum, spinal cord, and peripheral nerves can result in excessive detrusor contractions or the absence of contractions altogether depending on whether one has upper or lower motor neuron involvement.

Signs and symptoms reflecting bladder and sphincter dysfunction are classically discussed in relation to irritative and obstructive symptomatology. Unfortunately, the correlation between patient complaints and the pathophysiology of the underlying problem is clouded by secondary symptoms arising from the lesion itself, and there is a marked crossover of symptomatology such that one must be very careful to avoid making conclusions based on the history alone.

Obstructive symptoms include hesitancy, straining, dribbling, nocturia, and an intermittent urinary stream. Irritative symptoms are those complaints resulting from changes of the bladder lining (and wall), and include dysuria (painful or difficult urination), frequency of urination, and urgency.

On physical examination a distended bladder can be palpated above the pubic symphysis. Neurologic examination of the saddle region can certainly suggest impairment of bladder innervation. Lack of buttock sensation is indicative of neurological pathology, and anal sphincter tone may indicate the degree of perineal striated muscle integrity. The presence of the bulbocavernosus reflex demonstrates that the sacral reflex is intact, although this reflex is commonly absent in normal individuals. (In determining presence of the bulbocavernosus reflex, the glans penis or clitoris is squeezed and the external anal sphincter is felt to contract on the previously inserted examining finger.)

## Diagnostic Procedures

The diagnostic procedures available to the physician are myriad and include urinalysis, intravenous pyelogram (IVP), voiding cystourethrogram, and cystoscopy. Urodynamic studies serve to quantify the two major bladder functions. Data are collected by various techniques describing what occurs as the bladder is filling (storage) and emptying (micturition). The bladder outlet (vesical neck) is studied by modalities including a *urethral pressure profile*, which gives a picture of the functional length of the sphincter and its ability to contract and relax. *Cystometry* adds information as to sensation and accommodation during filling, and contractility of the detrusor musculature during both filling and emptying, and results can indicate the anatomic level of an extrinsic lesion or the irritability caused by intrinsic disease. Emptying is also evaluated by *uroflowmetry* (urine flow rate). Thus, urodynamic studies enable one to study bladder and sphincter activity as well as measure the activity of voiding. The results of cystometry, uroflowmetry, and the urethral pressure profile can suggest the underlying lesion especially when studies are performed by well-qualified personnel, although results are sometimes subjective even in the best of hands.

## Classification of Impairment

Signs and symptoms resulting from a bladder impairment vary with the nature of the injury or illness, its anatomic location, and its response to treatment. The AMA *Guides* has classified bladder impairment into four broad functional categories. The following is a rating system (adapted from the AMA *Guides*) using disorders seen by an examiner as a reference point, as well as the resultant scope of complications caused by disease and injury. Impairment ratings are assigned to each category commencing with a 0% to 15% impairment of the whole person for Class I impairments that result in intermittent symptoms without incontinence to 40% to 60% for Class IV impairments where the patient is totally incontinent.

## Class I

There are some disorders that only intermittently affect the filling and/or expulsion of urine from the bladder (Class I). These entities allow the patient to function normally between episodes, and have only limited ability to disrupt their work or home environment. Thus, these injuries or illnesses have limited impact and are associated with a low percent of impairment to the whole person.

**Example:** A middle-aged male has dysuria and frequency. An IVP and voiding cystourethrogram demonstrates a large bladder diverticulum. This becomes infected at varying intervals, causing symptoms consistent with a urinary tract infection, and responds rapidly to antibiotic therapy. The patient is asymptomatic between events. This example is indicative of a *low functional impairment*. The diverticulum may have been caused by bladder outlet disease; the patient may be best served by treating the underlying cause of the diverticulum as well as by performing a diverticulectomy. However, if symptoms are easily controlled with a course of antibiotics and the patient is asymptomatic in the interim, little time is lost from work and quality of life does not suffer. A 0% to 15% impairment rating is given based on the disturbance in their activities of daily living (ADL), time lost from work, frequency of infections, need for hospitalization, and the evaluator's summarization of these events.

## Class II

Many urologic conditions require continuous treatment to control ongoing signs and symptoms of bladder irritability. Chronic cystitis can be suppressed with appropriate long-term antibiotics. A second example of a Class II impairment would be a patient with a small, contracted, irradiated bladder resulting in frequent voiding due to a small storage capacity. Here, neurologic innervation of the bladder has been preserved, and urodynamics would not indicate a neurogenic bladder. However, the irritable bladder results in frequent voiding that disrupts work activities and interferes with the patient's sleep pattern.

Illnesses and injuries resulting in a frequent voiding pattern must be analyzed as to cause, extent, and whether pain is associated with micturition. Interstitial cystitis, radiation cystitis, and other causes of a small-capacity bladder may be best treated by cystectomy and urinary diversion rather than by ongoing intensive medical care, which does little to alleviate incapacitating symptoms. The functional impairment evaluation of these patients should reflect disruption of work and social patterns notwithstanding their designated Class II category. The appropriate response to surgical treatment with alleviation of many genitourinary symptoms should trigger reevaluation of the original impairment. Bladder extirpation would serve to restore quality of life, although urinary diversion with its associated stomal complications and problems must be analyzed.

## Class III

Class III impairments result in intermittent urinary incontinence and refer especially to disorders involving the bladder neck and sphincter where reflex activity is reduced and voluntary control is impeded by the anatomic nature of the lesion. Female stress incontinence would fall into this category as also would clinical complications from prostatic procedures. These types of impairments are described below.

**Example:** A middle-aged man underwent a transurethral prostate resection for benign prostatic hyperplasia. Excessive bleeding necessitated additional resection at the vesical neck. His postoperative course was complicated by urinary incontinence primarily associated with coughing and sneezing, but also occurring at other times and requiring pads to remain dry.

## Class IV

Neuromuscular dysfunction of bladder control can result from lesions and injuries affecting the cerebrum, brain stem, spinal cord, nerve roots, and peripheral nerves. It is necessary to study the patient carefully, perform required urodynamic studies, classify the type of neurogenic bladder present, and determine, if possible, the underlying cause of the problem.

The history may suggest the level of injury. The patient may have had a cerebrovascular accident or have a systemic disease such as multiple sclerosis or diabetes mellitus. Trauma to the spinal cord is frequently associated with bladder dysfunction. Vesical function is centered in the S2-4 regions of the spinal cord, and injuries here (corresponding to the level of the T11-L1 vertebrae) are most likely to result in a flaccid neurogenic bladder. Lesions cephalad usually result in a spastic or mildly spastic neurogenic bladder because inhibitive pathways from the cerebrum and brain stem have been disrupted. Flaccid bladders result in incontinence by overflow, whereas spastic bladders are associated with uninhibited detrusor contractions with frequent expulsion of small amounts of urine. The contractions are no longer dampened by ongoing upper-motor neuron inhibition. Spastic bladders are usually associated with irritative bladder symptoms. Physical examination can help define the anatomic site of injury. Preserved anal sphincter tone (bulbocavernosus reflex) in the presence of incontinence indicates a suprasacral lesion, while absence of tone suggests a sacral or peripheral nerve lesion. The presence of saddle anesthesia and an enlarged bladder further suggest bladder flaccidity. Deep tendon reflexes are hypoactive or absent when the lumbosacral spinal cord or nerve roots are compromised. Spastic bladders result in dimin-

ished urinary capacity. Diagnostic studies including IVP, voiding cystourethrogram, and endoscopy are useful in the evaluation, and urodynamic studies are used to quantitate and define the degree of bladder dysfunction. Uroflowmetry and cystometry are especially useful and results are easily correlated with findings.

**Example:** A young man fell 20 feet, sustaining several mid-dorsal compression fractures. He required operative intervention to ensure spinal stability, and did well in the postoperative period. He was noted to have urinary incontinence after removal of the urethral catheter. Studies revealed a spastic neurogenic bladder that improved after use of drugs, bladder training, and intermittent self-catheterization.

The complication of a neurogenic bladder resulting from injury or disease can have immeasurable consequences to the patient. The aim of the treating physician is to prevent deterioration of renal function (by protecting the kidneys from the high pressure generated by spasticity and by controlling urinary tract infection) and to keep the patient dry. Patients who can void to some degree either spontaneously or with various trigger techniques may have significant postvoiding residual urine remaining in the bladder. These patients do well with intermittent self-catheterization (every 4 to 6 hours). Urinary tract infections are reduced and the patient remains dry. Pharmacologic intervention with such drugs as oxybutynin, propantheline, or bethanechol is used to manipulate the bladder musculature and either increase or reduce vesical contractions. The result of urodynamic studies will suggest the underlying neuromuscular pathology, and the appropriate drug can then be chosen to reduce the level of urinary incontinence.

Trigger mechanisms, drug therapy, and intermittent self-catheterization may control the problem, although it is mandatory for the afflicted individual to remain dry. Persistent incontinence is associated with a high level of impairment (40% to 60%) and can prevent or deter employment, at the very least, as well as disrupt the home environment. Electrostimulation and various surgical procedures are available when incontinence is refractory to all treatments.

## Summary

The impairment resulting from either bladder trauma or disease must be carefully evaluated by the examiner. Incontinence may have a devastating effect. On the other hand, mild stress incontinence associated only with a transient marked increase in intra-abdominal pressure may be little more than a nuisance. Urinary frequency may completely disrupt a patient's life-style. Cystitis may be intermittent and mild, or may be constant and severe, resulting in one or two voidings per hour, disrupting the work day. Frequent nocturia interferes with sleep patterns and results in fatigue, tiredness, and generalized malaise. Efficiency in the workplace is decreased. Each entity has its specific impact on the daily living habits of the individual, and must be carefully assessed to render a fair impairment estimate. The patient with urinary incontinence may require diapers or pads at the very least and risk embarrassment from stains and odors. It is not unusual to resort to an external collection device. There is a wide disparity between Class I and Class IV impairments, reflecting the wide range of symptomatology and degree of functional impairment.

## URETHRA

### Anatomy and Function

The male urethra is a conduit for both urine and seminal fluid. It commences at the vesical neck and is totally surrounded by the prostate in its most proximal portion, receiving seminal emissions here, and continuing to the external urethral meatus enclosed through most of its course by the prostate. The female urethra is much shorter than the male urethra and represents the entire sphincter mechanism of the bladder. It also extends from the vesical neck and opens in the vaginal vestibule below the clitoris.

### Disorders Resulting in Impairment

Obstruction of the urethra interferes with the passage of urine, while injury or disease may result in the loss of voluntary control of urine. Signs and symptoms reflecting urethral pathology include dysuria, a slow or weak urinary stream, postvoiding dribbling, pain, incontinence, urinary retention, and urethral discharge. Physical examination may disclose an ectopic or stenotic urethral meatus or distended bladder. The urethra is easily evaluated by diagnostic techniques. Retrograde and excretory urethrography, cystoscopy (urethroscopy), and a voiding cystourethrogram easily visualize the urethra, and urodynamic studies (including cystometrogram) delineate loss of voluntary control. Distal urethral stenosis in the female is defined by urethral calibration using instruments, which when introduced into the urethra, measure the size of the lumen. Significant stenosis is commonly dilated in an attempt to alleviate obstruction.

### Classification of Impairment

Impairment is measured by the degree of symptomatology experienced by the patient and its overall impact on his or her usual and customary life-style. Testing will usually document a degree of severity commensurate with symptoms. These symptoms are alleviated in many cases by minimal therapeutic measures and represent only a minor impairment to the whole person. However, some symptoms may demand ongoing treatment or require significant surgical intervention in an effort to relieve patient distress and discomfort. These lesions would obviously result in a higher degree of impairment and would most likely impact on the patients' ability to function in the work place.

The AMA *Guides* describe two classes of urethral impairments: those urethral disorders that require intermittent treatment and those entities that are not effectively controlled despite therapy.

### Class I
There are many disorders of the urethra requiring only periodic treatment. The impact on the individual is usually not great and treatment can control the ongoing problem effectively, resulting in minimal time away from work or disruption of other activities.

Urethral stricture disease in the male is a complication of disease or injury or is acquired during instrumentation and is usually controlled by periodic dilation. The patient is symptom-free for varying intervals between dilations.

**Example:** A middle-aged man had a vesical neck injury requiring prolonged urethral catheterization. The lesion healed, but dysuria and a weak urinary stream six months later prompted evaluation. The patient had a bulbous urethral stricture according to endoscopy and voiding cystourethrogram studies that responded to dilation at three or four month intervals. He is asymptomatic for several months followed by gradually increasing obstructive symptoms until treatment.

The level of impairment is directly related to the frequency and severity of symptoms caused by stricture disease and ranges from 0% to 10%. Patients requiring monthly dilation would obviously receive a higher level of impairment that those patients requiring one or two dilations yearly with relatively long symptom-free periods.

### Class II
Lesions affecting the urethra and resulting in ongoing refractory symptoms represent a much more

serious threat to normal patient routine. Work may be disrupted on a regular basis, and the examiner must carefully question the patient regarding urinary and sexual (see next section) function. Refractory strictures, urethrocutaneous fistulas, abnormalities resulting from radical surgical procedures, and lesions caused by injuries that are refractory to reconstructive surgery all fall into the more severe degree of urethral impairments (10% to 20% impairment). The examples below represent urethral disorders that are refractory to treatment modalities.

**Example:** An elderly woman with carcinoma of the vulva required a radical resection with excision of a significant portion of her urethra. She has remained totally incontinent and has required an indwelling catheter as she refused urinary diversion. The indwelling catheter results in recurrent urinary tract infections that can lead to renal deterioration and bladder stones, and tends to be psychologically and socially debilitating. Her mental status may be adversely affected by the permanent urethral/suprapubic catheter, and her degree of impairment should reflect these obvious side effects (10% to 20%).

**Example:** A middle-aged man sustained a profound straddle injury disrupting the bulbomembranous urethra. He required reconstructive surgery as the injury was extensive and he could no longer void voluntarily. The patient has required long-term suprapubic diversion. Again, the presence of an indwelling catheter due to refractory urethral trauma results in an impairment that affects organ systems other than the urethra. The degree of functional disability must reflect all aspects of the injury as well as its resulting complications (e.g., lack of sexual function, renal dysfunction, psychological disorders).

### Summary

The urethra can be affected by disease or injury. Instrumentation of the male urethra can result in a wide variety of strictures, and injuries can result in urinary incontinence or retention. The facts of each individual case must be weighed with regard to its impact on work, home, and other activities. It becomes obvious that other organ systems and functions can be affected by refractory urethral lesions or by its subsequent treatment. Bladder, sexual function (see next section), renal disorders, and mental and behavioral disorders may need to be considered by the examiner before the impairment estimate is provided. This estimate needs to reflect the entire impairment, rather than a rating based solely on the localized urethral lesions.

## II. MALE REPRODUCTIVE SYSTEM

### PENIS

#### Anatomy and Function

The penis is an erectile organ largely consisting of three corporal bodies composed of erectile tissue with the anterior urethra coursing through the ventrally-situated corpus spongiosum and the two corpora cavernosa on either side in their dorsal position. Erection is caused by a complex interaction of neurologic, vascular, and hormonal factors that result in engorgement of the vascular spaces in the paired corpora cavernosa with blood. Parasympathetic and sympathetic stimulation of the penis along with the presence of adequate vascular channels determine the effectiveness of tumescence. The cause of dysfunction may be obscure and difficult to diagnose and may be the result of a lesion anatomically far removed from the penis or from psychological factors.

Ejaculation occurs after emission of semen into the posterior urethra. The ejaculate is then propelled through the anterior urethra and actively expelled from the external urethral meatus. The ejaculate is composed of spermatozoa from the vas deferens and epididymis and seminal fluid from the prostate and seminal vesicle. Erections are possible even when ejaculation is not and when penile sensation is minimal or absent. Injury and disease of the penis can also affect the anterior urethra, and urinary dysfunction caused by penile disorders is assessed by the criteria in the preceding section.

#### Disorders Resulting in Impairment

Sexual dysfunction resulting from penile disorders includes abnormalities of erection, ejaculation, and sensation. Erectile dysfunction is by far the most common abnormality stemming from disorders of the penis. However, various injuries, surgical procedures, and certain illnesses resulting in neurologic dysfunction can lead to retrograde ejaculation or even loss of emission and ejaculation or sensation.

An adequate medical history including detailed psychosexual evaluation may uncover an obvious cause for sexual dysfunction. The patient may have received treatment for priapism or Peyronie's disease (induration of corpora cavernosa producing fibrous chordae), or may have required a retroperitoneal procedure resulting in retrograde ejaculation. Examination of the groin and penis may uncover diminished peripheral pulses, absence of male escutcheon or the presence of Peyronie plaques. Of course, blood tests (testosterone, prolactin, LH, FSH), nocturnal penile tumescence, and urodynamics are meaningful. Tests for chemicals are discussed in the section in this chapter on Testes, Epididymides, and Spermatic Cords. Endocrine evaluation may suggest a hormonal etiology for impotence, and abnormal results should be carefully followed up to avoid overlooking an important cause of male sexual dysfunction. Hypogonadism, pituitary failure, diabetes mellitus, and thyroid disease can all result in impotence. Nocturnal penile tumescence is a useful adjunct, and measurement of penile blood flow, intracorporeal injection, and penile angiography can be considered. Unfortunately, many studies of erectile dysfunction lack the precise end results physicians have become accustomed to, and invalid interpretation, unsatisfactory technique, and lack of controls only serve to cloud understanding and add little to our knowledge of the underlying mechanisms of disease.

## Classification of Impairment

The AMA *Guides* lists criteria for sexual dysfunction due to penile lesions resulting in abnormalities of erection, ejaculation, and sensation. These range from Class I disorders where sexual function is possible with varying degrees of difficulty to Class III impairments with the loss of all sexual function with impairment ratings of 0% to 20%. Urethral dysfunction, if present, should be evaluated according to the criteria in the previous section. The total functional impairment should reflect both urethral and sexual dysfunction.

### Class I

Penile disorders affecting erection, ejaculation, or sensation include such disparate entities as Peyronie's disease, priapism, and diabetes mellitus. Penile trauma may diminish erection, although ejaculation and sensation can remain intact. Surgical procedures resulting in loss of ejaculation may not affect erection or sensation. Class I impairments involve one modality of sexual function and allow for some degree of sexual function. Many medications (antihypertensives) can cause a Class I impairment. However, this is a reversible problem and should not lead to a "permanent impairment" rating unless no other medication can be successfully substituted.

Retrograde ejaculation can occur in patients who have had surgical procedures involving the retroperitoneum.

**Example:** A 30-year-old male had an embryonal carcinoma of the left testis. He required an orchiec-

tomy and ultimately underwent retroperitoneal lymph node dissection. His postoperative course was unremarkable except that he was no longer able to ejaculate. Semen was obtained from the bladder during an infertility workup. Again, sexual function was possible but impaired. Erection and sensation remained intact while ejaculation was impossible. He belonged in a Class I category with a 0% to 10% impairment rating.

### Class II

Class II impairments involve both ejaculatory function and sensation while erection is intact. Injuries affecting the posterior urethra resulting in disruption of emission may not have a similar effect on erection. In addition, various surgical procedures interrupt the sympathetic fibers with consequent loss of ejaculation and sensation, leaving erectile potential intact. These problems are rated at 10% to 19% whole person impairment.

**Example:** A young man sustained a straddle injury with disruption of the posterior urethra. He required several reconstructive procedures in an effort to restore urethral continuity. Unfortunately, the patient eventually required urinary diversion due to marked complications at the wound site. In addition, ejaculation and penile sensation were lost, although erectile ability remained intact. His level of impairment must reflect both urethral and sexual dysfunction. Renal as well as mental and behavioral function would require assessment if indicated.

### Class III

Direct penile injuries may profoundly interrupt erectile potential and impair ejaculation and sensation. Penile amputation, severe crush and laceration injuries to the penis, and diseases requiring significant penile resection may preserve urethral integrity with the loss of all sexual function (Class III impairment, 20% impairment rating).

**Example:** A psychotic patient amputated his penis. The organ was reattached and retained urinary function. However, erection was no longer possible (20% impairment for penis alone that should be combined with the psychological impairment).

Radical genitourinary surgery in an effort to extirpate cancer from the region surrounding the ejaculatory duct (e.g., surgery for carcinoma of the prostate, posterior urethra, bladder, or rectum) will result in loss of ejaculation and sensation (see Prostate section). In addition, the significant disruption of sympathetic and parasympathetic nerve fibers frequently results in loss of erectile potential with the absence of all sexual function. Profound injuries to the same area may similarly result in loss of sexual function.

**Example:** A 59-year-old man had a malignant lesion involving the posterior urethra. He required radical surgery including cystoprostatectomy and urinary diversion with loss of all sexual function. The patient was fitted with a penile prosthesis six months later. His impairment should reflect both loss of sexual (20%) and urinary (40% to 60%) function as well as loss of the prostate and seminal vesicle (15% to 20%). (These values are combined to define the whole person impairment.)

Disorders affecting the penis are devastating to the male psyche and require an adequate impairment rating. Unfortunately, we have no effective method to quantitate the degree of erectile dysfunction, and one must frequently rely on the history and physical examination. Both urinary and sexual function must be taken into account when assessing impairment, and daily life activities need to be closely considered. An adequate sexual history is essential. The psychophysiologic effects of erectile dysfunction with its attendant loss of satisfactory sexual performance diminishing quality of life will markedly affect the patient. Work capacity may suffer due to associated depression. Age factors are measured by adding or subtracting 50% of the impairment for those men younger than 40 years of age or older than 65 years of age, respectively.

## SCROTUM

### Anatomy and Function

The scrotum is a cutaneous pouch containing and protecting the testes, epididymides, and structures of the spermatic cord. The layers of the scrotum are extremely distensible, responding to temperature extremes or exercise in order to maintain the testes at their optimum physiological temperature.

The scrotum is most easily examined by observation and palpation. The normal scrotal skin is contracted and thickened in cold temperature with rugae easily visible. The skin relaxes and is much smoother and thinner in warm temperature. On physical examination, masses and skin lesions may be appreciated. The skin itself may be tender or edematous. Evaluation of testicular mobility is germane to function and must be carefully assessed.

### Classification of Impairment

The extent of tissue loss associated with scrotal injuries may define whether the testes need to be transplanted into subcutaneous thigh pockets. There is usually sufficient scrotal skin to protect the testes

even if testicular mobility is compromised (AMA *Guides*, Class I impairment). However, if loss of scrotal skin is great, then implantation should be accomplished in order to preserve testicular function (AMA *Guides*, Class II impairment). Unfortunately, there are disorders involving the scrotum that cannot be adequately treated despite aggressive medical management (AMA *Guides* Class III impairment).

Thus, there is a spectrum of scrotal diseases and injuries. Each case much be carefully assessed especially with regard to testicular function and mobility, as well as response to treatment, with significant emphasis placed on ongoing symptoms resulting in limitation of physical activity. The following examples will serve to illustrate the range of scrotal involvement by disease or injury.

### Class I

**Example:** A young man sustained a gunshot wound to the scrotum requiring wide debridement followed by reconstruction. He did well but experienced occasional scrotal pain and discomfort associated with activity. Physical examination did reveal a small scrotum with tenderness on palpation of the testes and diminished testicular mobility.

**Example:** An elderly man with squamous cell carcinoma of the scrotum required extensive scrotal resection to obtain unaffected margins. The defect was closed after a conscious decision was made to avoid testicular transplantation. The patient did reasonably well but complained of a "pulling sensation" especially associated with prolonged sitting or accompanying heavy exercise. Physical examination again revealed a small scrotum with minimal testicular mobility.

The above two examples illustrate loss of scrotal skin by disease and injury. The smaller reconstructed scrotum was large enough to accommodate the testes but could not afford adequate mobility. Pain and discomfort were associated with various positions. There is obviously some impact on the work habits of the individual. Lifting, stooping, or prolonged sitting may be compromised, and this must be accounted for when estimating impairment. However, the level of impairment remains low (0% to 10%). There is a possibility that further scarring may necessitate testicular transplantation in the future.

### Class II

Scrotal impairment is greater if the ability to contain the scrotal contents is lost due to injury or disease. The loss of a critical portion of the scrotum, such that reconstruction will not contain the scrotal contents, necessitates testicular transplantation to adjacent subcutaneous thigh pouches. The examples given above can be used to illustrate Class II impairments. If sufficient scrotal skin were destroyed by the gunshot wound in the first example, or if lack of proper margins had resulted in sacrifice of most of the scrotum in the second example, it would then have been necessary to close the scrotal defects after implanting the testes into the subcutaneous tissue of the thighs to preserve function. There is sufficient discomfort and loss of mobility resulting from testicular implants to affect adversely many activities. Sexual function may be impaired by constant trauma to the testes during intercourse, and sports and other extracurricular activities may be reduced. Constant lifting, bending, or stooping can be associated with testicular pain. The impact on specific work activities must be considered carefully.

### Class III

There are few entities that result in ongoing signs and symptoms of scrotal disease uncontrolled by treatment (Class III). Medical and/or surgical intervention can usually result in successful management of a difficult clinical problem involving the scrotum. Certain congenital disorders defy treatment. Radiation dermatitis may present a serious dilemma in management. However, lymphedema is by far the most common refractory chronic disorder involving the scrotum. Surgery, radiation, and disease can all cause scrotal lymphedema. It may be impossible to hide marked scrotal enlargement, and little can be done to preserve appearance or lessen the associated symptoms.

**Example:** A middle-aged man required a groin dissection after the appearance of metastatic lymph nodes one year following treatment for penile carcinoma. He did well and subsequently remained free of disease. Unfortunately, massive scrotal lymphedema progressively developed and has hampered physical activity, as well as remaining unsightly and embarrassing to the patient. This patient has sustained a serious impairment that can grossly impact work performance. There is no way to hide his disability. Sports and extracurricular activities are markedly limited, and his entire life-style has been severely affected by the affliction. Impairment ratings should reflect his degree of discomfort and the physical limitations caused by his disability. Class III impairment is listed at a level of 20% to 35%.

### Summary

The scrotum's location protects it from injury, and it is not likely to be involved by disorders that affect other genitourinary organs. Nonetheless, devastating results can occur when its ability to contain and protect the testes is limited or removed. Scrotal pain and discomfort limit physical activity both at home and at work. An enlarged scrotum is unsightly and reduces patient mobility. Consideration must be made for ongoing distress and the possibility that symptoms may worsen, resulting in additional surgery.

## TESTES, EPIDIDYMIDES, AND SPERMATIC CORDS

### Anatomy and Function

The testis is a mobile ovoid organ lying at the lower end of the scrotal sac and responsible for the production of spermatozoa as well as various male hormones. Ninety-five percent of the body's production of testosterone originates in the Leydig cells of the testes. These cells, situated in the interstitial tissue of the testes, are directly influenced by LH (luteinizing hormone). Low levels of blood testosterone serve to increase anterior pituitary production of LH. FSH (follicle-stimulating hormone), also secreted by the anterior pituitary, is responsible for spermatogenesis, and acts directly on the Sertoli cells situated in the seminiferous tubules of the testis. The germinal epithelium lining the tubules produces spermatozoa. FSH and LH are both under the control of hypothalamic-secreted gonadotropin-releasing hormone (GnRH).

The epididymis, attached to the posterolateral surface of the testis, is responsible for the maturation of spermatozoa, which gain mobility and fertility prior to transport through the vas deferens to the ejaculatory duct. Sperm maturation takes up to 75 days, and transportation lasts another 10–15 days.

The testis is firm and rubbery, while the epididymis has a bulbous head at the superior aspect of the testis and can be traced by an easily palpable groove between the testis and the body of the epididymis to its tail lying inferiorly. The cord-like vas deferens, a continuation of the tail of the epididymis, is palpable as it travels in the spermatic cord to the external inguinal ring at the most cephalad portion of the scrotum. The spermatic cord itself consists of the vas (ductus) deferens as well as various nerves, lymphatics, arteries, and veins anchoring the testis in the most dependent portion of the scrotum.

### Examination and Diagnostic Studies

Physical examination should include palpation of the testis between the thumb and index finger, noting alterations in size, shape, and consistency. The epididymis should be evaluated, and abnormalities such as unusual induration, masses, or nodules noted. Disruption of the normal architecture has special significance when assessing functional impairment.

There are various diagnostic studies that may be of value and assist in defining functional abnormalities of the testes, epididymides, and spermatic cords. Semen analysis is used to assess the presence or absence (azoospermia) of sperm. Azoospermia or severe oligospermia may suggest obstruction during sperm transport. The motility and morphology of the spermatozoa itself may reflect ongoing testicular disease. Fructose, synthesized in the seminal vesicle, is normally present in semen. Testicular biopsy is rarely necessary but can document unusual causes of azoospermia. Scrotal ultrasound is used to clarify testicular lesions or other masses palpable in the spermatic cord or epididymis. It has become a very important noninvasive diagnostic tool with excellent imaging of the scrotal contents. In fact, it is the procedure of choice and primary imaging technique used to evaluate the scrotal contents. Scrotal ultrasound can accurately distinguish between testicular and extratesticular masses, as well as between solid and fluid-filled lesions. Vasography and vasoepididymography can reveal a site of obstruction when azoospermia is noted on semen analysis. Lesions involving the vas deferens, epididymis, and seminiferous tubules may be visualized. Testicular venography is also available. In addition, the various blood hormone levels (FSH, LH, and testosterone) should be obtained when assessing male infertility.

## Classification of Impairment

Diseases involving the scrotal contents, that is, testis, epididymis, and spermatic cord, may be unilateral or bilateral, require intermittent or continuous treatment, and may or may not result in alteration of seminal (spermatogenesis) or hormonal (testosterone) function. There is a range of severity of involvement by disease or injury. Signs and symptoms must be elicited by the examiner. Physical examination is important and anatomic alteration is a prerequisite for inclusion into Class I–III categories as listed in the AMA *Guides.*

### Class I
Patients with Class I impairments have signs and symptoms with physical evidence of anatomic alteration. However, treatment is only intermittent, and seminal and hormonal function remain intact. The loss of one testis falls into this category. In addition, trauma or disease affecting one testis, epididymis, or spermatic cord where the contralateral side is unaffected is a Class I impairment when anatomic alteration is defined and symptoms are present but respond to treatment. The presence of a normal contralateral organ ensures normal seminal and hormonal function. It is rated at a level of 0% to 10%.

**Example:** A young man sustained an injury to the right testis. He was treated conservatively but continued to complain of ill-defined discomfort while lifting heavy objects and follow-up examination documented unilateral testicular atrophy.

**Example:** A man was hospitalized for acute epididymitis shortly after he was required to lift a heavy computer at work. He required intensive antibiotic therapy but continued to have intermittent testicular pain, and physical examination revealed marked induration in the region of the epididymal head. Additional treatment did not change the nature of his complaints.

Class I impairments are frequently the result of trauma or infection to the testis or epididymis. Physical examination may reveal induration or enlargement of the epididymis or a soft small (atrophic) testis. The areas of involvement will be tender to palpation. The contents of the contralateral hemiscrotum are usually normal. The injuries and illnesses causing Class I impairments frequently result in lingering discomfort worsened by undue physical activity both at work and at home. Jogging, lifting heavy objects, and sexual intercourse all may exacerbate symptoms, and it becomes imperative to avoid those actions known to precipitate complaints.

### Class II
The presence of signs and symptoms as well as evidence of anatomic alteration is seen in both Class I and II patients, although treatment is continuous or not possible with Class II patients. In addition, seminal and hormonal abnormalities are detectable.

Bilateral testicular involvement is necessary to alter male hormonal levels, while bilateral involvement of the testes, epididymides, or spermatic cords are required to affect the production, maturation, or transport of spermatozoa. Disorders involving both testes may affect Leydig cell production of testosterone and/or germ cell production of spermatozoa, while disorders of the epididymides and vas deferens can obstruct or retard the motility and fertility of sperm. Impairment rating is set at 10% to 15%.

**Example:** A young man sustained a pelvic fracture with injury to the prostatomembranous urethra. He required long-term urethral catheterization, and his course was complicated by bilateral epididymitis. A workup for infertility several years later revealed evidence of bilateral chronic epididymitis with marked oligospermia on sperm analysis. His impairment would be 10% to 15% for the chronic epididymitis combined with a Class II impairment of the urethra at 15% to 20%.

The effects of bilateral involvement can be devastating, especially when fertility is important, and the lack of available treatment only adds to frustration. Low testosterone levels with possible loss of secondary sex characteristics and libido require immediate attention and hormonal levels need frequent monitoring. These changes may not be as nearly dramatic in the elderly, and any impairment assessment must take into account the patient's age. A comprehensive history will probably uncover prior workup, and expensive tests can be avoided when ancillary studies are documented by the examiner. The impact on the patient's life can be fully understood only when the impairment is assessed and delineated. A fair assessment is made when all aspects of disability are considered; almost always this is not the physician's responsibility.

### Class III

Class III impairments are the result of anatomic loss of the testes or the absence of detectable seminal or hormonal function. Significant trauma to both testes resulting in bilateral orchiectomy obviously results in complete loss of spermatogenesis and testosterone production. Bilateral vasectomy similarly results in azoospermia, although it is unusual for diseases affecting the testes to result in undetectable levels of spermatozoa on semen analysis or complete loss of testosterone production by the Leydig cells. The loss of both testes has broad psychological implications. Prostheses should be considered, and counseling is helpful. Hormonal replacement should be instituted immediately. The impairment is considerable at any age, and obviously worse if the patient is young and has not yet begun a family. It is rated at 15% to 20%.

### Summary

In assessing impairment, it is necessary to take into account ongoing symptoms. Testicular or epididymal discomfort that increases in severity during physical activity may be a significant hindrance in performing certain work activities. It may be necessary for a patient to lead a much more sedentary life-style and forego various extracurricular and sports activities he once enjoyed. Infertility must be documented and addressed, while loss of hormonal function demands replacement therapy to avoid signs of testosterone deficiency.

## PROSTATE AND SEMINAL VESICLES

### Anatomy and Function

The prostate is a fibromuscular, glandular, chestnut-sized, firm structure lying at the base of the bladder and enclosing the posterior urethra as it leaves the vesical neck. The two seminal vesicles are lobulated sacs lying on the posterior surface of the prostate representing outpouchings of the terminal portion of the vas deferens. The ejaculatory duct is formed by the coalescence of the seminal vesicle and the vas deferens, and traverses the prostate to empty into the prostatic urethra.

The seminal vesicle provides most of the fluid in semen, which is responsible for spermatozoa survival, and the prostate adds fluid and nutrients to the seminal fluid. The location of the prostate surrounding the urethra as it leaves the bladder frequently results in urinary obstructive symptoms, and this is addressed in the section describing urethral impairments. Infertility resulting from abnormalities of seminal emission is addressed in the section on Testes, Epididymides, and Spermatic Cords.

### Disorders Resulting in Impairment

Prostatic enlargement can result in obstructive urinary symptoms such as a slow or weak urinary stream, dribbling, dysuria, or nocturia. Prostate and seminal vesicle disease can result in infertility with concomitant abnormalities of semen analysis. In addition, diseases of the prostate (and seminal vesicle) can result in hemospermia, perineal and rectal pain and discomfort, low-back pain, and generalized malaise. Rectal examination may disclose a tender, boggy prostate. It is difficult to palpate the seminal vesicles. Diagnostic studies include urinalysis, split-urine techniques, cystoscopy, prostatic biopsy, and the modalities described previously to explore infertility and urinary obstruction. Prostatic ultrasonography has become an invaluable tool with high-resolution visualization of the prostate and surrounding structures.

### Classification of Impairment

The AMA *Guides* list three classes of impairment with respect to disorders of the prostate and seminal vesicles. Class I and II impairments are used primarily to grade levels of prostatitis. It is extremely rare to identify clinically infections of the seminal vesicle, and involvement by prostate carcinoma is usually the only time this organ is appreciated on physical examination.

Class I impairments (0% to 10%) require signs, symptoms, and evidence on physical examination indicating the presence of prostate or seminal vesicle disease. Continuous treatment is not a prerequisite for a Class I impairment but is necessary for a Class II impairment (10% to 15%). Again, evaluation may result in findings suggesting urethral obstruction or infertility, and assessment must take into account these problems.

Patients with recurrent episodes of acute prostatitis responsive to intermittent treatment who have an abnormal prostate on rectal examination fall into the Class I category. Patients with longstanding, smoldering, chronic prostatitis who require ongoing suppressive antibacterial therapy and who also have an abnormal prostate on digital evaluation fall into the Class II category.

Class III impairments (15% to 20%) are reserved for those patients requiring ablation of the prostate and seminal vesicle. Patients with prostatic carcinoma requiring radical retropubic or perineal prostatectomies are in this category. In addition, patients with carcinoma of the bladder undergoing radical cystectomy necessarily fall into Class III, as do patients requiring other radical pelvic exenterations where en bloc prostatic resection is performed. The ramifications of these surgical procedures are enormous. Urinary incontinence, a urinary stoma, erectile dysfunction, and infertility are some of the complications faced by men undergoing operative intervention. The functional assessment must account for all of these problems, and the impairment must reflect the devastating, ongoing consequences requiring treatment over the years.

## Summary

The involvement of the prostate and seminal vesicle by disease or injury can have far-reaching effects. Urinary obstructive symptoms and infertility are discussed in previous sections. Local pain and discomfort caused by intermittent or ongoing prostatitis is easy to diagnose and hard to treat. Systemic symptoms such as fever and malaise can result in frequent absenteeism, and the pain and discomfort associated with prostatitis can diminish efficiency in the workplace. Quality of life suffers, and chronic prostatitis can have a major adverse impact on the life-style of the afflicted patient.

## III. FEMALE REPRODUCTIVE SYSTEM

### VULVA AND VAGINA

#### Anatomy and Functions

The external female genitalia include the following structures: labia majora and minora (collectively the "vulva"), clitoris, hymen and vestibule, mons pubis, urethral meatus, and underlying perineal structures.[4,5] Disorders of the urethra have been described earlier and will not be discussed further.

The vulva and mons pubis function to protect the entrance to the vagina and urethral meatus.[5] The vulva and underlying structures have specific importance in the function of urination and urinary incontinence. The clitoris serves as a "nerve center" for coitus.[5] Sexual stimulation results in vascular engorgement and enlargement. When the penis is inserted, the clitoris is particularly sensitive to contact and orgasm may result by this stimulation. The vagina functions to receive the penis during coitus and protect and contain the seminal fluid and sperm.[5] The vagina also functions as the lowermost portion of the birth canal during parturition and as a conduit for menstrual discharge.[5]

#### Disorders Resulting in Impairment

Impairment of function of the external genitalia includes chronic irritations resulting in pain or discomfort, loss of sensation, atrophic or hypertrophic conditions, disorders leading to impairment of sexual intercourse or sexual response, difficulties with urinary function, vaginal parturition, and preneoplastic or neoplastic conditions.[2,4]

There are numerous causes for irritation of the external genitalia, including temporary causes such as infections or allergies, which are easily treatable. However, chronic irritation, as a result of systemic or autoimmune disease, may result in more severe and long-term impairment.[2,5]

Injuries or conditions that lead to loss of sensation in the vulvar and clitoral areas have far-reaching effects. These may include lack of sexual satisfaction and orgasm as well as adverse psychological effects such as depression.[3,6]

Impairment of sexual intercourse and sexual response might result from trauma to or surgery on the external genitalia. This can lead to scarring and stenosis, resulting in loss of sensation and pain or discomfort when walking, sitting, or engaged in other ordinary activities. Urinary function, particularly sensation to void, as well as urinary incontinence, may be affected by injury to or surgery on the external genitalia and urethral meatus.[3,6]

Severe injuries or disorders could result in lack of vaginal function altogether. This would prevent parturition and necessitate Cesarean section.

Disorders of vaginal support, depending on degree of loss, can cause impairment of sexual function, urination, or defecation. Cystocele, rectocele, enterocele, and vaginal vault descensus may occur separately or in various combinations. Severe loss of support results in pelvic discomfort and can lead to total prolapse, requiring continuous pessary use or surgery.

Finally, preneoplastic and neoplastic conditions and their various treatments certainly are obvious causes of impairment to genital function and discomfort. Surgery and radiation therapy for neoplasia may result in scarring and stricture formation, with a lack of pliability and painful intercourse.

### Physical Examination

Physical examination of the external genitalia is performed by both observation and palpation. Normal vulvar tissue is soft and cushioned by underlying adipose tissue. The labia majora is normally covered with pubic hair. The labia minora should be pink and pliable. The minor and major vestibular glands are contained in the vestibule and should exhibit no inflammation, discharge, or enlargement. The vaginal mucosa should also be pliable and should contain no other lesions or discharge. Anterior and posterior wall support should be good and there should be no uterine or vaginal descensus.[3,5]

### Diagnostic Procedures

Diagnostic procedures include pap smear for cytology, wet prep and/or culture for various infectious diseases, colposcopy, and biopsy.

Ultrasonography, CT scan, and MRI may be useful in the differential diagnosis of various tumors. Testing to exclude various systemic, endocrine and autoimmune disorders may also be helpful.[5]

Wise medical practice calls for a female staff member to be present if a male physician carries out examinations of, or a procedure involving, a female patient's genitalia.

### Classifications of Impairment

#### Class I

A patient belongs in the Class I category if (1) symptoms and signs of disease or deformity of the

vulva or vagina are present but do not require continuous treatment, and (2) sexual intercourse is possible, and (3) vagina is adequate for childbirth (if patient is premenopausal). This is rated at 0% to 15% impairment of the whole person.

**Example:** A 34-year-old, gravida II, para II has twice given vaginal birth and suffers periodically from chronic vestibulitis and urethritis. Sexual intercourse is possible and pleasurable when her vestibulitis and urethritis are under control. She responds well to a prolonged course of antibiotic therapy. Estimated impairment is 10%.

#### Class II

A patient belongs in the Class II category if (1) symptoms and signs of disease or deformity of the vulva or vagina are present that require continuous treatment, and (2) sexual intercourse is possible only with some degree of difficulty, and (3) potential for vaginal delivery is limited in the premenopausal patient. This is rated at 15% to 25% impairment of the whole person.

**Example:** A 36-year-old, gravida III, para II is pregnant in the second trimester with her third child. She had undergone multiple therapies including carbon dioxide ($CO_2$) laser vaporizations of the vagina and vulva for human papilloma virus (HPV) and dysplasia. This has resulted in scarring and some vaginal stenosis, making sexual intercourse painful. Cesarean section is planned for delivery for fear of vaginal lacerations with vaginal childbirth. Estimated impairment is 20%.

#### Class III

A patient belongs in the Class III category if (1) symptoms and signs of disease or deformity of the vulva or vagina are present that are not controlled by treatment, and (2) sexual intercourse is not possible, and (3) vaginal delivery is not possible for the premenopausal patient. This is rated at 25% to 35% impairment of the whole person.

**Example:** A 35-year-old, gravida II, para II had malignant melanoma of the vulva and lower vagina that required radical vulvectomy and partial vaginectomy. Stenosis of the vagina subsequently developed, resulting in total inability to achieve sexual intercourse or vaginal delivery. Estimated impairment is 35%.

### Evaluation of Impairment

There are multiple aspects to consider when evaluating the degree of impairment of the external genitalia. It is important to take into account the age of the patient, considering her reproductive potential, as well as the overall impact of the impairment to the whole person, including all physical, sexual, reproductive, and psychological dysfunctions resulting from the disorder.

## CERVIX AND UTERUS

### Anatomy and Functions

The cervix is the narrowed most-caudad portion of the uterus. It is somewhat conical in shape, measuring 2.5 × 3.0 cm in length in the adult nulligravida. The cervix is contiguous above with the inferior aspect of the uterine corpus and below with the vaginal apex. The cervix is divided into two segments: the upper or supravaginal portion and a lower vaginal portion.[2,4,5]

The primary physiologic function of the cervix is the secretion of mucus that facilitates transportation of spermatozoa. The mucus also serves as a plug to seal off the gravid uterus from the vagina after fertilization. Levels of circulating ovarian hormones produce extreme changes in the consistency of the cervical mucus.[2,4,5]

The cervix dilates gradually and functions as a segment of the birth canal. The cervix also functions as a conduit for the emission of menstrual discharge.[5]

The uterine corpus extends upward from the cervix and is composed of three distinct layers: (1) The perimetrium (serosa) is an outer peritoneal covering, which continues laterally as the leaves of the broad ligament, bladder, and rectal reflections. (2) The myometrium is an inner layer of smooth muscle and connective tissue. (3) The endometrium is the mucus membrane lining the uterine cavity and is the sensitive end organ that reflects the effects of the ovarian hormones estrogen and progesterone.[2,5] The endometrium, therefore, also reflects the stability of the hypothalamic-pituitary-ovarian axis. Dysfunction of any of the aforementioned organs usually results in abnormalities of menstrual flow, anovulation, or amenorrhea.[4,5]

The function of the uterus is to contain and nurture the products of fertilization. If the process of ovulation is not followed by fertilization, menstruation results, since the endometrial lining breaks down and is expelled.[2,5]

The uterus also serves as a means of transportation for spermatozoa, and initiates and is the driving force behind the process of labor and parturition.[5]

### Disorders Resulting in Impairment

Impairment can result from a variety of abnormalities of the cervix. These include cervical stenosis, which may lead to cramping and low-back pain as well as hematometria. Stenosis may result from congenital structural abnormalities, surgery, inflammation, atrophy, or radiation.[5,6] The absence of cervical mucus resulting from the above entities may impair fertility.[5] An incompetent cervix may result from surgery or congenital absence of cervical stroma, and usually results in second trimester pregnancy loss. Cervicitis may produce discharge and impair fertility as well as result in discomfort. However, most infectious processes are treatable and, therefore, do not lead to long-term impairment.[2,6]

Benign masses may result in either stenosis or discomfort to the patient. Nabothian or congenital cysts may become quite large and leiomyomata may also affect the cervix.[3,4,6] Preneoplastic and neoplastic masses may cause impairment or lead to treatment measures that may render a patient infertile or prevent the opportunity for vaginal birth.[3,5,6]

The uterine corpus is more often predisposed to leiomyomata, which may lead not only to lack of fertility but also pregnancy loss and occasionally difficulty with parturition.[3,5,6] Adenomyosis may lead to uterine hypertrophy, dysmenorrhea, and menometrorrhagia.[5] Congenital anomalies of the uterus may also result in either infertility or early-pregnancy loss.[2,3]

Malpositions of the uterus such as retroflexion or uterine prolapse may lead to dyspareunia, dysmenorrhea, and low-back pain.[3,6]

Infection and inflammation of the uterine corpus may result from an extension of cervicitis and can lead to salpingitis. These infections are also common in the postpartum period. Scarring may occur in the endometrial cavity, which can contribute to infertility.[2,5]

Disorders of menstruation may result either from local factors (i.e., uterine leiomyomata or adenomyosis) or ovarian or pituitary-hypothalamic dysfunction. This may result in anovulation with subsequent infertility.[4,5]

Malignant neoplasms of the uterine corpus generally require measures that render the patient infertile and may lead to some degree of chronic discomfort. Surgery and radiation therapy are generally used.[3,5,6]

### Physical Examination

The cervix is examined by direct visualization. The cervical os should be open and one should be able to obtain a mucous specimen for examination (Papanicolau, or pap, smear) from both the endocervical and ectocervical areas. Palpation is then performed to evaluate the size, shape, symmetry, and consistency of both the cervix and uterus.[5]

## Diagnostic Studies

Ancillary procedures that may offer additional information are colposcopy with directed biopsy and endocervical curettage, endometrial biopsy, pelvic ultrasonography, CT scan and MRI.[5] Occasionally, laparoscopy, fractional dilation and curettage, and hysteroscopy are helpful. Determining serum levels of various hormones including LH, FSH, estradiol, progesterone and thyroid function studies is useful in the workup of infertility and disorders of menstruation.[4,5]

## Classifications of Impairment

### Class I

A patient belongs in the Class I category if (1) symptoms and signs of disease or deformity of the cervix or uterus are present that do not require continuous treatment, or (2) cervical stenosis, if present, requires no treatment, or (3) there is anatomic loss of cervix or uterus in a post-menopausal patient. This is rated at 0% to 15% impairment of the whole person.

**Example:** A 37-year-old, gravida II, para I, AB I, was noted to have an enlarged uterus of approximately 11 weeks-pregnancy size, and multiple uterine fibroids, with at least three of the fibroids measuring 2.0 cm. The patient had moderate dysmenorrhea and menorrhagia but otherwise no major symptoms. Her complaints were controlled with analgesics and periodic courses of iron therapy. Estimated impairment is 5%.

### Class II

A patient belongs in the Class II category if (1) symptoms and signs of disease or deformity of the cervix or uterus are present that require continuous treatment, or (2) cervical stenosis, if present, requires periodic treatment. This is rated at 15% to 25% impairment of the whole person.

**Example 1:** A 29-year-old, gravida I, para I has undergone cervical cone biopsy on two occasions for recurrent cervical dysplasia. She has subsequently had severe dysmenorrhea from cervical stenosis and requires cervical dilation every six to nine months. Estimated impairment is 15%.

**Example 2:** An 81-year-old, gravida VIII, para VIII, who had a previous vaginal hysterectomy and anterior repair, now has total vaginal prolapse. She requires continuous pessary support in order to ambulate and function normally. Estimated impairment is 25%.

### Class III

A patient belongs in the Class III category if (1) symptoms and signs of disease or deformity of the cervix or uterus are present that are not controlled by treatment, or (2) cervical stenosis is complete, or (3) there is complete anatomic or functional loss of the cervix or uterus in the premenopausal patient. This is rated at 25% to 35% impairment of the whole person.

**Example:** A 36-year-old, gravida 0, had an adenocarcinoma of the endometrium. She underwent an exploratory staging laparotomy, total abdominal hysterectomy, and bilateral salpingo-oophorectomy. The patient has complete loss of cervix and uterus. Childbearing is obviously not possible. Estimated impairment is 35%.

## Evaluation of Impairment

It is important to weigh heavily the age of the patient when assessing the overall impairment of disorders involving the cervix and uterus.[1] Preservation of reproductive function is obviously of paramount importance and the subsequent psychological impact that may result from an inability to bear children may be devastating.

## OVARIES AND FALLOPIAN TUBES

### Anatomy and Functions

The fallopian tubes are paired muscular canals extending from the uterus to the ovaries.[2,4] Each measures approximately 12.0 cm in length. Their function is to transport the ova from the ovary to the uterine cavity for purposes of implantation.[5] In addition, spermatozoa are transported for the purpose of conception.[5]

The ovaries provide ova for reproduction and also function as an endocrine gland to produce sex hormones.[5] They are influenced by pituitary and placental hormones.[4,5]

### Disorders Resulting in Impairment

The fallopian tube is commonly affected by pelvic inflammatory disease. This may result in scarring and either dysfunction or blockage of the fallopian tube, which may result in infertility and chronic pelvic pain.[2,5] At times, a pregnancy may implant in a portion of the fallopian tube, eventually resulting in its rupture, loss of the pregnancy, and a surgical emergency due to hemorrhage.[5]

Benign neoplasms of the fallopian tubes such as cysts from congenital remnants or salpingitis isthmica nodosa may result in infertility secondary to obstruction or pelvic pain.[2,4,5]

Malignant neoplasms of the fallopian tube are rare in comparison to malignancies involving other female organs and usually require therapy that renders the patient infertile.[3,5,6]

Inflammation and infection affecting the ovary can result in infertility, although involvement is unusual. Ovarian pregnancy does occur but is rare.[5,6] Anovulation secondary to either pituitary hypothalamic dysfunction or other endocrine disorders (i.e., thyroid or adrenal dysfunction) can occur and may result in infertility as well as menstrual dysfunctions.[4,5]

Benign neoplasms of the ovary are common and frequently result in pelvic discomfort. The neoplasms may arise from the ovary itself, congenital remnants, or may be the result of benign conditions such as endometriosis.[2,4] These disorders frequently result in pelvic discomfort, occasionally require medical or surgical therapy and may also render the patient infertile.[5]

Malignant neoplasms of the ovary are common and result not only in pain but also in infertility. Some ovarian tumors produce highly abnormal levels of sex hormones, resulting in unpleasant systemic symptoms.[2,4,5]

## Physical Examination

The traditional evaluation of the ovaries and fallopian tubes is performed by bimanual pelvic examination.

## Diagnostic Studies

Cytologic testing, hysterosalpingograms, ultrasonography, CT and MRI studies, basal body temperature, laparoscopy, and ovarian biopsy are used to define further underlying pathology.[5,6] The impairment of the ovarian endocrine function can be assessed with serum FSH, LH, estradiol, and progesterone levels.[4,5]

## Classification of Impairment

### Class I

A patient belongs in the Class I category if (1) symptoms and signs of disease or deformities of the fallopian tubes or ovaries are present that do not require continuous treatment, or (2) only one fallopian tube or ovary is functioning in a premenopausal patient, or (3) there is a bilateral loss of function of the fallopian tubes or ovaries in a postmenopausal patient. This is rated at 0% to 15% impairment of the whole person.

**Example 1:** A 26-year-old, gravida 0, desired to become pregnant after two years of marriage but had

been unable to conceive. A hysterosalpingogram revealed a blockage in the left fallopian tube. Estimated impairment is 10%.

**Example 2:** A 32-year-old, gravida I, para I, who was wanting more children was admitted for sudden severe pelvic pain and underwent a laparotomy and right oophorectomy for a large dermoid tumor that had undergone torsion and necrosis. Estimated impairment is 5%.

### Class II

A patient belongs in the Class II category if (1) symptoms and signs of disease or deformity of the fallopian tubes or ovaries are present that requires continuous treatment, but (2) tubal patency persists and ovulation is possible. This is rated at 15% to 25% impairment of the whole person.

**Example:** A 25-year-old, gravida I, para I, has had regular but severely-painful menses since the birth of her child. A laparoscopy was diagnostic of pelvic endometriosis. She does not desire pregnancy at this time. Continuous oral contraceptive medication and analgesics are necessary to control her symptoms. Estimated impairment is 20%.

### Class III

A patient belongs in the Class III category if (1) symptoms and signs of disease or deformity of the fallopian tubes or ovaries are present and there is a total loss of tubal patency or total failure to produce ova in the premenopausal years, or (2) bilateral loss of the fallopian tubes or ovaries occurs in a premenopausal patient. This is rated at 25% to 35% impairment of the whole person.

**Example:** A 34-year-old, gravida 0, was married recently and desirous of childbearing. A pelvic mass was found during a routine gynecologic examination. Pelvic ultrasound demonstrated bilateral complex masses suggestive of ovarian neoplasms. A laparotomy confirmed bilateral borderline mucinous ovarian tumors and a bilateral oophorectomy was performed. Estimated impairment is 35%.

## Evaluation of Impairment

The ovary is a complex organ, and one must always take into account the overall impact of the impairment to the patient as a whole. Consideration should include not only impairments from physical symptoms but also hormonal dysfunction that may require periodic or continuous treatment, sexual dysfunction, loss of reproductive capability, and psychological dysfunction. The age of the patient and whether or not the patient is premenopausal or postmenopausal must be considered.

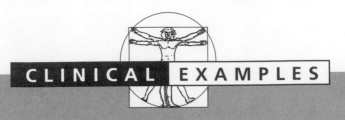

## UROGENITAL SYSTEM

EDITOR'S NOTE—Impairment assessment of the urogenital system involves the evaluation of several different structures. Examples provided here will address several of these structures; examples are also given in the text within specific discussions. Impairment caused by the urogenital system is generally infrequent.

### EXAMPLE 1
#### Bladder
**History:** A middle-aged woman presents with urinary incontinence occurring especially with sneezing, coughing, and lifting heavy objects. She had undergone a hysterectomy three years earlier.

**Physical Examination and Test Results:** Evaluation including cystoscopy and urodynamics (urethral pressure profile) documents stress incontinence.

**Assessment Process:** The level of impairment is related to the degree of urinary incontinence and its effect on the individual. Although intermittent incontinence, especially that resulting from elevation of intraabdominal pressure (as in coughing, sneezing, or straining), can be treated with diapers or pads, devastating psychological consequences can occur and markedly impact the patient's life-style and work habits.

**Evaluation:** The American Medical Association *Guides* rate this problem at a 25% to 40% whole person impairment (WPI), with the actual value left to the discretion of the evaluator, who measures the impact on the activities of daily living, job performance, and psyche.

### EXAMPLE 2
#### Urethra
**History:** A 33-year-old man requires frequent urethral dilations to void and has chronic urinary tract infections with ascending pyelonephritis secondary to the urethral obstruction and frequent urethral instrumentation. Two years previously he was struck by a motor vehicle

and suffered a pelvic fracture, fracture dislocation of the symphysis, and laceration of the prostatomembranous and bulbomembranous urethra. The pelvic fracture was stabilized and healed. The urethral lacerations were repaired but postoperative fibrosis resulted in extensive urethral strictures that were not corrected by further procedures. He has been diagnosed with traumatic urethral stricture disease with chronic pyelonephritis.

**Test Results:** The man's creatinine clearance has declined to 65 L/24 h (45 ml/min).

**Assessment Process:** A 20% impairment would be due to the urethral stricture, and a 25% impairment would be found to result from the upper urinary tract damage.

**Evaluation:** The combined impairment is 40% WPI (see Combined Values Chart, p. 322 of American Medical Association *Guides.*)*

### EXAMPLE 3
#### Penis
**History:** A young man with recurrent priapism requiring both medical and surgical intervention on several occasions is seen with an inability to gain more than a minimal erection. The glans penis enlarges, but the shaft does not engorge with blood. Ejaculation and sensation are unimpeded.

**Physical Examination and Test Results:** A workup reveals fibrosis of the corpora.

**Evaluation:** Sexual dysfunction is impaired solely by incomplete erection, a disability resulting in a low degree of functional impairment, rated at 0% to 10%.

### EXAMPLE 4
#### Testes, Epididymides, and Spermatic Cords
**History:** A 19-year-old man comes in for evaluation. He was injured by a farm machine

*All *tables* referred to in this discussion are found in AMA *Guides to the evaluation of permanent impairment,* ed 4, Chapter 11—The Urinary and Reproductive Systems, American Medical Association, Chicago, 1993.

*Continued.*

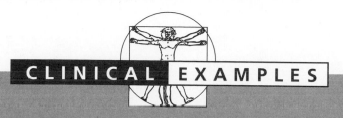
two years earlier sustaining amputation of the scrotum and its contents. His condition is stable at this time.

**Assessment Process:** His diagnosis is traumatic orchiectomy. Estimates of impairment are 20% due to gonadal loss, 15% due to scrotal loss (which considers the patient's young age), and 5% due to lack of an endocrine gland.

**Evaluation:** The impairment values would be combined (using the Combined Values Chart, p. 322 of the American Medical Association *Guides*) to give an estimated 35% WPI.

### EXAMPLE 5
#### Prostate and Seminal Vesicles

**History:** A 34-year-old man has on-going signs and symptoms of prostatitis following drainage of a prostatic abscess 15 months earlier. He can tolerate his complaints only through constant use of antibacterial medications.

**Physical Examination:** He has perineal pain, a low-grade fever, and hemospermia. A diagnosis of recurrent acute and chronic prostatitis is determined.

**Evaluation:** A 14% WPI is determined, which includes an allowance for the patient's age.

### EXAMPLE 6
#### Vulva and Vagina

**History:** A 34-year-old married woman developed a rectovaginal fistula after vaginal delivery of her second child. Although this was surgically corrected, she developed severe vaginal stenosis and required intermittent dilatation of the vagina under anesthesia and the continuous use of vaginal creams. These measures made sexual intercourse possible but painful and lacking in sexual sensation or enjoyment for the patient. A third pregnancy ended with a cesarean section because vaginal delivery was felt to be dangerous. She has been diagnosed with severe postoperative vaginal stenosis.

**Evaluation:** A 20% WPI is recommended, taking into consideration the patient's age.

### EXAMPLE 7
#### Cervix and Uterus

**History:** This 60-year-old married woman has developed vaginal vault prolapse. She noticed pelvic pressure and a large bulge protruding from the vulva. Twenty years previously she had a vaginal hysterectomy for adenomyosis.

**Physical Examination:** Clinical examination discloses the vaginal vault prolapse without significant rectocele, cystocele, or descent of the uterine-vaginal angle.

**Assessment Process:** The patient prefers a nonoperative approach to treatment of the bulge and a doughnut pessary is placed, which reduces the vaginal prolapse. Her symptoms resolve. She changes the pessary twice weekly and uses a povidone-iodine douche to diminish vaginal discharge.

**Evaluation:** Based on her status as having a Class I impairment, a 10% WPI is assessed.

### EXAMPLE 8
#### Ovaries and Fallopian Tubes

**History:** A 32-year-old mother of two children has severe pelvic infection.

**Physical Examination and Test Results:** Diagnostic studies reveal total proximal and distal occlusion of the fallopian tubes and the presence of bilateral 6 cm hydrosalpinx. A bilateral salpingectomy is performed.

**Evaluation:** The patient is determined to have a 30% WPI.

*Martin Fritzhand*
*Eric L. Jenison*

## References

1. American Medical Association: *Guides to the evaluation of permanent impairment*, ed 4, Chicago, 1993.
2. Gompel C, Silverberg SG: *Pathology in gynecology and obstetrics*, ed 3, Philadelphia, 1985, JB Lippincott.
3. Nichols DH: *Gynecologic and obstetric surgery*, St. Louis, 1993, Mosby–Year Book.
4. Novak ER, Woodruff JD: *Novak's gynecologic and obstetric pathology*, ed 8, Philadelphia, 1979, WB Saunders.
5. Ryan KJ, Berkowitz R, Barbieri RL: *Kistner's gynecology: principles and practice*, Chicago, 1990, Year Book Medical Publishers.
6. Thompson JD, Rock JA: *TeLinde's operative gynecology*, ed 7, Philadelphia, 1992, JB Lippincott.

## Suggested Readings

Ryan KJ, Berkowitz R, Barbieri RL: Kistner's gynecology: principles and practice, St. Louis, 1990, Year Book Medical Publishers.

## Bibliography

American Medical Association: *Guides to the evaluation of permanent impairment*, ed 4, Chicago, 1993.

Chisholm GD, Fair WR: *Scientific foundations of urology*, ed 3, Chicago, Year Book Medical Publishers, 1990.

Corriere JN, editor: *Essentials of urology*, Churchill Livingstone, 1986, New York.

Gillenwater JY, editor: *Adult and pediatric urology*, ed 2, St. Louis, Mosby–Year Book, 1991.

NIH: *Consensus statements on impotence*, Vol. 10, No. 4, Dec. 7–9, 1992, National Institutes of Health, Washington, DC.

Smith SW, Murphy TR, Blair JSG, Lowe KG: *Regional anatomy illustrated*, New York, 1983, Churchill Livingstone.

Snell RS: *Clinical anatomy for medical students*, Boston, 1973, Little Brown.

Tanagho EA, McAninch JW: *Smith's general urology*, ed 12, Pasadena, 1988, Appleton and Lange.

Walsh PC, editor: *Campbell's urology*, ed 5, Philadelphia, 1986, WB Saunders.

# CHAPTER 36

# DERMATOLOGY

*James S. Taylor*

## PREVALENCE: DISABILITY AND SKIN CONDITIONS

In the United States an estimated 35 to 43 million persons have a disability, costing the nation an estimated $176.7 billion annually.* According to US Census data from 1990, an estimated 12.8 million persons aged 16 to 64 years had a work disability of 6 months or longer.[1,2] Applications for federal disability benefits are "exploding" with 6.3 million Americans drawing checks in 1993. In contrast to 4.6 million in 1988.[3] In 1993 the Centers for Disease Control and Prevention (CDC) published data on the prevalence of selected chronic conditions in the United States for the period 1986–88, based on the National Health Interview Surveys. Rates per thousand persons for 10 skin conditions and the percentage of each causing limitation of activity, one or more hospitalizations, and one or more physician visits are listed. Dermatitis leads the list with a rate of 38.1 per 1000 persons, of which 1.2% caused limitations of activity. In contrast, chronic ulceration of the skin had the lowest rate affecting 0.9 per 1000 persons, but had the highest percentage (24.1%) causing limitation of activity.[4]

## DISABILITY PROGRAMS

Impairment caused by skin disorders, as with other organ systems, is rated using an accurate diagnosis; documentation of its effects on a person's occupation, activities of daily living (ADL), occupational risks and demands, response to treatment(s), and avoidance of precipitating factors; an estimation of the prognosis based on these factors; and a careful review of the information contained in the body of medical knowledge concerning the specific disorder.

Disability caused by skin disorders, as with other organ systems, is decided using the rating system spe-

cific to each patient's case and is usually based on who the referring source is or the conditions of employment and exposure associated with the development of the skin disorder. Many of the rating systems and referring sources have peculiarities inherent to the style, format, or purpose of the source and are discussed in this chapter.

### Workers' Compensation

Occupational skin disease cases under workers' compensation account for most of the impairment evaluations performed by dermatologists. According to figures from the U.S. Bureau of Labor Statistics, work-related skin disorders were the second-most-common cause of occupational disease in the United States in 1992.[17,18] In 1984, when federal statistics were last available on time lost from work, approximately 25% of workers with occupational skin disease lost time from work, averaging 10 to 12 days each.[19]

Most claims based on occupational skin disease involve temporary total or permanent partial disability. Temporary total occupational disability occurs when an occupational disorder prevents an individual from performing his or her job. This determination is usually made by the treating physician, and the disability may last a number of weeks and rarely a few years. In my experience the most common skin disorders resulting in temporary total disability are severe cases of irritant and allergic contact hand eczema in workers such as machinists and hairdressers.

It is important for the examining and treating physicians to know when temporary total impairment ceases. In Ohio (personal communication, Jon Starr, M.D., September 9, 1988) this occurs with one of the following events: (1) the patient has reached maximum medical improvement, or is "medically stationary"; (2) the condition has become permanent; (3) the patient has a valid job offer within his or her physical capabilities; (4) the patient states that he or she is capable of returning to work; or (5) the patient returns to work. In my experience the burden of this

---

*This paper is adapted, expanded, and reprinted in significant part from Taylor JS: Impairment due to work-related skin disease. *Occup Med* 9:1–9, 1994.

decision-making frequently is left to the treating physician. Some employers in Ohio, a state where workers are covered by a state insurance fund or through employer self insurance, utilize third-party consulting firms to review all claims or "outlying" claims. Typical examples include workers with frequent recurrences of dermatitis, those with chronic hand eczema, or those whose dermatitis persists despite a job change. Permanent partial disability claims are often reviewed, with employers seeking the lowest possible percentage when rating impairment and employees the highest possible percentage. Other problematic cases are those with transient skin complaints with few objective physical findings, cases of chronic urticaria with a putative occupational connection, and cases of putative multiple chemical sensitivity with complaints involving the skin and multiple organ systems. In my experience most cases of chronic urticaria or recurrent acute urticaria are not occupationally related. The clear exception are those workers with latex urticaria, whose disease may range from contact and generalized urticaria to angioedema and anaphylaxis.

Some states allow third party liability suits arising out of workers' compensation cases. As an example, a machinist who received workers' compensation for patch-test-proven allergic contact dermatitis to a coolant germicide also sued the manufacturer of the germicide for damages from the injury.

## Social Security Disability

The *Disability Evaluation under Social Security Handbook*[6] states: "Skin lesions may result in a marked, long-lasting impairment if they involve extensive body areas or critical areas such as the hands or feet and become resistant to treatment. These lesions must be shown to have persisted for a sufficient period of time despite therapy for a reasonable presumption to be made that a marked impairment will last for a continuous period of at least 12 months." Only five specific categories of skin impairments are listed, but "medically equivalent" impairments will also be considered. Skin impairments are also considered in the determination of "residual functional capacity", which is "what you can still do despite your limitations" (written communication, Ronal D. Fisher, Social Security Administration, Baltimore, May 10, 1994.)

## Department of Veterans Affairs

The Department of Veterans Affairs' *Physician's Guide for Disability Evaluation Examinations*[7] has now been formatted into the Automated Medical Information Exchange (AMIE) System. This system covers eleven types of benefit categories, ranging from VA disability, compensation, and pensions to former prisoners of war, Persian Gulf veterans, and a number of miscellaneous categories including some VA employees and veterans exposed to environmental hazards. Results of the VA Compensation and Pension Examination are then rated by a Rating Board at a VA regional office in accordance with the Veterans Benefits Administration Schedule for Rating Disabilities, which is included in Title 38, *Code of Federal Regulations.*

Specific skin conditions are listed by the VA, especially scars, eczema, various infections, psoriasis, and tumors. Other skin conditions can be considered (written communication, Teresa R. Oster, Department of Veterans Affairs, Atlanta, May 6, 1994). Specific Department of Veterans Affairs regulations relate to Agent Orange. Recently porphyria cutanea tarda and Hodgkin's disease have been added to chloracne, non-Hodgkin's lymphoma, and soft-tissue sarcoma as diseases with presumptive service connection, based on exposure to Agent Orange and other herbicides in Vietnam veterans.[8]

## Military Services and Department of Defense

The military services have standards for induction and retention into the armed services (written communication, William D. James, M.D., Walter Reed Army Medical Center, June 2, 1994.) These standards include medical conditions. Those involving the skin include severe acne and eczema as well as a number of other inflammatory and malignant conditions such as psoriasis, collagen vascular diseases, chronic urticaria, and lymphomas. Also included are "any other chronic skin disorder of a degree or nature that requires frequent outpatient treatment or hospitalization or interferes with the satisfactory performance of duty."[9] The Department of Defense also has specific disability separation guidelines that will often tie in with specific VA benefits.[10]

## Federal Employees Compensation Act

The Federal Employees Compensation Act pays for impairment causing loss of earnings without any lump-sum settlements. Skin conditions interfering with work may be compensable, although skin conditions are not included in any scheduled loss lists (personal communication, George Smith, M.D., Bethesda, MD, April 1994).

## Longshore and Harborworkers Act

Under the Longshore and Harborworkers Act, the government adjudicates claims that include conditions contained in scheduled lists, not including skin conditions, and that are paid by the employer through self insurance or private insurance coverage. Lump-sum benefits, but not continuation of pay, may be awarded. Fewer claims are now made for skin conditions because of the more frequent use of container ships. Some examples of skin-related conditions are dermatitis from cocoa and hemp (personal communication, John McClellan, J.D., June 1994).

## Americans with Disabilities Act (ADA)[5,15,16]

Nethercott has recently reviewed fitness to work under the ADA. Only a few skin conditions make a potential employee excludable under specific job requirements as regulated by the ADA. An example is an individual with chronic hand dermatitis that may affect grip strength. Topical therapy for the hand dermatitis may also interfere with job function, such as driving heavy machinery. Other conditions that may exclude a worker under certain circumstances include infectious disease of the skin, skin diseases affecting thermoregulation and physical agent intolerance. Work-aggravated skin diseases such as psoriasis and lichen planus, vitiligo, and eczema may require accommodation of the worker under the ADA.

## Dermatological Disability Proposals

Disability in specific skin diseases, psoriasis and acne, has been studied by Finlay and his colleagues.[11,12] In psoriasis, a sickness impact profile and psoriasis disability index have been studied and validated. The sickness impact profile allowed comparison of the impairment of some of the activities of daily living experienced by psoriasis patients with that experienced by patients with other systemic diseases; the disability index gave a rapid overall measure of psoriasis impairment based on responses to 15 questions about daily activities, work or school activities, personal relationships, leisure activities, and treatment. The responses were graded on a 7-point, linear analogue scale.[12]

General guides to the evaluation of cutaneous impairment have been proposed by Sauer, Canizares, Kanof, and Robinson between 1962 and 1968.[13] However, it was not until 1971, with the publication of the first edition of the AMA *Guides*, that a set of guidelines was proposed for all body systems, including the skin.[5] The basic definitions and concepts of permanent impairment and disability proposed by the members of the AMA Committee on Cutaneous Impairment still stand.

## OCCUPATIONAL DERMATOSES

Direct causes of occupational skin disorders include exposure to chemical, physical, mechanical, and biological agents. Injuries (lacerations, cuts, abrasions, burns, etc.) cause the overwhelming majority of cases. Chemicals cause 90% of occupational skin diseases. Of these, 70% to 80% is irritant contact dermatitis. Twenty percent to 30% is allergic contact dermatitis. The hands are involved in 90% of patients with contact dermatitis. The remaining 10% of occupational skin disease cases includes folliculitis and acne (e.g., oil acne, chloracne), pigmentary disorders (e.g., postinflammatory hyper- or hypopigmentation, contact leukoderma), granulomas (e.g., foreign body, infectious), ulceration (e.g., chrome holes), neoplasms (butchers warts, arsenic induced squamous cell carcinoma), and miscellaneous disease of the hair and nails.[20]

Studies of the prognosis for occupational skin disease indicate that persistent disease ranges from 32% to 75% of cases. Improvement in the persistent cases has been seen in some reports. Frequent factors causing these conditions to persist include the presence of atopic dermatitis, allergy to chromate, and cases of chronic irritant contact dermatitis. Other reasons for persistence of dermatitis include: misdiagnosis, secondary or iatrogenic allergic contact dermatitis, insufficient advice to workers, nondermatologic factors, and endogenous and multifactorial hand dermatitis. Other statistics, outcomes, factors that affect outcome, and social consequences of occupational disability have been discussed by Nethercott and Hogan.[19,21,22]

## EVALUATION OF PUTATIVE OCCUPATIONAL DERMATOSES

### Dilemmas for the Physician[25]

Medical determinations in workers' compensation involve a number of issues for the examining and treating physician:

1. Patient assertions and demands concerning work-relatedness of their disease, job changes, and job modifications.
2. Social gate-keeping concerning time off from work, date for return to work ("why can't it be

on Friday?"), and determination of work-relatedness of disease.

3. Lack of adequate workplace data, such as detailed job descriptions, lists of work contacts and exposures, including material safety data sheets, and in some cases samples of workplace chemicals. This is probably the major deficiency facing the physician. A plant visit is ideal but not often practical.

4. Clinical judgement versus technology (e.g., determining whether a machinist with hand eczema and negative patch tests has an occupational irritant contact dermatitis or endogenous hand eczema).

5. Conceptual differences in medical versus legal concepts of causation. Absolute proof fulfilling Koch's postulates is not required in workers' compensation cases. Determination by the physician that a cause-and-effect relation exists between a disease and a job "within a reasonable medical certainty or probability" is usually adequate. Statement of a "possible" relationship is not adequate.[25]

## Medical Evaluation

The patient's history is an integral part of the evaluation. Published history forms may be used by physicians or their assistants or adapted for self-administration by patients.[26,27] An initial examination of the area of chief complaint often helps to direct the questioning. The history of the present illness should focus on the following:

1. Patient's description of the chief complaint(s).
2. Chronology, including previous treatments and frequency of occurrence.
3. Location of the lesions at onset.
4. Spread of the lesions, if any.
5. Morphology of the lesions.
6. Time away from work, including weekends, vacations, sick leave, and disability.
7. Unintended overexposure versus usual exposure to the precipitating chemical(s) or agent(s).

Determination of the timing of the reaction also is important. Onset of symptoms within minutes or one to two hours points more to contact urticaria or irritation. Onset after one or two days or as long as one week suggests contact allergy, especially in first-time cases of dermatitis or in recurrent, intermittent acute dermatitis. This distinction is blurred in chronic cases. It is also important to remember that irritation, contact urticaria, and contact allergy may coexist. The interval between initial exposure and onset of occupa-

tional acne or pigmentary disturbance is usually several weeks; for tumors, several years.[28]

The course of occupational contact dermatitis is usually improvement away from work for a few days and exacerbation on reexposure, unless there is a common contact both at home and at work. Exceptions to this rule clearly exist. Outcome studies in workers with industrial dermatitis, as reviewed by Nethercott,[19,21] show persistent dermatitis in one third or more of cases; reasons for this were previously discussed. A list of drugs and other medications should be included. Systemic contact dermatitis is possible from the systemic administration of a number of drugs to which an individual is sensitive or cross-sensitive. The frequency and effect of systemic corticosteroids should be determined, especially for reports of improvement away from the job.

Work history should include:

1. A description of job and job title(s).
2. List of work contacts.
3. Review of material safety data sheets.
4. Dates of employment, hours worked per week, shift, and dates and effects of any job or task changes.
5. Similar complaints of other workers, if any.
6. Methods and frequency of cleaning the skin, including use of waterless hand cleaners and workplace solvents.
7. Protective creams and protective clothing, especially gloves.

Direct questions about specific causes of flares and improvements may be helpful.[26]

Past history should include:

1. List of previous compensation claims and skin conditions.
2. Allergies such as childhood eczema, asthma, and hay fever.
3. Overt reactions to the major contact allergens, including metals, medicaments, cosmetics, dyes, and preservatives.
4. Past medical history.
5. Review of systems.
6. Family and social history.
7. Hobbies and second jobs.[26]

In some instances a review of old medical and hospitalization records is important.[5]

The physical examination should include the location, description, and distribution of the eruption as well as a listing of other important cutaneous findings. A complete skin examination is often indicated. In contact allergy the area of most intense dermatitis usually corresponds to the site of the most intense contact with the allergen. Exceptions to this rule exist, as when allergens are transferred to distant sites. Volatile airborne chemicals may cause dermatitis on exposed body areas. Contact dermatitis may be symmetrical or asymmetrical, uniform or confluent, or may involve discrete patchy areas.

Results of diagnostic tests should be recorded, especially scrapings for microorganisms (a potassium hydroxide preparation for cutaneous fungal infections is the most common such procedure performed by dermatologists), cultures, laboratory tests, biopsies, and patch tests. Specific comments about their relevance should be included.[5]

Of the thousands of chemicals in commercial use today, only about 200 are commonly recognized as allergic contact sensitizers, while several thousand other potential contact allergens exist.[29] Valid positive patch tests are generally accepted as the gold standard for the diagnosis of allergic contact dermatitis. Thus patch testing plays a crucial role in the evaluation of patents with occupational hand dermatitis. Patch testing may yield false-positive and false-negative results. Selecting the proper concentration of the suspected chemical, vehicle, site of application, and type of patch is critical to assure the validity of the procedure; workers should be patch tested for all relevant allergens to which they are exposed at work and at home.[22] "Making such selections and determining the relevance of test results requires considerable skill and experience. A positive or negative patch test result should not be accepted at face value until the details of the testing procedures have been evaluated," and the direct clinical relevance of the test results to the workplace is accurately determined.[5]

## Diagnosis and Treatment

The diagnosis should be listed along with other significant cutaneous findings. Associated diagnoses, such as asthma or significant systemic illness, also should be recorded. Other major symptoms purported by the patient to be occupationally related should be included, and recommendations made for appropriate evaluation by an occupational physician or other specialist. An assessment of the current medical status and statement of further medical plans and treatment also should be included.[5]

## CAUSATION

Determination of the precise cause-and-effect relation between a skin disorder and an occupation is not always easy. Key[28] lists five criteria to consider for the diagnosis of occupational skin diseases:

1. Appearance of the lesions.
2. Site of the eruption.
3. History.
4. Course of the disease.
5. Diagnostic tests.

Mathias[30] has adapted these criteria for establishing occupational causation and aggravation in contact dermatitis. He proposes that a positive answer to four of the following seven questions would generally be adequate to establish probable cause:

1. Is the clinical appearance compatible with contact dermatitis?
2. Are there workplace exposures to potential irritants or allergens?
3. Is the anatomic distribution of the eruption compatible with job exposure?
4. Is the temporal relationship between exposure and onset consistent with contact dermatitis?
5. Have nonoccupational exposures been excluded as causes?
6. Does the dermatitis improve away from work exposure to the suspected irritant or allergen?
7. Do patch or provocation tests identify a probable cause?

## Work Aggravation of Skin Diseases[31]

Although terminology may vary, some states make a legal distinction between *work-connected* and *work-aggravated* conditions. Pre-existing skin conditions will often be disqualified for workers' compensation. Clear-cut exceptions should be accepted as work related or aggravated. An example would be work-aggravation such as a health-care worker with a history of remote or current atopic eczema who develops allergic contact dermatitis to a chemical in the work place, such as glutaraldehyde, or latex allergy from contact with rubber gloves.

## EVALUATION OF TEMPORARY TOTAL IMPAIRMENT AND RETURN TO WORK GUIDELINES

As a prelude to impairment evaluation, the physician must determine the impact of the medical condition on life activities and whether the condition is stable and unlikely to change. If the worker has a new recent condition that significantly precludes working on the current job, then temporary total impairment may exist, and an appropriate amount of time away from work may be warranted under most workers' compensation laws. Physicians should consult their own state's guidelines, if any, for temporary total disability or return to work. The State of Minnesota publishes a permanent partial disability schedule and the Minnesota Medical Association previously published a temporary total impairment guide.

The *Medical Disability Advisor*[32] lists a large number of medical diagnoses with suggested ranges of time away from work. These estimates were compiled by consensus and are diagnosis-dependent without specific guidelines for estimating time away based on factors such as disease severity, functional impairment, and extent or frequency of treatment. A number of dermatological diagnoses are included in the *Advisor,* which seem more useful to personnel departments than to physicians.

Other return to work guides are included in an extensive set of *Health Care Management Guidelines.*[33] Few dermatological diagnoses are included.

Unduly restrictive limitations upon return to work, such as avoiding all contact with a particular substance, may jeopardize a worker's job. Before writing such recommendations they must be discussed with the worker and occasionally with the employer. This is especially important because of the chronicity of some cases of occupational skin disease in which a change in jobs does not always result in the clearing of a worker's dermatitis. Some union management contracts may also restrict worker placement.

## USE OF THE *GUIDES TO THE EVALUATION OF PERMANENT IMPAIRMENT*[5]

The AMA *Guides to the Evaluation of Permanent Impairment* may be used to evaluate *permanent* impairment of any body system, from both occupational and nonoccupational causes; they are not designed for use in evaluating *temporary* impairment. The *Guides* are a set of guidelines, not absolute recommendations, and are designed to bring objectivity to an area of great subjectivity by providing clinically-sound and reproducible criteria useful to physicians, attorneys, and adjudicators. They espouse the philosophy that all physical and mental impairment affects the whole person. "A 95% to 100% whole-person impairment is considered to represent almost total impairment, a state that is approaching death." Before using the *Guides* for evaluating cutaneous impairment, the physician should read the two introductory chapters, the glossary, and then Chapter 13, The Skin. Chapter 2, "Records and Reports," lists a suggested outline for a medical evaluation report.

1. Medical history.
2. Clinical evaluation.
3. Diagnoses.
4. Stability of the medical condition.
5. Impact of the medical condition on specific activities of daily living, including occupation.
6. Explanation for concluding that the individual is or is not likely to suffer further impairment by engaging in usual activities.
7. Explanation for concluding that accommodations or restrictions related to impairment are or are not warranted.
8. A listing of specific impairment percentages.

The *Guides* chapter on skin lists five classes of impairment, ranging from 0% to 95%. The impact of the disorder on the activities of daily living should be the major consideration in determining the class of impairment. The frequency and intensity of signs and symptoms and the frequency and complexity of medical treatment should guide the selection of an appropriate impairment percentage and estimate within any class.

The activities of daily living (ADL) include self-care and personal hygiene, communication, physical activity, sensory function, hand functions (grasping, holding, pinching, percussive movements, and sensory discrimination), travel, sexual function, sleep, and social and recreational activities. Since most occupational skin disorders involve the hands, chronic hand dermatitis may have a significant impact on ADLs. Other examples of specific ADLs are listed in the glossary of the *Guides.*

The examples within each class are very important guides for the first time user. The AMA *Guides* divide skin impairment into five classes. Diagnoses of the following examples, by class, includes:

- *Class 1 (0%–9%):* argyria; mycosis fungoides; allergic contact dermatitis (two examples); skin grafts from burns (two examples); chronic urticaria
- *Class 2 (10%–24%):* chronic hand eczema; hypertrophic burn scar; atopic dermatitis; chemical burn; chemically induced nail dystrophy
- *Class 3 (25%–54%):* persistent occupational contact dermatitis; follicular occlusive triad with scarring; thermal burn scar; severe photosensitivity reaction; pemphigus vulgaris; systemic lupus erythematosus
- *Class 4 (55%–84%):* stasis dermatitis and ulceration; scleroderma, pustular psoriasis, thermal burn scars; mycosis fungoides
- *Class 5 (85%–95%):* xeroderma pigmentosum, epidermolysis bullosa dystrophica

The fourth edition of the *Guides* contains new examples of impairment from urticaria and skin grafts as well as refinement of some of the previous examples. Most are not workers' compensation cases but

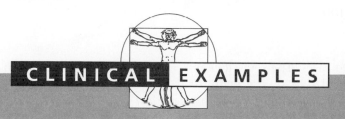

# CLINICAL EXAMPLES

## DERMATOLOGY

Editor's Note—Section 13.7 of the AMA *Guides* includes several pages of examples that illustrate impairment evaluation of the skin.* In addition to the example given here, the reader is directed to this section of the *Guides* for further information.

### EXAMPLE

#### History

A 25-year-old woman, whose job involved performing outdoor utility repairs, sustained a thermal burn on the left side of her face and arm that required a 6 by 10 cm skin graft of the left forearm. She complains that numbness in the graft interferes with certain non-specialized hand activities. In addition, she experiences intermittent pain of the left ear when she is outdoors in cold weather, especially when the temperature is below 20° F.

*This Clinical Example is from AMA *Guides to the evaluation of permanent impairment*, ed 4, American Medical Association, Chicago, 1993; with permission.

The pain requires warming of the ear with a cap or application of warmth to the area. The hypopigmentation requires that she wear sunscreen with a high sun-protection factor. The atrophy and scar on the left forearm requires the regular use of a moisturizer.

#### Physical Examination

The forearm graft is completely healed and shows only a protective reaction; it is atrophic and scaly, but normal range of motion is present. The rest of the skin on the left forearm and left side of the face, including the ear, is hypopigmented, but sensation is normal.

#### Assessment Process

The patient's numbness is related to the residual effects of the burn and graft, not to a peripheral nerve injury. Therefore neurologic assessment of the peripheral nerves is not needed.

#### Evaluation

The skin graft and hypopigmentation secondary to thermal burn lead to a determination of 5% whole person impairment (WPI).

are clearly applicable to such cases. The revised chapter also contains examples of two severe pediatric dermatological conditions in Class 5. It is critically important to remember that impairment is not determined by diagnosis alone but by the effect of the disease on ADL along with the frequency and intensity of the disease and the frequency and complexity of therapy; thus there are examples of the same disease in several different classes. Most cutaneous impairment falls within the first three classes ranging from 0% to 54%.

Certain therapies, such as PUVA (bath or systemic) for psoriasis or hand eczema and calcipotriol ointment for psoriasis, may have such a significant impact on disease outcome that the author believes they should be employed before making a final determination of permanent impairment.

Unique to the skin chapter are the discussions of pruritus, disfigurement, and scars and skin grafts. The evaluation of pruritus is based on its interference with the activities of daily living (ADLs) and the extent to which the description of pruritus is supported by objective findings, such as lichenification, excoriation, or hyperpigmentation. Disfigurement usually involves no loss of body function and little or no effect on the ADLs. Disfigurement may well impair self-image, cause life-style alteration, and result in social rejection. These changes are best evaluated in accordance with the criteria in the chapter on mental and behavioral conditions. Evaluation of scars and skin grafts is made according to the impact on ADLs. When impairment is based on peripheral nerve dysfunction, loss of range of motion, or caused by scarring, it should be evaluated in accordance with the criteria in the chapters on the nervous system and musculoskeletal system.

## CONCLUSIONS AND RECOMMENDATIONS

All diagnoses should be listed and summarized. A summary statement regarding causation is then made; for example, "Within a reasonable degree of medical certainty, the disease is or is not related to work." A physician is not required to have such an opinion and in some cases may not be able to make a determination of "probable cause". The diagnosis should include a description of specific clinical findings related to the impairment, and how they relate to and compare with the criteria in the *Guides*. The impairment value should also be explained. Specific recommendations for therapy should be included along with a brief explanation of the treatment. Recommendations for prevention including work restrictions are made next; this includes suggestions for en-

vironmental modification (exhaust ventilation, splash guards) and personal protective equipment. The effect of future exposures to chemical, physical, and biologic agents should be addressed, along with any need for rehabilitation.[5] Some states and insurance carriers provide rehabilitation services, several of which may be applicable to individuals with skin diseases; vocational evaluation, occupational therapy, and retraining programs may be helpful to motivated workers. Finally, the basis for the conclusions should be discussed, such as personal observations of the treating physician with specified dates, a one-time independent medical evaluation, and findings from history, old records, physical examination, and patch tests, alone or in combination. Inconsistencies and other disclaimers should be listed.[5]

## References

1. Prevalence of work disability–United States, 1990. *MMWR* 42:757–759, 1993.
2. Prevalence of mobility and self-care disability–United States, 1990. *MMWR* 42:760–761, 767–769, 1993.
3. Panetta warns of disability disaster. *The Plain Dealer*, November 11, 1993, Cleveland, Ohio.
4. *Prevalence of selected chronic conditions: United States (1986–88)—Vital and health statistics*, National Center for Health Statistics, Centers for Disease Control and Prevention, Series 10, No. 182, Feb. 1993, Atlanta.
5. American Medical Association: *Guides to the evaluation of permanent impairment*, ed 4, Chicago, 1993.
6. *Disability evaluation under Social Security*, Social Security Administration, U.S. Department of Health and Human Services, Washington, DC, SSA Pub. No. 64–039, Oct. 1992.
7. *Physician's guide for disability evaluation examinations*, Department of Medicine and Surgery, Veterans Administration, Washington, DC, March 1, 1985.
8. VA adds benefits for Agent Orange. *US Med*, April 1994.
9. *Physical standards of enlistment, appointment, and induction*, Department of Defense, Washington, DC, AR 40–501, Update Issue 1.
10. *Disability separation*, American Forces Information Service, Department of Defense, Washington, DC, July 1, 1988.
11. Finlay AY, Kelly SE: Psoriasis: An index of disability, *Clin Exp Dermatol* 12:8–11, 1987.
12. Finlay AY, Khan GK, Luscombe DK, Salek MS: Validation of sickness impact profile and psoriasis disability index in psoriasis. *Brit J Dermatol* 123:751–756, 1990.

13. Sauer GC: A guide to the evaluation of permanent impairment of the skin. *Arch Dermatol* 97:566–69 and 98:202–204, 1968.

14. Martin RA: *Occupational disability*, Springfield, 1975, Thomas.

15. Nethercott JR: The Americans with Disabilities Act. *Am J Contact Derm* 4:185–6, 1993.

16. Nethercott JR: Fitness to work with skin disease and the Americans with Disability Act of 1990. *Occup Med* 9:11–18, 1994.

17. Kane J: *Selected occupational illness data by category of illness, private industry, 1992*, Bureau of Labor Statistics, U.S. Dept of Labor, Dec. 1993.

18. *Occupational injuries and illnesses in the United States by industry—1990*, Bulletin 2399, Bureau of Labor Statistics, U.S. Department of Labor, 1992.

19. Nethercott JR: Disability due to occupational contact dermatitis, *Occup Med* 1:199–203, 1986.

20. Taylor J: Occupational dermatoses. Chapter 15 in *Clinical medicine for the occupational physician*, Alderman MH and Hanley MJ, New York, 1982, pp 299–304, M. Dekker.

21. Cooley JE, Nethercott JR: Prognosis of occupational skin diseases *Occup Med* 9:19–24, 1994.

22. Hogan DJ: The prognosis of occupational contact dermatitis. *Occup Med* 9:53–58, 1994.

23. *Analysis of Workers' Compensation Laws*, U.S. Chamber of Commerce, Washington, DC, 1992.

24. Fisher TF: New developments in workers' compensation law, *Annals NY Acad Sci* 572:256–260, 1989.

25. Leavitt SS: Defining and implementing medical standards for workers' compensation. Syllabus. Course on Workers' Compensation. Teknekron Inc., 2118 Milvia Street, Berkeley, CA, American Society for Law and Medicine, Washington, DC, Oct. 1975.

26. Freeman S: *Diagnosis and differential diagnosis.* Chapter 12, pages 194–214. In Adams RM, *Occupational skin disease*, Philadelphia, 1990, WB Saunders.

27. Goldstein A: Writing report letters for patients with skin disease resulting from on-the-job exposures. *Derm Clinics* 2:631–41, 1984.

28. Key M: Confusing compensation cases. *Cutis* 3:965–996, 1967.

29. Davidson CL: Occupational contact dermatitis of the upper extremity. *Occup Med:* 9:56–74, 1994.

30. Mathias CGT: Contact dermatitis and workers' compensation: criteria for establishing occupational causation and aggravation, *J Am Acad Dermatol* 20:842–8, 1989.

31. *Specialized skills of clinical practice*, Appendix 2 in LR Rosenstock and MR Cullen editors: *Clinical Occupational Medicine*, Philadelphia, 1986, page 273, W.B. Saunders.

32. *The medical disability advisor*, Reed Pressly.

33. Doyle RL: *Health care management guidelines*, San Diego, Millaman and Robertson.

# CHAPTER 37

# ENDOCRINOLOGY

*Philip Levy*
*David L. Horwitz*

## DEFINITIONS

The endocrine system is composed of a group of glands that secrete hormones that regulate the activity of various organ systems or tissues distant from the endocrine glands. The system is composed of the hypothalamic-pituitary complex, the thyroid, the parathyroids, the adrenals, the testes, the ovaries, and the islet cells of the pancreas. The endocrine glands are frequently interrelated, and a disorder of one gland may affect, or be interrelated with, another gland.

Impairments of the endocrine system are usually related to altered secretion by one or more glands, but they can also be due to distortion of adjacent anatomical structures by altered morphology of endocrine tissue. Abnormal levels of hormones can sometimes be associated with abnormal production by nonendocrine glands such as ectopic ACTH production secondary to malignancy. Morphologic changes can include atrophy, hypertrophy, hyperplasia, hypoplasia, or neoplasia. The neoplasia can be functional, such as a growth hormone-secreting tumor of the pituitary causing acromegaly. Neoplasia can also be nonfunctional, such as with a tumor of the adrenal gland or a benign follicular adenoma of the thyroid gland.

In the case of decreased secretion of a hormone, the hormone can often be replaced, allowing for a person's normal function and no obvious impairment. The hormone, however, must be replaced for the rest of the patient's life. In some cases, such as thyroid insufficiency, replacement can be given orally. In other cases, such as insulin-dependent diabetes, replacement hormones must be given by injection and may not completely restore normal secretory patterns.

Although physiologic replacement is usually possible under normal conditions, a patient's normal response to stress may not be possible at all times. The patient with Addison's disease, for example, may not be able to function under extreme stress in the workplace or at home without parenteral steroid supplementation and intravenous fluids. An impairment, therefore, exists because of the inability to handle the normal stresses of life.

Endocrine deficiencies do not always exist in isolation and may be associated with dysfunctions of other organ systems. In order to evaluate and determine impairment caused by endocrinologic diseases, the impairment in each of the secondary organ systems must also be assessed.

Hormone secretion excesses can generally be treated by removing the source of the excessive hormone (e.g., removal of a parathyroid adenoma). In some cases, however, the source cannot be removed, and the patient may require a lifetime of therapy with medications to control the problem (e.g., a prolactin-secreting pituitary tumor that is nonresponsive to surgery and irradiation).

Finally, diabetes mellitus, one of the most common endocrine disorders, is associated with complications that affect many organ systems. Diabetic neuropathy, retinopathy, and nephropathy are frequently related to Type I or insulin-dependent diabetes mellitus (IDDM). Type II diabetes or non–insulin-dependent diabetes mellitus (NIDDM) is frequently associated with hypertension, dyslipidemia, obesity, and premature atherosclerosis of the coronary, cerebral, and peripheral blood vessels. Coronary artery disease is the leading cause of morbidity in diabetes mellitus.

## CONDITIONS CAUSING IMPAIRMENT AS RELATED TO THE ENDOCRINE SYSTEM

### Hypothalamic-Pituitary Axis

Deficiencies in secretion of the pituitary can lead to hypothyroidism, adrenal insufficiency and hypogonadism since the anterior pituitary controls all of these target organs. Multiple endocrine deficiencies are to be expected when there is pituitary insufficiency. This section will consider those impairments that may result due to disorders of specific pituitary factors.

## Growth hormone deficiency

If pituitary insufficiency occurs before puberty, lack of growth hormone will result in short stature, which must be treated with growth hormone supplementation by injection. Delays in diagnosis or insufficient treatment may result in short stature and diminished muscle mass, and should be evaluated as any other musculoskeletal disorder. Short stature is included under the Social Security Evaluation System as an independent source of impairment. After epiphyses are closed, growth hormone therapy is not recommended and will not cause additional growth. One controlled, double-blind study has suggested that growth hormone therapy in adults with growth hormone deficiency may improve the patient's sense of well-being, and lead to increased mental alertness, improved physical capacity, and subjective muscle strength, although no objective increase in isokinetic muscle strength was observed.[1]

## Prolactin deficiency

Prolactin is necessary for lactation, and no replacement therapy is available at this time. Generally, no work or other type of disability results from prolactin deficiency.

## Antidiuretic hormone (ADH)

The posterior pituitary lobe is an extension of hypothalamic neurons and produces an antidiuretic hormone. A deficiency in antidiuretic hormone results in diabetes insipidus. This is normally controlled with antidiuretic hormone given intranasally or by injection and, if an adequate dose is given, any impairment such as that related to occupation is fully corrected. If the patient with diabetes insipidus has impaired consciousness or an impaired thirst mechanism, intensive in-hospital therapy will probably be required.

## Pituitary hormone excess

Hypersecretion by the anterior pituitary can occur from tumor or hyperplasia. Prolactin hypersecretion can lead to galactorrhea and gonadal insufficiency. If untreated, hyperprolactinemia can lead to osteoporosis. Growth-hormone hypersecretion can lead to gigantism in children and acromegaly in adults. Acromegaly can be associated with degenerative arthritis, diabetes, and premature cardiovascular disease especially if it goes unrecognized and untreated for long periods. Corticotrophin excess can lead to Cushing's disease,

which can be associated with diabetes, osteoporosis, hypertension, and premature cataracts, as well as avascular necrosis of the hip. Each of these impairments should be evaluated individually.

## Anatomical pituitary-hypothalamic disorders

Space-occupying lesions of the pituitary and hypothalamic area can cause alterations in hormone output as discussed above but can also cause problems because of their anatomic location. Visual field impairment, frontal lobe abnormalities, temporal lobe seizures, and obstructive hydrocephalus can all occur. The extent of permanent impairment will depend on the ability to remove, debulk, or irradiate these mass lesions. Sometimes drug therapy can help (e.g., the use of bromocriptine in treating a prolactin-secreting tumor). A study of patients with treated (by stereotactic surgery) craniopharyngiomas showed that at the 10- to 23-year follow-up, such patients were generally able to work full-time and had a low rate of intercurrent disease; in most cases, with substitution therapy for pituitary insufficiency, the patients were seldom disturbed subjectively by their disease.[2]

In general, evaluation of pituitary disease includes measurement of baseline hormonal levels, stimulation and suppression studies, and diagnostic radiographic techniques.

## Thyroid

Thyroid dysfunction usually results from undersecretion or oversecretion of thyroid hormone. In general the treatment of hyperthyroidism, thyroid nodules or thyroid carcinoma by surgery or radioiodine often leads to hypothyroidism, which then must be managed with replacement thyroid hormone. Most of the manifestations of hypothyroidism and hyperthyroidism are reversible with treatment and lead to no permanent impairment. An adequate time must be allowed after thyroid hormone substitution is begun before impairment is evaluated. A study by Hylander and Rosenqvist indicated that maximal working capacity on a bicycle ergometer was not observed until 6.2 to 9.0 weeks of therapy.[3]

Occasionally, because of coexisting disease in other organ systems (particularly heart disease), full replacement doses of thyroid hormone are not tolerated. In such cases, there may be impairment of work tolerance and symptoms of hypothyroidism will persist (such as cold intolerance, constipation, dry skin, and menstrual abnormalities).

The eye disease sometimes associated with Graves' disease and Hashimoto's thyroiditis (thyroid ophthalmopathy) does not always improve after the therapy of the thyroid dysfunction and can sometimes get worse, causing cosmetic disfigurement, recurrent eye infections, eye muscle dysfunction, and in some cases, permanent impairment of vision.

Thyroid carcinoma is generally localized to the thyroid and surrounding neck structures but can sometimes behave aggressively, causing respiratory problems and spinal cord dysfunction secondary to tumor involvement.

### Gonads

Hypofunction of the gonads can occur in either sex. In prepubertal females, hypogonadism will lead to permanent infertility. Testicular hypofunction will result in eunuchoidism and infertility when it occurs in prepubertal males. Osteoporosis can occur if hormonal replacement is not instituted. If the gonads are hyperfunctional in the prepubertal state, precocious puberty and short stature occur after a period of premature growth acceleration.

In postpubertal females, gonadal hypofunction can lead to premature menopause with the classical symptom complex including hot flashes and sweats. Premature menopause is also a risk factor for osteoporosis and may lead to accelerated atherosclerosis.

In postpubertal males, gonadal hypofunction can also lead to osteoporosis. Anemia can be a manifestation of hypogonadism. Males can also develop a symptom complex similar to the menopausal symptom complex in females.

While established osteoporosis with recurrent fractures and atherosclerosis with coronary, cerebral, or other vascular diseases are obvious sources of impairment, it is difficult to determine the degree of impairment due solely to the increased risk of these disorders in the younger individual. The most immediate impairment is loss of reproductive capacity.

### Parathyroid Glands

The parathyroids regulate calcium and phosphorus metabolism. Hyperfunction, or hyperparathyroidism, can be associated with nephrocalcinosis, renal calculi, bone pain, polyuria, and constipation. If the serum calcium level gets high enough, coma can result. In general, surgical removal of the abnormal parathyroid gland or glands fully corrects the problem, although hypoparathyroidism may sometimes ensue. When surgical treatment is not possible or not successful, medical management is necessary and some residual impairment may persist. This may be evaluated as in Table 37-1.

Hyposecretion can produce hypoparathyroidism with tetany, paresthesias, seizures, and sometimes cataracts, cutaneous moniliasis, and alopecia. Treat-

**TABLE 37-1     IMPAIRMENTS RELATED TO HYPERPARATHYROIDISM**

| SEVERITY | % IMPAIRMENT OF THE WHOLE PERSON |
| --- | --- |
| Symptoms and signs easily controlled with medical therapy | 0–14 |
| Persistent mild hypercalcemia with mild nausea and polyuria | 15–29 |
| Severe hypercalcemia with nausea and lethargy | 30–90 |

**TABLE 37-2     IMPAIRMENTS RELATED TO HYPOPARATHYROIDISM**

| SEVERITY | % IMPAIRMENT OF THE WHOLE PERSON |
| --- | --- |
| Symptoms and signs easily controlled by medical therapy | 0–9 |
| Intermittent hypercalcemia or hypocalcemia; symptoms more frequent than with above category, despite careful medical attention | 10–20 |

ment should reverse some of these abnormalities in most people. Impairment may be evaluated, as in Table 37-2, according to the symptoms that remain after treatment is optimized.

### Adrenal Cortex

Hypofunction of the adrenal cortex is commonly referred to as Addison's disease. Lack of glucocorticoids and mineralocorticoids forms the clinical basis of the syndrome, which can include severe problems with lack of sodium retention. Oral replacement therapy is adequate except at times of stress when the hypofunctioning adrenal cortex is unable to respond. If hormone replacement is not adequate, acute adrenal insufficiency can occur with severe hypotension and vascular collapse. Death can occur if immediate therapy is not instituted. Adrenal insufficiency can occur from autoimmune failure as well as destruction of the adrenals by tumor, infection, or chemotherapy.

In evaluating impairment due to adrenal insuffi-

**TABLE 37-3    IMPAIRMENTS RELATED TO HYPOADRENALISM**

| SEVERITY | % IMPAIRMENT OF THE WHOLE PERSON |
|---|---|
| Symptoms and signs controlled with medical therapy | 0–14 |
| Symptoms and signs controlled inadequately, especially during acute illnesses | 15–29 |
| Severe symptoms of adrenal crisis during major illnesses* | 30–90 |

*This would be considered a permanent impairment only if the episodes recurred and could not be controlled with therapy.

**TABLE 37-4    IMPAIRMENTS RELATED TO HYPERADRENOCORTICISM***

| SEVERITY | % IMPAIRMENT OF THE WHOLE PERSON |
|---|---|
| **Minimal,** as with hyperadrenocorticism that is surgically corrected by removal of a pituitary or adrenal adenoma or due to moderate pharmacologic doses of glucocorticoids | 0–14 |
| **Moderate,** as with bilateral hyperplasia that is treated with medical therapy or adrenalectomy or due to large pharmacologic doses of glucocorticoids | 15–39 |
| **Severe,** as with aggressively metastasizing adrenal carcinoma | Variable+ |

*This table should be used to evaluate impairments resulting from general effects of adrenal steroids, such as myopathy, easy bruising, and obesity. The estimated percentages should be *combined* with those related to specific impairments, such as diabetes or fractures due to osteoporosis.

+The degree of estimated impairment will depend on the effects of the tumor on other organ systems.

ciency, the impaired ability to respond to stress must be considered, as described in Table 37-3. With regard to occupational disability, jobs requiring heavy exertion and exposure to hot climates pose greater risk.

Hypersecretion by the adrenals can produce Cushing's syndrome, hyperaldosteronism, and androgen excess or estrogen excess due to hyperplasia or tumor. Although these hypersecretion states can be treated by surgery, irradiation, and drug therapy, residual conditions such as osteoporosis, hypertension, cataracts, skin changes, and diabetes mellitus may remain. Premature atherosclerosis may be present as a complication of long-standing adrenal hyperplasia. Table 37-4 may be used to evaluate impairments due to hyperadrenocorticism.

### Adrenal Medulla

The adrenal medulla produces catecholamines. Hypofunction does not cause any difficulty. Hyperfunction can occur from adrenal hyperplasia or from a tumor called pheochromocytoma. If the tumor is removed, no permanent impairment should remain. Pheochromocytomas, however, can be associated with massive cerebrovascular accidents and hypertension if undiagnosed, and one could have residual neurologic dysfunction. Table 37-5 may be used to evaluate permanent impairment.

### Endocrine Pancreas (Islets of Langerhans)

Hyposecretion of the islet cells of the pancreas leads to diabetes mellitus. In Type I or insulin-dependent diabetes mellitus (IDDM), complete islet cell ex-

**TABLE 37-5    PERMANENT IMPAIRMENT RELATED TO PHEOCHROMOCYTOMAS**

| SEVERITY | % IMPAIRMENT OF THE WHOLE PERSON |
|---|---|
| **Minimal,** as when the duration of hypertension has not led to cardiovascular disease and a benign tumor can be removed surgically | 0–14 |
| **Moderate,** as with an inoperable malignant pheochromocytoma; the signs and symptoms of catecholamine excess can be controlled with blocking agents | 15–29 |
| **Severe,** as with a widely metastatic malignant pheochromocytoma, in which symptoms of catecholamine excess cannot be controlled | 30–90 |

haustion occurs after the disease has been present for some months and insulin therapy is required for sustenance of life. In Type II or non–insulin-dependent diabetes mellitus (NIDDM), hyperinsulinemia and insulin resistance occur but, eventually, islet cell exhaustion can be present. Initially, insulin therapy is not necessary, but about 50% to 60% of patients with NIDDM will ultimately require insulin therapy.

One complication of therapy in diabetes is an unawareness of hypoglycemia (especially in patients receiving beta-blockers) leading to loss of consciousness in a small percentage of people on insulin therapy. These individuals may present a risk to other people as well as to themselves. Every effort should be made to manipulate therapy in an attempt to eliminate severe hypoglycemia. The occurrence of hypoglycemia, especially when it occurs without warning symptoms, is of particular concern when evaluating the ability of an insulin-taking patient to operate a motor vehicle safely. The *medical* decision, which is distinct from any administrative decision governed by specific state or federal laws, will generally depend on whether the patient has had any episodes of unconsciousness in the past six to twelve months, and on whether the patient is compliant with recommended regimens of medication and self-monitoring blood glucose levels.[4]

The major source of impairment caused by diabetes mellitus is its ability to cause vascular disease. Retinopathy and macular degeneration can lead to impaired vision or blindness. Before a determination of disability for retinopathy is made, physicians should urge maximum efforts to use low-vision aids and to undergo rehabilitative training. With use of such aids and training, it has been estimated that up to 89% of patients can return to work.[5] Nephropathy can lead to end-stage renal disease requiring chronic dialysis or kidney transplantation and therapy with immunosuppressive drugs. Patients with even slight increases in urinary albumin excretion may have an appreciably impaired aerobic work capacity that cannot be explained by autonomic neuropathy or by duration of diabetes.[6] Peripheral neuropathy with attendant lack of sensation can lead to ulceration of the feet with danger of amputation, as well as a Charcot foot due to repeated trauma. Paresthesias due to diabetic neuropathy may be symptomatically disturbing but are objectively difficult to evaluate. Nerve conduction studies have been recommended for this purpose.[7]

The above complications occur in IDDM and NIDDM. In addition, premature atherosclerosis can occur with involvement of larger blood vessels. Premature heart disease and stroke are important causes of medical impairments. NIDDM is associated with other risk factors for atherosclerosis including hyper-

tension, obesity, dyslipidemia, and hyperinsulinemia. In a study of 1707 persons with diabetes receiving disability compensation, functional handicaps and symptoms related to clinically advanced diabetes were regarded as the basis for a disability pension in 20% to 25% of the patients; in the remaining cases, neither diabetes nor its late complications could be held responsible for the reduced work capacity.[8] In these other cases, problems such as angina pectoris, obesity, and alcoholism were important. In a study comparing adults with and without diabetes, 13% of adults with diabetes were found to be permanently disabled compared with only 2% of other adults.[9]

The Diabetes Control and Complications Trial (DCCT) showed that microvascular complications of IDDM including retinopathy, neuropathy, and nephropathy could be decreased by 50% to 75% with intensive control of diabetes.[10] In boys with IDDM, but not in girls, good metabolic control is also associated with better physical fitness as measured by physical work capacity.[11] It is reasonable to assume that these same conclusions will carry over to NIDDM. Intensive control, however, can be associated with an increased incidence of hypoglycemia, and treatment goals may have to modified in the subset of the population that is prone to hypoglycemia.

The impairment evaluation of the patient with diabetes mellitus must include an evaluation of any coexisting risk factors and will require laboratory evaluation and assessment of cardiovascular status as well as a complete history and physical examination. In most cases, the impairment in diabetes is related to the complications of diabetes rather than to the presence of diabetes per se.

Hyperfunction of the pancreas due to hyperplasia or tumor can produce significant hypoglycemia, which can be remedied by removing the source of insulin production. In the case of malignancies, management may be extremely difficult.

## GENERALIZATIONS AND CONCLUSIONS

The impairments associated with endocrine diseases can be caused by the hormonal abnormality itself or by damage to distant organ systems from complications of the endocrinopathy. Endocrine abnormalities do not exist in vacuum; they are often associated with other endocrine abnormalities. For example, Hashimoto's thyroiditis and hypothyroidism are frequently associated with IDDM. Another example would be hypoparathyroidism, which is often associated with other primary endocrine failures such as adrenal insufficiency and ovarian failure.

Multiple endocrine neoplasia (MEN) is a group of

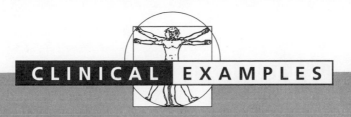
## ENDOCRINOLOGY

### EXAMPLE

#### History

An 18-year-old man came for an impairment evaluation related to diabetes mellitus, which he has had since he was 8 years old. He was considered "brittle," with frequent episodes of hyperglycemia and hypoglycemia requiring admittance to the medical service on numerous occasions due to abnormalities in blood sugar control. He was receiving 12 units of a long-acting insulin once a day and regular insulin three times a day, based on blood sugar test results.

#### Physical Examination

His physical examination, including both cardiovascular and ophthalmologic evaluations, was normal.

#### Test Results

His hemoglobin A1C was at the upper limits of normal at 6.8% (normal, 4.2% to 7%).

#### Assessment Process

This individual was assigned a Class IV impairment because he is an insulin-dependent diabetic with episodes of "hyperglycemia or hypoglycemia despite the conscientious efforts of both the patient and the physician." Therefore, he has a 20% to 40% whole person impairment (WPI). Since there is no evidence of diabetic vascular disease, a 20% impairment would be appropriate.

#### Repeat History

Ten years later this individual had an insulin pump inserted into his abdomen that produced excellent control of his blood sugar levels. He has not been hospitalized for diabetic control since the operation. A medical evaluator is asked to see him 1 year after his surgery for an impairment assessment. Over the past 6 months he has developed chest pain that was clinically diagnosed as angina pectoris. He also complains of coolness of his feet, stating that at times they become cold, and that he occasionally will have a burning sensation on his soles.

#### Physical Examination

All the pulses in the feet and legs are normal, but he does have sensory loss for light touch and temperature in a stocking distribution in both lower extremities. Numerous microaneurysms are seen on funduscopic examination. He is evaluated by an ophthalmologist who reports no visual impairment.

#### Test Results

The hemoglobin A1C level is now 5.0%. A treadmill stress test produces a 2 mm ST segment depression at the 5.5 METS level. A coronary angiogram is normal. Capillary refill time is mildly prolonged.

#### Assessment Process

Diabetes would place this individual in Class III. The American Medical Association *Guides* state that "a patient belongs in this Class when insulin-dependent (Type I) diabetes mellitus is present with or without evidence of microangiopathy."* His insulin pump controls the episodes of hyperglycemia and hypoglycemia, so he has only a 10% to 20% WPI. Considering his clinical course, the 20% value would be more appropriate.

From a cardiovascular standpoint, he is evaluated using the coronary heart disease model (Section 6.2 of the *Guides*). The abnormalities on his ECG stress test would place him in Class III. His coronary angiogram is negative because the diabetes has produced microvascular disease only. He exercised only to 5.5 METS. Therefore, with a possible range of 30% to 49% impairment, a 45% to 49% impairment would be considered appropriate.

From a peripheral vascular disease standpoint, this individual does not qualify for an impairment rating. Table 69 (page 189) states that a person has a 0% to 9% impairment (Class I) if there are no symptoms of claudication, if the individual has transient edema, and if there are subtle abnormalities on the physical examination. Anything higher than a Class I impairment implies the presence of

---

*All *tables* and *sections* referred to in this discussion are found in AMA *Guides to the evaluation of permanent impairment,* ed 4, Chapter 12—The Endocrinologic System and Chapter 6—The Cardiovascular System, American Medical Association, Chicago, 1993.

*Continued.*

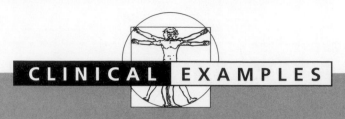

## ENDOCRINOLOGY—cont'd

claudication pain. This individual has no claudication, perhaps because he cannot walk far enough to produce this type of abnormality. However, he should be carefully watched for this development.

The patient does have sensory abnormalities in a stocking distribution, but the *Guides* produce sensory impairment ratings for peripheral nerves only, not covering stocking and/or glove distributions, so extrapolation is needed. If nerve roots are used to assess impairment, the L4, L5, S1, and S2 roots would be considered affected. Table 3 (page 130) produces sensory impairment percentages for nerve roots L3, L4, L5, and S1. Therefore extrapolation would use 5% (as for these nerve roots) for S2 as well. Section 3.1k is used to derive the impairment. Table 11 places this individual in Grade IV because there is decreased sensation with causalgia. This produces an 80% sensory deficit. Using an intermediary figure of 70%, one would multiply 5% by 70% to produce 3.5%. The 3.5% impairment of L4, L5, S1, and S2 are all combined, then multiplied by 0.4 to convert a lower extremity impairment to a WPI. To do this, the 3% is combined with 4%, with 3%, and with 4%, since 3.5% is not found on the values chart. This produces a 14% impairment of the lower extremity, which is then multiplied by 0.4, producing a 6% WPI based on the sensory deficit.

If the specific nerves are used instead of the nerve roots (a more correct approach), there are eight nerves affected, including the saphenous, lateral sural cutaneous, superficial peroneal, sural, deep peroneal, medial plantar, lateral plantar, and medial calcaneal (see Figure 9, page 93). Table 68 (page 89) only lists four of these nerves specifically, and these four nerves produce WPIs of 2%, 1%, 2%, and 2%. When combined, this produces a 7% WPI. However, this is only 50% of the nerves involved, so it should be doubled to yield a 14% WPI. No account, however, is given for the fact that the sensory abnormality is incomplete. Therefore, this must be diminished by an appropriate factor. Because of the multiple extrapolations required, the result is unsatisfactory. Therefore, while anatomically incorrect, the nerve root method would probably be most appropriate in this individual.

No impairment is given for visual abnormalities because visual acuity is normal.

### Evaluation

When combined, this individual's impairment caused by the diabetes (20%), coronary disease (45%), and sensory abnormalities (6%) gives a total value of 59% WPI.

*Stephen L. Demeter*

disorders associated with multiple endocrine tumors that may be functional. MEN-I is associated mainly with gastrinomas and tumors of the parathyroid and pituitary. MEN-II includes the presence of medullary carcinoma of the thyroid and multiple pheochromocytomas. Both of these syndromes can be associated with other endocrine tumors as well.

Hormone replacement usually will reverse most hormone deficiencies secondary to hypofunction. Treatment, however, is not always successful and some individuals may be resistant to therapy, thus allowing the impairment to continue. Response to therapy must always be evaluated on an individual basis.

## References

1. Degerblad M, Almkvist O, Grunditz R, et al: Physical and psychological capabilities during substitution therapy with recombinant growth hormone in adults with growth hormone deficiency. *Acta Endocrinologica* 123:185–193, 1990.
2. Sääf M, Thorén M, Bergstrand CG, et al: Treatment of craniopharyngiomas—the stereotactic approach in a ten to twenty-three years' perspective. II. Psychosocial situation and pituitary function. *Acta Neurochir (Wien)* 99:97–103, 1989.
3. Hylander B, Rosenqvist U: Peripheral responses to thyroxine in hypothyroid subjects as a function of dose and duration of substitution. *Acta Med Scand* 214:317–23, 1983.
4. Horwitz DL: Diabetes mellitus and other disorders. Chapter 5 in Doege TC, Engelberg AL, editors: *Medical conditions affecting drivers*, American Medical Association, pp 22–28, 1986.
5. Nilsson UL: Visual rehabilitation of patients with advanced diabetic retinopathy. *Doc Ophthal* 62:369–382, 1986.
6. Jensen T, Richter EA, Feldt-Rasmussen B, et al: Impaired aerobic work capacity in insulin dependent diabetics with increased urinary albumin excretion. *Br Med J* 296:1352–1354, 1988.
7. Dyck PJ: Detection, characterization, and staging of polyneuropathy: assessed in diabetics. *Muscle Nerve* 11:21–32, 1988.
8. Morén-Hybbinette I, Moritz U, Scherstén B: Diabetes mellitus and disability pension. *Scand J Soc Med* 17:193–201, 1989.
9. Goldman DL, Fulton JP, Perry DK, et al: Activity reduction and disability among persons with diabetes. *R I Med* 77:120–121, 1994.
10. The Diabetes Control and Complications Trial Research Group: the effect of intensive treatment of diabetes on the development and progression of long-term complications in insulin-dependent diabetes mellitus, *N Engl J Med* 329:977–986, 1993.
11. Huttunen NP, Käär ML, Knip M, et al: Physical fitness of children and adolescents with insulin-dependent diabetes mellitus. *Ann Clin Res* 16:1–5, 1984.

## Recommendations for General Reading

American Diabetes Association: Standards of medical care for patients with diabetes mellitus. *Diab Care* 17:616–623, 1994.

Sussman KE, Draznin B, James WE, editors: *Clinical guide to diabetes mellitus*, New York, 1987, Alan R. Liss.

Wilson JD, Foster DW, editors: *Williams textbook of endocrinology*, ed 8, Philadelphia, 1992, WB Saunders.

# SECTION C
## Neurological Assessment

# CHAPTER 38

## DIAGNOSTIC TESTS

*Scott Haldeman*

The nervous system is the most complex system of the body for the determination of impairment and disability. Disorders of the nervous system can influence virtually every organ function. The nervous system is responsible for the movement of limbs, the sensing of the environment, and the coordinated response to changes in the environment. It is the center for cognitive, intellectual, and behavioral functions. It is also an integral part of the control of visceral organs. Furthermore, disturbances in neurologic function can result in an extremely wide variation in the degree of impairment of body function. Minor changes in neurologic function such as coordination and sensation may be adapted to completely without significant impairment. On the other hand, serious disturbances of the spinal cord and central nervous system can cause total loss of use of a limb or specific organ function and lead to, in the worst case, a chronic vegetative state with, a total reliance on nursing care.

Since disturbances of the nervous system can cause different degrees of dysfunction, it is essential that methods be developed to differentiate the levels of neurologic impairment. Many impairment systems, including those in the AMA *Guides to the Evaluation of Permanent Impairment,* and California guidelines, list the major neurologic functions and then attempt to organize them using specific whole person impairment percentages. The Social Security Administration, on the other hand, lists specific diagnoses and symptom patterns. It is left up to the clinician to reach conclusions on the ability of a patient to perform certain activities or control bodily functions.

Testing is sometimes mentioned as a basis for diagnosing potentially-disabling neurologic deficits. The AMA *Guides* state that "the electrodiagnostic evaluation may provide useful information." The Social Security Administration requires the listing of laboratory results to justify a diagnosis. For example, the Social Security handbook specifically mentions EEG as one method of diagnosing epilepsy.[65]

## RATIONALE FOR TESTING

The clinical history and physical examination are the primary tools for neurologic impairment evaluation. It is, however, very difficult to complete the neurological examination in many individuals without relying to some extent on testing. This is especially true when the examination findings are equivocal or where different diseases present with similar clinical patterns. The testing should be considered complementary to or the extension of the neurological examination and not as the sole justification for an impairment rating. Testing is classically used for the reasons given below.

### Determination of Diagnosis

Without a specific diagnosis, it is very difficult to reach conclusions regarding neurologic impairment. Different disorders of the nervous system have different prognostic outcomes and responses to treatment. For example, multiple sclerosis may go through exacerbation and remitting phases while carpal tunnel syndrome may improve with surgery. Spinal cord injuries and stroke may leave significant permanent impairment and disability while a pure sensory radiculopathy may cause very minimal decreases in functional capacity. Each one of these disorders can present as numbness or weakness in an extremity but with a markedly different prognosis and potential impairment. Neurodiagnostic testing as an adjunct to the clinical examination is often essential in determining the diagnosis and prognosis on which the impairment is based. The electrodiagnostic tests that may be of value in localizing a neurologic lesion affecting the extremities are noted in Figure 38-1.

### Documentation of Loss of Function

The same disease can cause a marked variability in loss of neurologic function in different patients. Mul-

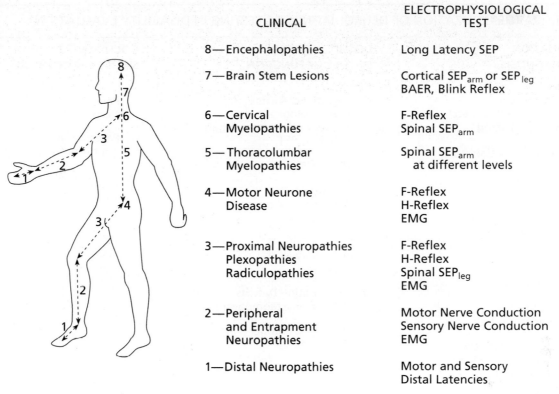

|  | CLINICAL | ELECTROPHYSIOLOGICAL TEST |
|---|---|---|
| 8 | Encephalopathies | Long Latency SEP |
| 7 | Brain Stem Lesions | Cortical SEP$_{arm}$ or SEP$_{leg}$ BAER, Blink Reflex |
| 6 | Cervical Myelopathies | F-Reflex Spinal SEP$_{arm}$ |
| 5 | Thoracolumbar Myelopathies | Spinal SEP$_{arm}$ at different levels |
| 4 | Motor Neurone Disease | F-Reflex H-Reflex EMG |
| 3 | Proximal Neuropathies Plexopathies Radiculopathies | F-Reflex H-Reflex Spinal SEP$_{leg}$ EMG |
| 2 | Peripheral and Entrapment Neuropathies | Motor Nerve Conduction Sensory Nerve Conduction EMG |
| 1 | Distal Neuropathies | Motor and Sensory Distal Latencies |

**FIGURE 38-1**    Example of electrodiagnostic tests used for localizing a neurological deficit in the extremities.

tiple sclerosis, for example, may cause dysfunction ranging from a reversible minor symptom of numbness or blurred vision to a combination of incapacitating deficits of cognitive function, coordination, and motor and sensory function. A spinal radiculopathy can result in a nondisabling reflex loss, partially disabling pain with certain activities, paralysis of specific muscles, or a cauda equina syndrome with loss of bowel and bladder function. The simple determination of a diagnosis, therefore, is not sufficient, by itself, to decide a level of impairment or disability. It is necessary to determine the nature and extent of any neurologic loss that is caused by a disease. Testing may be necessary to document the nature and degree of neurologic deficits caused by a specific diagnosis.

### Confirmation of Subjective Complaints

A number of patients have neurological symptoms that are based primarily on subjective statements or poorly-documented clinical observations by the clinician. Symptoms such as pain, muscle tenderness, vague feelings of weakness and fatigue, paresthesias, dizziness, and changes in memory are often difficult to confirm through the clinical examination. Most impairment evaluation systems, nonetheless, require some degree of objective verification of these clinical

symptoms. Neurodiagnostic testing has been advocated to confirm these subjective complaints.

The tests included in this chapter that illustrate these points are listed in Table 38-1.

### SENSITIVITY AND SPECIFICITY OF NEURODIAGNOSTIC TESTING

The determination of the sensitivity and the specificity of neurologic testing has posed one of the most difficult challenges facing neurologists. This is particularly true when considering impairment testing. The problem in defining the sensitivity and specificity of a test is the selection of the gold standard test against which any other test is judged. The classic neurologic gold standard is the clinical examination but only recently has intraobserver and interobserver reliability of the clinical examination been investigated, and in many cases it has been shown not to be reliable.[7,26] Neurodiagnostic testing has also been compared with radiographic imaging tests such as CT, MRI, and myelography.[58] This comparison suffers from the wide variation in imaging findings in most diagnoses and the observation that many abnormal findings on imaging can exist without neurological deficits.[6,8,11,13] The third factor against which neurodiagnostic testing has been

**TABLE 38-1** THE UTILIZATION OF NEURODIAGNOSTIC TESTING IN DISABILITY EVALUATION*

| DETERMINATION OF THE DIAGNOSIS | DOCUMENTATION OF LOSS OF FUNCTION | DOCUMENTATION OF SUBJECTIVE COMPLAINTS |
|---|---|---|
| 1. Brain Disorders<br> a) Imaging (MRI, CT, etc)<br> b) Cognitive testing<br> c) EEG<br> d) Evoked potentials (VEP, BAEP)<br> e) Spinal tap | 1. Cognitive Deficits<br> a) Psychological test<br> b) Event related potentials<br> c) SPECT, PET | 1. Pain<br> None |
| 2. Spinal Cord Disorders<br> a) Imaging (CT, MRI)<br> b) Evoked potentials<br> c) Spinal tap | 2. Motor Deficits<br> a) EMG<br> b) Motor NCV<br> c) Cortical motor evoked potentials | 2. Paresthesias<br> ? Sensory NCVs? |
| 3. Radiculopathy<br> a) Imaging<br> b) EMG<br> c) Reflex studies<br> d) Evoked potentials | 3. Sensory Deficits<br> a) Sensory NCV<br> b) SEP | 3. Muscle Spasms<br> ? Surface EMG?<br> ? Muscle evoked potentials? |
| 4. Peripheral Neuropathies<br> a) NCVs (motor, sensory)<br> b) Reflex studies<br> c) EMG | 4. Coordination Deficits<br> a) Electronystagmography | 4. False Positive Testing on EMG/NCV/SEP<br> EEG<br> Imaging |
| 5. Bowel, Bladder, and Sexual Disorders<br> a) Cystometry<br> b) Evoked potentials<br> c) Anal EMG<br> d) Penile tumescence | 5. Bowel and Bladder Deficits<br> a) Cystometry<br> b) Evoked potentials<br> c) Penile tumescence | |
| 6. Muscle Disorders<br> a) Blood analysis<br> b) EMG<br> c) Repetitive stimulation<br> d) Biopsy | | |

*MRI: magnetic resonance imaging, CT: computed tomography, VEP: visual evoked potential, BAEP: brain stem auditory evoked potentials, EMG: electromyography, NCV: nerve conduction velocity, SPECT: single photon emission computed tomography, PET: positron emission tomography, SEP: somatosensory evoked potential, EEG: electroencephalography.

compared is the results of surgery. The nonblinded observation of a surgeon, however, can be subjective and difficult to quantify. When reviewing the sensitivity and specificity of any test, it is therefore important to understand the quality of the standard against which it has been compared.

The majority of research that has been done to assess the specificity and sensitivity of testing has been in the area of the diagnosis of specific disease entities. Thus, brain MRI scans have been shown to have a high degree of sensitivity for the diagnosis and prognosis of multiple sclerosis but not for the degree of impairment.[8,27,43] A combination of tests such as evoked potentials with MRI may increase the sensi-

tivity in the diagnosis of multiple sclerosis when compared with MRI alone.[8] In the same way, spinal abnormalities such as degenerative changes, spondylolisthesis, disc herniation, and stenosis have been found in large numbers of asymptomatic patients.[10,11,13,51,66] Imaging and pathological tests (biopsy, blood tests) may present relatively accurate anatomic diagnoses for many diseases but may not give information as to the symptoms or functional status of the nervous system.

Electrodiagnostic testing procedures have different problems. Nerve conduction and evoked responses measure the function of a peripheral nerve or central pathway but are nonspecific for the nature of the disease process causing an abnormality. Somatosensory evoked potentials, for example, can be abnormal in any disease affecting the spinal cord including demyelination, neoplasms, degenerative disorders, and central disc herniations.

There have also been few, if any, well-constructed studies that have specifically addressed the relationship of neurological tests to impairment and to the loss of functional capacity. Therefore, when reading this chapter and other papers on the sensitivity and specificity of neurodiagnostic tests, one must be very careful to determine whether the test is being used for pathological diagnosis, loss of neurologic function, or impairment and recognize that these factors are not interchangeable.

## DETERMINATION OF DIAGNOSIS

The AMA *Guides* state: "Before evaluating and estimating the extent of an impairment, the physician should attempt to establish an accurate diagnosis."[4]

The primary requirement in determining a diagnosis is the confirmation of the presence or absence of specific pathology or loss of organ function. Neurodiagnostic testing is an integral part of this process. The choice of testing procedures is dependent upon the part of the nervous system that is presumed to be affected by the particular injury or disease. It is not possible in this chapter to describe the vast array of diagnostic tests used by neurologists for diagnostic purposes. The following is a simple outline of certain testing procedures that may be used to document neurologic diseases when impairment is an issue. The details concerning the methods of performing these tests, their accuracy and idiosyncrasies will be left to the textbooks on neurology.

Most neurologic diseases are classified according to the area of the nervous system that is affected. In this manner, the nervous system is commonly divided into the forebrain, brain stem, spinal cord, nerve roots, peripheral nerves, visceral nervous system, and muscles. Disorders of each of these subdivisions of the nervous system have specific tests that are used to document the nature and extent of pathology.

### Brain Disorders: Forebrain and Brain Stem

The number of diseases that can affect the brain fills multiple textbooks on neurology. It is not appropriate or possible in this setting to discuss specific diseases except as examples. Each brain disorder is diagnosed by a combination of clinical findings and diagnostic tests. Each test has different degrees of sensitivity and specificity depending on the nature and severity of the disease entity. The tests that are used to confirm the presence of pathology, however, can be divided into the following categories.

### Imaging studies

Diseases of the brain that result in structural lesions can often be visualized by means of imaging studies. Magnetic resonance imaging, computed tomography, angiography, and a variety of radiographic procedures fall under this heading. The accuracy of these studies is often enhanced by the infusion of intravenous contrast media. Chapter 15 describes the relative value of these tests as well as their sensitivities and specificities in the diagnoses.

These imaging studies are used to document anatomic and pathoanatomic structural changes in tissue that can result in neurologic impairment. For example, the location of a cerebral infarct or hemorrhage will guide the clinician as to the type of dysfunction that can be anticipated. If there is a lesion of the brain affecting the dominant motor strip and Broca's area, one can anticipate marked deficits in speech and motor function. On the other hand, if there is an infarct in the cerebellum, one can anticipate a coordination and balance impairment. Imaging is also important in documenting multiple sclerosis plaques, the presence and size of neoplastic lesions, as well as abscesses and infection.

Certain findings on imaging, however, are of questionable importance in the determination of neurologic impairment. For example, in the normal older population there can be multiple nonspecific punctate white-matter lesions reflecting asymptomatic vascular changes.[15,16] These white-matter lesions have been noted in over 50% of elderly volunteers free of neuropsychiatric or general disease.[54] Imaging, therefore, should be considered a tool for diagnosis rather than a mechanism for determining the degree of impairment in neurologic disorders.

### Cognitive neuropsychological tests

Significant psychological, cognitive, and psychiatric disorders can exist in the absence of any documentable intracranial pathologic condition as determined by imaging studies. On the other hand, certain findings commonly seen in asymptomatic patients such as white matter hyperintensities may be associated with subtle cognitive changes on neuropsychological testing.[54] Minor head injuries have been reported to cause disturbances in memory and personality while substantial parts of the brain can be destroyed by infarction or tumor without obvious loss of cognitive or intellectual abilities. There can also be considerable overlap between psychiatric disorders and cognitive functions. Furthermore, cognitive test scores can be influenced by mood, alertness, concentration, and nature of the test.[29] These factors often result in confusing differences in medical opinion when determining cognitive impairment. Neuropsychological and cognitive testing is an attempt to measure and document many higher brain functions. The use of specific cognitive testing and the psychiatric evaluation is outlined in Chapter 43.

## Electroencephalography

Electroencephalography (EEG) is one of the more established neurological tests of brain function. EEG abnormalities can be differentiated into nonspecific (slowing) and specific (epileptiform and disease specific) patterns that may be focal or generalized. The sensitivity and specificity varies with each disease entity.

In the evaluation of episodic neurologic disorders, the primary diagnostic tool for seizure disorders is the clinical examination, with the EEG often utilized as a confirmatory test. Epilepsy carries very specific disability connotations and legal responsibilities for physicians (e.g., driving, working at heights). The documentation of spikes and sharp waves from specific parts of the brain can confirm the diagnosis of seizures. It must be recognized, however, that many patients with seizure disorders, especially when controlled by medication, may have a perfectly normal electroencephalogram. When there is difficulty in differentiating between true seizures and pseudoseizures, it may be necessary to do simultaneous EEG recording and video monitoring. This may require hospitalization and observation during one of the epileptic events. Electroencephalography may also be of value in confirming a diagnosis of a generalized encephalopathy or coma. Depressed brain function following trauma, metabolic disturbances, and many degenerative brain diseases may cause a generalized slowing of background activity. Certain encephalopathies such as those caused by Jakob-Creutzfeldt disease and hepatic failure can result in specific EEG patterns. The EEG may aid in differentiating between organic coma and catatonia in comatose patients.

In recent years, the computer analysis of the EEG has become increasingly popular. So called "brain mapping" and computer assisted EEGs can be found in many neurophysiological laboratories. The use of computer-assisted EEGs to enhance the sensitivity of this test is gaining acceptance. The concern, however, has been raised that minor abnormalities found with computer-generated frequency analysis and event data have been assigned greater significance than ongoing research warrants. These procedures remain controversial and there remain problems in the differentiation between artifacts and true abnormalities.

The EEG and, particularly, brain mapping must be interpreted with care when attempting to confirm a condition related to impairment. Minor changes in background activity and asymmetries can exist as a normal variant. However, well-defined localized abnormalities and specific generalized activity changes can sometimes be the deciding factor in the diagnosis of cerebral disorders.

## Evoked potentials

Over the past two decades, with the development of computerized analysis of cerebral potentials, there has been a marked increase in the interest and utilization of evoked potentials in the evaluation of primary sensory pathways within the central nervous system. These tests may, under certain circumstances, provide unique information.

Visual evoked potentials (VEPs) are most useful in documenting demyelinating or compressing lesions on the optic nerve or optic tracks. Nath et al[46] note delays in 45% of patients with macular pathology. On the other hand, although the electroretinogram has been used to test the overall function of the retina, it has been noted to be normal or near normal in macular disease. A combination of pattern visual evoked potentials together with the electroretinogram has therefore been recommended to differentiate optic nerve from retinal disorders.[39] Visual evoked potentials have been used to differentiate hysterical blindness from true organic blindness but only in conjunction with a more complete examination. Furthermore, visual evoked potentials have been noted to be delayed in Friedreich's ataxia, Parkinson's disease, B12 deficiencies, and diabetes. Abnormal potentials are therefore not disease specific, although they are considered the hallmark of optic nerve demyelination. VEPs also do not correlate well with impairment. Chiappa[18] noted that when these potentials are normal, the examination is always normal but in patients with multiple sclerosis, the test is commonly abnormal despite clinically normal vision. There is also a wide variation in the reported sensitivity of visual evoked potential testing in demyelinating disease with published values ranging between 47% and 96%.[19]

Brain stem auditory evoked potential (BAEP) can be an important adjunct to the testing and localization of problems related to hearing. Together with cochlear potentials, BAEPs may help distinguish cochlear from auditory nerve pathology. This test measures potentials from the cochlea through the auditory nerve to the brain stem as a series of well-defined peaks that are thought to be generated in different structures through this neural pathway. Lesions at different locations in the auditory pathway show different patterns of abnormality. The sensitivity and specificity is, again, disease specific. For example, there is a reported false-negative rate of 5% in the diagnosis of acoustic neuromas and cerebellopontine angle tumors.[21] On the other hand, in brain stem demyelinating lesions, a positive test is reported in only 32% to 64% of patients.[18]

### Spinal tap and blood analysis

The analysis of cerebrospinal fluid and blood is an essential part of the diagnosis of certain central nervous system disorders. For example, determination of the organism responsible for most nervous system infections is dependent upon blood and spinal fluid analysis. Testing cerebrospinal fluid for immunoglobin abnormalities and specifically determining oligoclonal bands has become an integral part of making the diagnosis of multiple sclerosis. Many inherited metabolic disorders may similarly be confirmed by isolating specific abnormal proteins or polysaccharides. The tests are mentioned here simply for completeness. The sensitivity and specificity of these tests are disease specific.

### Spinal Cord Disorders

Disturbances in spinal cord function can cause substantial degrees of disability and impairment. Spinal cord lesions may result in loss of coordination, motor dysfunction, and sensory dysfunction below the level of the lesion as well as loss of control of bowel, bladder, and sexual function. Disorders that cause spinal cord dysfunction include spinal trauma, central disc herniation, neoplasm, congenital malformations, infection, and demyelinating disease. Many of these disorders can be documented on clinical examination but often they require other testing to determine the location and type of lesion causing the impairment.

### Imaging studies

Imaging has been covered in detail in Chapter 15 and will only be mentioned here briefly. The use of MRI scans, CT scans with and without contrast, and myelography are the most commonly used tests used for documenting spinal cord lesions. As in the case of brain disorders, there can be a significant discrepancy between lesions visualized on imaging studies and the symptoms and disability experienced by a patient. Significant degenerative changes, disc herniations, and even central stenosis may be found in patients who are asymptomatic and having normal functioning.[11,12,66]

### Evoked potentials

Somatosensory evoked potentials (SEPs) are commonly used in the evaluation of spinal cord lesions. These potentials are generated on stimulation of major nerves in the upper and lower extremities (Fig. 38-2). The pathways that are stimulated travel

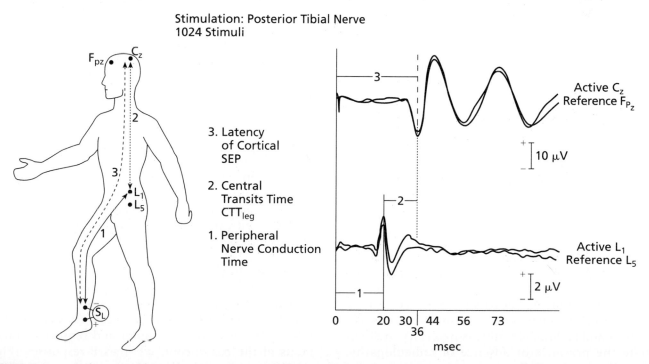

Stimulation: Posterior Tibial Nerve
1024 Stimuli

3. Latency of Cortical SEP

2. Central Transits Time $CTT_{leg}$

1. Peripheral Nerve Conduction Time

**FIGURE 38-2**    Pathways and form of somatosensory evoked potentials from the lower extremities.    *(From Haldeman S: Spine 9:42, 1984.)*

through the posterior column-meniscal system of the spinal cord and then through the brain stem to the thalamus. The usefulness of the test, therefore, is limited to lesions in that system. Patients with altered pain and temperature sensation usually have normal SEPs.[5,47] There is also a much weaker correlation between SEP abnormalities and cortical lesions. About 75% of all patients with suspected or definite multiple sclerosis have been reported to have SEP abnormalities on lower limb nerve stimulation.[49] SEPs may also be abnormal in other forms of myelopathy including trauma and spinal cord tumors. Restuccia[52] recently noted abnormal SEPs in 10 of 12 patients with confirmed lesions of the lumbosacral cord. These tests are of limited value in patients with cervical spondylosis in the absence of clinical myelopathy. However, if there is evidence of myelopathy, then lower-limb somatosensory evoked potentials may be abnormal.[25]

### Motor evoked potentials

Since somatosensory evoked potentials record only dorsal column function, it has been proposed that motor evoked potentials obtained on magnetic stimulation of the cerebral cortex be utilized to demonstrate lateral column function within the primary motor pathways.[24] Nogues et al[48] found that motor evoked potentials increased the sensitivity of somatosensory evoked potentials in patients with syringomyelia, whereas Tavy et al[63] reported abnormalities in 27 of 28 patients with cervical spondylitic myelopathy. This test, however, has not been approved for general use in the United States.

### Spinal tap and blood analysis

The indications for spinal tap and specific blood tests in the diagnosis of spinal cord disease are similar to those for brain diseases. These tests may be of particular importance in the diagnosis of infectious diseases and multiple sclerosis. There are numerous tests of cerebral spinal fluid and blood, each with its unique diagnostic criteria, sensitivity, and specificity. It is not possible to address these tests in a short chapter and they are only included for completeness.

### Radiculopathy

Many patients with radiculopathy have well-defined motor, sensory, and reflex abnormalities and a clinical pattern that does not require confirmation electrodiagnostically. Other patients, however, have a confusing clinical pattern of diffuse numbness or weakness and additional testing is necessary to differentiate the presence or absence of radiculopathy. Electrodiagnostic studies and cystometry are perceived as important differentiators when assessing categories of impairment under the AMA *Guides*.

### Imaging studies

The imaging of lesions that impinge on the nerve root is covered primarily in Chapter 15. An important point to be reiterated is that the presence of compressive lesions seen on imaging studies does not necessarily document the presence or absence of radiculopathy, because such lesions can exist in the asymptomatic population.[13,37,66] This observation has increased the importance of electrodiagnostic testing to determine the significance of an anatomical lesion seen on imaging studies.[59,60] Increasingly, a combination of imaging and electrodiagnostic studies is being advocated to determine the nature and clinical importance of a suspected lesion.[12,32]

### Needle electromyography

Needle electromyography remains the mainstay in the electrodiagnostic evaluation of radiculopathy. Aiello et al examined the sensitivity and specificity of needle EMG in a series of patients with clinical evidence of radiculopathy and surgically-confirmed disc herniations.[2,3] They found that all patients with confirmed disc herniation had abnormal EMGs, but that the ability of EMG to predict the level of involvement varied. True positive rates were 100% at the L3-L4 level, 96% at the L4-L5 level, and 71% at the L5-S1 level. Localization of the level of radiculopathy by needle electromyography, however, is only as accurate as the innervation of the muscles that are tested. Most muscles in the lower extremities are innervated by two or more nerve root levels and it is necessary to sample multiple muscles. Young et al[67] found that by using needle EMG the test correctly predicted the level of radiculopathy in 84% of patients with clinical findings of nerve root pathology. The test was negative in all patients without root pathology but missed the level in 16% of cases. It is important to realize that needle electromyography only becomes abnormal after three to four weeks of denervation. The acute signs of denervation including positive sharp waves and fibrillation potentials gradually give way to reinnervation over a nine- to twelve-month period. At that point, polyphasic potentials may be evident.

### Reflex studies

Reflex studies have the advantage of becoming abnormal immediately after the onset of radiculopathy. H-reflexes (Fig. 38-3) and bulbocavernosus reflexes (Fig. 38-4) measure both motor and sensory components of the nerve root, whereas F-responses (Fig. 38-5) measure only the motor root function. The

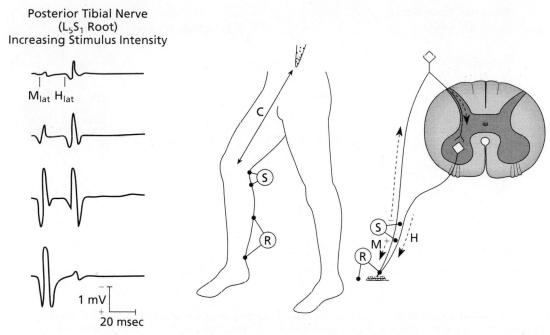

Posterior Tibial Nerve
($L_5S_1$ Root)
Increasing Stimulus Intensity

$M_{lat}$ $H_{lat}$

1 mV

20 msec

**FIGURE 38-3** Pathways and form of an H-reflex providing the electrical equivalent of a stretch reflex. *S*, stimulus electrode; *R*, recording electrode; *M*, direct motor response; *H*, H-reflex. *(From Haldeman S: Spine 9:42, 1984.)*

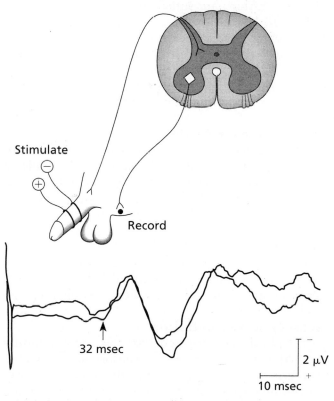

Stimulate

Record

32 msec

2 µV

10 msec

**FIGURE 38-4** Pathways and form of a bulbocavernosus reflex. *(From Haldeman S: Spine 9:42, 1984.)*

most commonly utilized reflex study is the H-reflex from the soleus-gastrocnemius muscle, which has been shown to have a very high correlation with S1 radiculopathies. Both Braddom[14] and Aiello[3] noted a 90%–100% true positive rate and a 0% true negative rate in S1 radiculopathies.

The bulbocavernosus reflex response has been correlated with lower sacral nerve lesions at the S2-S3 level, and it is useful in documenting cauda equina syndrome and pudendal nerve injuries, although the sensitivity is not known.[32,34] F-responses, on the other hand, measure only the function of proximal motor pathways both orthodromically and antidromically, and the major mixed nerves commonly have multiple root innervation. Abnormal F-wave latency prolongation has been reported in 14% to 47% of patients with radiculopathy and may be the only electrophysiologic abnormality in the first week following injury.[22,23,28]

## Evoked potentials

The major difficulty with needle electromyography is the inability to measure sensory radicular changes. Attempts have been made to complement electromyography with somatosensory evoked potentials. There is some controversy as to the sensitivity of these potentials and they can be technically difficult to record or interpret. Large mixed nerve somatosensory evoked potentials have multiple root innervations and do not appear to be of any value in

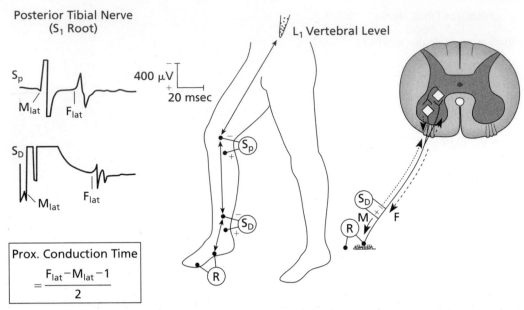

**FIGURE 38-5** Pathways and form of an F-response, measuring conduction in the proximal portions of a motor nerve and the ventral root of the spinal cord. *SD,* distal stimulus; *SP,* proximal stimulus; *R,* recording electrode. *(From Haldeman S: Spine 9:42, 1984.)*

documenting radiculopathy. However, Stolov[62] found abnormal SEPs in 17 of 18 patients with surgically demonstrated spinal stenosis. Snowden et al,[58] using independent evaluation of dermatomal somatosensory evoked potentials in spinal stenosis, demonstrated a sensitivity of 78% for multiple root disease and 93% for multiple plus single root disease. There were 3 false positive cases out of the 58 patients studied.

## Peripheral Neuropathy

Peripheral nerves can be injured or affected in a number of metabolic disorders including diabetes mellitus and hypothyroidism. These nerves are highly vulnerable to toxic exposure, especially by prolonged alcohol use and exposure to lead and other heavy metals and industrial chemicals. In the industrialized nations, there has been a rapid growth in repetitive trauma injury to nerves as they pass through narrow canals. Carpal tunnel syndrome, tardive ulnar palsy, and tarsal tunnel syndrome are among the most common of these entrapment neuropathies. Furthermore, peripheral nerves can be subjected to direct injury by a blow or penetrating wound. Radial and peroneal neuropathies are amongst the most common of these peripheral nerve injuries. In addition, there are a number of hereditary peripheral polyneuropathies as well as postinfectious polyneuropathies such as Guillain-Barré syndrome and the brachial and sciatic plexopathies. All of these disorders can result in functional impairment and disability.

In many of these conditions, the clinical examination and history are sufficient to make a diagnosis. However, testing is often necessary in individuals with feelings of numbness and/or pain in the extremities, especially if such symptoms are progressive and not well-delineated on the clinical examination. The following are the more commonly utilized neurodiagnostic tests for peripheral neuropathies.

### Motor nerve conduction

Motor nerve conduction has the advantage of recording a large potential when a nerve is stimulated at various sites along its course (Fig. 38-6). It is possible, for example, to record a response from the thenar muscle in the hand on stimulation of the median nerve at the wrist, above the elbow, in the axilla, and at Erb's point. The localization of a lesion is made considerably easier by means of these tests, which are commonly utilized in the diagnosis of all forms of peripheral and entrapment neuropathies.

### Sensory nerve conduction

Peripheral sensory neuropathies are commonly studied by means of recording sensory nerve conduction velocities and amplitudes in the upper and lower extremities. Changes in sensory nerve conduction across the median nerve appear to be the earliest detectable abnormality in carpal tunnel syndrome. With more sophisticated techniques and computer averaging, it is possible to record sensory nerve conduction through most of a peripheral sensory pathway and, when combined with somatosensory evoked poten-

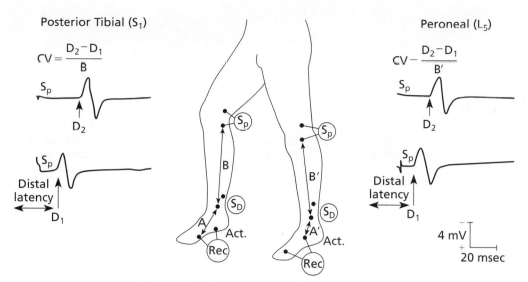

**FIGURE 38-6**    Pathways and form of standard motor nerve conduction studies in the posterior tibial and peroneal nerves.    *(From Haldeman S: Spine 9:42, 1984.)*

tials, the techniques can be used to record impulses throughout the somatosensory neuraxis.

### Reflex studies

Studies of H and F responses in peripheral neuropathies are less common than motor and sensory nerve conduction studies. Tests for F-responses, however, are often the easiest available for studying proximal neuropathies such as Guillain-Barré syndrome and plexopathies.

### Needle electromyography

The detection of denervation may be important in documenting traumatic peripheral nerve injuries. Localization of the injury by means of the level of denervation in a muscle can be most helpful. It is also of value to know whether a nerve injury is complete or partial by recording muscle responses on stimulation of the nerve proximal to an area of injury.

## Bowel, Bladder, and Sexual Disorders

Often the most significant and distressing symptoms in certain cerebral disorders, partial myelopathies, and cauda equina syndrome are the associated disturbances in bowel, bladder, and sexual function. Since complaints of bowel or bladder urgency, sexual impotency, and anorgasmia are difficult to confirm in the clinical examination, testing is often important in order to make the diagnosis.[32]

### Cystometry and urodynamics

The utilization of the cystometrogram and urodynamic studies to investigate bladder function has become increasingly sophisticated (see Ch. 35). Figure 38-7 demonstrates the testing that may be of value in isolating neurologic lesions affecting bowel, bladder, or sexual functioning. The cystometrogram has the capacity to differentiate peripheral from central nervous system disorders affecting the bladder. Peripheral neuropathies and injuries to the cauda equina are more likely to cause an areflexic cystometrogram, often with symptoms of urinary retention and overflow incontinence. Lesions affecting the central nervous system, and particularly the spinal cord, are more likely to cause hyperreflexia with symptoms of urinary urgency and frequency. Urodynamic studies can assist in determining the presence of dyssynergia of the urethral sphincter, which can result in urinary retention. Although 24-hour monitoring of bladder and urethral pressure has been reported, this remains an experimental procedure.[9]

### Electrodiagnostic studies

Somatosensory evoked potentials of the pudendal nerve test the neurogenic pathways within the S2-S4 nerve roots, cauda equina and spinal cord. This nerve follows pathways similar to the pelvic nerves to the bladder and bowel. Abnormalities anywhere along the pudendal somatosensory neuraxis can result in an inability to record a cortical response. These tests have been noted to be abnormal in patients with bowel, bladder, or sexual dysfunction due to diabetes, multiple sclerosis, and spinal cord injuries.[33-35] The test, however, does not differentiate between peripheral and central neurogenic pathways in most patients, because a spinal response is difficult to obtain.

The presence of bulbocavernosus reflex responses allows differentiation from central and peripheral lesions when combined with somatosensory pudendal

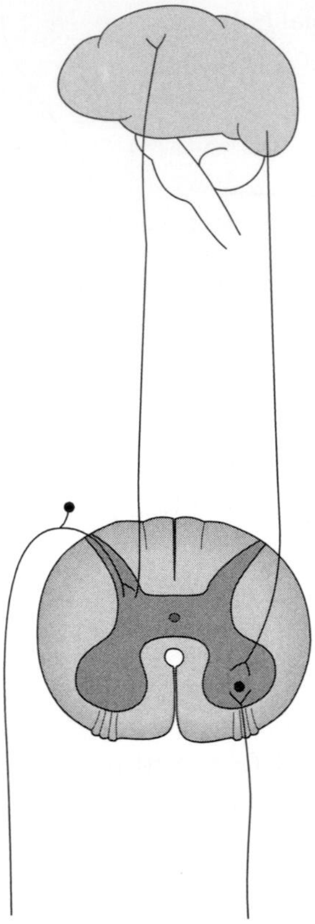

CENTRAL SENSORY

Cortical Evoked Responses
Electroencephalography

CENTRAL MOTOR

Cystometry
Colonometry
Nocturnal Penile Tumescence

PERIPHERAL SENSORY

Sensory Conduction
Spinal Evoked Response
Cystometry
Bulbocavernosus Reflex

PERIPHERAL MOTOR

Bulbocavernosus Reflex
Cystometry
Colonometry
Sphincter EMG

**FIGURE 38-7**    Tests used to evaluate neurologic lesions affecting bowel, bladder, or sexual dysfunction. *(From Haldeman S, Bradley WE, Bhatia NN: Bull LA Neurol Soc 47:76, 1983.)*

evoked potentials. The bulbocavernosus reflex response records a reflex loop through the sacral spinal cord and the cauda equina. It is noted to be abnormal in disorders affecting these structures including diabetes mellitus and tethered cord syndrome.

### Anal EMG and colonometry

The testing of neurologic dysfunction to the bowel is in its infancy. Needle electromyography of the anal sphincter does allow for the detection of denervation potentials. Colonometry has been utilized in the same manner as cystometry for the bladder. In this situation, bowel pressure is recorded on filling of the bowel. Hyperreflexia has been noted in spinal cord injuries and multiple sclerosis, whereas areflexic colonometry has been noted in diabetes mellitus.[30] These tests, however, have not been widely utilized and their sensitivity is not known.

### Penile tumescence and rigidity

It is difficult, on clinical grounds, to differentiate organic from nonorganic causes of impotence. The differentiation commonly requires the measurement of penile erectile function by means of nocturnal penile tumescence testing over a period of one to three nights. More recently the Rigi scan, which measures both tumescence and rigidity of the penis in the home setting, has replaced classic nocturnal penile tumescence testing in most routine settings.

### Muscle Disorders

The primary myopathies include congenital and inflammatory changes within the muscle that result in the breakdown of muscle tissue and decrease in muscle strength. Inflammatory myopathies may also result in generalized pain or tenderness within the muscles. Myasthenia gravis and similar disorders have their primary effect on the neuromuscular junction and result in unique patterns of weakness.

### Blood analysis

The inflammatory and infectious myopathies are most commonly diagnosed by blood evaluation. The measurement of sedimentation rate, creatine phosphokinase, and aldolase may suggest breakdown of muscle tissue. More specific biochemical tests of blood and urine may be necessary for the diagnosis of congenital and rheumatologic muscle diseases. Immunologic tests may be necessary to detect parasitic and other infections affecting muscles.

### Needle electromyography

Needle electromyography in generalized muscle diseases shows a unique pattern. In amyotrophic lateral sclerosis, the diffuse nature of the denervation and fasciculations may be the determining factors for making the diagnosis. In the primary myopathies, unique patterns such as bizarre high frequency potentials and myopathic motor units may help make the diagnosis.

### Repetitive stimulation

Myasthenia gravis is a unique neuromuscular junction disease with a high level of impairment, especially in its advanced stages. One of the most important diagnostic tools for myasthenia gravis is the response to repetitive stimulation of the muscle.[42] This test combined with the tensilon test and immunologic studies are the basis for the diagnosis. Single fiber electromyography for the measurement of jitter has been reported to be more sensitive than repetitive stimulation for the diagnosis of neuromuscular junction disorders.[55,61] (Electromyographic jitter is an assessment of neuromuscular transmission by recording the variation in latency between the potentials generated in two muscle fibers within the same motor unit.) Stalberg et al[61] even state that if jitter is normal, one can rule out myasthenia.

### Biopsy

The primary hereditary myopathies often require biopsy for differential diagnosis. The biopsy findings include the analysis of the staining characteristics as well as the morphology of the muscles. Muscle biopsy may also be important in the diagnosis of amyotrophic lateral sclerosis.

## DOCUMENTATION OF LOSS OF FUNCTION

The documentation of loss of neurologic function is best determined by the clinical examination and can often be extrapolated from testing used in making the diagnosis. The diagnosis is of particular importance in determining prognosis (i.e., Is the condition reversible, stable, or progressive?). In conditions where the diagnosis is clear from the examination, imaging and/or pathological studies (blood tests, spinal tap, biopsy), it may not, however, be clear whether a specific neurological function has been affected or impairment has been caused by the disease. This may require further testing.

Neurodiagnostic testing may be utilized to document the degree of loss of function resulting from a specific diagnosed disease. This infers a quantitative ability to the testing and a correlation between testing and the degree of disability and impairment. Attempts at quantification of the neurodiagnostic testing have generally led to very vague descriptive 4 or 6 point scales of abnormality. These scales commonly describe normal, mild or minimal, slight or moderate, severe, and profound abnormalities or complete loss of the ability to record a test or perform a function.

It is, however, difficult to transfer the concept of neurodiagnostic testing directly into an impairment rating. Most of the tests utilized have very poor sensitivity for the degree of loss of function. Nonetheless, the AMA *Guides* and other rating systems often require that sensory and motor loss and other abnormal neurological function be quantified in rough terms. To a large extent this is dependent upon the clinical evaluation and subjective considerations of the patient and physician. Testing may assist in determining the extent of loss of function but it should be interpreted with caution.

## Cognitive Deficits

Cognitive and intellectual deficits following an injury or illness can vary throughout a scale from normal to comatose. There is also a strong overlap between psychiatric illness and organic cognitive deficits. Although broad estimates of cognitive ability are easy to assess, it may be difficult in a basic clinical examination in a physician's office to define minor or specific degrees of loss of cognitive function. The neurologist is often dependent upon cognitive testing by a neuropsychologist to determine which higher functions are intact and which show significant dysfunction. These concepts are discussed in Chapter 43.

Attempts to correlate objective testing with cognitive deficits have met with mixed results. The so-called "event related potentials" are based on the premise that it is possible to measure disturbances in the neuronal processes accompanying cognition.[31,36,45] These studies, although statistically significant, have not proven to be sufficiently sensitive for diagnostic purposes.

The use of SPECT and PET scanning as a diagnostic tool for Alzheimer's disease has shown a statistical relationship between dementia and metabolic changes in the brain as measured by these procedures.[17,20,50] The sensitivity noted by Claus et al[20] was 42% in mild, 56% in moderate, and 79% in severe Alzheimer's disease. They suggest that the use of SPECT be limited to cases of mild Alzheimer's disease where there is considerable diagnostic doubt on clinical grounds.

## Motor Deficits

The documentation of weakness and the determination of the degree of weakness are primarily dependent upon functional capacity assessments. This is outlined in Chapter 18. Specific neurodiagnostic testing is not very helpful in this regard.

The measurement of interference patterns on needle electromyography gives a crude estimation of the degree of denervation but this is not easily transferred to the amount of weakness. Motor nerve conduction abnormalities can be noted as mild, moderate, or severe but again are not readily transferrable to degrees of weakness. These tests, however, can be of value in documenting complete neurogenic loss of function. Under these circumstances it is not possible to obtain a motor response past an area of nerve injury or record active motor unit potentials during attempts to contract muscles.

Muscle responses evoked by stimulation of the cortical motor strip have been noted to be abnormal in diseases of the primary motor pathways but, at the present time, quantification and the relationship of these tests to the degree of impairment have not been studied.

## Sensory Deficits

Sensory deficits are often rated during impairment examinations. Sensory deficits are, however, difficult to assess on a functional capacity evaluation. Nonetheless, the AMA *Guides* specifically rate pain with sensory loss as a greater impairment than pain without sensory loss.

Sensory nerve conductions in peripheral nerve injuries and peripheral neuropathies can be of value in documenting whether such injuries exist and whether a clinical finding of sensory loss can be verified. They are, however, very crude methods of determining severity or the degree of loss of sensory function. These responses can be described as normal, slightly abnormal, moderately abnormal, severely abnormal, or unobtainable. The relationship of these terms to impairment, however, is not known.

Somatosensory evoked potentials have the ability to document a lesion within the somatosensory system, both peripherally and centrally. They are notably abnormal in peripheral neuropathies and spinal cord lesions. It is, however, not possible to extrapolate a level of impairment from the degree of abnormality of the test. These tests also tend to be normal in patients with impairment caused by pain and altered temperature sensation.[5,47]

## Coordination Deficits

Coordination deficits may exist as a result of motor or sensory deficits from spinal cord, brain, or peripheral nerve injuries. They can also occur from disturbances of equilibrium and balance including vertigo. This may reflect diseases of the vestibular apparatus, brain stem, or cerebellum.

Assessment of coordination therefore requires a diagnosis as well as an understanding of vestibular, auditory visual, and proprioceptive function. The testing of hearing and vision are discussed in other sections of this chapter. Gait and coordination tests are described in other chapters.

In the presence of vertigo, electronystagmography may be helpful in determining the presence of a vestibular lesion or a central disturbance in vestibular function. A tremorgram on EMG may help document and differentiate certain types of tremor but is rarely necessary. The primary test for impairment as a result of incoordination is the clinical examination.

## VERIFICATION OF SUBJECTIVE COMPLAINTS

The strong emphasis of most disability systems on objective findings rather than subjective complaints has resulted in a proliferation of testing procedures in an attempt to confirm subjective complaints. Social Security Administration guidelines specifically state that subjective complaints of impairment must manifest themselves in signs or laboratory tests confirming anatomical, physiological, or psychological abnormalities.[65]

The primary nonspecific subjective complaints that can present with a normal clinical examination are pain, muscle spasm, dysesthesias, and vague feelings of weakness and fatigue. Minor cognitive and psychological symptoms are addressed in Chapter 43.

## Pain

One of the major causes of perceived impairment among patients is pain. Unfortunately, pain cannot be measured at this time or quantified by means of any neurologic testing. It remains a subjective sensation on the part of the patients with variable psychological and emotional responses.

The AMA *Guides* do rate pain associated with sensory deficits higher than pain with normal sensation. This has raised the importance of sensory nerve conduction and somatosensory evoked response testing beyond their diagnostic value. It has yet to be shown, however, that these tests relate in any way to the sensation of pain. Testing to assess pain is discussed in Chapter 47.

Previous attempts at relating thermographic changes to pain have been unsuccessful. Although thermography can measure skin temperature, most independent agencies, on review of the literature, have concluded that the test does not add sufficient diagnostic information to be useful. The observation that thermography is abnormal in reflex sympathetic dystrophy and causalgia is one possible exception (see Chapter 16).

## Weakness and Paresthesias

Subjective statements of weakness and paresthesias in the absence of documentable pathology on imaging and other studies may lead the clinician on a long search for an explanation. It is very easy to over-interpret or abuse neurologic testing in this setting. Minor abnormalities can be found in multiple tests that may in fact have no correlation with the clinical symptom patterns.

The EMG has a significant subjective interpretive component to its analysis that is dependent on the skill and experience of the physician. The test is rarely transferred to hard copy and the experience of clinicians in differentiating potentials can vary greatly. The AMA *Guides* recommend that technicians be certified by the American Board of Electrodiagnostic Medicine and that testing should be done in a laboratory meeting the guidelines of the American Association of Electrodiagnostic Medicine. Minor EMG changes such as slight increase in insertional potentials, mild polyphasia, and the misinterpretation of motor end plate potentials as fibrillations may be falsely reported as abnormal. The EMG should be considered an extension of the neurological examination and other testing and should not stand alone as a documentation of organic weakness.

## Muscle Spasm

One of the more controversial clinical findings in patients seeking disability is the presence of muscle spasm or tenderness. The AMA *Guides* recognize the presence of muscle guarding and nonuniform range of motion but consider this only in the category of minor impairment.

Attempts to objectify muscle spasm have not been very rewarding. Needle EMG has shown that areas of muscle tenderness are electrically silent.[40] Certain experimental techniques such as the direct recording of muscle spindle activity and the recording of cortical evoked responses on magnetic stimulation have shown some promise in looking at this issue.[38,68]

Surface EMG has also been proposed as a method of recording muscle guarding and unequal muscle contraction leading to nonuniform balance. Ahern[1] noted changes in surface EMG during dynamic flexion and extension in 89% of patients with low-back pain but also in 13% of asymptomatic patients. There was also no difference at rest between symptomatic and asymptomatic patients. Sihvonen[56] similarly found abnormalities in chronic back pain but also in a significant number of control subjects, which suggests that the sensitivity of that test is low.

## False-Positive Testing

The interpretations of abnormalities on nerve conduction tests are dependent upon the perceived normal values. There is variation between published normal values by different authorities and such values are not always transferable to a specific clinical laboratory. Factors that influence measurements include stimulus strength, inaccurate calibration or measurement, age and temperature.[41,44,57] The ideal situation is for each clinical laboratory to establish normative values based on age, sex, and skin temperature. This, however, is not always practical. Most electrodiagnosticians use normative values published from an academic laboratory. The problem is that this can leave some doubt as to the cutoff points for abnormality. Extreme care must be taken when dealing with values at the borderline between normal and abnormal. The comparison between a symptomatic and asymptomatic limb may be of assistance but even in this situation there can be fairly high variations between normal subjects.

Reflex and evoked responses can show significant variations between sides of the body, according to age, and with repeated study. In addition, the reflex and somatosensory evoked potentials show marked variation according to patient height. Amplitude variation in H-reflexes also can be extremely variable and dependent upon the location of electrodes. Anything less than a 50% reduction in side-to-side amplitude of H-reflexes should be considered within normal limits. Amplitude variation on somatosensory evoked potentials can be marked even when reproduced in the same individual on stimulation of the same nerve. Amplitude variations must be interpreted with extreme caution and probably should not be taken into account when interpreting somatosensory evoked responses.

Differentiating between normal and abnormal evoked responses requires considerable experience and understanding of the testing. Although brain stem auditory evoked potentials are the most stable of these tests,[53] there are significant variations in interpeak latencies in the same patient when comparing one ear with the other or reproducing the test in the same ear after a two-year interval.[64] Latency measurements depend on the point where a peak is assumed to begin or be maximum. These points can vary and are influenced by interference from muscle contraction or movement of the patient. Minor side-to-side differences should not be considered significant unless there are very tight controls on technique. Oken and Chiappa[49] reiterate the fact that when a normal value is taken as the mean plus two standard deviations, then 5% of normal patients may be considered to have abnormal test results. It is therefore recommended that mean plus three standard deviations be considered the basis of measuring normal values.

Electroencephalographic findings may be over-interpreted. Phantom spike, wave, and mu patterns, as well as movement artifact, may appear as abnormalities to the unsophisticated electroencephalographer. Asynchronous, intermittent, focal, temporal slow delta transient potentials can be found in 30% to 60% of normal controls, yet have the appearance of being abnormalities. Simultaneous recording of procedures that can explain potential artifacts, such as EKG, eye movement, and muscle contraction, can explain some of the artifactual changes and help reduce the misinterpretation of wave forms.

The correlation of imaging studies with neurologic disability and impairment is not always accurate. Numerous small white-matter lesions can be seen in the brain of normal individuals and do not always correlate with clinical symptoms or impairment. Similarly, extensive degenerative changes and disc herniations in the cervical, thoracic, and lumbar spine have been documented to be present in the absence of symptomatology or disability.

## CONCLUSION

Neurodiagnostic testing is extremely important in the evaluation of patients with neurological diseases that can lead to disability and impairment. The primary importance of neurodiagnostic testing is in the diagnosis of a potentially disabling disease or injury. The documentation and localization of a lesion is the basis for most diagnoses and is dependent on the correlation of the history, physical examination, and appropriate testing. At all times, however, the choice of testing and the interpretation of test results is dependent upon the suspected diagnosis. All diagnostic tests must be correlated with the history and physical examination before a diagnosis is reached.

Neurodiagnostic testing is only of slight value in the documentation of loss of neurologic function and the quantification of such losses. The correlation between test results and the degree of impairment in most diseases and injuries has not been adequately studied. However, when closely correlated with the patient's clinical examination, the degree of abnormality of a test may help the clinician reach a conclusion as to the presence and amount of loss of function.

Neurodiagnostic testing is of minimal or no value in confirming nonspecific subjective complaints. Neurodiagnostic testing cannot confirm the presence of pain symptomatology, dysesthesias, or muscle weakness in the absence of a well-defined disease entity. Extreme care must be taken to avoid abuse based on minor abnormalities or false-positive results in neurodiagnostic testing due to poor understanding or interpretation of a test. A full understanding of the factors causing variability in test results and the normal variations between laboratories and between patients is essential before giving credence to a test, if the patient has no other corresponding objective clinical findings.

## References

1. Ahern DK, Follick MJ, Council JR, et al: Comparison of lumbar paravertebral EMG patterns in chronic low back pain patients and non-patient controls. *Pain* 34(2):153-160, Aug 1988.
2. Aiello I, Serra G, Migliore A, et al: Diagnostic use of H-reflex from vastus medialis muscle. *Electromyogr Clin Neurophysiol* 23:159-166, 1983.
3. Aiello I, Serra G, Tugnoli V, et al: Electrophysiological findings in patients with lumbar disc prolapse. *Electromyogr Clin Neurophysiol* 24(4):313-320, May 1984.
4. American Medical Association: *Guides to the evaluation of permanent impairment*, ed 4, Chicago, 1993.
5. Anziska B, Cracco RQ: Short latency somatosensory evoked potentials. Studies in patients with focal neurological disease. *Electroencephalogr Clin Neurophysiol* 49:227-239, 1980.
6. Awad IA, Spetzler RF, et al: Incidental subcortical lesions identified on magnetic resonance imaging in the elderly: I—Correlations with age and cerebrovascular risk factors, *Stroke* 17:1084-1989, 1986.
7. Baldereschi M, Amato MP, Nencini P, et al: Cross-national interrater agreement on the clinical diagnostic criteria for dementia. *Neurology* 44:239-242, 1994.

8. Baumhefner RW, Tourtellotte WW, et al: Quantitative MS plaque assessment with MRI. Its correlation with clinical parameters, EPs, and intra blood-brain barrier. *Arch Neurol* 47:19-26, 1990.

9. Bhatia NN, Bradley WE, Haldeman S, et al: Continuous monitoring of bladder and urethral pressure, a new technique. *Urology* 18:207-210, 1981.

10. Biering-Sorenson F, Hansen FR, Schroll M, et al: The relation of spinal x-ray to low back pain and physical activity among 60-year-old men and women. *Spine* 10(5):445-451, June 1985.

11. Bigos SJ, Hansson T, Castillo RN, et al: The value of pre-employment roentgenographs for predicting acute back injury claims and chronic back pain disability. *Clin Orthop Rel Res* 283:124-129, Oct 1992.

12. Bischoff C, Meyer BU, et al: The value of magnetic stimulation in the diagnosis of radiculopathies, *Muscle Nerve* 16:154-161, 1993.

13. Boden SD, Davis DO, Dina TS, et al: Abnormal magnetic resonance scans of the lumbar spine in asymptomatic subjects. *J Bone Joint Surg [Am]* 72(3):403-408, 1990.

14. Braddom RI, Joynson EW: Standardization of H reflex and diagnostic use in S1 radiculopathy. *Arch Phys Med Rehabil* 55:161-166, 1974.

15. Bradley WG Jr, Waluch V, Brant-Zawadzki M, et al: Patchy, periventricular white matter lesions in the elderly: a common observation during NMR imaging, *Noninv Med Imag* 1:35-41, 1984.

16. Brant-Zawadzki M, Fein G, et al: MR imaging of the aging brain: patchy white matter lesions and dementia, *AJNR Am J Neuroradiol* 6:675-682, 1985.

17. Burns A, Philpot MP, et al: The investigation of Alzheimer's disease with single photon emission tomography, *J Neurol Neurosurg Psychiatry* 52:248-253, 1989.

18. Chiappa KH: *Evoked potentials in clinical medicine*, New York, 1989, Raven Press.

19. Chiappa KH, Jayakar P: Evoked potentials in clinical medicine. In Joynt RJ, editor, *Clinical neurology 1*, Philadelphia, 1992, J.B. Lippincott.

20. Claus JJ, van Harskamp F, Breteler MMB, et al: The diagnostic value of SPECT with Tc-99m HMPAO in Alzheimer's disease: a population-based study, *Neurology* 44:454-461, 1994.

21. Eggermont JJ, Don M, Brackmann DE: Electrocochleography and auditory brain stem electric responses in patients with pontine angle tumors, *Ann Otol Rhinol Laryngol (Suppl)* 89:75, 1980.

22. Eisen A, Schomer D, Melmed C: The application of F-wave measurements in the differentiation of proximal and distal upper limb entrapments. *Neurology* 27:662-688, 1977.

23. Eisen A, Schomer D, Melmed C: An electrophysiological method for examining lumbosacral root compression. *Can J Neurol Sci* 4:117-123, 1977.

24. Eisen A, Shtybel W: Experience with transcranial magnetic stimulation. *Muscle Nerve* 13:995-1011, 1990.

25. El Negamy E, Sedgwick EM: Delayed cervical somatosensory potentials in cervical spondylosis. *J Neurol Neurosurg Psychiatry* 42:238-241, 1979.

26. Farrer LA, Cupples LA, et al: Interrater agreement for diagnosis of Alzheimer's disease: the MIRAGE study. *Neurology* 44:652-656, 1994.

27. Filippi M, Horsefield MA, et al: Quantitative brain MRI lesion load predicts the course of clinically isolated syndromes suggestive of multiple sclerosis. *Neurology* 44:635-641, 1994.

28. Fisher MA, Shivde AJ, Teixera C, et al: Clinical and electrophysiological appraisal of the significance of radicular injury in back pain, *J Neurol Neurosurg Psychiatry* 41:303-306, 1978.

29. Galasko D, Abramson I, et al: Repeated exposure to the Mini-Mental State Examination and the Information-Memory-Concentration Test results in a practice effect in Alzheimer's disease, *Neurology* 43:1559-1563, 1993.

30. Glick ME, Meshkinpour H, Haldeman, S et al: Colonic dysfunction in patients with thoracic spinal cord injury. *Gastroenterology* 86:287-294, 1984.

31. Goodin DS, Squires KC, Starr A: Long latency event-related components of the auditory evoked potential in dementia, *Brain* 101:635-648, 1978.

32. Haldeman S: The neurodiagnostic evaluation of spinal stenosis. In Andersson GBJ, McNeil TW, editors: *Lumbar Spinal Stenosis,* St. Louis, 1992, Mosby–Year Book.

33. Haldeman S, Bradley WE, Bhatia NN, et al: Neurologic evaluation of bladder, bowel and sexual disturbances in diabetic men. In Goto Y, Horiuchi A, Kogure K, editors: *Diabetic neuropathy: Proceedings of the International Symposium on Diabetic Neuropathy and Its Treatment,* Tokyo, Sept 1981, Amsterdam, 1982, Excerpta Medica.

34. Haldeman S, Bradley WE, Bhatia NN, et al: Pudendal evoked responses in neurologic disease. *Neurology* 32:A67, 1982.

35. Haldeman S, Bradley WE, Bhatia NN, et al: Pudendal evoked responses. *Arch Neurol* 39:280-283, 1982.

36. Hillyard SA, Kutas M: Electrophysiology of cognitive processing, *Annu Rev Psychol* 34:33-61, 1983.

37. Hitselberger WE, Witten RM. Abnormal myelograms in asymptomatic patients. *J Neurosurg* 28:204-208, 1968.

38. Hubbard DR: Sympathetic spindle spasm. Presented at the annual meeting of the California Medical Association, March 1992, Anaheim, California.

39. Ikeda H, Tremain E, Sanders MD: Neurophysiological investigation in optic nerve disease: Combined assessment of the visual evoked response and electroretinogram. *Br J Ophthalmol* 62:227-239, 1978.

40. Johnson EW: The myth of skeletal muscle spasm. *Am J Phys Med Rehabil* 68:1, 1989.

41. Kaplan PE: Sensory and motor residual latency measurements in healthy patients and patients with neuropathy: Part I. *J Neurol Neurosurg Psychiatry* 39:338, 1976.

42. Kimura J: *Electrodiagnosis in diseases of nerve and muscle: principles and practice,* Philadelphia, 1983, FA Davis.

43. Koopmans RA, Li DKB, et al: Benign versus chronic progressive multiple sclerosis; magnetic resonance imaging features. *Ann Neurol* 25:74-81, 1989.

44. Mayer RF: Nerve conduction studies in man. *Neurology* 13:1021, 1963.

45. Michalewski HJ, Rosenberg C, Starr A: Event-related potentials in dementia. In Cracco RQ, Bodis-Wollner I, editors: *Evoked potentials,* New York, 1986, Alan R. Liss.

46. Nath S, Sherman J, Bass S: VEP delays in macular disease (ARVO Suppl). *Invest Ophthalmol Vis Sci* 22(3):60, 1982.

47. Noel P, Desmedt JE: Somatosensory cerebral evoked potentials after vascular lesions of the brain-stem and diencephalon. *Brain* 98:113-128, 1975.

48. Nogues MA, Pardal AM, Merello M, Miguel MA: SEPs and CNS magnetic stimulation in syringomyelia. *Muscle Nerve* 15:993-1001, 1992.

49. Oken BS, Chiappa KH: Somatosensory evoked potentials in neurologic diagnosis. In Cracco RQ, Bodis-Wollner I, editors: *Evoked potentials,* New York, 1986, Alan R Liss.

50. Perani D, De Piero V, Vallar G, et al: Technetium-99m HMPAO SPECT study of regional cerebral perfusion in early Alzheimer's disease. *J Nucl Med* 19:1507-1514, 1988.

51. Powell MC, Wilson M, Szypryt P, et al: Prevalence of lumbar disc degeneration observed by magnetic resonance in symptomless women. *Lancet* 13; 2(8520):1366-1367, 1986.

52. Restuccia D, Di Lazzaro V, Valeriana M, et al: N24 spinal response to tibial nerve stimulation and magnetic resonance imaging in lesions of the lumbosacral spinal cord. *Neurology* 43:2269-2275, 1993.

53. Robinson K, Rudge P: The stability of the auditory evoked potentials in normal man and patients with multiple sclerosis. *J Neurol Sci* 35:147-156, 1978.

54. Schmidt R, Fazekas F, et al: Neuropsychologic correlates of MRI white matter hyperintensities: a study of 150 normal volunteers, *Neurology* 43:2490-2494, 1993.

55. Schwartz MS, Stalberg E: Myasthenia gravis with features of the myasthenic syndrome: an investigation with electrophysiologic methods including single-fiber electromyography. *Neurology* 25:80, 1975.

56. Sihvonen T, Partanen J, Hanninen O, et al: Electric behavior of low back muscles during lumbar pelvic rhythm in low back pain patients and healthy controls. *Arch Phys Med Rehabil* 72:1080-1087, 1991.

57. Simpson JA: Fact and fallacy in measurement of conduction velocity in motor nerves, *J Neurol Neurosurg Psychiatry* 27:381, 1964.

58. Snowden ML, Haselkorn JK, Kraft GH, et al: Dermatomal somatosensory evoked potentials in the diagnosis of lumbosacral spinal stenosis; comparison with imaging studies, *Muscle Nerve* 15:1036-1044, 1992.

59. Spengler DM, Freeman CW: Patient selection for lumbar discectomy: an objective approach. *Spine* 4(2):129-134, 1979.

60. Spengler DM, Ouellette EA, Battie M, et al: Elective discectomy for herniation of a lumbar disc: additional experience with an objective method, *J Bone Joint Surg [Am]* 72(2):230-237, 1990.

61. Stalberg E, Trantelj JV, Schwartz MS: Single-muscle-fiber recording of the jitter phenomenon in patients with myasthenia gravis and in members of their families. *Ann NY Acad Sci* 274:189, 1976.

62. Stolov WC, Slimp JC: Dermatomal somatosensory evoked potentials in lumbar spinal stenosis, in *Proceedings,* Am Assoc Electromyography and Electrodiagnosis/Am Electroencephalography Soc Joint Symp, 1988: 17-22.

63. Tavy DLJ, Wagner GL, Keunen RWM, et al: Transcranial magnetic stimulation in patients with cervical spondylotic myelopathy: clinical and radiological correlations. *Muscle Nerve* 17:235-241, 1994.

64. Tusa RJ, Stewart WF, Shechter AL, et al: Longitudinal study of brainstem auditory evoked re-

sponses in 87 normal human subjects. *Neurology* 44:528-532, 1994.

65. United States Department of Health, Education and Welfare: *Disability evaluation under Social Security: a handbook for physicians*, HEW Publication No. (SSA) 79-10089, Aug. 1979.

66. Wiesel SW, Tsourmas N, Feffer HL, et al: A study of computer assisted tomography: I—The incidence of positive CAT scans in an asymptomatic group of patients. *Spine* 9(6):549-551, 1984.

67. Young A, Getty J, Jackson A, et al: Variations in the pattern of muscle innervation by the L5 and S1 nerve roots. *Spine* 8(6):616-624, 1983.

68. Zhu, Y, Haldeman S, Starr A, et al: Paraspinal muscle evoked cerebral potentials in patients with unilateral low back pain. *Spine* 18(8):1096-1110, 1993.

# CHAPTER 39

# CENTRAL NERVOUS SYSTEM

*Mark N. Ozer*

## NATURE OF THE PROBLEM

Impairments of the central nervous system, that is, the brain, brain stem, and spinal cord, are a major source of disability. As an example, the number of persons in the United States with cerebral vascular disease has been estimated as 2.5 million.[12] A substantial proportion of persons who have had a stroke are in the working-age group. The number of persons with spinal cord injury, most of whom are young, is in the range of 200,000.[13] Injury due to vascular disease affecting the cerebrum and brain stem is usually considered to be focal in nature but actually affects the actions of the entire central nervous system rather than merely the side affected. Trauma is the other major cause of cerebral impairment with a particularly high prevalence rate in the working-age population. The effects of trauma on the spinal cord are specific to the level of lesion whether in the cervical, thoracic, or lumbar cord. Demyelinating disease, most also frequently found in persons of working age, may be diffuse in its effects involving cerebrum, brain stem, and spinal cord segments.

Trauma may be acute in onset and is generally nonprogressive. However, there are changes that occur with time that can modify the initial effects of the trauma. The effects of cerebrovascular disease are acute in onset with improvement frequently found during the first several months after onset. There is considerable likelihood that there will be recurrent episodes with greater degree of subsequent impairment given that the underlying disease process tends to be progressive. The natural history of demyelinating disease is one of either progressive disease or remittently progressive disease with improvement after each acute episode. Thus the degree of impairment must take into consideration the time in the natural history of the disease process when the assessment takes place.

The impairments found vary with the site of involvement in the nervous system. Those arising from the cerebrum can bring about major impairments in language and communication, mental status and integrative function as well as emotional behavioral disturbances. General impairment of consciousness or episodic impairment of consciousness, such as with epileptic seizures, can occur. Major effects are also due to visual disturbances due to involvement of the visual system. Impairments due to brain stem involvement usually create dysfunction of the cranial nerves and can manifest as diplopia and disturbances in hearing and balance as well as swallowing and dysarthria. Impairments related to the spinal cord involve disturbances in physical mobility, and the use of the upper extremities, as well as control of urine, bowels, and sexual function.

Although the degree of impairment is defined by the site and the severity of involvement of that site, the ultimate effects go beyond this to the character of the nervous system as a whole and the person in whom the injury has occurred. The effects are not only due to the injury but the context in which the injury has occurred, such as previous level of training and personality traits as well as, most particularly, the ease with which new learning can occur to compensate in some way for the effects of the existing injury. Thus the overall degree of impairment for the entire person with difficulties arising from any single impairment will reflect the totality of impairments in that person. Particularly critical is the combined effect of motor and/or sensory loss with disturbance of consciousness or emotional and behavioral problems. Difficulties in mental status and integrative functioning can limit the availability and use of new strategies for improvement and may serve to exaggerate the effects of the motor/sensory problems.

The central nervous system is the organ system of adaptation. For example, there is coordination of sensory inputs and motor behavior to produce locomotion. Moreover, such actions are in accordance with the goals of the organism. Complex sets of actions are carried out to produce activities such as eating or dressing to meet the needs of the organism.[2] The central nervous system processes information from the external environment. Monitoring of actions must go on as conditions change. In addition, adaptation by the learning of the new patterns of activities requires the assimilation of information from the external environment. The end result is a stable internal environment despite changes in the external environment. Each of these several major activities will be discussed in this chapter in relation to functional impairments arising from the brain stem, spinal cord, and cerebrum.

## CENTRAL NERVOUS SYSTEM AS ORGAN FOR MAINTENANCE OF INTERNAL ENVIRONMENT

The maintenance of adequate fluid and energy supplies can be considered as an example providing a stable internal environment. The requirements include the safe ingestion of liquids and other food, with the cranial nerves in the brain stem responsible for the swallowing mechanism. Also contributory to the maintenance of a stable internal environment is the excretion of wastes via the urinary system or gastrointestinal tract at the appropriate time and place. These excretory activities are the function of the spinal cord modified by the cerebrum. These several actions represent an example of the total system for maintaining stability of internal environment. The actions taken for both ingestion and excretion provide a model of a feedback system that monitors deviation from what may be considered a relatively-fixed set point for fluid and energy balance. Evidence of deviation from the goal or set point will then lead to action which, once again, achieves the desired end point. This portion of the chapter will deal with maintaining the internal homeostatic environment.

### Ingestion

Impairments in swallowing are quite common in persons with cerebrovascular disease directly affecting the brain stem structures and the several cranial nerves. Alternatively bilateral involvement of the cerebral hemispheres can in turn affect the ability of the brain stem structures to carry out their coordinating function. Less commonly, dysphagia may also result from unilateral cerebral hemispheric involvement. The effects of the impairment may be amplified by preexisting changes due to aging already compromising the swallowing mechanism.[4]

Table 39-1 from the AMA *Guides*[5] describes the degree of impairment of the "whole person" attributable to difficulties relating to swallowing. Although

**TABLE 39-1    IMPAIRMENT CRITERIA FOR CRANIAL NERVES IX AND XII**

| IMPAIRMENT DESCRIPTION | % IMPAIRMENT OF THE WHOLE PERSON |
|---|---|
| Mild dysarthria or dysphagia with choking on liquids or semisolid food | 1–14 |
| Moderately-severe dysarthria or dysphagia with hoarseness, nasal regurgitation, and aspiration of liquids or semisolid foods | 15–39 |
| Severe inability to swallow or handle oral secretions without choking, with need for assistance and suctioning | 40–60 |

From AMA *Guides*, ed 4, 1993, American Medical Association, Chicago.

described in the context of cranial nerves IX and XII, the functional difficulties reflect the wide range of coordinated activities to be described below. The severity of the dysphagia tends to be reflected more readily in problems with liquids. Aspiration consists of material actually entering the respiratory tract (averaging 27% impairment), whereas symptoms such as choking or coughing might serve to protect the respiratory tract and thus the rating of degree of impairment is significantly less (averaging 7%). Requirement for assistance or suctioning leads to major impairment of the entire person (averaging 50%).

The swallowing mechanism involves several steps starting with the ingestion of food.[4] The *oral preparatory phase* includes mastication and salivary lubrication leading to cohesive bolus formation and placement of the bolus on the tongue preparatory to the actual process of swallowing. Neural control of mastication is thought to be provided by a neural pattern generator in the reticular formation of the brain stem. Peripheral sensory feedback provided by intraoral receptors and transmitted via the trigeminal nerve is believed to play a role in the initiation and ongoing modification of this process. Lower motor neuron innervation for the muscles of mastication is provided by the trigeminal nerve, whereas the labial and buccal musculature is supplied by the facial nerve and the intrinsic lingual musculature by the hypoglossic nerve. The requirements of this phase include adequate sealing by the lips and coordinated oral manipulation of the bolus. Pocketing of food in the cheek of the affected side can be a problem. All of these problems can occur with impairments of the facial musculature and tongue as well as bilateral cerebral involvement.

The *oral phase* is the actual voluntary initiation of swallowing. The tongue is used to squeeze the bolus into the upper portion of the pharynx with concomitant elevation of the palate to close off the nasopharynx to prevent leakage. Both these actions can be compromised by poor control of the cranial nerves carrying out these actions.

The *pharyngeal phase* is a complex series of motor actions normally completed in one second. The reflex is triggered by the stimulation of sensory receptors by the bolus. Triggering of the swallowing reflex generally occurs on transfer of the bolus to the oropharynx, at which time facial, glossopharyngeal, and vagus nerves transmit afferent messages to the swallowing center in the reticular substance of the medulla from sensory receptors in the faucial arches, tonsils, velum, base of the tongue, and posterior pharyngeal wall. Lower motor neuron innervation of the pharyngeal and laryngeal musculature originates in the ipsilateral nucleus ambiguus and travels through glossopharyngeal and vagus nerves. A number of events occur simultaneously. For example, the larynx is pulled upward; the vocal folds are adducted and the epiglottis tilted. All serve to protect the airway. Contraction of the pharyngeal walls results in initiation of a peristaltic wave propelling the bolus to pass into the upper esophagus through the now-open cricopharyngeal sphincter. Delay in initiation of the reflex and reduced peristalsis can occur with increased likelihood of aspiration. Other actions necessary for airway protection are also compromised by the delay. Cricopharyngeal sphincter dysfunction may also prevent complete passage of the bolus into the upper esophagus with resultant increased risk of aspiration.

The *esophageal phase*, lasting 8 - 20 seconds, completes the movement of the bolus by way of peristalsis through the segments of the esophagus to the stomach through the lower esophageal sphincter. Neural control of the esophageal phase is independent from that for the preceding phases and involves interaction between central and peripheral neurons. The striated muscles of the upper one-third of the esophagus are supplied by the lower motor neurons of the nucleus ambiguus, whereas innervation of the smooth muscle of the more caudal end of the esophagus is believed to involve parasympathetic pathways originating in the dorsal motor nucleus of the vagus nerve. The effect of cerebral or brain stem injury on the action of the esophagus may be to worsen the effects of preexisting esophageal reflux caused by a hiatal hernia by the above mentioned compromise of pharyngeal mobility and reduced airway protection.

## Excretion

The other aspect of the system for energy supply illustrative of maintenance of the internal environment is the excretion of waste products via the urinary and gastrointestinal system. The excretion of waste via the urinary tract will serve as a primary example. Defecation follows a similar neural pattern. Both involve the coordination within both the spinal cord and cerebrum of sensory input and outflow both to smooth and striated muscles.

Impairments in the urinary system are frequently found in persons with spinal cord injury.[9] The character of the disturbance will vary with the level of the spinal cord at which the injury has occurred as well as the extent of the injury. Disturbance of urination is also common in those with cerebral involvement. Once again the impact of the impairment due to the involvement of the central nervous system is amplified by preexisting problems in the person. For example, preexisting prostatic obstruction of the outflow tract may lead to worsening of urinary retention following injury to the brain. Another example is when preexisting frequency due to a small capacity bladder may lead to actual incontinence once the person is no longer able to get out of bed to urinate due to motor weakness.

Tables 39-2 and 39-3 from the AMA *Guides*[5] reflect the degree of whole person impairment attributable to the degree of voluntary control available for bladder and bowel. The development of reflex type bladder and bowel activity can substitute in part for the lack of voluntary control. Thus the presence of good bladder reflex activity permits a significantly lower level of impairment as exemplified by reduction in degree of impairment averaging 18% rather than 32% in the absence of satisfactory reflex control. The equivalent level of reflex regulation of the bowel in the absence of any voluntary control leads to a higher degree of whole person impairment. The degree of impairment averages 30% whereas it is an average of 18% for those with bladder reflex control. This, of course, reflects the higher social consequences of failure to maintain satisfactory bowel control and the greater likelihood of accidents in the content of reflex control alone. The physiologic background for these functional areas is exemplified by the following discussion of micturition.

Micturition at the appropriate time and in the appropriate place requires both adequate storage of urine and emptying. Urine storage and excretion require a coordinated action of the bladder wall and the

**TABLE 39-2      CRITERIA FOR NEUROLOGIC IMPAIRMENT OF BLADDER**

| IMPAIRMENT DESCRIPTION | % IMPAIRMENT OF THE WHOLE PERSON |
|---|---|
| Patient has some degree of voluntary control but is impaired by urgency or intermittent incontinence | 1–9 |
| Patient has good bladder reflex activity, limited capacity, and intermittent emptying without voluntary control | 10–24 |
| Patient has poor bladder reflex activity, intermittent dribbling, and no voluntary control | 25–39 |
| Patient has no reflex or voluntary control of bladder | 40–60 |

From AMA *Guides,* ed 4, 1993, American Medical Association, Chicago.

**TABLE 39-3      CRITERIA FOR NEUROLOGIC ANORECTAL IMPAIRMENT**

| IMPAIRMENT DESCRIPTION | % IMPAIRMENT OF THE WHOLE PERSON |
|---|---|
| Anorectum has reflex regulation but only limited voluntary control | 1–19 |
| Anorectum has reflex regulation but no voluntary control | 20–39 |
| Anorectum has *no* reflex regulation or voluntary control | 40–50 |

From AMA *Guides,* ed 4, 1993, American Medical Association, Chicago.

sphincter systems consisting of both striated and doubly innervated smooth muscles. Normally, an emptying contraction occurs when the bladder is full. The external striated muscle (urethral) urinary sphincter, usually in a state of tonic contraction throughout filling, now relaxes. The emptying mechanism involves the detrusor smooth muscle, which is mainly but not entirely cholinergic. The contraction of the bladder opens the bladder neck, and urine passes out through the relaxed external urinary sphincter until the bladder is empty. The closing mechanism consists of the striated external sphincter of the urethra, other striated muscles of the pelvic floor, and the smooth muscle bundles of the bladder neck (mainly alpha-adrenergic). This normal alternating activity between the bladder detrusor and the sphincters is the under the control of the brain stem micturition center.

In respect to micturition, the parasympathetic detrusor center arises from the intermediolateral cell column of S2-S4, with a major portion arising one segment higher than the more anterior pudendal nuclei innervating the body of the bladder. Conversely, the sympathetic outflow from the thoraco-lumbar intermediolateral cell column T11-L1 is inhibitory and promotes urine storage. Beta-adrenergic receptors in the bladder body lead to detrusor relaxation with epinephrine release. Conversely, the bladder base and proximal urethra contain more alpha-adrenergic receptors. Sympathetic stimulation produces smooth muscle contraction, described as the smooth muscle sphincter, aiding in urine storage.

Normal micturition is a brain stem reflex rather than a simple sacral reflex. Afferent discharges resulting from a full bladder travel through the pelvic nerve and pathways within the spinal cord to synapse in a supravesical micturition center thought to be in the rostral pons. It is at this level that the coordination between bladder contraction and sphincter relaxation is accomplished.

Disconnection between the brain stem micturition center and the sacral cord due to transection of the spinal cord above the level of S2-S4 leads to poor coordination between the action of the detrusor and the sphincter. During bladder emptying there may be dyssynergia in that the sphincter will fail to open completely, with simultaneous contraction of the bladder detrusor. The bladder wall may, however, contract independently of the control of the brain stem micturition center. The disconnection permits the development of a reflex type bladder wherein emptying can occur with various forms of external stimulation of the abdominal wall. However, the dyssynergia that frequently accompanies the reflex bladder arising from a lesion above the level of the sacral cord limits effective emptying.

A lesion of the sacral cord at the level of the parasympathetic detrusor center leads to denervation of the parasympathetic cholinergic outflow. The effect is to reduce the contractility of the detrusor. Other effects depend on the continued intact sympathetic outflow arising from the thoraco-lumbar cord above the level of lesion. The now unopposed sympathetic action continues to maintain closure of the alpha-adrenergic internal sphincter. Once again, there is resultant lack of complete emptying as in the case of a lesion above the level of the sacral cord.

Furthermore, it is thought that volitional control of voiding depends on communication between the frontal cortex and the brain stem micturition center. When these lines of communication are disturbed, as is often seen in cerebral dysfunction, the most common occurrence is loss of cortical inhibition, resulting in detrusor hyperreflexia with incontinence.[10]

## CENTRAL NERVOUS SYSTEM AS ORGAN FOR ADAPTATION TO EXTERNAL ENVIRONMENT

The interaction between the organism and the external environment must lead to the assimilation of appropriate sensory input that must then be acted upon. The action taken must be in accordance with the goals of the individual and progress must be monitored in relation to the degree to which goals are being achieved. One can then change such actions in accordance with the changing environmental conditions and goals. The model is of a feedback loop monitoring progress in accordance with a changing set of points. The three components are then the sensory input, motor control, and integrative output.

### Sensory Input

Basic to the proper operation of this adaptive system is the adequacy of the sensory input. The ability of the organism to carry out motor actions in the absence of consistent sensory input is a major impairment illustrated by production of skin ulcers in persons with spinal cord injury. The receipt of adequate information as to ischemia of the skin evidenced by pain in dependent areas is disrupted by the neural disconnection in spinal cord injury. The loss of awareness of that portion of the body below the level of the lesion deprives the person of the input, ordinarily unconscious, that permits the constant monitoring and subsequent fine-tuning of motor actions. A sense of discomfort can no longer be counted on to signal ischemia of the skin and muscle when one position is maintained for long periods, and it becomes necessary to develop a new set of procedures for the relief of pressure. Instead of relying on the signals of ischemia, one may use a clock to indicate when to change positions. What has previously been a closed loop in which input to the central nervous system had brought about an adaptation without conscious awareness must now become an open loop in which, at least initially, a deliberate decision to act on conscious input must occur in accordance with a schedule.

The type of sensory impairment may also affect the availability of sensory input for particular motor actions. The determination of the type of sensory loss particularly significant to the disruption of function differs from the usual tests used in the neurological examination. Examinations of pinprick and temperature, touch with cotton wool, and vibratory sense with a tuning fork are useful in localizing neurologic lesions. Quite different, however, is the significant sensory finding in relation to function in hand. In order to plan appropriately to reduce disability, Moberg[7] found the relevant afferent input to be that of "tactile gnosis"—the ability of the fingers and hand to "see" what they are doing. The fingers must "feel what they are holding, how they are holding it, and how strongly they are holding it." Being able to differentiate the two blunt ends of a paper clip 10 mm apart establishes the availability of cutaneous sensibility for learning and control. In its absence, visual input is the only alternative. A person dependent on vision can use only one hand at a time, which has significant implications for the degree of impairment in grasp and other hand actions. (This also affects work, recreational, personal, and social acts and goals—that is, "ability" and "disability.")

Proprioceptive disturbance can also be associated with problems in motor control. In the absence of feedback about the position of a limb in space or the lack of a sense of movement, it becomes necessary for the patient to depend on visual input. Such processing can be slow, compounding any difficulties introduced by the slowing of motor output.

### Motor Control

A major and common result of cerebral injury is hemiparesis in which the motor control of the affected extremities is impaired as the result of loss of supraspinal effects on the anterior horn cell. The factors hindering functional motor control are not merely weakness but the lack of selectivity of action and coordination at a joint. The balance of motor control that allows agonists and antagonists to work in concert is no longer present. The rapidity of release and contraction of the muscles operating at a joint is frequently compromised. In addition, the upper motor neuron dysfunction impairs selective motor control, which may lead to a mass synergy pattern. Selectivity of normal muscle action is a function of cortical motor control guided by proprioceptive feedback. In the presence of injury to the central nervous system, both the central motor and sensory tracts are disrupted.

"Patterned motion" refers to the primitive stereotyped synergies of mass flexion and mass extension, initiated when the person with hemiplegia attempts to perform a task. The muscles that participate and the strength of their responses are the same regardless of the demand. Particularly problematic is the effect of such a patterned response on the actions of the upper extremity. The functional actions of the upper extremity require considerable flexibility and maneuverability. In the lower extremity the primitive patterns are discrete and prominent, and most persons with hemiparesis regain considerable mobility. They can initiate the extensor pattern for standing and use the flexor pattern to take steps. The extension and flexion patterns can be used to provide a safe means of walking although the refinements of normal gait are not achieved.

Fundamental to our understanding of the nervous system has been the principle of vertically-distributed functional systems.[1,2] This principle states that functions are rerepresented at different levels of the nervous system. Progressively higher levels in the nervous system correspond to increasingly refined control with greater adaptive capacity. Higher levels inhibit the lower levels in the process of development. Lower levels function in a more automated fashion than higher levels. Thus damage at the higher level releases the lower levels to function, although in a less differentiated fashion. The type of motor recovery that occurs in the presence of neural injury is supported by this notion of vertical organization with the pyramidal or corticospinal tract reflecting the neocerebral, or highest, level of organization. The actions controlled by this level are those most affected by injury.

For example, distal weakness (particularly of the hand) is most likely to persist after cerebral injury be-

cause of the relatively large component dealing with the hand in the pyramidal corticospinal tract. The predilection for the recovery of strength in the flexors of the upper extremity also reflects the lesser contribution of the pyramidal tract to control these "antigravity" muscles in the upper extremity. A major clinical implication is the high frequency of recovery of the ability to stand (and possibly walk) in those with even severe damage to the motor cortex and lateral corticospinal tract. This is based on the relatively-larger contribution by the subcortical extrapyramidal motor system to the antigravity extensor muscles of the lower extremity. A greater degree of functional recovery of the leg versus the arm and of the antigravity musculature in the leg results. It is postulated that the reticulospinal and rubrospinal motor tracts participate in the process of recovery despite the continued injury of the corticospinal tracts.

Table 39-4 from the AMA *Guides*[5] illustrates the degree of impairment of the whole person attributable to difficulties in use of the upper extremities. The severity of impairment is greater in the preferred over the nonpreferred extremity with an approximately 10% greater impairment assessed for the preferred extremity. (The "handedness" concept applies only to impairment of the upper extremity caused by central nervous system or spinal cord lesions.) The impairment rating ranges from 0% to 15%. The automatic addition of 10% for the dominant hand was issued in previous editions of the AMA *Guides*. Section 3.1 states "little evidence exists that there is a significant difference in grip strength between the dominant and the nondominant hand. The *Guides* does not recognize such a difference." In Section 4.3b, the AMA *Guides* state that "impairment of the preferred ex-

**TABLE 39-4     CRITERIA FOR ONE IMPAIRED UPPER EXTREMITY**

| IMPAIRMENT DESCRIPTION | % IMPAIRMENT OF THE WHOLE PERSON | |
|---|---|---|
| | PREFERRED EXTREMITY | NONPREFERRED EXTREMITY |
| Patient can use the involved extremity for self care daily activities and holding, but has difficulty with digital dexterity | 1–9 | 1–4 |
| Patient can use the involved extremity for self care, can grasp and hold objects with difficulty, but has *no* digital dexterity | 10–24 | 5–14 |
| Patient can use the involved extremity but has difficulty with self care activities | 25–39 | 15–29 |
| Patient cannot use the involved extremity for self care and daily activities | 40–60 | 30–45 |

From AMA *Guides*, ed 4, 1993, American Medical Association, Chicago.

tremity...should be evaluated periodically, because the nonpreferred extremity eventually may become as capable of functioning as the preferred extremity." Thus there is a major policy shift away from the concept of "handedness" since, with time, individuals can and will adapt (if possible) by increasing the function of the nondominant extremity to minimize long-term impairment. One may carry out many of the self care activities relatively satisfactorily with only one hand intact. The relative severity of impairment is greatest when the upper extremity cannot participate in any way even in self care activities. This is assessed at an average of 50% whole person impairment whereas the availability of the hand for self care activities without dexterity averages 16% impairment. The use of the hand itself in grasping objects and then in carrying out activities actually requiring dexterity per se reflects the unique contribution of the hand to the whole person.

This same relationship is reflected in Table 39-5 derived from the AMA *Guides*,[5] which attaches greater degree of impairment of the whole person to the loss of both upper extremities rather than a single upper extremity. Once again the severity of impairment reflecting difficulty with self care (average 60%) reflects the relative importance of participation in self care and its retention over that of grasp and dexterity (average 10%).

The level of the nervous system at which the injury has occurred determines the initial degree of dis-

organization and the degree of reorganization that may take place. Of equal importance is the degree to which the neural injury is unilateral or bilateral. The differential effects on proximal versus more distal actions in both the arm and leg reflect the relative contribution of the components of the lateral corticospinal tract decussating at the level of the medullary pyramid in the control of more lateralized actions distal from the midline. The earlier return of axial and proximal limb activities reflects the relatively greater bilateral contribution to the innervation of these more midline structures. The greatest deficit is in the muscles acting as prime movers rather than stabilizers. In the lower extremities, upper motor neuron weakness is greater with flexion than with extension at the hip, knee, and ankle. Although there may be sufficient spinal circuitry to generate the cyclic activation of flexor and extensor muscle groups, the initiation of locomotion also requires a willful activation of muscles that may be absent.

Table 39-6 from AMA *Guides*[5] describes the degree of whole person impairment attributable to difficulties in mobility and ambulation. The higher degree of impairment permitted by the ability only to stand without actual ambulation reflects the common pattern of corticospinal injury. There is maintenance of antigravity extensor action of more proximal muscles.

---

**TABLE 39-5**      CRITERIA FOR TWO IMPAIRED UPPER EXTREMITIES

| IMPAIRMENT DESCRIPTION | % IMPAIRMENT OF THE WHOLE PERSON |
|---|---|
| Patient can use both upper extremities for self care, grasping, and holding, but has difficulty with digital dexterity | 1–19 |
| Patient can use both upper extremities for self care, can grasp and hold objects with difficulty, but has no digital dexterity | 20–39 |
| Patient can use both upper extremities but has difficulty with self care activities | 40–79 |
| Patient cannot use upper extremities | 80+ |

From AMA *Guides*, ed 4, 1993, American Medical Association, Chicago.

---

**TABLE 39-6**      STATION AND GAIT IMPAIRMENT CRITERIA

| IMPAIRMENT DESCRIPTION | % IMPAIRMENT OF THE WHOLE PERSON |
|---|---|
| Patient can rise to a standing position and can walk but has difficulty with elevations, grades, stairs, deep chairs, and walking long distances | 1–9 |
| Patient can rise to a standing position and can walk some distance with difficulty and without assistance but is limited to level surfaces | 10–19 |
| Patient can rise to a standing position and can maintain it with difficulty but cannot walk without assistance | 20–39 |
| Patient cannot stand without help of others, mechanical support, and a prosthesis | 40–60 |

From AMA *Guides*, ed 4, 1993, American Medical Association, Chicago.

What is less likely to occur is the more complex alternating of flexion and extension required for ambulation. Even in the presence of ambulation on a level surface, one may still have lesser degrees of difficulty evidenced only when hip flexion becomes a more significant factor such as in its contribution to activities like stair climbing. The various levels of impairment reflect the usual pattern of retained function. The degrees of impairment attributed to the successive degrees of standing (30% average), walking (15% average), and stair climbing (average 5%) reflect the degree of disruption of one's life. The highest degree of impairment of the whole person is seen when independent stance is unavailable (average 50%) or when the crucial ability to get out of bed to transfer to a wheelchair and from the wheelchair to toilet are impaired and limit independent function.

An injury that affects the upper motor neuron (pyramidal tract) has traditionally been considered to have several kinds of effects. One type is the weakness and loss of dexterity described earlier that can affect gait and use of the upper extremities. Another type of effect includes production of abnormal posture, exaggerated proprioceptive reflexes, spasticity, and exaggerated cutaneous reflexes of the limbs that produce flexion withdrawal spasms and the Babinski response. For example, additional time was required when persons with spasticity carried out alternating flexion and extension of the elbow.[11] This reflected difficulty in reversing the direction of movement. In normal subjects flexor activity ceased before the peak of flexion was reached. In the paretic limb the electromyogram (EMG) activity of the biceps muscle persisted throughout flexion and even during extension. There was also limited and prolonged recruitment of agonist contraction. Thus the motor abnormality is a disorder of the selection of muscles to be activated and inhibited and is not a simple consequence of the elevated stretch reflex.

## Integrative Output

Thus far, this chapter has considered the sensory-motor system in relation to its response to sensory input signalling changes in the external environment and the degree of motor control. The other level of organization is the development of new patterns of activity in relation to changing requirements. An intact subcortical diencephalon supports the coordination of the complex motor behaviors such as ambulation and grooming even without connection made with the overall goals of the organism and its changes. An intact forebrain is, however, necessary to carry out analytic and planning functions to monitor the activities in relation to the goals of the organism

and learn new patterns.[2] These "executive" type functions are those impaired in the presence of cerebral disease particularly when there is diffuse or bilateral involvement. Difficulties in learning thus can affect the entire person and be added to the level of other impairments.

The impact of alterations in mental status and behavior is far-reaching, leading to the general need for supervision in daily living and social situations. For example, Table 39-7, derived from the AMA *Guides*,[5] lists degrees in the amount of supervision required with some supervision leading to an average of 22%, but supervision of a more complete nature averaging 40% impairment. This same relationship is illustrated in Table 39-8 in AMA *Guides*[5] dealing with interpersonal and social situations with moderate limitation of some daily living situations averaging 22% whole person impairment and more severe limitations producing 30% to 70% impairment.

The effects of brain injury, affecting learning in persons with cerebrovascular disease, are compounded by the underlying quality of the brain and the person in whom the injury has occurred. The normal aging process brings about changes in cognitive functioning that may not be problematic in a familiar, predictable environment but may complicate adaptation to the demands of an unfamiliar environment. Generally signs of increased frontal lobe dysfunction such as reduced flexibility, abstract reasoning, and initiative may affect the ability to solve problems generated by new environments. Less effi-

---

**TABLE 39-7    MENTAL STATUS IMPAIRMENTS**

| IMPAIRMENT DESCRIPTION | % IMPAIRMENT OF THE WHOLE PERSON |
|---|---|
| Impairment exists, but ability remains to perform satisfactorily most activities of daily living | 1–14 |
| Impairment requires direction and supervision of daily living activities | 15–29 |
| Impairment requires directed care under continued supervision and confinement in home or other facility | 30–49 |
| Individual is unable to care for self and be safe in any situation without supervision | 50–70 |

From AMA *Guides*, ed 4, 1993, American Medical Association, Chicago.

**TABLE 39-8**    EMOTIONAL OR BEHAVIORAL IMPAIRMENTS

| IMPAIRMENT DESCRIPTION | % IMPAIRMENT OF THE WHOLE PERSON |
|---|---|
| Mild limitation of daily social and interpersonal functioning | 0–14 |
| Moderate limitation of some but not all social and interpersonal daily living functions | 15–29 |
| Severe limitation impeding useful action in almost all social and interpersonal daily functions | 30–49 |
| Severe limitation of all daily functions requiring total dependence on another person | 50–70 |

From AMA *Guides*, ed 4, 1993, American Medical Association, Chicago.

cient strategies for solving problems may be the result of, as well as an inability to generate, alternative solutions when the initial strategies do not work.[3]

A basic principle is that the nervous system is plastic; it changes from moment to moment. Plasticity is the term given to the adaptive capacities of the central nervous system to modify its own structural organization and functioning. It is an adaptive response to a functional demand. It requires feedback on whether environmental demands are being met.

Acceptance of this notion requires a change to a perception of the brain as a malleable rather than a fixed organ. Although individual cells do not regenerate, the cell processes, axons, and dendrites are responsive to functional demands. A large component of the process of maturation is an increase in cell processes and in glial cells. Such reorganization is not necessarily precluded by old age.

The frontal lobe is involved mostly in planning and carrying out other integrative functions. For example, patients with frontal lobe lesions have particular difficulty drawing a floor plan of their own apartment or house. They do poorly when asked to create a floor plan of a "dream house" that would be ideally suited for them and their family. They usually fail to place bathrooms next to bedrooms and misalign the kitchen, dining area, and living rooms. Such a floor plan takes forethought, organization, and planning. Copying of figures is usually normal in patients with frontal lobe lesions since it requires no initiative or planning.

Apraxia is the term given to impairments in motor planning without weakness. For example, persons with apraxia of speech show a marked difference in performance between volitional and automatic tasks. There is significant difficulty counting backwards from 10 to 0 (a volitional, purposeful task), whereas counting from 1 to 10 is usually done well (automatic nonvolitional task).

Lesions that affect the deep regions of the left temporal lobe, particularly when including structures such as the hippocampus and amygdala, can produce a significant deficit in the ability to remember and learn verbal information, while at the same time resulting in minimal or no aphasia. Lesions in the left frontal lobe anterior to Broca's area also typically produce minimal or no aphasia, but they can cause substantial impairment in concept formation ability, mental flexibility, verbal abstraction, verbal fluency, and overall verbal facilities.

The aphasia caused by left hemisphere lesions represents various forms of impairment in managing the denotative components of language. Some degree of difficulty in listening, talking, reading, and writing is common to all persons with aphasia. In short, to one degree or another, stroke victims with aphasia have difficulty processing symbols receptively and expressively. Receptively, the person with aphasia may have minimal or massive difficulty comprehending written or spoken words, phrases, sentences, and paragraphs. Expressively, the persons with aphasia may have difficulty expressing themselves in writing or speech.

Table 39-9 from the AMA *Guides* provides impairment ratings for aphasia and dysphasia. Once again the degree of impairment is assessed in the context of daily living wherein moderate impairment yields an average whole person impairment rating of 16% whereas more severe degrees of inability to communicate in daily living produces impairment ratings of 25% to 60%.

The right hemisphere supports parallel systems for managing the connotative components of language and communication.[3] Such connotative components of communication include interpreting the emotional tone of verbal and nonverbal communication, generating emotional tone in verbal and gestural communication, using inflection and prosody to add nuance to verbal communication, and accurately perceiving the emotional expression of visually-presented human faces. The disruptive potential of such right hemisphere deficits is apparent if one considers that

**TABLE 39-9**    IMPAIRMENT RELATED TO APHASIA OR DYSPHASIA

| IMPAIRMENT DESCRIPTION | % IMPAIRMENT OF THE WHOLE PERSON |
|---|---|
| Minimal disturbance in comprehension and production of language symbols of daily living | 0–9 |
| Moderate impairment in comprehension and production of language symbols of daily living | 10–24 |
| Inability to comprehend language symbols; production of unintelligible or inappropriate language for daily activities | 25–39 |
| Complete inability to communicate or comprehend language symbols | 40–60 |

From AMA *Guides*, ed 4, 1993, American Medical Association, Chicago.

**TABLE 39-10**    IMPAIRMENTS RELATED TO EPILEPSY, SEIZURES, AND CONVULSIVE DISORDERS

| IMPAIRMENT DESCRIPTION | % IMPAIRMENT OF THE WHOLE PERSON |
|---|---|
| Paroxysmal disorder with predictable characteristics and unpredictable occurrence that does not limit usual activities but is a risk to the patient or limits performance of daily activities | 0–14 |
| Paroxysmal disorder that interferes with some activities of daily living | 15–29 |
| Severe paroxysmal disorder of such frequency that it limits activities to those who are supervised, protected, or restricted | 30–49 |
| Uncontrolled paroxysmal disorder of such severity and constancy that it totally limits the individual's daily activities | 50–70 |

From AMA *Guides*, ed 4, 1993, American Medical Association, Chicago.

most people have several ways with which to say "yes" and that at least one of these ways actually communicates a very clear message of "no." The patient with such deficits can completely miss the true content of a communication and, indeed, can derive the opposite meaning of what was intended. Given that much of everyday communication relies heavily on gesture, inflection, and other connotative aspects of speech, deficits in this realm are important to identify to help the family and staff understand the need to communicate with the patient in ways in which the denoted content is the truly intended content.

These various impairments concerned with accurate communication as well as the integrative functions are crucial to the process of learning of new modes of behavior in response to the presence of the injury. The level of permanent impairment secondary to injury in the central nervous system is thus a reflection not only of the severity of the initial injury but the adaptive capabilities of the uninjured brain and the person in whom that injury has occurred.

### Epilepsy

The degree of impairment related to episodic disturbances of consciousness relates to the factors emphasized throughout this chapter. The degree of impairment depends not only upon the severity of neurological dysfunction but the context in the life of the person in which the seizures occur.

The average degree of impairment is least when unpredictability of seizure occurrence is modified by predictability of characteristics as illustrated in Table 39-10 from the AMA *Guides*.[5] For example, a consistent pattern of prodromal symptoms can provide enough warning for the person to seek safety to avoid injury if a seizure does occur. The unpredictability of time of occurrence can, however, lead to disruption in one's life despite the predictability of prodromal symptoms. Consistently nocturnal seizures occurring in bed can contrarily be of little risk and not limit performance of daily activities. The higher degree of disruption of normal activities is reflected in both the frequency of seizures and their unpredictability requiring increasing degrees of supervision and a protected environment to ensure against injury. The highest degree of impairment reflects not only the frequency and unpredictability but the effects of such on general cognitive function so as to interfere with living independently and everyday activities.

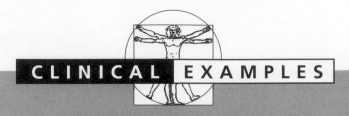

## CENTRAL NERVOUS SYSTEM

EDITOR'S NOTE—Impairment evaluation of the central nervous system is infrequent. It can be difficult because multiple abnormalities can exist as a result of the myriad functions of this system.

### EXAMPLE

**History**

A 28-year-old man has asked for an impairment evaluation. He has a history of seizures dating from a traumatic head injury suffered in a motor vehicle accident two years ago. He now takes three antiepileptic medications after proving intolerant to, or not improved by, other medications. Presently, he is averaging one seizure every three months. These occur unpredictably with little prodromal warning signs. No other abnormalities are reported.

**Physical Examination**

The physical examination is normal.

**Assessment Process**

Using Table 5 on p.143,* findings in this patient would place him in either Category II or

*All *tables* referred to in this discussion are found in AMA *Guides to the evaluation of permanent impairment,* ed 4, Chapter 4—The Nervous System, American Medical Association, Chicago, 1993.

Category III based on the frequency of the seizures and on interruption of activities of daily living.

However, the physician is also liable for the results of this determination. Therefore, recommendations for return to work must include an assessment of the risk at which he places both himself and others. For example, if his job is driving a taxi or a truck, he would be 100% disabled. He would be at risk to himself, his passengers, and other individuals on the highway. If he is a telephone operator, he could be returned to work safely, since he would only be at risk to himself. However, as the evaluator, the physician needs to make the risks known in the report.

**Evaluation**

The spread for the category chosen is 15% to 49%; the physician's experience as an evaluator would determine the exact percentage assigned. The physician should also add a recommendation regarding the possibility of returning to work based on the patient's occupation.

*Stephen L. Demeter*

## References

1. Bach-y-Rita P: Brain plasticity as a basis for therapeutic procedures. In Bach-y-Rita P, editor: *Recovery of function: theoretical considerations for brain injury rehabilitation*, Baltimore, 1980, University Park Press.
2. Gallistel CR: The organization of action: a new synthesis, *Behav Brain Sci* 4:609, 1981.
3. Garmoe W, Newman AC, Bleiberg J: *Neuropsychologic aspects of normal aging and stroke rehabilitation*. In Ozer MN, editor: *The management of persons with stroke*, St. Louis, 1994, Mosby.
4. Goldsmith TM, Baron CR: *Dysphagia and its management*. In Ozer MN, editor: *The management of persons with stroke*, St. Louis, 1994, Mosby.
5. *Guides to the evaluation of permanent impairment*, ed 4, Chicago, 1993, American Medical Association.
6. Jenkins WM, Merzenich MM, Recauzone G: Neocortical representation dynamics in adult primates: implications for neuropsychology, *Neuropsychologia* 28:573, 1990.
7. Moberg E: Criticism and study of methods for examining sensibility in the hand, *Neurol* 2:8, 1962.
8. Moore S: Neuroanatomical considerations relating to the recovery of function following brain injury. In Bach-y-Rita P, editor: *Recovery of function: theoretical considerations for brain injury rehabilitation*, Baltimore, 1980, University Park Press.
9. Ozer MN: *The management of persons with spinal cord injury*, New York, 1982, Demos.
10. Phillips MH: *Bladder management*. In Ozer MN, editor: *The management of persons with stroke*, St. Louis, 1994, Mosby.
11. Sahrmann SA, Norton BJ: The relationship of voluntary movement to spasticity in the upper motor neuron syndrome, *Ann Neuro* 4:460, 1977.
12. Stineman MG, Granger CV: Epidemiology of stroke related disability and rehabilitation outcome, *PM&R Clin North Am* 2:457, 1991.
13. Young JS, et al: *Spinal cord injury statistics: experience of the regional spinal cord injury systems*, Phoenix, 1982, Good Samaritan Center.

# CHAPTER 40

# PERIPHERAL NERVOUS SYSTEM

*Christopher A. Sheppard*

## PERIPHERAL NERVOUS SYSTEM

The peripheral nervous system (PNS) includes all neural structures lying outside the brain stem and spinal cord, excluding the cranial nerves. It includes the nerve roots within the spinal canal, along with various plexuses and peripheral nerves extending into the extremities. These nerves, composed of both motor and sensory fibers, carry motor impulses prodromically (from the brain to the spinal cord, to the peripheral nerves, to the muscles) to the muscle fibers and sensory impulses antidromically (from the muscles to the brain) back to the central nervous system in response to various stimuli. Sympathetic and parasympathetic nerves are part of the PNS and make up the autonomic nervous system, sending fibers via the peripheral nerves to innervate viscera, blood vessels, and sweat glands.

Anatomically, impairment of the peripheral nervous system can occur anywhere along the course of a nerve, from the cell bodies to the terminal portions of the nerve, either at a sensory nerve ending or at the motor end plate in the muscle fiber. In pathologic terms, PNS impairment may be due to entities that affect the nerve cells themselves, their processes, their myelin sheaths, or a combination of these components. Common examples include degenerative conditions of the nervous system such as motor neuron disease, injury to the nerves with trauma, metabolic injury to the nerves such as in diabetes mellitus, or demyelinating processes such as Guillain-Barré syndrome.

The prognosis for a neuropathic disease is dependent upon the cause of the neuropathy. If the neuropathy is caused by a degenerative condition such as motor neuron disease, or genetically-determined disorders, it is likely to worsen. There are presently few options of treatment of these conditions. The genetically-determined polyneuropathies are also likely to progress. The prognosis for the acquired polyneuropathies is largely dependent upon the underlying cause of the neuropathic process. For example, the neuropathies associated with such conditions as diabetes mellitus, connective tissue disease, amyloidosis, and uremia are likely to be progressive because of the difficulty of treating or handling the underlying disease process. Neuropathies associated with more treatable conditions, such as hypothyroidism or vitamin B-12 deficiency, may stabilize or improve with successful control of the illness. Traumatic injury to the peripheral nervous system, once maximal healing has occurred, is likely to be static. The majority of patients with Guillain-Barré syndrome recover.

The determination of impairment caused by peripheral neuropathies should not be assessed during the acute phase of the illness, during treatment, or prior to rehabilitation and maximal recovery. It is also not dependent on the etiologic causation of the neuropathic process although diagnosing the specific disorder provides important information regarding the stability or level of expected progression or regression of the disease process. Impairment determination is performed only when a residual impairment is fixed and is not amenable to further therapeutic interventions. Progressive disorders may also be assessed with proper notations made regarding present and extrapolated future impairments.

The patient's history is important in determining the etiology and prognosis of the patient's deficit. The main symptoms relating to permanent impairment of the peripheral nervous system include weakness, sensory abnormalities, and pain. Processes that affect the autonomic nervous system usually cause end-organ disorders (evaluation of which are covered elsewhere). Reflex sympathetic dystrophy causes combinations of pain and weakness akin to the processes that affect motor and sensory nerves. The varying symptoms of peripheral neuropathy may be confined to the distribution of a single nerve, as in a mononeuropathy, may affect multiple nerves in a single limb, as with a brachial plexopathy, or may present as a more generalized condition, as in a polyneuropathy.

Inherent to the determination of the degree of impairment due to any process affecting the peripheral nervous system is the assumption that the impairment and the process causing it are stable or not amenable to further treatment. This determination may require further diagnostic testing, but it also can be accomplished by review of historical data, both from the patient and from the previous evaluations.

Careful examination of the peripheral nervous system involves observation of muscle bulk looking for atrophy, and examination of muscle tone, deep tendon reflexes, and strength. Sensory examination is also important, although this is recognized as being the most difficult portion of the neurologic examination. Accurate examination of sensation requires a cooperative, attentive subject. Examination should localize and grade the magnitude of the decreased strength for each affected muscle, the type and site of altered sensation, and the presence of pain for each nerve found to be affected. This involves examining all muscle groups, describing which are weak and

identifying the nerves that innervate those muscles (Figs. 40-1 and 40-2). With altered sensation or pain, the examination focuses on and documents the topographic areas involved and identifies the nerve roots or peripheral nerves that innervate these areas (Figs. 40-3 to 40-5).

Strength is rated by a 5 point scale with Grade 5 representing full strength, Grade 4 representing normal movement against gravity with the ability to provide some but not normal resistance, Grade 3 representing normal movement against gravity but inability to provide any resistance, Grade 2 representing normal movement with gravity eliminated, Grade 1 representing the ability to contract the muscle but without movement and Grade 0 representing the complete inability to contract the muscle.[3] Table 12 and Table 21 of the AMA *Guides* in Sections 3.1k and 4.4b respectively provide an impairment rating for motor strength deficits, using the above scheme, for disorders of the peripheral nervous system (Tables 40-1 and 40-2).

The method of rating the degree of impairment due to sensory loss or pain is less well standardized and is usually judged on a 5 point scale with Grade 5

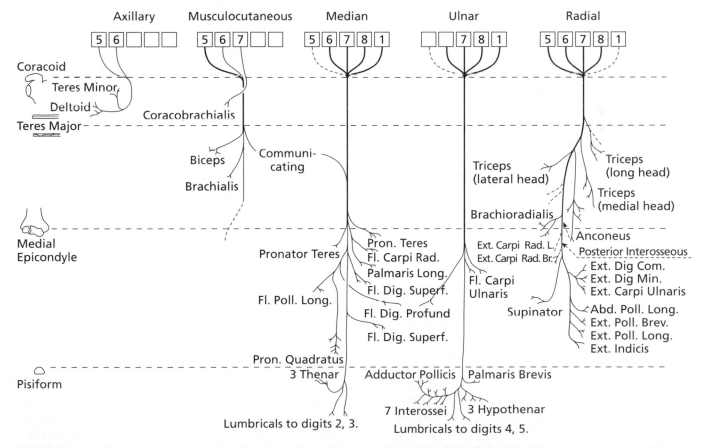

**FIGURE 40-1**    Motor innervation of the upper extremity.    *(From American Medical Association:* Guides to the evaluation of permanent impairment, *ed 4, Chicago, 1993.)*

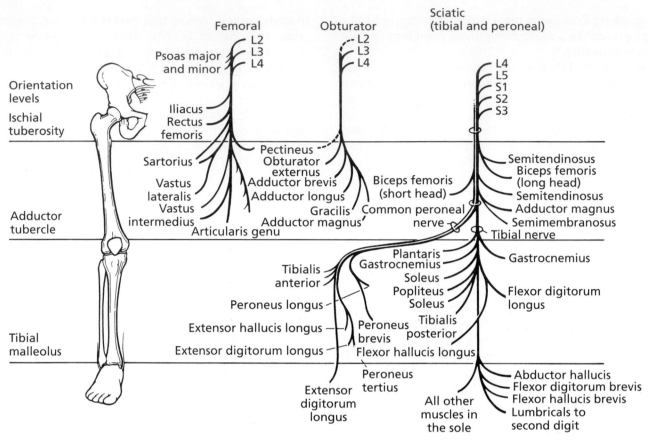

**FIGURE 40-2**    Motor innervation of the lower extremity.    *(From American Medical Association:* Guides to the evaluation of permanent impairment, *ed 4, Chicago, 1993.)*

representing normal sensation with no pain, Grade 4 representing decreased sensation or pain noted only at rest, Grade 3 representing decreased sensation or pain that interferes with activity, Grade 2 representing decreased sensation or pain that prevents some but not all activity, Grade 1 representing decreased sensation with severe pain preventing certain activity, and Grade 0, which represents decreased sensation with severe pain that prevents all activity. Tables 11 and 20 of Sections 3.1k and 4.4b of the AMA *Guides* provide an impairment rating for those problems similar to the scheme used when assessing strength. In general, when it is performed by an experienced clinician, the physical examination is believed to be a sensitive tool. Unfortunately, it lacks specificity. It does not identify all who have no abnormality. Also, as with carpal tunnel syndrome, other disorders, such as radiculopathies or tendinitis, may have similar signs and symptoms or may coexist with the condition being investigated. In the evaluation of a lumbar radiculopathy, leg pain and paresthesias can occur with irritation of many structures of the lumbosacral spine, including muscles and liga-

ments, and they may not always be indicative of nerve root abnormalities. The testing of a patient's strength may be influenced by pain and conscious effort and cooperation. Both increased and decreased sensation can be embellished or feigned by the subject consciously or subconsciously.

It must be remembered therefore that many abnormalities found on neurologic examination are subjective. Except in the most obvious cases where motor, sensory, and reflex changes are unequivocal, definable, and consistent, the task of delineating the presence and extent of a suspected abnormality is heavily dependent on electrodiagnostic procedures. Electromyography and nerve conduction studies provide objective evidence of nerve injury. Electromyography demonstrates objective evidence of denervation in conditions affecting motor nerves. Nerve conduction studies reveal abnormalities in conditions causing significant axonal loss or demyelination of the peripheral nerves. Extensive literature review reveals that sensitivities for electromyography have been systematically measured in only a limited number of specific conditions (Table 40-3). As with most

**TABLE 40-1    DETERMINING IMPAIRMENT OF THE UPPER EXTREMITY DUE TO LOSS OF POWER AND MOTOR DEFICITS RESULTING FROM PERIPHERAL NERVE DISORDERS BASED ON INDIVIDUAL MUSCLE RATING***

**A. CLASSIFICATION**

| GRADE | DESCRIPTION OF MUSCLE FUNCTION | % MOTOR DEFICIT |
|---|---|---|
| 5 | Active movement against gravity with full resistance | 0 |
| 4 | Active movement against gravity with some resistance | 1-25 |
| 3 | Active movement against gravity only, without resistance | 26-50 |
| 2 | Active movement with gravity eliminated | 51-75 |
| 1 | Slight contraction and no movement | 76-99 |
| 0 | No contraction | 100 |

**B. PROCEDURE**

1. Identify the motion involved, such as flexion, extension, etc.

2. Identify the muscle(s) performing the motion and the motor nerve(s) involved.

3. Grade the severity of motor deficit of individual muscles according to the classification given above.

4. Find the maximum impairment of the upper extremity due to motor deficit for each nerve structure involved: spinal nerves (Table 13, p. 51), brachial plexus (Table 14, p. 52), and major peripheral nerves (Table 15, p. 54).

5. Multiply the severity of the motor deficit by the maximum impairment value to obtain the upper extremity impairment for each structure involved.

*Modified from *Guides to the evaluation of permanent impairment,* ed 4, American Medical Association, 1993, Chicago.

**TABLE 40-2    CLASSIFICATION AND PROCEDURE FOR DETERMINING NERVOUS SYSTEM IMPAIRMENT DUE TO LOSS OF MUSCLE POWER AND MOTOR FUNCTION RESULTING FROM PERIPHERAL NERVE DISORDERS***

**A. CLASSIFICATION**

| GRADE | DESCRIPTION OF MUSCLE FUNCTION | % MOTOR DEFICIT |
|---|---|---|
| 5 | Active movement against gravity with full resistance | 0 |
| 4 | Active movement against gravity with some resistance | 1-25 |
| 3 | Active movement against gravity only, without resistance | 26-50 |
| 2 | Active movement with gravity eliminated | 51-75 |
| 1 | Slight contraction and no movement | 76-99 |
| 0 | No contraction | 100 |

**B. PROCEDURE**

1. Identify the motion involved, such as flexion or extension.

2. Identify the muscle(s) performing the motion and the motor nerve(s) involved.

3. Grade the severity of motor deficit of the individual muscles according to the classification given above.

4. Find the maximum impairment due to the motor deficit for each nerve structure involved, as listed in Chapter 3: upper extremity (Table 15, p. 54), brachial plexus (Table 14, p. 52), lower extremity nerves (Table 68, p. 89); and lumbosacral nerves (Table 83, p. 130).

5. Multiply the severity of the motor deficit by the percentage associated with the nerve(s) identified in procedure 4 (above) to obtain the estimated impairment from strength deficit for each structure involved.

*Modified from *Guides to the evaluation of permanent impairment,* ed 4, American Medical Association, 1993, Chicago.

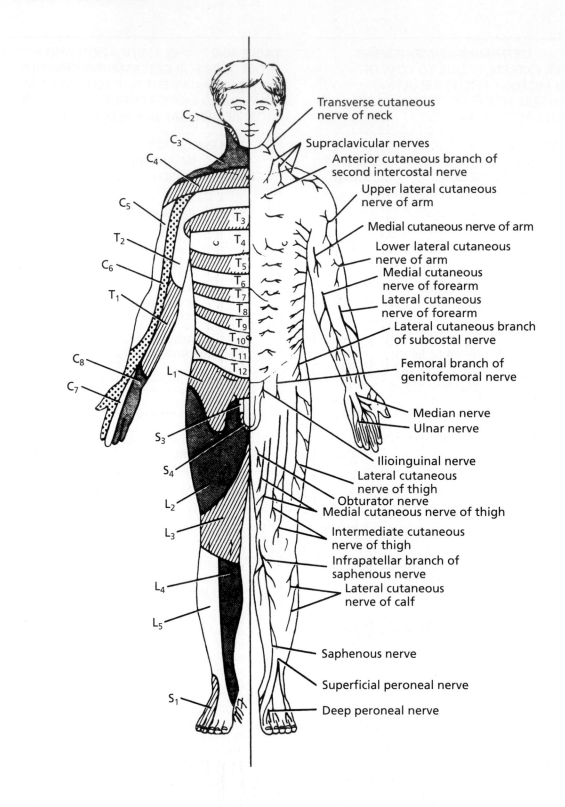

**FIGURE 40-3** Dermatomes and distribution of cutaneous nerves on the **(A)** anterior and **(B)** posterior aspects of the body. *(From Snell R, Smith M: Clinical Anatomy for Emergency Medicine, St. Louis, 1993, Mosby.)*

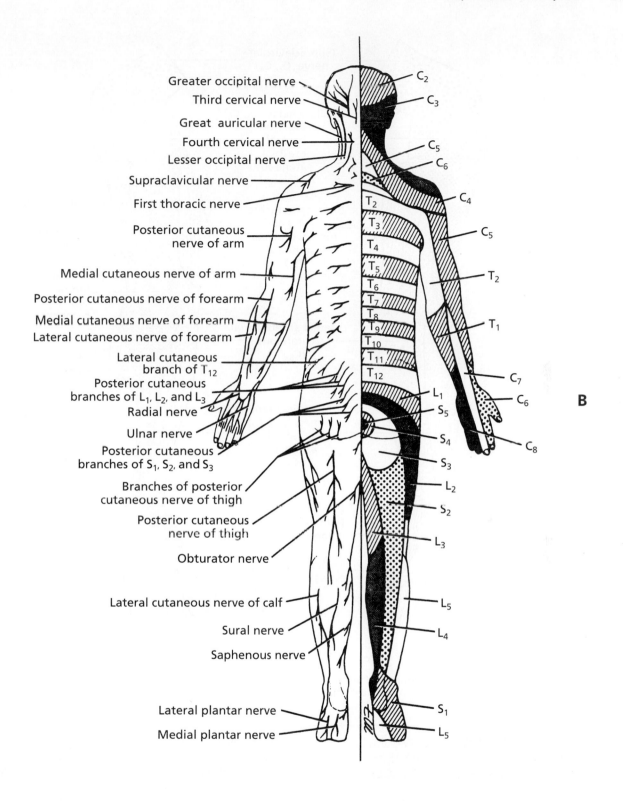

Greater occipital nerve
Third cervical nerve
Great auricular nerve
Fourth cervical nerve
Lesser occipital nerve
Supraclavicular nerve
First thoracic nerve
Posterior cutaneous nerve of arm
Medial cutaneous nerve of arm
Posterior cutaneous nerve of forearm
Medial cutaneous nerve of forearm
Lateral cutaneous nerve of forearm
Lateral cutaneous branch of $T_{12}$
Posterior cutaneous branches of $L_1$, $L_2$, and $L_3$
Radial nerve
Ulnar nerve
Posterior cutaneous branches of $S_1$, $S_2$, and $S_3$
Branches of posterior cutaneous nerve of thigh
Posterior cutaneous nerve of thigh
Obturator nerve
Lateral cutaneous nerve of calf
Sural nerve
Saphenous nerve
Lateral plantar nerve
Medial plantar nerve

$C_2$
$C_3$
$C_5$
$C_6$
$C_4$
$C_5$
$T_2$
$T_2$
$T_3$
$T_4$
$T_5$
$T_6$
$T_7$
$T_8$
$T_9$
$T_{10}$
$T_{11}$
$T_{12}$
$T_1$
$L_1$
$S_5$
$S_4$
$S_3$
$L_2$
$S_2$
$L_3$
$L_5$
$L_4$
$S_1$
$L_5$
$C_7$
$C_6$
$C_8$

**B**

**FIGURE 40-3, cont'd**    For legend see opposite page.

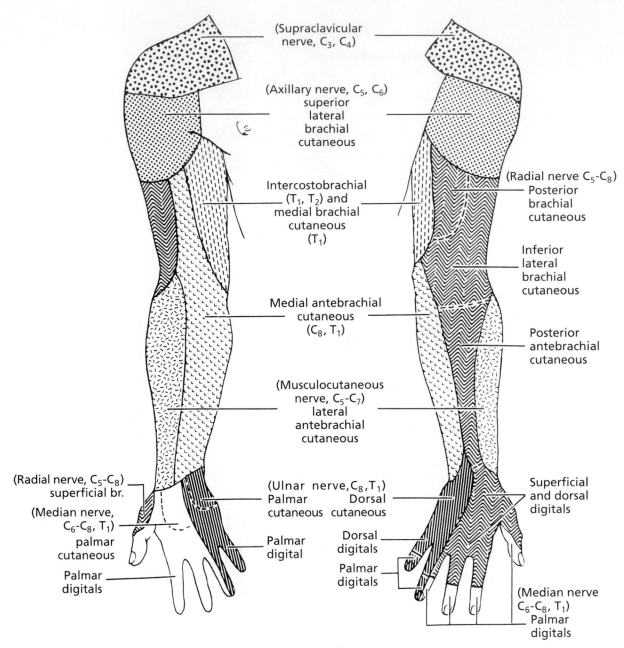

**FIGURE 40-4** Cutaneous sensory dermatomes of upper extremity and related peripheral nerves and roots. *(From American Medical Association:* Guides to the evaluation of permanent impairment, *ed 4, Chicago, 1993.)*

**TABLE 40-3    REPORTED SENSITIVITY OF ELECTROMYOGRAPHY IN VARIOUS PERIPHERAL NERVOUS SYSTEM DISORDERS**

| | |
|---|---|
| Carpal tunnel syndrome | 87%[10] |
| Guillain-Barré syndrome | 85%[11] |
| Hereditary neuropathies | 90%[11] |
| Lumbar radiculopathies | 60-85%[7] |
| Ulnar neuropathy | 77%[9] |

tests, electromyography is not infallible, and obtained results must be correlated with the findings from clinical examination. Once the exact anatomic location, type of tissue involved, and severity of the neuropathy is determined, the maximum percentage of lost function due to weakness, loss of sensation, or pain can be estimated. Various guidelines have been published listing the maximum percentage of loss of function due to diminished power or sensation or due to pain for spinal nerve roots, brachial or lumbosacral plexuses, or peripheral nerves (Tables 40-4 through 40-6). One of the most widely used is that

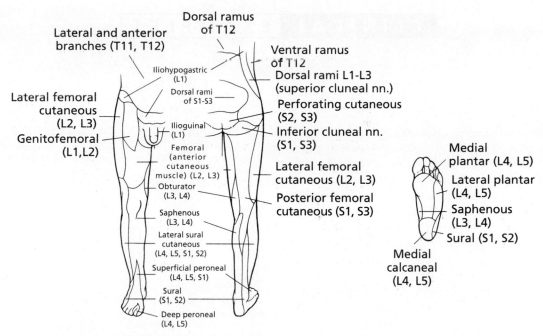

**FIGURE 40-5**    Sensory nerves of the lower extremity and their roots of origin.    *(From American Medical Association:* Guides to the evaluation of permanent impairment, *ed 4, Chicago, 1993.)*

**TABLE 40-4    MAXIMUM LOST FUNCTION DUE TO NERVE ROOT IMPAIRMENT (PERCENTAGE)**

| NERVE ROOT | DECREASED SENSATION OR PAIN | DECREASED POWER |
|:---:|:---:|:---:|
| C-5 | 5 | 30 |
| C-6 | 8 | 35 |
| C-7 | 5 | 35 |
| C-8 | 5 | 45 |
| T-1 | 5 | 20 |
| L-3 | 5 | 20 |
| L-4 | 5 | 34 |
| L-5 | 5 | 37 |
| S-1 | 5 | 20 |

Modified from *Guides to the evaluation of permanent impairment,* ed 4, American Medical Association, 1993, Chicago.

**TABLE 40-5    MAXIMUM LOST FUNCTION DUE TO PLEXUS IMPAIRMENT (PERCENTAGE)**

| | DECREASED SENSATION OR PAIN | DECREASED POWER |
|:---|:---:|:---:|
| Brachial plexus | 100 | 100 |
| Upper trunk | 25 | 25 |
| Middle trunk | 5 | 35 |
| Lower trunk | 20 | 70 |
| Lumbosacral plexus | 40 | 50 |

Modified from *Guides to the evalution of permanent impairment,* ed 4, American Medical Association, 1993, Chicago.

found in the AMA *Guides.* The values assigned each root, plexus, or nerve are somewhat arbitrary but are based upon the relative strength of the sensory or motor functions of each nerve and, in the case of motor nerves, the muscles innervated and their rela-

tive importance in determining the strength and function of the involved extremity. The value from the appropriate table is then multiplied by the degree of decreased strength or decreased sensation or pain as determined from physical examination. For example, if strength is graded at a level of 3 (26% to 50% motor deficit) and the inferior gluteal nerve is affected (25% maximum impairment of the lower extremity), the maximum loss is multiplied by the grade (25% × 26% to 50%) and then converted into a whole person impairment.

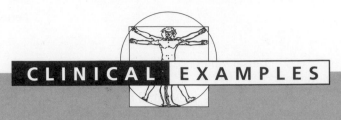

## PERIPHERAL NERVOUS SYSTEM

EDITOR'S NOTE—Peripheral nervous system impairment generally follows one of four patterns: nerve root lesions, plexus lesions, disturbances of single or multiple peripheral nerves, or abnormalities of a "stocking" and/or "glove" distribution. The impairment assessment of nerve root lesions is usually associated with a spinal pathologic process. When spinal impairment is assessed using the DRE model (see Chapters 24 and 25 herein), the radiculopathy is a part of the impairment process of the spine lesion. This will change an individual's impairment category from a Class II to higher values. The DRE Categorization scheme components are found in Tables 72, 73, and 74 of the AMA *Guides*.*

When using the "functional" or "range of motion" model, the contribution caused by the nerve root lesion is independently assessed and combined with the range of motion impairment. The dermatomes of the upper limb are found in Figure 46. Values for C5-T1 nerve root lesions are found in Table 13 (page 51). Values for L3-S1 are found in Table 83 (page 130).

With respect to plexus injuries, the sacral plexus is not specifically addressed in the *Guides*. The brachial plexus is addressed in Table 14 (page 52). The nerves creating the brachial plexus are found in Figure 47. Table 14 addresses impairment caused by motor and sensory problems of nerves originating from the brachial plexus due to plexus injuries.

Specific peripheral nerve impairment is found in various tables and charts throughout the *Guides*, as outlined here:

| | |
|---|---|
| Fingers | Section 3.1c, starting on page 20; section 3.f (thumb); figures 4, 5; and Table 4 |

*All *tables, figures,* and *sections* referred to in this discussion are found in AMA *Guides to the evaluation of permanent impairment,* ed 4, Chapter 4—The Nervous System, American Medical Association, 1993, Chicago.

| | |
|---|---|
| Impairment of the upper extremity originating from the brachial plexus, including both sensory deficits and pain | Section 3.1k; Tables 11 and 12 (sensory or motor disturbance); Table 10 and Figure 45 (sensory contributions); Table 15 and Figure 48; Table 16 and section 3.1k (entrapment neuropathies) |
| Strength in the hand as determined by both grip strength and lateral pinch strength | Pages 64 and 65 and Tables 31 to 33 |
| Strength in the lower extremity | Table 37 (muscle atrophy), Table 39 (weakness), and Table 38 (grading scheme) |
| Lower extremity | Section 3.2k (only peripheral nerve injuries as opposed to sacral plexus abnormalities); Figures 59 and 60 |
| Peripheral nervous abnormalities | Section 4.4c, Tables 10 and 21 (impairment losses) |

"Stocking" and/or "glove" neuropathies are not discussed separately but are found with systemic diseases such as diabetes mellitus. The examiner must select the nerves found in that area and describe sensory losses for them as if the entire nerve were affected.

### EXAMPLE
#### History

A 48-year-old man has asked for an impairment evaluation. He works in a factory where batteries are made, specifically picking batteries up from an assembly line and placing them in cartons. However, he also states that he works near the area where the leaves for the batteries are produced. He says that dust, fumes, and smoke are constantly present in the plant. He has been advised to wear respiratory protection, but he states that he has never worn it because of problems with breathing and nasal congestion. He has smoked two packs of cigarettes per day since the age of 18.

*Continued.*

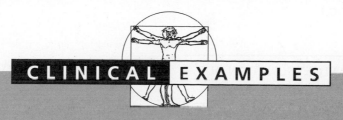
## PERIPHERAL NERVOUS SYSTEM—cont'd

In reviewing his records, the physician finds that his blood lead level was 64 mg% on a random screening, and he was referred to the company physician. He was treated with chelation and, over the next several months, his lead level fell to 15 mg%. The physician is asked to evaluate him for complaints of numbness and tingling in the first and second digits of both hands and weakness of the left upper extremity.

### Physical Examination

Tinel's and Phalen's signs are both positive in both hands, two-point discrimination is absent to 7 mm in the first and second digits in both hands, but motor strength is deemed normal in both hands. No other sensory abnormalities are present. Weakness is found in the left shoulder (Grade 3 to 4) but not the right. The remainder of the upper extremity motor examination is normal, as is the lower extremity motor and sensory examination. Deep tendon reflexes are all normal. However, he appears to have some difficulty remembering the exact description of his job, his medical history, and the names of his medications.

### Test Results

On the day of the examination, the lead serum blood level is 18 mg%. An EMG is positive for minor denervation in the region of the axillary nerve on the left. The remainder of the upper extremity EMG is normal. Nerve conduction test results are consistent with carpal tunnel syndrome in both hands. There is nerve conduction delay across the median nerve in both hands.

### Assessment Process

Lead can produce a peripheral neuropathy, but it is solely motor. Thus the diminished strength in the left shoulder and the positive EMG reveal an impairment consistent with lead intoxication. Carpal tunnel syndrome is primarily a sensory deficit and could not be attributed to the lead intoxication, although it may have been caused by the repetitive motion characteristic of his job. The physician also suspects a cognitive impairment, although this was not specifically tested.

Using Table 15, the maximum percent of upper extremity impairment caused by motor deficit in the axillary nerve is 35%. This individual has a Grade 3 to 4 strength assessment on physical examination and minor abnormalities in the EMG. Accordingly, a 20% to 25% impairment of the upper extremity due to the axillary nerve neuropathy would be considered appropriate. Using Table 3 on page 20, this yields a 12% to 15% whole person impairment (WPI). A value of 13% seems appropriate.

Because of the signs and symptoms as well as the nerve conduction test involving the median nerve at the wrists, the physician feels that a moderate impairment of the upper extremities is appropriate. For the median nerve, using Table 16 (page 57), a 20% impairment of the upper extremity results. This yields a 12% WPI using Table 3 (page 20).

### Evaluation

This individual has a 32% WPI based on the three separate neurologic abnormalities (13% combined with 12% combined with 12%). (With more than one nerve involved, the upper extremity impairments derived for each are combined using the Combined Values Chart.) If the evaluation is solely for lead intoxication, the impairment is only 13%. It should be noted that this individual should be referred for a psychiatric examination and neuropsychiatric testing to evaluate the presence of cognitive impairment. Lead intoxication can cause this type of abnormality and should be independently assessed.

*Stephen L. Demeter*

**TABLE 40-6     MAXIMUM LOST FUNCTION DUE TO SPINAL NERVE IMPAIRMENT (PERCENTAGE)**

| NERVE | DECREASED SENSATION OR PAIN | DECREASED POWER |
|---|---|---|
| Axillary | 5 | 35 |
| Musculocutaneous | 5 | 25 |
| Median | | |
| Above midforearm | 40 | 55 |
| Below midforearm | 40 | 35 |
| Ulnar | | |
| Above midforearm | 10 | 35 |
| Below midforearm | 10 | 25 |
| Radial | | |
| Triceps involved | 5 | 55 |
| Triceps uninvolved | 5 | 40 |
| Femoral | 5 | 35 |
| Inferior gluteal | 0 | 25 |
| Lateral femoral cutaneous | 10 | 0 |
| Superior gluteal | 0 | 20 |
| Sciatic | 25 | 75 |
| Common peroneal | 5 | 35 |
| Tibial | 15 | 35 |

Modified from *Guides to the evaluation of permanent impairment,* ed 4, American Medical Association, 1993, Chicago.

This process provides for calculating the degree of impairment of the involved extremity. If, as is usually the case, mixed motor and sensory fibers are affected, causing a mixture of symptoms, the estimated motor and sensory deficits can be combined as in the *Guides.* Once the degree of impairment of a limb has been calculated, it can be converted to an estimate that represents impairment of the whole person. If more than one limb is involved, the impairment value of each limb is calculated, and the values are combined and converted into a single whole person impairment estimate.

### References

1. Adams RD, Victor M: *Principles of neurology,* ed 5, New York, 1993, McGraw-Hill.
2. AAEM Quality Assurance Committee. Literature review of the usefulness of nerve conduction studies and electromyography for the evaluation of patients with carpal tunnel syndrome, *Muscle and Nerve,* 16:1392-1414, 1993.
3. American Medical Association: *Guides to the evaluation of permanent impairment,* ed 4, Chicago, 1993, American Medical Association.
4. Devinsky O, Feldmann E: *Examination of the cranial and peripheral nerves,* New York, 1988, Churchill Livingstone.
5. *Disability evaluation under Social Security,* U. S. Department of Health and Human Services, 1992.
6. Golding DN, Rose DM, Selvarajeh K: Clinical tests for carpal tunnel syndrome: an evaluation, *Br J Rheumatology,* 25:338-390, 1986.
7. Halderman S: The electrodiagnostic evaluation of nerve root function, *Spine,* 9:42-48, 1984.
8. Kimura J: *Electrodiagnosis in disease of nerve and muscle: principles and practice,* Philadelphia, 1989, F.A. Davis.
9. Raynor EM, Shetner JM, Preston DC, et al: Sensory and mixed nerve conduction studies in the evaluation of ulnar neuropathy at the elbow, *Muscle and Nerve,* 17:785-792, 1994.
10. Stevens JC: AAEE Minimonograph #26: The electrodiagnosis of carpal tunnel syndrome, *Muscle and Nerve,* 10:99-113, 1987.
11. Vinken PJ, Bruyn GW, Klavons AL, et al: *Handbook of clinical neurology,* vol 7-8, New York, 1970, American Elsevier.
12. Vinken PJ, Bruyn GW, Klavons AL, et al: *Handbook of clinical neurology,* vol 51, New York, 1987, Elsevier Science.

# CHAPTER 41

# THE VISUAL SYSTEM

*Arthur H. Keeney*

## DEFINITIONS: THE EYE AND THE VISUAL PATHWAYS

Vision is served by a highly complex end-organ apparatus—the eye and its appendages, a long neural pathway initiated by the optic nerve (cranial nerve II), the chiasmal crossing or partial decussation of the right and left nerves, and the optic tracts progressing to the first way-station or lateral geniculate ganglia. From this six-layered structure visual impulses proceed through the optic radiations to the primary visual projection areas or occipital poles of the cortex (Brodmann's area 17). Beyond this initial registration area are the visual association areas (Brodmann's areas 18 and 19) plus their interconnection of right and left sides through the splenium or posterior rounded end of the corpus callosum, to the ultimate interpretive areas of the temporoparietal lobes.

Visual impairment may occur from the most anterior or distal components such as the eyelids, the tear film, and the cornea, or elsewhere throughout the eyes and their long neural pathways to the visual cortex of the brain and the interpretive centers of the temporoparietal lobes. Thus visual impairments may be of optical origin at numerous locations connected with the eyes, or result from tissue alteration and physiologic disturbance of any of the cellular components of the visual pathways from the cornea to the brain. Cellular disturbances at any point along this route may lead to permanent visual impairment. It is neither necessary nor helpful to specify each detail of disease or malfunction that may strike the visual system in order to arrive at a quantitative, functional evaluation. Obviously, this does not obviate precise diagnosis, optimal therapeutic intervention, or careful prognosis.

The use of code schemes or guides to medical impairment or disability evaluation does not relate to acute illness, determining levels of visual function during treatment, or ascertaining visual status prior to optimal measures of correction and rehabilitation. Basic to disability evaluation is that all medical efforts have been exhausted, and a residual permanent impairment exists and is not amenable to the best of known therapeutic interventions at the current state of ophthalmologic science. Thus the examiner for medical impairment or disability evaluation is concerned with permanent reductions from normal physiological levels after consummation of all appropriate treatments aimed at restoring usual physiologic visual functions.

Some complex rehabilitative devices or optical systems may be invoked, creating apparent simulation of enhancement of specific visual parameters. Such systems include closed-circuit television readers, compound telescopic systems for specified distance ranges, infrared night-sight goggles, and miniature television circuitry worn in helmet configuration before the eyes. Although these devices may be in the vanguard of rehabilitative research, they are outside of the assessment system designed to measure residual permanent impairment. Similarly, medical care and rehabilitation do not aim toward "super sight" or acuity at the level of 20/10 or 6/3 when measured in feet or meters as is manifest in most U.S. astronauts, but rather gauges permanent loss after optimal therapy and correction with conventional spectacles, contact lenses, or interocular lens implants. These levels are then rated against average, normal physiologic function of the visual system.

## INDEX FUNCTIONS OF VISION

Because literally thousands of pathologic mechanisms may disturb visual function, it is both helpful and economical to look at index functions that in themselves reflect many specific disease disturbances.

## Central Visual Acuity

The prime index function of the visual system is central visual acuity or resolving power expressed since 1893 as a Snellen fraction, if needed, through optimal correction by conventional spectacles or contact lenses. This is based on the minimum detectable separation of two points in space or one minute of arc. The usual targets or optotypes devised for assessing this index function are based on components, each of which subtend one minute of arc or contain separation of one minute of arc between components. These are usually letters presented in nonserif design and high letter-to-background contrast. Visual acuity is usually tested at a distance of 20 ft or 6 m, which simulates infinity and does not require accommodative effort or convergence of the visual axes as in near-range evaluation. The Snellen notation 20/20 or 6/6 is accepted as average and normal, though many young and healthy eyes can resolve targets of 20/10 or 6/3 design with components subtending only ½ minute (30 seconds) of arc. Though with generally less precision and intertest reliability, central acuity is also evaluated in the near or reading range. For the presbyopic patient (that is, usually older than 40 years), this necessitates reading glasses or bifocals. The nearsighted or myopic individual of one to two diopters may demonstrate excellent near vision without reading glasses.

## Visual Field

The second major index function of the eye is the breadth of vision or visual field. This normally encompasses 180°-200° of arc in the horizontal plane with the two eyes together; with one eye alone the visual field is 90°-100° temporally and 45°-50° nasally, depending on the bony configuration of the orbit and the position of the eye, whether anatomically deep-set or prominent in the orbit. For an impairment analysis, a standardized Goldmann target designated III4e has been the accepted reference since the mid-1940s. This is equivalent to the earlier arc perimeter target specified as 3-33 white, or a 3 mm diameter white target moved kinetically along an arc located one-third of a meter or 33 cm from the patient's pupil. Conventionally, 8 radii or principal meridians are tested, and field loss is expressed in degrees of reduction from the normal or usual extent of field awareness in each radius.

Current automated test equipment, while excellent for following a patient with a specific ocular disease such as glaucoma, often assesses only the central 30°-60° of the visual field and thus cannot supply needed data in determining impairment of the far peripheral field. Thus a full bowl or full 180° arc perimeter is needed to calculate any reduction from the normal extent of the field. This poses a problem because automated central field analysis equipment has become very popular and is widely used in ophthalmic and optometric diagnoses, while Goldmann bowl perimeters are less commonly used.

As with measuring central visual acuity, it is diagnostically helpful to measure each eye separately, but there is also virtue at times in measuring the binocular or two-eyed fields.

Loss is calculated from the extent normally encompassed by the visual field for the given target stimulus in relation to a control group of similar age.

## Diplopia

The third index function is the presence or absence of diplopia, which is an increasingly significant impairment close to fixation. Diplopia only in extremes of rotation (beyond 30° from fixation) may cause little impairment, whereas diplopia within the near central fixation area (within 20° from fixation) may necessitate that the patient wears an occlusive patch for one eye, or has extraocular muscle surgery performed to reduce such diplopia. The significance of diplopia is also greater in lower than in upper fields of fixation.

## Defects Not Reflected in the Index Functions

Finally, there is a wide diversity of other and sometimes less serious impairments that may be evaluated by the examining ophthalmologist and suitable for an additional determination of 5% or 10% impairment. Such defects, not reflected in the index functions, include impaired color perception, poor adaptation to light, poor contrast sensitivity, impairment of stereopsis, tearing, and functional or cosmetic scars. The examiner may apply such judgmental additional impairment to an individual eye or to the visual system, or based upon an awareness of its effect(s) on the whole body.

## PERCENTAGE RATINGS OF IMPAIRMENTS

There are basically four separate components amenable to visual impairment rating: (1) the eye and its adnexa, (2) the two eyes conjointly as a visual system, (3) the reduction in whole body function created by visual impairment through the loss of one eye or reduction in the function of this system, and

(4) allowances specifically determined for more subtle functional impairments not reflected in the three major index functions.

## Determining Function of the Eyes

Function of eyes is usually calculated by striking an average between the reliable and precise measurements of resolving power or central visual acuity at distance, and the less reliable and less reproducible measurement made at the near range. Such distances are commonly taken to be 20 feet or 6 m for far regard, and 14 inches or 35 cm for near. The calculated loss of central acuity is then integrated with measured loss in degrees from the normal visual field by using a combined value table. This is done for each eye separately and then combined with any loss attributable to diplopia. The binocular or visual system impairment is then read from a different table utilizing a multiple value for the better eye and the impairment value of the less good eye. Such tables have been established from the mid-1950s and are well accepted in most jurisdictions of the United States. A separate table is used to convert the impairment of the visual system to impairment of the whole person.

Values established for impairment of the whole person as derived from impairment of the visual system have been well standardized and accepted, though fundamentally containing certain arbitrary decisions. For example, the total loss of vision in one eye corresponds to a 25% impairment of the visual system and is estimated to represent a 24% impairment of the whole person. Total loss of vision in both eyes corresponds to a 100% impairment of the visual system and is estimated to represent an 85% impairment of the whole person. Lesser visual losses descend from these values.

In general, the percentage values for losses in visual function have been widely published for nearly 40 years and should not be altered without overwhelming need. The resultant values have long been incorporated into principles of worker's compensation and Social Security disability determinations.

## Losses of Visual Function Not Represented in the Index Function

Certain specific and individual losses of function are not represented in the index function and, therefore, must be evaluated separately and clearly by the examining physician. This may be calculated for one eye or for the visual system. A maximum arbitrary value is usually established for such additional judgments, and these are to exclude any amount of impairment concurrently assigned for scars, deformities, and disorganizations extending from adjacent facial structures.

## LOSS OF VISUAL FUNCTION AND SAFETY

Though not strictly a function of disability evaluation, medical examiners must be aware of their fundamental roles as physicians to patients. By definition, a patient is "one who suffers" and is therefore in a dependent role to any physician involved in the care of his or her problems. The physician is not only the patient's advocate but is committed by oath to care, assist, and support the one who suffers. Because any impairment of the visual system produces some compromise in use of the eyes for operation of a motor vehicle, physicians have a responsibility to advise their patients or regulatory agencies about driving limitations, which are highly dependent on visual, perceptual, and motor functioning. The index visual functions necessary for operation of a motor vehicle depend on central visual acuity adequate for recognition and interpretation of Uniform Traffic Control Devices as governed by the Federal Highway Administration and a descriptive standard published by the American National Standards Institute. These generally are predicated on an optimally-corrected central visual acuity (with conventional spectacles or contact lenses) of at least 20/40 (6/12) and sizing of letters in nonserif design with high contrast of white letters on a dark background. Drivers are expected to recognize and interpret such uniform traffic control devices in clear weather, under maximum authorized speed limit for the road, and far enough in advance to permit interpretation and decision making.

The second index factor in safety is hazard awareness and detection, which is dependent on the breadth of the visual field. In essentially all U.S. states, a monocular driver is eligible for a private driving license; it is assumed or required by horizontal form field recognition in 20 states that a minimum of 140° is available in horizontal breadth of visual field in one eye for hazard detection.

The commercial driver, however, by administrative regulation, must have horizontal form field recognition of at least 140° in each of two eyes. Color perception or hue discrimination, at least in the red/green spectrum, seems to be logically related to safe vehicle operation. However, there are essentially no data supporting the need for hue discrimination in driving. This has been simplified by additional yellow in the red signal and blue in the green signal, so that the common red/green anomalies present in about

6% of American males and 0.5% of American females is engineered out of significance.

Though true stereopsis is important in near-range parking maneuvers, in estimation of road characteristics, and in activities of passing and gap judgment, this is a contingent function dependent on the coordinate use of the two eyes as a pair, and the level of acuity available in each of the two eyes. As acuity decreases, so does stereopsis or stereo-acuity. This function also decreases with reduction in illumination and distance from the observer. It is generally not measured separately.

## ROLE OF COMPENSATORY DEVICES, LOW VISION AIDS, AND VISUAL SUBSTITUTION SYSTEMS

### Spectacle or Contact Lens Correction

A spectacle correction is worn by approximately 51% of the U.S. population, and this increases from a very low percentage in early childhood to almost 100% in senior citizens. Contact lenses also have improved so much in the past few decades that they are now generally accepted as well-tolerated alternatives to spectacle correction. Contact lenses offer at times optical advantages not obtainable by spectacles. This occurs in eliminating the image–size reduction (minification) created by high minus power spectacles for myopia, and eliminating the problem of irregular stigmatism that is not amenable to spectacle correction. Extended-wear contact lenses have greatly reduced the optical problems of postsurgical aphakia and the encumbrance of such patients with thick spectacle lenses. For these patients, contact lenses provide a much broader field of vision, greatly reduced edge distortion, and afford nearly normal-sized relationships of seen objects. The examining physician must be aware that occasionally a patient cannot wear contact lenses and therefore, when ametropia is present, the patient may be committed to conventional spectacle lenses.

Spectacle lenses and contact lenses are no longer classified as prosthetic devices when employed to correct the normally large number of patients with physiologic refractive errors. They may be considered as prosthetic devices when correcting aphakia due to surgical removal of the lens from the eye. The latter procedure has been largely superseded by the implantation of a prosthetic or artificial lens within the globe after cataract extraction.

### Compound Lens Systems

Controversy exists concerning the use of compound lens systems or Galilean telescopes for individuals with subnormal visual acuity or resolving power. Such telescopes can provide a range of two- to five-power magnification but at the expense of proportionate reduction in available visual field and depth of focus. Thus, they do not convert a 20/70 or 20/100 best corrected spectacle visual acuity to 20/20 by the optical device of image size enlargement. The area of magnified visual field, through such devices, is reduced progressively, as the power of magnification rises to arcs of only 5° or 10° in diameter. Telescopic magnified fields are further hampered by a negative ring scotoma or blind ring that surrounds the small magnified area because of the device; the width of such rings of obscured vision varies from 7°-15°. Other optical limitations of vision through a telescope are well known and include decay of resolving ability because of vibration, contralateral movement of images with any movement of the head, loss of visual contact with the environment during shifting into or out of the telescopic area, and the need for altered head posture when such telescopes are placed in conventional spectacle lenses as carrier lenses.

### Additional Magnification for Close-up Work

Many individuals seek and use additional magnification in the near working range. This is most easily done by increasing the dioptric power of a bifocal above the usual maximum of plus 2.5 diopters to 4, 5, or 6 diopters. This can provide 1.5 power of magnification in the bifocal but of necessity reduces the depth of focus and requires that objects be brought closer to the bifocal for critical acuity. A common example of this type of device is the single-lens jeweler's loupe mounted at the edge of one lens in a pair of glasses. The jeweler flips this supplemental lens into the line of sight to gain magnification. The jeweler, of course, brings the item of inspection into very near range to attain this magnification.

### Intraocular Lens Implants

A longstanding optical problem following surgical removal of the crystalline lens from within the eye, as after cataract extraction, has been the need of a very high dioptric power (+10 to 12D) lens for distant acuity. Such lenses cause considerable distortion of the visual field, restriction in diameter of the field, and image magnification. These problems have been progressively eliminated by the increasing use of surgically implanted plastic lenses (pseudophakia). Approximately 1.2 million prosthetic lenses were implanted in eyes of cataract patients in the United States in 1992. This surgical process has greatly enhanced the near normalization of vision after cataract extraction.

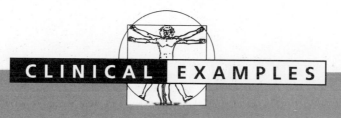

# CLINICAL EXAMPLES

## VISUAL SYSTEM

### EXAMPLE 1

#### History

A 28-year-old construction worker has come to be evaluated for permanent visual impairment one year after an injury to the right eye and orbit in a fall from scaffolding. Surgical repair was done on the day of injury, and appropriate medical and operative therapy have been carried out. An adequate length of time has elapsed since the accident for evaluation to take place.

#### Physical Examination and Test Results

Distance visual acuity in the right eye is 20/40 without glasses and is not improved by glasses or contact lenses. Distance vision in the left eye is 20/20 without glasses. Near visual acuity in the injured right eye is 14/28; the near-approximation of distance Snellen acuity is rated 20/40 and is not significantly improved by glasses. Near vision in the left eye is normal (14/14). There is a mild deficiency of hue discrimination in the right eye and none in the left. Goldmann visual field testing with the III4e target on the right eye shows irregular constriction of the visual field as follows:

| | |
|---|---|
| • Temporally | 40° |
| • Down and temporally | 35° |
| • Directly down | 30° |
| • Down and nasally | 10° |
| • Nasally | 25° |
| • Up and nasally | 10° |
| • Directly up | 10° |
| • Up temporally | 20° |

#### Assessment Process

These eight measurements add up to a total of 180 and, when this sum is divided by five, the result is 36, which is the percent of visual field loss. There was no loss of visual field for the uninjured left eye. In the right eye, total visual field retention is 64%. No additional loss is assigned on the basis of quadrantic loss.

Using the Combined Values Chart (p. 322),* the percentage of loss of central vision (11%) is combined with the percentage loss of visual field in the same eye (36%), to give an impairment rating of the right eye of 43%. Any significant loss of ocular motility is then rated on the basis of its presence and the location of diplopia with both eyes open. Here diplopia is found in depressed gaze between 30 and 40° from fixation. It is less in all other meridians of gaze. Taking the evaluation in the meridian of maximum impairment, according to Figure 3 (p. 217), motility impairment is evaluated as 30%. Again using the Combined Values Chart (p. 322), the diplopia rating of 30% is combined with the impairment of central vision and visual field of 43%, giving a 60% loss for the visual function of the right eye. Optic nerve damage is indexed by reduced acuity, visual field constriction, and impairment of hue or color discrimination. Using Table 7 (p. 219), visual system impairment for both eyes is derived by adding the impairment of the worst eye (60%) with that of the better eye (0%), which is read as a 15% impairment of the visual system.

#### Evaluation

The 15% impairment of the visual system is further extended in Table 6 (p. 218) to yield a 14% whole person impairment (WPI).

### EXAMPLE 2

#### History

A 40-year-old driver who had a history of normal vision in each eye has come for evaluation after being injured in an automobile accident. The injury involved a small penetrating wound through the cornea and lens of the right eye and multiple lacerations and ex-

---

*All *tables*, *figures*, and *charts* referred to in this discussion are found in AMA *Guides to the evaluation of permanent impairment*, ed 4, Chapter 8—The Visual System, American Medical Association, Chicago, 1993.

*Continued.*

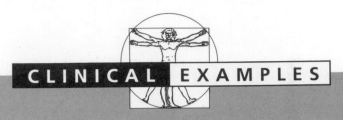
## VISUAL SYSTEM—cont'd

tensive disorganization of the left eye with no light perception. The left eye was surgically removed by enucleation the day after injury. The small wound in the right eye healed well, but a secondary (posttraumatic) cataract developed within the next two months. Cataract extraction was done three months after the accident using a pseudophakic implant; vision in the right eye was restored to 20/20+ at distance and 14/14 near vision. The visual field of the right eye is fully normal, as are pupillary reactions. A prosthesis was fitted to the left orbit about two months after the injury.

### Physical Examination and Test Results

Impairment of vision in the right eye shows no loss for distance vision, near vision, or visual field.

### Assessment Process

Because of monocular pseudophakia in the right eye, a 50% loss in remaining central vision is allowed for the pseudophakic eye despite normal Snellen acuity. Visual field loss is also zero in the right eye and 100% in the left. The loss of central vision in the right eye is calculated as 50% and loss of visual field as 0%. The Combined Values Chart (p. 322) is used to determine the combined value for loss in the right eye as 50% for central vision and 0% for visual field, yielding an estimated impairment of the right eye of 50%. On the left, there is 100% impairment of central vision and of fields, or a 100% impairment of the left eye (combined loss of 100%). Using the combined value from Table 7 (p. 221), to account for using the two eyes together, yields a 100% impairment plus a 50% impairment, or a 63% impairment of the visual system.

### Evaluation

Table 6 (p. 218) lists a 63% impairment of the visual system as equivalent to a 59% WPI.

*Arthur H. Keeney*

Complications from cataract surgery and lens implantation have been greatly reduced since the 1960s. Still there are occasionally interoperative complications, dislocations of the implant, and rarely inflammatory intolerance to the implant. Image size is essentially returned to normal by using such an implant as compared with even the modest image size enlargement produced by contact lenswear in the presence of aphakia. The procedure is now standardized, well accepted, and widely performed, particularly in the United States. However, because it is a prosthetic correction of surgically induced aphakia, nearly all impairment guides make some additional allowance in favor of the postoperative patient with such an implant and do not consider that visual function has been returned to a 100% normal status.

Postoperative cataract patients experience enhanced brightness of visual experience, with accentuated whiteness of objects and enhanced perception of the blue and violet end of the spectrum. These functions are best not explored even conversationally as their presence may become a source of worry and concern to the patient. In themselves, they do not merit evaluation of impairment, and in most patients there is successful adaptation postoperatively in a matter of months. With great improvements in contact lens material and fitting techniques now available, even the contact lens wearer, when well adapted, may wear the contact lens for extended—and unauthorized—periods of weeks or months without difficulty. This, of course, requires the wearer to be largely in a dirt-free environment and to have no corneal sensitivity to the monomer from which the contact lens is made. This is a reflection of widespread, individual differences in adaptation and in physiologic tolerance to contact lenses.

## References

1. American Medical Association: *Guides to the evaluation of permanent impairment*, ed 4, Chapter 8, The Visual System, Chicago 1993, American Medical Association.
2. Decina LE et al: *Evaluation of vision testing equipment, review of vision tests and the driving performance record, and recommendations for pilot vision screening program*, Malvern, Pa, Nov. 1988, Ketron.
3. Decina LE, Breton ME, Staplin L: *Visual disorders and commercial drivers*, Washington, D.C, Nov. 1991, Office of Motor Carriers, Federal Highway Administration.
4. Freytag E, Sacks JG: Abnormalities of the central visual pathways contributing to traffic accidents, *JAMA* 204(10):119-121, June 3, 1968.
5. Johnson CA, Keltner JL: Incidence of visual field loss in 20,000 eyes and its relationship to driving performance, *Arch Ophthalmol* 101:371-375, March 1983.
6. Keltner JL, Johnson CA: Visual function, driving safety, and the elderly, *Ophthalmology* 94:1180-1188, Sept. 1987.
7. *Manual on Uniform Traffic Control Devices for Streets and Highways*, New York, NY. American National Standards Institute, ANSI D6.1 and Washington, D.C., U.S. D.O.T., Federal Highway Administration, 1988 rev.

# AUDIOLOGICAL SYSTEM

*Aram Glorig*
*Robert Thayer Sataloff*

This chapter reviews impairment and disability resulting from dysfunction of selected structures in the head and neck. The head and neck are rich in sensory and motor structures that are important for communication, cosmesis, deglutition, olfaction, and other functions important to an individual's quality of life and ability to function in the workplace. This chapter does not discuss all aspects of otolaryngologic impairment and disability, but rather is limited to a few topics selected for their high incidence, important individual consequences, and complexity.

There are numerous methods of evaluating otolaryngologic impairment and disability. These can be classified as self-reporting or specific measurement. Self-reporting methods take two forms: questionnaires and personal interviews. Self-reporting methods are subject to many variables. For example, the results can be influenced by the objectives of the questioner and/or the interviewer. Unless the material used by the interviewer is well-standardized, inter-test results will not be comparable. Furthermore, unsupervised self-completed questionnaires will be influenced by the attitude and education of the subject who is completing the questionnaire. For example, young subjects and old subjects will respond differently. Older subjects are more forgiving of their impairments or loss of function. When the impairments are equal, older subjects describe themselves as being less affected than the young subjects.[17]

When specific measurements are used to rate impairment, the results are influenced by the measurement materials.[7] The shortcomings of assessment techniques have not been overcome for otolaryngologic impairments. Many of the practices described in this chapter have shortcomings, but they represent the best and most standardized approaches currently available. Research is constantly in progress exploring more precise assessment methodology.

## HEARING

The most common types of hearing dysfunctions are sensorineural, conductive, mixed, and central hearing loss. Sensorineural hearing impairment is caused by pathologic processes taking place in the cochlea, the acoustic nerve, or the brain stem. There are many causes of sensorineural hearing impairment including excessive noise exposure, ototoxic medications, childhood diseases, meningitis, tumors, and head injuries.[18,31] Conductive hearing impairment is due to pathology in the external or middle ear. Examples include otosclerosis, otitis media, congenital disorders, otitis externa, and impacted cerumen. Mixed hearing impairment occurs when there is combined sensorineural and conductive pathology. Examples include advanced otosclerosis and chronic otitis media. Central hearing loss involves the inability to process auditory signals; it may be seen and associated with multiple sclerosis, head trauma, brain tumors, and other conditions.

### Hearing Impairment

The need for some way of calculating or deriving impairment for patients with hearing loss became evident in the early 1940s. Perhaps the first useful formula was suggested by E.P. Fowler, Sr. in 1942. It tested hearing at 500 Hz, 1000 Hz, 2000 Hz, and 4000 Hz and weighted the losses in these frequencies.[6] Subsequently, the American Medical Association introduced a similar formula (1959) but with different weightings.

Various combinations of frequencies have been suggested since then (Table 42-1). These formulas were used to determine impairments for hearing and understanding speech under everyday conditions. All the original formulas were based on tests performed

**TABLE 42-1**      HEARING LOSS FORMULAS PROPOSED FOR EVALUATING IMPAIRMENT

| SOURCE | FREQUENCIES (kHz) | FORMULA | LOW FENCE (dB RE ISO 1960) |
|---|---|---|---|
| Fowler (1942) | 0.5, 1, 2, 4<br>0.4, 0.15 | Weighted 0.15, 0.3 | 10 |
| AMA (1947) | 0.5, 1, 2, 4 | Variable weights (depending on HTLs) | 20 |
| AAOO (1959) | 0.5, 1, 2 | Unweighted average | 25 |
| ISO (1971, 1975) | 0.5, 1, 2 | Unweighted average | 25 |
| NIOSH (1972) | 0.5, 1, 2 | Unweighted average | 25 |
| Macrae (1975-6) | 0.5, 1, 1.5, 2, 3, 4 | Weighted 0.2, 0.25<br>0.2, 0.15, 0.1 | < 3 kHz: 20<br>4 kHz: 25 |
| CHABA (1975) | 1, 2, 3 | Unweighted | 35 |
| BS 5330 (1976) | 1, 2, 3 | Unweighted average | 30 |
| Berney (Ginnold, 1979) | 0.5, 1, 2, 4 | Unweighted average | 25 |
| Oregon (Ginnold, 1979) | 0.5, 1, 2, 4, 6 | Unweighted average | 25 |
| ISO (1972a) | — | None standardized | — |
| AAO (1979) | 0.5, 1, 2, 3 | Unweighted average | 25 |
| Brit. Assoc. of Otolaryngologists (1983) | 1, 2, 4 | Unweighted average | 20 |

dB = Decibels
kHz = Kilohertz
HTL = Hearing Threshold Level
AMA = American Medical Association
AAO = American Academy of Otolaryngology
AAOO = American Academy of Ophthalmology and Otolaryngology
ISO = International Standards Organization
NIOSH = National Institute of Occupational Safety and Health
CHABA = Committee on Hearing and Bioacoustics of the American Standards Institute
BS = Bureau of Standards

while listening in a quiet environment. The original American Academy of Otolaryngology formula (1959) was modified in 1979 when 3000 Hz was added because it better represents speech perception and perception in noisy environments.

Why were all the formulas and assessment methods based on pure tones of various frequencies? Not because this provides the best representation of a person's ability to hear, but rather because pure tone audiometry is the best practical test available. It is standardized, valid, and reliable for determining the ability to detect soft sounds in a quiet environment in most cases. This provides a fairly useful guide to a person's ability to hear speech. Other common tests such as the speech reception threshold test (SRT),

which uses bisyllabic spondaic words (e.g., "baseball," "flytrap," "backstop"), and the speech discrimination score (SDS), which uses single-syllable phonetically-balanced word lists, provide additional information, but have important practical limitations that preclude their routine use in compensation formulas. Attempts to formulate useful and acceptable representative sentence lists and word lists have been unsuccessful, so far.

The human ear has a frequency range from about 20 to 20,000 Hz. It is so sensitive that it can almost hear the Brownian movement in the surrounding air. Pure tone measurements are made with an instrument called an audiometer. Earphones are placed over the ears and tones are controlled for level and frequency to determine the hearing threshold, which is the lowest sound pressure level that can be heard by the individual. Routine audiometry requires a voluntary response such as raising a finger or hand or pushing a button. Hearing is usually measured with pure tone signals at 250, 500, 1000, 2000, 3000, 4000, 6000, and 8000 Hz (Hz = cycles per second).

Standard zero hearing level is based on the hearing of a group of individuals whose age varied between 18 and 24 years and who had no history of previous ear problems. Pure tone tests may be done by air conduction or bone conduction. Air conduction tests measure the status of the external, middle, and inner ear, including the cochlea, acoustic nerve, brain stem, and cortex. Bone conduction tests measure sensorineural function directly, bypassing the external and middle ear. Speech is tested by using spondee and phonetically balanced words as described above.

There are more sophisticated and specialized tests such as brain stem audiometry, also called auditory brain stem response (ABR) or auditory evoked potential (AEP); electrocochleography; acoustic emission tests; and middle ear impedance measurement. These tests, along with other medical evaluations, are used by otologists to help determine the nature and specific cause of hearing impairment in selected individuals. They are often useful in differentiating noise-induced hearing impairment from other causes.

### Hearing Disability

Disability is defined as the auditory difficulties caused by hearing impairment. Examples of these are problems with communication by speech in work, social, or other settings, difficulties hearing warning signals, problems listening to music, and inability to localize sound sources or recognize different sounds. Communication by speech is considered to be the most important function of the auditory system. Therefore, communication difficulty is undoubtedly the most serious hearing disability.

Individuals with severe hearing loss may feel relegated to a second-class standard of living and status. In some cases, they may feel isolated and become introverted, refusing to go to parties, movies, religious services, and family gatherings. Participation in discussions may be limited. However, other individuals with similar hearing impairments may feel and function essentially normally, especially if they use amplification (hearing aids) effectively. Age has a deleterious effect. The same dysfunction in older individuals causes more difficulty than in the younger person, although this does not necessarily correlate with the individual's tolerance of the problems.[17]

In general, the effects of the hearing impairments on individuals vary as a function of the psychological make-up and particular daily activities. They are modified by the use of compensatory measures such as hearing aids, assistive devices, and speech reading (lip reading), as well as their self-confidence and willingness to request assistance from others.

### Handicap

A handicap caused by a hearing impairment is a disadvantage that prevents or limits an individual from completing a task that is normal or useful for that individual. These are nonauditory problems that arise because of hearing impairment or disability. According to the World Health Organization (WHO), hearing handicaps can be classified into the following categories:
1. Orientation handicaps (situational disorientation due to hearing losses, such as the inability to follow conversations).
2. Physical independence handicaps—inability to maintain a strictly independent existence.
3. Occupational handicaps—restriction of job or career choice.
4. Economic self-sufficiency handicaps.
5. Social integration handicaps—these cause numerous difficulties in carrying out ordinary daily activities, such as responding to warning signals and verbal messages.
6. Inability to cope with occupational requirements—loss of earning capacity.[38]

### Evaluation

Pure tone thresholds are used to quantify impairment and determine compensation. Various formulas average pure tone thresholds from various frequencies. Although this methodology is less than satisfactory, it is the current standard. A good example is the American Academy of Otolaryngology—American Medical Association formula based on the average of the thresholds at 500, 1000, 2000, and 3000 Hz. This formula (1) determines the average threshold at these four frequencies in one ear; (2) subtracts 25 dB, the point above which handicap is said to begin (low fence) (Figure 42-1); and (3) multiplies the difference by 1.5 to determine percent impairment in that ear. The average threshold in the remaining ear is treated the same way. This yields percent impairment in each ear. However, since one's possible handicap is based on binaural hearing, the percent impairment in each ear is combined by rating the better ear as 5 and the poorer ear as 1, then obtaining the average percent-

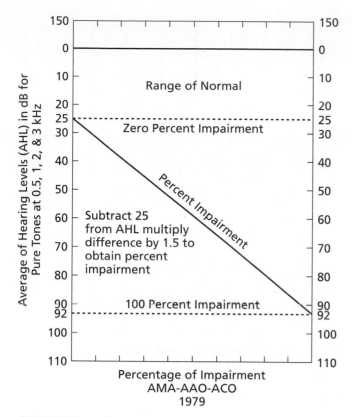

**FIGURE 42-1**    The present AMA formula for hearing impairment in graphic form. AMA = American Medical Association, AAO = American Academy of Otolaryngology, ACO = American College of Occupational Medicine (now ACOEM, American College of Occupational and Environmental Medicine).

may not truly represent speech intelligibility (Nilsson, 1993). Research is presently directed toward improving the presently accepted AMA method.[22] However, considerable additional research and experience will be needed before any change in the currently accepted, standardized methodology can be justified (Table 42-2).

## Other Considerations

In assessing any individual's disability from hearing loss, it is important to remember that there are millions of people in the United States with hearing loss from various causes unrelated to noise, injury, or other occupational cause. For medical and legal reasons, it is important to establish an accurate diagnosis in any individual with hearing loss or related dysfunction, such as tinnitus or vertigo.

It is also important to recognize that much can be done to ameliorate hearing disabilities and thereby mitigate the handicaps. Rehabilitative techniques include the use of (1) hearing aids, including in-the-ear, behind-the-ear, body aids, programmable aids, magnetic middle ear implants, cochlear and brain stem implants, and (2) assistive listening devices, including telephone amplifiers, infrared, microwave, and FM systems. With the proper amplification, counseling, and auditory training, most people with hearing impairments function extremely well, and many function normally.

## TINNITUS

### Introduction

The problems caused by tinnitus, its quantification, and its effect on human performance have been subjects of discussion and study for many years. A review of past and recent literature indicates that physicians have learned little of significance about tinnitus over the past century. Serious attempts are being made to develop animal models, measurement techniques, and self-scaling methods that should lead to a better understanding of the sources and mechanisms of the phenomenon. Such knowledge will undoubtedly also lead to better methods of management and treatment.

Tinnitus is not a disease. Rather, it is a symptom that may be the result of a disease or injury. However, tinnitus is so common that establishing causation is frequently difficult. The principal reason for the increasing interest in tinnitus within the context of a discussion of impairment and disability is its ef-

age of the two ears. This provides the percent binaural handicap. An average of 25 dB equals 0% impairment and an average of 92 dB equals 100% impairment.[12] An example is seen in Figure 42-2. The concept of using 25 dB as the cutoff point for hearing impairment is graphically demonstrated in Figure 42-3. This figure represents hearing losses in over a thousand patients who were tested by one of the authors (AG) and stratified by self-selection. The patients answered the question: "Do you think your hearing is good, fair, or poor?" and were then tested for hearing losses. All patients who stated that their hearing was "good" had intact 25 dB hearing. No patients with 25 dB hearing loss responded by saying their hearing was "good."

This formula has been widely adopted in the United States and in various other countries since it was proposed by the American Academy of Otolaryngology and approved by the American Medical Association in 1979. However, there has been controversy because the standard does not include frequencies above 3000 Hz. Recent studies have suggested that it

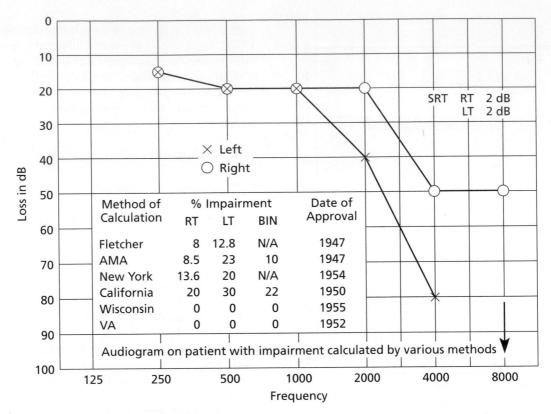

AMA = American Medical Association
VA = Veteran's Administration
SRT = Speech Reception Threshold Test
RT = Right ear
LT = Left ear
dB = Decibels
BIN = Binaural
↓ at 8000 = Arrow showing hearing level at 8 kHz is beyond limits of audiometer.

**FIGURE 42-2** Audiogram of sample patient. The inset table shows impairment of that patient by various rating systems. (Data compiled from Fletcher H: A method of calculating hearing loss for speech from the audiogram. *Acta Otolaryngology Suppl* (Stockh) 90:26-37; AMA, 1947; New York Workman's Compensation Board, 1954 (amended 1958); California Industrial Accident Commission, 1950 and March 1, 1962; Wisconsin Industrial Commission, 1955; Chief Medical Director, Veterans' Administration, Washington, D.C., 1952.)

fect on the daily activities of those individuals who have it. The major problem with tinnitus is that it is primarily a subjective phenomenon. Consequently, it is frequently difficult to verify even the presence of tinnitus, let alone its consequences.

**Definition and Prevalence**

Tinnitus, or noise in the ear, is one of the most challenging symptoms in otology. It has been speculated that tinnitus may be the result of a continuous stream of discharges along the auditory nerve to the brain caused by abnormal irritation in the sensorineural pathway. Though no sound is reaching the ear, the spontaneous nerve discharge may cause the patient to experience a false sensation of sound. Al-

though this theory sounds logical, there is as yet no scientific proof of its validity.

Tinnitus is a term used to describe perceived sounds that originate within a person, rather than in the outside world. Although nearly everyone has mild tinnitus momentarily and intermittently, continuous tinnitus is abnormal. However, it is not unusual: the National Center for Health Statistics reports that about 32% of all adults in the United States acknowledge having had tinnitus at some time.[21] Approximately 6.4% of the affected individuals characterize the tinnitus as debilitating or severe. The prevalence of tinnitus increases with age up until approximately 70 years and declines thereafter.[24] This symptom is more common in people with otologic problems, although tinnitus also

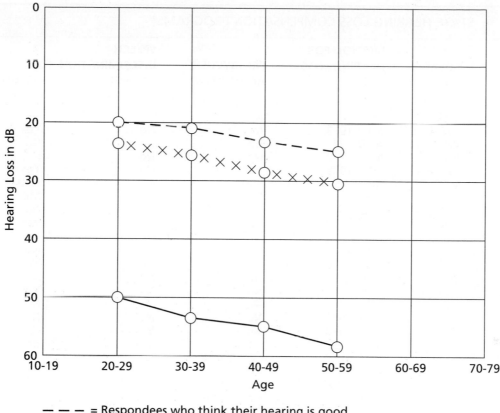

- - - = Respondees who think their hearing is good

× × × = Respondees who think their hearing is fair

———— = Respondees who think their hearing is poor

**FIGURE 42-3**    Rationale for choosing 25 dB as cutoff point for hearing impairment.

can occur in otologically-normal patients. Nodar reported that apparently 13% of school children with normal audiograms report having tinnitus at least occasionally.[23] Sataloff studied 267 normal elderly patients with no history of noise exposure or otologic disease and found that 24% have tinnitus.[25] As expected, the incidence is higher among patients who consult an otologist for any reason. Fowler questioned 2000 consecutive patients and 85% of them reported tinnitus.[5] Heller found that 75% of patients complaining of hearing loss reported tinnitus, and Graham found that approximately 50% of deaf children also complained of tinnitus.[11,13] According to Glasgold and Altmann, nearly 80% of patients with otosclerosis have tinnitus,[9] and House and Brackmann reported that 83% of 500 consecutive patients with acoustic neuromas had tinnitus.[15]

One of the surprising features about tinnitus is that not everybody has it. Consider that the cochlea is exquisitely sensitive to sounds, and relatively loud sounds are being produced inside each human head: the rushing of blood through the cranial arteries, as well as the noises made by muscles in the head dur-

ing chewing. That an individual rarely hears these body noises may be explained partially by the way that the temporal bone is situated in the skull and by the depth at which the cochlea is embedded in the temporal bone. The architecture and the acoustics of the head ordinarily prevent the transmission of these noises through the bones of the skull to the cochlea and thus to consciousness; yet, the cochlea is built and situated in such a way that normally it can respond to very weak sounds carried by the air from outside the head. Only when there are certain changes in the vascular walls—perhaps caused by arteriosclerosis—or in the temporal bone structure does the ear pick up these internal noises. The patients may say that they hear their own pulse as a result of a vascular disorder, and it may seem to be louder when the room is quiet, or at night when they are trying to go to sleep. Pressing on various blood vessels in the neck rarely stops this type of tinnitus, which is not associated with hearing loss.

Although it is frequently troublesome, tinnitus may serve as an early warning of auditory injury. For example, a high-pitched ringing or hissing may be

**TABLE 42-2**   STATE HEARING LOSS COMPENSATION PROGRAMS*

| JURISDICTION | LEGAL BASIS | METHOD FOR HEARING LOSS ASSESSMENT | PRESBYCUSIS ADJUSTMENT | SPEECH DISCRIMINATION CHANGE | TINNITUS | PROVIDE HEARING AIDS |
|---|---|---|---|---|---|---|
| Alabama | WC | ME | No | — | — | No |
| Alaska | WC | AAO 1979 | No | No | Yes | Yes |
| Arizona | WC | AAO 1979 | No | No | No | Yes |
| Arkansas | WC | ME | No | No | No | No |
| California | WC | AAO 1979 | Yes | No | Yes | Yes |
| Colorado | WC | ME | Poss | No | Poss | Yes |
| Connecticut | WC | ME | No | ME | ME | Yes |
| Delaware | WC | AAO 1979 | No | No | No | Yes |
| Dist of Col | WC | AAO 1979 | No | — | Yes | Yes |
| Florida | None | ME | No | — | — | — |
| Georgia | Statute | AAO 1979 | No | No | No | — |
| Hawaii | WC | AAO 1979 | No | No | Yes | Yes |
| Idaho | WC | ME | No | ME | ME | Yes |
| Illinois | Statute | Other | No | No | Yes | No |
| Indiana | None | — | — | — | No | No |
| Iowa | Statute | AAO 1979 | No | No | No | Yes |
| Kansas | WC | AAO 1979 | No | Yes | — | Yes |
| Kentucky | WC | ME | Yes | Yes | Yes | Yes |
| Louisiana | None | Only for simple traumatic accident | | | — | — |
| Maine | Statute | AAOO 1959 | Yes | — | No | Poss |
| Maryland | Statute | AAOO 1959 | Yes | No | No | Yes |
| Massachusetts | None | ME | No | Poss | Yes | No |
| Michigan | WC | — | — | — | — | Yes |
| Minnesota | WC | AAO 1979 | No | Yes | No | Yes |
| Mississippi | WC | ME | No | Yes | Yes | Yes |
| Missouri | Statute | AAO 1959 | Yes | No | No | Yes |
| Montana | Statute | AAO 1959 | Yes | No | No | Yes |
| Nebraska | WC | AAO 1979 | No | No | No | Yes |
| Nevada | WC | AAO 1979 | Yes | No | No | Yes |
| New Hampshire | WC | ME | No | ME | ME | Yes |
| New Jersey | Statute | Other | No | No | Yes | Yes |
| New Mexico | None | ME | — | — | — | Yes |
| New York | Statute | AAO 1979 | No | No | No | Yes |
| N. Carolina | Statute | AAO 1959 | No | No | No | Yes |
| N. Dakota | WC | AAO 1979 | No | No | No | Yes |
| Ohio | WC | ME | No | — | Yes | Yes |
| Oklahoma | WC | AAO 1979 | No | No | Yes | Yes |
| Oregon | WC | Other | Yes | No | Yes | Yes |
| Pennsylvania | WC | ME | No | ME | ME | No |
| Rhode Island | Statute | AAO 1959 | Poss | Poss | No | Yes |
| S. Carolina | WC | AAO 1979 | No | — | — | No |
| S. Dakota | WC | AAO 1979 | Yes | No | No | Yes |
| Tennessee | WC | AAO 1979 | No | No | No | Yes |
| Texas | WC | AAO 1979 | No | No | No | No |
| Utah | Statute | AAO 1979 | Yes | No | Poss | Yes |
| Vermont | WC | ME | No | Yes | Yes | No |
| Virginia | None | AAO 1959 | No | No | No | Yes |
| Washington | WC | AAO 1979 | No | No | Yes | Yes |
| W. Virginia | WC | Other | No | Yes | No | Yes |
| Wisconsin | Statute | Other | No | No | Yes | Yes |
| Wyoming | WC | AMA 1979 | No | Yes | Yes | Yes |

*WC = Workers' Compensation Law, ME = Medical Evaluation, AAO = American Academy of Otolaryngology, AAOO = American Academy of Ophthalmology and Otolaryngology, AMA = American Medical Association.

— = Not available, not applicable

(Data from American Academy of Otolaryngology-Head and Neck Surgery, Subcommittee on Medical Aspects of Noise, committee on Hearing and Equilibrium. In Osguthorpe JD (ed): Guide for Conservation of Hearing in Noise (rev ed). Washington, DC, USGPO, 1988; and From Fodor WJ. Oleinick A: Workers' compensation for occupational noise induced hearing loss: A review of science and the law, and proposed reforms. St. Louis University Law Journal 30:703, 1986.)

the first indication of impending cochlear damage from ototoxic drugs—a clear signal that the drug should be stopped or its dosage reduced. Generally, the tinnitus disappears and no measurable hearing loss results, though in some instances the head noises may persist for months or even years.

Among the common drugs capable of producing tinnitus are aspirin and quinine in large doses, and many antibiotics.[32] These drugs should be used with extreme caution, especially when kidney function is deficient.

Among the common misconceptions about tinnitus is that it is idiopathic and incurable. Neither of these assumptions is always correct. Awareness of conditions that cause tinnitus, however, has not been as helpful to tinnitus research as might be expected. Recognizing a causal relationship has not shed much light on the actual mechanisms by which internal sounds are created.

Tinnitus usually poses a difficult problem for the physician and patient. Tinnitus may be either subjective (audible only to the patient) or objective (audible to the examiner as well). Objective tinnitus is comparatively easy to detect and localize because it can be heard by the examiner using a stethoscope or other listening device. It may be caused by glomus tumors, arteriovenous malformations, palatal myoclonus, and other conditions. Subjective tinnitus is much more common; however, it cannot be confirmed by current tests. Consequently, it is usually difficult to document its presence and quantify its severity, although a few tests are currently available to help. Although the character of tinnitus is rarely diagnostic, certain qualities are suggestive of specific problems. A seashell-like tinnitus is often associated with endolymphatic hydrops, swelling of the inner-ear membranes associated with Meniere's syndrome, syphilitic labyrinthitis, trauma, and other conditions. Unilateral ringing tinnitus may be caused by trauma, but it is also suggestive of acoustic neuroma. Pulsatile tinnitus may be caused by arteriovenous malformations or glomus jugulare tumors, although more benign problems are more common.

## Evaluation and Rating

Tinnitus is found in large numbers of people, but it is not a frequent unsolicited complaint or a significant handicap. Nevertheless, workers' compensation boards in many states require a statement regarding tinnitus-related impairment. How does one rate or scale "annoyance" or "debilitating" subjective reactions to tinnitus? There is no way to do this scientifically from the information presently available. Consequently, since physicians are often required to rate

tinnitus, a variety of individually devised systems that seem reasonable based on available data are used. However, these are not standardized or generally accepted by any official medical organization such as the American Academy of Otolaryngology or the American Medical Association.

The rating scale used by one of the authors (AG) is presented here as an example. Tinnitus is scaled as slight, mild, mild-moderate, moderate, or severe.[39] The ratings are based on judgements, or perhaps more correctly, educated guesses, derived from the patient's reported complaints. These are derived through answers to a set of questions designed to determine whether tinnitus is present, and if so, how much of a problem it poses. The questionnaire is not sufficiently extensive to permit a diagnosis. In the following questionnaire, numerical values, indicated in parentheses, are used for rating quantification:

A. Do you have ringing or noises in your ears or head?
Yes ( )    No ( )
(If yes, continue to B)

B. Is the noise constant or intermittent?
Constant ( ) (3)    Intermittent ( )

If intermittent, is it:
On more than off ( ) (2)
Off more than on ( ) (1)

C. Does it prevent you from going to sleep?
Yes ( ) (2)    No ( ) (0)

D. Is it worse in quiet?  Yes ( ) (1)    No ( ) (2)

E. Is it worse when you are not busy doing something?
Yes ( ) (1)    No ( ) (2)

F. What does it sound like?
High-pitched tone                ( ) (2)
Low-pitched tone                 ( ) (1)
Rushing air                      ( ) (1)
Static                           ( ) (2)
Any other pitch problems (e.g.,
buzzing or humming)              ( ) (1)

G. How much does it bother you?
Mild                      ( ) (1)
Moderate                  ( ) (2)
Severe                    ( ) (3)

When this is adapted to the California scale, we have:

| | | |
|---|---|---|
| 5 | = | Slight |
| 6-7 | = | Mild |
| 8-9 | = | Mild-to-moderate |
| 10-11 | = | Moderate |
| 12 | = | Severe |

These ratings are based strictly on the patient's answers. If a physician has any reason to believe that the answers are not truthful and correct, supporting evidence must be presented.

Various other questionnaires and methods for tinnitus evaluation have been proposed. Most prominently, these include techniques for tinnitus matching. Although these are well described and widely used, and are in fact used by one of the authors (RTS), they may have significant shortcomings, as discussed below.

## Verification

Verification of the presence of tinnitus is an exceedingly difficult task, except in the uncommon cases of objective tinnitus. Measurements of tinnitus loudness and pitch can be made in some patients by matching techniques. It is argued that if the tinnitus can be matched to known signals, it must be present. However, numerous other studies have shown that measurements using these techniques are often unreliable for loudness and pitch, especially for pitch. In individual cases, this may be due to test artifact or fluctuation of the tinnitus. Research sponsored by the American Tinnitus Association has shown that such measurements are fraught with pitfalls, and in the hands of many, the results can be questionable. Nevertheless, in some cases, these studies are helpful. One of the authors (RTS) often uses tinnitus masking and matching studies on the same individual, repeated at subsequent evaluations over a period of months. If the individual consistently reports tinnitus at the same frequency and intensity, this is considered reasonably good supporting evidence that the tinnitus is present. All studies agree that subjective complaints of tinnitus do not correlate with measurement findings in most patients.

Experience suggests a direct correlation between compensation amounts and severity of tinnitus complaints. Consequently, it appears particularly important to devise criteria that will help sort out the merits of various claims. A set of criteria developed by a colleague working with tinnitus claims in the Veterans Administration provides interesting guidelines. Before such a tinnitus claim may be considered meritorious, the following conditions have to be met:

1. The complaint (or claim) that tinnitus was present and disabling must have been unsolicited. If the complaint was not present in the medical records before the claim, it seemed reasonable to assume that it arose as a consequence of the interview and medical history process.
2. The tinnitus must accompany a compensable level of hearing loss.

3. The treatment history must include one or more attempts to alleviate the perceived disturbance by medication, prosthetic management, or psychiatric interview.
4. There must be evidence to support the idea of personality change or sleep disorders.
5. There must be no contributory history of substance abuse.
6. The complaint of tinnitus must be supported by statements from family members, spouses, or others close to the patient.[40]

Although these criteria may seem somewhat severe, the difficulties of objective verification and the potential for abuse of the compensation system necessitate such rigor. In the experience of the authors, awards for tinnitus at jury trials have varied from $15,000 to $1,500,000. When compared, these cases show little, if any, difference in their descriptions of patients' hearing or tinnitus complaints, and some patients have had no compensable hearing loss. With this monetary potential, claimants alleging tinnitus are often familiar with the subject and are aware that its presence cannot be definitively confirmed or refuted in most cases.

The criteria listed above are designed to elicit some objective corroborating evidence that tinnitus is present. A medical record with tinnitus complaints and evaluations that substantially predates considerations of compensation litigation may be one such piece of evidence. However, at present, one must recognize the hazards of providing compensation for a totally subjective alleged complaint, the presence of which cannot usually be verified, and the personal consequences of which are also extremely difficult to measure. At present, compensation for tinnitus should be considered appropriate only in a very small percentage of alleged cases.

## DIZZINESS

Dizziness, like deafness and tinnitus, is a subjective experience and is a symptom, not a disease. Its cause must be sought carefully in each case. The term "dizziness" is used by patients to describe a variety of sensations, many of which are not related to the vestibular system. It is convenient to think of the balance system as a complex conglomerate of senses that each send information to the brain about one's position in space. Components of the balance system include the vestibular labyrinth, the eyes, neck muscles, proprioceptive nerve endings, and cerebellum. If all components of the balance system are providing accurate information, one has no equilibrium problem. However, if most of the components indicate to the brain that the body is standing still, for example, but one component indicates that the body is turning left, the brain becomes confused and a person will experience dizziness. It is the physician's responsibility to analyze systematically each component of the balance system to determine which component or components are providing incorrect information, or whether correct information is being provided and analyzed in an aberrant fashion by the brain. Typically, labyrinthine dysfunction is associated with a sense of motion. It may be true spinning, a sensation of being on a ship or of falling, or simply a vague sense of imbalance when moving. In many cases, it is episodic. Fainting, body weakness, spots before the eyes, general light-headedness, tightness in the head, and loss of consciousness are generally not of vestibular origin. Such descriptions are of only limited diagnostic help. Even some severe peripheral (vestibular or eighth nerve) lesions may produce only mild unsteadiness or no dizziness at all, as with many patients having acoustic neuromas. Similarly, lesions outside the vestibular system may produce true rotary vertigo, as seen with trauma or microvascular occlusion in the brain stem and with cervical vertigo.

Dizziness is a relatively uncommon problem in healthy individuals. In contrast to a 24% prevalence of tinnitus, Sataloff et al. found only a 5% prevalence of dizziness in their study of 267 normal senior citizens.[25] However, most of the population is not as healthy as the highly selected sample in this study. From 5% to 10% of initial physician visits involve a complaint of dizziness or imbalance, accounting for over 11 million physician visits annually.[36] Dizziness is the most common reason for a visit to a physician in patients older than 65 years. Approximately one-third to one-half of people age 65 years and older fall each year, and the consequences can be serious.[16] Falls result in approximately 200,000 hip fractures per year, and this injury carries a 10% mortality rate. Falls are the leading cause of death by injury in people 75 years and older.[16] Dizziness is also a common consequence of head injury. Over 450,000 Americans suffer serious head injuries annually.[37] A majority of these people complain of dizziness for up to five years after the injury, and many are disabled by this symptom.[8] Dizziness may also persist for long periods of time after minor head injury.[18]

In addition to deafness and tinnitus, vertigo is an important symptom associated with disorders of the ear. The intimate relationship of the vestibular portion of the labyrinth to the cochlea makes it easy to understand the reason why many diseases and lesions such as Meniere's disease, head trauma, and vascular conditions affect both balance and hearing. Some diseases such as mumps classically affect only the cochlea. Certain toxins and viruses affect only the vestibular portion without affecting the hearing. Intense noise damages only the cochlea.

Causes of dizziness are almost as numerous as causes of hearing loss, and some are medically serious, such as multiple sclerosis, acoustic neuroma, diabetes, and cardiac arrhythmia. Consequently, any patient with an equilibrium complaint needs a thorough examination. For example, although dizziness may be caused by head trauma, the fact that it is reported for the first time after an injury is not sufficient to establish causation without investigating other possible causes.

It is important to carry out a systematic inquiry in all cases of disequilibrium, not only because the condition is caused by serious problems in some cases, but also because many patients with balance disorders can be helped. Many people believe incorrectly that sensorineural hearing loss, tinnitus, and dizziness are incurable, but many conditions that cause any or all of these may be treated successfully. It is especially important to separate "peripheral", or noncentral, causes, which are almost always treatable, from more central causes, such as brain stem contusion in which the prognosis is often worse.[32]

## Balance Testing

The balance system is extremely complicated, and ideal tests have not been developed. Research is currently underway to develop tests that will assess accurately the entire composite functioning of the balance system and test each component in isolation. At present, the most commonly performed test is electronystagmography. Computerized dynamic posturography is just coming into use, and vestibular evoked potential testing is under investigation.

### Electronystagmography (ENG)

Electronystagmography is a technique for recording eye movements and detecting spontaneous and induced nystagmus. It allows measurement of eye movements with eyes open and closed, and permits quantification of the fast and slow phases, time of onset and duration, as well as other parameters. Although some centers use only horizontal leads, the use of both horizontal and vertical electrodes is preferable. Electronystagmography must be done under controlled conditions with proper preparation, which includes avoidance of drugs (especially those active in the central nervous system). Even a small drug effect may cause alterations in the electronys-

**Dix Hallpike Testing:** A part of the ENG that is specific for paroxysmal spasmodic vertigo.

**Romberg Testing:** A cerebellar test; individual with clumsiness of all movements of gait with the eyes closed can indicate peripheral ataxia; no change with the eyes open or closed indicates cerebellar dysfunction.

**Tandem Romberg Testing:** Gait is tested by asking patient to walk using heel to toe movements.

tagmographic tracing. The test is performed in several phases. These include calibration, which assesses cerebellar function; tests for gaze nystagmus, sinusoidal tracking, optokinetic nystagmus, and spontaneous nystagmus; Dix Hallpike (see box above) and positional testing; and caloric irrigations. The test may give useful information about peripheral and central abnormalities in the vestibular system. Interpretation is complex and difficult.[3,32] The performance of ENG is especially helpful when a unilateral reduced vestibular response is identified in conjunction with other signs of dysfunction in the same ear. In such cases, it provides strong support for a peripheral (eighth nerve or end organ) cause of balance dysfunction.

### Dynamic posturography

For approximately 15 to 20 years, platforms have been used to try to assess more complex integrated functioning of the balance system. Until recently, most were static posture platforms with pressure sensors used to measure body sway while patients tried to maintain various challenging positions, with the Romberg and Tandem Romberg maneuvers (see box above). Movement was measured with eyes closed and opened. The tests had many drawbacks, including inability to separate proprioceptive function and eliminate visual distortion. In 1971, Nashner introduced a system of dynamic posturography, which has been developed into a test system that is available commercially (Equitest).[20]

Dynamic posturography uses a computer-controlled moveable platform with a sway-referenced surrounding visual environment. In other words, both the platform and visual surround move, tracking the anterior-posterior sway of the patient. The visual surround and platform may operate together or independently. The system is capable of creating visual distortion or totally eliminating visual cues.

The platform can perform a variety of complex motions, and the patient's body sway is detected through pressure-sensitized strain gauges in each quadrant of the platform.

The typical test protocol assesses sensory organization through six test procedures and movement coordination through a variety of sudden platform movements. Balancing strategies and responses are assessed using both the sensory organization and movement coordination test batteries. Dynamic posturography provides a great deal of information about total balance function that cannot be obtained from using tests such as ENG alone. Research suggests that dynamic posturography is valuable in distinguishing organic from non-organic disequilibrium, an asset that is particularly valuable in some cases of alleged disability.

### Evoked vestibular response

Evoked vestibular response testing is analogous to brain stem auditory-evoked testing. However, vestibular evoked potentials are not being used clinically. Preliminary research indicates that this test is likely to be valuable in the near future, and clinical trials to assess its efficacy are already underway.

### Impairment and Disability

In many cases, it is possible to document an impairment in the balance system. In others, the subjective complaint of dizziness may be the only abnormality. When present, vertigo and other conditions of disequilibrium may be disabling, particularly for people working in hazardous job situations. Persons who lose their balance even momentarily may injure themselves or others severely when working around sharp surfaces, rotating equipment, driving a forklift, or working on ladders or scaffolding.

There are many other examples of occupations that are not possible for people with disequilibrium disorders. The problem is even worse in conditions that typically cause intermittent severe disequilibrium, such as Meniere's disease. Inability to test the balance system thoroughly makes it impossible in some instances to disprove objectively workers' contentions that they have spells of dizziness. For example, if a worker is struck in the head while performing his job and claims that he has intermittent "dizzy spells" afterward, even if he has a normal ENG, his assertion may be true. Even if malingering is suspected, in the absence of objective proof, if a physician contests this claim and declares him fit to return to work, both the physician and the industry may incur substantial liability if the worker has a period of disequilibrium and seriously injures himself or other workers. Considerable research is needed to develop more sophisticated techniques of assessing equilibrium.

## Treatment

It must be recognized that dizziness may be curable in some cases. A comprehensive discussion of treatment is beyond the scope of this chapter. However, medications, surgery, manipulation, physical therapy, and other modalities may be successful in some patients, especially when a specific etiology can be identified.[32]

## VOICE AND SPEECH

For many years, "voice" and "speech" were treated as one subject under the heading "speech." In the last 20 years, voice and voice science have evolved as subspecialties in the field of otolaryngology and speech-language pathology. Technology and standards of practice now permit appropriate consideration of both aspects of verbal communication. Voice refers to production of sound of a given quality, ordinarily using the true vocal folds. Speech refers to the shaping of sounds into intelligible words. The disability and handicap associated with severe impairment of speech are intuitively obvious: if a person cannot speak intelligibly, verbal communication in the home, workplace, and social setting is extremely difficult or impossible. However, voice disorders have been underappreciated for so long that their significance may not be as immediately apparent. Nevertheless, if a voice disorder results in hoarseness, breathlessness, voice fatigue, decreased vocal volume, or other similar voice disturbances, the worker may be unable to be heard in the presence of even moderate background noise, to carry on telephone conversations for prolonged periods, or to perform work-related and many other kinds of functions. Communication with hard-of-hearing family members and friends may be particularly difficult and frustrating for everyone involved.

Numerous conditions can result in voice or speech disturbances; such information is readily available in the literature.[1,10,25] Briefly, voice and speech afflictions may be due to injury of or trauma to the brain, face, neck, and chest, exposure to toxins and pollution,[30,33] adverse cerebrovascular events, voice misuse, cancer, psychogenic factors, and other causes. The following discussion concentrates on the consequences of voice and speech dysfunction.

## Evaluation

For the purposes of this chapter, it should be assumed that evaluation of voice and speech involves assessment of ability to produce phonation and articulate speech, and does not involve assessment of content, language, or structure. In 1995 there is no single, generally accepted measure to quantify voice or speech function. Therefore, the standard of practice requires the use of a battery of tests.

Various tests and objective measures of voice have become clinically available since the late 1970s and are used in specialized centers. However, because of limited availability and standardization, it is not yet appropriate to require their use for all impairment evaluations. However, tests such as strobovideolaryngoscopy, acoustic analysis, phonatory function assessment, and laryngeal electromyography are recognized as appropriate and useful in the evaluation of speech and voice disorders.[2,14,27,29]

Evaluation of voice requires visualization of the larynx by a physician trained in laryngoscopy, usually an otolaryngologist, and determination of a specific medical etiology for voice dysfunction. Assessment of quality, frequency range, intensity range, endurance, pulmonary function, and function of the larynx as a valve or airflow regulator can be performed easily and inexpensively. Normative values have been established.[41] When they become available, more sophisticated techniques to quantify voice function, such as spectrography and inverse filtering, may be helpful. Slow-motion assessment of vocal fold vibration using strobovideolaryngoscopy is an established procedure described over 100 years ago. This procedure often is necessary to establish a diagnosis.[26,28]

A battery of tests is required to determine the audibility, intelligibility, and functional efficiency of speech. Audibility permits the patient to be heard over background noise. Intelligibility is the ability to link recognizable phonetic units of speech in a manner that can be understood. Functional efficiency is the ability to sustain voice and speech for a period sufficient to permit useful communication.

There are many approaches available for speech assessment, most of which are described in standard speech-language pathology textbooks.[1] However, for the purposes of determining impairment and disability, the method recommended in the AMA *Guides* is used most commonly.[4] This assessment procedure uses "The Smith House" reading paragraph, which reads as follows:

Larry and Ruth Smith have been married nearly fourteen years. They have a small place near Long

Lake. Both of them think there's nothing like the country for health. Their two boys would rather live here than any other place. Larry likes to keep some saddle horses close to the house. These make it easy to keep his sons amused. If they wish, the boys can go fishing along the shore. When it rains, they usually want to watch television. Ruth has a cherry tree on each side of the kitchen door. In June they enjoy the juice and jelly.

The patient is placed approximately eight feet from the examiner in a quiet room. The patient is then instructed to read the paragraph so that the examiner can hear plainly and understand the patient. Patients who cannot read are asked to count to 100 (and should be able to do so in under 75 seconds). Patients are expected to be able to complete at least a 10-word sentence in one breath, sustain phonation for at least 10 seconds on one breath, speak loudly enough to be heard across the room, and maintain a speech rate of at least 75 to 100 words per minute.

The advantages of the system described in the AMA *Guides* are simplicity and wide use. However, this approach does not take advantage of many standardized speech evaluation tests available in the speech-language pathology literature, of technology for better quantification, or of techniques available to help identify psychogenic and intentional voice and speech dysfunction. These advanced methods should be used at least when the results of simple confrontation testing as described in the AMA *Guides* are unconvincing.

## NOSE, SINUSES, OLFACTION, AND TASTE

Rhinitis, rhinorrhea, allergic "sinus" conditions, and related maladies are so common that establishing a causal relationship between occupational exposure and these conditions is often difficult. Nevertheless, exposure to various pollutants and irritants, especially organic pesticides, can produce such symptoms, and it is possible for these symptoms to persist even after the patient has been removed from the causal environment. In most cases, mild nasal congestion and rhinorrhea are not serious health problems. However, exposure to some products, including sawdust and radium, may be associated with the development of cancers in the nose and sinuses. These may cause serious permanent impairment and even loss of life. No criteria have been established to measure impairment associated with rhinorrhea, and this condition is usually not a serious disability or handicap. However, when nasal abnormalities are also associated with loss of olfaction or taste, more important consequences may ensue.

Impairment of smell and taste may also be caused by exposure to inhaled pollutants or those absorbed into the body through points of entry other than the respiratory tract. Bilateral complete loss of either sense results in disturbing impairment and disability when there is loss of olfaction, causing an inability to detect toxic fumes and other hazards. In the past, taste and smell assessment have depended entirely upon subjective response. However, more sophisticated taste and smell testing is now available and capable of sorting out typical organic and non-organic responses. The AMA *Guides* suggests a value of 3% impairment of the whole person for patients in whom there is complete loss of olfaction and taste. However, partial loss or distortion of taste and smell may be a more serious impairment or disability for persons in certain industries, such as those involving food and fragrance. Impairment and disability assessment must be individualized in such cases. Complete loss of olfaction in some cases has led to serious psychiatric disorders and malnutrition.[34]

## OTHER AREAS OF OTOLARYNGOLOGY

Impairment of the face, oral cavity, temporomandibular joint, neck, lungs, and the systems for mastication and deglutition may also occur in some patients. The AMA *Guides* divide facial impairment and disfigurement into classes, citing percentage impairments of the whole person to each class.[4] The *Guides* also provide classification for respiratory impairment (dyspnea). Neck abnormalities are not widely discussed in terms of impairment. However, neck injury or surgery that produces cranial nerve injury may produce substantial disability in some occupations. This is especially true of injury to the eleventh cranial nerve in anyone who requires upper arm strength and the ability to work with arms above shoulder level. Assessment of mastication and deglutition has traditionally depended upon subjective assessment, such as reports on a patient's dietary tolerance. However, recent advances in the science of deglutition have produced better assessment techniques including swallowing assessment with flexible fiberoptic endoscopy, three-phase swallowing studies, and others. These techniques should be used to specify and quantify, when possible, the nature and severity of impairment of mastication and deglutition. There is little precedent and no agreement or standardization regarding quantification of impairment, disability, or compensation levels for most of these conditions. Consequently, until further research has been completed, disability judgements must be made taking the individual's impairment, response to this

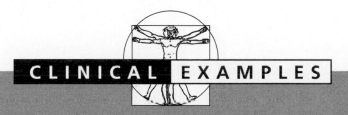

## AUDIOLOGIC SYSTEM

### EXAMPLE 1

#### History

A 50-year-old police officer complained of having difficulty hearing everyday communication, especially in noisy environments. He also complained of tinnitus in both ears, which he described as a constant, high-pitched tone. The tinnitus appeared to be worse in a quiet environment and bothered him when he was trying to go to sleep.

#### Physical Examination

Physical examination of his ears, nose, and throat was unremarkable except for a moderate high-frequency, sensorineural hearing loss demonstrated by pure tone audiometry. The past occupational history revealed that he had been a police officer for 25 years. His duties required him to practice with his .9mm handgun on a monthly basis and each time he would fire from 50 to 60 rounds of ammunition. He did not use ear protection for the first 15 years, but used it regularly for the remaining 10 years.

#### Evaluation

When impairment is calculated according to the present AMA *Guides* formula, the patient shows an 8.8% binaural handicap. His audiogram shows a pure tone hearing loss as follows:

| Hz | 500 | 1000 | 2000 | 3000 | 4000 | 6000 |
|---|---|---|---|---|---|---|
| Right ear | 15 | 15 | 30 | 60 | 70 | 60 |
| Left ear | 10 | 15 | 40 | 70 | 80 | 60 |

### EXAMPLE 2

#### History

A 20-year-old woman, a singer and artist, has come for an impairment evaluation of her audiological system. She had experienced no voice difficulties until she was exposed to fumes during art classes. Investigation of the site revealed that the room had no windows and poor ventilation. The students worked with acrylics, oil paints, and some materials that were heated in flames. Within the first week of classes she noticed a cough, shortness of breath, and headaches during class. Her requests for room ventilation went unanswered. By the end of the first semester, she could not sing or speak for prolonged periods without becoming hoarse. She also developed severe hoarseness and a headache within 30 minutes of exposure to acrylics and after exposure to other art supplies.

One year later, her symptoms persist. She becomes severely dysphonic and short of breath when she is exposed to acrylics, perfumes, and many other art supplies. Thus she is unable to continue her career as an artist. In addition, the pulmonary consequences of her exposure have left her with airway reactivity-induced asthma in singers (ARIAS syndrome), making it impossible for her to pursue a career as a singer or public speaker. In addition to singing, exercise, cold air, and exposure to smoke, dust, and fumes other than perfumes also induce her asthmatic symptoms, which included shortness of breath, wheezing, and coughing. She also becomes hoarse and develops a stuffy nose at these times.

Treatment has included the use of antihistamines and decongestants, which she still takes twice a day. When she does not use these medications, she notices the gradual onset of increasing nasal congestion, sinus drainage, and headaches within 24 hours. To help her breathing difficulties, she takes three puffs of ipratropium bromide three times a day, three puffs of beclomethasone dipropionate three times a day, and two puffs of cromolyn sodium three times a day. She is intolerant of theophylline, even at low doses. In addition, she uses an albuterol inhaler on an as-needed basis. She generally needs an average of two puffs per day.

Despite these medications, she has occasional episodes of respiratory infection. She averages one sinus infection (characterized by pain, fever, and the production of yellow to green discharge) approximately once every two to three months. She develops lower respiratory infections (characterized by increasing episodes of shortness of breath, wheezing, cough, and the production of yellow to green sputum) approximately once every four

*Continued.*

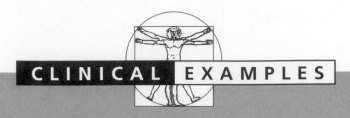
## AUDIOLOGIC SYSTEM—cont'd

months. On these occasions, she is treated with antibiotics and a 10-day course of oral steroids. In addition, she requires steroid injections two to three times a year for wheezing.

### Physical Examination and Test Results

Rhinomanometric studies of her nose reveal moderate resistance to airflow that is completely reversed with phenylephrine. Wheezes were heard in both lungs. A CT scan of her sinuses shows concha bullosa in both maxillary sinuses with generalized sinus mucosal thickening. A screening spirometry test is obtained after she has been off her medications for 24 hours. Her forced expiratory volume at one second is 44% of predicted. This improved to 62% after an aerosolized bronchodilator was administered. A methacholine challenge test is also obtained and shows a $PC_{20}$ mg/ml of 0.40.

### Assessment Process

Using Tables 29-2 to 29-5 (pp. 348–349) in Chapter 29 of this text, from a pulmonary perspective, she is in the Class III impairment category with a total score of 8. Using Table 8 (p. 162 of AMA *Guides*),* she has a 26% to 50% whole person impairment (WPI).

From the standpoint of rhinitis/sinusitis, her CT scan showed chronic inflammatory changes and a rhinomanometric study showed moderate abnormalities. Her medication need is as outlined. Extrapolating from and using Tables 1 through 4 of the pulmonary section,

she again belongs in the Class III impairment category. This is based on (1) being on four different medications for her sinus and rhinitis control; (2) occasionally needing systemic steroids; (3) having rhinomanometric study results in the "3 range" (using an analysis similar to the methacholine challenge test); and (4) having a CT scan (substituted for the postbronchodilator forced expiratory volume at one minute) that indicates she has chronic inflammatory changes.

In arriving at an impairment percentage for her chronic rhinitis/sinusitis, there are no tables in Chapter 9 similar to Table 8 in the pulmonary section. However, a Class III impairment of the sinuses/nasal membranes probably should not be assessed as high as a similar asthma impairment because the amount of impairment and disturbance in daily function are not as significant. A value of 25% to 30% of the pulmonary impairment might be more realistic.

### Evaluation

This individual would have a 26% to 50% whole person impairment (WPI) based on the pulmonary impairment (40% would be considered appropriate) and an additional 10% based on chronic rhinitis/sinusitis (25% × 40% = 10%). When 40% and 10% are combined, this individual would be assigned a 46% WPI. In addition, she is totally disabled for the occupations noted.

*All *tables* and *chapters* referred to in this discussion, unless indicated otherwise, are found in AMA *Guides to the evaluation of permanent impairment*, ed 4, Chapter 5—The Respiratory System, and Chapter 9—Ear, Nose, Throat, and Related Structures, American Medical Association, 1993, Chicago.

*Aram Glorig*
*Robert Thayer Sataloff*
*Stephen L. Demeter*

type of impairment, interference with daily activities, occupation or social and recreational requirements, and other factors into account.

## References

1. Aronson A: *Clinical voice disorders,* ed 3, New York, 1990, pp. 117-145, Thieme Medical Publishers.

2. Baken RJ: *Clinical measurement of speech and voice,* Boston, 1987, College Hill Press, Little, Brown.

3. Barbarh O, Stockwell CW: *Manual of electronystagmography,* St. Louis, 1976, CV Mosby.

4. AMA *Guides to the Evaluation of Permanent Impairment,* ed 4, Chicago, 1993, American Medical Association.

5. Fowler EF: Tinnitus aurium: its significance in certain diseases of the ear, *NY State J Med* 12:702-704, 1912.

6. Fowler EP Sr.: A simple method of measuring percentage of capacity for hearing speech, *JASA* 13:373, April 1942.

7. Gatehouse S: The role of non-auditory factors in measured and self-reported disability, *Acta Otolaryngologica* (Suppl. 476); 249-256, 1991.

8. Gibson WPR: Vertigo associated with trauma. In Dix, editor, *Vertigo,* Somerset, NJ, 1984, John Wiley and Sons.

9. Glasgold A, Altmann R: The effect of stapes surgery on tinnitus in otosclerosis, *Laryngoscope* 76:1642-1632, 1966.

10. Gould WJ, Sataloff RT, Spiegel JR: *Voice surgery,* St. Louis, 1993, C.V. Mosby.

11. Graham JM: Tinnitus in children with hearing loss, CIBA Foundation Symposium 85, *Tinnitus,* London, pp. 172-181, 1981.

12. Guides to evaluation of permanent impairment, *JAMA* 241:19, May 11, 1979.

13. Heller MR, Bergman M: Tinnitus aurium in normally hearing persons, *Ann Otol Rhinol Laryngol* 62:73-83, 1953.

14. Hirano M: *Clinical examination of the voice,* New York, 1981, pp. 1-98, Springer-Verlag.

15. House JW, Brackmann DE: Tinnitus: Surgical treatment, CIBA Foundation Symposium, *Tinnitus,* London, pp. 204-212, 1981.

16. Jenkins HA, Furman JM, Gulya AJ, et al: Dysequilibrium of aging, *Otolaryngol Head Neck Surg* 100:272-282, 1989.

17. Lutman ME: Hearing disability in the elderly, *Acta Otolaryngologica* (Suppl. 476); 239-248, 1991.

18. Mandel S, Sataloff RT, Schapiro S: *Minor head trauma: Assessment, management and rehabilitation,* New York, 1993, Springer-Verlag.

19. McFadden D: *Tinnitus facts, theories and treatments,* National Research Council, Washington, DC, 1982, National Academy Press.

20. Nashner LN: A model describing vestibular detection of body sway motion, *Acta Otolaryngol Scand* 72:429-436, 1971.

21. National Chapter for Health Statistics: Hearing status and ear examination: Findings among adults. Untied States, 1960-1962. Vital and Health Statistics, Series 11, No. 32, U.S. Dept. of HEW, Washington, DC, November 1968.

22. Nilsson M, et al: Development of the hearing in noise test for the measurement of speech reception thresholds in quiet and in noise, *J Acoust Soc Am* 95:2, February 1994.

23. Nodar RH: Tinnitus aurium in school-age children: survey, *J Aud Res* 12:133-135, 1972.

24. Reed GF: An audiometric study of two hundred cases of suspected tinnitus, *Arch Otol* 71:94-104, 1960.

25. Sataloff J, Sataloff RT, Lueneburg W: Tinnitus and vertigo in healthy senior citizens with a history of noise exposure, *Amer J Otol* 8(2):87-89, 1987.

26. Sataloff RT, Spiegel JR, Carroll LM, et al: Strobovideolaryngoscopy in professional voice users: results and clinical value, *J Voice* 1(4):359-364, 1988.

27. Sataloff RT: *Professional voice: the science and art of clinical care.* New York, 1991, Raven Press.

28. Sataloff RT, Spiegel JR, Hawkshaw MJ: Strobovideolaryngoscopy: Results and clinical value, *Annals of Otology, Rhinology and Laryngology* 100(9):725-727, 1991.

29. Sataloff RT: The human voice, *Scientific American* 267(6):108-115, 1992.

30. Sataloff RT: The impact of pollution on the voice, *Otolaryngol Head Neck Surg* 106(6):701-705, 1992.

31. Sataloff RT, Sataloff J: *Hearing loss,* ed 3, New York, 1993, Marcel Dekker.

32. Sataloff RT, Sataloff J: *Occupational hearing loss,* ed 2, New York, 1993, Marcel Dekker.

33. Sataloff RT: Vocal tract response to toxic injury: Clinical issues, *J Voice* 8(1):63-64, 1994.

34. Spiegel JR, Frattali M: Olfactory consequences of minor head trauma. In Mandel S, Sataloff RT, Schapiro SR, editors, *Minor head trauma: Assessment, management and rehabilitation,* New York, 1993, pp. 225-234, Springer-Verlag.

35. Stephens D: Impairment, disability, and handicap in audiology: Toward a consensus (Editorial), *Audiology* 30:185-200, 1991.

36. U.S. Department of Health and Human Services, Public Health Services, National Center for Health Statistics Series 13, No. 56, 1978.

37. U.S. Department of Health and Human Services: *Head injury: Hope through research.* National Institutes of Health Publication, No. 84-2478, 1989.

38. WHO: International classification of impairments, disabilities, and handicaps. Geneva, 1980, World Health Organization.

39. Physicians' Guide to Medical Practice in the California Workers' Compensation System, Industrial Medical Council, State of California, Chapter 3, page 37, 1994.

40. Knox: Personal communication, 1985.

41. Sataloff RT: *Professional voice: the science and art of clinical care,* New York, 1991, Raven.

# SECTION D
Psychiatric Assessment

# PSYCHIATRIC IMPAIRMENT AND DISABILITY

*David Robbins*
*Moshe Torem*

It has been said that physicians determine impairment and lawyers determine disability. (See Chapter 1.) In many respects, this is a true statement. The physician's role in determining impairment, as seen in the previous chapters in the clinical section, is one of arriving at diagnoses, describing the limitations that an individual has due to these diagnoses, and deriving an impairment rating based upon the severity of the illness and its limitations. That information is used to determine the limitations that individuals have in their activities of daily living and how this translates into limitations in the workplace.

By the very nature of their specialty, psychiatrists and other mental health professionals must be aware of the circumstances of a patient's life and job. These activities of occupational and daily living are integral parts of a person's psychiatric illness, treatment, and placement. For these reasons, those involved in the psychiatric profession often find themselves better equipped to assess the impact of a person's psychiatric illness upon the quality of both the occupational and daily living activities than do other members of the medical profession.

In 1993, the fourth edition of the AMA *Guides* departed from the traditional concept of impairment rating found in other sections of the book, as well as in previous editions of the AMA *Guides*, by stating that "unlike the situations with some organ systems, there are no precise measures of impairment in mental disorders. The use of percentages implies a certainty that does not exist; and the percentages are likely to be used inflexibly by adjudicators, who then are less likely to take into account the many factors that influence mental and behavioral impairment. Also, because no data exist that show the reliability of the impairment percentages, it would be difficult for the AMA *Guides* users to defend their use in administrative hearings. After considering this difficult matter, the Committee on Disability and Rehabilitation of the American Psychiatric Association advised AMA *Guides'* contributors against the use of percentages in the chapter on mental and behavioral disorders of the fourth edition."[1]

There are other reasons against the use of impairment percentages in the psychiatric impairment section. The first is a lack of external verification examinations. For an orthopedic impairment, for example, one starts with a diagnosis, measures a functional impairment by means of a variety of tests, and is then in a position of describing impairments and disabilities by using these validating tests. When a patient has arthritic pain in a shoulder caused by a prior rotator cuff injury, there will be limitation in the range of motion, and in some circumstances, in strength caused by these two disorders. The diagnosis is thus validated by means of the restriction of motion and diminished strength. The examination abnormalities are then assessed by testing many such individuals with similar diagnoses and restrictions and then measuring the amount of impairment in the activities of daily living or occupational functioning due to these conditions. Similar examples can be given for the remainder of the chapters of the clinical section of this book. A person who has shortness of breath and a diagnosis of emphysema will have certain degrees of abnormalities in pulmonary function testing. Many such individuals with this degree of abnormality on a pulmonary function test are then assessed in the activities of daily or occupational life and impairment percentages are applied. However, with psychiatric impairments, this middle step is missing. Diagnoses can be made and tests can be administered. Yet, for all their reliability and validity, these tests do not have good objective methods of validation. The disturbances in functional activities are driven by the diagnosis, rather than by test results.

A more subtle argument can be made against the use of impairment percentages by stating that only impairment is measured by physicians in all other areas save psychiatric. Disability (as defined in Chapter 1) is described more frequently by the psychiatric evaluator. In other words, impairment is translated in situational restrictions. As a result of a psychiatric evaluation, the evaluator may give a diagnosis and state that, because of the particular diagnosis, the severity of symptomatology, and the response to treatment that an individual is precluded from certain situational activities. Thus, psychiatric evaluations more often result in a true disability evaluation rather than an impairment rating.

The last argument is one of time course. Both the Social Security Guidelines[2] and the AMA *Guides*[1] restrict impairment evaluation for psychiatric patients to permanent disorders. The Social Security department defines disability as "the inability to engage in any substantial gainful activity by reason of any medically determinable physical or mental impairment(s) which can be expected to result in death or which has lasted or can be expected to last for a continuous period of not less than 12 months."[2] The AMA *Guides* state that "an impairment should not be considered "permanent" until the clinical findings, determined during a period of months, indicate that the medical condition is static and well stabilized."[1] By applying such criteria, many of the acute, situational difficulties that arise because of behavioral or psychiatric disorders will be eliminated. The evaluator of psychiatric impairment, from material developed on these patients previously, not only will be aware of a patient's diagnosis and restrictions upon both the activities of daily and occupational life, but should also be aware of the response to treatment (behavioral, drug, rehabilitative, and placement setting). This information will then be incorporated into the impairment evaluation. As such, greater opportunity is afforded the psychiatric evaluator to assess disability, as opposed to strictly impairment.

## DSM-IV

In 1994, the American Psychiatric Association published the fourth edition of the *Diagnostic and Statistical Manual of Mental Disorders,* DSM-IV.[3] This book is described as a "team effort. More than 1000 people (and numerous professional organizations) have helped us in the preparation of this document."[3] The book lists and describes the criteria necessary to arrive at various psychiatric diagnoses. The World Health Organization has published a similar classification titled *International Statistical Classification of Diseases and Related Health Problems,* ICD-10,[4] and the au-

thors of the DSM-IV state that the two systems are compatible.

In recent years, the number of people claiming disability due to psychiatric illness has been steadily rising. This phenomenon may be, in part, due to an increased public awareness and knowledge of the nature of mental illness as a result of regular patient education campaigns by professional organizations, such as the American Psychiatric Association, and the increased popularity of self-help publications. In addition, DSM-III introduced some new diagnostic categories, making it easier to identify psychiatric illness as a result of trauma (Posttraumatic Stress Disorder)[5] and added a new diagnostic category in DSM-IV, the Acute Stress Disorder.[3]

Moreover, DSM-III introduced a new system of diagnosing mental illness on a multi-axial paradigm. This approach has been continued and refined in the following editions of DSM-IIIR[6] and DSM-IV.[3] This multi-axial system requires that mental health professionals diagnose the patient's condition on five different axes or categories.

## Axis I: Clinical Disorders and Other Conditions That May Be a Focus of Clinical Attention

Axis I is for reporting all the various mental disorders or conditions except for personality disorders and mental retardation, which are reported on Axis II; If more than one mental disorder is diagnosed, the first and principal diagnosis listed will be the one that is the major cause of the patient's impairment.

## Axis II: Personality Disorders and Mental Retardation

Axis II is for reporting personality disorders and mental retardation. Here, the clinician is expected to assess patients' life-long behavioral patterns that define their character and personality. Many patients may have a diagnosis on both Axis I and Axis II; however, some patients may only have a diagnosis on Axis I and none on Axis II.

## Axis III: General Medical Conditions

Axis III refers to the patient's general medical health, determined by a review of medical records and examinations, and should include all coexisting medical diagnoses. When an individual has more than one clinical diagnosis on Axis III, all diagnoses should be reported. Here again, some patients may have no diagnosis on Axis III, suggesting that they are in good physical health.

## Axis IV: Psychosocial and Environmental Problems

In this section, the physician is expected to report any psychosocial and environmental problems that may reflect the patient's condition, treatment, and prognosis. A psychosocial or environmental problem may be a stressful life event, an environmental difficulty or deficiency, a family or other interpersonal stressor, an inadequacy of social support or personal resources, or any other problem relating to the context and setting in which the patient's difficulties have developed. Some patients have so-called "positive stressors," such as a job promotion, falling in love, getting married, having children, and getting a prestigious award. These should be listed only if they lead to a specific identified problem or contribute to the patient's maladaptive functioning.

In some cases, psychosocial problems may develop as a consequence of the person's psychopathology on Axes I and II as well as the patient's medical condition on Axis III. In some individuals, multiple psychosocial or environmental problems may be identified, and in these cases, clinicians are required to list as many as are judged to be relevant. The general guideline, according to DSM-IV,[3] is that clinicians should note only those psychosocial and environmental problems that have been present during the year preceding the current evaluation. However, DSM-IV states, "the clinician may choose to note psychosocial and environmental problems occurring prior to the previous year if these clearly contribute to the mental disorder or have become a focus of treatment—for example, previous combat experiences leading to Posttraumatic Stress Disorder." For convenience, DSM-IV has grouped the problems into nine categories (see box).

## Axis V: Global Assessment of Functioning

According to DSM-IV, Axis V was created for reporting the individual's overall level of functioning. This information is useful not only in assessing the severity of impairment, but also in planning treatment and measuring its impact and predicting outcome. Assessing the overall level of functioning in Axis V is done by using the Global Assessment of Functioning (GAF) Scale (found in the appendix of DSM-IV). The GAF Scale is to be rated with respect only to psychological, social, and occupational functioning. The instructions clearly specify, "do not include impairment in functioning due to physical (or environmental) limitations."[3] In many cases, it is useful to rate the patient's global level of functioning at the time of the examination and, separately, the

**DSM-IV - AXIS IV - PSYCHOSOCIAL AND ENVIRONMENTAL PROBLEMS**

1. Problems with primary support group.
2. Problems related to the social environment.
3. Educational problems.
4. Occupational problems.
5. Housing problems.
6. Economic problems.
7. Problems with access to health care services.
8. Problems related to interaction with the legal system and crime.
9. Other psychosocial and environmental problems.

Courtesy American Psychiatric Association, 1994.

highest level of functioning for at least three months during the past year preceding the examination.

The rating of the overall psychosocial functioning is done on a scale of 0 - 100 and was operationalized by Luborsky.[7] Endicott, Spitzer, and colleagues[8] developed a revision of Luborsky's Health-Sickness Rating Scale, which they called the Global Assessment Scale. The GAF is a modified version of the Global Assessment Scale (GAS).

Other than the GAF scale, Axis V also utilizes the Defensive Functioning Scale and the Social and Occupational Functioning Assessment Scale (SOFAS), which are also found in the appendixes of DSM-IV.[3]

## THE PSYCHIATRIC EXAMINATION

To determine psychiatric disability and impairment, a competent evaluation begins with a thorough psychiatric and medical history that includes the following items: the date that the patient's symptoms began, the existing environment in which the symptoms took place, the patient's level of stress or dissatisfaction in the personal life and work environment, what the patient thought was going on at the time that the symptoms started, to what did the patient attribute the source of the symptoms (for example, to being overworked, to a specific injury, to a harsh and critical boss, to the threat of losing one's job, to being required to do work without proper training, to family and marital conflicts, to a recent death in the family, to the abuse of alcohol and drugs, or being sinful to God). Such a history should also specify the patient's actions taken to relieve these symptoms including visits to previous physicians, psychiatrists, and other mental health professionals. This history should also describe the patient's response to any given treatments such as medications, their positive effects in controlling symptoms, side effects, and which medications created no significant changes. The history should also delineate past events prior to the beginning of the present illness symptoms or work impairment and should provide material regarding the patient's past treatment, hospitalizations (if any), suicide attempts, or personal losses. The history should also provide material about the patient as a person, including such significant elements as a history of childhood abuse, trauma, functioning in school, level of education, as well as personal habits, such as the use of caffeine, alcohol, non-prescription drugs, and a history of possible addiction such as the abuse of laxatives, smoking cigarettes or the use of other forms of tobacco, alcohol, and illicit drugs. The history should also portray the patient's current relationship in a marriage (if applicable) and any possible forms of stress and family dysfunction. It is also very important to inquire about the health of the patient's parents, grandparents, and siblings, since certain psychiatric conditions have a strong genetic component to them, such as bipolar mood disorders, obsessive-compulsive disorder, attention-deficit disorder, and certain forms of mental retardation, forms of communication disorders, forms of anxiety disorders, forms of alcoholism, forms of depressive disorders, and personality disorders.

Before a patient is seen, it is helpful to use a self-assessment questionnaire that is mailed to the patient in advance and instructs patients to use their own words to describe, in writing, the nature of their distress, what relieves it, what makes it worse, and their opinion about possible solutions including their desire for disability and their assessment of the degree of impairment. It is also important to include in such a self-assessment form a section that relates to the patient's wishes about the future, as well as concrete plans regarding their job and their plans for a source of income for themselves.

The examination of the patient is based on a thorough mental status examination that includes the following sections: general observations of the patient's appearance, including how well the patient is dressed and groomed, and how that is compatible with the patient's socioeconomic and professional status. General observations should also include the patient's general demeanor, to what extent the patient was spontaneous in describing perceived problems, to what extent the patient only responded to direct questioning, to what extent the patient was overtly negativistic, and hostile, mistrustful and suspicious, or to what extent the patient was pleasant and cooperative. Other important observations include items that are relevant to the patient's general behavior and activity during the interview and psychiatric examination. Such observations may include any of the following: hyperactive, hypoactive, silly, agitated, grimaces, mannerisms, ticks, compulsions, hypervigilance, boredom, tearfulness, sitting stooped, pacing, elation, or that simply the patient's facial expressions, body, and posture were appropriate to the interview. It is helpful to record the overall, comprehensive findings of the psychiatric examination on a structured form. An example is provided in Figure 43-1.

The general observations should also include the patient's level of eye contact, whether the patient avoids direct eye contact, stares into space, or watches suspiciously during the interview. Motor behavior, such as the existence of psychomotor retardation, excitement, or the existence of posturing, tremors, fidgeting, pacing, as well as the patient's gait are also relevant and important.

The psychiatric examination proceeds with the examination of the patient's mood and affect, the patient's thought processes, thought content, somatic functioning and concern, perception, sensorium, cognitive functions, judgement, insight and attitude toward illness, and the potential for self-injury, suicide, or violence.

The examination should also include the patient's attitude toward the examiner, as well as the possible barriers to communication including deficiencies in speaking English and the need of an interpreter, being deaf and the need for a sign language interpreter, poor quality of speech with severe stuttering, refusal to cooperate, or conscious falsification of information. All of the above determine the reliability and completeness of information that should be rated by the examiner.

The examiner should rate the overall severity of illness and the impact upon the patient's life on a scale of mild, moderate, marked, severe, or extremely severe. Once these are completed, the examiner should formulate the case, including the patient's strengths and assets.

## EVALUATING PSYCHIATRIC IMPAIRMENTS

As mentioned above, to meet the criteria for disability, patients must suffer from an impairment that disrupts their level of adaptive functioning in the activities of daily living at home or in the workplace.

*Text continued on page 509.*

Akron General Medical Center
Center for Psychiatry
and Behavioral Sciences

Section II

# Psychiatric History & Mental Status Examination

(To be completed by attending psychiatrist or psychiatric resident under direct supervision of the attending psychiatrist)

## Psychiatric History

Chief Complaint(s)

________________________________________

Present Illness(es) (Presenting symptoms, precipitating events, details of outpatient therapy, medications & pt.'s response)

________________________________________

Past Psychiatric History (Include previous mental illnesses, suicide attempts, hospitalizations, treatments, medications)

________________________________________

Habits (Include use of tobacco, caffeine, laxatives, alcohol & non-prescription drugs)

________________________________________

Personal History (Education, occupational functioning, military, legal, marital, history of childhood abuse, etc.)

________________________________________

Family History (Include all information relevant to this admission)

________________________________________

**FIGURE 43-1** Sample of a psychiatric history and mental status examination form. (Used with permission from the copyright holder, Akron General Medical Center, 1995.)

# Mental Status Examination

## General Observations

| | | | |
|---|---|---|---|
| General Appearance | ○ Neat/well-groomed | ○ Casually groomed & dressed | ○ Dishevelled/unkempt |
| General Demeanor | ○ Spontaneous ○ Overtly negativistic & hostile | | ○ Mistrustful & suspicious |
| | ○ Preoccupied ○ Regressed ○ Demanding & manipulative | | |
| Behavior/Activity | ○ Hyperactive ○ Hypoactive ○ Stuporous ○ Agitated ○ Silly | | |
| (Check all that apply) | ○ Grimaces ○ Mannerisms ○ Tics ○ Compulsions ○ Hypervigilant | | |
| | ○ Bored ○ Stooped ○ Tearful ○ Elated | | |
| | ○ Facial expression and body posture appropriate to interview | | ○ Other (specify) |

| | | | | |
|---|---|---|---|---|
| Eye Contact: | ○ Avoids direct gaze | ○ Most of the time | ○ Often | ○ Occasionally |
| | ○ Stares into space | ○ Most of the time | ○ Often | ○ Occasionally |
| | ○ Glances furtively | ○ Most of the time | ○ Often | ○ Occasionally |

**Motor Behavior**

| | | | | |
|---|---|---|---|---|
| Psychomotor Retardation | ○ None | ○ Mild | ○ Moderate | ○ Marked |
| Psychomotor Excitement | ○ None | ○ Mild | ○ Moderate | ○ Marked |
| Specific Observations | ○ Posturing | ○ Waxy Flexibility | ○ Catatonic Rigidity | ○ Catatonic Stupor |
| | ○ Pacing | ○ Fidgeting | ○ Tremors Gait: ○ Rigid | ○ Unsteady |

Comments on Behavior:

_____

_____

## Mood and Affect

| | | | | |
|---|---|---|---|---|
| Depression | ○ None | ○ Mild | ○ Moderate | ○ Severe |
| Anxiety | ○ None | ○ Mild | ○ Moderate | ○ Severe |
| Anger | ○ None | ○ Mild | ○ Moderate | ○ Severe |
| Anhedonia | ○ None | ○ Mild | ○ Moderate | ○ Severe |
| Loneliness | ○ None | ○ Mild | ○ Moderate | ○ Severe |
| Euphoria | ○ None | ○ Mild | ○ Moderate | ○ Severe |
| Diurnal mood variation | ○ None | ○ Worse in a.m. | ○ Worse in p.m. | |

**Affect**

| | | | | |
|---|---|---|---|---|
| Range | ○ Full | ○ Restricted | | |
| Inappropriate | ○ None | ○ Mild | ○ Moderate | ○ Severe |
| Flat | ○ None | ○ Mild | ○ Moderate | ○ Severe |
| Labile | ○ None | ○ Mild | ○ Moderate | ○ Severe |

Comments on Mood & Affect:

_____

_____

## Thought Processes

| | | | | |
|---|---|---|---|---|
| Quality of speech | ○ Clear, comprehensible ○ Blocking | | ○ Slow | ○ Slurred |
| | ○ Rapid ○ Pressured | | ○ Flight of Ideas | ○ Talkative |
| Incoherence | ○ None | ○ Mild | ○ Moderate | ○ Severe |
| Irrelevance | ○ None | ○ Mild | ○ Moderate | ○ Severe |
| Evasiveness | ○ None | ○ Mild | ○ Moderate | ○ Severe |
| Circumstantiality | ○ None | ○ Mild | ○ Moderate | ○ Severe |
| Loose Associations | ○ None | ○ Mild | ○ Moderate | ○ Severe |
| Concrete Thinking | ○ None | ○ Mild | ○ Moderate | ○ Severe |
| Other Findings: | ○ None | ○ Clang Associations | ○ Neologisms | ○ Flight of Ideas |
| | ○ Echolalia | ○ Perseverations | ○ Word play | ○ Excessive profanity |
| | ○ Unintelligible muttering | | | |

Comments on Thought Processes:

_____

_____

_____

FIGURE 43-1, cont'd   For legend see page 504.

# Mental Status Examination—cont'd

## Thought Content

Delusions   ○ Absent   ○ Present
            ○ Grandiose   ○ Persecutory   ○ Somatic   ○ Bizarre   ○ Religious   ○ Nihilistic

Other Findings   ○ Phobic Ideas   ○ Ambivalence   ○ Obsessive Ideas   ○ Autistic Thinking
                 ○ Guilt   ○ Self Reproach   ○ Ideas of Reference   ○ Suicidal Ideation
                 ○ Suspicious   ○ Self-derogatory   ○ Resentful of Others   ○ Preoccupation with death
                 ○ Preoccupied w/ self-harm

Comments on Thought Content:

_____

_____

## Somatic Functioning & Concern

| | | | | |
|---|---|---|---|---|
| Appetite Disturbance: | ○ None | ○ Poor | ○ Excessive | |
| Energy Disturbance: | ○ None | ○ Easily Fatigued | ○ Excessively Energetic | |
| Libido Disturbance | ○ None | ○ Decreased | ○ Markedly increased | |
| Insomnia | ○ None | ○ Diff. falling asleep | ○ Early a.m. awakening | ○ Awakening at night |
| Incontinence | ○ None | ○ Occasional | ○ Often | ○ Very Often |
| Seizures (past week) | ○ None | ○ One | ○ Several   ○ Daily | ○ Several/day |
| Sensory impairment (organic) | ○ None | ○ Visual | ○ Hearing | |
| Preoccup. with physical health | ○ None | ○ Mild | ○ Moderate   ○ Marked | |

Somatic concerns (e.g., constipation, diarrhea, GI disturbance, short of breath, headaches, backaches, sweating, itching, etc):

_____

_____

## Perception

| | | | | |
|---|---|---|---|---|
| Hallucinations | ○ Unknown | ○ None | ○ Suspected | ○ Definite |
| Auditory | ○ Slight | ○ Mild | ○ Moderate | ○ Marked |
| Visual | ○ Slight | ○ Mild | ○ Moderate | ○ Marked |
| Olfactory | ○ Slight | ○ Mild | ○ Moderate | ○ Marked |
| Gustatory | ○ Slight | ○ Mild | ○ Moderate | ○ Marked |
| Tactile | ○ Slight | ○ Mild | ○ Moderate | ○ Marked |
| Visceral | ○ Slight | ○ Mild | ○ Moderate | ○ Marked |
| Belief that hallucinations are real | | ○ Knows unreal | ○ Unsure | ○ Convinced they are real |

Hallucinatory content (threatening, accusatory, self-derogatory, grandiose, flattering, reassuring, sexual, religious):

_____

| | | | |
|---|---|---|---|
| Illusions | ○ None | ○ Mild | ○ Moderate | ○ Marked |
| Depersonalization | ○ None | ○ Mild | ○ Moderate | ○ Marked |
| Derealization | ○ None | ○ Mild | ○ Moderate | ○ Marked |

Misperceptions of Role & Meaning:

_____

_____

## Sensorium

| | | | |
|---|---|---|---|
| Orientation Disturbances | ○ Tested | ○ Too disturbed to test | |
| Time | ○ None | ○ Mild | ○ Moderate | ○ Marked |
| Place | ○ None | ○ Mild | ○ Moderate | ○ Marked |
| Person | ○ None | ○ Mild | ○ Moderate | ○ Marked |
| Clouded Consciousness | ○ None | ○ Mild | ○ Moderate | ○ Marked |
| | ○ Fluctuating | ○ Continuous | |
| Dissociation | ○ None | ○ Mild | ○ Moderate | ○ Marked |

Comments on Sensorium:

_____

_____

FIGURE 43-1, cont'd   For legend see page 504.

# Mental Status Examination—cont'd

## Cognitive Functions

| Memory Disturbances | ○ Tested | ○ Too disturbed to test | | ○ Confabulations | |
|---|---|---|---|---|---|
|    Immediate | ○ Unknown | ○ None | ○ Mild | ○ Moderate | ○ Marked |
|    Recent | ○ Unknown | ○ None | ○ Mild | ○ Moderate | ○ Marked |
|    Remote | ○ Unknown | ○ None | ○ Mild | ○ Moderate | ○ Marked |

| Attention Disturbances | ○ None | ○ Mild | ○ Moderate | ○ Marked | |
|---|---|---|---|---|---|
| Distractibility | ○ None | ○ Mild | ○ Moderate | ○ Marked | |
| Intelligence (estimated) | ○ Unknown | ○ Retarded | ○ Borderline | ○ Average | ○ Bright |

Comments on Cognitive Functions:

_____

_____

## Judgment

| Family Relations | ○ Poor | ○ Fair | ○ Healthy | |
|---|---|---|---|---|
| Other social relations | ○ Poor | ○ Fair | ○ Healthy | |
| Employment | ○ Poor | ○ Fair | ○ Healthy | |
| Future Plans | ○ No Plans | ○ Poor | ○ Fair | ○ Realistic |

Comments on Judgment:

_____

_____

## Insight & Attitude Toward Illness

Recognition of one's illness
  ○ Unknown    ○ Too sick to be tested    ○ Physically ill only
  ○ None    ○ Little    ○ Fair    ○ Full recognition

Awareness of one's contribution to problem
  ○ Unknown    ○ Too sick to be tested    ○ Not applicable
  ○ None    ○ Little    ○ Fair    ○ Full awareness
  ○ Blames others    ○ Blames circumstances

Motivation for getting well
  ○ Unknown    ○ Too sick to be tested
  ○ None    ○ Little    ○ Fair    ○ Highly motivated
  ○ Accepts offered treatment    ○ Refuses offered treatment

Comments on insight:

_____

_____

## Potential for Self-Injury, Suicide and Violence

| Self-Injury | ○ Unknown | ○ Absent | ○ Minimal | ○ Potentially present | ○ Marked (specify precautions) |
|---|---|---|---|---|---|
| Suicide Risk | ○ Unknown | ○ Absent | ○ Minimal | ○ Potentially present | ○ Marked (specify precautions) |
| Assaultiveness | ○ Unknown | ○ Absent | ○ Minimal | ○ Potentially present | ○ Active (specify interventions) |

Comments on self-injury, suicide/violence potential (e.g., plan, history, behavior):

_____

_____

_____

_____

## Reliability and Completeness of Information:

  ○ Very good     ○ Good     ○ Only Fair     ○ Poor     ○ Very Poor

**FIGURE 43-1, cont'd**   For legend see page 504.

# Mental Status Examination—cont'd

Barriers to Communication/reliability due to (Complete only if reliability rated poor/very poor):

    ○ Dialect/Foreign language   ○ Quality of speech   ○ Deafness   ○ Physical Illness
    ○ Refuses to give information   ○ Massive Denial   ○ Conscious falsification
    ○ Pt. psychopathology    Other (explain) _____

_____
_____

**Attitude Toward Examiner:**

   ○ Positive   ○ Neutral   ○ Ambivalent   ○ Negative   ○ Unknown

**Overall Severity of Illness:**

   ○ Mild   ○ Moderate   ○ Marked   ○ Severe   ○ Extremely Severe

**Discussion & Formulation** (include description of patient's strengths/assets)

_____
_____
_____
_____
_____
_____

**Diagnoses (DSM-IV)**

   Axis I _____
   Axis II _____
   Axis III _____
   Axis IV (assessment of psychosocial/environmental problems) _____
   Axis V (Global Assessment of Functioning score) Current _____ Past year _____

**Recommendations:**

_____
_____
_____
_____
_____
_____
_____
_____

_____    _____
Examiner's Name, Title                             Date

_____    _____
Examining Psychiatrist Signature                     Date

**FIGURE 43-1, cont'd** For legend see page 504.

**TABLE 43-1      ASSESSMENT OF MENTAL IMPAIRMENT SEVERITY**

| AREA OR ASPECT OF FUNCTIONING | CLASS 1: NO IMPAIRMENT | CLASS 2: MILD IMPAIRMENT | CLASS 3: MODERATE IMPAIRMENT | CLASS 4: MARKED IMPAIRMENT | CLASS 5: EXTREME IMPAIRMENT |
|---|---|---|---|---|---|
| Activities of daily living Social functioning Concentration Adaptation | No impairment is noted | Impairment levels are compatible with most useful functioning | Impairment levels are compatible with some, but not all, useful functioning | Impairment levels significantly impede useful functioning | Impaired levels preclude useful functioning |

From U.S. Department of Health and Human Services: Disability evaluation under social security. Social Security Administration Publication No. 64-039, 1994, Washington, D.C.

According to the U.S. Department of Health and Human Services Disability Evaluation Under Social Security,[2] the assessment of severity of mental impairment includes four different aspects: (1) limitations in activities of daily living; (2) social functioning; (3) concentration, persistence, and pace; and (4) deterioration or decompensation in work or work-like settings (see Table 43-1). These are discussed in detail in that source.[2]

## PSYCHOLOGICAL TESTS

There are many psychological tests. Some of the tests that are helpful in performing a thorough psychiatric examination are listed below. Some are given to the patient to be self-administered and later interpreted by the examining psychiatrist.

1. *Zung Scales to Assess Anxiety and Depression*
   These two scales consist of twenty questions each with four possible answers on a Lickert-type scale. The interpretation is simple and provides information as to the patient's level and severity of anxiety and depression.[9-14]

2. *Hamilton Scale for Assessing Anxiety and Depression*
   Hamilton[15-17] developed specific scales that assist in the assessment of anxiety and depression. However, they require the active assessment by the examiner of the patient's mental state. The patient is rated on a specifically structured rating scale as a result of a thorough psychiatric examination. The Hamilton Rating Scales for anxiety and depression have become a standard in the practice of patient assessment in the field of psychiatry, in clinical and research settings.

3. *Incomplete Sentences Blank—Adult Form*
   This is a projective test. The patients project their thoughts and feelings into words that are interpreted by the examining psychiatrist. This specific instrument has been used and found helpful by psychologists and psychiatrists. It instructs the patients to complete a list of 40 sentences that begin with one to three words and allow patients indirectly to reveal some of their inner feelings, ambivalence, thought content, thought processes, and richness of vocabulary in communicating in written form. The psychiatrist looks for the existence of internal inconsistencies and contradictions within each sentence as well as the overall content of the full 40 sentences, looking for central themes that emerge from the written material.

4. *Assessing the Patient's Strengths*
   Here, patients are asked to complete a questionnaire focusing on their strengths and health, rather than psychopathology, illness, and symptoms. This assessment provides information on such items as their hobbies, health habits, strength of social support systems, favorite foods, favorite movies, use of leisure time, religious practices, ability for imaginary capacity and daydreaming, personal style of relating to the external world, ability to manage and handle finances, and ability to activate and use external available resources.

5. *Minnesota Multiphasic Personality Inventory (MMPI)*
   This particular test has been widely used in the United States and consists of over 500 declarative statements that the person has the choice of answering "true", "false", or "I can't say." The results are scored by a computer and provide general hypotheses for the psychologist to follow-up with more specific testing. A new version of this test has recently been introduced, called the MMPI-II.

6. *Tests of Intellectual Functioning*

These tests measure the person's apparent level of intellectual functioning, as well as intellectual capacity. Commonly, they are known as the IQ tests. The most reliable and best validated test for intellectual functioning are the Wechsler Tests. The one commonly used for adults is called the Wechsler Adult Intelligence Scale-Revised (WAIS-R).

7. *Neuropsychological Testing*

In the last decade, a growing awareness has developed of a not–uncommon presence of impaired higher functioning originating from within the neocortex. Some authors[18] believe that about 20% of individuals previously diagnosed as having a psychogenic disorder actually are suffering from some type of organic brain syndrome. Neuropsychological tests are performed by psychologists with special training in the field, and are designed to measure a wide range of cortical functions influencing the patient's behavior. Some of these brain-behavior functions assessed by neuropsychological testing include the following: (1) the capacity for learning new skills and ideas; (2) the ability for complex conceptual cognitive processing without being distracted; (3) the capacity to make fine sensory discriminations; (4) the capacity to perform fine motor coordination; (5) the adequacy of perceptual-motor functions; (6) the adequacy of perception and perceptual reasoning; (7) the adequacy of short-term memory; (8) the adequacy of constructional skills; (9) the capacity to persist in performing difficult tasks without being distracted in the face of environmental pressure; (10) the ability to flexibly shift one's expectations, focus, and efforts in the face of a change in the conditions of the external environment; (11) the adequacy of language-related functions; and (12) the ability to control one's impulses, especially during a stressful situation. It is important to note that these neuropsychological tests are useful in detecting impairment in cortical brain functions, especially in patients in whom the CT scan, MRI, or EEG may be within the normal range and do not reveal a specific disorder or impairment. Filskov and Boll[19] provide an excellent resource for learning more about neuropsychological testing and its place in the assessment of functional impairments of the brain.

8. *Projective Personality Tests*

These tests systematically measure a person's psychological strengths and weaknesses by assessing how well the patient copes when emotionally aroused. The person taking the test is required to respond to ambiguous and vague stimuli, such as inkblots. The most commonly used tests are the Rorschach Inkblot[20] and the Thematic Apperception Test (TAT).[21]

9. *Global Assessment of Functioning*

Axis V requires the psychiatrist to assess the patient on a Global Assessment Functioning (GAF) Scale that provides a score on a scale of 0 - 100; zero meaning inadequate information, 1 - 10 meaning "persistent danger of severely hurting self or others (for example, recurrent violence) or persistent inability to maintain minimal personal hygiene or serious suicidal act with clear expectation of death," while a rating of 91 - 100 means "superior functioning in a wide range of activities, life's problems never seem to get out of hand, is sought out by others because of his or her many positive qualities. No symptoms."[3]

Another scale that has been found helpful is the Jenkins Activity Survey (JAS),[22] which is a 52-item self-report that evaluates an interaction measure of stress since it focuses on the cognitive and perceptual characteristics of the individual that mediate the responses to stress. The JAS has shown predicted validity in populations of patients with coronary heart disease.

The Social Adjustment Scale-Self Report (SAS-SR) is composed of 42 questions rated on a 5-point scale of severity and was developed by Weissman and Bothwell.[23] It covers such issues as emotional and instrumental qualities in role performance, social and leisure activities, relationships with the extended family, marital role, parental role, family unit, and economic independence. Norms are available for non–patient community samples, acute and recovered depressed patients, patients with schizophrenia, and patients with drug addiction.

## PSYCHIATRIC RATING SYSTEMS

Since disability determination is basically a social decision, with medical input, various jurisdictions have different rules and requirements. For example, Social Security Disability Insurance determinations are binary; the patients are either qualified or they are not.[2,24,25,26] In the Veterans Administration and workers' compensation systems, disability may range from mild, partial to marked, total.[27-29] Obviously disability measurements must consider the specific system requirements as well as the assessed psychiatric impairments.

The New York State Department of Social Services, Office of Disability Determinations, requests semiquantitative ratings in the following "work related mental activities":[25,26,30]

1. understanding and memory

2. sustained concentration and persistence
3. social interaction
4. adaptation (that is, adaptation to environmental change and demand)

In California, the division of Industrial Accidents Medical and Chiropractic Advisory Committee, Subcommittee on Permanent Psychiatric Disability, devised a list of eight work functions with five degrees of impairment:[31]

1. the ability to comprehend and follow instructions
2. the ability to perform simple and repetitive tasks
3. the ability to maintain a work task appropriate to a given work load
4. the ability to perform complex or varied tasks
5. the ability to relate to other people beyond giving and receiving instructions
6. the ability to influence people
7. the ability to make generalizations, evaluations, or decisions without immediate supervision
8. the ability to accept and carry out responsibility for direction, control, and planning

The Social Security System[2] organizes behavioral and psychiatric impairment into the following categories: organic mental disorders, schizophrenic, paranoid and other psychotic disorders, affective disorders, mental retardation and autism, anxiety related disorders, somatoform disorders, personality disorders, and substance addiction disorders. Additionally, a special section is devoted to mental disorders for children and young adults (under the age of 18). There are 11 diagnostic categories for these individuals: organic mental disorders; schizophrenic, delusional (paranoid), schizoaffective, and other psychotic disorders; mood disorders; mental retardation; anxiety disorders; somatoform, eating, and tic disorders; personality disorders; psychoactive substance dependence disorders; autistic disorder and other pervasive developmental disorders; attention deficit hyperactivity disorder; and developmental and emotional disorders of newborn and younger infants.

The AMA *Guides* follow the Social Security guides very closely. However, there are special notations made about substance abuse, personality disorders, mental retardation, and pain. The subject of pain will be covered in Chapter 45.

## MAJOR CATEGORIES OF DISABLING PSYCHIATRIC CONDITIONS

The various criteria used to establish inclusion in the categories used by the Social Security System are found in References 2 and 3. Some of these categories will be described in greater detail below due to their pervasive inclusion within the rating systems.

## Organic Brain Diseases

Organic brain diseases are expressed clinically as either dementias or deliria. By definition, delirium is an acute brain disorder characterized by clouding of consciousness. Delirious patients are almost universally unable to function vocationally or socially. They are usually hospitalized and require intensive medical treatment for the underlying condition, for example, delirium tremens or gram-negative septicemia. Most disability decisions for organic brain disease involve dementias that are chronic disorders with impairment of intellectual functioning. In the appraisal of disability related to dementia, accurate quantification of specific impairment in cognitive functions is essential. In addition to the standard battery of psychological tests, including the Wechsler Adult Intelligence Scale, detailed neuropsychological tests may be indicated. These results should be integrated with workplace appraisals. If an employee cannot function in the usual assignment, other jobs should be considered before disability is determined. (See Clinical Example 1 on p. 513.)

## Schizophrenia

The diagnostic category of schizophrenia includes a diverse group of disorders, some with a formal subtype designation such as catatonic or paranoid. Impairments range from moderate, with ability to work in carefully-controlled environments, to profound, with chronic institutionalization.[32] Although there is good interrater agreement about global function assessment, there is no generally-accepted list of critical functions, let alone techniques for their quantitative measurement.[26,28,30,31,33,34] The principal impairments associated with schizophrenia that interfere with work capacity are cognitive functions and social skills. Cognitive-intellectual functioning can be accurately measured in the mental status examination and in psychometric tests such as the WAIS-R. Social skills often vary from one setting to another, and therefore are best measured in specific situations such as a workplace or sheltered workshop.[28,29,35] In occupational environments, managers can offer the best appraisal of a patient/employee's work capacity.[36]

In quantifying the degree of disability associated with schizophrenia, the patient's job skills must be weighed and considered as thoroughly as cognitive and social impairments. (See Clinical Example 2 on p. 513.)

## Affective Disorders

Affective disorders vary significantly in severity, chronicity, and periodicity. The range of impairment runs from mild, chronic dysthymia to severe, rapid-cycling bipolar disorder or to refractory major depression. Many of these patients have prolonged periods of well-being with normal social and vocational functioning. For these individuals with intermittent illness, disability is often measured by the amount of time lost from work. (See Clinical Example 3 on p. 513.)

Patients with chronic, non-cyclical affective disorders usually manifest impairments in cognition, initiative, and mood.[35,36] The mental status examination and psychometric testing can provide a measure of impairment in work-related skills and capacities. But the measurement of disability is best served by accurate and thorough work appraisal, for example, comparing the patients' contribution to that of their peers. Usually the degree of impairment due to chronic depression is reflected in a reduction of productivity that can be quantified by management.[27,35,36]

## Anxiety Disorders and Dissociative Disorders

Current standard nomenclature, for example, DSM-IV and ICD 10,[3,4] groups anxiety disorders together, based in part on a psychodynamic conviction that all of them stem from anxiety and maladaptive defenses. But the behavioral manifestations of these disorders range from internal preoccupations with no external signs, as in mild obsessions, to severe anxiety or panic attacks with secondary agoraphobia. A housebound, markedly phobic person may appear cognitively intact on formal examination and yet deserve a very high or total disability rating because such a person cannot maintain regular attendance in the workplace.[35,36] For each of these anxiety disorders, specific impairments may compromise vocational and social functions:

> *Generalized anxiety disorder*—concentration, attention, and memory
> *Panic disorder*—episodic interruption of cognitive capacities
> *Phobic disorders*—avoidance, including inability to travel
> *Obsessive-compulsive disorder*—inability to make decisions
> *Dissociative disorders*—inconsistent cognitive performance and interpersonal problems with peers and managers

The quantitative measurement of disability depends on the nature of the patient's disorder as well as the requirements of their work. (See Clinical Example 4 on p. 513.)

## Somatoform Disorders

Somatoform disorders encompass a wide variety of physical complaints for which little or no organic pathology can be discovered.[29] Many individuals with somatoform disorders have pain or fatigue, two perceptions or experiences that cannot be measured or externally validated. In other words, they have symptoms without signs. How then can disability be evaluated? The question is urgent because of the extensive absence from work or their life responsibilities associated with these conditions.

At the present time there is no consensus in measuring disability related to somatization. The Social Security Administration, taking a "functional" approach, has awarded full disability benefits to patients with Chronic Fatigue Syndrome. Many private corporations have argued that they cannot award benefits to people with symptoms in the absence of physical, laboratory, or psychometric pathology. Other companies have been willing to consider disability awards after unsuccessful treatment, including integrated pain clinics. Some employees with Chronic Fatigue Syndrome, Multiple Environmental Allergies, Multiple Chemical Sensitivities Syndrome, or Chronic Benign Intractable Pain Syndrome have sued corporations after rejection of disability applications. They claim that their inability to perform activities of daily living, because of fatigue and/or pain, should be accepted despite the lack of corroborating evidence. In the absence of definitive legislation, psychiatrists must await an appellate level court decision to clarify this critical question. (See Clinical Example 5 on p. 514.)

## Personality Disorders

Personality disorders are characterized by aberrant behavior, usually in the absence of major affective or intellectual disturbances. The most definitive diagnostic information is derived from the patient's history, rather than the mental status examination or formal psychological tests.[28,29,36] Valuable data can be discovered in the personal history, especially subsections devoted to school, military, employment, and criminal performance and behavior. Interviewing family members is very useful.

The question of disability determination is as thorny for personality disorders as it is for substance abuse. Many jurisdictions hold to a long established position equating personality disorders with character traits, that is, they develop early, are relatively immutable, and do not represent a disease or illness. Therefore personality disorders are processed

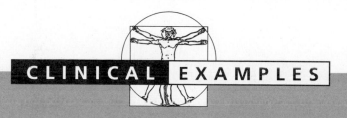

## PSYCHIATRIC DISORDERS

### ORGANIC BRAIN DISEASES

**EXAMPLE 1**

W.C. was a bright, competent accountant prior to an automobile crash in which he sustained damage to the frontal and temporal lobes. Neuropsychological testing revealed substantial loss of short-term memory and appreciable interference with attention, concentration, tracking, and set. These impairments were also obvious during a trial of work in his usual profession. As an accommodation the patient was given an administrative assignment. He remained employed until clerical and administrative work was taken over by a contractor. His employer, unable to find a suitable place for this patient, then determined that he was totally disabled. W.C.'s story illustrates the relationship between impairment and disability, that is, he became vocationally disabled when the workplace no longer could provide work that he could perform despite his chronic, cognitive impairments.

### SCHIZOPHRENIA

**EXAMPLE 2**

D.S., a 50-year-old chronic schizophrenic computer programmer, has remained employed despite severe introversion and bizarre appearance because of his superior technical skills and a protective manager. Occasionally, because of concerns expressed by other employees, he has needed counseling with the company employee assistance program. His programming talent has enabled him to maintain a job despite marginal social capacity. An unusually empathetic manager has buffered him from many corporate environ-

mental pressures. Despite his impairment, he is not considered disabled.

### AFFECTIVE DISORDERS

**EXAMPLE 3**

C.E., an electrical engineer-programmer, remained employed despite several episodes of mania. His contribution to the mission of his department was considered acceptable by his management. But the Veterans Administration, comparing his position and pay with that expected of a person with his education and experience, awarded him a permanent, partial disability (~33%).

### ANXIETY DISORDERS

**EXAMPLE 4**

E.M., a gifted research scientist with obsessive-compulsive disorder, developed an original technique in computer science. But he delayed too long in applying for a patent and in publishing his work because of an obsessive inability to limit the literature citations in his paper. What began as a research disclosure grew as complex as a review article, then a monograph, and finally a textbook. During this long period of obsessive rumination, other scientists published similar work, thereby diminishing the value of his effort to the scientific community and to his company. Although he remained employed, in some jurisdictions he could have been awarded a disability proportional to his reduced effectiveness. Here, again, the most salient measures derive from the workplace rather than from the physician's office.

*Continued.*

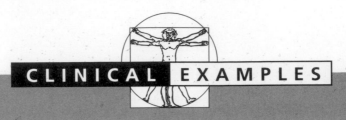

## CLINICAL EXAMPLES

### PSYCHIATRIC DISORDERS—cont'd

## SOMATOFORM DISORDERS

### EXAMPLE 5

M.N., a 35-year-old, single, female manager is in her second episode of chronic fatigue syndrome, currently lasting 13 months. She has been absent from work more than five months. Repeated examinations, including extensive laboratory tests, have failed to reveal physical abnormalities. Despite a healthy, robust appearance, she describes profound fatigue following minimal exertion. Antidepressant medication has not been efficacious. Her first episode, following a period of unusually heavy workload, lasted almost one year. She has joined a support group of fellow sufferers who are convinced that they are afflicted with chronic fatigue immune dysfunction syndrome, a mysterious physical disease only recently gaining understanding within the medical community. Since her disorder has been present for a prolonged period of time and there is no expectation that it will remit in the near future, she is considered totally impaired/disabled for the workforce. A notation should be made in the report, however, that her condition did remit in the past and that periodic reassessments are appropriate.

## PERSONALITY DISORDERS

### EXAMPLE 6

L.M. worked for several years as an administrative assistant despite her claims of possessing two advanced degrees and unusual creative gifts. Her behavior was characterized by impulsiveness, grandiosity, suspiciousness, and somatization. Repeated mental status examinations uncovered significant distortions in reality testing, with primitive ego defenses (that is, splitting and projection). Treatment with several psychiatrists was unsuccessful. On the verge of her forced separation from the business for unsatisfactory performance and insubordination, she was reviewed for medical disability and adjudicated unable to function because of severe borderline personality pathology. Here again her behavior was the determining factor, not intellectual impairments measured by formal tests. Psychiatric examinations did establish that her unacceptable behavior was derived from the impairments of severe character pathology.

*David Robbins*

through administrative channels and patients are separated from these organizations without disability benefits.[35,36]

Recent research and clinical interest in severe personality disorders, such as borderline and narcissistic disorders, have led to a reopening of the disability issue and have cast doubt on the exclusion of these disorders from other psychiatric diseases. Some companies will review personality disorders on a case-by-case basis, using functional criteria rather than diagnosis, for disability determinations. If approved, most of these patients are awarded total disability, since their behavior is considered incompatible with the needs of the organization. (See Clinical Example 6 on p. 514.)

## SUBSTANCE ABUSE

Substance abuse and drug addiction is one of the most controversial topics in the disability area. Should people, whose impairments appear to be self-induced, derive benefits, especially if their economic support can be used to prolong their "disease" and disability? Why cannot these people maintain abstinence and sobriety? Should society reward relapse by providing benefit programs?

People recovering from substance abuse, who are able to maintain sobriety with continued community support, may be able to resume their customary activities of daily living, including work. In the absence of comorbid disorders, that is, a mentally-ill substance-abusing patient, substance abuse in remission is not a disabling condition.

What, then, of alcohol-drug abusers or addicts who frequently relapse or who remain chronically drug-dependent? Under mandate of federal regulations, business and government organizations must be drug-free. Consequently, individuals who continue to use drugs cannot be employed.[36] Exemptions include sheltered workshops and medically supervised methadone maintenance programs.

Various organizations and entitlement programs differ dramatically in the determination of disability for substance abusers. Private industry usually separates employees after two or three unsuccessful rehabilitation efforts; this is an administrative separation rather than medical disability. Conversely, the Society Security system considers substance abuse, unresponsive to rehabilitation techniques, a totally disabling condition.[2] Obviously there are no elements of partial disability or measures of degree of disability. Because of legal social sanctions, chronic, relapsing substance abuse is not compatible with employment.

## References

1. American Medical Association: *Guides to the evaluation of permanent impairment*, ed 4, Chicago, 1993, American Medical Association.
2. U.S. Department of Health and Human Services: *Disability evaluation under social security*, Washington, D.C., Social Security Administration, 1994. SSA Publication No. 64-039.
3. American Psychiatric Association: *Diagnostic and statistical manual of mental disorders*, ed 4, Washington, D.C., 1994, American Psychiatric Association.
4. World Health Organization: *Manual of the international statistical classification of diseases, injuries, and causes of death; International classification of diseases* (ICD). Geneva, 1992, World Health Organization.
5. American Psychiatric Association: *Diagnostic and statistical manual of mental disorders—III*, Washington, D.C., 1982, American Psychiatric Association.
6. American Psychiatric Association: *Diagnostic and statistical manual of mental disorders—IIIR*, Washington, D.C., 1987, American Psychiatric Association.
7. Luborsky L: Clinicians' judgments of mental health, *Arch Gen Psychiatry* 7:407-417, 1962.
8. Endicot J, Spitzer RL, Fleiss JL, et al: The Global Assessment Scale: A procedure for measuring overall severity of psychiatric disturbance, *Arch Gen Psychiatry* 33:766-771, 1976.
9. Zung WWK: A self-rating depression scale, *Arch Gen Psychiatry* 12:63-70, 1965.
10. Zung WWK: Evaluating treatment methods for depressive disorders, *Am J Psychiatry* 124(suppl): 40-48, 1968.
11. Zung WWK, Wonnacott TH: Treatment prediction in depression using a self-rating scale, *Biol Psychiatry* 2:321-329, 1970.
12. Zung WWK: A rating instrument for anxiety disorders, *Psychosomatics* 12:371-379, 1971.
13. Zung WWK: From art to science: The diagnosis and treatment of depression, *Arch Gen Psychiatry* 29:328-337, 1973.
14. Zung WWK: Prevalence of clinically significant anxiety in a family practice setting, *Am J Psychiatry* 143:1471-1472, 1986.
15. Hamilton M: The assessment of anxiety states by rating, *Br J Med Psychol* 32:50-55, 1959.
16. Hamilton M: A rating scale for depression, *J Neurol Neurosurg Psychiatry* 23:56-61, 1960.
17. Hamilton M: Development of a rating scale for primary depressive illness, *Br J Soc Clin Psychol* 6:278-296, 1967.
18. Strub RL, Black FW: *The mental status examination in neurology*, Philadelphia, 1977, F.A. Davis.

19. Filskov SB, Boll TJ, editors: *Handbook of neuroclinical psychology.* New York, 1981, John Wiley & Sons.

20. Rorschach H: *Psychodiagnostics,* New York, 1949, Grune and Stratton.

21. Murray HA: *Thematic apperception test manual,* Cambridge, MA, 1943, Harvard University Press.

22. Jenkins CD, Rossman RH, Friedman J: Development of a psychological test for the determination for the coronary-prone behavior pattern in employed men, *J Chronic Dis,* 20:371-379, 1967.

23. Weissman MM, Bothwell S: Assessment of social adjustment by patient self report, *Arch Gen Psychiatry* 33:111-115, 1976.

24. Goldman HH, Runck B: NIMH Report. Social Security Administration revises mental disability rules, *Hospital and Community Psychiatry* 36:343-345, 1985.

25. New York State Department of Social Services, Office of Disability Determination: *Reporting requirements for psychiatric consultative examinations,* Albany, NY, July, 1985.

26. Pincus HA, Kennedy C, Simmens SJ, et al: Determining disability due to mental impairments: APA's evaluation of Social Security Administration guidelines, *Amer J Psychiatry* 148:1037-1043, 1991.

27. Grant B, Robbins D: *Disability, workers' compensation, and fitness for duty.* In Kahn J, editor: *Mental health in the workplace: A practical psychiatric guide.* New York, 1993, Van Nostrand Reinhold, pp. 83-105.

28. Massel HK, Liberman RP, Mintz J, et al: Evaluating the capacity to work of the mentally ill, *Psychiatry* 53:31-43, 1990.

29. Robbins D: *Medical disability absence from work,* Valhalla, NY, 1989, New York Medical College.

30. Nussbaum K, Schneidmuhl AM, Shaffer JW: Psychiatric assessment in the Social Security Program of disability insurance, *Amer J Psychiatry* 126:897-899, 1969.

31. Enelow AJ: Assessing the effect of psychiatric disorders on work function, *Occupational Medicine: State of the Art Reviews* 3:621-627, 1988.

32. Reich J: DSM-III diagnoses in Social Security disability applicants referred for psychiatric evaluation, *J Clin Psychiatry* 47:81-82, 1986.

33. Bonder BR: Disease and dysfunction: the value of Axis V, *Hosp and Community Psychiatry* 41:959-60, 1990.

34. Rosen A, Hadzi-Pavlovic D, Parker G: The life skills profile: a measure assessing function and disability in schizophrenia, *Schizophr Bull* 15:325-337, 1989.

35. Robbins D: Psychiatric conditions in worker fitness and risk evaluation, *Occupational Medicine: State of the Art Reviews* 3:309-321, 1988.

36. Robbins D: The psychiatric patient at work, *Occupational Medicine: State of the Art Reviews* 1:549-558, 1986.

# CHAPTER 44

# STRESS

*Brian Schulman*

"The single most remarkable historical fact concerning the term stress is its persistent widespread usage in biology and medicine in spite of almost chaotic disagreement over its definition."[1]

## CONCEPT OF STRESS IN MEDICAL PRACTICE

It is widely agreed among physicians that excessive stress contributes to the development of mental and psychosomatic disorders. There is less consensus on what constitutes stress. Although stress has been the subject of much psychiatric and social science research, little is known about the mechanisms that link psychological and physiological stress to the development of mental or physical illness and disease.

Theoretical problems abound. For the researchers in the area of psychosocial behavior, stress is an elusive concept to measure. The causal nexus between objective environmental stressors (such as life events, hassles of daily living, and losses) and the development of pathophysiological change and illness is hampered by the inherent difficulty of defining and quantifying stressful conditions, as well as accounting for individual variability of response. Stressful conditions rarely occur independently of other aggravating or modifying events in life. How does the researcher account for the passage of time or the idiosyncratic nature of people? How does one account for personal characteristics such as defense, coping, and hardiness? Variability of response is the rule, not the exception in stress research. Haan has noted, "Stress is whatever stresses people, but its essential properties are not clear."[2]

Many psychosocial studies have demonstrated the proximate association of objective life events with the later development of illness,[3-6] but those, as well as numerous other comparable studies, rely on the retrospective analysis of events. It has been far easier to rate the severity of an environmental event or condition than to demonstrate in a prospective study that such a stressor produces an illness or a disability. In this regard, the absence of reproducible scientific data has not diminished or altered the widely-held belief among physicians and their patients that such a causal nexus exists and is a significant factor in the development of illness and disability.

Although stress lacks an objective clinical standard of measurement, the adverse consequences of stress (as well as the recommendation to manage stress better) are conspicuous in many clinical assessments. Clinically, stress seems to have a binary quality; it is either contributory or noncontributory to the medical or psychiatric diagnosis. In many instances, the basis for the determination of that contribution is subjective. The individual may perceive an implicit internal threshold for tolerating stress. When that threshold is exceeded, the discomfort is attributed to stress. In practice, the assessor's objective standard for determining the existence of stress is limited and often too dependent on the patient's subjective history.

In part, the primary problem for the assessor of stress is understanding the subjective history of the patient, in an objective context, that allows for a meaningful and scientific attribution of causality. The language of stress[7] bridges the gap between the patients' perception of the source of their distress and the medical basis of their suffering. For the patient, stress language has the utility of attribution. Stress language is a lexicon of cause. The utility is obvious: to find the cause of one's distress and reverse it.

For the modern physician, attributing a wide variety of clinical problems to "stress" is a common and well accepted means of gaining some closure to the clinical assessment. For the patients, otherwise unable to understand the cause of their distress, "stress" is, at times, an acceptable and welcome explanation. It is an attribution of cause that links unpleasant environmental experiences with life events. It provides individuals with a plausible, although not necessarily medically-accurate, explanation for feeling poorly. The language of stress seeks to bridge the gap between personal experience and "common sense" and the biomedical model of illnesses, where all pathological change has a specific molecular cause.

## UTILITY OF STRESS IN MEDICAL COMMUNICATION

In pragmatic terms, one may observe that an internal state of stress is necessary to recognize real and potential dangers in the environment. Stress serves a protective function as it alerts the organism to danger and provides the mechanisms of survival. The experience of stress mediates man's relationship with the psychosocial environment. Thus, mediating stress is an integral factor in the preservation of health and the avoidance of disease. In an effort to validate this hypothesis, numerous models of health and disease have been proposed to illustrate the interactive relationship of man in the biopsychosocial environment.[8,9] It has not proven easy to provide the modern physician with a pragmatic and functionally operative model to complement the current biomedical model. Engel has worked to expand the understanding of illness by proposing a biopsychosocial model that depicts the illness affecting concentric and overlapping systems from the submolecular elements to the social and cultural system.[10] He emphasizes the interaction of biological with environmental systems, where illness has a ripple effect disrupting all aspects of a person's life. Cassel urges the physician to appreciate the multiple dimensions of what he describes as the "personhood."[11] Only by acknowledging and then therapeutically addressing the multiple and complex dimensions of the person can a physician assist in the relief of suffering. The ultimate "transcendence" of suffering expands medical therapeutics to include psychological, cultural, and even spiritual issues.

Stress language communicates a perception of personal strain, reminding the modern physician that human suffering is not always objective nor does it readily conform to measurable medical standards. Stress is deeply rooted in the subjective experience of living. The language of stress hopes to identify the interface between life events, subjective response, and, on occasion, illness. When patients speak of being under stress, they are advising the physician that the circumstances of their lives are not quite right. In a comparable way, when the physician speaks of stress to their patients, they are cautioning the patient that factors related to life-style are affecting the patients' state of health and contributing to their suffering. This explicit communication connecting the experience with the therapeutic recommendation is conveyed through the language of stress.

## BIOLOGICAL CONCEPT OF STRESS

In its most elementary sense, the concept of human stress encompasses the study of stimulus and response. The history of human stress research began with studies of physiological response, but now includes psychological as well as social investigations.

The history of stress is as old as life. Beginning with the Neanderthal who was forced to find water and shelter from the cold to the modern commodities trader attempting to shout orders into two telephones simultaneously, stress has been part of the survival mechanism. Threats to security or the anticipation of danger produce marked stimulation of the central nervous system, hormonal secretion, and alterations in behavior. It makes evolutionary sense that the original cavemen needed a good dose of adrenalin to escape the predatory animals roaming the tundra. Over millions of years, little has changed. Commodities traders still relish the "thrill of the pit," as they barter to make a profit. Man is dependent upon, perhaps even addicted to, stress. The stress response is at the fulcrum of survival; its adaptive utility is precariously balanced by its destructive potential.

The ability to regulate stress internally is critical to the survival of even the most primitive biological system. An intuitive awareness of stress (as well as the individual's ability to cope with stress) is as old as recorded civilization. Socrates offered that our way of life is a major key to our sickness and our health. Hippocrates, the father of modern medicine, spoke of the body's intrinsic healing powers and the ability of the body to restore health naturally.

The biological understanding of the interaction of systems unfolded in the eighteenth century. The French physiologist Claude Bernard advanced the concept of living beings existing in a "harmonious whole," and emphasized that survival under difficult external conditions was dependent on the maintenance of a constant internal environment.[12]

The American physiologist Walter Cannon advanced the principles by which living systems survived in nature, noting that only when cells grow in masses and selectively differentiate into specialized functional units could they maintain internal stability capable of separating them from disturbances due to shifts in the external environment.[13] The maintenance of internal stability in the face of changing external conditions is biological homeostasis. Any factor or condition that alters the state of homeostasis creates a condition of stress.

The mediation of biological homeostasis is largely a function of the autonomic nervous system. Cannon correctly identified the critical role of sympathetic activation as a signal alerting the body to the physiological dangers of cold, hemorrhage, lowered blood sugar, or toxins. Activation of the sympathetic system initiated a "fight versus flight" response with resultant activation of the hypothalamic-pituitary-adrenal (HPA) axis and biochemical reactions designed to restore homeostasis.

Cannon proposed that the concept of homeostasis could be expanded to social systems as well. "Only when human beings are grouped in large aggregations is there an opportunity of developing an internal organization which can offer mutual aid and the advantage, to many, of special ingenuity and skill." Stress could be generated by shifts in the social as well as the biological environment. Expanding the concept of biological homeostasis to include human stability in the social order served to integrate the biological with the psychological condition. Human adaptation bridges the dichotomy of mind and body. Adaptation is the ultimate antidote for stress, seeking to conceptualize the processes by which humans actively seek to restore internal and external stability. The study of adaptation encompasses coping, defense, and mastery—processes by which man seeks to maintain stability in the face of difficult conditions.

Hans Selye, considered by many as the father of modern stress medicine, described the physiological impact of chronic stress.[14] In 1936, Selye published an article in *Nature* entitled, "A syndrome produced by diverse nocuous agents." The Syndrome was the General Adaptation Syndrome (GAS) in which he delineated three distinct physiological stages: alarm, resistance, and exhaustion. For Selye, stress was a nonspecific response to essentially the wear and tear of life . . . "the unconscious, wired in stress responses mediated by the neurohumoral system." The deleterious effect of stress was chronic activation of the HPA axis, resulting in biochemical and structural tissue changes and the clinical syndrome of "just being sick." Stress is a state of chronic activation of interdependent physiological events initiated by virtually any toxic demand. He was less concerned with defining the first mediator of the alarm process than understanding the physiological consequence of organ exhaustion. "Whatever the nature of the first mediator, however, its existence is assured by its effects, which have been observed and measured."

The relationship between stress and the development of physical illness has proved to be a fascinating area for speculation. Historically, there have been many theories attempting to link life events, personality, and illness, but little in the way of scientific evidence to elucidate the causal nexus. Many theories of psychosomatic specificity have been largely aban-doned in favor of a more broadly based, albeit less precise, acceptance of the World Health Organization's recognition of the interdependent role of biological, psychological, and social variables in health and disease.

What can be said with certainty is that acute intense psychological stress activates the HPA[15-17] and that significant activation of the HPA is evident in posttraumatic stress disorder (PTSD)[18] and depression,[19,20] and possibly in various chronic illnesses. An accumulating body of data indicates that HPA alterations do represent a measure of severity in psychiatric illness (albeit difficult to assess quantitatively) and produce cognitive dysfunction and behavioral impairment.

The role of environmental stress in the pathogenesis of physical illness is less clear. The connection between events and illness is elusive. However, some interesting studies have hypothesized about specific life events such as the "goal frustrating" event and the subsequent development of peptic ulcer disease,[21] "negative life events" and myocardial infarction,[22] and "severe life events" prior to the onset of multiple sclerosis.[23]

Although it is widely assumed among laypeople (as well as many physicians) that emotional stress is a significant factor in the precipitation and aggravation of hypertension, the available literature does not support the etiologic role of stress in the development of hypertension.[24]

The finding that stress—whether associated with a single or repeated exposure to an experimentally designed stressor—increases neurochemical activity in the brain may have important implications for understanding pathophysiology, but at present has little direct clinical correlation with the pathogenesis of specific physical illnesses.

## PSYCHOLOGICAL DIMENSION OF STRESS

Selye saw stress as an inevitable consequence of living,[14] that essentially anything that disrupted the state of adaptive balance could cause stress. His frequently-quoted advice to business executives seemed to imply the inevitability and unescapable nature of stressful events, "It's not what happens to you that matters but how you take it." Indeed, he cautioned, "the only condition where there is no stress is death."

A major difficulty hampering the assessment of psychological stress is reaching consensus among investigators on definitions and meaning. Stress reaches to the heart of the subjective experience. Definitional boundaries must encompass issues of personal variability. Consequently, most studies of stress are highly sensitive to individual differences and tend to produce broad, inclusive criteria.

The requirement for investigational objectivity in assessment must, of necessity, limit the subjective perceptions of respondents. Not everything is stressful. Mikhail[25] has surveyed the early literature and highlights consensus in the historical development of the stress concept. To summarize, the following are considered important aspects of the stress concept:

1. Individuals show considerable variability in their reactivity to stress.
2. Stress is largely determined by an individual's perception of the stressful situation, or the individual's anticipation of the inability to respond adequately to a given demand rather than the situation itself.
3. The extent of stress depends partly on the capability of an individual to cope.

The operative psychological model of stress reactivity is predicated on the awareness, which is presumed to be cognitively assessed, of a demand-capability imbalance. The psychological model is particularly concerned with both the qualitative nature and quantitative weighing of the demand. The study of life events, daily hassles and uplifts, and conditions of living provide a framework for assessing and standardizing demand. The hypothesis of psychological stress models is that the dimension of environmental events correlates with the individual's perception of stress.

## POSTTRAUMATIC STRESS AND PANIC DISORDER SYNDROMES: A NEURAL MODEL

The most compelling clinical evidence linking environmental events with psychiatric symptomatology has been found in studies of individuals intensely exposed to extreme situations such as exposure to natural disasters, concentration camps, and the horrific aspects of war.[26-28]

Exposure to intense severe trauma is likely to produce a clinically identifiable syndrome of posttraumatic stress disorder (PTSD). PTSD is characterized by intense, recurrent, and intrusive (upon consciousness) revivification of the traumatic environmental event. Various perceptual stimuli can trigger these states for decades after the event. The clinical syndrome is characterized by a state of hypervigilance, avoidance of stimuli likely to trigger revivification, and possibly a variety of less specific findings of anxiety, sleep disturbance, and diminished motivation.[29]

The current neurobiological assumptions that underlie the PTSD model are derived from investigational studies of fear and electrical shock conditioning primarily conducted with laboratory animals.[30,31] Few investigational studies have been conducted in humans. Nonetheless, it is thought that the intensity and persistence of memory are related in part to the activation of certain neuromodulatory systems.[18] For example, the initial intense environmental stimulus activates the adrenergic system, which facilitates the encoding of memories in the amygdala, hippocampus, locus ceruleus, and the sensory cortex. The amygdala, which has extensive connections throughout the cortex, is thought to play a central role by attaching fear and anxiety behaviors to a number of neural stimuli. Repeated environmental exposures are thought to reactivate these fear conditioning networks in the central nervous system (CNS). Presumably, the process of fear extinction, which would normally occur over time, is inhibited.

PTSD is a response to intense, severe, environmental events that activate neurobiological responses throughout the CNS that are, at least initially, essential for survival. Whether PTSD is an accurate neurobiological model for less severe environmental stressors is arguable and will require far more investigational study. Examples of these less severe environmental exposures are those events that are presently described as a variety of phobias (for example, fear of heights, crowds, and leaving home) and produce responses that are considered together as panic disorder. What can be said with relative certainty is that the CNS is designed to identify changes in the internal and external environment and through highly evolved neural pathways effect protective mechanisms. Acute neurobiological responses serve an adaptive function and ensure survival. The chronic activation of neural networks that is thought to occur in PTSD is maladaptive and leads to illness. At this time, little is known about issues of vulnerability, predisposition, or the contribution of other psychiatric or medical conditions to the development of PTSD.

## DIAGNOSIS AND MEASUREMENT OF STRESS

The process of assessment is initiated by clinical exploration of the proximate life history of the patient. A history of recent events may provide important information about events that caused significant changes in a person's life. The degree of change occasioned by an event may be sufficiently great to prevent adaptation and possibly contribute to the onset of either psychological or physical illness.

In recent years there has been much interest in environmentally-induced illness, particularly illness precipitated by exposure not only to psychologically traumatic events but events that precipitate measurable life change.

Psychiatrists and clinicians have long been most interested in the correlations of life events with the development of illness. This association has been most clearly identified in widows who have shown high morbidity in the twelve months following the death of a spouse.[3] The vulnerability occasioned by bereavement was shown to relate to reduction in cell mediated and humoral immune functions.[32]

In the life events model, events have psychological significance because they have a propensity to initiate social change and cause disruption of the adaptational balance. The relation between life events and social change can be quantified. In 1967, Holmes and Rahe devised and published the Social Readjustment Rating Scale (SRRS), which, in survey form, defined 42 life-change events ranging from the severe, such as the loss of a spouse, to the more commonly experienced issues of job changes or financial difficulties.[33] Rater groups, serving as judges, assigned values to each event on the list, producing a hierarchy of stressful events. The result was a standardized survey that could be widely administered to assess the magnitude of social readjustment.

There are many critics of the life event–social readjustment scaling. The essential problem has been the utility of considering an event, any event, "out of context." Many environmental and constitutional factors influence the psychological impact of a given event. The timing, sequencing, and social circumstances play modifying roles.[34] Moreover, personality factors, as well as the broadly-defined abilities of coping, defense, and mastery, are critical determinants. Social support and cultural factors play a critical role in determining the all-important response of the individual to the event.

Consequently, investigators have refined measuring systems for life events that encompass both the quantitative and the various qualitative aspects of the event. Dohrenwend and Dohrenwend devoted considerable effort to assessing the applicability of a life-event scale to a particular population. They developed the Psychiatric Epidemiological Research Interview–Life Event Scale (PERI-LES) as part of a study in New York City to develop methodology to study life change and psychiatric illness in a particular community.[35] Paykel in New Haven developed assessment instruments to correlate life events that occurred within six months of illness. In an effort to gain greater specificity, they categorized life events by activity (work, school, family), whether the event was socially desirable or undesirable, and whether the life change occasioned by the event represented an entrance or an exit from a person's social field.[36]

Better delineation of life events, with specific regard to the multiple variables that determine the response to an event, is critical in psychosocial research of stress. Dohrenwend et al have designed their research to delineate group variability within event categories.[37] The authors felt that any scale designed to understand the nature of stressful events must appreciate the variables influencing the respondent's reaction to the event. For example, when a person "stopped working," did they have anticipation of the event, was it desirable, and what was the sequence of prior events that led to that event?

It is abundantly clear from numerous investigations that the impact of life events is variable across cultural, educational, and socioeconomic groups.[38,39] Numerous factors may modify the impact of a particular life event. Clearly, a specific event must be appreciated in the context of a person's life. The face value of an event has little correlation to the degree of life change. For example, the birth of a child may be planned and anticipated or, conversely, unplanned and unwanted. Moreover, the expectation for child-rearing and the life change created by childbirth is variable across cultural, ethnic, and sociocultural groups. The most elusive aspect to assess may be the "desirability" of the event. Events that are perceived as undesirable or events over which an individual has little control may have disproportionate impact and create significant life change. The variability of response to a life event can best be assessed through careful history.

Moreover, a life change event is not the only source of environmentally-induced stressors. Investigators have examined the etiological role of many qualitative and quantitative aspects of living such as everyday problems,[40] the absence of uplifting events,[41] and the occurrence of hassles[41] as sources of stress. Burks identified everyday problems, defined as ongoing often chronic situations, which produced recurring unpleasantness and distress, and developed an inventory for assessment.[40] Everyday problems that include financial problems, poor health, or unsatisfactory living conditions are ubiquitous and can, like life change events, have an interactive effect on psychological symptoms. The Hassles Scale was designed to assess the impact of ongoing life situations from both a quantitative and qualitative perspective. It consists of 117 items that are commonly experienced in the course of life that cover a full range of work, family, social, and practical considerations such as time pressures, absence of opportunity, and losing things. The results are tabulated on the basis of frequency, intensity, and cumulative severity. Results from application of the Hassles Scale support the finding that variance in reported psychological symptoms can be accounted for by hassles considered independently of major life change events. Early work with the Hassles Scale suggested that the broadly-defined concept of life hassles may be more strongly associated with adaptational outcomes and presumably the development of illness than life events.

A final consideration in assessing the nexus between life events and life change is the independence of occurrence of events. Independence of events refers to a life event occurring independently of the predisposition of the individual. Events that occur as a function of a person's psychiatric illness or as a consequence of disordered personality functioning are dependent events. The degree of independence of an event may be difficult to determine. A thorough history is useful. For example, if a person has a history of impulsive, angry, or disruptive behavior, and then has a serious automobile accident because of driving irresponsibly at an excessive speed or in an intoxicated state, the accident event would be rated dependent, not independent, of the psychological state.

In summary, the assessment of recent life events as well as ongoing life hassles will provide important information about the contribution of stress to disability. In taking a history, it is important to elicit information regarding the degree to which an event is unexpected, negative, and outside the control of the individual; the extent to which the timing of events produces transient conditions of stimulus overload; whether the life event is uniquely problematic, by virtue of the existence of personal vulnerability, personality disorder, psychiatric illness, or the absence of social support to cushion the impact of the event; and the degree to which the persistence of the event exceeds the adaptive capacity of the individual and produces a state of chronic distress.

## STRESS AND THE DSM-IV

The stress concept has only recently been introduced into the psychiatric nomenclature. The current *Diagnostic and Statistical Manual of Mental Disorders (DSM-IV)* acknowledges the etiologic role of intense stress in the pathogenesis of PTSD (309.81) and now identifies a new entity on Axis I of Acute Stress Disorder (308.3). Both of these conditions are considered Anxiety Disorders. Adjustment Disorders, considered separately, are defined as excessive symptomatic reactions to identifiable psychosocial and environmental stressors. The multidimensional axis model allows for the inclusion under Axis IV for psychosocial and environmental factors that may contribute to the pathogenesis of conditions listed on Axis I and II.

The essential feature of PTSD is the development of the characteristic features following exposure to an extreme traumatic stressor. The criteria allow for the delayed onset of symptoms, noting that clinical symptoms may not appear for up to six months following exposure to the stressor. The definition of extreme stressor is quite broad and encompasses virtually all serious negative events. The characteristic symptoms include the reexperiencing of the event in any of four ways: intrusive distressing recollections, recurrent distressing dreams, acting or feeling as if the distressing event was recurring, and intense distress to internal or external cues. Other primary symptoms include persistent avoidance of the stimuli associated with the trauma, numbing of general responsiveness, and persistent symptoms of arousal. The syndrome is considered acute if the duration of the symptoms is less than three months, or chronic if the symptoms are still present more than six months after the trauma.

Acute Stress Disorder (ASD) is a new diagnosis in DSM-IV. The essential features of this disorder are the development of characteristic anxiety, dissociation, and other symptoms that occur within one month after exposure to an extreme traumatic stressor. The diagnosis requires the presence of at least three dissociative symptoms as well as reexperiencing of the trauma, marked avoidance of the stimuli that arouse recollections of the trauma, marked symptoms of anxiety, and increased arousal. The disturbance lasts for at least two days and does not persist beyond four weeks after the traumatic event.

These clinical stress syndromes are considered a neurobehavioral model of an excessive and protracted arousal state that is initiated by a profound stimulus to the central nervous system. The neurobehavioral model, which is believed to be the biological substrate of PTSD and ASD, strongly suggests that the initial cognitive, affective, and behavioral response following exposure to extreme environmental events or conditions is an instinctive protective mechanism. The excitation of neural protective mechanisms initiated by the sensory cortex produces a state of heightened arousal and alertness. By extension of this hypothesis derived from experimental animal models,[18] it is felt that the persistence of this acute state of activation, beyond the time frame of its protective function, may produce the syndrome of PTSD—a state of chronic, maladaptive arousal. The neurobehavioral hypotheses and the research designs linking animal models with the clinical syndromes of PTSD and ASD are intriguing but, as yet, still unproven. Far more human research is necessary to explain the psychopathology of the syndrome and delineate the pathogenesis of the human condition.

In the DSM-IV, Adjustment Disorder is considered as a separate Axis I disorder—a syndrome characterized by the development of clinically significant emotional or behavioral symptoms in response to an identifiable psychosocial stressor or stressors. The clinical significance of the reaction is indicated by the severity of the clinical response, which is greater than would be expected given the nature of the stressor.

Adjustment disorder is considered a distinct Axis I disorder (not a situational disturbance or transient psychological overreaction) that is manifest by a maladaptive reaction that occurs as a proximate response to the effect of either a single severe stressor or cumulative effect of numerous lesser stressors. The disorder is presumed to exist until the stressor is removed or, if the stressor persists, until the individual develops sufficient coping skills to adapt to its presence. A time limit of six months is placed on the duration of the Adjustment Disorder. The Adjustment Disorder has heuristic value suggesting a possible nexus between psychosocial stressors and transient psychological distress.

The severity of the functional impairment contributes to the diagnosis of Adjustment Disorder. To make a diagnosis, the maladaptive nature of the symptomatic and behavior response must be in excess of an expectable reaction to the stressor. Rating the severity of the stressor was assumed to have predictive validity to the Axis I disorder and led to the development of Axis IV.

Care must be applied in the diagnosis of the adjustment disorders. There may be considerable symptom overlap with other Axis I and II disorders. The presence of an identifiable psychosocial or environmental stressor does not, in and of itself, indicate that the stressor is the cause of the psychological condition. Reliance on the presence of psychosocial and environmental factors alone may divert attention from other factors that may produce psychological distress, including biological diatheses, preexistent psychiatric illnesses, and personality disorders. Further, the presumption of a unitary relationship between the presence of psychosocial stressors and the development of adjustment disorder is potentially reductionistic. A simple cause-effect relationship between identifiable psychosocial stressors and the manifestation of symptoms does not address the very nature of variability of response, personal vulnerability, and the all-important issue of personality dysfunction—all of which are powerful determinants of human adaptation.

Finally, the multiaxial dimension of the DSM IV allows Axis IV for reporting psychosocial and environmental problems that may affect the diagnosis, treatment, and prognosis of mental disorders. Axis IV allows for the listing of a broad range of problems that can be considered stressors including problems with the primary support group, problems related to the social environment, educational problems, occupational problems, housing problems, economic problems, problems with access to health care, problems related to interaction with the legal system, and any other psychosocial or environmental problems.

This simple listing of events represents a departure from the DSM III-R, where the clinician was asked to code the overall severity of a psychosocial stressor or multiple psychosocial stressors that occurred in the year preceding the evaluation and may have contributed to development of a new mental disorder, recurrence of a prior mental disorder, or exacerbation of an existing mental disorder.

Previously, the clinician was required to consider the effect of the psychosocial events based on the theoretical consideration of the "average person," and not on the reaction of a particular vulnerable person. The judgement involves consideration of the degree of change occasioned by the stressor, whether the change was desired, the number of stressors and the amount of control the individual had over the events. Questions about the validity of the "average person" perspective resulted in the current revision.

## STRESS AND IMPAIRMENT

The contribution of stress to medical impairment is best made when the conditions of stress are abundantly apparent and the timing and duration of those factors show clear and proximate relationship to the onset of symptoms and illness. The etiological significance and quantitative contribution of environmental factors is further validated by rapid clinical improvement when an individual is removed from the noxious agent.

In practice, the astute clinician usually appreciates the role of stress as a factor in the pathogenesis of illness, but may be minimally able to use medical standards to define or measure the stress contribution. Consequently, the clinical assessment of the stress contribution may be broadly defined and attributed to various general, nonspecific conditions or events in a person's life such as "job stress," "marital conflict," or "financial problems."

Commonly this subjective designation of stress lacks a medical standard and serves the clinical utility of pseudo-clarifying what may be an ill-defined, poorly understood clinical problem. Stress is held cul-

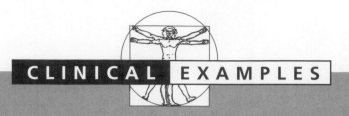
## STRESS

EDITOR'S NOTE—The severity of a stressor-generated impairment can best be assessed by evaluating changes in occupational, social, and interpersonal function. On clinical examination, the examiner may find evidence of attentional impairment such as increased distractibility, hypervigilance, and diminished span of attention. Associated cognitive changes include pseudo-rationality (idiosyncratic thinking), obsessional ruminations, preoccupation with the event, and diminished mental acuity. Anxiety is almost always present and accompanied by a persistent fear of recurrence, revivifications, and disturbed sleep. Finally, there are behavioral and adaptive alterations as evidenced by the individual's inability to resume and reinstitute usual activities such as work, social activities, and recreation. Determining the impact of these symptoms on social, occupational, and interpersonal function is critical in assessing the severity of a stressor-generated disability. Furthermore, assessing the resolution of functional impairments, which can be considered a measure of restored adaptation, is an indication that the stressor-generated condition is resolving.

### EXAMPLE
#### History

A 34-year-old married woman is referred for evaluation of a permanent psychiatric impairment with specific concern over the extent that sexual harassment and exposure to a hostile work environment may have contributed to her impairment. The woman married at age 15 and has three teenage children. She reports that the marriage has always been "badly troubled." Her husband is a construction worker with a history of recurrent alcohol abuse. When his drinking escalated, his "personality changed." On several occasions, he has been physically abusive. The woman's eldest son has been charged with several larcenous acts and faces incarceration. The woman reports that, "feeling stressed-out," she sought help from the county mental health agency. Family therapy was suggested but her husband refused to attend any sessions. He saw a counselor only briefly.

Over the past two years her husband has not worked because of a back injury, and financial pressures forced the woman to get a job. She dropped out of school in ninth grade and has acknowledged trouble with basic academic skills. Her previous work experience was at minimum wage doing food service and housekeeping. However, she found a job as a security officer doing security checks in an office building. The job required a 90-mile commute from her rural home, so she moved into her own apartment. She enjoyed the job because it "made me feel like I was worthwhile," and she enrolled in an evening program for remedial reading "so I could do my job better."

After six months on the job, she was handed a paper by a security supervisor who worked in another building in the same complex. On the paper was drawn a picture of large male genitalia and a note suggesting that the supervisor might be able to satisfy her more than her husband. "Disgusted," she reported the incident. She had no further contact with the supervisor until six months later when she was transferred to work directly under his supervision. He created a hostile work environment by making suggestive sexual comments almost daily. He commented on how well she "filled out her uniform," grunted when she bent over, and made disparaging remarks about her husband's inability to perform sexually. The woman became fearful of seeing the supervisor and requested a transfer because she "didn't want to work around him." The transfer was denied.

The woman suffered a depression and received both psychotherapy and antidepressive medication. After several months of treatment, her psychiatrist reported improvement, but her attendance at work and her ability to concentrate on assignments were poor. She was frequently absent, and when her allotted medical leave was exhausted, she was terminated. She has now sued her employer on the

*Continued.*

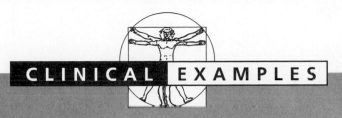
grounds that sexual harassment had created a permanent psychiatric impairment.

**Assessment Process**

The woman's depression was treated aggressively and resolved within four months, but it appears that a combination of stressors contributed to and possibly formed the proximate cause of the depression. Furthermore, there is the indication that occupational stressors contributed to the disability and may have occasioned her dismissal.

The woman also has long-standing marital and family problems, chronic stressors that caused considerable disruption in her lifestyle. However, in and of themselves, they have not compromised her ability to function at her job (have not caused an occupational disability). The impairment that led to occupational disability was precipitated by the hostile work environment and the reasonable expectation that she would be continually subjected to sexual harassing comments from the supervisor. This chronically stressful condition has resulted in the development of anticipatory anxiety. To avoid the stressor, she became less able to concentrate, developed affective lability, and behaved impulsively. This avoidance behavior also contributed to her excessive absenteeism. The resultant inability to perform her job, which had previously been a source of stability in her life, increased her anxiety and added to the severity of her impairment.

**Impairment**

Because she has no identifiable personality disorder and previously demonstrated reasonably sound adaptive mechanisms in her efforts to cope with her family and occupational problems, it is felt that the hostile work environment is a major contributor to the stressors predisposing her to the onset of depression and anxiety.

*Brian Schulman*

prit when other, more objective, medical findings are lacking.

The response to stressful conditions is modified by many factors. The assertion that life events play an unambiguous causal role in the development of personal stress has not been scientifically demonstrated in even the most extreme states. Personal variability is the rule, not the exception. Individual differences are determined by multiple factors including genetic, familial, cultural, ethnic, occupational, and social factors.

Every assessment of stress should focus on an individual's ability to manage difficult and challenging life conditions—a process involving coping skills. Mechanic[42] emphasizes three components at the individual level. A person must have the abilities and skills, the motivation to respond to demands, and, perhaps most significantly, the capability to maintain a state of psychological equilibrium to direct their energies to meeting external in contrast to internal needs.

The assessment of stress is a balanced exploration of stressful psychosocial conditions, as well as an examination of the person, that includes an identification of the change or changes that gave rise to stress. The assessment of stress should include the following items:

1. A thorough identification of the age, gender, marital and familial status, occupational status, and living condition.
2. A detailed response history to the recent stressful conditions, an accounting of the manifest life changes, and an assessment of the impact of those changes on the adaptive state.
3. A history of the recent medical and psychiatric treatment. The extent of treatment and response to treatment should include both objective evidence of efficacy and the individual's perception of benefit or harm. Treatment history should include a complete medication and prescription history including current drug usage.
4. A substance and ethanol history. The Michigan Alcohol Screening Test (MAST), or similar profile, is helpful.
5. An educational and occupational history that includes the history of all relevant training and acquired skills. Inquiry into the employment history, length of employment, reasons for changing employment, and assessment of occupational progression provides valuable information in response to external demand.
6. A relevant marital and familial history, including the occupational status, health, and quality of relationship. The history of social and community support systems is contributory.
7. A detailed analysis of the routine activities of daily living, including assessment of the circadian pattern, quality and duration of sleep, nutrition, avocation, recreation, social interaction, and ability to perform activities of daily living.
8. An assessment of the mental status that includes attention, span of attention, mental acuity, affective stability, mood, level of depression or depressive equivalents, and anxiety. The utilization of the mini-mental status examination, Hamilton Rating Scales for Depression and Anxiety, the Luria-Nebraska Brief Neuropsychological Screening, and the Beck Depression Inventory are useful adjunctive tools.
9. A clinical and, if possible, self-administered assessment of personality function. The clinical examination relies on elements of history, response to important historical figures, response to the examiner and examining situation, and a reliance on the criteria for personality disorder described in the DSM-III-R. The Minnesota Multiphasic Personality Inventory-II is, without dispute, the most widely-utilized and reliable instrument to augment the clinical examination. The Millon Multiaxial Clinical Inventory II provides psychologically explicit information in a narrative context that may, if not appropriately correlated with the clinical findings, overstate the influence and extent of personality function.
10. An assessment of occupational, phase of life, transcultural, and financial factors including the issues of gain and protracted effect of current and potential litigation.

## SUMMARY

Stress is a common complaint that brings patients to a physician. Stress is a subjective state of distress. The medical assessment lacks a clear, reliable, and valid methodology for assessing the contribution of stress to the development of symptoms and ultimately disability.

## References

1. Mason J: Historical view of the stress field: Part I, *J Human Stress* 1:6-12, 1975.
2. Haan N: *The assessment of coping, defense, and stress.* In Goldberger L, Breznitz S: *Handbook of stress: Theoretical and clinical aspects,* New York, 1993, Free Press.
3. Parkes CM, Benjamin B, Fitzgerald RG: Broken heart: a statistical study of increased mortality among widowers, *Br Med J* 1:740-743, 1969.
4. Cohen S, Tyrell DA, Smith AP: Psychological stress and susceptibility to the common cold, *New Engl J Med* 325:606-612, 1991.

5. Stone AA, Reed BR, Neale JM: Changes in daily event frequency precede episodes of physical symptoms, *J Human Stress* 2:70-75, 1987.

6. Cooper CL, Cheang A: Psychosocial factors in breast cancer, *Stress Medicine* 1:61-65, 1985.

7. Schulman B: Lingual techniques avoid confusion in office communication, *Occ Health and Safety*, vol 3, no 12, 1987.

8. Dubos R: *Man adapting*, New Haven, Conn, 1965, Yale University Press.

9. Menninger K: *The vital balance*, New York, 1963, Viking.

10. Engel G: *The need for a new medical model: a challenge for biomedicine*. In Caplan AL, Engelhardt HT, McCartney JJ: *Concepts of health and disease: Interdisciplinary perspectives*. Reading, Mass, 1981, Addison-Wesley.

11. Cassell E: *The nature of suffering*, New York, 1991, Oxford University Press.

12. Bernard C: *Introduction to the study of experimental medicine*. In Caplan AL, Engelhardt HT, McCartney JJ: *Concepts of health and disease: Interdisciplinary perspectives*. Reading, Mass, 1981, Addison-Wesley.

13. Cannon WB: *Relations of biological and social homeostasis*. In Caplan AL, Engelhardt HT, McCartney JJ: *Concepts of health and disease: Interdisciplinary perspectives*, Reading, Massachusetts, 1981, Addison-Wesley.

14. Selye H: *History and present status of the stress concept*. In Monat A, Lazarus RS: *Stress and coping, an anthology*, New York, 1985, Columbia University Press.

15. Axelrod J, Reisenet D: Stress hormones, their interaction and regulation, *Science* 224:452-59, 1984.

16. Mason J, Giller EL, Kosten TR: Elevated norepinephrine/cortisol ratio in PTSD, *J Ment Nerv Dis* 176:498-502, 1988.

17. Yehuda R, Giller EL, Southwick SM, Mason JW: Hypothalamic-pituitary-adrenal dysfunction in PTSD, *Biol Psychiatry* 30:1031-1048, 1991.

18. Charney DS, Deutch AY, Krystal JH, et al: Psychobiological mechanisms of posttraumatic stress disorder, *Arch Gen Psychiatry* 50:294-302, 1993.

19. Ranga Rama Krishnan, K: Pituitary and adrenal changes in depression, *Psych Ann* 23:671-675, 1993.

20. Stein M, Miller AH, Trestman RL: Depression, the immune system, and health and illness: findings in search of meaning, *Arch Gen Psychiatry* 48:11-119, 1991.

21. Craig JT, Brown GW: Goal frustrating aspects of life events stress in the etiology of GI disorders, *J Psychosom Research* 28:411-421, 1984.

22. Siegrist J, Dittman KA, Rittner K, et al: The social context of active distress in patients with early myocardial infarction, *Social Science and Med* 16:443-454, 1982.

23. Creed F: Stress and psychosomatic disorders. In Goldberger L, Breznitz S: *Handbook of stress: Theoretical and clinical aspects*, New York, 1993, Free Press.

24. National Heart, Lung, and Blood Institute: *Fifth report of the joint national committee on detection, evaluation, and treatment of high blood pressure*. NIH Publication No. 93-1088, 1993.

25. Mikhail A: *Stress: A psychophysiological conception*. In Monat A, Lazarus RS: *Stress and coping, an anthology*, New York, 1985, Columbia University Press.

26. Terr LC: Chowchilla revisited: the effects of psychic trauma four years after a school-bus kidnapping, *Am J Psychiatry*, 140:1543-1550, 1983.

27. Pitman RK, Or SP, Forgue DF, et al: Psychophysiological assessment of posttraumatic stress disorder imagery in Vietnam combat veterans, *Arch Gen Psychiatry* 44:970-975, 1987.

28. Pynoos RS, Frederick C, Nader K, et al: Life threat and posttraumatic stress disorder in school-age children, *Arch Gen Psychiatry* 44:1057-1063, 1987.

29. American Psychiatric Association: *Diagnostic and statistical manual of mental disorders IV*, Washington, D.C., 1994, American Psychiatric Association.

30. Hitchcock JM, Davis M: Efferent pathway of the amygdala involved in conditioned fear as measured with the fear-potentiated startle paradigm, *Behav Neuroscience* 105:826-842, 1991.

31. Davis M: Animal models of anxiety based upon classic conditioning, *Pharmacol Ther* 47:147-65, 1990.

32. Bantrop RW, Lazurus L, Luskhurst E, et al: Depressed lymphocyte function after bereavement, *Lancet* 1:834-836, 1977.

33. Holmes TH, Rahe RH: The Social Readjustment Rating Scale, *J Psychosom Res* 11:213-218, 1967.

34. Levine S: The influence of social factors in the response to stress, *J Psychother Psychsom* 60:33-38, 1993.

35. Dorhenwend BS, Krasnoff L, Dohrenwend BP: Exemplification of a method for scaling life events, the PERI life events scale, *J Health Soc Behavior* 19:205-229, 1978.

36. Paykel ES, Prusoff BA, Uhbenhuth EH: Scaling of life events, *Arch Gen Psych* 25:340-347, 1971.

37. Dohrenwend BP, Dohrenwend BS: Socioenvironmental factors, stress and psychopathology. Part I: Quasi-experimental evidence on social causation-social selection issue posed by class differences, *Amer J Com Psychology* 9:129-146, 1981.

38. Skodol AE, Dohrenwend BP, Link BG, et al: The nature of stress: problems of measurement. In Noshpitz JD, Coddington RD: *Stressors and the adjustment disorders,* New York, John Wiley & Sons.

39. Dohrenwend BS, Dohrenwend BP: Some issues on research on life stress events, *J Nerve Mental Dis* 153:207-234, 1978.

40. Burks N, Martin B: Everyday problems and life change events: ongoing versus acute sources of stress, *J Human Stress* 11:27-35, 1985.

41. Kanner AD, Coyne JC, Schaefer C, et al: Comparison of two modes of life stress measurement: daily hassles and uplifts versus major life events, *J Behav Med* 4:1-39, 1981.

42. Mechanic D: *Social structure and personal adaptation: some neglected dimensions.* In Coelho GV, Hamburg DA, Adams JE: *Coping and adaptation,* New York, 1974, Basic Books.

# CHAPTER 45

## PAIN

*Gerald M. Aronoff*

Chronic pain is a major public health problem that inflicts not only tremendous personal suffering but also economic loss to individuals and society. If the pain remains intractable, the health care professional and the patient become increasingly uncertain as to the appropriate course of treatment and both develop a sense of impotence and helplessness. As each becomes frustrated and disappointed in the other, their interaction becomes more strained and less direct.[1]

Pain is a complex personal, subjective, unpleasant experience involving sensations and perceptions that may or may not be related to physical injury, tissue damage, or nociception (the perception of pain based on organic pathology, transmitted from peripheral receptors to the central nervous system). Its expression may be influenced by psychosocial, ethnocultural, genetic, biochemical, religious, and other factors.[2] Some people will actually take the definition further and say chronic pain per se is what an individual says it is.[3] It is a subjective experience that cannot adequately be measured. However, studies have found that there is no direct relationship between tissue damage and the severity of pain.[4]

Loeser's paradigm[5] in conceptualizing chronic pain syndromes is useful. He suggests that the initial noxious stimulus leading to nociception seems to be less important in the management of chronic pain syndromes than the suffering, which is an emotional experience, and the pain behaviors that the patient exhibits. This is not meant to discount that nociception may have initiated the pain process. It does, however, suggest that in chronic pain syndromes, central more than peripheral factors may be prolonging the suffering and disability. Nociception, if still present, may not be directly treatable by conventional techniques (such as peripherally acting analgesics, nerve blocks, or surgery).

Clinically, physicians cannot prove or disprove the existence of pain in a given individual. A person complaining of pain may or may not have nociception, suffering, pain behavior, impairment, or disability. Pain behaviors are any and all actions that communicate to an observer that an individual is in pain. Examples include grimacing, groaning, limping, using visible pain relieving or support devices, and requesting pain medications, among others. Pain behaviors are often conditioned, learned, and goal directed. As such they are amenable to behavioral interventions and psychotherapies and can be modified or replaced by wellness behaviors that are more adaptive.

## CHRONIC PAIN AND PSYCHIATRIC ILLNESS

Pain is an extremely common complaint in patients with known emotional disorders and may be an associated symptom in virtually any psychiatric illness. There has been extensive clinical research indicating the tendency for affective and personality disorders to occur with intractable chronic pain.[6-10] DSM III listed the term Psychogenic Pain Syndrome.[11] The revision, DSM III-R, deleted the preceding term and substituted Somatoform Pain Disorder.[12] The latest revision, DSM IV, uses the term Pain Disorder.[13] These terms apply to only a relatively small percentage of the chronic pain population. Many of the remainder have underlying organic pathophysiology as well as an emotional disorder.

The box on page 530 lists emotional disorders associated with chronic pain syndromes.

### Somatoform Disorders

Somatoform Disorders are those in which physical symptoms suggest a physical disorder for which there is evidence of underlying psychopathology but not demonstrable organic findings or known physiologic mechanisms. It should be emphasized that the creation of the physical symptom in a Somatoform Disorder is not intentional.

## EMOTIONAL DISORDERS ASSOCIATED WITH CHRONIC PAIN SYNDROME[1a]

A) Somatoform Disorders
   1. Somatization Disorder
   2. Conversion Disorder
   3. Pain Disorder
   4. Hypochondriasis
   5. Undifferentiated Somatoform Disorder
B) Affective Disorders
C) Personality Disorders
D) Psychological Factors Affecting Medical or "Organic" Conditions
E) Malingering
F) Schizophrenia
G) Substance Use Disorders

### Somatization Disorder

Somatization Disorder, formerly known as Briquet's Syndrome and often referred to as hysteria, is a chronic, polysymptomatic disorder generally with onset early in life before age 30 years. Chiefly affecting women, the condition's main feature is a repetitive or chronic concern with physical symptoms without objective findings to substantiate the subjective complaints. These individuals tend to consult many physicians in an attempt to validate their symptoms and frequently have surgical procedures with minimal pathologic findings. They often have prolonged phases of incapacity, are at high risk for iatrogenic complications, and should be managed conservatively unless there are clear signs of objective pathology warranting more aggressive treatment.

### Conversion Disorder

Individuals said to have underlying hysterical personality patterns are prone either to exaggerate the magnitude of their complaints or to present these complaints in a melodramatic fashion. It should be emphasized, however, that in no way do these statements imply the patient's pain is not real or that it is not organically based. Working with these patients, one learns that their choice of words as descriptors for their pain usually involves emotionally laden and flamboyant language that often prejudices the clinician. Therefore, it should be emphasized that some symptoms initially felt to represent conversion may later be found to have a neurologic basis. The diagnosis requires an astute diagnostician. Conversion symptoms are those that result from an emotional conflict, are not related to bodily disease directly, and

are ultimately in accordance with the patient's concept of functional loss of a part rather than actual anatomy or physiology. If the symptoms affect the body, they are called conversion symptoms. Comparable symptoms not affecting the body, such as hysterical loss of memory, are known as dissociative symptoms. When pain is the only conversion symptom, the term Somatoform Pain Disorder should be used. Several factors are noteworthy. Patients with Conversion Disorder truly believe that they have the deficits they claim. Their inability to move or appropriately use body parts often leads to secondary impairments through, for example, disuse atrophy or joint contractures. An ominous combination is that of individuals with Conversion Disorders and dependent personality traits (or Dependent Personality Disorder) because they are at increased risk to develop a chronic sick role or chronic disability syndrome.

### Pain Disorder

Pain Disorders are not infrequent occurrences among patients going to pain centers. Clinically, the primary feature is the complaint of pain without adequate physical findings but associated with evidence of the etiologic role of psychological factors. It is not, however, a diagnosis of exclusion. Patients with nondiagnosed chronic pain or chronic pain of uncertain etiology should not be presumed to have psychogenic pain. To do so is incorrect and does the individual with pain a disservice. It should be established that no other mental disorder is contributing to the disturbance. It has been the author's impression that the premorbid personalities of these individuals commonly reveal evidence of neurotic functioning and, less often, borderline personality organization preceding the trauma of an injury or painful medical illness. These patients often become quite incapacitated and are at risk to become invalids unnecessarily.

Pain itself may become the focal aspect within a neurotic conflict. It is then called a Pain Neurosis and it may be linked with the possibility of financial compensation as with a Compensation Neurosis. Sometimes a core issue involves unmet dependency needs and both primary and secondary gain. The diagnosis of Somatoform Pain Disorder must be made cautiously and periodically reexamined to rule out the possibility that the pain may be explained on an organic basis.

If a specific treatment for a pain disorder is available and if the potential benefits to the patient outweigh the risks, that treatment should be suggested. If, however, invasive treatment offers no distinct advantage over conservative treatment, and carries an increased risk, conservative treatment should be suggested.

### Hypochondriasis

Hypochondriasis implies a fascinated absorption and preoccupation with physical symptoms. It is quite common among pain patients. That is not to say that these individuals may not have underlying organic pathology and mechanical causes of pain, but rather that their degree of somatic preoccupation becomes an obsession. They fail to be reassured by clinical or laboratory evaluations and remain fixated in their belief that they need more diagnostic tests and evaluations. Arguing with these individuals and trying to dissuade them from their convictions is generally futile. The degree of their concern often causes significant psychosocial dysfunction and may impair occupational functioning, depending upon the extent of psychopathology and the extent to which their lives revolve around the sick role. One must, of course, exclude true organic disease. However, it should be emphasized that the presence of true organic disease does not rule out the possibility of coexisting hypochondriasis. These patients are at increased risk for iatrogenic complications because of the excessive diagnostic procedures they undergo, as well as the multiple medication trials they attempt.

### Undifferentiated Somatoform Disorder

Undifferentiated or Atypical Somatoform Disorder is a category used to describe physical symptoms or complaints not explained by demonstrable organic findings or a known pathophysiologic mechanism and apparently linked to psychologic factors but without adequate symptoms to make a diagnosis of Somatoform Disorder.

### Psychologic Factors Affecting Medical Conditions

According to DSM IV the category Psychologic Factors Affecting Medical Condition can be used to describe disorders that in the past have been referred to as either psychosomatic or psychophysiologic. The author's experience indicates that a very common problem with pain patients is a tendency to suppress emotional expression and internalize feelings. The physiologic expression of these tendencies is manifested in autonomic hyperactivity and muscle tension, both of which directly contribute to the pain. Included in this category are tension and migraine headaches, angina pectoris, painful menstruation, sacroiliac pain, neurodermatitis, arthritis, peptic ulcers, and other conditions.

### Malingering

Malingering implies a conscious and voluntary fabrication of a physical or psychological symptom for personal gain. This may involve financial compensation, drug seeking, personal manipulation, vocational disability, or other attempts to manipulate the individual's environment through the use of pain. To be classified as a malingerer, the person must be consciously feigning illness. These individuals are often difficult to treat because the obvious gain is so overwhelming. Frequently they perceive themselves as having more to gain by retaining the symptom than by relinquishing it. There is commonly a great deal of underlying psychopathology, and the primary treatment of malingering, if amenable to treatment at all, must be psychiatric. It is the author's belief that whereas malingering in the general medical population involves relatively few patients, it is a significantly greater issue among workers' compensation or personal injury pain patient population, both of which may involve active litigation. That is not to imply that all or even most of these patients are malingerers. Experienced pain clinicians can generally distinguish the patient's underlying motivation.

### Schizophrenia

Patients with schizophrenia attending a pain center with primary pain complaints are uncommon, but this can occur. Symptoms are often discussed as part of a bizarre somatic delusion. A British study[14] of 78 hospitalized schizophrenic patients found 29 to have pain complaints. Of these, 13 had an appropriate physical cause. The remainder were felt to have somatoform pain. The head, leg, and back were the most common sites of pain. Complaints were most often described in sensory terms. The report summary indicated that patients with schizophrenia may have less pain than those with anxiety or depression but may experience pain from physical and psychological causes.

### Substance Use Disorders

Patients with chronic pain are often very experienced in the use of medication. When evaluating psychoactive substance use disorders one needs to recognize that for some the pattern is sporadic and intermittent with medication taken only by prescription from one primary physician. For others there are many physicians writing many prescriptions, each unaware of the actions of the others. Some patients receive medication from illicit sources outside the medical system. These are individuals whose illicit use of medications may have preceded the onset of their pain and who now hope to have this use legitimized by physicians. Other persons who never would have considered illicit drugs are now faced with chronic pain and are unable to obtain what they feel is adequate medication. The problem is complex and the physician is often in a compromised position in the midst of ethical dilemmas. The author has suggested guidelines for maintenance opioid use in chronic pain.[15]

## CHARACTERISTICS OF CHRONIC PAIN SYNDROME PATIENTS

With chronic pain syndromes there are often complex interactions between physical and psychological factors. These patients share many of the characteristics listed below.

- Preoccupation with pain
- Strong and ambivalent dependency needs
- Feelings of isolation and loneliness
- Characterological masochism (meeting others' needs at their own expense)
- Inability to take care of self needs
- Passivity
- Lack of insight into patterns of self-defeating behavior
- Inability to deal appropriately with anger and hostility
- Use of pain as a symbolic means of communication

The pain-prone individual, initially described by Engel,[16,17] and later by Blumer and Heilbronn,[18,19] has a significant developmental history notable for unhappiness and trauma during childhood, often involving physical and sexual abuse, emotional neglect, high incidence of alcoholism in the family, and a personal and family history of illness, disability, and chronic pain. These individuals often had to assume early adult responsibilities and are described as having been hyperresponsible children. They may have had many early unmet dependency needs. Later in life following an injury or illness, pain may be their way of saying "I would like someone to take care of me now."

There is growing evidence that depression lowers pain tolerance, increases analgesic requirements, and adds to the debilitating effects of pain.[20] Studies of the relationship between chronic pain and depression in hospital patients in whom there was no organic lesion[21] found consistently that a greater percentage of patients seen in hospital or pain clinic consultation with what was called chronic indeterminate pain have clinical depression, than in a comparative population who had chronic pain explained by underlying pathophysiology. A high percentage of subjects with chronic indeterminate pain were found

to have a family history of depression and depressive spectrum disease.

Currently, tricyclics are the most common nonanalgesic medications used in the management of chronic pain syndromes. Their usage for the treatment of chronic pain has been summarized by Aronoff and Evans,[22] Oxman and Denson,[23] Atkinson,[24] and Monks.[25] The newer class of serotonin reuptake inhibitors including fluoxetine, sertraline, and paroxetine are less-well studied with the chronic pain population but should also be considered as they have been found to be useful in the management of depression and appear to have a favorable side effect profile. The author has found that in patients with chronic pain, depression, and insomnia the use of sertraline in the morning combined with a sedating tricyclic in the evening often achieves excellent efficacy with a lower incidence of side effects than a higher dose of the sedating tricyclic alone.

Are there distinguishing personality characteristics in individuals prone to develop chronic pain syndrome or become disabled by pain? Although studies suggest that there may be, there are no clear findings indicating to what extent well-defined personality traits are associated with the development of a chronic pain syndrome as opposed to having the pain amplify traits that are then maintained by operant mechanisms. In addition to pain-prone personality characteristics, other common personality characteristics include being antisocial, passive-dependent, histrionic, and masochistic self-neglectful.[26] The latter refers to individuals who meet others' needs at their own expense and whose behaviors, therefore, can be considered self-defeating.

## DISABILITY INTERVENTION

There is no linear relationship between the degree of medical or psychiatric impairment and the resulting disability rating. The findings of a multidisciplinary medical panel from the Boston University Medical Center emphasize this.[27] In this study, 111 consecutive chronic low-back pain patients referred by the Office of Workers Compensation Programs (OWCP) were assessed. The mean age of the cohort was 49.4 years of age with an average length of predetermined disability of 4.92 years. Of these, only 13 (11.7%) were found to have evidence of significant objective impairment that, by itself, warranted total disability. Of the 13, roughly half were physically impaired and half were psychiatrically impaired. One finding was that in none of the six patients granted psychiatric disability was the psychiatric impairment found to be work-related. In other words, in each of these cases (100%), the insurance carrier for the employer was paying for a claim that was not their responsibility. Among those found not to be totally disabled, only 5 of the 98 patients (5.1% or 4.5% of the total sample) had returned to work at least part-time by the time of their evaluation. It was noted that of the 98 patients with a partial or full work capacity, 93 patients (94.9% or 83.8% of the total sample) had incorrectly overestimated their own impairments from a narrow and strict medical perspective and had not returned to work.

Strang discusses the "chronic disability syndrome" in which individuals who are capable of working choose to remain disabled.[27] They lack motivation to recover and return to productivity. The disability is often the result of a fairly minor injury but actually represents an inability to cope with other life problems.

Brena and Chapman[28] describe the "5 D's," a cluster of symptoms often seen in chronic pain patients: *d*ramatization (of vague, diffuse, nonanatomic pain complaints); *d*rug abuse (misuse of habit-forming pain medications); *d*ysfunction (bodily impairments related to various physical and emotional factors); *d*ependency (passivity, depression, and helplessness); and *d*isability (pain contingent on financial compensation and pending litigation claims). The latest AMA *Guides* add other "D's" including *d*uration (longer than is considered normal for a given process); *d*iagnostic dilemma (clinical impression are often inconsistent, inaccurate, and vague despite extensive evaluations); and *d*isuse (from prolonged inactivity). The AMA *Guides* suggest the need for at least four of these eight characteristics to establish a presumptive diagnosis of chronic pain syndrome.[68]

Several authors have contributed to an understanding of why pain-related disability and litigation are such major problems. Brena and Chapman[29] reviewed several studies of the disability process, indicating that certain patient characteristics made them prone to be involved in a disabling injury. In one study, Weinstein[30] noted these factors: 1) low self esteem in a dependent person, 2) inability to deal competently with stress, 3) demanding job, and 4) tension at home. The injury was viewed as a socially acceptable way out of a stressful situation.

Ellard[31] enumerates some significant characteristics of patients who have psychological reactions to injury. 1) They lack the usual objective signs of suffering (a disparity between verbal pain complaints and untroubled manner). 2) Objective clinical findings do not correlate with the complaint (for exam-

ple, no atrophy of the paralyzed limb). 3) Poor motivation is exhibited (the patient remains a passive sufferer, vehemently asserting a problem and a desire to get well, yet failing to effectively participate in the treatment). 4) The patient exhibits unusual treatment responses. Initially, these patients may not actively seek treatment; once treated, they fail to benefit from it, although they continue to pursue it. Ellard notes that, in many of these patients, there is no evidence of a stated psychopathological condition preceding the injury episode. He summarizes the diagnostic and treatment dilemma these patients create, stating that the symptoms may represent a conscious or unconscious desire for the person to establish that he or she is sick, "not so much because of his personal pathological condition, but because of the social consequences of the sick role." He notes that, when financial gain is involved, the complaints are more often remedied by legal rather than medical processes. Brena and Chapman[29] noted the demoralized behavior of many patients in chronic pain management programs when consistently confronted with situations in which they could not control the outcome. They demonstrated elements of depression, passivity, and lack of initiative in attempting to affect situation outcomes. They point to the common features between these behaviors and those previously noted in workers prone to chronic disability following a work-related injury.

Disability is more difficult to treat once it has continued for six months or longer. Thus, early recognition of features predicting poor prognosis and prompt intervention are important. Seres and Newman[32] note that 80% to 90% of workers with back injuries return to work within days or weeks of the injury. Of the remaining injured, 5% to 15% have prolonged or permanent disability. This author has found that the latter group do not necessarily have more significant impairment than the former group that returned to work earlier.

McGill[33] noted in his study of industrial back problems that a lengthy period of disability predicted a low likelihood of ever returning to work. Those out of work longer than six months had a 50% probability of return, those out of work for over one year had a 25% chance of return, and those out of work longer than two years were extremely unlikely to return.

The author has written on the "disability epidemic"[1,34] that is most prominent in the United States and other countries where entitlement programs are viewed as appealing alternatives to gainful employment. If this epidemic is to be reversed, the compensation and disability systems must be changed so that they encourage early intervention, prevention of chronicity with incentives toward rehabilitation, and early return to work.

Often the patient's attitude and motivation, coupled with the support system, are likely to determine whether the patient allows pain to be totally disabling. It is especially a reflection of the patient's underlying personality style and life goals. Physicians at the Boston Pain Center have found these to be far better predictors for a successful outcome than the medical diagnosis.

Chronic pain research indicates that decreased function depends not only on pathophysiology but also on "illness behaviors" or "pain behaviors" (such as inactivity, drug misuse, and learned helplessness).[35] Patients with lengthy disabilities are special in several respects. Snook[36] found that patients receiving workers' compensation for back injuries were less likely to have objective findings or definitive diagnosis than those with back injuries who were not receiving compensation.

In discussing patients with chronic low-back claims, Carron[37] indicated the three most striking factors were 1) 78.7% of the subjective complaints were not supported by objective findings; 2) 60% were taking dependency-inducing drugs; and 3) 49.3% had a previous back injury. In those injuries (occult) that were neither witnessed nor reliably documented and with pain as the major manifestation of injury, he noted a high incidence of previously compensable injury, drug dependency, obesity, low income, and nonsupervisory work. In one study by Leavitt et al,[38] 70% of workers receiving compensation for back injuries reported that a specific work activity or event triggered the pain or injury, but only 35% of workers not receiving compensation for low-back pain reported a clear-cut work-related event.

Catchlove and Cohen's[39] retrospective review of two groups of chronic pain patients receiving workers' compensation emphasizes the importance of return to work as a goal of pain management programs. When a directive return-to-work approach was incorporated into their treatment, 60% of patients returned to work, and 90% of them continued to work an average of 9.6 months later. They were also receiving fewer compensation benefits and less additional pain treatment than a group of patients similarly treated, but for whom a return-to-work directive was not included. Although the improvements may have been related both to selection factors (a treatment contract that patients had to affirm) and to treatment efficacy, the results were significant.

The author strongly believes that one should not underestimate the importance of physicians' authoritarian guidance, which can be offered as supportive paternalism. Patients will either live up to medical expectations that they need not be disabled or, conversely, become invalids unnecessarily through learned helplessness. Their physical, emotional, social, and spiritual well-being is more likely to be realized with the self-esteem that results from feeling useful because of gainful employment than with a disability award.

Of back-pain patients treated at pain programs, many have undergone multiple pain-related surgeries. In Waddell's[40] study of failed lumbar disc surgery in workers' compensation patients following industrial injuries, 97% had some persistent pain complaints, 77% continued with impaired functioning, and of those who had third or fourth operations, outcomes were progressively worse, with increased psychological dysfunction.

The author has evaluated several thousand patients who would meet criteria for post-surgical failed-back syndromes. These are patients who claim to be no better following one or more surgical procedures, have limitations in functional activities of daily living, have behavioral sequelae consistent with the term chronic pain syndrome, and often have significant associated depression. Common denominators for many of these problems include a well-intentioned but perhaps overzealous surgeon who may feel guilty or responsible for the patient's persistent pain and suffering, a demanding and persistent patient who insists on being fixed or cured, a health care system that is procedure-driven, and the enormous inefficiency of a disability system that often reinforces disability rather than rehabilitation. Based on chart reviews spanning more than 15 years, the author has recommended the following criteria for patients who should have a second opinion prior to elective surgery:

- Two or more pain-related surgeries without beneficial results.
- One or more pain-related surgeries with negative findings.
- Attorney-referred patients involved in pain-related litigation.
- Known or highly-suspected major psychopathology.
- History of unjustified overuse of health care system.

Seres and Newman[32] indicate that low-back injuries are the most frequently litigated claims and represent the most common type of "cumulative trauma" injury. Many studies[33,36,41] indicate that pain treatment is less successful for those receiving workers' compensation or with pending litigation than for those not receiving it. However, other studies have reported contradictory results.

Dworkin et al.[42] found that in 454 chronic pain patients, only the employment status at initial evaluation predicted treatment response (employed patients had better outcomes than those not employed). Neither litigation nor compensation was a significant predictor of treatment outcome. Similarly, Peck, Fordyce, and Black[43] found no significant effects of either litigation or representation by attorney on the pain behavior of patients with pending workers' compensation claims.

In evaluating workers' compensation or personal injury-related pain patients, the screening process is extremely important, especially when the issue of disability compensation is involved. If, on the basis of the initial evaluation, it is thought that the patients' motivation toward behavioral change is marginal or that they are content to collect compensation and to have others in attending roles, thus assuming a passive-dependent attitude, treatment at a pain program should generally be deferred. This must be clearly expressed to the patients in a nonjudgmental way. It should be the patients' right to continue with the pain and suffering if they so choose. An interpretation and clarification should address the issues very candidly. The primary concerns should not be with the patients' reaction, but rather assisting the patients to recognize motivational and attitudinal deficits, psychological factors complicating the disability, and issues of primary, secondary, and tertiary gain.

One should attempt to clarify life stressors, traumatic life events, past patterns of disability in the patient or other family member, repetitive patterns of self-defeating behaviors, a family history of chronic pain, illness, or disability, unmet dependency needs, childhood deprivations, and substance abuse. Having information about all of these is important in understanding how the patient became the person who is now seeking treatment. This information is essential in formulating a treatment plan and understanding prognosis, as well as in making statements about vocational matters and disability.[44]

## IMPAIRMENT AND DISABILITY ASSESSMENT

In performing an impairment evaluation, it is essential to take a detailed medical, developmental, behavioral, and psychosocial history to assess an individual's current and premorbid level of functioning. Only then can one try to understand the impact of an injury or illness with subsequent pain. It is not enough to see an individual who is suffering and demonstrating pain behaviors. In attempting to address issues of causality or to apportion all or a part of an impairment to a specific incident or injury, one must know how the individual was functioning prior to the incident in question. Turk and colleagues have suggested three essential questions useful in assessing chronic pain.[45,46]

1. What is the extent of the patient's disease or injury?
2. What is the magnitude of the illness? That is, to what extent is the patient suffering, disabled, and unable to enjoy usual activities?
3. Is the illness behavior appropriate to the disease or injury, or is there evidence of amplification of symptoms for psychological or social reasons?

In addition to the above questions, the author has found the following questions useful in performing evaluations related to chronic pain and psychiatric illness:

1. Was your childhood happy, difficult, stressful, or traumatic? (Unless it was happy, get details. Specifically, look for dysfunctional family issues, physical or sexual abuse, emotional neglect, and unmet needs.)
2. Were there any traumas during childhood, adolescence, or later in adulthood? (This can often add clarification to an understanding of post traumatic stress disorders, phobias, and other psychopathology.)
3. How did you do in school? Were there specific problems? (If an individual dropped out of school at an early age or repeated grades, get details. If you get a sense that the individual was driven to excel to the point of its becoming pathological, get details.)
4. Is there any prior history of emotional problems or past treatment? (If so, get details including use of medications, duration of drug trials, and dosages.) Did treatment help? What precipitated prior problems? Specifically, attempt to evaluate the developmental, psychosocial, and family histories for pain-prone characteristics.
5. Have you been able to make friends easily in the past? Do you have close friends now? (Other than the nuclear family, what type of support system has there been? Is there evidence of inadequacies in personality development?)
6. If there were abnormalities in usual developmental transitions, inquire. For example, what led to your leaving home at 16? To never leaving home by 50? To your 5 divorces?
7. Do any family members have emotional problems now or have they had these in the past? (Other than the details, obtain an understanding

of the impact on the person you are evaluating. Does the patient believe they are just like that relative and will develop the same problems? What was it like growing up in the home with the ill relative? Who did the caretaking?)

8. Is there a personal or family history of substance dependence or abuse? (Medical illness or chronic pain can occasionally be used for secondary gain to perpetuate a preexisting substance use problem. Also evaluate the possibility that substances may be diverted to other family members.)

9. Is there a history of prior psychosomatic illness or unexplained physical symptoms? Evaluate the role of stressors. Is there any insight by the individual?

10. Have there been prior medical problems or injuries similar to the current ones? Specifically, get details regarding a prior history of similar complaints of pain. What was the location of symptoms? types of treatment? duration of treatment? severity? response to treatment? Was there any pain prior to the present illness? Were you in treatment? With whom? When did you last see this individual prior to the present illness? Were you taking any medication for pain prior to the present illness? If you had pain prior to the present illness, were there any limitations of restrictions? Did the pain interfere with normal activities of daily living?

    Be able to comment with a reasonable degree of medical certainty whether the current injury or illness has exacerbated or aggravated a preexisting condition. Aggravation indicates a permanent worsening of a preexisting condition. Exacerbation indicates a temporary recurrence of the prior symptoms that can be expected to subside with the individual's returning to baseline premorbid functioning.

11. Has disability been an issue in the past? (Has the person either been disabled or applied for disability? Have a good understanding of the many issues that may have precipitated the request for disability status.)

12. Is litigation pending related to the present illness or injury? Has there been prior litigation related to other health issues or injuries? (The extent to which litigation can prolong physical and emotional symptoms and complicate disability is discussed in detail in other works.[1,38,45-50])

The above list is not all-inclusive but rather is meant to give the reader guidelines for some of the subjects that should be explored. In evaluating the responses to the above questions it is the author's experience that the likelihood of psychosocial issues influencing disability is as follows:

0-2 positive responses: not suggestive
3-5 positive responses: suggestive
6+ positive responses: highly suggestive/probable

Occasionally the author has encountered resistance from the individual being evaluated who cannot or will not appreciate the relevance of the questions to the current evaluation. The author clarifies the importance of understanding past events and behaviors to assess accurately current as well as future functioning.

## MEASURING AND RATING PAIN

One of the more difficult questions asked of the evaluating physician will relate to the measurement or rating of pain. Since clinical pain is a subjective process there are no purely objective physiological measures currently available to measure pain and the best methods use subjective reports by the individual with pain. Although there are inherent limitations in relying on self-report measures, these ratings are felt to be the most reliable tool available.[51] However, it must be recognized that some individuals may bias their reporting for personal gain.

One of the simplest, single dimension measures of pain intensity is the verbal scale in which an individual is asked to estimate pain on a continuum from no pain, mild, moderate, severe, to horrible or excruciating.

Perhaps the most commonly-used pain rating scale is the linear visual analog scale (VAS) shown below. The individual places a mark on the line indicating the pain estimate between no pain to the worst imaginable pain. The rater can measure the distance from 0-10 and form a quantified measure. The advantage of the VAS is its simplicity, the disadvantage is its oversimplicity, treating pain as if it were unidimensional. Revill et al[52] found that patients produce estimates on the VAS that are reliable over time. It has also been shown that the scale can predict outcome six months later,[53] while others have found that the VAS only reflects a single point in time.

NO PAIN ⟵⟶ WORST PAIN IMAGINABLE

A similar method is used in the AMA *Guides* relating pain intensity with pain frequency (Fig. 45-1).[68] Since pain is known to be multidimensional in nature, other self-report tools commonly used in pain management programs include pain drawings and pain diaries. Pain drawings are assessed in terms of being appropriate (corresponding to the pathophysiological process), inappropriate (not corresponding to the pathophysiological process), or, depending upon how bizarre the drawing, suggestive of various types

| | | Frequency | | | |
|---|---|---|---|---|---|
| | | Intermittent | Occasional | Frequent | Constant |
| Intensity | Minimal | | | | |
| | Slight | | | | |
| | Moderate | | | | |
| | Marked | | | | |

**FIGURE 45-1**    Pain intensity-frequency grid.[68]

of psychopathology (see Fig. 25-1, page 278). Pain diaries, which monitor pain intensity as well as daily activities, medication usage, sleep patterns, and pain behaviors, are helpful in assessing the frequency, intensity, and duration of pain and how it affects activities of daily life.

The McGill Pain Questionnaire (MPQ)[54] was developed to measure clinical pain as a multidimensional experience. Specifically looking at sensory and affective components, intensity, as well as miscellaneous dimensions of the pain experience, the MPQ also includes a pain drawing. A review by Hinnant[55] indicates that although the MPQ shows reliability and validity, there is significant disagreement over the accuracy of the test and its ability to discriminate diagnostic groups of patients.

The Dartmouth Pain Questionnaire (DPQ)[56] is used as an adjunct to the MPQ because its authors believe that the MPQ neglects measurements of somatic interventions, impaired function, remaining positive aspects of function, and changes in self-esteem since the onset of pain. Cronbach[57] notes that the DPQ can be used to differentiate between patients who have and have not benefited from pain treatment.

The Pain Disability Index (PDI)[58] is a self-reporting inventory that is useful in assessing the degree to which chronic pain interferes with daily activities. According to Tait et al. high scores on the PDI relate to "time spent in bed, psychosomatic symptoms, stopping activities because of pain, work status, pain duration, usual pain intensity, quality of life, pain extent, and education." Hebben[51] notes that the measure appears to possess both test-retest reliability and validity with regard to pain-based disability.

The Vanderbilt Pain Management Inventory (VPMI)[59] evaluates patients' response to pain in terms of their use of active versus passive coping styles, noting that the more active copers had less pain, depression, helplessness, and impairment.

The West Haven-Yale Multidimensional Pain Inventory (WHYMPI)[60] focuses on the "impact of pain on the patient's life, the responses of others to the patient's communication of pain, and the extent to which patients participate in common daily activities."

Several psychological tests that are not specific to either pain or disability evaluation and have achieved popularity in clinical evaluation of both include the Minnesota Multiphasic Personality Inventory (MMPI)[61] and the updated revision the MMPI-2,[62] the Symptom Checklist 90-revised (SCL-90R),[63] and the Millon Behavioral Health Inventory (MBHI).[64] These are used to measure psychopathology in medical and psychiatric populations with attention to various personality characteristics that may influence treatment outcome and prognosis. None of these should be used as definitive tests of psychogenicity or organicity of a specific pain problem. In the well-known and often quoted Boeing study, Bigos et al[65] found the MMPI useful in predicting subjects most likely to report back injuries at work. For a detailed discussion of clinical pain measurement the reader is referred to chapters by Hebben,[51] White,[66] and Hinnant.[67]

## SOCIAL ISSUES

It can be anticipated that issues such as unemployment during an economic recession, job dissatisfaction, and financial or job insecurity may influence the patient's demands on the treating physician to recommend temporary or permanent disability as a way of coping with economic stressors. As difficult as it may be, physicians must, with understanding and compassion, objectively assess impairment, not confuse their role as the patient's advocate with their responsibility for objectivity. Perhaps it is an independent physician rather than the treating physician who can most objectively, accurately, and unemotionally rate impairment, thus maintaining the uniqueness of the treating physician's relationship with their patient.

Physicians must realize that rehabilitation is preferable to disability, and that there is a need to improve the ability to reinstate people with pain so that they remain functional and productive. Invalidism is a process that can and must be addressed by the health care system. It remains the author's conviction that the individuals who must endure chronic pain suffer less when their lives have purpose and meaning. Gainful employment frequently can serve as a distraction from pain. Rehabilitation and occupational health personnel can help facilitate the process of returning the injured worker to employment by creatively devising employment opportunities geared toward the limitations of the patient.

## IMPAIRMENT FROM CHRONIC PAIN

The most recent edition of the AMA *Guides*[68] recognizes that chronic pain involves altered perceptions and maladaptive behaviors; that pain per se cannot be validated objectively or quantitated; that the subjective complaints may be disproportionate to objective findings, which may be lacking; that "chronic pain is a self-sustaining, self-reinforcing, and self-regenerating process;" and that there may be no ongoing nociception. The AMA *Guides* note, however, that chronic pain is a medical and not a psychiatric disorder.

On the issue of impairments, the AMA *Guides* take the position that "chronic pain and pain-related behaviors are not, per se, impairments, but they should trigger assessments with regard to ability to function and carry out daily activities. The *Guides* also state that other rating systems (Social Security, private insurance companies, Veterans Administration) take similar positions that pain, per se, is not a cause of impairment but that the underlying medical (both organic and psychiatric) conditions are.

The critical issues for there to be impairment are that the pain or pain-related condition has become stabilized and is unlikely to change substantially within the next year with or without medical treatment (defines Maximum Medical Improvement); and there is significant diminished capacity to carry out activities of daily living (not merely that the daily activity is painful). Both of these issues appear to be problematic for physicians not accustomed to treating chronic pain patients, and there can be an overestimation of its contribution to impairment. As noted earlier in this chapter, pain behavior is learned and goal-directed. As such it is modifiable. Since pain behavior often is the reason for diminished activities of daily living, physicians should not consider someone as having a permanent impairment solely on the basis of pain behavior. The author, therefore, has great difficulty with the Pain Intensity-frequency Grid (see Fig. 45-1) in the AMA *Guides,* because, if used by the inexperienced rater, it allows for a pain rating based on modifiable pain behaviors.

Individuals with chronic pain should not be considered to have reached Maximum Medical Improvement unless they have (1) been evaluated by physicians knowledgeable about chronic pain, (2) had a multidisciplinary evaluation, and (3) had an adequate trial of adjuvant analgesics (for example, many patients with chronic pain and comorbid depression lose their symptoms when adequately treated with antidepressants, and similarly for some patients with neuropathic pain treated with anticonvulsants).

Brena[70] has noted that according to the World Health Organization's definition of impairment, chronic pain could be rightly viewed as a sensory impairment affecting at least two bodily systems: the musculoskeletal system through altered pattern of daily activity, and the nervous system, through altered central neuronal activity. Chronic pain also affects psychological functioning as pain-perceived emotional difficulty. Impairments could be classified as primarily resulting from a demonstrable pathological lesion affecting organ systems and secondarily resulting from the consequences of the painful experience (such as from inactivity or substance dependence and abuse).

The AMA *Guides* allow for emotional factors resulting in alterations in mental health, although it should be recognized that "psychogenic pain is not the same as chronic pain, but it is a psychiatric disorder that should be treated by specialists in that field."

## CONCLUSION

Pain perception may be distorted by psychiatric illness. It is very important to evaluate motivation which the AMA *Guides* note cannot be ignored as a connecting link between impairment and disability. Impairment may lead to an almost total or minimal disability depending upon motivational factors. In studies at the Boston and Presbyterian Pain Centers physicians found that attitude, motivation, and support systems were more important prognosticators than any one physical finding.

There may be concurrent impairment related to the etiology of pain and to the psychiatric condition. Chronic pain may or may not affect daily activities, social functioning, concentration, or adaptation to stressful circumstances. It is important to defer evaluation of impairment from chronic pain until it has been appropriately evaluated and managed including by a physician specializing in pain medicine, if necessary. Multidisciplinary pain-center treatment may reverse the effects of chronic pain syndromes by diminishing suffering, increasing functional daily activities, decreasing pain behaviors, improving coping skills, and decreasing or eliminating disability.

The AMA *Guides* note that with chronic pain there may or may not be impairment, variable amounts of disability, but there is almost certainly a handicap.

Physicians must rate impairment by objective criteria. However, it is the author's belief that chronic pain behaviors and psychopathology can contribute to and result from the suffering that coincides with the chronic pain syndrome. These can impede an individual's ability to function and carry out activities of daily living. Evaluation of these factors should be performed by those experienced and trained in pain medicine and impairment evaluation.

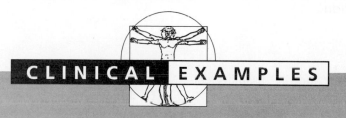

## CLINICAL EXAMPLES

### EXAMPLE

#### History

A 33-year-old divorced secretary has come to the Pain Therapy Center with complaints of chronic low-back pain, cervical pain, and diffuse myalgias for approximately the past two years. Most notable is the fact that symptoms developed insidiously, and, although no specific antecedent trauma was noted, the symptoms were concurrent with strenuous activity while moving furniture into her new home. When her symptoms persisted after several days of rest, she consulted her primary care physician, who put her on a regimen of NSAIDs, muscle relaxants, and several days off work. Pain continued and gradually increased despite medication and a trial of physical therapy, including TENS and massage. The initial diagnostic impression was acute cervical and lumbar strain. Over the next three to six months, the patient missed increasing numbers of workdays, and currently her symptoms include generalized myalgias and arthralgias.

Significant associated history includes her mother having had a cardiovascular accident one year before the patient's symptoms began. The patient was involved in her mother's ongoing care until her death approximately nine months before the onset of symptoms. Also of note are significant marital stress and work-related stress with anxiety over possible layoffs.

Initial evaluation indicates the patient developed increased somatic preoccupation associated with depression and gradually progressive life disruption, including diminished efficiency at work, increased absenteeism, and increased pain with prolonged sitting, lifting, bending, or typing. She is already on medical leave and has applied for disability. She spends approximately half of her day recumbent, using a heating pad for her various myalgias. She claims an inability to perform usual household activities as a result of pain and debilitating fatigue and requires assistance for shopping. Associated with her complaints of neck and upper back pain are complaints of constant headaches of increasing severity. The patient feels she is unable to maintain herself vocationally and has considerable difficulties with other activities of daily living. She is also having increasing difficulties in her marital relationship.

#### Physical Examination

Musculoskeletal examination notes 14 of 18 fibrocystic tender points. Neurologic examination is normal. Mental status evaluation reveals depression with matching affect and vegetative symptoms, including insomnia, complaints of fatigue, and diminished appetite and libido.

#### Test Results

Laboratory evaluation is essentially normal, including a normal sedimentation rate and rheumatoid factor levels. Cervical MRI indicated a mild bulging disc without nerve root compression.

#### Assessment Process

The patient is not rated because she has not yet reached Maximum Medical Improvement (MMI). She is felt to have chronic pain and meets the diagnostic criteria for both fibromyalgia and major depression, single episode. Although she has not responded to conventional approaches with conservative treatment, her symptoms do not seem stable and are likely to change in the future despite therapy. She is referred for an outpatient pain management approach through a pain center.

At the time of discharge from this pain center, her symptoms are considerably improved. Pain is now occasional and intensity slight. The patient is increasingly aware of a psychophysiologic component to her symptoms that increase during stressful times. She has become more aware of personality characteristics that often interfere with her getting her own needs met, as well as her tendency to become increasingly passive and dependent with greater reliance on the health care system.

#### Evaluation

The pain center evaluation indicates that, although she continues to complain of pain, there are no objectively-validated limitations in daily activities. Therefore at discharge she is felt to be at MMI and has no impairment.

*Gerald M. Aronoff*

## References

1. Aronoff GM: Chronic pain and the disability epidemic, *Clin J Pain* 7:330-338, 1991.

1a. Aronoff GM. Psychological aspects of nonmalignant chronic pain: a new nosology. In Aronoff GM: *Evaluation and treatment of chronic pain*, pp 399-408, Baltimore, Williams & Wilkins, 1992.

2. Aronoff GM, McAlary PW: Pain centers: Treatment for intractable suffering and disability resulting from chronic pain. In *Evaluation and treatment of chronic pain*, ed 2, Baltimore, p. 416, 1992, Williams & Wilkins.

3. Crue BL: Personal Communication,

4. Beecher HK: Relationship of significance of wound to the pain experienced, *JAMA* 161:1609, 1956.

5. Loeser J: In Stantin-Hicks M, Boas R, editors: *Chronic low back pain*, pp 145-148, New York, 1982, Raven Press.

6. Blazer D: Narcissism and the development of chronic pain, *Int J Psych Med* 10(1):69-77, 1980-1981.

7. Blumer D, Heilbronn M: Chronic pain as a variant of depressive disease: The pain-prone disorder, *J Nerv Ment Dis* 170:381-406, 1982.

8. Kramlinger KG, Swanson DW, Maruta T: Are patients with chronic pain depressed? *Am J Psych* 140:747-749, 1983.

9. Romano JH, Turner JA: Chronic pain and depression: Does the evidence support a relationship, *Psych Bull* 97:18-34, 1985.

10. Turner JA, Roman JM: Review of prevalence of coexisting chronic pain and depression. In: Benedetti C, Chapman CR, Moricca G, editors: *Advances in pain research and therapy*, vol 7, New York, 1984, Raven Press.

11. American Psychiatric Association: *Diagnostic and statistical manual of mental disorders*, ed 3, Washington, D.C., 1982, American Psychiatric Association.

12. American Psychiatric Association: *Diagnostic and statistical manual of mental disorders*, rev ed 3, Washington, D.C., 1987, American Psychiatric Association.

13. American Psychiatric Association: *Diagnostic and statistical manual of mental disorders*, ed 4, Washington, D.C., 1993, American Psychiatric Association.

14. Watson GD, Chandarana PC, Mersky N: Relationships between pain and schizophrenia, *Br J Psychol* 138:33-36, 1981.

15. Aronoff GM, Evans WO: Pharmacological management of chronic pain: a review. In Aronoff GM: *Evaluation and treatment of chronic pain*, ed 2, p 361, Baltimore, 1992, Williams & Wilkins.

16. Engel G: Psychogenic pain and the pain-prone patient, *Am J Med* 899-918, June 1959.

17. Engel G: Guilt, pain, and success, *Psychosom Med* 24:37-48, 1962.

18. Blumer D, Heilbronn M: Chronic pain as a variant of depressive disease: the pain prone disorder, *J Nerv Ment Dis* 170:381-406, 1982.

19. Blumer D, Heilbronn M: The pain-prone disorder: A clinical and psychological profile, *Psychosomatics* 22:395-402, 1981.

20. Merskey H: The effect of chronic pain upon the response to noxious stimuli by psychiatric patients, *J Psychosom Res* 8:405-419.

21. Magni G, Arsie D, DeLeo D: Antidepressants in the treatment of cancer pain: A survey in Italy, *Pain* 29:347-353, 1987.

22. Aronoff GM, Evans WO: Doxepin as an adjunct in the treatment of chronic pain, *J Clin Psych* 43(8/Sec 2):42-45, 1982.

23. Oxman T, Denson DD: Antidepressants and adjunctive psychotrophic drugs. In Raj RP, editor: *Practical management of pain*, pp. 528-538, Chicago, 1988, Year Book Medical Publishers.

24. Atkinson JH: Psychopharmacologic agents in the treatment of pain syndrome. In Tollison CD, editor: *Handbook of chronic pain management*, pp. 69-99, Baltimore, 1989, William & Wilkins.

25. Monks R: Psychotropic drugs. In Bonica JJ, editor: *The management of pain*, p. 1677, Lea & Febiger, Philadelphia, 1990 Response to Anti-Depressants, *Psychosomatics* 22:571-577, 1981.

26. Rutrick D, Aronoff GM: Combined psychotherapy for chronic pain syndrome patients at a multidisciplinary pain center. In Aronoff GM, editor: *Evaluation and treatment of chronic pain*, pp. 491-492, Baltimore, 1985, Urban & Schwarzenberg.

27. Strang JP: The chronic disability syndrome. In Aronoff GM, editor: *The evaluation and treatment of chronic pain*, ed 1, Baltimore, 1985, Urban & Schwarzenberg.

28. Brena SF, Chapman SL: The learned pain syndrome, *Postgrad Med* 69:53-62, 1981.

29. Brena SF, Chapman SL: Pain and litigation. In Wall PD, Melzack R, editors: *Textbook of pain*, pp 832-839, New York, 1984, Churchill Livingstone.

30. Weinstein MR: The concept of the disability process, *Psychosomatics* 19:94-97, 1978.

31. Ellard J: Psychological reactions to compensable injury, *Med J Aust* 349-355, August 1970.

32. Seres JS, Newman RI: Negative influences of the disability compensation system: Perspectives for the clinician, *Semin Neurol* 3:4, 1983.

33. McGill CM: Industrial back problems: A control program, *J Occup Med* 10:174-178, 1968.

34. Aronoff GM: The disability epidemic (Editorial), *Clin J Pain* 1:187-188, 1986.

35. Brena SF, et al: Chronic pain states: Their relationship to impairment and disability, *Arch Phys Med Rehab* 60:387-389, 1979.
36. Snook SH, et al: A. Study of three preventive approaches to low back injury, *J Occup Med* 20:478-481, 1978.
37. Carron H: Compensation aspects of low back claims. In Carron H, McLaughlin RE, editors: *Management of low back pain*, Boston, 1982, PSG.
38. Leavitt SS, Beyer RD, Johnson TL: Monitoring the recovery process: Pilot results of a systematic approach to case management, *2nd Med Surg* 41(4):25-30, 1972.
39. Catchlove R, Cohen K: Effects of a directive return to work approach in the treatment of workers' compensation patients with chronic pain, *Pain* 14:181-191, 1982.
40. Waddell G, et al: Failed lumbar disc surgery following industrial injuries, *J Bone Joint Surg* 61:201-1207, 1979.
41. Leavitt SS, Beyer RD, Johnston TL: Monitoring the recovery process: Pilot results of a systematic approach to case management, *2nd Med Surg* 41(4):25-30, 1972.
42. Dworkin RH, Handin DS, Richlin DM, Brand L, Vanucci C: Unraveling the effects of compensation, litigation and employment on treatment response in chronic pain, *Pain* 23:49-59, 1985.
43. Peck JC, Fordyce WE, Black: The effect of pendency of claims for compensation upon behavior indicative of pain, *Wash Law Rev* 53:257-278, 1978.
44. Aronoff GM: The role of the pain center in the treatment of intractable suffering and disability from chronic pain, *Semin Neurol* 3(4):377-81, 1983.
45. Turk DC, Rudy TE: Persistent pain and the injured worker: Integrating biomechanical, psycholosocial, and behavioral factors in assessment, *J Occup Rehab* vol 1, no 2, 1991.
46. Turk DC: Evaluation of pain and disability, *J Disability* 2:24-43, 1991.
47. Brena SF, Turk DL: Vocational disability: A challenge to pain rehabilitation programs. In Aronoff GM, editor: *Pain centers: A revolution in health care*, New York, 1988: 167-180, Raven Press.
48. Seres JS, Newman RI: Negative influences of the disability compensation system: Perspectives for the clinician, *Semin Neurol* vol 3-4, 1983.
49. Walsh NE, Dumitru D: Financial compensation and recovery from low back pain, *Spine* 2:109-121, 1987.
50. Krusen EM, Ford DE: Compensation factors in low back injuries, *JAMA* 166:1128-1133, 1958.
51. Hebben N: Toward the assessment of clinical pain in adults. In Aronoff GM, editor: *Evaluation and treatment of chronic pain*, Baltimore, p. 384-93, 1992. William & Wilkins
52. Revill SI, Robinson JO, Rosen M, et al: The reliability of a linear analogue for evaluating pain, *Anesthesia* 31:1191-1198, 1976.
53. Yang JC, Wagner JM, Clark WC: Psychological distress and mood in chronic pain and surgical patients: a decision theory analysis. In Bonica JJ editor: *Advances in pain research and therapy*, Florida: American Pain Society, (5):901-906, 1983.
54. Melzack R: The McGill Pain Questionnaire, *Pain* 1:277-299, 1975.
55. Hinnant DW: Psychological evaluation and testing. In Tollison CD, editor: *Handbook of Pain Management*, ed 2, Baltimore, pp. 18-35, 1994, Williams & Wilkins.
56. Corson JA, Schneider MJ: The Dartmouth Pain Questionnaire: an adjunct to the McGill Pain Questionnaire, *Pain* 19:59-69, 1984.
57. Cronbach LJ: Test validation. In Thorndike RL, editor: *Educational measurement*, Washington, D.C., American Council on Education, 1971, p. 462.
58. Tait RC, Chibnall JT, Krause S: The Pain Disability Index: psychometric properties, *Pain* 40:171-182, 1990.
59. Brown GK, Nicassio PM: Development of a questionnaire for the assessment of active and passive coping strategies in chronic pain patients, *Pain* 31:53-64, 1987.
60. Kerns RD, Turk DC, Rudy TE: The West Haven-Yale Multidimensional Pain Inventory (WHYMPI), *Pain* 23:345-356, 1985.
61. Strassberg DS, Reimherr F, Ward M, et al: The MMPI and chronic pain, *J Consult Clin Psychol* 49:220-226, 1981.
62. Ahles TA, Yunus MB, Gaulier B, et al: The use of contemporary MMPI norms in the study of chronic pain patients, *Pain* 24:159-163, 1986.
63. Kinney R, Catchell RJ, et al: *The SCL-90R: An alternative to the MMPI for psychological screening of chronic low back pain patients.* Presented at the Annual Meeting of the International Society for the Study of the Lumbar Spine, Kyoto, Japan, May, 1989.
64. Millon T, Green CJ, Meagher RB: Millon Behavioral Health Inventory, ed 3, Minneapolis, 1982, Interpretive Scoring System.
65. Bigos SJ, Battie MC, Spengler DM, et al: A prospective study of work perceptions and psychosocial factors affecting the report of back injury, *Spine* 16:1-6, 1991.
66. White P: Pain measurement. In Warfield CA, editor: *Principles and practice of pain management*, pp 27-42, New York, 1993, McGraw-Hill.

67. Hinnant DW: Psychological evaluation and testing. In Tollison CD: *Handbook of pain management*, ed 2, Baltimore, pp 18-35, 1994, Williams & Wilkins.

68. American Medical Association: *Guides to the evaluation of permanent impairment*, ed 4, 1993, American Medical Association.

69. Ibid #63, p. 310.

70. Brena SF, Turk DC: Vocational disability: A challenge to pain rehabilitation programs. In Aronoff GM: *Pain centers: A revolution in health care*, New York, p. 171, 1988, Raven Press.

# PART III

# RESOURCES IN DISABILITY EVALUATION

# PHYSICAL REHABILITATION

*Jeffrey A. Saal*
*Joel S. Saal*

## INTRODUCTION

Rehabilitation of patients with musculoskeletal disorders is a comprehensive process that requires both accurate diagnosis and early intervention. Although pain may be a patient's initial chief complaint, the primary goal of rehabilitation is to optimize function. Patients may state that they are unable to participate in their normal activities because of pain and that their quality of life has suffered. They may no longer be able to work, take care of their household or pursue their usual recreation.

The focus of a rehabilitation program is to improve function and quality of life instead of treating pain. Control of pain frequently follows the change in function. The treatment program should teach patients to assume control of their musculoskeletal dysfunction instead of allowing their condition and pain to dictate their lives. Patients who are not adequately and effectively rehabilitated will be left with a greater degree of disability (that is, with functional loss) than their underlying medical condition dictates.

The rehabilitation process should begin as soon as possible after the onset of an illness or injury and should be terminated only at the point when the patient can successfully return to the maximal realistic level of active function. A careful outlining of the rehabilitation goals prior to embarking upon the program will eliminate frustration and discouragement. Early diagnostic intervention with the establishment of a precise diagnosis is the key to establishing an effective rehabilitation plan. An improper or imprecise diagnosis can lead to mistaken paths in the treatment regimen. Early intervention will lead to control of the inflammatory processes and speed the recovery of normal articular and soft tissue ROM. Adequate control of inflammation plays a critical role in allowing the patient to participate actively in the rehabilitation program.

In order to facilitate progress and outline its milestones, short- and long-term goals must be set for each individual. The short-term goals will require continual monitoring and adjustment as the clinical progression is monitored during rehabilitation. It is imperative that the patient be integrally involved in the goal-setting process. The patient must fully understand the realistic goal for improving their clinical condition. Additionally, the patient must understand the length of time required and the methods to be used to achieve this outcome. If the physician and patient do not agree in these respects, the outcome will be less than optimal.

Both the patient and the physician must be aware that the musculoskeletal system's maladaptations to certain conditions, such as muscle and soft tissue contractures, muscle weakness, flexibility asymmetries, and segmental motion limitations, require an extended period to develop. A rehabilitation plan must allow sufficient time to reverse these processes. The principles of exercise and connective tissue physiology dictate the length of time required to establish new length in shortened tissues, strengthen weakened muscle groups and improve flexibility and segmental spinal motion. The patient and the physician must understand that there are no quick fixes. Successful rehabilitation requires sufficient time to permit the patient to optimize physical function and control any outstanding psychosocial barriers to recovery.

A treatment program typically requires 8 to 18 visits of supervised active physical therapy followed by a transition to an independent exercise program either at home or in a health club. In order to achieve an adequate level of strength and coordination, the patient's participation in the exercise regimen three to four times per week will be necessary. The chronicity and extent of the functional deficit coupled with the patient's improvement schedule will determine the exact period required for each individual case. Careful monitoring of the rehabilitation program is necessary to determine when alterations in the exercise regimen or treatment to control pain or inflammation may be necessary to facilitate progress. Careful monitoring will avoid unnecessary treatment, overtreatment, or inappropriate resource allocation.

The physical rehabilitation process may be divided into the eight phases shown below, each of which is part of the overall plan to restore function:

1. Control the inflammatory process
2. Control pain
3. Restore joint ROM and soft-tissue extensibility
4. Improve muscular strength
5. Improve muscular endurance
6. Develop specific biomechanical skill patterns (coordination retraining)
7. Improve general cardiovascular fitness and endurance
8. Begin maintenance exercise programs

The utilization of therapeutic exercises in physical rehabilitation is guided by physiologic principles. Training muscular strength and endurance are two different and specific activities, and their incorporation into coordinated, automatic patterns of movement requires special emphasis. An essential concept in rehabilitation programs is the principle of specific adaptation to imposed demands, which states that the body responds to a given demand with a specific and predictable adaptation.[1] If one can define the specific goals of the rehabilitation process, then the designed program may be tailored to meet that need.

The non-operative rehabilitation and treatment program has many potential tools available to the provider. This program may include the following elements:

- Anti-inflammatory medications
- Pain-modulating medications
- Physical modalities for pain control
- Detoxification from addictive medications acting on the CNS
- Therapeutic exercises to control pain (flexion range vs. extension range); improve flexibility; improve ROM; improve muscle strength and endurance; improve balance; improve proprioception and coordination; improve cardiorespiratory aerobic and anaerobic capacity; reacquaint with sustained effort or work ("work harden"); and train for a particular sport, job, or activity.
- Use of braces and orthoses
- Ergonomic evaluation and workplace modification
- Body mechanics instruction
- Psychosocial evaluation and intervention

- Psychiatric intervention when necessary and appropriate
- Family counseling
- Vocational counseling
- Nutritional counseling and weight reduction
- Smoking cessation
- Establishing a successful doctor-patient relationship

The decisions for implementation of the specific components of the program include the factors of timing and goal-setting (after taking into account the clinical type of injury or pain), the pattern of development of clinical findings, the extent of structural pathology, the patient's age, the perceived outcome, as well as the patient's activity level, motivation to improve, level of physical conditioning, and psychosocial barriers to recovery.

## PERIPHERAL JOINT TREATMENT PROGRAMS

Examples of treatment plan algorithms for the shoulder, knee, and ankle are found in Figs. 46-1 through 46-6. Similar programs have been developed for other musculoskeletal injuries.

## STRENGTH TRAINING: BASIC PHYSIOLOGIC PRINCIPLES

The major principle to keep in mind is one of progressive resistance exercise.[17] This type of exercise must be performed on a regular basis a minimum of three times per week. The initial programs involve progressive resistance exercise to the muscle groups designated as the prime movers of that particular injured area. Programs using daily adjusted progressive resistance exercise (DAPRE) techniques appear to achieve maximum resistance. The DAPRE technique is based on the principle that strength can be redeveloped more quickly after injury than it was developed initially.[18] The key component of the program consists of performing maximal repetitions during the third and fourth sets, with the number of repetitions performed used as a basis for adjusting the resistance used during the fourth set and on the next day.[4,7]

Maintenance strength programs are begun once the patient has achieved 90% to 95% of the expected strength gains. The limits of performance must be persistently extended to improve muscle strength. The rate of improvement appears to depend upon the willingness of the subject to overload.[11,16]

To achieve maximum intensity of muscle contrac-

*Text continued on p. 551.*

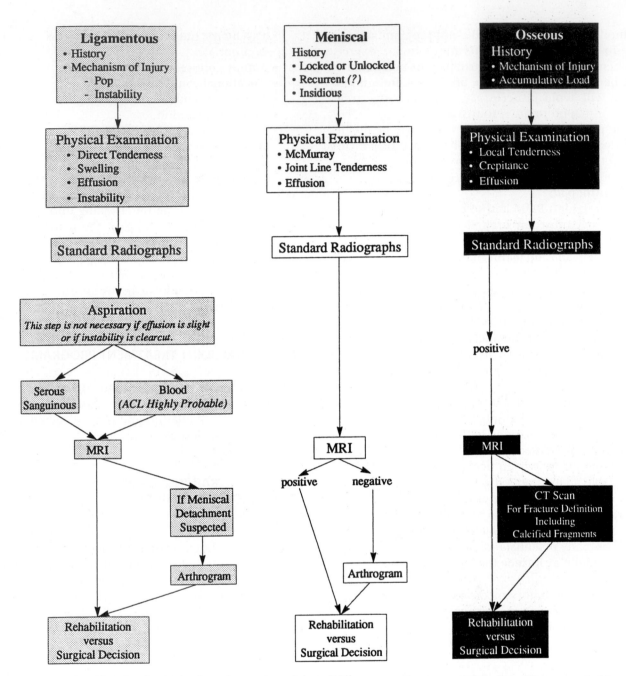

**FIGURE 46-1** Algorithm for the evaluation of acute knee injury. (MRI = magnetic resonance imaging, CT = computed tomography, ACL = anterior cruciate ligament.)

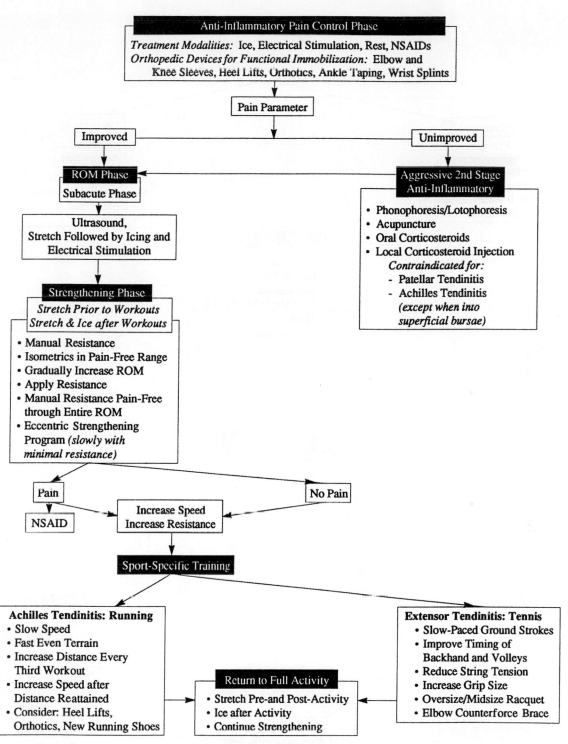

**FIGURE 46-2**    Algorithm for the rehabilitation of tendinitis. (NSAIDs = nonsteroidal anti-inflammatory drugs, ROM = range of motion.)

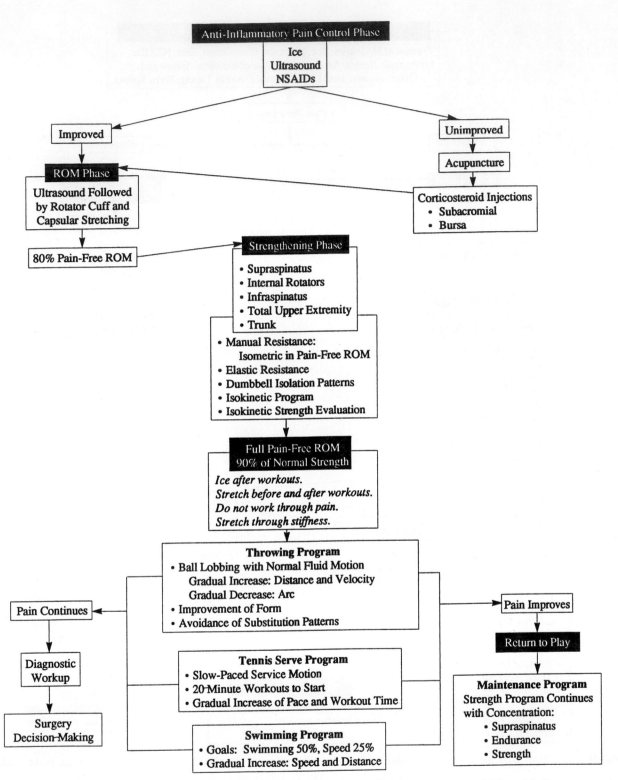

**FIGURE 46-3** Algorithm for the rehabilitation of shoulder impingement. (NSAIDs = nonsteroidal anti-inflammatory drugs, ROM = range of motion.)

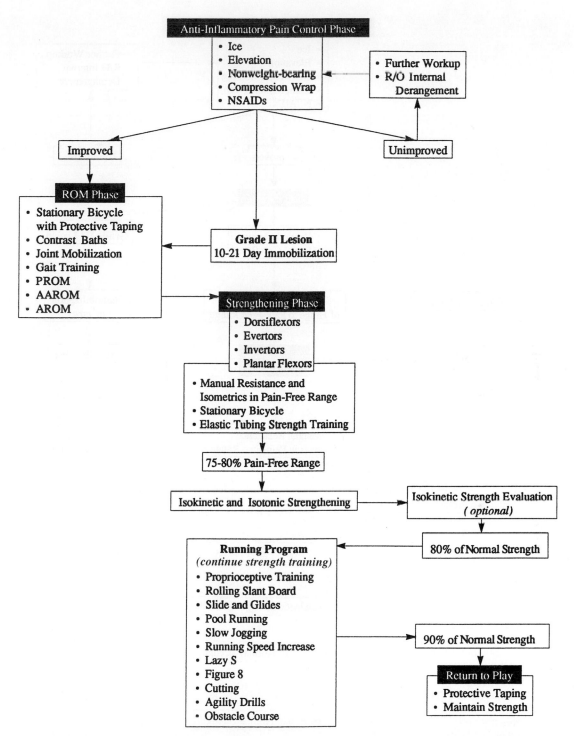

**FIGURE 46-4**    Algorithm for the rehabilitation of ankle ligament injury. (NSAIDs = nonsteroidal anti-inflammatory drugs, ROM = range of motion, AAROM = assisted active range of motion, AROM = active range of motion.)

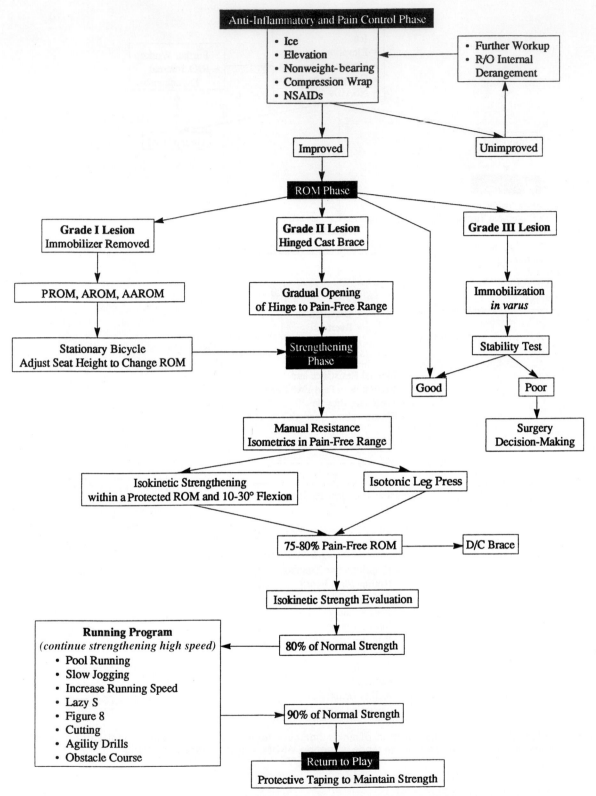

**FIGURE 46-5** Algorithm for the rehabilitation of collateral ligament injury of the knee. (NSAIDs = nonsteroidal anti-inflammatory drugs, ROM = range of motion, AROM = active range of motion, AAROM = assisted active range of motion.)

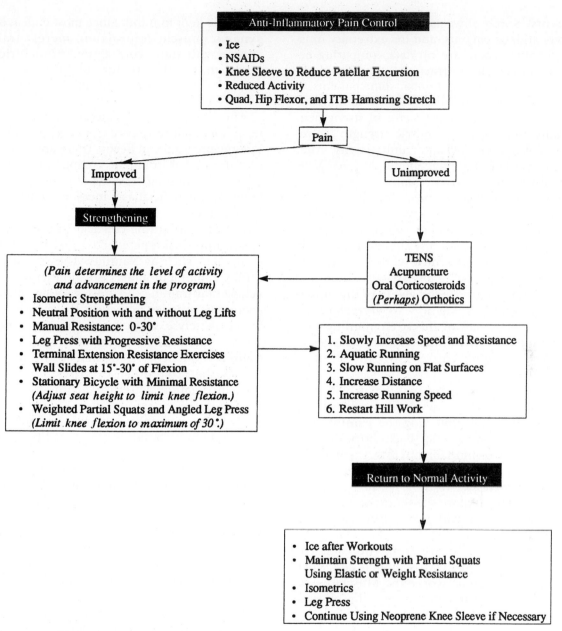

**FIGURE 46-6**    Algorithm for the rehabilitation of the patellofemoral pain syndrome. (NSAIDs = nonsteroidal anti-inflammatory drugs, ITB = iliotibial band muscles, TENS = transcutaneous electrical nerve stimulation.)

tion, the highest possible percentage of muscle mass should be involved in any given moment.[5,7] To achieve this end, good form is of utmost importance. The resistance should be accelerated in a smooth fashion and briefly halted at the position of full muscle contraction. The speed used in raising and lowering the weight may also train the muscle to develop the appropriate speed of contraction for the types of activity designated.[12,32,34] Concentric exercise programs are the most frequently used in rehabilitation. Eccentric training programs have been developed for the treatment of tendinitis.[37] Eccentric programs are felt to be beneficial in increasing load. The speed of

the contraction is modified during the specialized eccentric program that gradually increases the speed of movement while increasing the load on the tendon. This type of eccentric loading program parallels normal musculotendinous unit functions in movement patterns. It has been suggested that concentric programs may place greater stress on the musculotendinous unit and are unable to increase the length of the soft tissues. Some authors have reported that patients will often report increased symptoms with concentric contraction and decreased symptomatology with eccentric programs. Eccentric exercises for trunk and abdominal muscles may be uncomfortable for most back patients. Some physicians prescribe them in higher-level athletic patients, and for extremity muscle strengthening. There are no data comparing eccentric and concentric contractions specifically applied to the trunk muscles in lumbar spine patients.

The use of overload to attain muscle fatigue appears to be the most important factor in strengthening programs. Initial gains in muscle strength are related to improved levels of motor unit activity. After the first two weeks of training, additional force gains are made through muscle hypertrophy.[10,16,20]

The ability to synchronize the firing ratios of the motor units is a consequence of weight-training programs. Improvement in strength correlates with increased synchronization patterns. Therefore, carefully concentrated exercise performed at the proper skill level and proper speed will allow synchronization of the motor units and improve the ability of the muscle to gain strength more rapidly.[2,7,8,16] Overzealousness during the initial phases of the strengthening program can result in reactive inflammatory changes or joint synovitis. Carefully progressing the strength program is imperative.

The strengthening program may begin with isometric exercises. The isometric phase can be carried out early on while still protecting the painful area. Manual resistance exercises may begin once the area can be moved more comfortably. In this situation, the therapist uses a carefully-graded manual resistance that acts as the progressive resistor. As the patient accomplishes this with comfort, the therapist and physician can note the range within which it will be appropriate to exercise.

Strength programs advance from the isometric state and are used when ROM is limited and when pain accompanies isotonic workouts. Muscle weakness and fatigue are pinpointed during the physical examination and concentrated upon in the rehabilitation process.

Once the patient has carefully progressed through the manual resistance program and isometric program, pain-free ranges can be carefully adjusted. Isometric contractions are optimally held for five or six seconds with a rest period of between 10 and 20 seconds. This ensures a proper muscle blood flow and removes the substrate products of muscular contraction. The isometric contraction should be carried out frequently during the day, in sets of 10 to 12 repetitions.[1] The goal is to transfer this isometric strength development to the isotonic program. Individuals who carry out isometric exercises of a greater frequency develop greater endurance, which transfers better to progressive resistive exercises.

The concept of specificity of exercise should constantly be kept in mind. Since most endeavors rely on dynamic muscle contraction, merely training the muscle with static contractions (isometric contractions) may not transfer to the dynamic activities[1,23,26,27] even though this method can increase absolute static strength.[35]

After the patient can successfully perform isometric and manual resistance exercises, progression to an isotonic program can begin. There are no data to support the use of isokinetic equipment for strength or endurance training. This type of equipment appears to be most beneficial as a measurement tool, not as a training tool.

Isotonic programs can use free weights, elastic bands, universal type exercise machines, or cammed equipment such as Nautilus. The recently-designed MEDX equipment allows isolation patterns to be developed for training the erector spinae and the rectus abdominis muscles. However, the muscle groups can be adequately exercised without special equipment. There are no data to support the contention that specialized equipment strengthens trunk muscles more rapidly than traditional exercises. Free weights are used in isolation patterns, such as using dumbbells for the upper extremity after a rotator cuff injury. With heavier weights, the free weights should be used only in a "buddy system" and by patients who are skilled lifters.

For the novice, weight machines such as the Cybex and Nautilus are especially useful. Isolation patterns are difficult to obtain, but the ease of use of the machine and the multiple stations make this type of equipment extremely practical. The use of cammed equipment such as the Nautilus has many distinct advantages. This type of equipment varies the resistance offered by a given load to try to match the average torque curves for each of a large number of muscle groups. This theoretically eliminates the dead areas that are noted in certain portions of the ROM when an individual trains with free weights. Another advantage to cammed equipment is that individualized stations allow adjustment of foot rests and seat height.

The use of elastic bands is extremely practical, especially for home strengthening programs. Elastic bands may be used not only to supply resistance, but also for flexibility programs. Isolation patterns can be accomplished with the use of elastic bands. This type of exercise is extremely practical because the patient is able to travel with the exercise equipment. Maintenance programs using elastic bands can be helpful.

Occasionally, the buoyancy associated with water is useful during the initial phase of strengthening programs. An individual may be placed in the pool and, with use of a life vest, can begin to use water and body weight as resistance for strengthening. These "hydro programs" allow the individual to maintain lower extremity strength and ROM as well as aerobic endurance. This satisfies not only physiological goals, but also the psychological goals of the patient. Performing stabilization exercise in water allows some lower-level patients to advance more easily and quickly. Additionally, clinicians teach patients proper swimming techniques to avoid repetitive injuries.

Costill has demonstrated the necessity for combining strength and endurance programs into the muscle rehabilitation portions of the program.[25] Because there is a specific program response to the type of exercise performed, an exercise program must be tailored to meet the needs of the individual.[21] Steadman has employed a group of exercises that challenge the muscles in three different ways.[38] High-repetition, moderate-weight sets are performed initially, followed by a rapid, low-resistance repetition until fatigue. The last step is to hold an isometric contraction for approximately one minute. This type of program improves not only absolute strength but also endurance. This program also stresses the anaerobic pathway that is necessary for burst-type activities.[10]

Gaining muscle endurance necessitates stressing the aerobic pathways and improving the oxidative enzyme capacity of slow-twitch muscle fibers,[16] which results in higher repetition work at lower weight levels.[5,7] These types of muscle endurance sets are useful as maintenance programs also. Isolating the specific muscle contractions necessary for endurance training is based upon the activity in which the individual is engaged.

The threshold of change in the development of muscular endurance is unclear. Therefore, the degree of intensity placed upon the muscle cannot be clearly defined. In one study, strength scores improved significantly when preceded by a program using high-repetition work. Therefore, it would seem appropriate to start the patient on a high-repetition, low-weight program before embarking on a higher resistance program.[18] This would appear to allow time for cellular adaptation to occur and would enhance the eventual strength gains of the program participant.

The use of the stationary bike with variable resistance is extremely beneficial in lower-extremity muscle-endurance programs. Additionally, stair steppers and climbing machines are also beneficial. Swimming and other hydro exercises are useful in upper-extremity muscular-endurance programs. The maintenance of muscle endurance has been demonstrated to be a significant factor in the prevention of sporting injury. This appears to be related to depletion of oxidative enzymes in slow-twitch fibers leading to fatigue of the musculature and inability of the musculature to protect the joints.[19]

## FLEXIBILITY TRAINING

Training for flexibility is another essential component of programs for spine stabilization. For passive trunk flexion to occur at the hips rather than about the axis of the lumbar spine, adequate flexibility in the hip and leg extensors, hip abductors and external rotators, flexors and knee extensors is important. The hamstrings, gluteus medius, the short hip rotators, quadriceps, iliopsoas, and gastroc-soleus complex are specific sites that should be targeted for training. It is critical that stretching exercises be performed in a spine-safe manner. Loaded trunk flexion and torsion are the primary risks. Many of the flexibility techniques taught in school athletic programs and popular exercise video tapes are less than ideal for this reason, and should be avoided. It is important that these stretches be carried out passively in a spine-safe manner.

When prescribing flexibility exercises, clinicians need to keep in mind certain facts. Flexibility exercises increase the elasticity of connective tissue, not only that of loose connective tissue, but of the connective tissue of muscle and muscle contractile units.[36] Connective tissue behaves viscoelastically.[22] This means that it will deform in response to applied force, and if the force is large enough, it will return to a slightly longer length once the force stretching it is removed.[29] In addition, a tissue's viscoelasticity will be enhanced in the presence of increased temperature.[29,31] Its increase in length will be greater if force is applied slowly. Thus, one should apply a stretch slowly, for an adequate period, after warming the tissue.

Actual lengthening of the muscle contractile units is accomplished by slightly different physiologic principles, but both the sets of principles for tissue elasticity and those for muscle contractile unit lengthening can be applied to good advantage together. The relationship of muscle fibers to each other is governed by neural factors as well as physical principles. Relaxation of incoming neural input is essential for lengthening a contractile unit.[39] This relaxation is best accomplished by a stretch that occurs slowly and evenly and is accompanied by gentle contraction of the antagonist muscles. For example, gentle contraction of the ankle dorsiflexors while passively stretching the gastrocnemius-soleus facilitates a better stretch.[27] Performing stretching exercises both before and after an exercise period has been demonstrated to result in increased flexibility gains.[33] The ideal length of time for an individual to hold an isolated stretch is probably 15 to 30 seconds. Continuation of the stretch for a period longer than this will not generate any greater flexibility gains except in the case of pathologic contracture.[28,36]

For many years, flexibility training was an ignored aspect of injury rehabilitation and injury prevention.[36] Now, however, the literature supporting flexibility training continues to grow, as it repeatedly demonstrates how to reduce sports injury in various environments.[3,6,9] There are no data specifically regarding prevention of lumbar injuries. Flexibility programs with a sound scientific foundation should be incorporated into rehabilitation training programs.[14,15] One such program, the proprioceptive neuromuscular facilitation (PNF) procedure, is a proven, effective means of passive stretching.[39] A PNF procedure involves an initial passive static flexibility maneuver of the agonist, followed by a three-second-maximum voluntary contraction, and then static stretching. This type of flexibility program has been found to be more effective than use of passive static flexibility methods alone.[39]

Flexibility programs can enhance the concentric contraction velocities of muscles. These programs can also reduce the subjective symptoms of muscle soreness after vigorous exercise.[24]

## AEROBIC TRAINING

During the entire physical rehabilitation program the patient is not allowed to remain sedentary. At the earliest possible moment the patient should begin aerobic training with walking; if necessary, this can be performed on a treadmill. When the patient is physically capable the stationary bike or stair stepper can be used for training. Depending on the ability of the patient to stabilize the spine, the patient may be advanced to many forms of aerobic conditioning. Knee, hip, and foot problems will also be factors in determining the preferred type of aerobic conditioning. Performing exercises in the pool is another way to keep the patient active without stressing the affected area. The aerobic capacity of the patient should not be allowed to diminish in the early postinjury period and during the initial phases of the rehabilitation program.

Aerobic conditioning can increase the patient's endorphin levels.[13] This will improve the patient's sense of well-being and increase the pain thresholds. This increase in pain threshold will allow the patient to perform at higher levels of function before perceiving pain. However, one should not rely on aerobic conditioning as the sole form of exercise training. Aerobic conditioning can physiologically improve cardiorespiratory endurance but cannot enhance muscular strength, muscular endurance, balance, or body mechanics specific to the function of the patient.

Contrary to some popular opinion, no direct or inferential scientific evidence exists that running is injurious to the spine or hip. Recent studies have shown that running does not adversely affect the articular cartilage of the hip and does not either create arthritic degeneration or cause it to progress.[30] If the hip is not adversely affected by the loads to which it is subjected during running, it is likely that the spine is uncompromised as well.

## DISCHARGE PLANNING AND EXERCISE TRANSITION

The decision to discharge the patient from the supervised exercise program to begin a maintenance program must be a team decision. Because of their athletic background and motivation, some patients can learn the program quickly (in 6-8 visits), and thereby complete the supervised portion of the program. However, the deconditioned nonathletic individual may need 18 sessions of supervised physical therapy to reach a level that will allow the transitional program to begin.

Exercise training is not finished in the physical therapy gymnasium. All patients must be transitioned to home programs. The patient must receive detailed and clear information regarding the precise program at the time of discharge. The program should be updated four to six weeks after discharge. In many circumstances the exercise program will continue at a neighborhood gym. In this case the physical therapist or trainer must accompany the patient to the gym to instruct the patient about the program and proper weight training activities using the specific equipment available in the gym. In some circumstances the duration of supervised physical therapy can be shortened by having a trained exercise instructor work with the patient in the gym. The exercise trainer may monitor the program progression and act as the patient's coach during the recovery process. The exercise trainer should give progress reports to the treating physician to allow for smooth program progression.

## SUMMARY

Physical rehabilitation when appropriately applied can make a tremendous impact upon the functional outcome of patients with painful musculoskeletal disorders. The program must be specifically prescribed and carefully monitored, and follow sound physiologic principles.

Appropriately applied, physical rehabilitation can optimize function and limit residual disability. The degree of residual disability will be unnecessarily severe if the rehabilitation process is inadequate.

## References

1. Allman FL: Exercise in sports medicine. In Basmajian JV, editor: *Therapeutic exercise,* Baltimore, 1984, Williams & Wilkins, pp. 485-509.
2. Basmajian JV, Harden TP, Regenos EM: Integrated actions of the four heads of quadriceps femoris: An EMG study, *Anat Rec* 172:15-20, 1972.
3. Beck JL, Day RW: Overuse injuries, *Clin Sports Med* 4(3):553, 1985.
4. Blackburn TA: Rehabilitation of anterior cruciate ligament injuries, *Orthop Clin North Am* 16(2):241-269, 1985.
5. Bonde-Petersen F, Grandal H, Hansen JW, et al: The effect of varying the number of muscle contractions on dynamic muscle training, *Eur J Appl Physiol* 18:468-473, 1966.
6. Borms J: Importance of flexibility in overall physical fitness, *Int J Phys Ed* 21:15-26, 1984.
7. Burger RA: Optimal repetitions for the development of strength, *Res Q* 33:334-338, 1962.
8. Chu DA: *Comparisons of selected electromyographic data under isokinetic and isotonic stress load,* Menlo Park, Calif., 1974, Stanford University Press.
9. Cornelius WL: A flexibility method designed to establish suitable internal environment for strength, *Int Gymnast Techn* (Suppl) 2:33-34, 1981.
10. Costill DL, Coyle EF, Fink WF, et al, Adaptations in skeletal muscle following strength training, *J Appl Physiol* 46:149, 1976.
11. Costill DL, Fink WJ, Habansky AJ: Muscle rehabilitation after knee surgery, *Phys Sports Med* 5:71-74, 1977.
12. Coyle EF, Feiring DC, Rotkis TC, et al: Specificity of power improvements through slow and fast isokinetic training, *J Appl Physiol* 51(6):1437-1442, 1981.
13. Davies JE, Gibson T, Tester L: The value of exercise in the treatment of low back pain, *Rheumatol Rehab* 18:243, 1979.
14. de Vries HA: Electromyographic observations of the effect of static stretching upon muscle distress, *Res Q* 32:468-480, 1961.
15. de Vries HA: Evaluation of static stretching procedures for improvement flexibility, *Res Q* 33:222-230, 1962.
16. DeLateur BJ: Therapeutic exercise. In Basmajian JV editor: *Exercise for strength and endurance,* Baltimore, 1984, Williams & Wilkins.
17. DeLorme TL: Restoration of muscle power by heavy-resistance exercises, *J Bone Joint Surg* 27A:645-667, 1945.
18. Dickinson AD, Bennett KN: Therapeutic exercise, *Clin Sports Med* 4(3):417-429, 1985.
19. Ericksson E: Anatomical, histological, and physiological factors in experienced downhill skiers, *Orthop Clin North Am* 7:159-165, 1976.
20. Ghosh P: Influence of drugs, hormones, and other agents on the metabolism of the disc and the sequelae of its degeneration. In Ghosh P, editor: *The biology of the disc,* Boca Raton, Florida, 1988, CRC Press.
21. Hanai K: Conservative treatment for lumbar spinal canal stenosis. In *Spine across the sea,* Maui, Hawaii, 1994.
22. Haut R, Little R: A constitutive equation for collagen fibers, *Biomech* 5:423-430, 1972.
23. Holland DP: Exercise prescription and therapeutic rehabilitation in sports medicine, *Athletic Training* 17:283-286, 1982.
24. Hortobagyi T, Faludi J, Tihanyi J, et al: Effects of intense "stretching" flexibility training on the mechanical profile of the knee extensors and on the range of motion of the hip joint, *Int J Sports Med* 6:317-321, 1985.
25. Kelemen MH, Stewart KJ: Circuit weight training: A new direction for cardiac rehabilitation, *Sports Med* 2:385-388, 1985.
26. Knapik JJ, Wright JE, Mawdsley RH, et al: Isokinetic, isometric, and isotonic strength relationships, *Arch Phys Med Rehabil* 64:77-80, 1983.
27. Knott M, Voss DE: *Proprioceptive neuromuscular facilitation,* New York, 1956, Harper & Row.
28. Kottke F, Pauley D, Ptak R: The rationale for prolonged stretching for correction of shortening of connective tissue, *Arch Phys Med Rehab* 47:345-352, 1966.
29. LaBan M: Collagen tissue: Implications of its response to stress in vitro, *Arch Phys Med Rehab* 43:461-466, 1962.
30. Lane NE, Buckwalter JA: Exercise: A cause of osteoarthritis, *Rheum Disc Clin North Am* 19(3):617-633, 1993.
31. Lehman JF, DeLateur BJ: Therapeutic heat. In Lehman JF, editor: *Therapeutic heat and cold,* Baltimore, 1982, Williams & Wilkins, p. 531.
32. Moffroid M, Whipple R: Specificity of speed of exercise, *Phys Ther* 50(12):1692-1700, 1970.
33. Moller M, Oberg B, Gilquist J: Stretching exercise and soccer: Effect of stretching on range of motion in the low extremity in connection with soccer training, *J Sports Med* 6:50-52, 1985.

34. Murray MP, Baldwin J, Gardner G, et al: Maximum isometric knee flexor and extensor muscle contractions: normal patterns of torque versus time, *Phys Ther* 57(6):637-643, 1977.

35. Rasch PJ, Morehouse LE: Effect of static and dynamic exercises on muscular strength and hypertrophy, *J Applied Physiol* 11:29, 1957.

36. Saal JS: Flexibility training. In Saal JA, editor: *Physical medicine and rehabilitation: State of the art reviews*, vol 1, 1987, Philadelphia, Hanley and Belfus, pp. 537-554.

37. Stanish WD, et al: Tendinitis analysis and treatment, *Clin Sports Med* 4:593-608, 1986.

38. Steadman JR: Rehabilitation after knee ligament surgery, *Am J Sports Med* 8(4):294-296, 1980.

39. Tanigawa MC: Comparison of the hold-relax procedure and passive mobilization on increasing muscle length, *Phys Ther* 52:725-735, 1972.

# CHAPTER 47

# VOCATIONAL REHABILITATION

*John Allen*

## WHAT IS VOCATIONAL REHABILITATION?

Vocational rehabilitation is a process that assists individuals with impairments to overcome their handicaps to employment and to return to work at their maximum physical and intellectual capacities at or near their previous earning level. The use of vocational rehabilitation depends on the severity of injury or illness and the likelihood that employment in a new occupation will be necessary due to a significant loss of the individual's functional abilities. Vocational rehabilitation is achieved by carrying out a comprehensive program of services that is mutually planned by the practitioner and client and involves a series of short-term goals that result in appropriate reemployment and reintegration into the community.

## HISTORY OF VOCATIONAL REHABILITATION

The need to provide services to World War I veterans returning with impairments resulted in the Smith-Hughes Act (1917) that authorized the first vocational rehabilitation services, defined as "the development of residual capacities needed for vocational effectiveness." The federal Civil Vocational Rehabilitation Act, also known as the Smith-Fess Act (1920), authorized a range of vocational rehabilitation services for civilians with physical disabilities who were either "totally or partially incapacitated for remunerative occupations." The New Deal that followed the Great Depression resulted in the Social Security Act (1935), which established, as permanent, the federally- and state-supported Vocational Rehabilitation Program. The Bardon-LaFollette Act (1943) extended vocational rehabilitation services to persons with mental retardation and mental illness. The eligibility for and the range of services provided through vocational rehabilitation were further expanded through the Rehabilitation Act of 1973; the Rehabilitation, Comprehensive Services, and Developmental Disabilities Amendments of 1978; and the Technology-Related Assistance for Individuals with Disabilities Act of 1988—all of which promoted research and development, education and training, consumer involvement, and program evaluation. Finally, the Americans with Disabilities Act of 1990 linked disability rights to civil rights and prohibited discrimination against persons with disabilities in all aspects of employment.

## VOCATIONAL REHABILITATIONISTS

Vocational rehabilitation practitioners, or vocational rehabilitationists, come from diverse educational backgrounds and are employed in a wide variety of work settings. The activities performed and the services provided by vocational rehabilitationists encompass the breadth of needs experienced by their clients in their efforts to return to suitable gainful employment after physical rehabilitation. However, whether in the public or the private sector and whether employed by a nonprofit or a for-profit organization, the focus of the vocational rehabilitationist is assisting the client in maximizing employability and thus full participation in society.

Vocational rehabilitationists include vocational evaluators, vocational counselors, and rehabilitation counselors. Their educational preparation includes coursework in the following subjects: principles of counseling, theories of vocational counseling and career development, psychometric testing and vocational assessment, medical and psychosocial aspects of disability, community resources, legislation affecting persons with disabilities, and supervised field work. Bachelors, Masters, and Doctoral degree programs are available throughout the country. Training programs are accredited by the Counsel on Rehabilitation Education (1972).

Vocational rehabilitationists practice in many different employment situations: state vocational rehabilitation agencies, private rehabilitation case management firms, insurance companies, private industry, national physical rehabilitation companies, rehabilitation facilities, hospitals, half-way houses, independent living centers, social service agencies, and schools. Clients may be involved with a host of delivery systems: the federal-state Vocational Rehabilitation Program, the federal Office of Workers' Compensation Programs, individual state workers' compensation systems, Social Security Disability Insurance benefits, long-term disability policies, catastrophic injury provisions of group health insurance, automobile liability insurance coverage, and special education plans. In addition, vocational rehabilitationists may be involved in the following activities: forensic rehabilitation (expert testimony) in benefit entitlement, medical malpractice, employment discrimination, personal injury and divorce cases, life care planning, outplacement, employee assistance programs, and health and wellness promotion.

Two distinct roles are basic to the practice of vocational rehabilitation regardless of the setting—those of counselor and of coordinator of services. As counselors, the vocational rehabilitationists are called on to perform personal adjustment, family, and group counseling, as well as offer educational and vocational guidance. As coordinators of services, rehabilitationists must identify, evaluate, and effectively manage medical, educational, vocational, and community resources. Melding these two roles into a continuum of services, vocational rehabilitationists must identify and assess client needs, develop a plan to meet these needs, research and arrange for the services necessary to achieve the plan's goals, and monitor the program and follow up on its successful completion. The vocational rehabilitationists' specific roles will be defined by their employment situation.

Many individual states maintain licensure for vocational rehabilitationists, and requirements for such licenses vary from state to state. However, the credential process developed by the Commission on Rehabilitation Counselor Certification (1973) and the subsequent Certified Insurance Rehabilitation Specialist Commission (1984), which includes specific educational and employment requirements as well as an examination, serve as a good measure of those who are adequately prepared to function as vocational rehabilitationists.

## WHAT VOCATIONAL REHABILITATIONISTS DO

Like other health care providers, vocational rehabilitationists perform an evaluation and develop a plan for the remediation of obstacles to the client's maximum recovery of function. Consistent with the general principles of rehabilitation, the vocational rehabilitation client must be encouraged and supported in setting personal goals and in determining the best ways to achieve those goals. The vocational rehabilitationist serves many roles throughout this process—sounding-board, coach, information provider, and reality tester. All roles must be grounded on the same premise: unconditional positive regard for the client.

The first step in the vocational rehabilitation process is gathering comprehensive medical records and arranging specialty evaluations as necessary to (1) document the client's impairment, (2) identify handicaps to employment and (3) define functional limitations and work capacities. Next, the client's background is analyzed, focusing on education, work history, and avocational interests. Based on these factors, the vocational rehabilitationist can determine the client's transferable skills, leading to an identification of alternate occupational goals for the client's consideration. A number of computerized job-matching systems are available to facilitate this process.

Occupational goals are described by job titles as defined in the *Dictionary of Occupational Titles (DOT)*, published by the U.S. Department of Labor. The *DOT* specifically describes the physical and intellectual demands of the more than 20,000 jobs found in the economy and is supplemented by *Selected Characteristics of Occupations Defined Within the Dictionary of Occupational Titles*. Information found in the *DOT* then forms the basis for occupational exploration by the client in determining which of the alternatives is most appropriate. This determination will take into consideration a variety of factors such as job opportunities available, wages, benefits, need for training or retraining, time-frame for same, opportunities for advancement, and promise of long-term security. Baseline data can be found in the *Occupational Outlook Handbook* or accessed through the local Division of Employment Security and data from the Bureau of Labor Statistics. Research on these factors is best done through a hands-on labor market survey of employers in the client's local area offering the jobs under consideration. Additional information can then be obtained by networking through family and friends to talk directly to people performing or knowledgeable about the jobs under consideration.

After the selection of a new job, the client may need to pursue an academic skill or on-the-job training. Sources of funding should be thoroughly researched to determine the client's eligibility. Careful consideration should be given to any course of training so that it does not delay the client's reentry to work without significantly increasing opportunities for hire, pay, or advancement. Upon completion of any necessary training, the client moves into the job placement phase of vocational rehabilitation. As with any other job seeker, the client must be focused, well-organized, well-prepared, and follow through; perseverance will result in success. During job placement the vocational rehabilitationist can play many roles: helping the client prepare for the application and interview procedures (job seeking skills training); targeting specific employers and identifying job leads (job development); arranging job interviews and helping process specific employer experiences (job placement); and, most of all, providing encouragement and support throughout (job club).

Job seeking is essentially a numbers game—the more jobs applied for, the better the chances of obtaining one. Nevertheless, job seeking must always be targeted to the jobs for which the client is best suited. The more experiences the client has in job seeking, the more effective the presentation will become. Although first jobs after rehabilitation are always hard to obtain, the client should not be wary of asking questions of the potential employer, because no job situation will be productive unless there is an employer-employee match. Follow-up with the client, and in some cases with the employer, by the vocational rehabilitationist at 30 and 90 days helps to ensure a vocational success. The vocational rehabilitation process is summarized in the box on this page.

## WHEN TO REFER A PATIENT TO A VOCATIONAL REHABILITATIONIST

Early identification and referral of potential clients is the key to successful vocational rehabilitation. In cases of catastrophic or serious injury or illness, it may be evident from the outset that patients will not be able to return to their former jobs, even with reasonable accommodation by the employer through workplace modification. In other cases, recovery of function through recuperation and rehabilitation may not meet initial projections, thus leaving patients unable to return to their former jobs. Consequently, whenever it becomes clear that patients will not be capable of resuming regular, modified, or alternate duties with their employers, vocational rehabilitation should be initiated and proceed concurrently with physical restoration measures. Whether facility-based or agency-based, the vocational rehabilitationist should be a member of the treatment team (including physicians, nurses, physical therapists, occupational therapists, and psychologists), which should have a clear picture of the patient's functional capacities. With this information, a plan is developed for the patient to return to productive and rewarding work. To

### VOCATIONAL REHABILITATION PROCESS

**INTAKE**
Receipt and review of referral information
Description of impairment, functional limitations, work capacities
Vocational interview
Determination of labor market data

**EVALUATION**
Vocational assessment
  Educational, vocational, or psychological testing
  Transferable skills analysis
Establishment of tentative job goals

**PLANNING**
Vocational exploration
Selection of targeted job goals
Labor market survey

**TRAINING (IF NECESSARY)**
Evaluation of training resources
Educational, vocational, or on-the-job training

**JOB PLACEMENT**
Job-seeking skills training
Job development
Job placement
Job club
Employer consultation
Job modification
Job coaching
Follow-up

**RELATED SERVICES**
Assistance with benefit entitlement
Identification and coordination of support services
  Architectural and vehicular modifications
  Tools and equipment
Referral for family and social services

do so the vocational rehabilitationist should receive copies of all medical reports and regularly attend any case staffings. Consultation with team members may precede direct intervention with the patient.

Efforts by care providers to wish away or minimize the extent of a patient's limitations or to extend the course of physical rehabilitation beyond the time when there is no longer progress toward functional goals are misguided. Each patient should be given the benefit of the doubt and encouraged to achieve maximum improvement. However, the longer caregivers avoid recognizing the reality of permanent impairment, the more false hope the patient assumes and the harder the adjustment will be when reality must be faced. If the vocational rehabilitationist has been introduced as a part of the treatment team and has begun to build a relationship with the patient before the patient must deal with the reality of future limitations, the easier and more effective will be the patient's transition to focusing efforts on new vocational goals.

The longer such a delay goes on, the greater the likelihood the patient may develop a negative style in adjusting to his impairment. Misunderstanding or outright rejection of such information is commonplace and is often preceded by the phrase "but you said . . ." Disappointment in the results of rehabilitation to date can lead some patients to quit on their future and even focus their energy on bitterness or anger. Other patients may adopt a disability mentality toward the rest of their lives, with an outlook characterized by "I can't." Still others whose lives may have been less than fulfilling at the onset of their illness or injury may, consciously or not, focus their efforts on maintaining their new role as impaired and become unable to resume their previous roles and responsibilities. This behavior is often described as symptom magnification or malingering, especially when economic benefits are associated with the continuing disability. Thus, without a smooth, uninterrupted transition to vocational rehabilitation, the achievements and momentum of physical rehabilitation can be lost, sometimes forever.

Often the early work of the vocational rehabilitationist involves listening to the client's lengthy history—almost as a period of testing or hazing of the professional so the client can be sure the vocational rehabilitationist can be trusted. Interestingly, this feeling-out period seems to transpire even when the injured client has made use of psychological and social services earlier in the rehabilitation process. A recounting of past events can become a chronic and self-destructive behavior unless the vocational rehabilitationist moves the client forward to begin thinking about and planning for the future. Allowing clients to remain fixated on past events may be perceived by them as a message that this is what they are supposed to do or that there is no hope for their future.

Acceptance, support, and encouragement by the vocational rehabilitationist will enable clients to move on to this phase of their rehabilitation. They will begin to believe in themselves if someone else believes in them. The job of the vocational rehabilitationist then becomes that of helping clients to establish a series of short-term, obtainable goals to speed them on their way back to meaningful work. Success breeds success and with it clients gain greater confidence and independence. With each experience, clients increase their understanding of and ability to cope with their situation and develop the skills that allow them to take charge of their own lives once again without depending on others to do for or show them how. See the Clinical Example for a description of a vocational rehabilitation plan.

## HOW TO REFER A PATIENT TO A VOCATIONAL REHABILITATIONIST

Vocational rehabilitation does not require a physician's prescription nor is it covered by health insurance, because it is not considered medically necessary. However, in many cases vocational rehabilitation assistance may be critical to patients resuming active and productive life-styles. Nothing is sadder than the situation of patients who have expended enormous energy in achieving maximum physical rehabilitation and then find that they are unable to return to work and, consequently, to their regular social activities.

Any member of the treatment team, including the patient and family members, can initiate a referral for vocational rehabilitation. The vocational rehabilitationist will require the patient's diagnosis, a clear and objective description of functional limitations and work capacities, and the purpose of the referral. Information on the patient's medical history and current medical status is necessary to understand the patient's overall needs. Background data concerning the following serve to give a more complete picture of the individual: age, sex, race, marital and family status, dependents, residence, transportation, and financial support. Any special considerations that may impact on the individual's return to work should be noted, such as architectural barriers, need for modified vehicles, or family members who will require assistance.

The aforementioned materials should be sent to the vocational rehabilitationist in advance of the initial client meeting. A call by the physician to review the materials, to highlight the unique needs of the case, and to establish lines of communication is most helpful. However, nothing can take the place of a personal meeting of patient, physician, and vocational rehabilitationist to ensure mutual understanding of the referral and a smooth transition to this new phase of rehabilitation. The box on page 561 lists the many factors that affect vocational rehabilitation.

## FACTORS AFFECTING VOCATIONAL REHABILITATION

**I. REALITY FACTORS**

Timing of referral: must be early to be effective; all necessary information provided

*Medical*

Handicaps to employment: functional limitations

Complicating medical conditions, such as hypertension, diabetes, obesity

Coping skills: ability to adapt and change; adjustment to impairment

*Educational and Vocational*

Educational achievement: grade level completed

Academic skills: current functioning

Acquired skills: job specific

Transferable skills: part of, or needed to learn, new job

Employment history: types of jobs, number of employers

Job performance: evaluations and references

*Personal and Family*

Age: if over 50

Area of residence: if urban, many unskilled jobs; if rural, few local employers

Transportation available: automobile, car pool, public transportation

Communication barrier: English as a second language, mutism, deafness, or blindness.

Family and community reaction: provide support, employment opportunities

Family responsibilities: child care, dependent relative

*Systems*

Benefit status: economic loss

Litigation pending: seeking financial windfall

**II. BEHAVIORAL FACTORS**

Denial of disability and limitations

Fixation on reliving past events

Blaming of others for condition

Avoidance of responsibility for own recovery

Dependency

Anger or depression

Overprotection by caregivers and family

Identification of self by job role

Disability mentality

Symptom magnification

Malingering

Plaintiff mentality

## WHAT TO EXPECT FROM A VOCATIONAL REHABILITATION PROGRAM

The physician and other members of the rehabilitation team receive a full report in writing and, if possible, in person from the vocational rehabilitationist immediately after their initial evaluation. This report provides a clear picture of the client's education, work history and avocational interests, as well as an analysis of these facts in regards to employment potential and recommendations for any further evaluations, such as educational, psychological, or vocational testing, and functional or work capacity evaluation.

After the vocational assessment of the client is completed, the vocational rehabilitationist presents a written vocational rehabilitation plan established in conjunction with the client. The rationale for the plan is explained, and the plan's goals, action steps, timeframes, assigned responsibilities and projected costs are stated. The plan should be based on specific job goals that have been determined as most suitable for the client in consideration of all accumulated information. The vocational rehabilitation plan is based on an individualized approach to meeting a client's needs and provides for options for achieving the job goals.

It is imperative that the job goals develop from the client's ideas and initiative as much as possible. The process of involving clients in planning their vocational rehabilitation may require a series of counseling sessions focusing on identifying information needs and then reviewing the results of research the clients may need to perform in order to make an informed choice. Eventually, job goals must be agreed on by the client and the vocational rehabilitationist. A written document or signed contract can formalize this process and serve as a guide for future activities. Some clients will require stronger direction or will need to model behavior first demonstrated by the vocational rehabilitationist in research tasks and will

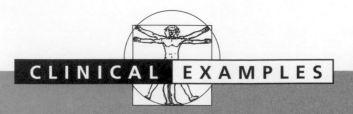

# CLINICAL EXAMPLES

## VOCATIONAL REHABILITATION

EDITOR'S NOTE—The following is an example of a typical cost and time-line analysis provided to an insurer by a vocational rehabilitationist.

**EXAMPLE**
**History**

A 45-year-old high school graduate, journeyman maintenance electrician, earning $23.50 per hour, suffered an on-the-job injury to his left ankle after a 60-foot fall. His injury required a tibiotalar fusion. Restrictions precluding his return to his previous occupation include no climbing, balancing, or working at heights; no overhead lifting exceeding 30 pounds; and no prolonged standing or walking. He was referred for a vocational rehabilitation evaluation by his employer before the last of his three surgeries.

**Vocational Rehabilitation Plan**

*Job goal:* Electronics Technician
*Projected wage:* $16-$20/hour

1. Three semesters training in electronics technology at a technology institute leading to certificate as an electronics technician:
   Tuition $2750
   Books, supplies, and fees 450

2. Transportation costs (18 months):
   Mileage $1150
   Tolls 160
   Parking 0

3. Educational guidance and supportive counseling by vocational rehabilitationist:
   7 hours @ $70 per hour $490

4. Job development and job placement by vocational rehabilitationist in conjunction with career placement office:
   $500 per month for up to 3 months $1500

5. Follow-up with client and employer at 30 and 90 days to ensure vocational success:
   2 hours @ $70 per hour $140

   TOTAL COST: $6640

   *John Allen*

gain confidence or motivation as they become immersed in the process. Other clients may fight or undermine vocational rehabilitation because of unresolved issues concerning their disability or simply to hold on to the secondary financial gain of various benefit programs.

Once a vocational rehabilitation plan has been established, it must be communicated to all members of the treatment team and to the family. Approval by funding sources such as the state vocational rehabilitation agency, the insurance company, or the employer may be necessary. Then the plan should be initiated on a timely basis to ensure that clients can maximize their interest and motivation and not slip backward into focusing on their disability and limitations. Throughout the course of the vocational rehabilitation, contact should be maintained with the physician and other members of the treatment team to anticipate or solve any new client needs. Family members should be consulted periodically to ensure that clear understanding and support of the client's activities remains strong. A good plan will only succeed through a well-coordinated effort of all persons involved in the client's rehabilitation.

## Suggested Reading

Commission on Rehabilitation Counselor Certification: *Guide to rehabilitation counselor certification*, Rolling Meadows, IL, 1990,

Council on Rehabilitation Education: *Accreditation manual for rehabilitation counselor education programs*, Champaign-Urbana, IL, 1991,

LaFon RN: The past, present and the future: How can we avoid the pitfalls and realize the potential of vocational rehabilitation? *J Private Sector Rehab* 3:75-84, 1988.

McGowan JF, Porter TL: *An introduction to the vocational rehabilitation process*. Washington, D.C., 1967, U.S. Department of Health, Education, and Welfare; Rehabilitation Services Administration.

Parker RM, Szymanski EM, editors: *Rehabilitation counseling basics and beyond*, ed 2, Austin, TX, 1992, PRO-ED.

Rubin SE, Roessler RT: *Foundations of the vocational rehabilitation process*, ed 3, Austin, TX, 1987, PRO-ED.

U.S. Department of Labor, Employment and Training Administration: *Dictionary of occupational titles*, ed 4 rev, Washington, D.C, 1991, U.S. Government Printing Office.

U.S. Department of Labor, Employment and Training Administration: *Guide for occupational exploration*, Washington, D.C, 1979, U.S. Government Printing Office.

U.S. Department of Labor, Employment and Training Administration. *Selected characteristics of occupations defined within the dictionary of occupational titles*, Washington, D.C, 1981, U.S. Government Printing Office.

# CHAPTER 48

# OCCUPATIONAL THERAPY

*Karen Jacobs*
*Rowland G. Hazard*

## DEFINITION OF OCCUPATIONAL THERAPY

Occupational therapy is a health profession that helps people to be as independent as possible in performing socially defined skills that broadly relate to self-care, work, play, and leisure activities. Occupational therapy practitioners use goal-directed or purposeful activities in treatment to enhance or maintain occupational performance, and to prevent or overcome occupational dysfunction. Purposeful activities are defined as tasks or experiences in which an individual actively participates; these activities are used as the primary therapeutic instruments of change by occupational therapy practitioners.[1] Purposeful activities may include homemaking or work tasks, exercise, sports, games, or arts and crafts activities. Other agents of change include therapeutic interaction, patient education, and adjunctive treatments, such as splinting, seating, facilitation, and inhibition procedures.

## EDUCATIONAL REQUIREMENTS FOR REGISTERED OCCUPATIONAL PRACTITIONERS

There are three different levels of occupational therapy personnel: (1) the Registered Occupational Therapist, (2) the Certified Occupational Therapy Assistant, and (3) the Occupational Therapy Aide. The term *occupational therapy practitioner* refers to those practioners who are certified by the American Occupational Therapy Certification Board as a Registered Occupational Therapist or a Certified Occupational Therapy Assistant.[1] As of 1995, 49 states, the District of Columbia, and Puerto Rico have enacted laws regulating the practice of occupational therapy. The American Occupational Therapy Association believes that licensure is an effective method for preventing unnecessary and inappropriate health care expenditures.

The American Occupational Therapy Association represents the professional interests of over 50,000 occupational therapy practitioners and students. The Association is headquartered in Bethesda, Maryland.

The Registered Occupational Therapist has completed a four-year baccalaureate or two years masters degree in an accredited occupational therapy program as well as six to nine months of supervised fieldwork experience. The academic curriculum includes courses in anatomy, neurology, neurophysiology, psychology, and the social sciences. Once academic and fieldwork experiences are completed, the individual is eligible to take a national certification examination that is administered under the auspices of the American Occupational Therapy Certification Board. Also, postprofessional masters and doctoral programs for Registered Occupational Therapists are available. Many of these prepare the therapist for specialized practice, teaching, or research.

The Certified Occupational Therapy Assistant has completed a two-year college program and two months of supervised fieldwork experience. The academic curriculum focuses on human physiology and tasks and skills used in daily life. Once academic and fieldwork experiences are completed, the individual is eligible to take a national certification examination administered by the American Occupational Therapy Certification Board.

The Occupational Therapy Aide typically does not have any formal academic education in occupational therapy but has received on-the-job training that equips him/her to assist with routine procedures in occupational therapy programs.[2]

## ROLES AND FUNCTIONS OF REGISTERED OCCUPATIONAL THERAPY PRACTITIONERS IN SPECIFIC PRACTICE FIELDS

Occupational therapy may be provided to people of all ages who have physical, psychosocial, or developmental disabilities. These may include individuals with work-related injuries; people who have had a stroke or have arthritis, cancer, or other debilitating illnesses; children with congenital defects, birth trauma, or brain dysfunction; individuals with mental illness or with a substance abuse condition; individuals with burns, spinal cord injuries, head injuries, or other traumatic injuries; individuals with diseases such as multiple sclerosis, Guillain-Barré disease, or amyotrophic lateral sclerosis; and individuals with orthopedic or sports-related injuries.

Impairment of the functional components of occupational performance, such as sensory-motor, cognitive-perceptual, and socio-emotional, can be a result of disease, trauma, excessive stress, maladaptive lifestyle, or developmental abnormalities. According to the AMA's *Guides to the evaluation of permanent impairment*,[3] impairment is considered permanent once sufficient time has passed for tissue repair to have taken place, the impairment has ceased to continue changing, and further medical or surgical intervention is not likely to produce beneficial results.[1] The role of the occupational therapy practitioner is to intervene with an individual to enhance development, recovery, and learning.[4] They also intervene with an individual and interact with the environment to enhance adaptation and learning that promote a satisfactory individual-environment interaction.[4] Intervention to enhance the individual's access within society and to facilitate political and attitudinal changes in society and culture is also possible.[4]

The major function of an occupational therapist is to provide quality occupational therapy services, including assessment, intervention, program planning and implementation, discharge-planning-related documentation, and communication. Occupational therapists use a variety of standardized and nonstandardized evaluation procedures to gain an accurate historical and clinical picture of functional capacities in the spheres of: (1) independent living and daily living skills and performance; (2) physical skills and performance; (3) cognitive skills and performance; (4) psychosocial skills and performance; (5) therapeutic adaptations; and (6) specialized evaluations (special training is required for administration) (see box on this page). Specific approaches vary from setting to setting. Subsequent services may include direct, monitored, and consultative approaches.[1]

### FUNCTIONAL ASSESSMENTS USED BY OCCUPATIONAL THERAPISTS IN MENTAL HEALTH PRACTICE

Allen Cognitive Level Test
Bay Area Functional Performance Evaluation
Comprehensive Evaluation of Basic Living Skills
Comprehensive Occupational Therapy Evaluation
Independent Living Skills
Milwaukee Evaluation of Daily Living Skills
Parachek Geriatric Rating Scale
Routine Task Inventory
Kolman Evaluation of Living Skills
Scorable Self-care Evaluation
Azima Battery*
Comprehensive Assessment Process*
Goodman Battery*
Shoemyen Battery*

*Projective Tests

The major function of a Certified Occupational Therapy Assistant is to provide quality occupational therapy services to assigned individuals under the supervision of a Registered Occupational Therapist. The level of supervision is related to the ability of the Certified Occupational Therapy Assistant to provide safely and effectively those interventions delegated by an Registered Occupational Therapist.[1]

There is a fundamental difference between occupational therapy and physical therapy. This difference is in the means of the therapeutic intervention. Occupational therapy stresses work, self-care, and leisure activities, that is, purposeful activity that will promote functional independence. Physical therapy emphasizes exercise and movement to increase physical interaction with the environment. Overlap exists between the two disciplines and will continue to grow with the trend toward the adoption of a transdisciplinary approach in many treatment settings.

Occupational therapy practitioners provide services in many settings, such as acute-care hospitals, comprehensive outpatient and inpatient rehabilitation centers, long- and short-term psychiatric facilities, skilled nursing facilities, outpatient clinics, community mental health centers, day care centers, private and public schools, independent practices, home health agencies, and business and industry.

## Acute-Care Settings

In an acute-care setting, the purpose of occupational therapy is to assist the client in achieving a maximum level of independent living by developing those capacities that remain after injury or illness. The occupational therapist's initial focus is on identifying those pathologic conditions or impaired functions that preclude independence and productivity. Occupational therapists evaluate and treat:

- impaired muscle strength, range of motion, and endurance
- impaired concentration, attention span, organizational skills, problem solving, and endurance
- impaired visual-spatial relationships, body schemes, figure-ground discrimination, eye-hand coordination, and motor skills/coordination
- impaired ability to perform daily activities such as self-care skills, work activities, and play or leisure skills

Occupational therapists also seek to prevent or inhibit muscle atrophy, prevent or minimize deformity, increase pain tolerance, and enhance interaction with the environment. They are also vitally concerned with the psychosocial impairments and deficits that frequently result from the client's physical or mental illness or trauma.

## Functional Restoration

The provision of services in functional restoration has been one of the most common specialty areas for occupational therapy practitioners. However, within this area there has been a trend for practitioners to become specialized in subjects and activities such as hand therapy or work disability prevention and management. In hand therapy, for example, the occupational therapists guide clients through a comprehensive rehabilitation program including:

- wound care
- techniques to improve range of motion, sensation, or strength
- fabricate an orthosis or splint to protect, strengthen, or increase function
- evaluate the ability to perform tasks required on the job
- training in the use of an artificial hand
- instruction in joint protection and energy conservation

- arrange for special equipment to improve function

A sampling of procedures used in evaluation includes:

- manual muscle testing to ascertain the strength of a muscle by manual evaluation
- goniometry to measure passive and active range of motion (ROM)
- dynamometry to measure hand strength
- sensory testing for light touch, pain, temperature, or stereognosis
- manual dexterity and motor function testing, including use of the Crawford Small Parts Dexterity Test or Purdue Pegboard. In addition, the occupational therapist assesses the client's level of functional independence in activities of daily living. Performance testing—that is, observing the client engaging in an activity such as lacing a leather wallet—may be used to measure problem-solving ability or eye-hand coordination.

## Work Disability Prevention and Management

Occupational therapists use work-related activities in the assessment and treatment of persons whose ability to function in a competitive work environment has been impaired by developmental abnormalities, physical or emotional illness, or injury. Examples of assessment procedures include physical capacity evaluation, functional capacity evaluation, ergonomic work site analysis, post-offer screening, endurance and tolerance testing, range of motion and muscle strength testing, and interest inventories. The physician oversees the evaluation of the individual's functional capacity. This functional capacity evaluation assesses the individual's ability to perform certain activities associated with the work environment in a structured setting (see Chapters 18 and 51). Assessment of functional capacity may be one of many duties carried out by the occupational therapists in this setting. Other roles and responsibilities of the occupational therapist in work disability prevention and management are:

1. Obtain a comprehensive history of the individual's occupational performance related to activities of daily living, work, play, and leisure, and identify the individual's work-related behaviors, interests, abilities, needs, and goals.
2. Assess the sensorimotor, cognitive, and psychological skills and deficits of the worker and potential worker while considering future goals.
3. Analyze resources, constraints, demands, and ex-

pectations in home, school, work site, or community environment of worker or potential worker to facilitate progress toward identified goals.[5]

Occupational therapy's ideal goal is injury or disability prevention. When this goal is not attainable and the client sustains an injury or becomes impaired, occupational therapists focus attention on assessing individual needs and follow that with any form of intervention deemed appropriate.[5] Intervention might include work hardening, work conditioning, or transition programs. In addition, occupational therapy practitioners have been active in the implementation of the Americans with Disabilities Act by providing services to employers and individuals with disabilities, such as delineating the essential functions of a job, writing job descriptions, and recommending reasonable accommodations (see Chapter 50).

## Mental Health Practice

With the increasing emphasis on a continuum of care for psychiatric services, clients may begin with short-term inpatient hospitalization and proceed to residential, then outpatient care. The diagnostic categories frequently treated by occupational therapy practitioners cover a wide range including schizophrenia, depression, manic depression, borderline personality, stress reactions, chemical dependency, eating disorders, antisocial personality, autism, and adolescent adjustment reaction.

An important trend in mental health has been the focus on functional assessment. From a psychiatric viewpoint, functional assessments are used to predict community adjustment, to select appropriate housing, and to assist with vocational placement."

The goal of mental health occupational therapy is to aid in:

- improving the cognitive, social, and organizational skills required for success in work, school, and leisure activities
- increasing the ability to perform self-care activities, such as personal hygiene, which improve health and social acceptance
- increasing skills in community living, such as use of public transportation to improve self-sufficiency
- increasing recognition of stress indicators and developing coping skills[3]

Simulated or real activities, such as a job interview, that provide individuals the opportunity to practice life skills, recognize difficulties, and learn ways to improve performance are examples of treatment activities.

## Practice with Developmental Abnormalities

It is important that individuals with developmental abnormalities receive occupational therapy beginning at birth and continuing throughout the life span if the need still exists. The ideal program offers a family-centered approach in which the individual is treated within the environment, which includes the family, caregivers, or an independent living situation. The environment is evaluated by the occupational therapist, who can provide adaptations to aid functional performance, such as providing adapted seating or assistive technology. Occupational therapists provide screening for developmental delay and evaluate developmental abilities and adaptive functioning. Standardized tests such as the Bayley Scales of Infant Development and the Peabody Developmental Motor Scales are used to measure gross and fine motor abilities and skills such as stacking blocks and drawing. To assess fine and gross motor abilities, adaptive language, and psychosocial areas, occupational therapists use the Gesell Developmental Scales. The Erhardt Developmental Prehension Assessment is used to measure involuntary and voluntary arm-hand patterns. Many nonstandardized tests are used by occupational therapists to measure muscle tone, reflex patterns, motor development, and sensory status as well as the observations of spontaneous behavior.

Using purposeful activity, occupational therapy practitioners seek to minimize the effects of disease, injury, congenital deficit, disability, developmental delay, or deprivation in infants and children. Occupational therapists use a variety of screenings and comprehensive assessments. Some commonly-used instruments are listed in the top left-hand box on page 568. In general, the goal of occupational therapy for infants and children is to assist them, to the greatest degree possible, to achieve age-appropriate self-help and play and leisure skills. Examples of specific goals are listed in two boxes on page 568.

## Practice with the Elderly

The OTR provides services for the elderly in settings such as hospitals, home health programs, community-based health care centers, hospices, congregate living facilities, outpatient rehabilitation facilities, senior centers, adult day- and long-term care facilities, community service agencies, and retirement housing.

## INSTRUMENTS COMMONLY USED BY OCCUPATIONAL THERAPISTS IN SERVICES FOR INFANTS AND CHILDREN

Pediatric Evaluation of Disability Inventory (PEDI)
Miller Assessments for Preschoolers (MAP)
Sensory Integration and Praxis Test (SIPT)
Marianne Frostig Developmental Test of Visual Perception
Motor-Free Visual Perception Test
Berry-Buktenica Developmental Test of Visual Motor Integration (VMI)
Bayley Scales of Infant Development*
Brazelton Behavioral Assessment Scale*
Brigance Screen*
Denver Developmental Screening Test*
Developmental Screening*
Gesell Developmental Tests*

*Developmental Tests

## EXAMPLES OF SPECIFIC OCCUPATIONAL THERAPY GOALS FOR INFANTS

- Improved feeding skills
- Improved behavioral state, organization, and regulation
- Prevention of deformities through therapeutic positioning and splinting
- Promotion of age appropriate mobility and motor skills
- Facilitation of developmental skills and play behaviors

## EXAMPLES OF SPECIFIC OCCUPATIONAL THERAPY GOALS FOR CHILDREN

- Prevention of deformities
- Facilitation of normal developmental sequence
- Decreasing the effect of pathologic conditions on functional abilities
- Improvement of motor development, self-concept, and emotional maturation
- Promotion of independence in activities of daily living
- Fabrication of, or adjustment and training in the use of, assistive, prosthetic, or orthotic devices
- Environmental adaptation to enable increased independence

"Occupational therapists who work with the elderly assess the older person's environment as well as his or her functional performance to evaluate the match between environment and person."[6] The assessment of the environment should include physical features, such as accessibility and design, as well as cultural and social aspects of the environment as they relate to behavior.[6]

Functional performance tests, such as the Barthel Self-Care Index, assess self-care tasks, such as feeding, transfer skills, personal hygiene, toileting, bathing, ambulation, dressing, using stairs, and bowel and bladder continence.[7] In other functional performance scales, daily activities are divided more hierarchically into: self-maintaining activities of daily living and instrumental activities of daily living. The ADL include the basic self-care tasks mentioned previously, and the IADL are more complex tasks, such as managing medications.[8]

Treatment goals in occupational therapy for the elderly include the promotion of functional independence, prevention of impairment, and maintenance of wellness. Examples of services provided by occupational therapy practitioners include:

- education and retraining in activities of daily living
- therapeutic adaptations, such as assistive equipment and design to promote mobility in home and community
- sensorimotor treatment for strengthening, endurance, range of motion, coordination, and balance
- adaptation to sensory loss such as impaired vision or hearing
- therapeutic activities for memory, orientation, cognitive integration, and the life-review process
- prevention and health promotion through retirement planning for leisure time, self-management skills, socialization, energy conservation, body mechanics, and joint protection
- care of the terminally ill through maintenance of independent living skills and meaningful activity

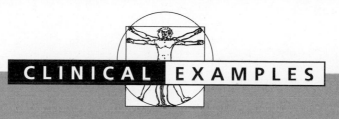

## OCCUPATIONAL THERAPY

### EXAMPLE

#### History

An 8-year-old girl's arms and hands were severely burned with scalding water. The severity of the injury has made it virtually impossible for her to flex or extend the fingers or wrists. On admission to the hospital, the occupational therapist viewed the wounds during initial procedures on the ward to determine areas of involvement that could require positioning splints. Also during the initial assessment, a complete active and passive range of motion (ROM) test was performed and a strength evaluation provided. This was compared to the preinjury level of function as determined through an interview with the patient and her parents.

#### Therapy

Treatment includes the following:

- Activities to increase hand coordination, range of motion, and strength
- Splinting and application of compression garments to restore movement and reduce scarring
- Intensive functional retraining using school work and daily living simulation models

#### Progression of Impairment

Over the next three years, the patient had numerous operations for skin grafting and transplantation, as well as tendon lengthening. The occupational therapist assisted with psychological counseling and physical rehabilitation. Currently, at age 14 years, the patient is considered to have reached maximum medical improvement. She has persistent impairment of her hands with respect to motor skills, sensory levels, and fine manipulation. Discomfort and psychological difficulties are also present. The occupational therapist continues to work with her to increase her functional adaptation for the activities required at home, socially, and recreationally as well as assisting with school and training programs directed toward a realistic career goal.

*Karen Jacobs*
*Rowland G. Hazard*

## REFERRAL PROCESS

### Traditional Medical Model

Patients with disabling medical conditions visit their physicians with certain expectations. Generally, their major goal is to have their symptoms diagnosed and treated. This process involves deduction and testing of hypothetical pathoanatomic lesions that might produce the symptoms and that can be cured or palliated through appropriate therapy. While many diseases resolve spontaneously or respond to medical interventions, a wide variety of medical conditions persist despite the physicians' best efforts, leaving patients with impaired functional abilities.

It is in this setting that the physician can get the most help from an occupational therapist. Faced with increasing pressures on time and resources, many physicians find it harder and harder to look beyond the basic business of diagnosis and treatment to the often complicated issues of matching functional capacities and environmental demands. Furthermore, relatively few physicians are well-trained in assessing function and translating such assessments into clear and realistic statements about feasibility of activities and prognosis. This inadequacy is reflected in the frustration many physicians feel when patients with chronic musculoskeletal pain present work return forms requesting estimations of capacity for activities such as lifting, sitting, standing, climbing, and crawling. Physicians require the help of other professionals with such estimations. Physicians may be further taxed by patients who have chronic illnesses that elude operational diagnosis or who do not respond to treatment. When such patients ask the physician how they are supposed to deal with their predicaments, a referral to an occupational therapist may well be in order.

### When and Why to Refer

Whenever the physician decides the patient's condition is likely to lead to significant loss of function, a referral should be considered. Initially, a referral may be required for secondary prevention of disability. For example, early mobilization and reactivation through partial work return may be a critical step in avoiding prolonged sick leave. As the patient's condition reaches maximal medical improvement, careful evaluation of the patient's physical and psychosocial capacities becomes a cornerstone of advice regarding return to work and other activities. Functional evaluation can also be essential in estimating the patient's qualification for workers' compensation, third party settlements, Social Security Administration sup-

port, and vocational rehabilitation. Occupational therapists generally are trained and equipped to evaluate broad categories of human capacities. Their facilities for measuring and promoting people's functioning may be a great boon to physicians and their patient with impairments.

### References

1. American Occupational Therapy Association: *Occupational therapy roles,* Rockville, Md, 1993, American Occupational Therapy Association.
2. Punwar A: *Occupational therapy: Principles and practice,* ed 2, Baltimore, 1994, William & Wilkins, p 49.
3. American Medical Association: *Guides to the evaluation of permanent impairment,* ed 4, Chicago, 1993, American Medical Association.
4. Boston University: *Philosophical statements: Department of Occupational Therapy,* Boston, 1994, Boston University.
5. Jacobs K, Bettencourt C, Ellsworth P, et al: Statement: occupational therapy service in work practice, *Am J Occ Ther* 46:1086-1088, 1992.
6. Hasselkus B: Functional disability and older adults. In Hopkin H, Smith H, editors: *Willard and Spackman's occupational therapy,* Philadelphia, 1993, JB Lippincott, pp 742-752.
7. Mahoney F, Barthel D: Functional evaluations: The Barthel Index, *Maryland State Med J* 14:61-65, 1965.
8. Lawton M, Brody E: Assessment of older people: Self-maintaining and instrumental activities of daily living, *Gerontologist* 9:179-186, 1969.

### Suggested Readings

American Occupational Therapy Association: *Facts about occupational therapy: Occupational therapy in mental health,* Rockville, Md, 1992, Occupational Therapy Association.

American Occupational Therapy Organization: *Facts about occupational therapy: Occupational therapy and long term care in mental health,* Rockville, Md, 1992, American Occupational Therapy Association.

American Occupational Therapy Association: Purposeful activities, *Am J Occ Ther* 37:805-806, 1983.

Azima F: Diseases of the nervous system. Monograph Suppl 22 and in Hemphill BJ, editor: *The evaluative process in occupational therapy,* Thorofare, NJ, 1961, 1982, Slack.

Bair J: *How do you describe occupational therapy? Administration and Management Special Interest Section Newsletter,* Rockville, Md, 1991, American Occupational Therapy Association.

Ehrenberg F: Comprehensive assessment process. In Hemphill BJ, editor: *The evaluative process in occupational therapy,* Thorofare, NJ, 1982, Slack.

Evaskus M: *Goodman battery.* In Hemphill BJ, editor: *The evaluative process in occupational therapy,* Thorofare, NJ, 1982, Slack.

Llorens L: How do you describe occupational therapy? *Administration and Management Special Interest Section Newsletter,* Rockville, Md, 1991, American Occupational Therapy Association.

Shoemyen C: Occupational therapy orientation and evaluation: A study of procedure and media, *Am J Occ Ther* 24:276, 1970.

Smith H: Assessment and evaluation: An overview. In Hopkins H, Smith H, editors, *Willard and Spackman's occupational therapy,* Philadelphia, 1993, JB Lippincott, pp 176-179.

# HUMAN RESOURCE MANAGEMENT: THE INTERFACE FOR GETTING DISABLED EMPLOYEES BACK TO WORK

*Michael Cooper*
*Margaret Bryant*

An injury or illness that prevents an employee from working creates a loss both for the individual and for the employer. For the individual, it means a dramatic change in day-to-day activity, including a course of evaluation and treatment by a team of medical providers who may not fully understand the needs, resources, and limitations of their patient. For the employer, it often means a loss of control in the information-gathering and decision-making process concerning the nature of the medical condition, and its impact on the individual's employability, the expected duration of the absence, the conditions of the employee's return, and the employee's status in the interim.

A disability-related interruption in the normal employment relationship may be aggravated by underlying problems that exist between employees and their managers. On a larger scale, employee-relation problems as a result of a lack of consistent and effective policy implementation may also exist throughout the organization. If the quality of management-employee relations suffers from unresolved human resources issues, employees may be predisposed to request disability leaves more often and to stay out on leave longer.

Tension between a particular employee and manager may manifest itself in the disability leave process through an adversarial "stand-off" between the employer and the employee's medical care providers. Moreover, general dissatisfaction and hostility among employees may nurture an environment where "getting everything you can out of the employer" is part of the corporate culture. In such instances, obtaining a leave of absence with income may be viewed as a prize.

Notwithstanding the fact that real needs drive most requests for disability leaves, employees who feel they have "beaten the system" can infect an already disgruntled staff with hostility, resentment, or apathy. In such cases, the employer suffers a loss disproportionate to the absence of the individual employee who is on leave. Identifying and resolving the underlying employee relations issues will serve to build a more positive and healthy human resources environment and to discourage unnecessary and prolonged disability leaves.

The role of the Human Resource Manager/Department is discussed herein. This role is often combined with others in small businesses. In this chapter, the term "employer" will be used to conform to the language of various laws but it should be assumed to be in that role as the employer in an employing capacity (hiring, firing, and defining or changing the role of the employed individual). This role requires the active intervention of the skills of human resources management and involves the human resource manager as an advisor or director to the person who is in charge of these decisions for the business.

## ASSESSING THE HR ENVIRONMENT AND THE QUALITY OF MANAGEMENT/EMPLOYEE RELATIONS

Even before the employment relationship begins, the human resources (HR) function has opportunities and obligations with respect to prospective employees. The more thorough, informative, and controlled the recruiting and selection process, the more likely an employer is to attract, hire, and retain individuals who are qualified for the job and well-matched with the organization. To that end, recruitment and selection policies and practices should be tailored to the particular needs of the organization, as well as that of the position to be filled. Through these policies and practices, the employer has the opportunity to establish an employee relations environment that emphasizes fairness, consistency, and the importance to the organization of getting the job done within reasonable expectations for reliability and attendance.

There are many tools that are used in the recruitment and selection process to aid the human resources function in the placement of individuals who are well qualified and compatible with the goals and expectations of the organization. Job applications, preemployment skills tests, and preemployment psychological and medical examinations routinely have been used to screen and help select employees from a pool of job applicants.

These and other screening devices may be subject to certain restrictions imposed by anti-discrimination laws, such as Title VII of the Civil Rights Act of 1964 (Title VII) and the Americans with Disabilities Act (ADA) (see Chapter 50). Specifically, preemployment aptitude tests, psychological profiles, and other job-specific testing procedures must be validated as meeting certain requirements formulated by the Equal Employment Opportunity Commission (EEOC). Moreover, the EEOC has established specific guidance under the ADA prohibiting preemployment medical and psychological inquiries.

One of the most important tools in the selection and hiring process is the job description, which is discussed in greater detail later in this chapter. While not required by law, job descriptions for a particular job category are extremely useful at a variety of stages in the employment relationship and can be the foundation for performance expectations that are concrete and objective for all individuals in that job category.

In terms of screening and selecting qualified applicants, job descriptions are a written explanation of the tasks and duties of that particular job. They should identify the essential and nonessential functions of the job, indicating which functions are essential, and they must be reviewed periodically to insure that any changes in the actual duties, tasks, training, skills, or expectations for the job have been incorporated into the written description.

During the course of the employment relationship, performance should be monitored periodically to measure how well the employee is meeting job expectations. Performance appraisals, evaluations, and reviews should be done on a regular basis in a logical and orderly fashion, using standardized and objective criteria. When performance is reviewed sporadically, insincerely, or not at all, employees lack the feedback they need to know how they are doing on the job. This can lead to dissatisfaction, discontent, and disappointment both for the employee and for management. Perhaps even more damaging is the lack of any documentation for counseling, discipline, or discharge should such adverse personnel actions become necessary.

With respect to training, advancement, and promotion, corporate policies and procedures must reflect the same sensitivity to fairness, consistency, and objectivity as other personnel actions. Employees should be judged on the basis of established criteria that are applied evenhandedly to all similarly situated candidates. When employees perceive that favoritism, bias, or other subjective factors have played a role in the selection process, management is discredited and employees begin to distrust the decision-making process.

Perhaps the most volatile personnel actions involve reprimand, counseling, discipline, and ultimately discharge when employees fail to meet performance, conduct, or attendance expectations. The establishment and consistent application of fair and effective policies on discipline and discharge are essential to preserve management's ability to take adverse personnel actions while minimizing the risk of incurring charges, complaints, or lawsuits. When such actions become necessary, it is critical that employees perceive the process and the procedures as neutral, fairminded, and based on job-related concerns.

Not uncommon among organizations is a lack of adequate training for managers and supervisors, not only regarding how to manage the injured or disabled employee, but in employment laws generally. Managers should be knowledgeable about good human resources management practices and about the various anti-discrimination laws, their impact on corporate policies and personnel actions, and the rights that they accord to their subordinates. Supervisors and managers should also have a working knowledge of workers' compensation, family and medical leave laws, and disability rights laws, including the Americans with Disabilities Act (see Chapter 50), and state disability laws. Layered over a solid understanding of the applicable laws should be training in basic employee relations skills that are essential for every management and supervisory position.

Another potential source of employee relations difficulties is the misinterpretation or misapplication of personnel policies. All too often the policies contained in an employee handbook, supervisory manual, or other collection of rules and procedures are unknown, misunderstood, misapplied, or simply ignored. From an employee-relations viewpoint, this can be very damaging, as management's credibility, fairness, and consistency may be questioned. Also, the organization may be needlessly exposing itself to the potential for a claim of discrimination, or perhaps breach of contract or wrongful termination. If aggrieved employees can point to an applicable written policy or standard operating procedure for discipline that was not followed, they have significantly bolstered a potential discrimination claim.

Related to this are the problems that may result from *ad hoc* decision-making by managers or supervisors. Again, without following prescribed procedures and policies for workplace conduct, management is vulnerable to charges that personnel actions are arbitrary, unfair, inconsistent, or discriminatory. It is important for management's response to a problem to be viewed as predictable, even-handed, and consistent with prior actions. This not only provides employees with an understanding of the consequences for misconduct or poor performance, but it also protects management against charges that an individual was singled out for unfair treatment because of sex, race, religion, disability, age, or other protected characteristics.

Sometimes there is a weak link in the management chain that cannot be corrected by training or even flawless personnel policies and procedures. When a manager or supervisor has failed to grasp the need for sensitivity to employee-relations issues or lacks the ability to overcome deficiencies in communicating with employees, management may have to remove that individual and repair the damage by installing a manager with the necessary skills and knowledge to create a positive employee relations environment.

## THE BASICS OF EQUAL EMPLOYMENT OPPORTUNITY

The concept of equal employment opportunity (EEO) is a by-product of the struggle for civil rights during the 1950s and 1960s. As it is known today, equal employment opportunity is a creation of federal and state statutes that prohibit certain conduct by employers. It encompasses a wide range of employment-relations concepts, such as disparate treatment, affirmative action, workplace harassment, glass ceiling, and wrongful discharge, to name a few. A brief overview of the major federal EEO laws follows:

1. *Title VII of the Civil Rights Act of 1964* prohibits discrimination based on race, color, religion, sex, or national origin. In 1978, the Pregnancy Discrimination Act amended Title VII to include pregnancy and related conditions, and in 1991 Title VII was amended to allow for jury trials, punitive damages, and compensatory damages (for example, for pain and suffering). The amendment places a monetary cap on combined punitive and compen-

satory damages per claimant depending on employer size. The amendment also makes it easier for claimants to bring certain kinds of claims.

2. *Equal Pay Act of 1963* prohibits pay differentials based on sex. Employers may not pay employees of one sex less than they pay employees of the opposite sex for work that requires equal skill, effort, and responsibility and is performed under similar working conditions.

3. *Age Discrimination in Employment Act* prohibits discrimination against individuals age 40 or older.

4. *Americans with Disabilities Act* makes it unlawful for employers to discriminate against employees on the basis of disability. Reasonable accommodation to enable a disabled individual to perform the essential duties of a job must be provided unless it would pose an undue hardship to an employer.

5. *Executive Orders 11246 and 11141* ban discrimination on the basis of race, sex, disability, and veterans' status, and require affirmative action on the part of certain federal government contractors. Executive Order 11141 prohibits discrimination on the basis of age by government contractors.

6. *Vocational Rehabilitation Act of 1973, Sections 503 and 504* bans discrimination against disabled persons by federal contractors and grant recipients, who also are required to take affirmative action in hiring qualified disabled individuals.

7. *Vietnam Era Veterans' Readjustment Assistance Act of 1974* calls for affirmative action by federal contractors to employ and advance in employment qualified veterans of the Vietnam era and all disabled veterans.

8. *Civil Rights Act of 1966* prohibits racial discrimination in certain areas of private employment.

9. *Immigration Reform and Control Act of 1986* bans intentional discrimination on the basis of citizenship or national origin. These anti-discrimination provisions do not apply to illegal aliens or in the limited circumstances when U.S. citizenship is required by law.

10. *Fair Labor Standards Act* requires minimum rates of pay and overtime for most employees.

11. *Employee Polygraph Protection Act* generally prohibits private employers from requiring or requesting that any employee or job applicant take a lie detector test (except in very limited circumstances) and from discharging, disciplining, or discriminating against an employee or prospective employee for refusing to take a test.

12. *State Laws* Many state fair-employment-practice laws prohibit job discrimination on the basis of age, race, creed, color, national origin, sex, marital status, or disability. Some also prohibit discrimination on the basis of sexual preference.

## BASIC PRINCIPLES OF EQUAL EMPLOYMENT OPPORTUNITY

In addition to the statutes, there are some basic rules of conduct for employers to follow to minimize the risk of intentional and inadvertent discriminatory actions:

1. Applicants and employees with equal qualifications, skills, and abilities must be treated equally.
2. Employers must be able to provide valid business-related reasons for adverse employment actions against applicants and employees in a protected class.
   a. Employers must show that policies and rules are enforced uniformly.
   b. Employers must show, by documentation, that the supervisor followed policy, whether written or established by practice, on warnings or corrective counseling prior to taking any action (except for serious problems or infractions).
3. Standards that appear to be neutral and apply to all applicants or employees may still be discriminatory if they have an adverse impact on a protected class (that is, when compared to the impact of the standard on those not in the protected class).
4. Employment decisions based on stereotypes usually lead to unlawful results. Individual applicants or employees must be evaluated on their abilities; and never on unjustified assumptions or stereotypes about them as members of a group.
5. Exceptions to the rule of equal treatment: "reasonable accommodation" is required for religious practices and the disabled, that is, if the accommodation can be made without undue hardship on the employer.

## THE ROLE OF HR IN EVALUATING THE "EMPLOYABILITY" OF INJURED AND DISABLED WORKERS

The human resources function has an important role to play in setting the tone for managing employees while on disability or workers' compensation leave and in getting them back to work as quickly as possible. By focusing on business necessity as the driving force behind policy implementation and decision-making based on job placement needs, the organization will be better able to control the disability evaluation, leave, and return-to-work process.

Key components of this process are the job description and the performance appraisal. A well-drafted, thorough, and accurate job description should reflect the job-related qualifications necessary to perform the position. It should also clearly describe both the "essential" and the "nonessential" functions of the job. Essential functions are those tasks that are necessary to fulfill the purpose of the job. While it is important to evaluate what percentage of the time an individual will spend performing each task, this does not necessarily determine essential versus nonessential. For example, an airplane pilot spends a relatively small amount of time landing an aircraft; however, no one would dispute that this is an essential function of the job.

Nonessential functions are those tasks that may ordinarily be done in the course of performing a particular job, but they are not required to be accomplished to perform the job adequately. For example, while a legal secretary may occasionally deliver documents from the office to the attorney's home, this is probably not an essential task in performing the job of legal secretary. Such determinations must be made about each task that is done in the course of performing a particular job.

## LEGAL CONCEPTS GOVERNING DECISIONS ABOUT DISABLED EMPLOYEES

The distinction between essential and nonessential functions becomes especially critical when the ill or injured worker meets the definition of a disabled individual under the Americans with Disabilities Act and is protected from discrimination based on disability. Under the ADA, a "disability" is a physical or mental impairment that substantially limits one or more major life activities, or a record of having such an impairment, or the perception of having such an impairment. The ADA prohibits discrimination against "otherwise-qualified" individuals who can perform the essential functions of the job with or without reasonable accommodation.

While job descriptions are not required by the ADA or any other law, their importance cannot be overstated. When properly developed, they establish an objective standard by which to measure qualifications of candidates and by which to evaluate performance. In connection with disability evaluation, an existing job description that defines the essential and nonessential job functions may be used to defend a charge of discrimination under the ADA. Where the essential job functions are defined before the charge is filed, the employer may rest on its determination that an otherwise-qualified individual must be able to perform those functions with or without reasonable accommodation. Where the individual is unable to do so, that employee does not meet the definition of a qualified individual with a disability.

The Rehabilitation Act of 1973 and various state disability rights laws generally provide similar protection to qualified individuals with disabilities. Some differences do exist, and it is essential that the HR function recognizes which laws apply and understand their particular requirements and restrictions.

Traditionally speaking, workers' compensation statutes are the main source of legal rights and remedies for employees who have suffered work-related injuries or illnesses. Each state has its own workers' compensation laws and administrative system, and in most cases, it has been the exclusive forum for injured workers to seek redress for their injuries (see Chapter 6). With the enactment of the ADA, however, some injured workers also meet the definition of qualified individuals with disabilities and are entitled to ADA rights.

Generally, as explained in Chapter 6, workers' compensation systems provide income replacement for employees who, because of an injury or illness arising in and out of the course of employment, are temporarily totally disabled and unable to continue to earn wages. In addition, workers' compensation systems provide additional benefits for permanent partial disability, usually defined as resulting from the residuals of an injury after the individual has recovered maximally.

There is a fundamental difference between the concepts underlying the ADA and workers' compensation systems. As explained in Chapters 2 and 6, workers' compensation systems evolved as a social construct to compensate injured workers who lost wages, both in the short term and the long term, for reasons beyond their control. The emphasis is clearly economic, and characteristically, when an injured worker does not return to the job being performed at the time of injury, workers' compensation systems have been concerned with restoration of a worker's functional capability through physical and vocational rehabilitation as a benefit. Nevertheless, while an employer may be obligated to furnish and pay for this benefit, workers' compensation laws do not require an employer to return an injured worker to work, nor do they require that the employer make an effort to do so, at any time during the course of a claim, even if the worker wishes to return to employment.

When, however, a claimant wishes to return to work and is covered under the ADA as a "qualified individual with a disability," the ADA requires that an employer attempt to return that individual to employment through consideration of reasonable accommodation.

Although the ADA appears to make up for a deficiency in the workers' compensation systems, an odd paradox arises. Before a claim is closed, claimants may their defend status as "disabled" while the employer, although unwilling to return the claimants to work (usually because there are unresolved employee relations problems), asserts that the claimants are not "disabled" and, therefore, not entitled to a temporary total disability benefit. On the other hand, when the claim is closed, the roles could reverse: the employees may claim to be "qualified persons with a disability" and, consequently, entitled to reasonable accommodation, whereas the employer, still unwilling to return the individuals to work (for the same reasons), may assert that the claimants are unemployable. This paradox cannot arise, however, if the employer follows appropriate human resource management practices from the outset and does not attempt to use the workers' compensation system to avoid dealing with administrative matters or disciplinary problems.

Compounding the tension between workers' compensation and the ADA are the federal and state family and medical leave laws. Under the federal Family and Medical Leave Act (FMLA), eligible employees are entitled to up to 12 weeks of unpaid leave during a 12-month period (see Chapter 50). A covered employer under the FMLA must provide an employee who has a "serious medical condition" with up to 12 weeks of leave that may, if indicated, be taken intermittently, rather than all at once.

Under the FMLA, a "serious medical condition" has a lower threshold than the requirements of either the ADA or workers' compensation. To qualify, an employee must submit a doctor's certificate as documentation of a disabling medical condition that requires inpatient treatment or absence from work for a period of more than three calendar days with continuing treatment by a health care provider.

Upon completion of the leave, employees are entitled to restoration to the same job or an equivalent position. While employers are not required to provide paid leave under the FMLA, they are required to continue any existing health insurance benefits to the same extent as if the employee had not taken the leave.

Employers are required to notify employees of their FMLA rights: a poster must be displayed in the workplace and notice must be given at the time an employee requests leave that would qualify as FMLA leave. It is not necessary that the employee specifically ask for FMLA leave; if the employer knows or has been put on notice that the employee qualifies for FMLA leave, the employer must provide information about the employee's rights and obligations while on FMLA leave. If an employer fails to do this, it may not count the leave period against the employee's FMLA entitlement.

## THE INTERPLAY OF THE INJURED EMPLOYEE, THE HR FUNCTION, AND THE HEALTH CARE PROVIDER

Whether an employee is injured or becomes ill on the job or for a nonwork related reason, the effect is the same: the employee is unable to work. For this reason, the human resource function has an interest in the validity of the reasons for the employee's absence and the expected duration of the absence. This interest arises out of the employer's need to manage the employee's position. As such, HR should not turn over the process of managing that employee's absence from work to a workers' compensation insurance carrier or health-care providers.

An employee who takes FMLA leave for a serious medical condition regardless of whether the injury or illness is work-related may be required to submit a medical certification from the health-care provider of the necessity for the leave. If the employer has reason to doubt the validity of the certification, it may require the employee to obtain a second and even a third opinion at the employer's expense. The employer may select the health-care provider for the second opinion, and from a mutually agreeable provider for a third opinion. The employer may also require recertification of the employee's medical condition on a reasonable basis (usually no more than every 30 days). Upon return from FMLA leave, the employer may require the employee to submit a medical certification if it has a uniformly applied policy of doing so. While the employer may not contest the return to work certification, it may deny reinstatement to an employee who fails to provide one.*

It appears that workers' compensation systems focus on an applicant's impairment and loss of function as primary issues. However, this appearance arises out of administration of the claims management process rather than out of direct requirements of workers' compensation laws. The usual role of the medical practitioner *vis-à-vis* impairment and disability is to evaluate a patient's overall functioning and capabilities, and those of the multiple organ systems that contribute to an effective and useful life. Some physicians, however, in their work responsibilities and practices, may become more involved with matters such as disability and employability.

Under the provision of workers' compensation laws, an indemnity benefit is paid when the individual is able to prove a disability and is unable to work because of an injury or illness arising in and out of the course of employment, and as a result has lost wages. While this approach appears to be quite straightforward, problems and disputes arise because the laws do not provide a definition of "disabled." Furthermore, the proof, quite commonly, consists of an unexplained and unsupported statement of opinion by a physician that the individual is disabled (see Chapter 1). When the foundation of the physician's opinion is not explained or clearly supported by medical information, the opinion amounts to little more than a testimonial statement that is subject to challenge by the other party as the beginning of an escalating confrontation between "dueling doctors." The problem is compounded by the fact that, strictly speaking, disability, is not the ultimate issue: workers' compensation laws compensate injured workers for lost wages, not for disability *per se*.

A shift in orientation to look at employability rather than disability points the way out of this dysfunctional situation.[1] An individual is quite clearly employable when the medical condition does not preclude:

- travel to and from work
- being at work
- assignment of appropriate tasks and duties with or without accommodation

If a medical condition does not preclude travel to and from work, and if the employer is willing to pay full wages for work assigned within the boundaries of the employee's medical condition and job, then the employer cannot justify approval of the absence and may order the employee to report to work at a particular time and place. If, on the other hand, the employer can determine that the medical condition does preclude travel to and from work, there is no question about approving the absence and supporting the award of a benefit.

This approach appropriately separates the determination of duty status from determination of pay status. While workers' compensation, short- and long-term disability, and sick pay, for example, provide a benefit to replace an individual's lost wages when particular criteria are met, none of these systems has the machinery for determining whether or not an employee should be at work. A decision not to pay an indemnity benefit should be based on management's decision to pay wages, not a medical assertion that the employee is not disabled. When retention at work and return to work are approached in this way, the trade-off for the injured worker is between payment of wages or payment of a benefit, and not, as commonly occurs in workers' compensation claim administration, between a benefit or no benefit, which places the employee at a serious disadvantage. The employer does not deny the employee anything by saying, in effect, "Come to work, and we will pay you full wages for what you are capable of doing."

---

*The rules are somewhat different for an employee who takes leave because of a work-related injury not covered by the FMLA. In those cases state rules apply. See Chapters 6 and 50.

Management is able to retain a good measure of control over the outcome of a claim starting at the very beginning by taking steps to ensure the following: (1) that the claim is filed promptly and that the submitted information is accurate and complete; (2) by monitoring the employee's medical condition and employability with an eye toward not letting the employee stop work, if at all possible; and (3) by enabling an employee whose absence could not be avoided to return to work as quickly as is practical through assignment of appropriate tasks and duties with due consideration of reasonable accommodation. To achieve this type of result, management should appropriately ask, "Would there be a medical reason to recommend that the employee not return to work (to work at appropriately assigned tasks and duties, with accommodation if necessary), if the employee wanted to do so?" instead of asking the doctor "When will the employee return to work?"

Keeping the focus on what the injured employee is capable of doing is an essential part of maintaining control of the basic business objective, that is, to maintain the productivity of the employee's position. Implementation of well-structured policies and procedures for managing medically based absence and accommodation, rather than managing disabled employees, will allow the employer to manage the employee's absence and return to work from the standpoint of business necessity. For example, a policy with procedures for managing medically based absence should allow only as much time for an employee's absence from the job as needed for the employee to recover to the degree that the medical condition no longer precludes travel to and from work. This may be accomplished through a requirement that the employee periodically continue to document the medical necessity for the absence. When such medical necessity ceases to exist, management may offer the employee the options either to return to work or to leave employment.

Appropriately structured communication between the human resources function or others responsible

---

## SAMPLE LETTER TO A DOCTOR WHO HAS RECOMMENDED WORK RESTRICTIONS

Dear Doctor X:

We have received your letter indicating that Ms. Jones is unable to return to work for an unspecified period because of her back injury. We would like to receive some additional information:

1. Does this employee's medical condition prevent travel to and from work? If so, what is the medical reason?
2. Does this employee's medical condition prevent her from being at work? If so, what is the medical reason?
3. To your knowledge, has the employee's medical condition affected her life activities such as driving, shopping, self-care, or recreational activities? If so, how? What is your basis for this information?
4. Does the employee's medical condition preclude assignment of any of the tasks and duties I have enclosed on the attached list? If so, identify the tasks and duties, and the medical reason for your conclusion.
5. Is there a medical reason to believe that the employee is likely to experience injury, harm, or aggravation of the medical condition by performing or attempting to perform any of the described tasks and duties? If so, what is the degree of injury, harm, or aggravation that should be expected, and what is the likelihood that it will occur? What is the time frame within which it is likely to occur? What is the expected duration of the risk? What is the medical reason for your conclusions?
6. Is there a medical reason to believe that, because of the medical condition, the employee is likely to experience sudden or subtle incapacitation? If so, to what degree could the employee be incapacitated, and what is the likelihood that this will occur? What is the expected duration of the risk? What is the medical reason for your conclusions?
7. Is the employee likely to recover sufficiently to perform the tasks and duties described to you? If so, what is the time frame? If not, what is the medical reason?
8. If any restrictions for the employee are warranted because of a significant risk of substantial harm to the employee or to others, what kinds of measures should be considered in identifying possible accommodations to eliminate the reason for the restrictions?

for managing the injured employee and the treating physician or health-care provider is essential. While the health-care provider is responsible for providing the medical evaluation and treatment, and for helping the employer to understand the impact of the medical condition on the employee's functional abilities, it is the employer that must make the decisions regarding the employability of that individual. For that reason, it is extremely helpful for the employer to ask appropriate questions of the health care provider. The box on page 578 is a sample letter designed to elicit specific information about the employability of an injured employee.

## ASSESSING RETURN TO WORK OPTIONS

Getting the employee back to work is the name of the game for those who are on leave either for work- or nonwork-related medical reasons. While in general employers are willing to bring injured employees back to work as early as possible, in some cases, especially when there were employee-relations problems prior to the injury, the employer may take the position that the employee may not return to work until classified as "100%." This is invariably a costly mistake. First and foremost, it delays the employee's return to work, increases workers' compensation costs, and forces additional replacement costs. Most likely such an approach will violate the ADA for covered disabilities, under which employers are required to make reasonable accommodations that enable employees to perform the essential functions of their jobs. Beyond this, the effect of such an approach is to emphasize the employee's lost abilities and to define employees by their impairments. Eventually, this kind of approach causes employees to feel much less capable than they really are.

Unless an employee's medical condition precludes travel to and from work, being at work, or being able to perform assigned appropriate tasks and duties, the employer is not legally required to approve the employee's absence. Even if the employee is unable to resume normal job duties, however, there are several options that employers should and, in some cases, must consider.

Under the ADA, an employer must consider reasonable accommodations that will enable an employee covered by the ADA to perform the essential functions of the job while not creating an undue hardship for the employer. A reasonable accommodation may mean providing a stool to allow an employee to sit while working, or it could mean providing an interpreter for a hearing-impaired worker. It may also mean rescheduling the employee's working time to accommodate the need for physical therapy or permitting an employee to work at home. There are many possibilities, and an employer has an obligation to an individual with a disability who is protected by the ADA to consider any accommodation request presented by that individual. Where the employer determines in good faith that it would create an undue hardship for the business, such as a complete rearrangement of a production schedule, the employer may reject the request. If a less burdensome alternative is available, however, the employer must consider it.

The ADA does not require an employer to create a light duty or other alternative position for an employee or to reassign the employee to another permanent position. Reasonable accommodation under the ADA does not include accepting lower production standards. To the contrary, a reasonable accommodation enables the employee to perform the essential job functions up to standard. Coworkers should be educated to view reasonable accommodation as a benefit, rather than a detriment.

While not required under the ADA, alternative duty assignments otherwise different from the employee's original assignment may be an effective medical management and recovery tool to increase productivity and profit by reducing and controlling workers' compensation costs. By getting the employee back to work in some capacity, the cycle of unproductive time, doctor's appointments, and patient mentality is broken. Once the employee is back in the work environment, the chances that the employee will resume regular job responsibilities are increased.

This focus on returning the employee to work in some capacity need not take the form of a mere request to report to work. If the employee is medically able to travel to and from work and to be at work, and the employer is willing to assign the employee tasks that the employee's medical condition does not preclude the employee from performing, then the employer may direct the employee to report to work at a specific time and place. If, in such circumstances, the employee does not report to work, the employer may terminate the employment of the employee, provided that the employee has exhausted any remaining FMLA leave. Note, however, that the workers' compensation laws in a few states (such as California) may preclude termination of employment when the employee is on a workers' compensation leave at the time the employee is directed to return to work.

An employee may not be required to accept alternative duties if qualified for FMLA leave. Under the FMLA, the employee is entitled to be restored to the same or an equivalent position at the end of the leave period, and the employer cannot force the employee either to accept the alternative duty assignment or terminate employment until the period of FMLA leave expires. Once the FMLA leave expires, however, the employee can be directed to return to work in the circumstances discussed above.

While permanent reassignment to another position may be an alternative to restoring the employee to the regular position, an employer is under no legal obligation by reason of the ADA (unless there is an open, available position for which the employee is qualified), workers' compensation laws, or the FMLA. Additionally, permanent reassignment may become a problem if it is provided for one disabled employee but not another. After considering the consequences of establishing a precedent of permanent reassignment, an employer may nonetheless decide that bringing the employee back to work will solve more problems than it will create.

## TERMINATING THE EMPLOYMENT OF A DISABLED EMPLOYEE

Termination of employment may become an issue if the employee is unable or refuses to return to work in any capacity with or without reasonable accommodation. If permitted under state law, an employer may enforce a neutral attendance policy against a disabled employee and discharge that employee who is absent the required amount of time. A neutral attendance policy is one that states that any employee who is absent from work for more than an established period of time as specified in the policy, regardless of the reason, will be terminated. Such a policy must be enforced uniformly and consistently for all covered employees. It should be noted that under some state workers' compensation laws, neutral attendance policies cannot be applied to terminate the employment of an employee who qualifies for workers' compensation benefits. Some state workers' compensation laws run counter to these policies by prohibiting discharge of an employee who has filed for or is receiving benefits. Also, a neutral attendance policy may not be enforced against an employee who qualifies for FMLA leave until the maximum period of FMLA leave has been exhausted.*

---

*A neutral attendance policy is one which states that any employee who is absent from work for more than an established period of time as specified in the policy, regardless of the reason, will be terminated. Such a policy must be enforced uniformly and consistently for all covered employees. It should be noted that, under some state workers' compensation laws, neutral attendance policies cannot be applied to terminate the employment of an employee who qualifies for workers' compensation benefits.

If an employee is protected by the ADA, which prohibits discrimination against qualified individuals who can perform the essential functions of the job with or without reasonable accommodation, the decision to terminate employment requires demonstration of the individual's failure to meet job demands and conditions of employment.

Other issues arise when the discipline or termination of an employee who is on disability leave is for cause. If an employee had performance or other work-related problems prior to the request for disability leave, the employer may proceed with the disciplinary process even though the employee may be absent from work. However, the employer must follow its own established and uniformly-applied procedures for discipline and termination and must thoroughly document its actions as job-related and consistent with how it has handled other similar situations. Here, the bottom line is establishing through a record of lawful policies and written documentation that the employer would have taken the same action against the employee regardless of the medical condition or absence from work.

## THE BENEFITS OF KEEPING THE FOCUS ON RETURNING EMPLOYEES TO WORK

The conceptual difference between a system of disability evaluation and management that emphasizes an individual's incapacities and limitations and one that focuses on ability and accommodation is significant for all employers who want to reduce their benefits costs and increase productivity. By focusing on ability rather than incapacity, employers will be more likely to get injured or disabled employees back to work sooner. For the employee, this means a restoration of at least partial earnings and benefits. It also means the employee is back in the running for any advancement or lateral job opportunities that may arise. A return to work, even in a light-duty position or with accommodation, also means the transition from incapacitated "patient" to productive "employee."

For employers, the speedy return to work of injured or disabled employees means a reduction in workers' compensation benefits and disability payments and a halt to rising workers' compensation and health insurance premiums that are based on usage or experience. Thus, by directing employees to return to work when it is legally appropriate to do so, employers will see an overall decrease in the cost of benefits. Assisting injured or disabled employees in returning to work as quickly as possible also reduces the likelihood that they will file a charge of discrimination against the employer under the ADA, Title VII, or state or local fair-employment-practice laws.

The adoption of a business-necessity approach to the evaluation of medical and disability leaves will enable the employer to retain control of the decisions about the employee's absence from and return to work. Employees must be accountable to management for meeting the demands of their jobs within reasonable limits, notwithstanding the restrictions or recommendations of a doctor or other health-care provider. When business necessity is the driving factor in making determinations about employee-leave requests, the focus is on managing the job rather than the individual. The end result is an even flow of work and products and a management tone that promotes productivity and morale while discouraging employees from attempting to abuse the disability management system.

## Reference

1. Pimentel R, Bell C, Smith G, Larson H: The workers' compensation ADA connection, Milt Wright & Associates, Inc., 1993.

# CHAPTER 50

# OVERVIEW OF THE AMERICANS WITH DISABILITIES ACT AND THE FAMILY AND MEDICAL LEAVE ACT

*Christopher Bell*

Since 1990, Congress has enacted two major pieces of legislation prohibiting discrimination on the basis of disability and providing for family and medical leave.* The Americans with Disabilities Act of 1990 (ADA) and the Family and Medical Leave Act of 1993 (FMLA) radically affect the practice of occupational medicine and, in addition, both the medical and nonmedical aspects of managing employment-related disability matters.

The ADA protects persons with disabilities from discrimination and mandates accommodations for disabled employees, customers, clients, and patients. The ADA affects the provision of health care in many ways including: architectural design of a health care provider's office; how the health-care provider communicates with patients with impaired cognitive or communication skills; the scope and timing of a medical examination requested for an employee by an employer; and the timing and nature of the medical information an employer may require of a treating physician.

The ADA has also spawned a considerable volume of claims of disability discrimination. For example, from July 26, 1992, through November 30, 1994, 38,250 charges of employment discrimination have been received by the Equal Employment Opportunity Commission (EEOC), the federal agency that enforces the ADA. Twenty percent of these charges are filed by individuals claiming to have a disabling back impairment and another 25% of the charges are filed by persons with some other form of impairment not administratively catalogued by the EEOC. Approximately 50% of the charges allege a discriminatory discharge from employment.

The FMLA is not quite so sweeping in its impact on health care providers. The FMLA provides unpaid time off for eligible employees of a covered employer for up to 12 weeks for a variety of family and medical

reasons. These employees are guaranteed job restoration and the continuation of health benefits while on leave. Leave may be taken because of a serious health condition of employees that prohibits them from doing their job for more than three days; the care of a spouse, child, or parent with a serious health condition; and the birth, adoption, or placement in foster care of a child. Employers are provided only certain limited rights of access to medical information by the FMLA with respect to authorizing employee absences and return to work.

This chapter briefly explores the impact of the ADA and the FMLA on the business and practice of medicine. In particular, the chapter will discuss how these two laws affect the health care providers in their obligations to patients and the nature and timing of medical input an employer may obtain to comply with these new legal mandates.[1]

## THE ADA

This section provides a general overview of the ADA and explores the patient's new rights *vis-à-vis* the doctor, the patient's employer, and the employer's relationship with the doctor.

### Overview of the ADA

The ADA is a civil rights law that prohibits discrimination in public and private employment, governmental services, public accommodations, public transportation, and telecommunication. Its prohibitions apply to employers with 15 or more employees and to state and local governments and public services of any size. The ADA's protections apply to an individual with a "disability." A disability is defined by the AOAAS as a mental or physical impairment that currently substantially limits an individual in any major life activity including working, that did so at some documented time in the past, or that is now per-

---

*"Disability" in this chapter will be used in the context of the ADA, rather than in the context used throughout the book.

ceived by the employer as doing so. The ADA's employment provisions protect an applicant or an employee with a disability if the employee is a "qualified individual with a disability." A qualified individual is defined by the ADA as a person with a disability who satisfies certain job prerequisites such as knowledge, skills, abilities, education, and experience and who has the capacity to perform the "essential functions" of a job with or without reasonable accommodation.[2] The ADA prohibits discrimination against a "qualified individual with a disability" in all aspects of the employment relationship including recruitment, hiring, compensation, training, discharge, and benefits.[3]

An employer is required to provide a reasonable accommodation to enable a qualified individual with a disability to perform the essential functions of the job and to otherwise meet the demands of the job and conditions of employment, unless the specific accommodation would impose an undue hardship on the employer's business.[4]

The "essential functions" of a job are the fundamental rather than the marginal duties of a position, considering factors such as the job description, the time spent doing a function, the number of people available to do the function, and the consequences if the function is not performed.[5] A reasonable accommodation is a modification or adjustment to the work environment or to the manner or circumstances under which a job is customarily performed, that enables a qualified individual with a disability to perform the essential functions of that position, to be considered for employment, or to receive equal benefits provided to other similarly-situated employees.

The ADA's definition of disability is, at once, both broader and narrower than traditional definitions of disability used in benefits systems (see Appendix A). The ADA adopts a functional approach to disability but also recognizes that societal attitudes may define when a particular medical condition is considered to be disabling. A "person with a disability" is defined in three ways by the ADA:

1. Any person who has a physical or mental impairment that substantially limits one or more of the individual's major life activities.[6]
2. Any person who has a "record of" a substantially-limiting impairment.[7]
3. Any person who is "regarded as" having a substantially-limiting impairment, regardless of whether the person is in fact disabled.[8]

Major life activities include caring for oneself, performing manual tasks, walking, seeing, hearing, speaking, learning, and working.[9] Other common daily activities such as sitting, standing, bending, reaching, grasping, concentrating, reasoning, and basic socialization skills would also be included.

Minor, nonchronic impairments of short duration with little or no permanent or long-term impact do not constitute an ADA-covered disability.[10] This includes common workplace injuries such as a broken leg or sprained joints.[11]

However, according to the EEOC, even a temporary condition, such as a broken leg, can become a disability when the recovery period is significantly longer than normal and if, during the healing period, the individual is unable to walk, or if the impairment heals but leaves a permanent residual impairment, such as a limp, that substantially limits the individual's ability to walk.[12]

An applicant or employee may also be protected because of a "record of" a disability. An injured worker has a "record of" a disability when that employee has recovered in whole or in part from an impairment that is documented as having substantially limited a major life activity in the past. For example, according to the EEOC, an injured worker who had been unable to work for one year because of a personal injury or workplace injury would probably have a record of a disability. If an employer refused to hire or return this person back to work because of this record alone, this action would violate the ADA if the worker were otherwise qualified for the position sought. Note, however, that a mere record of having filed a workers' compensation claim or a claim for other disability benefits does not automatically give a person a "record of" a substantially-limiting impairment.[13]

An applicant or employee also may be "regarded as" disabled, that is, have no current or past "disability" but still be protected by the ADA because of the subjective perception of an employer that the individual is disabled. When an employer perceives that an individual is significantly restricted in the ability to perform manual tasks or any other major life activity, the individual is, thereby, regarded as disabled by the employer.[14] This is true regardless of whether the individual is, in fact, substantially limited by the impairment.

The "regarded as" part of the ADA's definition of disability is expansive and depends upon the attitude of the employer, not the nature of the medical condition. Many injured workers may potentially be protected by the ADA as a result of an employer's fears concerning the risk of future injury, increases in workers' compensation premiums, or the cost of accommodation. These common employer concerns about an injured worker create ADA coverage when it can be shown that the employer took an adverse employment action because it regarded the individual as being substantially limited in a major life activity such as performing manual tasks or performing a class of jobs.[15]

Physicians may unwittingly provide a trigger for

ADA coverage by recommending broad work restrictions without addressing an applicant's or employee's ability to perform particular job functions with or without a reasonable accommodation. If a physician recommends work restrictions by simply focusing on what he or she believes an employee is unable to do and does not relate these restrictions to the particular functions of the job at issue, and if the employer accepts the restrictions, it will be easier for an employee or applicant to claim that he or she was regarded as a person with a disability by the employer.

Suppose, for example, an employer accepts and implements a doctor's recommended work restrictions permanently prohibiting repeated bending and stooping, sitting for more than two hours at a time, and standing for more than one hour at a time. Even if the employer had no way of knowing that the restrictions were not medically warranted, it may be difficult for the employer to successfully argue that it did not regard the applicant or employee as having a disability under the terms of the ADA. Accordingly, to avoid inadvertently creating a potential ADA liability, it is important for both the physician and the employer to review critically the physician's recommendations, to verify that there is, in fact, a medical basis for recommending restrictions, and to verify the expected duration of the restrictions.

Case law developed under the ADA and its precursor, the Rehabilitation Act of 1973, however, continues to be more favorable to employers in limiting claims by persons who profess to have a disability. Courts are interpreting both laws to exclude from disability status persons who merely are unable to perform or are regarded by an employer as being unable to perform one job for one particular employer.[16] Rather, to be covered by the ADA because of a medically-related limitation in working, an individual must be disabled from a class of jobs or broad range of jobs in many classes.[17]

In addition, because a growing number of courts are interpreting that the ADA and the Rehabilitation Act do not cover "temporary" or perceived "temporary" disabilities,[18] many more injured workers will be excluded from ADA protection.

### Qualified Individual with a Disability

Operationally, the ADA requires that an applicant or employee be simultaneously disabled and qualified. These twin standards put a potential ADA claimant in a different "Catch-22;" if the claimant emphasizes the severity of limitations resulting from disability, the claimant is likely to prove not to be qualified for the job. On the other hand, if the claimant emphasizes ability, this may defeat the claim of being disabled. However, being simultaneously disabled yet qualified is not necessarily an insurmountable burden. For example, an individual is protected from discrimination based on a past record of a disability, such as a history of severe back problems, and also on being perceived as being more disabled than one actually is. The impediments for employment for such a qualified person are addressed by the ADA without that individual being caught in the law's "Catch-22," when the person has recovered from a disability or when the disability is in the perception of an employer. Reasonable accommodation also can turn an unqualified person with a disability into a qualified individual with a disability by reducing or eliminating the effects of the individual's functional limitation on the job by changing some features of the job, without affecting the person's disability status.

However, when an individual cannot be effectively accommodated and the job's essential functions require the use of physical or mental functions that the individual cannot perform because of impairments, the individual is not likely to be qualified.

The tension between being disabled and qualified is increased when an employee files for disability benefits. A current employee who files for permanent total disability benefits is claiming an inability to perform on the job but might, at the same time, seek reasonable accommodation. A claim of permanent and total disability, however, may undercut that employee's claim of being a "qualified individual with a disability," and thus able to perform the essential functions of a job in spite of a disability. Courts have used the sworn factual statements on an application for long-term disability benefits as a basis for finding that an employee is not qualified to perform the essential functions of a job.[19]

To avoid this problem, some individuals with disabilities have asserted that their only disability stems from an employer's perception that they are not qualified for a position because of an impairment. This emphasis on being qualified rather than disabled also has doomed claims for workers because some courts have concluded that such individuals are not truly disabled.[20]

Accordingly, health-care providers need to be aware that their statements attesting to a disability claimant's inability to perform a job may well be used against the claimant, if the claimant later pursues a claim of disability discrimination. Health-care providers should recognize that the eligibility requirements for most disability benefits do not take into account either an employee's essential job functions or the possibility that the employee might be somehow accommodated to perform in the original job or in another job to which an employee might be reassigned. Overly-broad assertions regarding an employee's inability to work or perform in the customary occupation without regard to these ADA refinements may not be in the employee's or employer's best interest.

## Restrictions on Medical Examinations and Inquiries

The employment provisions of the ADA severely restrict disability-related medical inquiries and examinations in ways that affect medical practice. Before a job offer is made, an employer may not inquire about an applicant's impairment or medical history. Inquiries concerning past on-the-job injuries or workers' compensation claims are expressly prohibited.[21] This includes inquiries to third parties about an applicant's workers' compensation history.

An employer may, however, conditionally offer a position based on the satisfactory completion of a medical examination or medical inquiry, but only if such examinations or inquiry is made of all applicants for the same job category and the results are kept confidential with a few narrow exceptions.[22] For example, an employer may choose to require all postoffer candidates to complete a medical history questionnaire and to selectively require medical examinations of those candidates whose medical history justifies a more thorough medical evaluation concerning a particular issue.[23] Postoffer medical examinations and inquiries do not have to be job-related. Questions concerning recent medical treatment, hospitalization, prescription drug use, past workers' compensation claims, and on-the-job injuries are expressly permitted.

A job offer may be withdrawn only if the findings on medical examination, when reviewed in conjunction with a job's essential functions, support a conclusion that individuals are either (1) unable to do the essential functions of a job even with reasonable accommodation or (2) the individuals would pose a direct threat to their own health or safety or the health or safety of others that cannot be eliminated or acceptably reduced by reasonable accommodation.[24]

Medical examinations and inquiries of current employees are required to be job-related and consistent with business necessity.[25] Accordingly, in connection with current employees, an employer may not require a medical examination or make inquiries to determine if an employee has an impairment or to ascertain the nature or severity of an impairment unless the employer can demonstrate that there is a substantive basis for such an inquiry or examination. For example, a medical inquiry, including medical examination, when warranted, may be carried out if

medical issues arise when an employee is having difficulty performing on the job or an employer has reason to believe that an employee may pose a risk to the health or safety of the employee or others in the workplace.

The postemployment medical examination also is narrower in scope than the postoffer, preemployment medical examination. While an employer is permitted to require a full medical examination during the postoffer stage, it may not require a general medical examination once an employee has commenced work. Rather, the examination must focus on ascertaining whether and to what degree an employee has a medical condition impacting the ability to perform, safely and satisfactorily, the essential functions of the position the employee occupies. Thus, for example, a hospital employee whose essential functions include lifting and transferring patients and who is complaining of back pain could be evaluated to determine the employee's current capacity to continue safely lifting and transferring patients. However, that medical examination cannot include bloodwork for HIV disease because this would not relate to the employee's essential job functions.

Lastly, return-to-work medical evaluations, in addition to addressing the capacity of the employee to perform the essential duties of the job, must also consider the possibility that an employee may return to work with a reasonable accommodation.

## Direct Threat to Health or Safety

In order to withdraw a job offer or restrict the return to work on health or safety grounds, an employer must show that the individual poses a high probability of causing substantial harm to their health or safety and that the risk of substantial harm cannot be eliminated or reduced below the direct threat level by reasonable accommodation.[26] This is a very stringent standard that employers rarely will be able to meet when attempting to screen for potential future injury. In fact, medical science will rarely have the data to demonstrate that there is a high probability that something bad will happen. Moreover, such claims cannot be speculative or based on potential future risk. Only the current abilities of the individual to perform essential job functions safely can be assessed.

The following examples were derived from the EEOC's Technical Assistance Manual. They demonstrate how the direct threat standard applies to common scenarios.

1. An applicant for a laborer job has had no back pain or injuries in his previous jobs that require heavy lifting. But a back x-ray reveals a back

anomaly. The company doctor worries that, because of the x-ray finding, but without any medical history or clinical findings that indicate a current back problem, there is a slight chance that the applicant could develop back problems in the future. The threat of future back injury in such a case is too slender to meet the direct threat standard, according to the EEOC.

2. A significant risk would exist for an individual with a back anomaly who has a history of repeated back injuries in similar jobs, and whose back condition has been aggravated further by injury, and where there are no accommodations that would eliminate or reduce the risk.

3. A physician's evaluation indicates that an employee has a disc condition that might worsen in eight to ten years. This is not a sufficient indication of imminent potential harm.[27]

## Reasonable Accommodation

Unlike most disability benefit systems, the ADA requires an employer to make reasonable accommodations for the known physical or mental limitations of an individual with a disability who is qualified for a job in all respects except for limitations imposed by the disability. The concept underlying reasonable accommodation is a deceptively simple one. Making adjustments in the job structure, work space, work schedule, or tools used on the job can enable a person with medically-based functional limitations to perform a job successfully. Of necessity, however, reasonable accommodation must be tailored to the specific abilities and limitations of the individual as well as the particular demands of the job. To this end, the ADA provides a list of nonexclusive examples of reasonable accommodations.

Reasonable accommodation under the ADA means:

1. Modifications or adjustments to a job application process that enable a qualified applicant with a disability to be considered for the position such qualified applicant desires; or

2. Modifications or adjustments to the work environment, or to the manner or circumstances under which the position held or desired is customarily performed, that enable a qualified individual with a disability to perform the essential functions of that position; or

3. Modifications or adjustments that enable a covered entity's employee with a disability to enjoy equal benefits and privileges of employment as are enjoyed by its other similarly situated employees without disabilities.[28]

The statute and regulations provide the following nonexclusive list of examples:

1. Making existing facilities used by employees readily accessible to and usable by individuals with disabilities; and

2. Job restructuring; part-time or modified work schedules; reassignment to a vacant position; acquisition or modification of equipment or devices; appropriate adjustment or modifications of examinations, training materials, or policies; the provision of qualified readers or interpreters; and other similar accommodations for individuals with disabilities.

Good communication between employer, employee, physician, and various occupational specialists (including industrial hygienists, safety specialists, and plant engineers) is essential to the provision of reasonable accommodation. Providing reasonable accommodation is an interactive process between an employer and a person with a disability requesting it. The EEOC has suggested that the following steps be taken when an employee is unable to suggest a reasonable accommodation that an employer is willing to provide:

1. Identify the purpose and functions of the job the individual is seeking to perform.

2. Identify barriers to employment by consulting with the individual with a disability to ascertain abilities and limitations as they relate to performance of the job's essential functions.

3. Identify possible accommodations by consulting with the individual and, where necessary, seek technical assistance.

4. Select a reasonable accommodation that is effective, and that provides an equal employment opportunity.[29]

Moreover, should an employer not grant a request for accommodation, the employer's failure to make an effort to identify possible accommodations in consultation with the person with a disability who requested accommodation results in denial of an employer's "good faith" defense to liability for compensatory and punitive damages.[30]

Medical input may be critical in any accommodation decision, and an employer has a right to medical information necessary to determine the nature and extent of a medical impairment and its expected duration, and to information regarding the impact of the impairment on an individual's daily life activities. The accommodation requested must be medically warranted and the employer is entitled to sufficient medical information to understand the medical basis for the accommodation. An employer has a legitimate interest in knowing, for example, the specific medical reasons for which an individual with diabetes could be expected to suffer injury, harm, or aggravation of the condition when they are precluded from rotating shifts. In addition, the employer may be entitled to obtain copies of medical records of an employee seeking reasonable accommodation in circumstances where the individual's disability status and need for accommodation are not obvious. An employer is not limited to accepting a treating physician's "doctor's note" as the only proof of the disability status or the medical necessity for the accommodation requested by the employee, and employers are allowed to seek guidance from an independent medical advisor.

## Undue Hardship

An employer does not have to provide a reasonable accommodation that would impose "significant difficulty or expense" on the employer in relation to its business and the resources available to provide the accommodation.[31] An accommodation is not required if it is "unduly costly, extensive, substantial, or disruptive, or that would fundamentally alter the nature or operation of the business."[32] In determining whether the cost of an accommodation would pose an undue hardship, the EEOC has apparently instructed its investigators to consider the cost of making the accommodation and the amount of money an employer would save in workers' compensation related expenses if an injured worker is returned to work with reasonable accommodations as opposed to the amount spent if that employee remained out of work and received benefits.[33]

## Role of Physicians in ADA-related Determinations

From the foregoing brief summary, it should be clear that medical input of various kinds can be critical to both an employee or applicant and an employer in making ADA-compliant employment decisions. Medical input may be necessary in assessing whether an individual has a physical or mental impairment and whether that impairment "substantially limits" the individual's major life activities. Medical input also may be needed to determine whether an applicant has the physical or mental capacity to perform a job and to do so safely without posing significant risk to the individual or others. In addition, an employer may need to understand how an individual's medical condition limits an employee's ability to perform essential job functions or otherwise meet job demands, so that the employer can consider possible reasonable accommodations.

Physicians can only provide medical information

and give recommendations. The quality of the information and recommendation is, of necessity, influenced by the quality of the questions asked by the employer, as well as by the knowledge and experience of the physician. Physicians do not make the employment decision. This is the employer's responsibility. Using this input, an employer can decide, consistent with applicable law and company policy, whether to hire, return to work, or accommodate a particular person. The ultimate decision is a management one, not a medical one. The EEOC makes this point clear in its ADA Technical Assistance Manual:

> A doctor who conducts medical examinations for an employer should not be responsible for making employment decisions or deciding whether or not it is possible to make a reasonable accommodation for a person with a disability. That responsibility lies with the employer.
>
> The doctor's role should be limited to advising the employer about an individual's functional abilities and limitations in relation to job functions, and about whether the individual meets the employer's health and safety requirements.[34]

However, while physicians play a significant role in many aspects of ADA compliance, the nature of the needed medical input may differ from the information a physician has provided to an employer. (See Chapters 1, 10, and 11.)

It will sometimes be necessary for an employer to know the diagnosis of the physical or mental impairment in order to determine whether an individual has a disability or to determine whether a requested accommodation is medically necessary. For example, suppose an applicant requests that an employer provide extra time for an employment test because of difficulty with reading. This could be a reasonable accommodation if the employee's need for accommodation is due to a medical condition such as dyslexia. On the other hand, if the employee simply never learned to read well, such an extension of time would not be required.

## Patient's Rights to Equal Access to Medical Services

Physicians, in the private and public practice of medicine, have new obligations toward patients with disabilities under the ADA. These obligations can be summarized as follows:
(1) provision of accessible facilities, (2) provision of effective communication for patients with communication impairments, and (3) nondiscrimina-

tion in the provision of medical services on the basis of disability.

## Provide accessible facilities

A physician or other health-care provider in private practice has an obligation to ensure that patients with disabilities, including patients with mobility impairments, have physical access to the health care facilities. Narrow doorways, steps, deep pile carpeting, and furniture-cluttered waiting rooms may prove obstacles to a person using a wheelchair or crutches. The ADA imposes an obligation on health-care providers who provide services from a "place of public accommodation," including a doctor's office, to take steps to remove architectural and communication barriers in existing facilities. After January 26, 1992, architectural barriers were to be removed if it was "readily achievable" to do so. This means, if the barrier can be removed without "significant difficulty or expense." The Department of Justice provides the following examples of barrier removal:[35]

1. Installing ramps
2. Making curb cuts in sidewalks and entrances
3. Repositioning shelves
4. Rearranging tables, chairs, vending machines, display racks, and other furniture
5. Repositioning telephones
6. Adding raised markings on elevator control buttons
7. Installing flashing alarm lights
8. Widening doors
9. Installing offset hinges to widen doorways
10. Eliminating a turnstile or providing an alternative accessible path
11. Installing accessible door hardware
12. Installing grab bars in toilet stalls
13. Rearranging toilet partitions to increase maneuvering space
14. Insulating lavatory pipes under sinks to prevent burns
15. Installing a raised toilet seat
16. Installing a full-length bathroom mirror
17. Repositioning the paper towel dispenser in a bathroom
18. Creating designated accessible parking spaces
19. Installing an accessible paper cup dispenser at an existing inaccessible water fountain
20. Removing high pile, low density carpeting
21. Installing vehicle hand controls.

However, in an existing facility, the ADA does not require extensive ramping of a flight of stairs or the installation of an elevator, because such extensive renovations would be burdensome and expensive to undertake and therefore would not be readily achievable. The ADA also does not require a health-care provider to lease only accessible space. However,

once space is leased, the obligation to undertake readily-achievable barrier removal applies to both landlord and tenant.[36]

Greater accessibility modifications are required once a health-care provider makes alterations to a facility. The alterations must be done in compliance with the ADA's Accessibility Guideline (ADAAG). Put simply, the altered space must be designed to be fully accessible.[37] This obligation covers a wide range of items too numerous to mention here. In addition, if a health-care provider alters patient service or work areas, there is an additional obligation that there be an "accessible path of travel" leading from the outside of the building through to the altered area of the facility. Along this accessible path of travel, various amenities including bathrooms, drinking fountains, and public telephones also may have to be altered to make them accessible and usable to persons with disabilities. A sufficient number of accessible parking spaces also would have to be provided if parking is made available for patients or employees. However, expenses associated with providing an accessible path of travel are capped at 20% of the cost of the original renovation.[38]

The greatest degree of accessibility is required of buildings designed for first occupancy after January 26, 1993. These buildings must be designed and built to be fully accessible in accordance with ADAAG.[39] There is no cost defense applicable to the construction of new public accommodations or commercial facilities. In some cases, an elevator may be required in order to provide accessible vertical access to health-care facilities and providers.[40]

## Provide effective communication

Patients or clients with communication impairments may have a right to an auxiliary aid or service from the health care provider to facilitate effective communication. Auxiliary aids or services include qualified interpreters or other effective methods of making aurally-delivered materials available to individuals with hearing impairments; qualified readers, taped texts, or other effective methods for making visually delivered materials available to individuals with visual impairments; acquisition or modification of equipment or devices; and other similar services and actions.[41] For example, in the past, a patient with a severe hearing impairment might have brought a relative who knew sign language when visiting a doctor. With the enactment of the ADA, the doctor may have an obligation to provide and pay for a sign language interpreter when requested.[42]

In some cases, effective communication is satisfied when the health-care provider and a hearing-impaired patient communicate by passing written notes.

However, when the complex interchange of medical information occurs, such as the patient's detailed description of symptoms or a physician's discussion of potential side effects of proposed medication, passing notes may not be sufficient. In addition, a physician may be required to read aloud a consent form to a visually-impaired patient.

## Nondiscrimination in the provision of medical services

A health-care provider is prohibited from discrimination on the basis of disability in providing health care. One area that is spawning litigation is the denial of medical or dental treatment to patients with HIV disease.[43] The ADA does not require a physician to expand into other areas of medical specialty. While the ADA would prohibit an ear, nose, and throat specialist from denying treatment to an AIDS patient with a throat infection, it would not require the ENT physician to treat the patient's broken leg. The ADA only requires equal access to the medical services by the physician provided to other patients.

## THE FAMILY AND MEDICAL LEAVE ACT (FMLA)[44]

The FMLA requires an employer of 50 or more employees to make provision for up to 12 weeks of unpaid leave, within a 52-week period, to FMLA-eligible employees for the birth and subsequent care of a child; for the placement of a child for adoption or foster care; for care of an employee's seriously-ill spouse, child, or parent; and for care of a serious health condition that makes an employee unable to perform a job.[45] An employee is entitled to the continuation of employer-provided health care benefits for the duration of the FMLA leave and must be restored to the same or equivalent position if able to return to work within the leave-entitlement period.

Health-care providers are being called upon to provide medical input concerning certain leave authorizations mandated by the FMLA. An employer may require an employee to provide medical certification when requesting leave because of the employee's or employee's spouse's, child's, or parent's serious health condition.[46] The FMLA defines a "serious health condition" as one that requires either inpatient care, or "continuing treatment" by a health care provider.[47] The term "serious health condition" is intended to cover conditions or illnesses affecting one's health to the extent that inpatient care is required, or absences are necessary on a recurring basis or for more than a few days for treatment or recovery. When inpatient care is not involved, the interim regulations require that the absence from work, or from

school, or incapacity in performing other daily activities in the case of a family member, be for a period of more than three days in addition to requiring the continuing treatment of a health-care provider.[48]

The health-care provider may be a doctor of medicine or osteopathy licensed to practice medicine, podiatrists, dentists, clinical psychologists, optometrists, and certain chiropractors, nurse practitioners, nurse-midwives, and Christian Science practitioners.[49]

The information that an employer may require an employee to provide includes explaining the reasons for which the employee is needed to care for the serious health condition of a covered family member, or for which the employee is unable to work at all or unable to perform at least one essential function of the position. The regulations anticipate that the employer will provide the health-care provider with a list of the employee's essential job functions. If no such job description is provided by the employer, then the health-care provider is to identify those functions through discussion with the employee.

If the employee requests intermittent or reduced leave, the health-care provider will be asked to certify as to the medical necessity for such leave. In addition, an employer may obtain the practitioner's name and type of medical practice or specialty, the date the serious health condition commenced, and the health-care provider's best medical judgment concerning the probable duration of the condition; the diagnosis;[50] a brief statement of the regimen of treatment including the estimated number of visits, nature, frequency, and duration of treatment, including treatment by another provider of health services on referral; and indication of whether inpatient hospitalization is required.

The U.S. Department of Labor, the agency that enforces the FMLA, has provided an optional certification form for employers to use. However, an employer is prohibited from seeking further medical information or from contacting the health-care provider directly.

If an employer has reason to believe that a medical certification provided by an employee is not valid, the employer may invoke the law's procedure for contesting medical certifications. This procedure permits the employer to refer an employee to a second health-care provider, of the employer's choosing, but not in the employer's regular employ or under contract with the employer, for issuance of a second medical certification. If the second certification disagrees with the employee's initial certification, the employer and employee may mutually agree upon a third health-care provider whose certification is binding on both the employer and employee.[51]

Significantly, the FMLA's restrictions on an employer's access to medical information apply only to authorization of FMLA leave and job restoration after an FMLA leave. The FMLA does not restrict an employer's access to medical records for determining benefit eligibility or processing a workers' compensation claim.

Interestingly, the FMLA establishes a leave entitlement that is not abrogated if an employer is willing and able to provide an employee with a serious health condition with reasonable accommodation or light duty that would enable the employee to return to work.[52] Although the employer is not obligated to pay the employee during the period of FMLA leave, the employer cannot require the employee to report to work.

An employer may adopt a uniformly-applied policy requiring an employee out on leave for a serious health condition to present a physician's certification stating that the employee is able to return to work.[53] As with the ADA, the medical certification must be related only to the employee's ability to perform, safely and effectively, essential job functions.

## CONCLUSION

The ADA and FMLA pose new challenges for health-care providers. The definition of "disability" used in many public and private benefit systems is not congruent with the ADA's concept of "disability" and a "qualified individual with a disability." Health-care providers are being required to focus more closely on an applicant's or employee's abilities, as well as medically based inabilities or risks, to take into account the "essential functions" of a job, and to consider the consequences and benefits of reasonable accommodation that the employer may be required to offer, including reassignment of an employee to a different job.

The FMLA, which imposes another demand for medical input, ironically does not permit consideration of the possibility of reasonable accommodation. Health-care providers will need to become familiar with these two laws in order to assist patients and employers in assessing how a medical condition impacts an applicant's or employee's employability.

## References

1. Portions of this chapter have been previously published.
2. 42 U.S.C. § 12111(8); 29 C.F.R. § 1630.2(m).
3. 42 U.S.C. § 12112(a); 29 C.F.R. § 1630.4.
4. 42 U.S.C. § 12112(b)(5)(A); 29 C.F.R. § 1630.9.
5. 1630.2(n).
6. 42 U.S.C. § 12102(2)(A); 29 C.F.R. § 1630.2(g)(1).
7. 42 U.S.C. § 12102(2)(B); 29 C.F.R. § 1630.2(g)(2).
8. 42 U.S.C. § 12102(2)(C); 29 C.F.R. § 1630.2(g)(3).
9. 29 C.F.R. § 1630.2(i).
10. 29. C.F.R. § 1630.2(j) App.
11. 29 C.F.R. § 1630.2(j) App.
12. See EEOC, Technical Assistance Manual on the Employment Provisions (Title I) of the Americans with Disabilities Act, January 1992 (TAM), p. IX-2.
13. TAM, p. IX-2.
14. See, e.g., Cook v. Rhode Island; E. E. Black, Ltd., v. Marshall, 497 F. Supp. 1088 (D. Haw. 1980).
15. TAM, p. IX-3.
16. E.g., Welsh v. City of Tulsa, 977 F.2d 1415 (10th Cir. 1992); Byrne v. Board of Educ., School District of West Allis-West Milwaukee, 979 F.2d 560 (7th Cir. 1992); Maulding v. Sullivan, 961 F.2d 694 (8th Cir. 1992); Dailey v. Koch, 892 F.2d 212 (2d Cir. 1989); Forrisi v. Bowen, 794 F.2d 931, 934 (4th Cir. 1986); Jasany v. United States Postal Service, 755 F.2d 1244 (6th Cir. 1985); Fuqua v. Unisys Corp., 716 F. Supp. 1201 (D. Minn. 1989); Elstner v. South Western Bell Telephone Co., 659 F. Supp. 1328 (S.D. Tex. 1987) aff'd, 863 F.2d 881 (5th Cir. 1988); and Tudyman v. United Airlines, 608 F. Supp. 739 (D. Cal. 1984).
17. Id. 1630.2(j)(3).
18. E.g., Evans v. Dallas, 861 F.2d 846, 852-853 (5th Cir. 1988); Grimard v. Carlston, 567 F.2d 1171, 1174 (1st Cir. 1978); Paegle v. Dept. of Interior, No. 91-1075 (D. D.C. Feb. 8, 1993); Visarraga v. Garrett, No. C-88-2828, 1992 U.S. Dist. LEXIS 9164 at *13 (N.D. June 16, 1992); Saffer v. Town of Whitman, No. 85-4470, 1986 WL 14090 at *1 (D. Mass. Dec. 2, 1986); Stevens v. Stubbs, 576 F.Supp. 1409 (D. Ga. 1983).
19. August v. Offices Unlimited, Inc., 2 AD Cases 401 (1st Cir. 1992); Reigel, M.D. v. Kaiser Foundation Health Plan of North Carolina, No. 93-556-CIV-5-F (June 29, 1994), slip op. at 24 ("[R]equiring the Medical Group to either permanently assign an existing physician assistant to work with plaintiff to perform the physical aspects of her position or hire a new assistant to do the same cannot be considered a reasonable accommodation. The [ADA] does not require an employer to hire two individuals to do the tasks ordinarily assigned to one."); Johnston v. Morrison, Inc., 849 F. Supp. 777, 780 (N.D. Ala. 1994) (Restaurant not required to assign another employee to help food server during her panic attacks as this would eliminate essential job functions); See also Gilbert v. Frank, 949 F.2d 637, 644 (2d Cir. 1991) (employer not re-

quired to assign coworker to do physically demanding tasks employee no longer able to do); *Treadwell v. Alexander,* 707 F.2d 473, 478 (11th Cir. 1983) (Assigning additional employees to cover plaintiff's physically-demanding duties was an undue hardship); *Coleman v. Darden,* 595 F.2d 533, 540 (10th Cir.), *cert. denied,* 444 U.S. 927 (1979) (Under the Rehabilitation Act, an employer may be required to have someone assist the disabled individual to perform the job, but the employer is not required to have someone perform the job for the disabled individual).

20. *Jasany v. U.S. Postal Service,* 755 F.2d 1244 (6th Cir.1985); *Forrisi v. Bowen,* 794 F.2d 931 (4th Cir. 1986).

21. 42 U.S.C. § 12112(d); 29 C.F.R. § 1630.13.

22. 42 U.S.C. § 12112(d)(3); 29 C.F.R. § 1630.14.

23. EEOC, Enforcement Guidance: Preemployment Disability-Related Inquiries and Medical Examinations Under the Americans with Disabilities Act of 1990, May 19, 1994.

24. 42 U.S.C. § 12112(d)(3); 29 C.F.R. § 1630.14(b) and .15.

25. 42 U.S.C. § 12112(d)(4); 29 C.F.R. § 1630.14(c) and 1630.15.

26. 42 U.S.C. § 12113(b); 29 C.F.R. § 1630.15(b)(2).

27. *See generally,* TAM, Chapter IV, "Establishing Non–discriminatory Qualification Standards and Selection Criteria."

28. 29 C.F.R. § 1630.2(o)(1).

29. 29 C.F.R. § 1630.9 App.

30. 42 U.S.C. § 1981a(a)(3).

31. 42 U.S.C. § 12111(10); 29 C.F.R. § 1630.2(p).

32. 29 C.F.R. Part 1630, App. at 413.

33. Letter from Evan J. Kemp, Jr., Chairman, EEOC to Christopher G. Bell dated.

34. EEOC, Technical Assistance Manual on Title I of the Americans with Disabilities Act, § 6.4.

35. 28 C.F.R. § 36.304(b).

36. The ADA's prohibition of discrimination in public accommodation applies to private entities who lease, own, or operate a place of public accommodation. 42 U.S.C. § 12182(a); 28 C.F.R. § 336.201(b).

37. 42 U.S.C. § 12183.

38. 28 C.F.R. §§ 36.402-36.404.

39. 42 C.F.R. § 12183.

40. *Id.*

41. 42 U.S.C. § 12102(1).

42. *Mayberry v. Von Valtier,* 3 AD Cases 39 (E.D. Mich. 1994); *Aikens v. St. Helena Hospital,* 3 AD Cases 29 (N.D. Cal. 1994).

43. *U.S. v. Morvant,* 2 AD Cases 51769 (E.D. La. 1994).

44. The definition of a "serious health condition" and other aspects of the Department of Labor's interim final regulations have been under review. Final regulations were issued by the Department of Labor on January 6, 1995, after the publication of this chapter. The reader is encouraged to consult an attorney or the final regulations directly when FMLA issues arise.

45. The FMLA applies to employers with 50 or more employees. It took effect on August 5, 1993, for nonunionized employers and no later than February 5, 1994, for employers with collective bargaining agreements. An individual must be an "eligible employee" in order to take FMLA leave. An employee must have at least one year of service with the employer, have worked 1,250 hours in the 12 months preceding the request for leave, and work at a worksite with 50 or more employees within a 75 mile radius.

46. 29 C.F.R. § 825.304.

47. 29 C.F.R. § 825.114.

48. 29 C.F.R. § 825.306.

49. 29 C.F.R. § 825.118.

50. Note that under the final FMLA rules issued January 6, 1995, an employer will not be entitled to receive the diagnosis of an employee's medical condition.

51. 29 C.F.R. § 825.307.

52. 29 C.F.R. § 825.792(b).

53. 29 C.F.R. § 825.310.

# CHAPTER 51

# FITNESS FOR DUTY

Richard E. Johns, Jr.
James M. Elegante
Paul D. Teynor
Leonard J. Swinyer
Donald S. Bloswick
Alan L. Colledge

## INTRODUCTION

Physicians are confronted daily with risk-management problems as part of employment decisions involving temporary or permanent medical disability. Safety, ergonomics, industrial hygiene, and supervisory personnel are likewise confronted with managing risk created by job tasks and the workplace environment. Social policy and employment law dictate that any attempt to manage individuals at risk for a health-related condition should involve a medical, legal, and ethical approach that protects the worker and the employer. While the methodology the authors propose in this section relates to the ADA, the authors believe it is also relevant under social employment law schemes in many countries. The methodology provides an analytical paradigm that can be adapted to employment regimes under virtually any legal system that takes into account fitness for duty as a criterion for action. This model establishes an analytical line of communication to be used by lawyers, health-care providers, employers and benefit adjudicators working together to protect the legal rights of the disabled worker. The methodology allows the current state of medical knowledge to be used effectively in the administration of legal principles governing workplace rights and responsibilities.

Interest in risk assessment and fitness for duty is not new. Investigators in the era predating the Americans with Disabilities Act (ADA)[1] developed several systems designed to assist practitioners in performing fitness for duty evaluations. Although somewhat complex, these programs remain useful for specific types of employment settings and medical decision making. For example, Koyl,[2] in 1974, devised a method for charting the worker's physical and environmental requirements for performing a specific task. The earlier idea of matching the worker to the job was objectified using a seven category scale such as the General Physique, Upper Extremity, Lower Extremity, Hearing, Eyesight, Mentality, and Personality (GULHEMP) evaluation to organize and rate the data obtained from a medical history and physical examination. The same scale is used to rate and profile the requirements of a specific job. The outcome produces objective criteria for matching the two.

Approximately 10 years later, Nylander and Carmean, working for the County of San Bernadino, published the Medical Standards Project.[3] This work promoted a method by which an organization could implement a complete and comprehensive job-related medical screening program based on assessing the physical demands of jobs and a physical abilities analysis. Further use of this updated system is now proprietary and must be obtained through agreements from the original authors. The U.S. Department of Labor (DOL) and Social Security Administration[4] have, for many years, classified jobs in terms of exertional level, skill level, and other categories. All jobs in the U.S. economy have been classified into the following five levels of exertion: sedentary, light, medium, heavy, and very heavy work. The DOL model is widely accepted and used in making legal determinations of disability and fitness for duty. A representative form used by the DOL system is shown in Table 51-1.

Although not a specific fitness for duty model, Himmelstein and Pransky[5] coedited a significant work on the medical, legal, and ethical aspects of worker fitness and risk assessment evaluations. Implementation of the ADA in 1992, however, requires that employers and health-care providers work more closely

**TABLE 51-1     PHYSICAL DEMAND CHARACTERISTICS OF WORK (©1992 LEONARD M. MATHESON)**

| PHYSICAL DEMAND LEVEL (PDL) | OCCASIONAL (0-33% OF WORKDAY) | FREQUENT (34-66% OF WORKDAY) | CONSTANT (66-100% OF WORKDAY) | TYPICAL ENERGY REQUIRED |
|---|---|---|---|---|
| SEDENTARY | 10 lbs | NEGLIGIBLE | NEGLIGIBLE | 1.5-2.1 METS |
| LIGHT | 20 lbs | 10 lbs (and/or walk/stand/ push/pull of arm/ leg controls | NEGLIGIBLE (and/or push/pull of arm/leg controls while seated) | 2.2-3.5   METS |
| MEDIUM | 50 lbs | 20 lbs | 10 lbs | 3.6-6.3 METS |
| HEAVY | 100 lbs | 50 lbs | 20 lbs | 6.4-7.5 METS |
| VERY HEAVY | >100 lbs | >50 lbs | >20 lbs | >7.5 METS |

This chart is based on the United States Department of Labor System for classifying the general strength demands of the occupations described in the *Dictionary of Occupational Titles* (1977 and Supplements). The "typical energy required" data are estimates of the metabolic demand (in terms of oxygen consumption) of the predominant job tasks at each PDC level.

together in matching workers with disabilities to the essential functions of their jobs.

By adapting the pioneering works mentioned above to a post-ADA era, the following method allows employers and health-care professionals to effectively manage risk assessment and fitness for duty issues in the workplace. The following three basic activities should form the framework of any post-ADA risk management model:

1. Evaluating job risk and essential job functions,
2. Evaluating worker (personal) risk and "direct threat," and
3. Evaluating legal risks involved with matching essential job functions with personal direct threat risks.

## EVALUATING JOB RISK AND ESSENTIAL FUNCTIONS

Equal Employment Opportunity Commission (EEOC) regulations and guidance[6] that implement the ADA recommend the following considerations be made in identifying the essential functions of a job:

1. Whether employees in the position actually are required to perform the function,
2. Whether removing that function would fundamentally change the job,
3. Whether the position exists to perform the function,
4. Whether there are a limited number of other employees available to perform the function, or

among whom the function can be distributed, and
5. Whether a function is highly specialized, and the person in the position is hired for special expertise or ability to perform it.

Other relevant factors might ultimately be considered, and while ADA leaves to the employer the judgement as to which functions are essential, the burden of proof remains on the employer to defend the requirements of a job as truly being "essential" in a contested case.

Evaluating job risk involves defining the relationship between the worker and the work environment to determine the "fit" between them. A poor fit can cause unnecessary stress, unfavorably affecting the worker through job-related injuries or illnesses. A poor fit may also adversely affect product quality and profits through reduced production efficiency. This fit may be pictured as the overlap between the capabilities of the individual and the essential functions of the task, as illustrated in Figure 51-1.

When the essential functions of a task fit within the capabilities of the individual, job-related stresses are minimized. When the essential functions exceed or do not match the capabilities of the individual, job-related stresses increase as does the potential for injury. The fit between the worker and the work environment can be enhanced by increasing the capabilities of the individual through, for example, physical conditioning or training or by decreasing the physical requirements of the essential functions through task analysis and redesign.

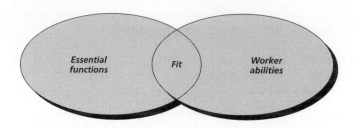

**FIGURE 51-1**   Matching worker abilities to essential functions of the job.

## EVALUATING WORKER (PERSONAL) RISK AND DIRECT THREAT

An employer may require that a worker not pose a "direct threat" to the health or safety of the worker or of others. To establish a direct threat however, the employer must show:

1. A significant risk or high probability of substantial harm to the worker or others in the workforce or public;
2. An identifiable and specific risk that considers the duration of the risk, the nature and severity of the potential harm, the likelihood that the potential harm will occur, and the imminence of the potential harm;
3. A current risk, not one that is speculative, remote, or based on future risk; and
4. An assessment of risk that is based on objective medical evidence related to a particular individual.

Thus, the determination of a "direct threat" to health or safety must be based on a reasonable medical judgement that relies on the most current medical knowledge and objective evidence that may include:

1. Input from the individual with a disability;
2. The experience of this individual in previous jobs; or
3. Documentation from physicians, psychologists, rehabilitation counselors, physical or occupational therapists, or others who have expertise in the disability involved, perhaps coupled with direct knowledge of the individual's impairment.

Decisions that affect an individual's employment and earning capacity carry heavy legal and ethical responsibilities. Furthermore, assessment of pre- or post-hire medical risk may be illegal if not performed within the guidelines established under the ADA and the implementing regulations of the EEOC.[1,6] Prior to a job offer, the ADA prohibits inquiry regarding health history problems that the job applicant may choose not to disclose. As discussed in Chapter 50, it is the employer, not the physician, who bears the responsibilities under the ADA.

## EVALUATING LEGAL RISKS OF MATCHING ESSENTIAL FUNCTIONS TO INDIVIDUAL DIRECT THREAT RISKS

The ADA closely regulates the medical inquiries made in connection with employment. The ADA regulates (1) inquiries made before a job is offered to an applicant, (2) inquiries made after a conditional offer of employment is tendered to the applicant, and (3) inquiries made of current employees of the company.

At any stage of employment, an employer may inquire about an applicant's ability to perform the essential functions of the job offered or held. At the preoffer stage, however, there must be no inquiry as to any underlying impairment, whether visible or hidden. Obvious limitations, such as poor range of motion, cannot lead to questions designed to elicit whether the applicant has chronic low-back pain. Regardless of the methodology chosen to evaluate the worker/job "fit," none are applicable to the preoffer stage of the employment process. Nonetheless, an offer of employment may be made conditionally to an applicant's being subject to a physical examination, provided that all entering conditional applicants in the same job category are subject to examination. Physical examinations must not be designed to screen out the impaired, unless the impairment tested for results in exclusion of individuals because of business necessity and job-related reasons. There may be no questions as to how the applicant became impaired, although questions about previous workers' compensation claims are allowed. Where a postoffer medical examination discloses an impairment, the results of the examination cannot be a reason for rejection unless the rejection is job-related and justified by business necessity. At this stage, however, the examining physician may probe without limit to determine and define the past history and severity of any medical condition and the extent of the conditional employee's ability to perform the essential functions of the job offered.

Thus, fitness for duty and risk assessment decisions in the worker with a medical condition will necessarily involve, from the legal standpoint, two inquiries. First, there must be a survey of the individual's physical abilities and of the job's essential functions. The second inquiry involves assessing and managing the direct threat risk associated with placing the worker in a job where there may be either aggravation of the physical condition or a threat of harm to fellow workers.

## FITNESS FOR DUTY: MATCHING THE WORKER TO THE JOB

A risk assessment methodology has been developed by which health practitioners could consider risk issues for several commonly-encountered medical conditions in the workplace. Application of the methodology, however, is appropriate to virtually any permanent, stable medical condition when related to appropriate job essential functions described by the employer. Such fitness for duty assessments, when reviewed critically under the prohibitions of the ADA, represent an objective method of categorizing and managing medical risk. The worker with an impairment can be examined by a physician and then matched by the employer to specific essential functions, although in some cases reasonable accommodations may be required. The methodology serves as a tool to help practitioners and employers as they work in cooperation to develop medical restrictions, if necessary, for individuals at risk within the confines of the ADA.

### Medical Criteria

All potential risk factors should be considered by the physician in building a medical risk profile for any given individual. However, in most cases, the medical history is the most practical and epidemiologically defensible finding in a qualitative assessment of medical direct-threat risk. The authors are aware of only a few epidemiologic models in the postemployment setting that have attempted to quantify the prospective risk of sustaining a work-related injury or illness while performing essential job functions.[7,8]

### Legal Criteria (see also Chapter 50)

The ADA protects qualified individuals with a permanent impairment from discrimination in connection with employment.[1] The worker who has the appropriate education, work experience, training, skills, licenses, or certificates necessary to perform the essential functions of the job offered is a qualified individual. "Essential functions of the job" is defined as those components which, if removed, will change the fundamental methodologies and/or outcomes of the job. Duties not strictly required to achieve the goal for which the job was created are not essential functions. The employer must accommodate the impairment of an otherwise-qualified person to aid performance of the essential functions of the job if to do so will not create an "undue hardship" on the employer.

An undue hardship is an action that requires "significant difficulty or expense" in relation to the size of the employer, the resources available, and the nature of the operation.

An employer is not required to make an accommodation if it would impose an "undue hardship" on the operation of the business. If a particular accommodation would impose an undue hardship, the employer must consider whether there are alternative accommodations that would not impose hardship. An accommodation that imposes no undue hardship is a "reasonable accommodation."

Whether a particular accommodation will impose an undue hardship must be determined on a case-by-case basis. An accommodation that poses an undue hardship for one employer at a particular time might not pose an undue hardship for another employer, or for the same employer at another time. In general, a larger employer would be expected to make accommodations requiring greater effort or expense than is required of a smaller employer. The concept of undue hardship includes any action that is unduly costly, extensive, substantial, or disruptive, or that would fundamentally alter the nature or operation of the business. Factors to be considered in determining whether an accommodation would impose an undue hardship on a particular business are reviewed in greater detail in the ADA Technical Assistance Manual.[6]

It is important to restate that it is not the responsibility of the physician to determine the essential functions of the job, to devise an accommodation for the impaired/disabled employee, or to determine the reasonableness of any accommodation proposed for the impaired/disabled employee. These decisions lie with the employer. This is not to say that the employer should disregard the input of the physician particularly with respect to the reasonable accommodation issues. The employer should arrive at a determination of the essential functions of the job and of the physical requirements needed for that job. The physician must objectively recommend appropriate medical restrictions based on knowledge of the patient's history, physical condition, and essential functions of the job. It is also appropriate for the physician to opine regarding future risk based on the risk criteria and risk categorization proposed in this chapter. Regardless of the physician's finding of risk from a medical point of view, it falls to management to analyze and determine whether the worker is, in fact, disabled according to ADA criteria and if so, whether the employee poses a direct threat to his or her own health or safety or to that of others. The physician's report is only one source of information necessary to make that assessment.

Obviously the physician is initially concerned with the issue of whether the individual would be injured further by accepting or continuing the employment offered. Here again, however, it is the physician's role only to make an assessment of medical factors. It is the employer's role to determine whether a direct threat exists. The criteria laid down by the ADA guide both the physician and the employer.[1,6]

The mere concern that individuals will harm themselves further does not provide a sufficient reason to deny employment. Furthermore, mere speculation that the employee, once on the job, could cause harm to others will not justify a denial of employment. As previously noted, a direct threat exists where there is a current specific risk that is significant in nature and threatens substantial harm, rather than a speculative or remote risk. The physician must demonstrate through objective medical data that a current risk exists. Speculation that in a number of years a medical condition is likely to deteriorate is insufficient with respect to the imminence of the potential harm. The employer must be able to show that the medical condition presents a significant risk with a high probability of substantial harm.

The worker found to be at high risk for certain medical conditions may, in some cases, pose a direct threat to others. For example, the direct threat posed by a worker with chronic, recurrent low-back pain (LBP) would most likely be apparent if such an individual were placed in a job that requires handling of hazardous materials, assuming awkward postures, or using moving machinery such as cranes or forklifts that might dump materials on or run into coworkers if the disabled worker were to experience the acute onset of LBP symptoms. Similarly, these individuals may pose a direct threat to others where the workers handle materials as a team without mechanical assistance. Again, for example, a high-risk LBP worker carrying materials in tandem with or side-by-side a coworker may cause injury to the coworker should a sudden onset of LBP cause the worker to drop the load.

The ADA Technical Assistance Manual[6] offers a hypothetical example: "A medical history reveals that the individual has suffered serious multiple reinjuries to his back doing similar work, which have progressively worsened the back condition. Employing this person in this job would incur significant risk that he would reinjure himself."

While the ADA[1] defines direct threat as a significant risk to the health or safety of others, the regulations implementing the ADA broaden the term to include a risk of substantial harm to the health or safety of the individual as well. Establishing direct threat to the impaired worker requires a greater degree of evidence demonstrating the imminence of potential harm.

Although it is possible that individuals considered at moderate risk could be found to present a direct threat to themselves or others, under most circumstances employees with a moderate risk profile should be managed only as a possible direct threat. The employee should be notified, however, of the risk category and possible fitness for duty decisions that might arise should another illness or injury occur creating a high risk and likely direct threat situation.

Obviously, the more detailed the medical history and the more objective the risk data provided by the physician, the more secure the employer may feel in a determination that an individual does or does not pose a direct threat. Again, at this stage, the employer must analyze the nature of the threat and determine whether there is a reasonable accommodation that could eliminate the threat. Here the physician can provide valuable input, without having to make ultimate employability decisions.

Based on the above medical and legal criteria, Figure 51-2 can be used as a mechanism for evaluating potential direct threat risk for individuals who do not appear to be appropriately matched to the essential functions of their jobs.

Once medical, ergonomic, legal, or other criteria are identified for any given health condition or disability, this categorization scheme will help provide guidance for professionals in implementing the ADA direct threat standard of "reasonable medical judgement that relies on the most current medical knowledge and/or the best available evidence."[1]

For illustration purposes, this methodology has been applied to the following commonly encountered medical conditions in the workplace that frequently require fitness for duty evaluations: (1) recurrent low-back pain (LBP), (2) postmyocardial infarction, (3) irritant and (4) allergic contact dermatitis. The risk criteria proposed for these conditions are neither absolute nor founded with exact scientific certainty. (Clearly other medical conditions affecting consciousness such as seizures, substance abuse, asthma, and others could have been chosen, but these four conditions are offered as examples. Appropriate extrapolations for other conditions can be made based on this model.) The important ADA requirement to remember is that health-care providers use objective data, reasonable medical judgement, current medical knowledge and best available evidence as noted above in adopting the high, moderate, or low risk category notations.

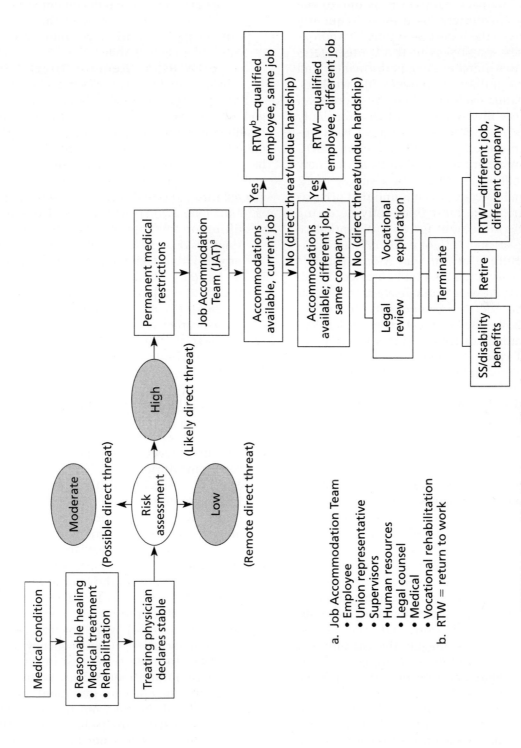

**FIGURE 51-2** ADA risk assessment/fitness for duty case management model. (SS = social security.)

a. Job Accommodation Team
- Employee
- Union representative
- Supervisors
- Human resources
- Legal counsel
- Medical
- Vocational rehabilitation

b. RTW = return to work

## RISK MANAGEMENT MODELS

### Recurrent Low-Back Pain

Occupational low-back pain (LBP) is one of the most commonly encountered and most frequently studied conditions in the industrial setting.[7,8] Approximately 10 million employees in the United States have back pain that impairs their performance, and an estimated one million employees file workers' compensation claims each year.[9] Of the more than 11,500 complaints filed with the EEOC from July 1992 to June 1993, 18.5% have been for back impairments, making them the most common EEOC complaint with monetary benefit awards having now reached $26.7 million in 1992.[10] In a survey of 12 states, the National Safety Council found that occupational back injuries, the most frequently occurring workplace disorder,[11] account for 22% of workplace injuries and illnesses and 32% of workers' compensation costs. The Bureau of National Affairs (BNA)[12] notes that about half of the 22.4 million cases of back pain reported in 1988 were work-related. In 1986, it was estimated that the total compensable cost of occupational low-back cases in the U.S. exceeded $10 billion.[13] An anatomic cause for LBP is identified in only 10-20% of cases.[14] Vague, nonspecific terms such as "musculo-ligamentous", "mechanical," "lumbar sprain/strain", or "lumbar syndrome" are frequently used to describe the patient without a specific identifiable lesion. Regardless of the cause, approximately 70% of affected individuals recover in two to three weeks and 90% in six weeks.[15,16,17,18] Low-back pain that persists for more than seven weeks is considered chronic.[19] The complex biological, psychological, and sociological variables involved in managing the chronic LBP patient in the workforce require an interdisciplinary approach. Unfortunately, studies suggest that patients who recover from an initial episode of LBP face a 60%-83% recurrence rate.[7,8,17,18] Since recurrent episodes of LBP in a material-handling setting are such a frequent problem, health care providers, industrial supervisors, rehabilitation specialists, claims adjustors, and other professionals work together in managing the back-injured employee with the goals of diminishing residual impairments and disability and returning the employee to work as soon as possible. Since recurrent LBP often involves fitness for duty and risk assessment issues, the following medical, ergonomic, and legal risk management approach, which takes into account the employer's obligation under the ADA,[1] is suggested:

**HIGH RISK (Likely Direct Threat):** Three or more documented LBP episodes in the medical history over the past five years involving lost work days and/or medical treatment for each episode.

**MODERATE RISK (Possible Direct Threat):** One to two documented LBP episodes in the medical history over the past five years involving lost work days and/or medical treatment for each episode.

**LOW RISK (Remote Direct Threat):** No documented LBP episodes in the medical history.

The authors have previously published specific, ergonomically based criteria related to typical material handling activities for individuals with high or moderate LBP risk.[20] Use of these criteria allows defensible medical restrictions to be recommended, although additional material handling tasks must also be considered through on-site ergonomic job analyses:

1. *Stationary Lifting—One Person:* No single-person lifting or carrying of more than 20 kg [44 lb] (high risk) or 30 kg [66 lb] (moderate risk) using proper lifting techniques. (The 20 kg [44 lb] and 30 kg [66 lb] limits are based on the midpoint of the 15-25 kg [33-55 lb] limit for "high risk" and 23-38 kg [51-84 lb] limit for "moderate risk" discussed earlier.)

2. *Stationary Lifting—Two Person:* No two-person lifting or carrying of approximately 77 kg [35 lbs] (high risk) or 110 kg [50 lbs] (moderate risk) using proper lifting technique. (Research suggests that in a lifting task performed by two persons, the load is not distributed evenly throughout the lift. A conservative estimate is that each person will lift between 55 and 60% of the total load at some time during the lift.[21]

3. *Stooping or Bending:* No repetitive stooping, bending, or twisting activities more than six times per hour (high risk) or nine times per hour (moderate risk) for less than one hour at a time involving loads not greater than those identified in the specifications for stationary lifting above and 76 cm [30 inches] from the floor at the beginning of lifting. (As restrictions for these type of activities are more difficult to derive, the reader is referred to the 1993 NIOSH Work Practices Guide for further guidance.[22,23,24] The frequency multiplier in the 1993 formula is defined by the number of lifts per minute (frequency), amount of time engaged in lifting activity (duration), and the vertical height of the lift from the floor. Our hypothetical restriction is based on lowest risk frequency of 12 lifts per hour, lift tasks of less than one hour duration, and vertical height at the beginning of the lift at 76 cm [30 inches] above the floor. Further, the restrictions continue

the authors' proposed use of a 50% reduction factor for high risk and 75% factor for moderate risk employees. See also Chapters 17 and 18.)

4. *Pushing/Pulling:* No single-person pulling activities requiring more than 50 kg [110 lb] of hand force (as measured by strain gauge equipment) to pull a load on a level surface with good traction at approximately a 109 cm [43 inch] grip height using appropriate posture. (Research indicates that pulling with 50 kg [110 lb] on a 109 cm [43 inch] high handle generates a back compressive force of approximately 1713 N [385 lb][25] or 50% of the 3427 N [770 lb] limit established by NIOSH.[22,24])

## Postmyocardial Infarction

Acute myocardial infarction (MI) is not an uncommon occurrence among workers, especially in an aging workforce. Hundreds of thousands of men and women survive an MI every year in the U.S. Restoring post-MI patients to their prior employment status is an appropriate goal that frequently involves risk assessment and fitness for duty issues.

There are three major determinants of occupational work potential after acute MI: (1) prognosis, (2) functional capacity, and (3) psychosocial status. The three determinants have important interactions. For example, clarification of prognosis, assessment of functional capacity, and provision of individualized guidelines for physical work will help improve psychosocial status and reduce many of the obstacles involved in returning to work after MI.[26] There are many nonmedical factors that influence decisions regarding return to work. Many of these reflect a lack of information on the true medical status, and therefore the occupational work potential, of the patient/employee. Consequently, some decisions may be made by employers in violation of the ADA. Only when prognosis and functional capacity have been clarified can these nonmedical obstacles be removed.

Due to mechanical assistance and engineering controls, the metabolic requirements of most occupations in industrialized countries have greatly decreased during the past century. Thus, most post-MI employees will have no difficulty returning to work when the essential job functions have low metabolic requirements (see Table 51-1 and Chapters 28 and 30). In patients with ischemic heart disease, the focus of the fitness for duty evaluation is to determine whether the increase in cardiac demands produced by physical, psychological, or environmental stressors will exceed the threshold for a "safe working capacity."[27] Prognosis in a cardiac disease patient is the key medical management issue that drives all other decisions. If a patient's functional capacity is poor, but prognosis is good, at worst the employee may fatigue easily. This is not a desirable outcome, for example, in a material-handling environment, but is, perhaps, more acceptable to the patient than constant fear and anxiety of sudden cardiac death.[28] Cardiac rehabilitation programs following acute MI can frequently improve poor functional capacity, especially in an individual with a good prognosis. Three major pathophysiological processes influence prognosis: left ventricular dysfunction, myocardial ischemia, and electrical instability. If significant abnormalities are found, medical or surgical therapy is required before risk assessment and fitness for duty recommendations can be made.[29]

Symptom-limited treadmill exercise stress testing (EST) is the most acceptable and frequently-used tool for evaluating prognosis and estimating functional capacity in persons without severe post-MI complications (for example, congestive heart failure or angina at rest or low levels of activity). The EST is helpful in objectively demonstrating that the post-MI employee has the functional capacity to perform the essential functions of the job.[26,27] The workload is measured in the metabolic unit, MET, with one MET being the required energy to stand quietly or the equivalent of approximately 3.5 ml oxygen consumption per minute per kilogram body weight.[30] The first stage of the Bruce EST protocol requires a 5 MET exercise capacity. The EST is best performed two to four weeks from the date of infarction.[26] Although the following risk categories and potential direct threat assessment is appropriate for any type of worker, physicians are most interested in the application to material-handling employees with ischemic heart disease.

**HIGH RISK (Likely Direct Threat):** Patients with such symptoms as positive or abnormal EST with activities at a measured or estimated low exercise level of less than 5 METS, low ejection fraction, and congestive heart failure. Individuals in this category require further evaluation, medical therapy, or revascularization to move them into the moderate or low-risk classification before return to work is allowed.[26]

**MODERATE RISK (Possible Direct Threat Risk):** Ability to perform a symptom-limited EST between 5 and 7 METS without evidence of ischemia; **or** average metabolic job requirements for an eight-hour shift exceed 40-45% of the individual's measured EST functional capacity and the peak energy job requirements are 20% lower than the EST functional capacity; **or** individuals do not meet criteria for high risk or low risk classifications. Individuals in this category require good control of their ischemic heart disease with medical therapy. The average and peak metabolic requirements of the job should be estimated or measured. Table 51-1 describes the Department of Labor job classification scheme for very heavy, heavy, medium, light, or sedentary work based on energy (MET) requirements.[4]

Specific occupational energy requirements have also been measured that may be helpful in estimating job energy requirements.[29] These studies were performed between 1940 and 1960 and probably represent overestimates of present occupational energy requirements.[26] If an employee's functional capacity is at least twice this value, no further job evaluation is needed. If the job requirements exceed 50% of the measured functional capacity, a more detailed job metabolic analysis should be performed. If the job requires a higher functional capacity, the individual should have an accommodation review based on direct-threat risk or undue hardship before returning to work (see also Chapters 18 and 28).

**LOW RISK (Remote Direct Threat):** There is a symptom-limited EST without ischemia and functional capacity greater than 7 METs. Individuals in this category may return to work in many jobs without limitations, as their risk of recurrent MI and sudden death may be as low as 1.0% and 2.5% respectively.[26] In some jobs, the threat to others may be too great even at this reduced level of sudden death risk. Individuals in strenuous occupations and low risk category may require EST to ensure adequate functional capacity to meet the essential functions of the job, regardless of ischemic heart disease history.

## Irritant Contact Dermatitis

Irritant contact dermatitis can occur in almost any individual independent of constitutional susceptibility. Various types of inciting irritants have been noted.[31] Irritant reactions have been characterized as acute, delayed, cumulative, traumatic, pustular, and acneiform, or nonerythematous. Regardless of the type, the basic underlying mechanism of any irritant contact dermatitis is loss of skin barrier function. This occurs when the barrier function of the skin has been damaged due to water, soaps, lotions, dryer sheets, phosphate detergents, alcohol or acetone, or other chemicals that can irritate the skin of any individual. The irritant reaction usually arises within minutes to hours of contact with the irritant. This frequently occurs in patients with a history of atopy. The treatment for atopic dermatitis that has been aggravated by some type of irritant is aimed at restoring the skin barrier function. Though medicated creams or ointments for two to three weeks may reduce or eliminate clinical symptoms, emollients should be used for at least four weeks after the reaction has resolved or the symptoms can recur immediately. In managing risk and fitness for duty issues for such individuals, the following criteria and restrictions are suggested:

**HIGH RISK (Likely Direct Threat):** Three or more documented episodes of recurrent irritant contact dermatitis that can be directly related to specific occupational exposures over the past three years. Individuals in this category should receive medical treatment and follow-up for at least six weeks. After skin barrier function has been reestablished, the individual should be permanently restricted from exposures to potentially-offending irritants or chemicals in the workplace. They should also be cautioned about similar exposures from hobbies, the home, or the environment. The physician should not rely on the patient history alone for this assessment but should involve management to determine the source of any potential occupational exposures, since the physician's judgement can have a major impact on the employer and employee in terms of compensability and worker fitness for duty.

**MODERATE RISK (Possible Direct Threat):** One to two documented episodes of recurrent irritant contact dermatitis that can be related to specific occupational exposures over the past three years. Individuals in this category should be temporarily restricted from potentially offending irritant exposures for at least six weeks. They should also receive appropriate medical treatment using nonirritating emollients and cleansers during this period. After skin barrier function has been reestablished and maximum medical improvement has been reached, individuals should be allowed to return to the workplace with specific precautions to use all appropriate personal protective equipment including clothing and gloves. Maintenance of skin care and personal hygiene must also be emphasized. Patients should be notified that further episodes of occupationally related dermatitis could move them into the high risk category, thus triggering permanent work exposure restrictions.

**LOW RISK (Remote Direct Threat):** No documented episodes of irritant contact dermatitis in the medical history. No specific restrictions are indicated for this risk category.

## Allergic Contact Dermatitis

Although allergic contact dermatitis comprises only a small percentage of occupational skin disease cases, its importance cannot be overemphasized. The condition has great significance to workers since typical personal protective clothing and equipment may be ineffective and many affected individuals must be accommodated in some other job or learn an entirely new trade. If near retirement age and unable to learn or qualify for a new job, the worker could potentially be permanently and totally disabled. Many individuals with this condition experience prolonged symptoms and periods of unemployment that frequently result in contested workers' compensation claims.

Allergic contact dermatitis is immunologically classified as a Type IV, delayed, or cell-mediated reaction. Most contact allergens produce sensitization in only a small percentage of workers after exposure to certain chemicals that have been used for an extended period. The reaction is usually delayed one to several days after exposure, but it continues to develop for several weeks and becomes worse after each exposure. Patch testing, with approved concentrations of antigens, is usually the best tool to discover potentially offending chemical(s).[32] Patients should not be patch tested to full-strength chemicals as they exist in the workplace but rather to tested concentrations made by a qualified laboratory. Treatment is accomplished by avoiding the offending chemical and restoring skin barrier function by using appropriate steroids and emollients. As with irritant contact dermatitis, emollients should be used for four weeks beyond the time when the skin appears normal to prevent recurrence. The more a patient comes in contact with an offending chemical the more exaggerated the reaction. In managing risk and fitness for duty issues for individuals with this condition, the following criteria and restrictions are suggested:

**HIGH RISK (Likely Direct Threat):** Two or more episodes of allergic contact dermatitis that can be directly related to specific occupational exposures. There should be objective medical evidence (such as a positive patch test) of immune system activation such as progressively severe symptoms on the second episode of dermatitis. In addition to six weeks of medical treatment, individuals in this risk category should be permanently restricted from any further exposures to known offending chemicals or

antigens. Job accommodation issues and/or vocational rehabilitation should also be addressed by management during this period.

**MODERATE RISK (Possible Direct Threat):** One episode of allergic contact dermatitis that can be directly related to specific occupational exposures. As in the high risk category, there should be objective medical evidence of immune system activation. The individual should be temporarily restricted from exposures to offending chemical(s) for the six-week treatment and healing period. After six weeks of treatment, the worker may be returned to the workplace and instructed in the proper use of all appropriate personal protective clothing and equipment. Meticulous work and personal hygiene habits need to be observed. Individuals should also be notified that further episodes of allergic contact dermatitis could place them in a high risk category with permanent restrictions.

**LOW RISK (Remote Direct Threat):** No evidence of allergic contact dermatitis in the medical history. No specific restrictions are recommended for this category.

A useful review of fitness to work with skin disease and the ADA is provided by Nethercott.[33] The reader is referred to Chapter 36 on Skin Disability for a more in-depth review of dermatologic impairment and rating guidelines.

## RECOMMENDATIONS

### Health Care Providers

Health care providers confronted with an employee or patient with a high or moderate risk medical condition have the responsibility of determining fitness for duty. Typically, treating physicians simply write return-to-work notes stating: "light duty," "no heavy lifting," and "no exposures to chemicals or noise," without regard to the individual's risk status or essential job functions. Such restrictions are meaningless in properly placing the individual or determining reasonable accommodations, because most physicians simply do not understand the patient's job or workplace. Thus, restrictions are usually based on what the physician subjectively thinks the patient can or cannot do. These restrictions are occasionally based on functional capacity evaluation reports or on what the patient tells the physician about the job requirements. They are rarely based on a description of essential job functions or visits to the workplace, two elements important to a thorough fitness for duty evaluation.

The primary responsibilities of a treating physician in a disability setting affecting compensability or work restrictions are to accurately and objectively:

1. Determine causation in terms of "reasonable medical probability" (usually greater than 50%). The rules of evidence as applied to causation should be considered, making sure that exposures (such as material handling work) and outcomes (such as low-back pain) are "consistent," "sequentially related," have a "dose-response" gradient, and "make sense."[34]
2. Provide appropriate medical treatment and monitor rehabilitation efforts.
3. Determine the end of a healing and rehabilitation period and provide a statement that medical stability or maximum medical improvement has been reached.
4. Rate permanent impairment using locally accepted guides or systems.
5. Assist the patient and employer with timely return-to-work decisions using objective risk assessment tools of the type described above as well as appropriate, quantitative medical restrictions by which fitness-for-duty decisions can be made.

Many physicians, however, perpetuate or prolong disability through inappropriate patient advocacy, which keeps the employee off work after maximum medical improvement (MMI) has been reached. Most progressive companies have early return-to-work policies and programs that will accommodate reasonable medical restrictions. Most restrictions are temporary until the patient has sufficiently healed to perform full duty. Occasionally, however, when a high risk medical condition is encountered, the physician may recommend permanent restrictions in an effort to protect the individual from aggravating a stable injury or illness. Under the ADA, a medical examination is permitted only when it is necessary to determine whether the individual has a disability, whether the individual can perform the essential functions of the job, and whether there is an effective accommodation that could assist the otherwise qualified individual with an impairment to perform the essential functions of the job. If the employee is obviously having difficulty performing the job, then the underlying medical condition can be ascertained through a physical examination and appropriate medical inquiry. Thus, assuming either a return-to-work situation after an individual has been injured on the job and reaches MMI or a fitness for duty analysis that determines that the applicant or the worker may be an individual with a disability, the following methods can be used to establish appropriate temporary or permanent medical restrictions for most employment settings:

1. Document all personal risk factors from the patient's history and past medical records, if available, noting previous work- or nonwork-related medical conditions, time off work, and extent of medical treatment.
2. Perform a pertinent, thorough physical examination of the patient with special attention to objective findings that correspond to potential risk criteria for a given medical condition.
3. Be aware of nonorganic symptoms and signs using appropriate distraction tests such as those recommended by Waddell[35] for chronic LBP conditions. Significant psychosocial stressors are also often overlooked in managing risk and performing fitness for duty evaluations. Bigos[36,37,38] has investigated the impact of nonphysical contributors to low-back disability. Factors such as low job enjoyment, personal and social unhappiness, unusual life stressors, and depression are strong contributors to prolonged disability and must be part of the health care practitioner's inquiry.
4. Whenever possible, and especially in difficult or delayed recovery cases, visit the workplace, or obtain good information about the workplace (from a video or objective workplace evaluation). Review usual and unusual material-handling activities as well as chemical exposures in terms of frequency, duration, and protective clothing or equipment required. Discuss potential accommodations that the patient and employer feel are appropriate.
5. Use the patient's history, objective examination findings, and job analyses with videotapes or Polaroid prints of specific tasks, chemical material safety data sheets (MSDSs), functional capacity reports, biomechanical models, essential job functions, and performance reports from supervisors to define appropriate medical restrictions for a given medical condition. The restrictions become the basis for the employer to analyze what, if any, reasonable accommodations can be made or if a direct threat or undue hardship condition exists. Physicians should not be coerced by the employer into offering an opinion as to whether or not the employee can perform the job.

## Employers

An employer faced with a disabled or potentially disabled employee with a likely direct threat risk has a distinct legal responsibility under ADA. In order to meet this challenge successfully, decisions must be made in accordance with all ADA guidelines, as described above. By creating a job accommodation team

(JAT), many of the difficult risk assessment and fitness for duty decisions can be successfully managed to legally-defensible conclusions as shown in Figure 51-2.

The JAT is a multidisciplinary team consisting of the disabled employee, union representative (if appropriate), company and treating physicians (if available), human resource personnel, key managers responsible for accommodation decisions, legal counsel, and vocational rehabilitation specialists if the employee may no longer be considered a "qualified employee" within the company. Accurate minutes of each JAT meeting (and there may be many) are kept by the human resource representative. While medical records are maintained separately under ADA requirements, JAT minutes can be maintained in personnel files to document the employee's input, the job accommodation review process, considerations of direct threat, concerns over undue hardship, and final decisions regarding employment status.

## CONCLUSIONS

Whether applicants for a position or workers seeking to continue employment, individuals whose medical condition limit a major life activity, thus rendering them disabled persons are protected by the ADA with respect to employment decisions. Management, health care providers, attorneys, ergonomic experts, and others should work together to provide a risk assessment and fitness for duty recommendation. Reassignment or termination actions should always be reviewed by legal counsel experienced in ADA law. A coordinated approach significantly reduces potential employer liability for increased risk of workers' compensation actions as well as for violations of the ADA while at the same time assures the patient/employee of a studied approach to full implementation of their legally protected rights.

## References

1. Americans with Disabilities Act of 1990 (ADA), 42 U.S.C. § 12101 et seq.
2. Koyl L: *Employing the older worker: Matching the employee to the job*, ed 2, 1974, National Council on the Aging.
3. Nylander A, Carmean G: *Medical standards project—Final report*, vols 1 and 2, 2nd rev ed, San Bernadino County, California, January 1983, Office of Personnel Management.
4. Appendix C—Physical demands. In *The classification of jobs according to worker trait factors: Addendum of occupational titles*, Roswell, GA, 1977, Vocational Services Bureau.
5. Himmelstein JS, Pransky GS: Worker fitness and risk evaluations. In *Occupational medicine, state of the art reviews*, Philadelphia, 1988, Hanley & Belfus.
6. Equal Employment Opportunity Commission Regulations and Guidelines (EEOC): 29 C.F.R. Part 1630; *A technical assistance manual on the employment provision* (Title I) of the Americans with Disabilities Act, U.S. Equal Employment Opportunity Commission (EEOC) Section VI-7, 1992.
7. Troup JDG, Martin JW, Lloyd DCEF: Back pain in industry: A prospective survey, *Spine* 6:61-69, 1981.
8. Chaffin DB, Park KYS: A longitudinal study of low back pain as associated with occupational weight lifting factors, *Am Indus Hyg Assoc J* 34:513-525, 1973.
9. U.S. Bureau of National Affairs: *Back injuries: Costs, causes, cases & prevention*, Washington, D.C, 1988:80, BNA.
10. EEOC National Database (as of 7-11-93): Office of Communication and Legislative Affairs, EEOC, Washington, D.C, 1993.
11. National Safety Council: *Accident facts.* Chicago: NSC; 1990: 38.
12. Bureau of National Affairs: *Occupational safety and health reporter*, June 10, 1992: 1226.
13. Webster B, Snook S: The cost of compensable low back pain, *J Occup Med* 32(1): 13-15, 1990.
14. Bigos SJ, Battie M: Overdiagnosis and overprescription of low back pain: Acute care to prevent back disability, *Clin Orthop* 221:121-130, 304, 1987.
15. Andersson GBJ, Svensson H-O, Oden A: The intensity of work recovery in low back pain, *Spine* 8:880-884, 1983.
16. Choler U, Larsson R, Nachemson A, et al: Back pain: Attempt at a structured treatment program for patients with low back pain (in Swedish), *SPRI Report* 188, Social Planerings-och Rational Isesingsinstitut Rapport, Stockholm, 1985:188.
17. Bergquist-Ullman M, Larsson U: Acute low back pain in industry, *Acta Orthop Scand (Suppl)* 170, 1977.
18. Nachemson AL: The natural course of low back pain. In White AA, Gordon SL, editors, *Idiopathic Low Back Pain*, St. Louis, 1982, C.V. Mosby.
19. Spitzer WO, Le Blanc FE, Dupuis M, et al: Scientific approach to the assessment and management of activity-related spinal disorders: A monograph for clinicians. *Spine* [suppl 1] 12:1-59, 1987.
20. Johns RE, Bloswick DS, Elegante JM, et al: Chronic recurrent low back pain: A methodology for analyzing fitness for duty and managing risk under the Americans with Disabilities Act, *J Occup Med* 36:537-547, 1994.
21. Karwowski W, Mital A: Isometric and isokinetic

testing of lifting strength of males in teamwork, *Ergonomics* 29(7):869-878, 1986.

22. Work practices guide for manual lifting, *NIOSH Pub. 81-122*, Akron, OH, 1983, and 1987, AIHA.

23. DeClercq NG, Lund J: NIOSH lifting formula changes scope to calculate maximum weight limits, *Occupational Health & Safety*, Feb 1993: 45-61.

24. Waters TR, Putz-Anderson V, Garg A, et al: Revised NIOSH equation for the design of manual lifting tasks, *Ergonomics* 36(7):749-776, 1993.

25. Lee KS, Chaffin DB, Waiker AM, et al: Lower back pain in pushing and pulling, *Ergonomics* 32(12):1551-1553, 1989.

26. Dennis C, Goins P, DeBusk RF: Working after heart attack, *Compr Ther* 15(11):3-6, 1989.

27. DeBusk RF, Davidson DM: The work evaluation of the cardiac patient, *J Occup Med* 22(11):715-721, 1980.

28. DeBusk RF: Report on Bethesda 20, *Trans Assoc Life Ins Med Dir Am* 74:65-68, 1990.

29. Haskel WL, Brachfeld N, Bruce RA, et al: Task Force II: Determination of occupational working capacity in patients with ischemic heart disease, *J Amer Coll Cardiol* (in press).

30. DeBusk RF: Specialized testing after recent myocardial infarction, *Ann Int Med* 110(6):470-481, 1989.

31. Lammintausta K, Maibach H: Contact dermatitis due to irritation. In Adams R, editor, *Occupational skin disease*, ed 2, Philadelphia, 1990, pp. 1-15, W.B. Saunders.

32. Fisher A: *Contact dermatitis*, ed 3, Philadelphia, 1986, pp. 9-29, Lea & Febiger.

33. Nethercott JR: Fitness to work with skin disease and the Americans with Disabilities Act of 1990. In *STAR's* Nethercott JR, editor: *Occupational medicine, occupational skin disease*, Philadelphia, 1994; 9(1):11-18, Hanley & Belfus.

34. Sackett DL, et al: *Applying the rules of evidence to causation*. In *Clinical epidemiology: A basic science for clinical medicine*, Boston, 1991, pp. 294-297, Little, Brown.

35. Waddell G, McCulloch JA, Kummel E, et al: Nonorganic physical signs in low-back pain, *Spine* 5(2):117-125, 1980.

36. Bigos SJ, Battie MC, Fisher LD, et al: A longitudinal, prospective study of industrial back injury reporting, *Clin Orthop* 279:21-34, 1992.

37. Bigos SJ, Battie MC, Fisher LD: Back pain among industrial workers, *Washington Public Health*, Winter 1990.

38. Bigos SJ: The practitioners guide to the industrial back problem, *Semin Spine Surg* 4:42-54, 1992.

# APPENDICES

## PRIMARY DEFINITIONS ACCORDING TO VARIOUS SOURCES

### DEFINITIONS USED IN THIS BOOK

**1. Disability**

A medical impairment that prevents remunerative employment, desired social or recreational activities, or other personal activities.

**2. Impairment**

The inability to complete successfully a specific task based upon insufficient intellectual, creative, adaptive, social, or physical skills.

**3. Medical Impairment**

An inability to complete a specific task successfully that the individual was previously capable of completing or one that most members of society are capable of completing, due to a medical or psychological deviation from an individual's prior health status or from the status expected of most members of a society.

### AMA GUIDES[1]

**1. Disability**

An alteration of an individual's capacity to meet personal, social, or occupational demands, or statutory or regulatory requirements, because of an impairment.

**2. Impairment**

Conditions that interfere with an individual's "activities of daily living," which include, but are not limited to, self-care and personal hygiene; eating and preparing food; communication, speaking and writing; maintaining one's posture, standing, and sitting; caring for the home and personal finances; walking, traveling, and moving about; recreational and social activities; and work activities.

A deviation from normal in a body part or organ system and dysfunctioning.

**3. Permanent Impairment**

One that has become static or stabilized during a period of time sufficient to allow optimal tissue repair, and one that is unlikely to change in spite of further medical or surgical therapy.

**4. Handicap**

An impaired individual is handicapped if there are obstacles to accomplishing life's basic activities that can be overcome only by compensating in some way for the effects of the impairment. Such compensation or accommodation often entails the use of assistive devices.

### WORLD HEALTH ORGANIZATION[2]

**1. Disability**

Any restriction or lack (resulting from an impairment) of ability to perform an activity in the manner or within the range considered normal for a human being.

**2. Impairment**

Any loss or abnormality of psychological, physiological, or anatomical structure or function.

### SOCIAL SECURITY ADMINISTRATION[3]

**1. Disability**

The inability to engage in any substantial gainful activity by reason of any medically determinable physical or mental impairment that can be expected to result in death or that has lasted or can be expected to last for a continuous period of not less than 12 months.

### AMERICANS WITH DISABILITIES ACT[4]

**1. Disability**

A physical or mental impairment that substantially limits one or more of the major life activities of the individual; or a record of such an impairment; or being regarded as having such an impairment.

**2. Impairment**

Any physiological disorder or condition, cosmetic

disfigurement, or anatomic loss affecting one or more of the following body systems: neurologic, musculoskeletal, special sense organs, respiratory (including speech organs), cardiovascular, reproductive, digestive, genital/urinary, hemic and lymphatic, skin and endocrine systems; or any mental or psychological disorder, such as mental retardation, organic brain syndrome, emotional or mental illness, and specific learning disabilities.

## References

1. American Medical Association: *Guides to the evaluation of permanent impairment,* ed 4, Chicago, 1993, AMA.

2. World Health Organization: *International classification of impairment, disabilities, and handicaps,* Geneva, Switzerland, 1980, World Health Organization.

3. Social Security Administration, U.S. Department of Health and Human Services: *Disability evaluation under Social Security.* Social Security Administration publication #64-039/ICN #468600, Washington, D.C, 1994.

4. EEOC Title One Regulations: An interpretive appendix (29 CFR 1630).

# "REASONABLE ACCOMMODATION" RESOURCE LIST

*Barbara Judy*

"Reasonable accommodation" of a qualified individual with a disability refers to a modification of the work situation or environment that enables the individual to meet the same job demands and conditions of employment as any other individual in the same job or a similar job.

In a recent survey conducted by the Job Accommodation Network, 78% of all accommodations cost less than $1,000. In addition employers, in response to another survey, reported that they believed the return on investment in an accommodation was more than 30 to 1.

The following list identifies resources at community, state, and national levels that provide both information and support regarding the Americans with Disabilities Act (ADA) and reasonable accommodation.

These resources span the spectrum of information and services and are available to individuals who are in need of information and assistance; to executives, staff, managers, and workers in the business and industrial communities; to claims adjusters and managers in the insurance industry; to professionals and consultants in all fields; and to any other interested parties.

They may be used when there is a particular problem to solve or to obtain general information. There are resources to help with all aspects of accommodation from analyzing the capabilities of a person with a disability to onsite job analysis and designing the accommodation in a particular case.

## Federal Agencies That Provide ADA Assistance

### Title I
*Equal Employment Opportunity Commission*
1801 L Street, NW, Washington, D.C. 20507
(800) 669-3362 (Voice); (800) 800-3302 (TDD)

### Titles II and III
*U.S. Department of Justice—Office on the Americans with Disabilities Act Civil Rights Division*
P.O. Box 66738, Washington, D.C. 20035
(800) 514-0301 (Voice); (800) 514-0383 (TDD)
*Department of Transportation*
400 Seventh Street, SW, Washington, D.C. 20590
(202) 366-1656 (Voice); (202) 366-4567 (TDD)

### Title IV
*Federal Communications Commission*
1919 M Street, NW, Washington, D.C. 20554
(202) 632-7260 (Voice); (202) 632-6999 (TDD)

### ADA Accessibility Guidelines
*Architectural and Transportation Barriers Compliance Board*
1311 F Street, NW, Suite 1000; Washington, D.C. 20004-1111
(800) 872-2253 (Voice/TDD)

### President's Committee on Employment of People with Disabilities
1331 F Street, NW, Third Floor; Washington, D.C. 20004-1107
(202) 376-6200 (Voice); (202) 376-6205 (TDD); (202) 376-6219 (Fax)

### President's Committee on Employment of People with Disabilities–Job Accommodation Network (JAN)
West Virginia University, 918 Chestnut Ridge Road, Suite 1, P.O. Box 6080
Morgantown, WV 26506-6080
(800) 526-7234 (Voice/TDD)
(800) 304-5407 (Fax)

**Regional Disability and Business Technical Assistance Centers (DBTACs)**
**1-800-949-4232 (Voice/TDD)**

A free call will ring through to the NIDRR DBTAC responsible for the region that contains your area code.

| Region | Address/Phone/Fax/TDD |
|---|---|
| **I-New England**<br>DBTAC<br>CT, ME, MA, NH, RI, VT | Univ. of South Maine-Muskie Inst. of Public Affairs<br>145 Newbury St, Portland, ME 04101<br>(207) 874-6535 (V/TDD); (207) 874-6529 (Fax) |
| **II-Northeast**<br>DBTAC<br>NJ, NY, PR, VI | United Cerebral Palsy Assoc./NJ<br>354 South Broad Street, Trenton, NJ 08608<br>(609) 392-4004 (Voice); (609) 392-7044 (TDD); (609) 392-3505 (Fax) |
| **III-Mid Atlantic**<br>DBTAC<br>DE, DC, MD, PA, VA, WV | Independence Center of No. Virginia<br>2111 Wilson Boulevard, #400, Arlington, VA 22201<br>(703) 525-3268 (Voice); (800) 232-4999; (703) 525-6835 (Fax) |
| **IV-Southeast**<br>DBTAC<br>AL, FL, GA, KY, MS, NC, SC, TN | United Cerebral Palsy Assoc. Inc./National Alliance of Business<br>1776 Peachtree Road, #310N, Atlanta, GA 30309<br>(404) 888-0022 (V/TDD); (404) 888-9091 (Fax) |
| **V-Great Lakes**<br>DBTAC<br>IL, IN, MI, MN, OH, WI | U. of Illinois at Chicago/U. Affiliated Program<br>1640 W. Roosevelt Road, M/C 626, Chicago, IL 60608<br>(312) 413-7756 (V/TDD); (312) 413-1326 (Fax) |
| **VI-Southwest**<br>DBTAC<br>AR, LA, NM, OK, TX | Independent Living Research Utilization/Inst. for Rehab. & Research<br>2323 S. Shepherd St, Suite 1000, Houston, TX 77019<br>(713) 520-0232 (Voice); (713) 520-5136 (TDD); (713) 520-5785 (Fax) |
| **VII-Great Plains**<br>DBTAC<br>IA, KS, NE, MO | University of Missouri at Columbia<br>4816 Santana Drive, Columbia, MO 65203<br>(314) 882-3600 (V/TDD); (314) 884-4925 (Fax) |
| **VIII-Rocky Mountain**<br>DBTAC<br>CO, MT, ND, SD, UT, WY | Meeting The Challenge, Inc.<br>3630 Sinton Road, #103, Colorado Springs, CO 80907-5072<br>(719) 444-0252 (V/TDD); (719) 444-0209 (FAX) |
| **IX-Pacific**<br>DBTAC<br>AZ, CA, HI, NV, Pacific Basin | Berkeley Planning Associates<br>440 Grand Avenue, #500, Oakland, CA 94610<br>(510) 465-7884 (Voice); (800) 949-4232 (TDD); (510) 465-7885 (Fax) |
| **X-Northwest**<br>DBTAC<br>AK, ID, OR, WA | Washington State Gov.'s Comm. on Disability Issues & Employment<br>605 Woodland Square, Loop S/E, Olympia, WA 98507-9046<br>(800) 949-ADA (V/TDD); (206) 438-4116 (V/TDD) |

# State Rehabilitation Agencies

**Alabama**
Rehabilitation Services
P.O. Box 11586
Montgomery, AL 36111-0586
(205) 281-8780 (Voice/TDD)

**Alaska**
Vocational Rehabilitation
801 West 10th St., Suite 200
Juneau, AL 99801-1894
(907) 465-2814 (Voice)
(907) 465-2440 (TDD)

**Arizona**
Dept. of Economic Security
Rehabilitation Serv. Administration
1789 W. Jefferson, 271 NW Wing
Site code 930A
Phoenix, AZ 85007
(602) 542-3332 (Voice)
(602) 542-6049 (TDD)

**Arkansas**
Arkansas Dept. of Human Resources
Division of Rehabilitation Services
P.O. Box 3781
Little Rock, AR 72203
(501) 682-6708 (Voice)
(501) 682-6667

**California**
Department of Rehabilitation
830 K. St. Mall
Sacramento, CA 95814
(916) 445-3971 (Voice)
(916) 323-4347 (TDD)

**Colorado**
Department of Social Services
Rehabilitation Services
1575 Sherman Street, 4th Floor
Denver, CO 80203-1741
(303) 866-5196 (Voice/TDD)

**Connecticut**
State Board of Education
Division of Rehabilitation
10 Griffin Road
North Windsor, CT 06095
(203) 289-2003

**Delaware**
Department of Labor
Div. of Vocational Rehabilitation
Elwyn Bldg., 4th Floor
321 East 11th Street
Wilmington, DE 19801
(302) 577-2850 (Voice/TDD)

**District of Columbia**
Dept. of Human Services
D.C. Rehab. Serv. Administration
Commission on Social Services
605 G. Street, NW, Route 1101
Washington, D.C. 20001
(202) 727-3227

**Florida**
Dept. of Labor & Employment Security
Div. of Vocational Rehabilitation
1709 A. Mahan Drive
Tallahassee, Florida 32399-0696
(904) 488-6210 (Voice)
(904) 922-2246 (TDD)

**Georgia**
Dept. of Human Resources
Div. of Rehabilitation Services
878 Peachtree Street NE
Room 706
Atlanta, GA 30309
(404) 894-6670 (Voice/TDD)

**Hawaii**
Department of Human Services
Div. of Vocational Rehabilitation
Bishop Trust Building
1000 Bishop St., Suite 605
Honolulu, HI 96813
(808) 586-5355 (Voice)
(808) 586-5381 (TDD)

**Idaho**
Div. of Vocational Rehabilitation
Len B. Jordon Building, Rm. 150
650 West State Street
Boise, ID 83720
(208) 334-3390 (Voice/TDD)

**Illinois**
Illinois Dept. of Rehab. Services
P.O. Box 19429
623 East Adams Street
Springfield, IL 62794-9429
(217) 782-2093
(217) 782-5734 (TDD)

**Indiana**
Indiana Dept. of Human Services
Div. of Rehabilitation Services
P.O. Box 7083
402 West Washington Street
ISTA Building
Indianapolis, IN 46207-7083
(317) 232-1433

**Kansas**
Dept. of Social & Rehabilitation Serv.
300 Southwest Oakley Street
Biddle Bldg., First Floor
Topeka, KS 66606

**Kentucky**
Dept. of Vocational Rehab.
500 Mero St., Capitol Plaza
Tower, 9th Floor
Frankfort, KY
(502) 564-4440

**Louisiana**
Dept. of Social Services
Div. of Rehabilitation Services
P.O. Box 94371
Baton Rouge, LA 70804
(504) 765-2310
(800) 256-1523

**Maine**
Department of Human Services
Bureau of Rehabilitation
35 Anthony Avenue
Augusta, ME 04333-0011
(207) 624-5300

**Maryland**
Division of Vocational Rehab.
Administrative Offices
2301 Argonne Drive
Baltimore, MD 21218
(410) 554-3000

**Massachusetts**
Massachusetts Rehabilitation Commission
Fort Point Place
27-43 Wormwood Street
Boston, MA 02210-1606
(617) 727-2172

**Michigan**
Department of Education
Michigan Rehabilitation Services
P.O. Box 30010
Lansing, MI 48909
(517) 373-2062

**Minnesota**
Dept. of Rehabilitation Services
390 North Robert Street
5th Floor
St. Paul, MN 55101
(612) 296-5616

**Mississippi**
Div. of Vocational Rehab. Services
P.O. Box 1698
Jackson, MS 39215
(601) 354-6825

**Missouri**
State Dept. of Elem. and Secondary Education
Division of Vocational Rehabilitation
2401 East McCarty Street
Jefferson City, MO 65101
(314) 751-4249

**Montana**
Dept. of Social & Rehab. Services
P.O. Box 4210; 111 Sanders
Helena, MT 59604
(406) 444-2590

**Nebraska**
State Dept. of Education
Vocational Rehab. Services
301 Centennial Mall South,
6th floor
Lincoln, NE 68509
(402) 471-3649

**Nevada**
Department of Human Resources
Rehabilitation Division
505 East King Street; 5th Floor
Carson City, NV 90710
(702) 687-4440

**New Hampshire**
State Department of Education
Division of Vocational Rehab.
78 Regional Drive; Bldg. #2
Concord, NH 03301
(603) 271-3471

**New Jersey**
NJ Dept. of Labor & Industry
Div. of Vocational Rehab. Services
John Fitch Plaza; CN 850
Trenton, NJ 08625
(609) 292-5987

**New Mexico**
State Department of Education
Division of Vocational Rehabilitation
604 West San Mateo
Santa Fe, NM 87503
(505) 827-3511

**New York**
NY State Education Dept.
Vocational Educational Services
One Commerce Plaza, Rm. 1606
Albany, NY 12234
(518) 473-9333

**North Carolina**
NC Dept. of Human Resources
Div. of Vocational Rehab. Services
State Office, P.O. Box 26053
Raleigh, NC 29611
(919) 733-3364

**North Dakota**
Department of Human Services
Office of Vocational Rehab. Services
400 East Broadway, Suite 303
Bismarck, ND 58501-4038
(701) 224-3999 (Voice)
(701) 224-3975 (TDD)

**Ohio**
Ohio Rehab. Serv. Commission
400 East Campus View Blvd.
Columbus, OH 43235-4604
(614) 438-1210 (Voice/TDD)

**Oklahoma**
Dept. of Human Resources
Rehabilitation Serv. Commission
2409 North Kelley
Oklahoma City, OK 73111
(405) 424-6006 (Voice)
(405) 424-2794
(800) 833-8973 (Voice/TDD)

**Oregon**
Dept. of Human Resources
Vocational Rehabilitation Division
2045 Silverton Road, NE
Salem, OR 97310
(503) 378-3830 (Voice)
(503) 378-3933 (TDD)

**Pennsylvania**
Dept. of Labor & Industry
Office of Vocational Rehab.
1300 Labor & Industry Bldg.
7th and Forster Sts.
Harrisburg, PA 17120
(717) 787-5244 (Voice)
(717) 783-8917 (TDD)

**Rhode Island**
Dept. of Human Services
Vocational Rehabilitation
40 Fountain Street
Providence, RI 02903
(401) 421-7005

**South Carolina**
Vocational Rehabilitation Dept.
P.O. Box 15, 1410 Boston Ave.
West Columbia, SC 29171-0015
(803) 734-4300

**South Dakota**
Div. of Rehabilitation Services
700 North Governors Drive
Pierre, SD 57501-2275
(605) 773-3195

**Tennessee**
Dept. Human Services
Div. of Vocational Rehabilitation
Citizen Plaza Bldg., 15th Floor
400 Deaderick St.
Nashville, TN 37219
(615) 741-2521

**Texas**
Texas Rehabilitation Commission
4900 North Lamar Blvd., Room 7102
Austin, TX 78751-2316
(512) 483-4001

**Utah**
Utah State Office of Rehab.
250 East 500 South
Salt Lake City, Utah 84111
(801) 538-7530

**Vermont**
Agency of Human Services
Vocational Rehabilitation Div.
Osgood Bldg., Waterbury Complex
103 South Main St.
Waterbury, VT 05671-2303
(803) 241-2189 (Voice/TDD)

**Virginia**
Commonwealth of Virginia
Virginia Dept. for the Visually Handicapped
397 Azalea Avenue
Richmond, VA 23227-3697
(804) 371-3140 (TDD)

**Washington**
Dept. of Social & Health Services
Division of Vocational Rehab.
P.O. Box 45340
Olympia, WA 9854-5340
(206) 438-8000 (Voice/TDD)

**West Virginia**
State Board of Rehabilitation
Division of Rehabilitation Services
State Capitol Complex
Charleston, WV 25305
(304) 766-4601 (Voice)
(304) 766-4970 (TDD)

**Wisconsin**
Dept. of Health & Social Services
Div. of Vocational Rehabilitation
P.O. Box 7852
1 West Wilson, 8th Floor
Madison, WI 53707
(608) 266-2186 (Voice)
(608) 266-9599 (TDD)

**Wyoming**
Department of Employment
Division of Vocational Rehab.
1100 Herschler Bldg.
Cheyenne, WY 82002
(307) 777-7385

## Commonwealths, Possessions, Territories

**American Samoa**
American Samoa Government
Dept. of Human Resources
Division of Vocational Rehab.
Pago Pago, AS 96799
(684) 633-2336

**Commonwealth of Puerto Rico**
Dept. of Social Services
P.O. Box 1118
Hato Rey, PR 00910
(809) 725-1792

**Commonwealth of the Northern
Mariana Islands**
Commonwealth of the Northern Mariana Islands
Vocational Rehabilitation Div.
P.O. Box 1521-CK
Saipan, CM
(607) 234-6538

**Guam**
Government of Guam
Dept. of Vocational Rehab.
122 Harmon Plaza, Rm. B201
Harmon Industrial Park
Harmon, GU 96911
(617) 646-9468

**Trust Territory of the Pacific Islands**
Bureau of Education
P.O. Box 189
Koror, Palua
Western, Carolina Islands 96940
(680) 488-1467

**Virgin Islands**
Department of Human Resources
Division of Disabilities & Rehabilitation Services
Barbel Plaza South
St. Thomas, VI 00892
(809) 774-0930

## PRIVATE ORGANIZATIONS

American Cancer Society, National Headquarters
1599 Clifton Road
Atlanta, GA 30329
(404) 320-3333

American Diabetes Association, Inc.
(800) 232-3472

American Foundation for the Blind
15 West 16th Street
New York, NY 10011
(212) 620-2000 (V); (212) 620-2158
or (800) 232-5463

American Speech-Language-Hearing Association
10801 Rockville Pk.
Rockville, MD 20852
(301) 897-5700 (V); (800) 638-8255 (V/TDD)

Arthritis Foundation
1214 Spring Street, NW
Atlanta, GA 30309
(404) 872-7100; (800) 283-7800

Asthma and Allergy Foundation of America
1125 15th St., NW, Ste. 502
Washington, DC 20005
(202) 466-7643; (800) ASTHMA

CDC National AIDS Clearinghouse
(800) 458-5231

Chronic Fatigue and Immune Dysfunction
    Syndrome Association
(800) 442-3437

Epilepsy Foundation of America
4351 Garden City Drive
Landover, MD 20785
(301) 459-3700; (800) EFA-1000 (V/TDD)

Gallaudet University-National Information
Center on Deafness, Kendall Green
800 Florida Avenue, NE
Washington, DC 20002
(202) 651-5051 (V); (202) 651-5052 (TDD)

National Cancer Information Service
(800) 422-6237

National Center on Employment of the Deaf/
National Technical Inst. for the Deaf
Rochester Institute of Technology
One Lomb Memorial Drive, P.O. Box 9887,
Rochester, NY 14623-0887
(716) 475-6834 (V); (716) 475-6205 (TDD)

National Center for Learning Disabilities
99 Park Avenue
New York, NY 10916
(212) 687-7211

National Easter Seal Society
70 East Lake St.
Chicago, IL 60601
(312) 726-6200 (V); (312) 726-4258 (TDD)

National Head Injury Foundation, Inc.
(800) 444-6443

National Institute on Deafness and Other
 Communications Disorders Clearinghouse
(800) 241-1044 (V); (800) 241-1055 (TDD)

National Leadership Coalition on AIDS
1730 M. St., NW, Ste. 905
Washington, DC 20036
(202) 429-0930

National Mental Health Association
1021 Prince St.
Alexandria, VA 22314
(703) 684-7722; (800) 969-6642 (V)

National Multiple Sclerosis Society
733 Third Avenue
New York, NY 10017
(212) 986-3240; (800) 532-7667

National Organization for Rare Disorders
(800) 999-6673

National Spinal Cord Injury Association
600 W. Cummings Park, Ste. 2000
Woburn, MA 01801
(617) 935-2722; (800) 962-9629

Paralyzed Veterans of America
801 18th St., NW
Washington, DC 20006
(202) 872-1300 (V); (202) 416-7622 (TDD)

Respiratory Disorders: Asthma and Allergy
 Foundation of America
(800) 727-8462

United Cerebral Palsy Association, Inc.
1522 K St., NW
Washington, DC 20005
(800) 872-5827